Morson and Dawson's
Gastrointestinal Pathology

This book is dedicated to the memory of two outstanding gastrointestinal pathologists, Professor Jeremy Jass and Professor Bryan Warren.

Morson and Dawson's Gastrointestinal Pathology

Edited by

Neil A. Shepherd, DM, FRCPath
Professor of Gastrointestinal Pathology and Consultant Histopathologist
Gloucestershire Cellular Pathology Laboratory
Cheltenham, UK

Bryan F. Warren, MB ChB, FRCP(London), FRCPath[†]
Professor of Gastrointestinal Pathology
John Radcliffe Hospital
Oxford, UK

Geraint T. Williams, OBE, BSc, MD, MRCR, FRCP(London), FRCPath, FMedSci
Professor of Pathology
Cardiff University
Cardiff, UK

Joel K. Greenson, MD
Professor of Pathology
University of Michigan Medical School
Ann Arbor, MI, USA

Gregory Y. Lauwers, MD
Vice Chair of Pathology, Massachusetts General Hospital
Professor of Pathology, Harvard Medical School
Boston, MA, USA

Marco R. Novelli, MB ChB, PhD, FRCPath
Professor of Gastrointestinal Pathology and Consultant Histopathologist
University College Hospital
London, UK

FIFTH EDITION

[†]Deceased

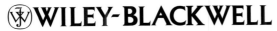

A John Wiley & Sons, Ltd., Publication

Library of Congress Cataloging-in-Publication Data

Morson and Dawson's gastrointestinal pathology. – 5th ed. / edited by Neil A. Shepherd . . . [et al.].

p. ; cm.

Gastrointestinal pathology

Includes bibliographical references and index.

ISBN 978-1-4051-9943-8 (hardcover : alk. paper)

I. Shepherd, Neil A.   II. Morson, Basil C. (Basil Clifford). Gastrointestinal pathology.

III. Title: Gastrointestinal pathology.

[DNLM: 1. Gastrointestinal Diseases–pathology.   WI 140]

616.3'3071–dc23

2012009760

A catalogue record for this book is available from the British Library.

Contents

Contributors

Richard L. Attanoos, BSc, MB BS, FRCPath
Consultant Histopathologist
Department of Histopathology
University Hospital Llandough
Penarth, UK

Shinichi Ban, MD, PhD
Head, Department of Pathology
Saiseikai Kawaguchi General Hospital
Saitama, Japan

Adrian C. Bateman, BSc, MD, FRCPath
Consultant Histopathologist and Honorary Senior Lecturer in Pathology
Southampton General Hospital
Southampton, UK

Lodewijk A.A. Brosens, MD, PhD
Chief Resident in Pathology
Department of Pathology
University Medical Centre Utrecht
Utrecht, The Netherlands

Ian Brown, FRCPA
Visiting Senior Specialist
Royal Brisbane and Women's Hospital;
Specialist Pathologist
Envoi Specialist Pathologists
Brisbane, QLD, Australia

Fiona Campbell, BSc, MD, FRCPath
Honorary Professor and Consultant Gastrointestinal Pathologist
Department of Pathology
Royal Liverpool University Hospital
Liverpool, UK

Frank A. Carey, BSc, MD, FRCPath
Consultant Pathologist and Honorary Professor in Pathology
Department of Pathology
Ninewells Hospital and Medical School
Dundee, UK

Fátima Carneiro, MD, PhD
Professor of Pathology and Head of Department of Pathology
Faculty of Medicine of the University of Porto
Centro Hospitalar de São João and IPATIMUP
Porto, Portugal

Andrew D. Clouston, MBBS, PhD, FRCPA
Associate Professor, Molecular and Cellular Pathology
University of Queensland;
Visiting Senior Specialist, Royal Brisbane and Women's Hospital;
Specialist Pathologist
Envoi Specialist Pathologists
Brisbane, QLD, Australia

Claude Cuvelier, MD, PhD
Head, Academic Department of Pathology
Ghent University
Ghent, Belgium

Paola Domizio, BSc, MB BS, FRCPath
Professor of Pathology Education
Barts and The London School of Medicine and Dentistry
Queen Mary University of London;
Department of Cellular Pathology
The Royal London Hospital
London, UK

Erinn Downs-Kelly, DO, MS
Staff Pathologist
Department of Anatomic Pathology
Cleveland Clinic
Cleveland, OH, USA

David K. Driman, MBChB, FRCPC
Professor of Pathology
Department of Pathology
Schulich School of Medicine and Dentistry
Western University and London Health Sciences Centre
London, ON, Canada

Robert P. Eckstein, MB, BS, FRCPA
Associate Professor of Pathology
Department of Anatomical Pathology
Pacific Laboratory Medicine Services
Royal North Shore Hospital
St Leonards, NSW, Australia

Nadine Ectors, MD, PhD
Professor in Histopathology and Coordinator
Translational Cell and Tissue Research
AC Biobanking
University Hospitals and University Leuven
Leuven, Belgium

Hala El-Zimaity, MD, FRCPC, MSc
Associate Professor
Department of Laboratory Medicine and Pathobiology
University of Toronto
Toronto, ON, Canada

Jean-François Fléjou, MD, PhD
Professor of Pathology
Department of Pathology
Hôpital Saint-Antoine, AP-HP;
Faculté de Médecine Pierre et Marie Curie
Paris, France

Karel Geboes, MD, PhD, AGAF
Professor of Pathology
Department of Pathology
University Hospital and Medical School KU Leuven
Leuven, Belgium

Muriel Genevay, MD
Consultant Gastrointestinal Pathologist
Service of Clinical Pathology
University Hospitals of Geneva
Geneva, Switzerland

John R. Goldblum, MD
Chairman, Department of Anatomic Pathology
Cleveland Clinic;
Professor of Pathology
Cleveland Clinic Lerner College of Medicine
Cleveland, OH, USA

Joel K. Greenson, MD
Professor of Pathology
University of Michigan Medical School
Ann Arbor, MI, USA

Thomas Guenther, MD, PhD, FRCPath
Honorary Consultant Histopathologist
St Mark's Hospital
North West London Hospitals NHS Trust
London, UK;
Professor of Pathology and Consultant Histopathologist
Otto-von-Guericke University
Magdeburg, Germany

Gordon Hutchins, BMedSci(Hons), MB BS
Academic SpR in Histopathology & Honorary Clinical Lecturer
Pathology and Tumour Biology
Leeds Institute of Molecular Medicine
University of Leeds
Leeds, UK

Dhanpat Jain, MBBS, MD
Associate Professor of Pathology and Medicine (Digestive Diseases)
Director, Program in Gastrointestinal and Liver Pathology
Department of Anatomic Pathology
Yale University School of Medicine
New Haven, CT, USA

Marnix Jansen, MD, MSc, PhD
Chief Resident, Pathology
Department of Pathology
Academic Medical Centre
Amsterdam, The Netherlands

Laura W. Lamps, MD
Professor and Vice-Chair
Department of Pathology
University of Arkansas for Medical Sciences
Little Rock, AZ, USA

Gregory Y. Lauwers, MD
Vice Chair of Pathology, Massachusetts General Hospital;
Professor of Pathology
Harvard Medical School
Boston, MA, USA

Laurence de Leval, MD, PhD
Professor of Pathology
Clinical Director, Institute of Pathology
Centre Hospitalier Universitaire Vaudois
Lausanne, Switzerland

Maurice B. Loughrey, BSc, MRCP, MD, FRCPath
Consultant Histopathologist and Honorary Lecturer
Royal Victoria Hospital
Queen's University Belfast
Belfast, UK

Joanne E. Martin, MA, MB BS, PhD, FRCPath
Professor of Pathology
Barts and the London School of Medicine and Dentistry
Queen Mary University of London;
Department of Cellular Pathology
The Royal London Hospital
London, UK

Raymond F.T. McMahon, BSc, MD, FRCPath
Professor and Hospital Dean
Central Manchester NHS Foundation Trust;
Honorary Consultant Pathologist
Manchester Royal Infirmary
Manchester Medical School, University of Manchester
Manchester, UK

Joseph Misdraji, MD
Associate Professor of Pathology
Director, Histopathology
Massachusetts General Hospital
Harvard Medical School
Boston, MA, USA

Elizabeth Montgomery, MD
Professor of Pathology, Oncology, and Orthopedic Surgery
Johns Hopkins Medical Institutions
Baltimore, MD, USA

Cian Muldoon, MB BCh, MRCPI, FRCPath, FFacPathRCPI
Consultant Histopathologist
Department of Histopathology
St James's Hospital
Dublin, Ireland

Amy E. Noffsinger, MD
Gastrointestinal Pathologist
Miraca Life Sciences
Camp Dennison, OH, USA

Marco R. Novelli, MB ChB, PhD, FRCPath
Professor of Gastrointestinal Pathology and Consultant
Histopathologist
University College Hospital
London, UK

Robert D. Odze, MD, FRCPC
Professor of Pathology
Harvard Medical School;
Chief, GI Pathology Division
Brigham and Women's Hospital
Boston, MA, USA

G. Johan A. Offerhaus, MD, MPH, PhD
Professor of Pathology
Department of Pathology
University Medical Centre Utrecht
Utrecht, The Netherlands

Scott R. Owens, MD
Assistant Professor
University of Pittsburgh Medical Center
Pittsburgh, PA, USA

Jeremy R. Parfitt, MD, FRCPC
Assistant Professor
Department of Pathology
Schulich School of Medicine and Dentistry
Western University and London Health Sciences Centre
London, ON, Canada

Do-Youn Park, MD, PhD
Professor
Department of Pathology
Pusan National University College of Medicine
Pusan National University Hospital
Busan, Republic of Korea

Robert E. Petras, MD
National Director for Gastrointestinal Pathology Services
AmeriPath, Inc.
Oakwood Village;
Associate Clinical Professor of Pathology
Northeast Ohio Medical University
Rootstown, OH, USA

Phil Quirke, BM, PhD, FRCPath
Yorkshire Cancer Research Centenary Professor of Pathology
Pathology and Tumour Biology
Leeds Institute of Molecular Medicine
University of Leeds
Leeds, UK

Robert H. Riddell, MD, FRCPath
Professor of Laboratory Medicine and Pathology
Mount Sinai Hospital
Toronto, ON, Canada

Brian P. Rubin, MD, PhD
Associate Professor of Pathology
Cleveland Clinic
Cleveland, OH, USA

Manuel Salto-Tellez, MD (LMS), FRCPath
Professor and Chair of Molecular Pathology
Clinical Consultant Pathologist
Centre for Cancer Research and Cell Biology
Queen's University Belfast
Belfast, UK

D. Scott A. Sanders, MD, FRCPath
Consultant Histopathologist
Coventry and Warwickshire Pathology Services
Warwick, UK

Kieran Sheahan, MB, BSc, FRCPI, FRCPath
Associate Clinical Professor
University College Dublin;
Consultant Pathologist
St Vincent's University Hospital
Dublin, Ireland

Neil A. Shepherd, DM, FRCPath
Professor of Gastrointestinal Pathology and Consultant
Histopathologist
Gloucestershire Cellular Pathology Laboratory
Cheltenham, UK

Michio Shimizu, MD, PhD
Professor
Department of Pathology
Saitama Medical University
Saitama International Medical Center
Saitama, Japan

Amitabh Srivastava, MD
Assistant Professor
Harvard Medical School;
Department of Pathology
Brigham and Women's Hospital
Boston, MA, USA

Kaiyo Takubo, MD, PhD
Team Leader
Research Team for Geriatric Pathology
Tokyo Metropolitan Institute of Gerontology;
Clinical Professor
Tokyo Medical and Dental University School of Medicine
Tokyo, Japan

Neal I. Walker, MD, BS, FRCPA
Specialist Pathologist
Envoi Specialist Pathologists;
Associate Professor
Molecular and Cellular Pathology
University of Queensland
Brisbane, QLD, Australia

Shaun V. Walsh, MB BCh BAO, FRCPath
Consultant Histopathologist
Department of Pathology
Ninewells Hospital and Medical School
Dundee, UK

†**Bryan F. Warren**, MB ChB, FRCP(London), FRCPath
Professor of Gastrointestinal Pathology
John Radcliffe Hospital
Oxford, UK

Kevin P. West, BSc, MB ChB, DMJ, FRCPath
Consultant Histopathologist
Honorary Senior Lecturer in Cancer Studies and Molecular
Medicine
University Hospitals of Leicester NHS Trust
Leicester Royal Infirmary
Leicester, UK

Nicholas P. West, BSc, PhD, MB ChB, PGCert
NIHR Academic Clinical Lecturer in Histopathology
Pathology and Tumour Biology
Leeds Institute of Molecular Medicine
University of Leeds
Leeds, UK

Geraint T. Williams, OBE, BSc, MD, MRCR, FRCP(London),
FRCPath, FMedSci
Professor of Pathology
Cardiff University
Cardiff, UK

Alison M. Winstanley, BSc, MB BS, FRCPath
Consultant Cellular Pathologist
University College Hospital
London, UK

†Deceased

Foreword

Since the first edition was published in 1972, there have been many changes in both the scope and the practice of gastrointestinal pathology.

Forty years ago gastrointestinal pathology as a subspecialty within general histopathology did not exist in contrast, for example, to gynaecological pathology and neuropathology. The picture today is very different. All academic departments will have one or more full-time gastrointestinal pathologists with time available for research and teaching in their subject. In the general hospitals serving large districts there is likely to be at least one pathologist with special expertise in gastrointestinal work. To what can these changes be attributed?

During the last 50 years there has been an increasing abundance of surgical specimens available for detailed examination. More important, perhaps, is the revolution in endoscopy. Virtually the entire gastrointestinal tract is now accessible to biopsy. As surgeons and gastroenterologists increasingly rely on biopsy interpretation for their practice, so the numbers of biopsies have escalated. The demand, therefore, for skilled gastrointestinal pathologists has hugely increased.

This book aims to provide an up-to-date contribution to training for this now fully acknowledged subspecialty of histopathology. It should also be helpful as a major point of resource in the practice of gastrointestinal pathology. The structure of this edition remains substantially the same as in previous ones except there are now six editors, including one lead editor. The inclusion of editors from North America and authors from North America, the European continent, Asia and Australia, is a deliberate attempt to internationalise the contributors.

The practice of gastrointestinal pathology has now reached a stage where there is sub-specialisation within our discipline, with the inclusion of authors who have a special diagnostic or research interest in particular parts and/or particular diseases of the gastrointestinal tract. This trend is likely to continue. Moreover, this further sub-specialisation is leading to rationalisation of pathology departments. One can also envisage the development of specialised technical support in the future for gastrointestinal pathologists.

It is extraordinary how, in contrast to other sub-specialties in general histopathology, molecular pathology has yet to make more than a very limited impact on day-to-day diagnostic work. Haematoxylin and eosin (H&E)-based technical support remains the mainstay of diagnosis but it is likely that new molecular analyses will break into the traditional approach, particularly in the management of colorectal cancer.

The gastrointestinal pathologist has an increasingly important part to play in the management of patients with gastrointestinal disorders. Surgeons, gastroenterologists and endoscopists know this and insist on access to the special skills of an experienced gastrointestinal pathologist as part of the team approach to patient care. It is important, therefore, that gastrointestinal pathologists take an active interest in the patient, not just the surgical specimen or biopsy. The view down the microscope should surely be interpreted with awareness that one is looking at part of a patient.

Basil C. Morson, CBE, VRD, MA, DM, FRCS, FRCP,
FRCPath, FRACS(Hon)
Consulting Pathologist at St Mark's Hospital
London, UK

Preface

This, the fifth edition of 'Morson & Dawson', marks a radical departure from previous editions. Gastrointestinal pathology has developed into such a large and diverse subject that it becomes very difficult for a small group of authors to write the entire book. So, the remaining editors decided that, not only should the book become multi-author, but it should also become international in its authorship. We make no excuses for this because we believe this is the best way for this unique title to survive in the face of much excellent competition.

There have been very considerable changes to the editorship. Very sadly, Professor Jeremy Jass died of a brain tumour in November 2008. Jeremy was one of the world's outstanding gastrointestinal pathologists and his incisive and creative writing and editing are very sorely missed. During production of this edition, Professor Bryan Warren also succumbed to cancer. Bryan was also one of the world's great gastro-intestinal pathologists and has been a highly influential member of the Morson & Dawson team for two editions. His death leaves a huge void in UK and international gastrointestinal pathology that just cannot be filled. Furthermore, no less than four of our editorial colleagues have retired from practice and authorship in the last few years. They, too, are greatly missed. They are David Day, Ashley Price, Jimmy Sloan and Ian Talbot. So, we were delighted to be joined by our friend and colleague, Marco Novelli, who brings a touch of relative youth to the team. In line with internationalisation of the title, we were also delighted when two of North America's top gastrointestinal pathologists, Joel Greenson and Gregory Lauwers, agreed to become editors. They have brought with them vitality, expertise and knowledge of the international scene that has been of very considerable value. They greatly complement the team at Morson & Dawson.

There have been other changes to Morson & Dawson. The title now features almost 100% colour photographs. In a lot of ways, we miss the striking quality and historical context of many of the black and white photographs that previous editions held but we cannot stand in the way of progress. The chapter titles have been standardised for the entire luminal gastrointestinal tract and we have restored the section on the 'peritoneum' to its rightful place in this book. The new edition also reflects the very considerable advances in molecular pathology, immunohistochemistry and pathological practice that have occurred since the fourth edition was published in 2003. Becoming multi-author and international does inevitably change a book. Nevertheless we are confident that the choice of authors, from four continents, has meant that the quality initiated by Basil Morson and Ian Dawson has been upheld.

We are delighted to report that Basil, now into his nineties, is well and still attends the lecture, bequeathed to him, each year at the British Society of Gastroenterology, amongst other attendances at UK functions. He has once again provided the Foreword and has told us how delighted he is to see the title he created, way back in 1972, still flourishing. In that regard, we were honoured when the fourth edition won First Prize in the 'Multi-author Text Book' section of the UK's Society of Authors/ RSM Medical Book Awards in 2004. No pressure on the fifth edition, then!

We would like to place on record our gratitude to all of our colleagues who have provided illustrations for this book. These are too numerous to mention individually but important acknowledgements have been made in the legends to the relevant illustrations. We would also record our grateful thanks to all of our colleagues and friends at Wiley-Blackwell, especially Oliver Walter, Elisabeth Dodds, Cathryn Gates, Julie Elliott, Annette Abel, Ruth Swan and Jane Sugarman for their endeavours. They have ensured safe passage of the book, through some stormy waters, and we wish to thank them all sincerely for their help, professionalism and bonhomie.

Neil A. Shepherd
Bryan F. Warren
Geraint T. Williams
Joel K. Greenson
Gregory Y. Lauwers
Marco R. Novelli

About the companion website

This book is accompanied by a companion website:

www.wiley.com/go/morsondawson

The website includes:

- Powerpoints of all figures from the book for downloading

PART 1

Oesophagus

The normal oesophagus: anatomy, specimen dissection and histology relevant to pathological practice

Kaiyo Takubo[1] and Neil A. Shepherd[2]

[1]Tokyo Metropolitan Institute of Gerontology and Tokyo Medical and Dental University School of Medicine, Tokyo, Japan
[2]Gloucestershire Cellular Pathology Laboratory, Cheltenham, UK

Anatomy

The adult oesophagus is a muscular tube some 250 mm long, which extends from the pharynx, at the cricoid cartilage opposite the sixth cervical vertebra, to the oesophago-gastric junction, about 25 mm to the left of the midline, opposite the tenth or eleventh thoracic vertebra. The oesophagus has longitudinal mucosal folds and, when empty, a very narrow lumen. For endoscopists, the distance from the incisor teeth to the upper end of the oesophagus is about 150 mm and to the oesophago-gastric junction about 400 mm, depending, clearly, on the height of the person. The oesophagus pierces the left crus of the diaphragm and has an intra-abdominal portion about 15 mm in length. Its principal relations, important to the pathologist in assessing the local spread of cancer, are with the trachea, left main bronchus, aortic arch, descending aorta and left atrium.

The arterial supply of the oesophagus is by the inferior thyroid, bronchial, left phrenic and left gastric arteries and by small branches directly from the aorta. Its veins form a well-developed submucosal plexus draining into the thyroid, azygos, hemiazygos and left gastric veins. It, thus, provides an important link between the systemic and portal venous systems. Lymphatic channels from the pharynx and upper third of the oesophagus drain to the deep cervical lymph nodes, either directly or through the paratracheal nodes, and also to the infrahyoid lymph nodes; from the lower two-thirds they drain to the posterior mediastinal (para-oesophageal) lymph nodes and thence to the thoracic duct. From the infra-diaphragmatic portion of the oesophagus, drainage is to the left gastric lymph nodes and to a ring of lymph nodes around the cardia. Some lymph vessels may drain directly into the thoracic duct. In its upper part the oesophagus is innervated by the glossopharyngeal nerve and, throughout its length, it is supplied by fibres from the vagus nerve and local sympathetic ganglia.

The lower end of the oesophagus is anchored posteriorly to the pre-aortic fascia and is surrounded by the phreno-oesophageal ligament, which blends into the muscularis propria of the oesophagus. This arrangement allows some degree of movement and rebound. Dissection studies indicate that no discrete anatomical sphincter is present but there are differences of opinion as to whether, and if so how, the muscle at the oesophago-gastric junction is modified. One careful anatomical study [1] has ruled out the presence of any thickening of the muscularis mucosae or of the circular muscle coat but has described the separation of obliquely arranged inner circular muscle fibres into fascicles, which continue into the stomach to form the circular muscle layer. However, another equally thorough investigation [2] describes a definite thickening of the inner circular muscle coat. Both studies have concluded that the arrangements that they describe might, and probably do, act as a functional sphincter.

The oesophageal wall in cross-section can be divided macroscopically into stratified squamous epithelium, lamina propria, muscularis mucosae, and the submucosa, muscularis propria and adventitia (Figure 1.1). Gross inspection of cut sections of tumours in the oesophagus generally reveals the depth of tumour invasion and this

Morson and Dawson's Gastrointestinal Pathology, Fifth Edition. Edited by Neil A. Shepherd, Bryan F. Warren,
Geraint T. Williams, Joel K. Greenson, Gregory Y. Lauwers and Marco R. Novelli.
© 2013 Blackwell Publishing Ltd. Published 2013 by Blackwell Publishing Ltd.

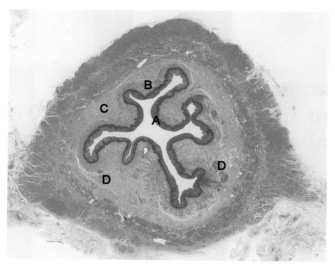

Figure 1.1 The microanatomy of the wall of the oesophagus: in this cross-section, A is the squamous epithelium-lined mucosa and B the muscularis mucosae, which is separated from the mucous membrane by the lamina propria. C is the submucosa, which contains the oesophageal submucosal glands (D), whereas the circular and longitudinal layers of the muscularis propria are outside the submucosa.

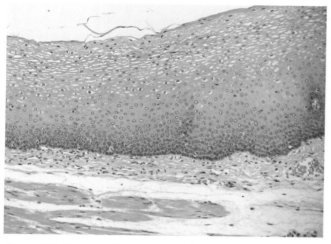

Figure 1.2 The normal squamous epithelium of the oesophagus: this is a stratified squamous epithelium with no keratinisation or a well-developed glandular layer. Note the thickness of the basal cell layer and the height of the papillae.

assessment of depth, through the various layers of the wall, is of critical importance for staging and prognostication.

Histology

Mucosa

The squamous-lined mucosa is about 500–800 μm thick and is composed of non-keratinising stratified squamous

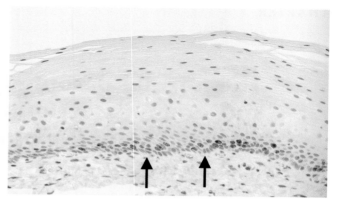

Figure 1.3 The normal oesophageal epithelium on Ki-67 immunostaining: the basal cells (arrows) on the basement membrane do not stain but parabasal cells are positive for Ki-67.

epithelium with a subjacent lamina propria resting on the underlying muscularis mucosae.

Epithelium

Resection specimens usually have a thinner squamous epithelium compared with biopsy specimens because the superficial layers are likely to be lost during surgical handling. The squamous epithelium (Figure 1.2) has a basal zone consisting of several layers of cuboidal or rectangular basophilic cells, with dark nuclei, in which glycogen is absent. It occupies about 10–15% of the thickness of the normal epithelium, although it may be thicker in the last 20 mm or so of the squamous-lined oesophagus. Occasional mitoses are evident in the basal and parabasal cell layers. Above the basal zone, the epithelial cells are larger and become progressively flattened but, even on the surface, they retain their nuclei. Keratohyaline granules are not usually present in the surface cells of the normal epithelium. However, glycogen is abundant. Ki-67 (monoclonal antibody MIB-1) immunostaining usually shows a negative reaction in the basal layer, on the basement membrane, and a positive reaction in the parabasal layers. Epithelial stem cells may be present in the basal layer. The presence of Ki-67-positive cells in more than three cell layers is an abnormal feature, consistent with gastro-oesophageal reflux disease (Figure 1.3).

Single intra-epithelial lymphocytes ('squiggle' cells) lying between the squamous cells are common, particularly in the lower half of the mucosa, and in this situation their convoluted nuclei may be confused with the nuclei of neutrophils. They are a normal feature. Characterisation using monoclonal antibodies has shown them to be T lymphocytes [3]. Langerhans' cells are antigen-presenting cells that are demonstrable, by electron microscopy and metal impregnation techniques, as sparsely distributed ovoid forms with radiating dendritic processes, occurring in all layers of the oesophageal epithelium [4]. They are positively stained with antibodies against S-100 protein and react with monoclonal antibodies against HLA-DR (major histocompatibility complex [MHC] class II) and OKT6 (CD1). They also contain calcitonin gene-related peptide (CGRP), which may serve as an immunomodulator. The number of Langerhans' cells and the intensity of their immunoreactivity for CGRP are increased in reflux oesophagitis [5]. They contain Langerhans' granules (Birbeck's granules), seen on electron microscopic examination.

Both melanocytes and non-melanocyte argyrophil cells are randomly distributed in the basal layer of the epithelium, the former usually as small groups and the latter singly [6,7]. These cell types are presumably the origin of primary malignant melanomas and small cell undifferentiated (oat cell) carcinomas, respectively, that occur at this site. Merkel's cells are also present in the epithelium.

Transmission electron microscopy (TEM) studies of the squamous epithelium have broadened our understanding of the micro-anatomy [8–13]. Basal cells are cuboidal or columnar with large, centrally placed nuclei and relatively simple cytoplasm containing few organelles. They are attached to the basement membrane by frequent hemidesmosomes. Prickle cells show numerous keratin filaments, relatively abundant glycogen, a prominent Golgi apparatus and more numerous desmosomes. The squamous cells of the superficial or functional zone become increasingly flattened towards the lumen, contain some phospholipid material and have a coating of acid mucosubstance which is likely to have a protective function. Scanning electron microscopy shows a complex pattern of micro-ridges lining the lumen. Membrane-coated granules, 0.1–0.3 μm in diameter, are present in the intermediate and superficial zones of the oesophageal epithelium. As well as being the source of mucosubstances, they also contain acid hydrolases which, when secreted into the intercellular space, may be responsible for the reduction of desmosomes exhibited by squamous cells as they approach the luminal surface.

Free-ending nerves are located in the intercellular spaces of the squamous epithelium and reach the subepithelial nerve plexus. These nerves probably mediate oesophageal pain. Cell proliferation studies have demonstrated a slower cell cycle time in basal cells overlying papillae, in comparison with the interpapillary basal cells [14]. The turnover time of the oesophageal epithelium is about 4–7 days in rats and mice. The corresponding period in humans is said to be 10 days or less, although no definitive data are available.

Lamina propria

The lamina propria consists of loose connective tissue containing a sprinkling of lymphocytes, mostly helper T cells, plasma cells, and occasional eosinophils and mast cells. Focal collections of lymphocytes and plasma cells may be aggregated around the ducts of the oesophageal submucosal glands. There are numerous vascular papillae (also known as intrapapillary vessels or intrapapillary capillary loops), associated with connective tissue, which project upwards for two-thirds of the total thickness of the epithelium. Changes in the vascular pattern are evident by magnifying endoscopy under various pathological conditions.

Relatively large vessels are observed more frequently in the lamina propria than in the submucosa in cross-sections of the lower oesophageal sphincter. These vessels are considered to be the longitudinal palisade vessels visible at endoscopy and helpful in defining the true oesophagogastric junction.

Muscularis mucosae

The muscularis mucosae shows a variable pattern. In its upper part it commonly consists of isolated or irregularly arranged muscle bundles, rather than forming a continuous sheet, but in the middle and lower thirds it forms a continuum of longitudinal and transverse fibres and may reach up to 300 μm in thickness at the squamo-columnar junction. In the resected oesophagus, thick collections of fine irregular muscle fibres are evident at sites of previous biopsy.

Submucosa

The submucosa contains the oesophageal submucosal glands (deep glands, oesophageal glands proper), Meissner's plexus and a ramifying lymphatic plexus within a loose connective tissue network, which accounts for the early and extensive submucosal spread of oesophageal carcinoma. The oesophageal submucosal glands tend to be arranged in rows parallel to the long axis [15] and, although scattered, they are relatively concentrated at the upper and lower ends of the oesophagus. The glands are compound tubulo-alveolar in type and resemble labial salivary glands, containing both mucous and serous secretory cells and oncocytes, with surrounding myo-epithelial cells, anchoring them to the underlying basement membrane. The mucous cells contain sulphomucins. Many glands do not contain serous cells. From two to five lobules drain into a common duct lined by a flattened cuboidal epithelium initially, which becomes stratified squamous in type, and surrounded by lymphocytes and plasma cells after passing obliquely through the muscularis mucosae (Figure 1.4). The presence of oesophageal submucosal glands and/or their ducts is presumptive evidence that any sampled biopsy material derives from the true anatomical oesophagus.

Muscularis propria

The muscularis propria consists of well-developed circular and longitudinal coats. In its upper part these are striated

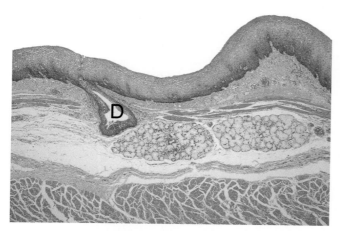

Figure 1.4 The submucosal gland of the oesophagus: the terminal portions consist of mucous cells. A duct (D) is evident.

and both oxidative (fast twitch) and glycolytic (slow twitch) fibres are present [16]. There is a gradual change to smooth muscle in the upper and middle thirds, although, in the lower third, both coats are entirely composed of smooth muscle with no clear evidence of sphincter formation. A well-defined myenteric nerve (Auerbach's) plexus is present at all levels but there appears to be no well-formed submucosal plexus. Three types of neuron are identifiable [17,18]. One is argyrophilic, multi-axonal and, probably, sympathetic, and sends out numerous dendrites and axons to surround other neurons in the same and adjacent ganglia but does not directly supply muscle. The second type is not argyrophilic but cholinergic and probably parasympathetic, supplying the muscle. It is likely that the former has a coordinating function and the latter a motor function. A third type of fibre, probably part of the communicating system, is rich in vasoactive inhibitory peptide (VIP). Such fibres are commonly associated with sphincteric mechanisms [18]. There are also numerous intrinsic fibres containing neuropeptide Y [19]. Ganglion cells decrease in number with age [20] but the smooth muscle does not appear to undergo corresponding atrophy.

Adventitia

The adventitia of the oesophagus is a thick layer of coarse connective tissue around the oesophagus and is seen to surround the oesophagus in resection specimens. It contains blood vessels, lymphatics and lymph nodes, multiple branches, anterior and posterior, of the vagus nerve and other neural structures. Its comprehensive examination is of particular importance in such resection specimens because here proximity of tumour to the circumferential surgical resection margin and the pleural surfaces will

be evident and assessable (see below). The adventitia is in continuity with the adjacent mediastinal connective tissues.

Tissues adjacent to the oesophagus, including the pleura

These are of some importance because they are or may be present in resected oesophagus specimens. The proximal stomach is almost universally present in such specimens whereas pharynx and spleen are occasionally seen in specimens resected with the oesophagus. The trachea, bronchus, lung, diaphragm, azygos vein, thoracic duct, thymus and aorta can also be present in oesophageal resection specimens. Although usually termed the *circumferential* resection margin of the oesophagus, it is important to note that, especially on the right but also on the left, a sizable proportion of the circumference of oesophageal resection specimens is actually invested not by adventitial connective tissues, thus constituting a true surgical margin, but by pleura, which all radical oesophago-gastrectomy specimens will possess. Involvement of the circumferential margin can be influenced by surgical quality but a surgeon can do little about pleural involvement. We advocate accurate identification of the pleura, on both sides, and painting, preferably by coloured gelatin, of only the true circumferential surgical margin to allow differentiation of these structures in histological sections.

Location of the oesophago-gastric junction

Precise definitions of the oesophago-gastric junction are essential before an accurate diagnosis of columnar-lined oesophagus (CLO) (see Chapter 5: Barrett's oesophagus) can be made. Anatomically, the definition of the oesophago-gastric junction is the line between the angles of the opened oesophagus and gastric curvature. This definition can be used for surgically resected materials. Clinically, however, the location of the oesophago-gastric junction is controversial [21]. The distance between the anatomical oesophago-gastric junction and the squamo-columnar junction, on macroscopic examination of postmortem specimens, has ranged from 0–10 mm with a mean of 3 mm [22] to 5–21 mm with a mean of 11 mm [23].

In North America and European countries, the endoscopic definition of the oesophago-gastric junction is the upper limit of the gastric folds. However, this upper limit shows considerable vertical movement during endoscopy [24]. When a small volume of air is present in the oesophagus, or at expiration, the upper end of the mucosal folds moves rostrally. When a large volume of air is present, or in deep inspiration, the upper end of the columnar mucosal folds moves caudally. Therefore, the upper limits of the columnar mucosal folds are not in a constant position. Palisade vessels are always evident within the oesophagus

[25], are observed within the lower oesophageal sphincter and can be used to define the oesophago-gastric junction. So, in Japan, the oesophago-gastric junction is defined endoscopically as the lower limit of the palisade vessels [22]. Based on this definition, many cases may actually be defined as representing ultra-short segment columnar-lined oesophagus (see Chapter 5 section 'Ultra-short segment Barrett's oesophagus'). Pathologists should always pay attention to the true origin of any biopsy specimen from the mucosa around the oesophago-gastric junction.

Oesophageal cardiac glands (superficial glands, mucosal glands) are small mucous glands in the lamina propria. They are branched simple tubulo-alveolar glands, located mainly in the lower and upper oesophagus. Oesophageal cardiac glands beneath the oesophageal squamous epithelium at the squamo-columnar junction show continuity with the gastric cardiac mucosa and can be observed at endoscopy through the squamous epithelium in about half of all patients examined. However, cardiac glands are histologically evident at or around the oesophago-gastric junction in almost all individuals (Figure 1.5). The maximum overlap of the squamous epithelium and cardiac glands extending continuously from the gastric cardia, as demonstrated by histological and endoscopic examination, may be up to 15 mm. Endoscopically, oesophageal cardiac glands beneath the squamous epithelium in the oesophago-gastric junction zone usually appear yellowish in colour, and are flat or slightly elevated. Columnar-lined islands are also observed endoscopically in squamous mucosa and are similar in colour to those of the gastric cardiac mucosa, being unstained with Lugol's iodine. Columnar islands can

often be found in the distal 10 mm of the oesophagus. They are observed in about half of all patients with oesophageal or gastric carcinoma.

In cardiac mucosa adjacent to the squamo-columnar junction, most of the gland cells are mucous in type and stain strongly with periodic acid–Schiff (PAS). Occasional cells near the upper ends of the glands, close to the squamous junction, may secrete both sialomucins and sulpho-mucins [26]. Parietal cells, morphologically identical to those in the fundic glands, are present in small numbers (oxyntocardiac glands) and occasionally chief cells are present as well. Numerous endocrine cells, some of which are argentaffin and others argyrophil, are found in this region [27]. Lymphoid follicles are also common in the deeper part of the mucosa, or extend through the muscularis mucosae into the submucosa.

Pancreatic tissue (Figure 1.6) may be seen in the mucosa at the oesophago-gastric junction: it is recognisable by the presence of variably sized nests or lobules of acinar tissue, 0.2–1.6 mm in diameter, admixed with cardiac glands, and composed of cells with basally located, small, round and uniform nuclei and abundant cytoplasm. These structures appear eosinophilic and granular in the apical and middle portions and basophilic in the basal area. Some mucous cells may be intermingled [28]. As a result of their resemblance to pancreatic exocrine cells and their immunopositivity for lipase, the term 'pancreatic acinar metaplasia' has been used to describe this feature. Some have suggested an association with gastritis but subsequently it has been recognised as a common feature in patients attending for elective upper gastrointestinal endoscopy and is not

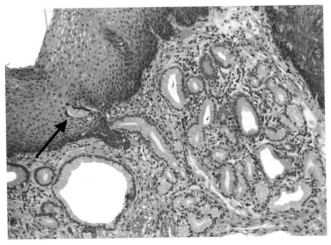

Figure 1.5 The oesophageal cardiac glands (also known as superficial or mucosal glands) beneath squamous epithelium in the oesophago-gastric junction zone. Mucous gland lobules are present. Part of a cardiac-type gland (arrow) is apparent in the squamous epithelium.

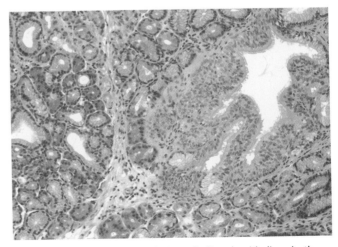

Figure 1.6 Pancreatic metaplasia and ciliated epithelium in the mucosa at the oesophago-gastric junction. Pancreatic acinar cells with eosinophilic cytoplasmic granules are present among cardiac-type glands. The ciliated epithelium is histologically similar to that of bronchial pseudo-stratified columnar epithelium.

specifically associated with any clinical or histological abnormalities of the oesophagus or stomach [29]. Similar foci have been described in the gastric antral and body mucosa but appear to be much less common at these sites, although they have been reported in some 3% of antral biopsies from children [30]. A pancreatic phenotype is also well recognised in Barrett's metaplastic tissue in the true oesophagus (see Chapter 5).

Multilayered epithelium (ME) or squamous metaplasia-like change may be evident in the oesophageal cardiac glands beneath the squamous epithelium and in cardiac mucosa adjacent to it (Figure 1.6). There may also be a pseudo-stratified (partly ciliated) columnar epithelium, often merging with the squamous metaplasia-like change [31,32]. When histological examination of a biopsy specimen reveals pancreatic acinar metaplasia, multilayered epithelium, squamous metaplasia-like change or pseudo-stratified columnar epithelium with occasional cilia, we firmly believe that the tissue can yet derive from the 'normal' mucosa of the oesophago-gastric junction zone and does not necessarily infer true glandular metaplasia of the lower oesophagus, alternatively known as Barrett's oesophagus (see Chapter 5).

Handling of endoscopic and resection oesophageal specimens

Endoscopic resection specimens (Figure 1.7)

Endoscopic mucosal resection (EMR) and endoscopic submucosal dissection (ESD) are relatively new techniques of increasing importance for the diagnosis and treatment of neoplasia in the oesophagus. They can be used for the removal of small benign tumorous nodules, such as granular cell tumours and other small connective tissue tumours

Tangent line

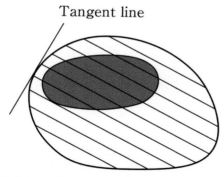

Figure 1.7 Schema illustrating one method for sectioning endoscopic mucosal resection (EMR) and endoscopic submucosal dissection (ESD) specimens advocated by the Japan Esophageal Society [33]. Fixed specimens that have been obtained by EMR and ESD are cut into slices 2–3 mm thick. (Reproduced with kind permission from Springer Science+Business Media: Esophagus, Japanese Classification of Esophageal Cancer, tenth edition: part I, vol 6, 2009, p.39, Japan Esophageal Society, © 2009.)

in the submucosa, but EMRs are also employed as a 'big biopsy', e.g. for the definitive diagnosis of well differentiated squamous cell carcinoma when multiple previous biopsies have been unable to fully confirm the diagnosis. Of increasing importance is their use in the management of early neoplasia complicating Barrett's oesophagus (see Chapter 5).

Although somewhat dependent on the endoscopic methodology used, before fixation they can be stretched to reflect the size and shape as in the body and then pinned to a board with the mucosal aspect uppermost. The specimen(s) should then be immersed in a large container of formalin and fixed for at least half a day or overnight. Either initially or after fixation, they can be painted to demonstrate peripheral and deep margins of excision. India ink, coloured paints and coloured gelatin can be used, depending on local laboratory preferences. For specimens that have been resected piecemeal, pinning and fixation should be performed by an endoscopist aware of the actual configuration of the lesion in vivo to enable more precise restructuring and assessment of ultimate (especially peripheral) resection margins.

It is recommended that fixed specimens obtained by EMR and ESD are cut into slices 2–3 mm thick for serial sectioning and microscopic examination. The lines of sectioning should be at right angles to the line forming a tangent to the resection margin close to the tumour [33].

Surgical resection specimens

Oesophagectomy and oesophago-gastrectomy operations are most commonly undertaken for carcinoma of the oesophagus. In the Far East, this is usually for squamous cell carcinoma whereas, in western countries, adenocarcinoma complicating Barrett's oesophagus is now overwhelming the most common indication for these operations. Increasingly neo-adjuvant chemo(radio)therapy has been used and this may make identification of the site of the tumour difficult and require extensive blocking of the oesophagus to ensure that the entire tumour site has been assessed histologically. This section will give guidance as to the appropriate macroscopic preparation and assessment of these specimens but the interested reader is referred to guidelines and protocols published by Japanese, UK and US authorities for a comprehensive guide to the assessment of such specimens [33–35].

Surgically resected specimens should be opened longitudinally in a standard way. We recommend standard opening ventrally. The part of the oesophagus containing the tumour may then be left unopened with an appropriate fixative-soaked wick to ensure internal fixation. Alternatively, that part can be opened in a standard way (ventrally) with the circumferential margin previously painted to aid accurate assessment of margins of excision. At this time, whether or not the tumour is opened, it is important for the prosector to identify the pleural surfaces and ensure that these can be accurately differentiated, at the time of histological assessment, from the true circumferential resection margin by appropriate painting (see above). Furthermore, these specimens undergo dramatic shortening immediately after surgery because of contraction of the muscularis propria such that the oesophageal segment is often only half the length it was *in situ*. Efforts should therefore be made to ensure that these specimens are received in the laboratory as soon as possible so that they can stretched and pinned on a corkboard to reflect the length at the time of resection.

Although some authorities recommend that oesophagectomy specimens should *always* be fixed unopened through the tumour, we believe that there are times, especially in early cancer, multifocal dysplasia and superficial cancer (particularly that complicating Barrett's oesophagus) and when neo-adjuvant therapy has effectively ablated the tumour, when opening the specimen is appropriate to allow accurate identification of those parts of the specimen for submission for histological assessment. After neo-adjuvant therapy, only an area of superficial scarring of the mucosa may be seen, on opening, and this may be less easy to appreciate in transverse sections of a specimen previously left unopened. Assessment of these specimens should not be beholden to blanket national and international 'rules' but should be determined by the requirements of the individual case and local laboratory practices.

In a specimen left unopened, a large sharp knife should be used to section the entire tumour area transversely with identification of the orientation achieved by differential painting or another method favoured by the laboratory. These slices can then be submitted for histology in their entirety, usually in big blocks, such that all adventitial tissues, para-oesophageal lymph nodes and pleural surfaces can be assessed, along with the true circumferential resection margin, previously identified by painting. We recommend coloured gelatin for this purpose because it adheres very effectively to the surface, is readily identified in histological sections and does not run or spread like other fluids used in laboratories for this purpose.

It is important to ensure that proximal and distal surgical resection margins are assessed histologically and separate doughnuts from these margins should always be submitted for histology in their entirety because oesophageal cancer, both squamous cell carcinoma and adenocarcinoma, can demonstrate discontinuous spread, often as a result of submucosal lymphovascular spread, with involvement of margins at some distance from the primary tumour. The proximal and distal resection margins can be assessed in sections taken parallel to the margins and/or in longitudinal sections perpendicular to them [33,34].

Superficial carcinoma can usually be distinguished from advanced carcinoma by macroscopic observation of cut surfaces of the tumour or by determining whether a super-

ficial tumour is fixed to the muscularis propria. If not fixed, the tumour will slide over the muscularis propria when only slight force is applied to the mucosa, indicating that it is probably a superficial carcinoma without invasion to the muscularis propria. We recommend that, in cases of superficial carcinoma, the specimen is sliced parallel to the long axis of the oesophagus. Whole step sections can then be prepared [33,35].

In more advanced carcinoma, be it squamous cell carcinoma or adenocarcinoma, it is clearly important to extensively sample the most deeply invasive tumour. One or more representative slices of the tumour at the site of deepest invasion, estimated by inspection and palpation, parallel and perpendicular to the oesophagus, should be blocked and submitted for histopathological examination to demonstrate the deepest aspect of the tumour and its relationship to the layers of the oesophageal wall, adventitial tissues and, critically, the circumferential resection margin and pleural surfaces [33–35].

References

1. Jackson AJ. The spiral constrictor of the gastro-esophageal junction. *Am J Anat* 1978;**51**:265.
2. Liebermann-Meffert D, Allgower M, Schmid P, Blum AL. Muscular equivalent of the lower esophageal sphincter. *Gastroenterology* 1979;**76**:31.
3. Mangano MM, Antonioli DA, Schnitt SJ, Wang HH. Nature and significance of cells with irregular nuclear contours in esophageal mucosal biopsies. *Mod Pathol* 1995;**5**:191.
4. Geboes K, DeWolf-Peeters C, Rutgeerts P, et al. Lymphocytes and Langerhans cells in the human oesophageal epithelium. *Virchows Arch A Pathol Anat Histopathol* 1983;**401**:45.
5. Singaram C, Sengupta A, Stevens C, Spechler SJ, Goyal RK. Localization of calcitonin gene-related peptide in human esophageal Langerhans cells. *Gastroenterology* 1991;**100**:560.
6. de la Pava S, Nigogosyan G, Pickren JW, Cabrera A. Melanosis of the esophagus. *Cancer* 1963;**16**:48.
7. Tateishi R, Taniguchi H, Wada A, Horai T, Tanaguchi K. Argyrophil cells and melanocytes in esophageal mucosa. *Arch Pathol* 1974;**98**:87.
8. Hopwood D, Logan KR, Coghill D, Bouchier IAD. Histochemical studies of mucosubstances and lipids in normal human oesophageal epithelium. *Histochem J* 1977;**9**:153.
9. Logan KR, Hopwood D, Milne G. Ultrastructural demonstration of cell coat on the cell surface of normal human oesophageal epithelium. *Histochem J* 1977;**9**:495.
10. Al Yassin TM, Toner PG. Fine structure of squamous epithelium and submucosal glands of human oesophagus. *J Anat* 1977;**123**:705.
11. Hopwood D, Logan KR, Bouchier IAD. The electron microscopy of normal human oesophageal epithelium. *Virchows Arch* (B) 1978;**26**:345.
12. Hopwood D, Logan KR, Milne G. The light and electron microscopic distribution of acid phosphatase activity in human normal oesophageal epithelium. *Histochem J* 1978;**10**:159.
13. Logan KR, Hopwood D, Milne G. Cellular junctions in human oesophageal epithelium. *J Pathol* 1978;**126**:157.
14. Jankowski J, Austin W, Howat K, et al. Proliferating cell nuclear antigen in oesophageal mucosa: comparison with autoradiography. *Eur J Gastroenterol Hepatol* 1992;**4**:579.

15. Goetsch E. The structure of the mammalian esophagus. *Am J Anat* 1910;**10**:1.

16. Whitmore I. Oesophageal striated muscle arrangement and histochemical fibre types in guinea pig, marmoset, macaque and man. *J Anat* 1982;**134**:685.

17. Smith B. The neurological lesion in achalasia of the cardia. *Gut* 1970;**11**:388.

18. Alumets J, Fahrenkrug J, Hakanson R. A rich VIP nerve supply is characteristic of sphincters. *Nature* 1979;**280**:155.

19. Aggestrup S, Emson P, Uddman R, et al. Distribution and content of neuropeptide Y in the human lower esophageal sphincter. *Digestion* 1987;**36**:68.

20. Eckardt V, Le Compte PM. Esophageal ganglia and smooth muscle in the elderly. *Am J Dig Dis* 1978;**23**:443.

21. American Joint Committee on Cancer. Esophagus and esophagogastric junction. In: *AJCC Cancer Staging Manual*, 7th edn. New York: Springer, 2009: 103.

22. Takubo K, Arai T, Sawabe M. Structures of the normal esophagus and Barrett's esophagus. *Esophagus* 2003;**1**:37.

23. Bombeck CT, Dillard DH, Nyhus LM. Muscular anatomy of the gastroesophageal junction and role of phrenoesophageal ligament. Autopsy study of sphincter mechanism. *Ann Surg* 1966;**164**:643.

24. Takubo K, Vieth M, Aida J, et al. Differences in the definitions used for esophageal and gastric diseases in different countries. Endoscopic definition of the esophagogastric junction, the precursor of Barrett's adenocarcinoma, the definition of Barrett's esophagus, and histologic criteria for mucosal adenocarcinoma or high-grade dysplasia. *Digestion* 2009;**80**:248.

25. De Carvalho CAF. Sur l'angio-architecture veineuse de la zone de transition oesophagogastrique et son interpretation fonctionnelle. *Acta Anat* 1966;**64**:125.

26. Gad A. A histochemical study of human alimentary tract mucosubstances in health and disease. 1. Normal and tumours. *Br J Cancer* 1969;**23**:52.

27. Krause WJ, Ivey KJ, Baskin WN, MacKercher PA. Morphological observations on the normal human cardiac glands. *Anat Rec* 1978;**192**:59.

28. Doglioni C, Laurino L, Dei Tos AP, et al. Pancreatic (acinar) metaplasia of the gastric mucosa: histology, ultrastructure, immunocytochemistry and clinicopathologic correlation of 101 cases. *Am J Surg Pathol* 1993;**17**:1134.

29. Wang HH, Zeroogian JM, Spechler SJ, Goyal RK, Antonioli DA. Prevalence and significance of pancreatic acinar metaplasia at the gastroesophageal junction. *Am J Surg Pathol* 1996;**20**:1507.

30. Krishnamurthy S, Integlia MJ, Grand RJ, Dayal Y. Pancreatic acinar cell clusters in pediatric gastric mucosa. *Am J Surg Pathol* 1998;**22**:100.

31. Glickman JN, Chen Y-Y, Wang HH, et al. Phenotypic characteristics of a distinctive multilayered epithelium suggests that it is a precursor in the development of Barrett's esophagus. *Am J Surg Pathol* 2001;**25**:569.

32. Takubo K, Vieth M, Honma N, et al. Ciliated surface in the esophagogastric junction zone: a precursor of Barrett's mucosa or ciliated pseudostratified metaplasia? *Am J Surg Pathol*, 2005; **29**:211.

33. Takubo K, Makuuchi H, Fujita H, et al. Japanese classification of esophageal cancer. Parts I, II and III. *Esophagus* 2009;**6**:1.

34. Mapstone N. *Dataset for the Histopathological Reporting of Oesophageal Carcinoma*, 2nd edn. London: Royal College of Pathologists, 2007. Available at: www.rcpath.org/resources/pdf/G006OesophagealdatasetFINALFeb07.pdf (accessed April 2011).

35. Washington K, Berlin J, Branton P, et al. *Protocol for the examination of specimens from patients with carcinoma of the esophagus*. College of American Pathologists, 2011. Available at: www.cap.org/apps/docs/committees/cancer/cancer_protocols/2011/Esophagus_11protocol.pdf (accessed April 2011).

CHAPTER 2

Normal embryology, fetal development and developmental abnormalities

Kaiyo Takubo[1] and Neil A. Shepherd[2]

[1]Tokyo Metropolitan Institute of Gerontology and Tokyo Medical and Dental University School of Medicine, Tokyo, Japan
[2]Gloucestershire Cellular Pathology Laboratory, Cheltenham, UK

Embryology and fetal development

There are a number of excellent accounts of the development of the trachea and oesophagus and its relationship to various malformations [1–6]. Between days 23 and 26 of embryonic development (3 mm, somite stage 10–11) a bud develops on the ventral (anterior) aspect of the foregut at the caudal end of the primitive pharynx; it grows to become a diverticulum and develops a lumen. This diverticulum will form the larynx, trachea, bronchi and lung buds. It grows caudally and becomes separated from the oesophagus, posteriorly by the craniocaudal ingrowth of two lateral folds, which fuse in the midline and separate the tracheal lumen from that of the oesophagus. As separation proceeds, the oesophagus elongates, due mainly to a rapid increase in growth at its cranial end rather than primary caudal positioning of the stomach. Separation is complete at 35–40 days, by which time the stomach has been carried down below the developing diaphragm. Anatomical studies [5] suggest that the tracheo-oesophageal septum may be the primitive floor of a respiratory outgrowth.

The epithelial lining is initially stratified columnar in type; ciliated cells develop by the 70-mm stage [7–9]. The ciliated epithelium in the middle third then changes to stratified squamous and this change extends both upwards and downwards [10] to form a complete squamous lining at term, although small islands of ciliated epithelium may remain in postnatal life [11]. The muscularis mucosae develops in the fourth to seventh months, beginning from the lower oesophagus and proceeding proximally. Oesophageal glands proper, in the submucosa, which develop

after squamous epithelialisation, appear late in gestation and much of their development is postnatal [8].

The circular muscle coat is present at 8 weeks but the longitudinal coat does not become apparent until approximately 13 weeks' gestation. Neurons can be recognised concomitantly with the circular muscle at 8 weeks and their density increases up to 16–20 weeks, when there is a rapid decrease, with a further reduction towards adult levels during infancy. Ganglion cells and nerve fibres in the myenteric plexus are also maximal at 16–20 weeks, with a subsequent decline in their density up to 30 weeks, when their numbers become constant, despite further oesophageal growth [12,13]. The ontogeny and distribution of neuropeptide expression in the human oesophagus from 8 weeks' gestation to 28 months after birth are characterised by the progressive appearance of immunoreactivity in fibres of the myenteric plexus at 11 weeks, and in cell bodies at 13–15 weeks, the patterns of expression of hormones and peptides being comparable to those in mature newborns and infants by 22 weeks' gestation [14].

Anomalies of development

Duplications, diverticula and cysts

In some descriptions of these oesophageal variations, the three conditions are separated but many embryologists and pathologists, ourselves included, now regard most of them as differing degrees of manifestation of a single embryological defect. A number of subgroups have been defined [15]. Most of these developmental cysts are found

Morson and Dawson's Gastrointestinal Pathology, Fifth Edition. Edited by Neil A. Shepherd, Bryan F. Warren,
Geraint T. Williams, Joel K. Greenson, Gregory Y. Lauwers and Marco R. Novelli.
© 2013 Blackwell Publishing Ltd. Published 2013 by Blackwell Publishing Ltd.

in children who present with respiratory distress or feeding difficulties. In adults, foregut duplication cysts are uncommon and may be an incidental finding in routine radiological studies. Endoscopic ultrasonography has been shown to be invaluable in their diagnosis and may eliminate the need for surgery in asymptomatic individuals [16].

Congenital duplication cysts

The most common oesophageal cysts are duplication cysts [17–19], which represent a doubling of the oesophagus to some degree. Dysphagia and retrosternal pain have been reported in patients with duplication cysts. Elevation of serum CA19-9 and CA-125 levels has been reported occasionally [20]. About 60% of duplication cysts are located in the lower part of the oesophagus and about 20% in the upper and lower parts, respectively [21]. They can be spherical or tubular: even triplication has been described. Large duplication cysts measuring up to 125 mm have been reported [22,23]. The lining epithelium may be ciliated or non-ciliated columnar, squamous or a mixture of these types. The wall of a congenital duplication cyst has the same structure as the wall of the normal digestive tract, having both muscularis mucosae and muscularis propria (Figure 2.1) and oesophageal glands proper.

Acute rupture [23] and massive mediastinal haemorrhage secondary to such cysts have been described [22,24]. *Mycobacterium avium* infection has also been described [25] and adenocarcinoma and squamous cell carcinoma arising in a duplication cyst are documented [26].

Oesophageal bronchogenic cysts

Bronchogenic cysts are the most common cystic lesion in the mediastinum, often being located in the anterior mediastinum. However, completely intramural, oesophageal bronchogenic cysts are very rare: 23 cases of oesophageal bronchogenic cyst have been reported between 1981 and 2007 [27]. Elevation of the serum CA-125 level has been reported. The inner surface is lined by a smooth mucosa, and the cyst wall contains cartilage, smooth muscle and bronchial glands; there is usually a lining of ciliated pseudostratified columnar epithelium but there is no muscularis mucosae in bronchogenic cysts. Although generally related to the bronchial tree, rare cases have been reported in the abdomen, including the stomach [28], or in the subcutaneous tissues of the neck or chest [29]. A case of oesophageal bronchogenic cyst measuring 90 mm in diameter has been reported [30].

Other cysts

Oesophago-bronchogenic cysts are rare cystic lesions in the mediastinum (Figure 2.2). They have the combined features of bronchogenic and oesophageal cysts (Figure 2.3). Ten cases of such cysts have been reported [31].

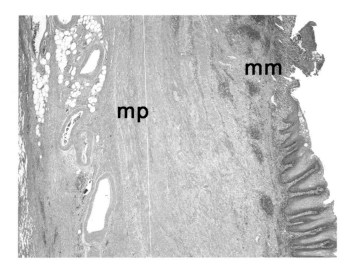

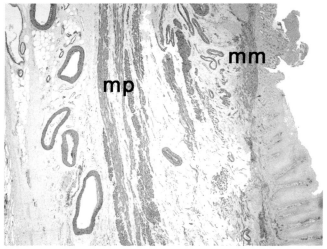

Figure 2.1 (a) The wall of an oesophageal duplication cyst. The wall is lined with acanthotic squamous epithelium with an erosion and has a lamina muscularis mucosae (mm) and tunica muscularis propria (mp). Prominent fibrosis and lymphocyte accumulation are seen in the wall. Haematoxylin and eosin (HE) stain. (b) Immunostaining of smooth muscle actin of the section serial to the H&E section. The lamina muscularis mucosae and tunica muscularis propria show a positive reaction. (Courtesy of Drs T. Nishisaka, C. Watanabe and H. Yamada, Hiroshima Prefectural Hospital, Hiroshima, Japan.)

Gastro-enteric cysts have a gastric or enteric mucosal lining and can secrete hydrochloric acid from gastric parietal cells. Gastro-enteric cysts are often associated with malformations of the vertebrae. Some cases of this type have been reported as neurenteric cysts [32–35].

Atresia, stenosis and tracheo-oesophageal fistula

Knowledge of the normal development of the trachea and oesophagus and the mode of separation of their lumina suggest a number of potential defects, some of which are found in practice [36]. There may be complete failure of division resulting in a single common trachea and oesophagus [37]. Division may be so unequal that the oesophagus is absent or represented only by a thin fibrous cord of variable length, without a lumen or with fistulous communication of the trachea. Part or all of the upper trachea may similarly be absent, although this extremely rare malformation is usually associated with distal tracheo-oesophageal [38] or broncho-oesophageal [39] fistula and a single umbilical artery. Tracheal dominance with oesophageal stenosis or atresia is the more common form of unequal division and a fistula is much more commonly present than absent.

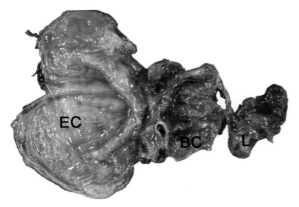

Figure 2.2 Macroscopic appearance of an oesophago-bronchogenic cyst. The resected specimen consists of three parts, an oesophageal cyst (EC), a bronchogenic cyst (BC) and the simultaneously resected upper pulmonary lobe (L). The inner surface is lined with white smooth mucosa in part of the oesophageal cyst and red, slightly rough mucosa in part of the bronchial cyst. (Courtesy of Drs K. Takaoka and Y. Fujioka, Nikko Memorial Hospital, Muroran, Hokkaido, Japan.)

Pure oesophageal atresia without fistula is extremely rare. However, stenosis without fistula occurs in about 13–16% of all infants with some form of oesophageal maldevelopment [40,41], is usually found in the mid-oesophageal region opposite the tracheal bifurcation and can be associated with maternal hyperhydramnios [42]. There are occasional reported cases of fusiform stenosis, usually occurring in the distal oesophagus and resulting from tracheo-bronchial remnants (chondroepithelial choristoma, cartilaginous oesophageal ring) deep below the normal squamous-lined mucosa [43–45].

Oesophageal atresia with tracheo-oesophageal fistula is a relatively common congenital anomaly with an incidence varying from 1 in 800 to 1 in 10 000 live births in different studies [46,47]. However, surgical pathologists rarely encounter material from patients with oesophageal atresia showing tracheo-oesophageal fistula. The atresia may extend over a variable length or, rarely, may consist of a single transverse diaphragm that may or may not be totally imperforate. It has occasionally been described in siblings [48] but hereditary factors probably do not normally play a part. Other congenital malformations are common [49]: some of these are described under the VATER syndrome, which links vertebral defects, anal atresia, tracheo-oesophageal and renal dysplasias [50]. It has subsequently been expanded to include cardiac anomalies and limb, especially radial, defects [51]. Congenital heart defects are also common [52], as are duodenal atresia with gastric distension [53,54]. When any of these are present in a neonate, the others should be sought. Infantile pyloric stenosis has been described as developing after surgical treatment [55]. There is no significant sex difference in incidence, and maternal hydramnios is more common in association with pure atresia.

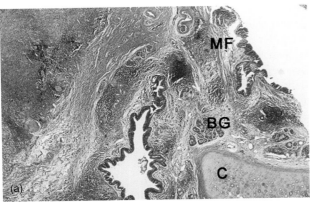

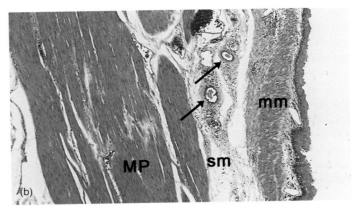

Figure 2.3 (a) Histology of part of a bronchogenic cyst from the oesophago-bronchogenic cyst in Figure 2.2. The inner surface is lined with ciliated pseudo-stratified squamous epithelium. Bronchial glands (BG), cartilage (C) and smooth muscle fibres (MF) are evident in the wall of a part showing a bronchogenic cyst. (b) Histology of part of the oesophageal cyst in Figure 2.2. The inner surface is lined by squamous epithelium. Oesophageal gland ducts (arrows) are present in the submucosa (sm). The muscularis mucosae (mm) is evident. MP: tunica muscularis propria. (Courtesy of Drs K Takaoka and Y Fujioka, Nikko Memorial Hospital, Muroran, Hokkaido, Japan.)

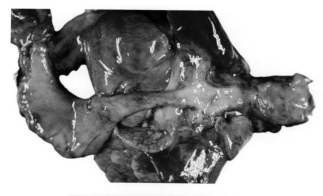

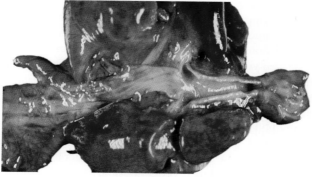

Figure 2.4 Upper: macroscopic appearance of oesophageal atresia and tracheo-oesophageal fistula. Oesophageal atresia and tracheo-oesophageal fistula are seen. Lower: the oesophagus and trachea are opened. (Courtesy of Dr H. Kishimoto, Division of Pathology, Saitama Children's Medical Center, Saitama, Japan.)

A number of anatomical varieties of oesophageal atresia have been described [56]. In the most common, accounting for some 85–90% of cases, the upper end of the oesophagus ends in a blind pouch (Figure 2.4). All coats of the oesophagus are present and the muscle is usually hypertrophic. The anterior wall of the pouch often fuses with the trachea but only rarely communicates with it. The lower oesophagus is normal at the cardia but becomes progressively narrowed proximally. It usually communicates with the trachea within 20 mm of the bifurcation but occasionally ends in one or other of the main bronchi, more often the right. The opening is slit-shaped or funnel-like and oesophageal and tracheal muscle are intimately blended. The gap between the blind upper pouch and the lower end varies from 10 mm to 50 mm and there is sometimes a fibrous cord uniting the two. Surgery is usually feasible but subsequent stenosis leading to recurrent respiratory infection is common, which may be due to stricture consequent on surgery or to an alteration of normal oesophageal physiological activity.

The pathogenesis of oesophageal atresia is uncertain. The most probable explanation is that, as dorsal structures elongate rapidly in weeks 4 and 5, cell proliferation in the foregut does not keep pace and both dorsally and ventrally situated cells differentiate into tracheal, rather than oesophageal, tissue. Failure of recanalisation is inherently unlikely, because the oesophageal lumen is probably never occluded and the condition has been described in a 9-mm embryo [57]. The presence of abnormal vessels running between the upper and lower parts of the oesophagus has been implicated but these are not present in most cases [58]. The lateral septa that separate the trachea from the oesophagus may meet on the posterior, rather than the anterior, wall of the foregut, or the posterior wall may be drawn forward with partial incorporation of the oesophagus into the trachea.

Radiological evidence of additional thoracic or lumbar vertebrae, often with supernumerary ribs, supports the idea of a disturbance of growth at this period of development [59]. The possibility of genetic factors or viral infection [47] has also been mooted but this is open to criticism in favour of a non-specific action of several teratogenic processes [60]. Deficiencies in Auerbach's (myenteric) plexus, with an extra plexus in the membranous part of the trachea, have been reported, ascribed to incomplete separation of the trachea from the oesophagus [61,62]. There is also clinical evidence that disorders of motility can be a problem after surgical repair [63]. Occasional examples of fistula without atresia (H-shaped tracheo-oesophageal fistula) have been recorded and are compatible with survival to adult life. In many the fistula is between the oesophagus and bronchus rather than the trachea.

Oesophago-bronchial fistula and pulmonary sequestration

A small number of cases have been reported in which a supernumerary lung bud appears to arise from the lower part of the foregut in association with a congenital diaphragmatic hernia: its bronchus may or may not retain a patent communication with the oesophagus [64–66]. The incidence of congenital broncho-oesophageal fistula is less than one-tenth that of tracheo-oesophageal fistula unaccompanied by oesophageal atresia [67]. The fistula usually opens into the right main bronchus. The fistulous tracts are lined by squamous epithelium which shows a transition to respiratory epithelium via transitional epithelium [68].

Heterotopias

Islands of ciliated epithelium, sometimes found in premature infants and more rarely in full-term babies [11], and very occasionally in adults [69] in any part of the oesophagus, are remains of the ciliated epithelium normally present at an early stage of development. They are therefore not true heterotopias.

Heterotopic gastric mucosa

The presence and frequency of heterotopic gastric mucosa in the upper oesophagus have long been appreciated from postmortem studies [70–72], but have only recently been observed in endoscopy surveys. These lesions, when carefully looked for, are found in up to 13.8% of patients [73]. They present as deep pink, translucent, velvety patches which contrast sharply with adjacent pearl-grey squamous oesophageal mucosa and occur just below the upper oesophageal sphincter (the inlet patch).

Measuring anything from 2 mm to 50 mm in maximum dimension, they are typically oval with the greatest diameter in the longitudinal oesophageal plane. Rarely, they may involve the whole circumference of the oesophagus. Multiple lesions are not uncommon. Some parts of the lesion are covered with squamous epithelium. The histology is that of gastric body-type mucosa with a normal appearance or a thinned body mucosa with equal proportions of foveolae and glands (Figure 2.5). Less commonly, a transitional type of mucosa and an antral pattern may be present. Very occasional intestinal metaplasia of the complete type has been documented [74].

Inflammation is not usually a feature, although the adjacent oesophageal squamous epithelium may show basal cell hyperplasia and elongation of papillae. Despite their ability to secrete acid [75] these lesions are rarely associated with clinical complications or even symptoms. Colonisation of heterotopic gastric mucosa by *Helicobacter pylori* has been reported [76]; this has occurred in association with *H. pylori* gastritis. There are occasional reports of high oesophageal stricture [77,78], ulcer, oesophago-tracheal fistula [79], upper oesophageal web [80], hyperplastic polyp and adenocarcinoma of the cervical oesophagus [81–83], attributed to heterotopic gastric mucosa. The current consensus favours a congenital origin and suggested associations with oesophageal reflux disease and Barrett's oesophagus have not been substantiated [84].

Heterotopic gastric epithelium has also been described in the lower oesophagus as islands surrounded by squamous epithelium [85] but, in practice, such changes are virtually always an acquired metaplasia (see Chapter 5) as a result of reflux of gastric contents. Heterotopic pancreas has also been described in the lower oesophagus [86].

Heterotopic sebaceous gland tissue

Heterotopic sebaceous glands in the oesophagus were first described at postmortem examination, where they were present in 2% of cases [87]. Some patients with heterotopic sebaceous glands in the oesophagus have been reported to have gastro-oesophageal reflux disease and symptoms of chronic oesophagitis. There have been subsequent reports in the endoscopy literature describing yellow, papular, oval and rounded lesions, sometimes multiple and 1–5 mm in dimension, at different levels of the oesophagus. They are observed in oesophagi resected for carcinoma (Figure 2.6) [88,89]. Histologically, mature sebaceous glands are present deep below the oesophageal epithelium, opening on to the surface via a duct in the lamina propria mucosae (Figure 2.7). Associated chronic inflammatory cells may be present [90].

Congenital diaphragmatic hernia

Congenital maldevelopment of the diaphragm may give rise to herniation of the abdominal contents into the thoracic cavity [91]. The ventral part of the diaphragm is derived from the septum transversum, which in the early embryo separates the heart from the abdominal contents. Normally it fuses with the rib cage and sternum but small canals, the foramina of Morgagni, remain lateral to the

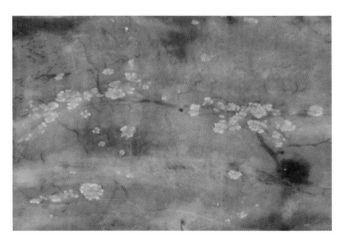

Figure 2.6 Macroscopic appearance of heterotopic sebaceous glands. Sebaceous glands appear yellow though the squamous epithelium and protrude slightly. (Courtesy of Dr T. Nemoto, Department of Pathology, Tokyo Metropolitan Komagome Hospital, Tokyo, Japan.)

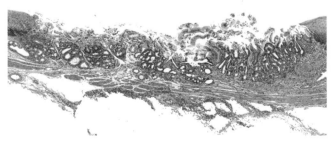

Figure 2.5 An islet of heterotopic gastric mucosa in the upper oesophagus. Fundic-type glands are seen and the gastric-type mucosa is surrounded by squamous epithelium. (Courtesy of Dr T. Nemoto, Department of Pathology, Tokyo Metropolitan Komagome Hospital, Tokyo, Japan.)

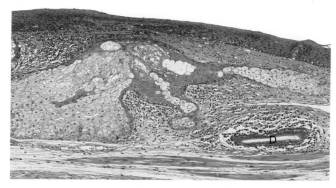

Figure 2.7 Sebaceous glands beneath the oesophageal squamous epithelium. Sebaceous glands are seen in the lamina propria mucosae. A duct (D) of an oesophageal gland proper is evident. (Courtesy of Dr T. Nemoto, Department of Pathology, Tokyo Metropolitan Komagome Hospital, Tokyo, Japan.)

sternum on either side. The dorsal part is formed from the dorsal mesentery but there are persistent posterolateral communications on either side, the canals of Bochdalek, between the pleural and peritoneal membranes. Later they are further separated by an ingrowth of muscle from the body wall. The oesophagus passes through a hiatus posterior and to the left of the central part.

Four main types of hernia occur in association with imperfectly closed foramina or with the oesophageal hiatus. These are:
• Left posterolateral (through the left Bochdalek canal): stomach, intestine and spleen herniated.
• Right posterolateral (through the right Bochdalek canal): the liver and intestine herniated.
• Retrosternal (through the Morgagni canals): these are much less common; the liver and intestine herniate.
• Hiatus hernia: the oesophageal hiatus enlarges and the stomach herniates. Rarely the central tendon of the diaphragm is absent.

There is a high incidence of congenital malrotations of the midgut with all types of congenital diaphragmatic hernia.

Anterior and posterior rachischisis

These conditions are associated with anomalies of the cervical and thoracic vertebrae, which are completely or partially divided into halves. There may be anomalies of diaphragm formation with herniation of abdominal contents into the thorax [92] and of the gastrointestinal tract, taking the form of a short oesophagus or neurenteric cysts lying between the tract and vertebrae, spinal cord or even dorsal skin.

Laryngo-tracheo-oesophageal cleft

Laryngo-tracheo-oesophageal clefts are rare developmental disorders of the upper aerodigestive tract. The complete type of the disease has a high mortality rate [93].

References

1. Lewis FT. Separation of the esophagus from the trachea. In: Keibel F, Mail FP (eds), *Manual of Human Embryology*. Philadelphia, PA: Lippincott, 1912.
2. Smith EI. The early development of the trachea and esophagus in relation to atresia of the esophagus and tracheo-esophageal fistula. *Embryology* 1957;**36**:41.
3. Gray SW, Skandalakis JE. *Embryology for Surgeons*. London: WB Saunders, 1972.
4. Moore KL. The developing human. In: *Clinically Orientated Embryology*. London: WB Saunders, 1974.
5. Zaw-Tun HA. The tracheo-esophageal septum – fact or fantasy? Origin and development of the respiratory primordium and esophagus. *Acta Anat (Basel)* 1982;**114**:1.
6. Montgomery RK, Mulberg AE, Grand RJ. Development of the human gastrointestinal tract: twenty years of progress. *Gastroenterology* 1999;**116**:702.
7. Johnson FP. The development of the mucous membrane of the esophagus, stomach and small intestine in the human embryo. *Am J Anat* 1910;**10**:521.
8. Johns BA. Developmental changes in the oesophageal epithelium in man. *J Anat* 1952;**86**:431.
9. Botha GS. Organogenesis and growth of the gastroesophageal region in man. *Anat Rec* 1959;**133**:219.
10. Menard D, Arsenault P. Maturation of human fetal esophagus maintained in organ culture. *Anat Rec* 1987;**217**:348.
11. Rector LE, Connerley ML. Aberrant mucosa in the esophagus in infants and in children. *Arch Pathol* 1941;**31**:285.
12. Smith RB, Taylor IM. Observations on the intrinsic innervation of the human foetal oesophagus between the 10-mm and 140-mm crown–rump length stages. *Acta Anat (Basel)* 1972;**81**:127.
13. Hitchcock RJ, Pemble MJ, Bishop AE, Spitz L, Polak JM. Quantitative study of the development and maturation of human oesophageal innervation. *J Anat* 1992;**180**(Pt 1):175.
14. Hitchcock RJ, Pemble MJ, Bishop AE, Spitz L, Polak JM. The ontogeny and distribution of neuropeptides in the human fetal and infant esophagus. *Gastroenterology* 1992;**102**:840.
15. Arbona JL, Fazzi JG, Mayoral J. Congenital esophageal cysts: case report and review of literature. *Am J Gastroenterol* 1984;**79**: 177.
16. Geller A, Wang KK, DiMagno EP. Diagnosis of foregut duplication cysts by endoscopic ultrasonography. *Gastroenterology* 1995; **109**:838.
17. Langston HT, Tuttle WM, Patton TB. Esophageal duplications. *AMA Arch Surg* 1950;**61**:949.
18. Maier HC. Intramural duplication of the esophagus. *Ann Surg* 1957;**145**:395.
19. Borrie J. Duplication of the oesophagus. *Br J Surg* 1961;**48**:611.
20. Goto T, Maeshima A, Oyamada Y, Kato R. Esophageal cyst producing CA19-9 and CA125. *Interact Cardiovasc Thorac Surg* 2010;**10**:448.
21. Yoshida T, Fukahara T, Inoue A, Sakurazawa K, Sasabe M, Iwabuchi K. Congenital esophageal duplication. *Gastrointest Endosc* 2005;**61**:350.
22. Pisello F, Geraci G, Arnone E, Sciutto A, Modica G, Sciume C. Acute onset of esophageal duplication cyst in adult. Case report. *G Chir* 2009;**30**(1–2):17.

23. Neo EL, Watson DI, Bessell JR. Acute ruptured esophageal duplication cyst. *Dis Esophagus* 2004;**17**:109.

24. Gatzinsky P, Fasth S, Hansson G. Intramural oesophageal cyst with massive mediastinal bleeding. A case report. *Scand J Thorac Cardiovasc Surg* 1978;**12**:143.

25. Kuwashima S, Chikatsu H, Kohno T, Fujioka M, Hagisawa S, Tsuboi T. Esophageal duplication cyst complicated by *Mycobacterium avium* complex infection. *Pediatr Int* 2005;**47**:592.

26. Lee MY, Jensen E, Kwak S, Larson RA. Metastatic adenocarcinoma arising in a congenital foregut cyst of the esophagus: a case report with review of the literature. *Am J Clin Oncol* 1998;**21**:64.

27. Turkyilmaz A, Eroglu A, Subasi M, Findik G. Intramural esophageal bronchogenic cysts: a review of the literature. *Dis Esophagus* 2007;**20**:461.

28. Sumiyoshi K, Shimizu S, Enjoji M, Iwashita A, Kawakami K. Bronchogenic cyst in the abdomen. *Virchows Arch A Pathol Anat Histopathol* 1985;**408**:93.

29. Bagwell CE, Schiffman RJ. Subcutaneous bronchogenic cysts. *J Pediatr Surg* 1988;**23**:993.

30. Pages ON, Rubin S, Baehrel B. Intra-esophageal rupture of a bronchogenic cyst. *Interact Cardiovasc Thorac Surg* 2005;**4**:287.

31. Takekawa H, Takaoka K, Fujioka Y. [Mediastinal esophago-bronchogenic cyst presenting as a single mass.] *Nihon Kyobu Shikkan Gakkai Zasshi* 1997;**35**:796.

32. Rhaney K, Barclay GP. Enterogenous cysts and congenital diverticula of the alimentary canal with abnormalities of the vertebral column and spinal cord. *J Pathol Bacteriol* 1959;**77**:457.

33. Fallon M, Gordon AR, Lendrum AC. Mediastinal cysts of foregut origin associated with vertebral abnormalities. *Br J Surg* 1954;**41**:520.

34. Smith JR. Accessory enteric formations: a classification and nomenclature. *Arch Dis Child* 1960;**35**:87.

35. Superina RA, Ein SH, Humphreys RP. Cystic duplications of the esophagus and neurenteric cysts. *J Pediatr Surg* 1984;**19**:527.

36. de Lorimier AA, Harrison MR. Esophageal atresia: embryogenesis and management. *World J Surg* 1985;**9**:250.

37. Zachary RB, Emery JL. Failure of separation of larynx and trachea from the esophagus: persistent esophagotrachea. *Surgery* 1961;**49**:525.

38. Sankaran K, Bhagirath CP, Bingham WT, Hjertaas R, Haight K. Tracheal atresia, proximal esophageal atresia, and distal tracheoesophageal fistula: report of two cases and review of literature. *Pediatrics* 1983;**71**:821.

39. Parameswaran A, Krishnaswami H, Walter A. Congenital broncho-oesophageal fistula associated with tracheal agenesis. *Thorax* 1983;**38**:551.

40. Guthrie KJ. Congenital malformations of the oesophagus. *J Pathol Bacteriol* 1945;**57**:363.

41. Rosenthal AH. Congenital atresia of the esophagus with tracheoesophageal fistula. Report of 8 cases. *Arch Pathol* 1931;**12**:756.

42. Scott JS, Wilson JH. Hydramnios as an early sign of oesophageal atresia. *Lancet* 1957;**273**:569.

43. Fonkalsrud EW. Esophageal stenosis due to tracheobronchial remnants. *Am J Surg* 1972;**124**:101.

44. Sneed WF, LaGarde DC, Kogutt MS, Arensman RM. Esophageal stenosis due to cartilaginous tracheobronchial remnants. *J Pediatr Surg* 1979;**14**:786.

45. Shoshany G, Bar-Maor JA. Congenital stenosis of the esophagus due to tracheobronchial remnants: a missed diagnosis. *J Pediatr Gastroenterol Nutr* 1986;**5**:977.

46. Belsey RH, Donnison CP. Congenital atresia of the oesophagus. *BMJ* 1950;**ii**:324.

47. Ozimek CD, Grimson RC, Aylsworth AS. An epidemiologic study of tracheoesophageal fistula and esophageal atresia in North Carolina. *Teratology* 1982;**25**:53.

48. Hausmann PF, Close AS, Williams LP. Occurrence of tracheoesophageal fistula in three consecutive siblings. *Surgery* 1957;**41**:542.

49. Holder TM, Cloud DT, Lewis JE. Esophageal atresia and tracheoesophageal fistula. A survey of its members by the surgical section of the American Academy of Pediatrics. *Pediatrics* 1964;**34**:542.

50. Quan L, Smith DW. The VATER association. Vertebral defects, anal atresia, T-E fistula with esophageal atresia, Radial and Renal dysplasia: a spectrum of associated defects. *J Pediatr* 1973;**82**:104.

51. Baumann W, Greinacher I, Emmrich P, Spranger J. [Vater or Vacterl syndrome (author's transl).] *Klin Paediatr* 1976;**188**:328.

52. Barry JE, Auldist AW. The Vater association: one end of a spectrum of anomalies. *Am J Dis Child* 1974;**128**:769.

53. McCook TA, Felman AH. Esophageal atresia, duodenal atresia, and gastric distension: report of two cases. *AJR Am J Roentgenol* 1978;**131**:167.

54. Crowe JE, Sumner TE. Combined esophageal and duodenal atresia without tracheoesophageal fistula: characteristic radiographic changes. *AJR Am J Roentgenol* 1978;**130**:167.

55. Qvist N, Rasmussen L, Hansen LP, Pedersen SA. Development of infantile hypertrophic pyloric stenosis in patients treated for oesophageal atresia. A case report. *Acta Chir Scand* 1986;**152**:237.

56. Willis RA. *Oesophageal Atresia. The borderland of embryology and pathology*. 2nd edn. London: Butterworths, 1962.

57. Fluss Z, Poppen KJ. Embryogenesis of tracheoesophageal fistula and esophageal atresia; a hypothesis based on associated vascular anomalies. *AMA Arch Pathol* 1951;**52**:168.

58. Gruenwald P. A case of atresia of the esophagus combined with tracheo-esophageal fistula in a 9mm human embryo, and its embryological explanation. *Anat Rec* 1940;**78**:293.

59. Stevenson RE. Extra vertebrae associated with esophageal atresias and tracheoesophageal fistulas. *J Pediatr* 1972;**81**:1123.

60. David TJ. The epidemiology of esophageal atresia. *Teratology* 1983;**28**:479.

61. Nakazato Y, Landing BH, Wells TR. Abnormal Auerbach plexus in the esophagus and stomach of patients with esophageal atresia and tracheoesophageal fistula. *J Pediatr Surg* 1986;**21**:831.

62. Nakazato Y, Wells TR, Landing BH. Abnormal tracheal innervation in patients with esophageal atresia and tracheoesophageal fistula: study of the intrinsic tracheal nerve plexuses by a microdissection technique. *J Pediatr Surg* 1986;**21**:838.

63. Romeo G, Zuccarello B, Proietto F, Romeo C. Disorders of the esophageal motor activity in atresia of the esophagus. *J Pediatr Surg* 1987;**22**:120.

64. Louw JH, Cywes S. Extralobar pulmonary sequestration communicating with the oesophagus and associated with a strangulated congenital diaphragmatic hernia. *Br J Surg* 1962;**50**:102.

65. Halasz NA, Lindskog GE, Liebow AA. Esophago-bronchial fistula and bronchopulmonary sequestration. Report of a case and review of the literature. *Ann Surg* 1962;**155**:215.

66. Frater RW, Dowdle EB. Congenital esophagobronchial fistula. Report of case and review of literature. *Arch Surg* 1964;**89**:949.

67. Blackburn WR, Amoury RA. Congenital esophago-pulmonary fistulas without esophageal atresia: an analysis of 260 fistulas in infants, children and adults. *Rev Surg* 1966;**23**:153.

68. Nakamura Y, Yamazumi T, Hatama T. Congenital bronchoesophageal fistula in adult. *Surg Diagn Treat (Geka Shinryo)* 1972;**14**:1067.

69. Raeburn C. Columnar ciliated epithelium in the adult oesophagus. *J Pathol Bacteriol* 1951;**63**:157.

70. Schmidt FA. De mammalium oesophago atque ventriculo. Halle: Inaugural dissertation, 1805.

71. Hewlett AW. The superficial glands of the oesophagus. *J Exp Med* 1901;**5**:319.

72. Taylor AL. The epithelial heterotopias of the alimentary tract. *J Pathol Bacteriol* 1927;**30**:415.

73. Kumagai Y. Incidence of heterotopic gastric mucosa in the upper esophagus (inlet patch). *Progr Dig Endosc* 2005;**66**:19.

74. Bogomoletz WV, Geboes K, Feydy P, Nasca S, Ectors N, Rigaud C. Mucin histochemistry of heterotopic gastric mucosa of the upper esophagus in adults: possible pathogenic implications. *Hum Pathol* 1988;**19**:1301.

75. Jabbari M, Goresky CA, Lough J, Yaffe C, Daly D, Cote C. The inlet patch: heterotopic gastric mucosa in the upper esophagus. *Gastroenterology* 1985;**89**:352.

76. Borhan-Manesh F, Farnum JB. Study of *Helicobacter pylori* colonization of patches of heterotopic gastric mucosa (HGM) at the upper esophagus. *Dig Dis Sci* 1993;**38**:142.

77. Steadman C, Kerlin P, Teague C, Stephenson P. High esophageal stricture: a complication of 'inlet patch' mucosa. *Gastroenterology* 1988;**94**:521.

78. McBride MA, Vanagunas AA, Breshnahan JP, Barch DB. Combined endoscopic thermal electrocoagulation with high dose omeprazole therapy in complicated heterotopic gastric mucosa of the esophagus. *Am J Gastroenterol* 1995;**90**:2029.

79. Kohler B, Kohler G, Riemann JF. Spontaneous esophagotracheal fistula resulting from ulcer in heterotopic gastric mucosa. *Gastroenterology* 1988;**95**:828.

80. Weaver GA. Upper esophageal web due to a ring formed by a squamocolumnar junction with ectopic gastric mucosa (another explanation of the Paterson–Kelly, Plummer–Vinson syndrome). *Dig Dis Sci* 1979;**24**:959.

81. Christensen WN, Sternberg SS. Adenocarcinoma of the upper esophagus arising in ectopic gastric mucosa. Two case reports and review of the literature. *Am J Surg Pathol* 1987;**11**:397.

82. Ishii K, Ota H, Nakayama J, et al. Adenocarcinoma of the cervical oesophagus arising from ectopic gastric mucosa. The histochemical determination of its origin. *Virchows Arch A Pathol Anat Histopathol* 1991;**419**:159.

83. Sperling RM, Grendell JH. Adenocarcinoma arising in an inlet patch of the esophagus. *Am J Gastroenterol* 1995;**90**:150.

84. Borhan-Manesh F, Farnum JB. Incidence of heterotopic gastric mucosa in the upper oesophagus. *Gut* 1991;**32**:968.

85. Haque AK, Merkel M. Total columnar-lined esophagus: a case for congenital origin? *Arch Pathol Lab Med* 1981;**105**:546.

86. Razi MD. Ectopic pancreatic tissue of esophagus with massive upper gastrointestinal bleeding. *Arch Surg* 1966;**92**:101.

87. De La Pava S, Pickren JW. Ectopic sebaceous glands in the esophagus. *Arch Pathol* 1962;**73**:397.

88. Salgado JA, Andrade Filho J de S, Lima GF Jr, et al. Sebaceous glands in the esophagus. *Gastrointest Endosc* 1980;**26**:150.

89. Bambirra EA, de Souza Andrade J, Hooper de Souza LA, et al. Sebaceous glands in the esophagus. *Gastrointest Endosc* 1983;**29**:251.

90. Bertoni G, Sassatelli R, Nigrisoli E, Conigliaro R, Bedogni G. Ectopic sebaceous glands in the esophagus: report of three new cases and review of the literature. *Am J Gastroenterol* 1994;**89**:1884.

91. Kiesewetter WB, Gutierrez IZ, Sieber WK. Diaphragmatic hernia in infants under one year of age. *Arch Surg* 1961;**83**:561.

92. Dodds GS. Anterior and posterior rachischisis. *Am J Pathol* 1941;**17**:861.

93. Chitkara AE, Tadros M, Kim HJ, Harley EH. Complete laryngotracheoesophageal cleft: complicated management issues. *Laryngoscope* 2003;**113**:1314.

CHAPTER 3

Neuromuscular and mechanical disorders of the oesophagus

D. Scott A. Sanders

Coventry and Warwickshire Pathology Services, Warwick, UK

Classification

The control of normal oesophageal motor function, entailing transport of a swallowed bolus from the oesophagus to the stomach, takes place at three levels: (1) intrinsic activity of oesophageal smooth and striated muscle; (2) intrinsic nerve pathways, mainly involving neurons containing neuropeptides; and (3) extrinsic nerves arising from the central nervous system which modulate intrinsic nerve or muscle function. It is not surprising, from this, that the exact aetiological mechanism for most oesophageal motor disorders remains unknown and classification is not clear cut [1]. In one classification [2], the main causes of motor dysfunction fall into four groups, namely: connective tissue disorders; neural, neuromuscular (motility abnormalities) and primary muscular disorders; metabolic and endocrine disorders; and miscellaneous conditions. The more important are described here and good reviews of selected aspects are available [3–7]. Gastro-oesophageal reflux disease, the most clinically significant motility disorder, is considered in Chapter 4.

Progressive systemic sclerosis (scleroderma)

Scleroderma in the oesophagus occurs as part of either a generalised systemic disease or a more localised systemic sclerosis confined to the alimentary tract. Oesophageal involvement is frequent in both [8]. Symptoms include dysphagia for solid foods and heartburn. Motor abnormalities of decreased or absent peristalsis are present,

predominantly affecting the lower two-thirds of the oesophagus, including the lower oesophageal sphincter. The resting tone of the latter is markedly decreased, with predisposition to gastro-oesophageal reflux and its complications (see Chapter 4). Strictures are not uncommon and tend to be intractable, leading to severe dysphagia, or even aphagia, and aspiration into the lungs. Adenocarcinoma arising in metaplastic columnar-lined (Barrett's) mucosa has been described [9,10]. Candidiasis has been reported in up to 30% of patients [11].

In the past, symptoms and histological features of scleroderma have been attributed to ischaemia and secondary fibrosis with reports, histologically, of gradual patchy atrophy and replacement fibrosis of smooth, but not striated, muscle, particularly the inner circular layer, submucosal fibrosis and non-specific inflammatory changes [12]. A prominent vascular component has been reported, consisting of elastosis and intimal fibrosis in the smaller arteries. The amount and degree of fibrosis reported vary markedly from patient to patient and have been taken to represent chronic ischaemia consequent on the arterial lesions [12,13]. Detection of circulating antibodies to myenteric neurons, in a considerable proportion of patients with scleroderma [14] and the association with Raynaud's phenomenon in up to 90%, have raised the possibility of a neural, rather than a vascular, pathogenesis. In a more recent and substantial case-controlled study of 74 patients, scleroderma was associated histologically with marked atrophy of circular smooth muscle distally, with no evidence of fibrosis [15] (Figure 3.1). Vascular intimal hyperplasia was noted in 38% of cases but this did not correlate

Morson and Dawson's Gastrointestinal Pathology, Fifth Edition. Edited by Neil A. Shepherd, Bryan F. Warren, Geraint T. Williams, Joel K. Greenson, Gregory Y. Lauwers and Marco R. Novelli.
© 2013 Blackwell Publishing Ltd. Published 2013 by Blackwell Publishing Ltd.

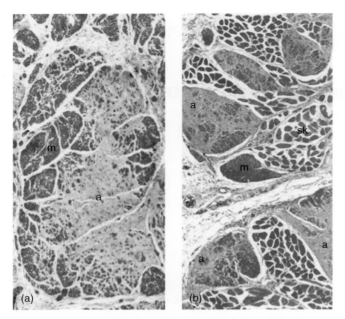

Figure 3.1 (a) The distal oesophagus in scleroderma showing the tendency of smooth muscle bundles to have central atrophy (a) with histologically normal smooth muscle at the periphery (m) (Masson trichrome). (b) In the proximal oesophagus, when smooth and skeletal muscle fibres are present in the same tissue specimen, skeletal muscle fibres (sk) are free of visible abnormalities, whereas interdigitating and closely apposed smooth muscle (m) is atrophic (a) (haematoxylin and eosin). (Republished from Roberts CGP, Hummers LK, Ravich WJ, Wigley FM, Hutchins GM. A case-control study of the pathology of oesophageal disease in systemic sclerosis (scleroderma). Gut, 2006; 55: 1697–1703 with permission from the BMJ Publishing Group.)

with atrophy. A key feature was atrophy of smooth muscle only when interdigitated with skeletal muscle, a feature not compatible with an ischaemic cause. No increase in inflammatory cells was found in the myenteric plexus. However, an interesting, but very preliminary, finding was reduced staining for the interstitial cells of Cajal (ICCs), with a proposed novel hypothesis of smooth muscle atrophy occurring secondary to damage to ICCs.

Similar motility disorders and abnormalities to those occurring in scleroderma have been described in patients with Raynaud's phenomenon alone, in patients with the latter condition and lupus erythematosus or mixed connective tissue disease [16,17], rarely in association with rheumatoid arthritis [18] and in infants breast-fed by mothers with silicone breast implants [19].

Primary muscle disorders

In theory, dysphagia can be a prominent feature of any primary muscle disorder. However, this feature tends to predominate in certain muscular dystrophies, such as oculopharyngeal muscular dystrophy and myotonic dys-

trophy, in rare advanced cases of Duchenne muscular dystrophy and in inflammatory disorders, such as polymyositis and inclusion body myositis [20]. In most cases dysphagia results from oropharyngeal and cricopharyngeal striated muscle weakness but, in some, there is an oesophageal element. In myotonic dystrophy (Steinert's disease, the most common form of adult-onset muscular dystrophy), there is impaired relaxation of muscle after forceful voluntary contraction, due to repetitive depolarisation of the muscle membrane. The predominant motor dysfunction is incomplete relaxation of the upper oesophageal sphincter. Oesophageal striated muscle shows marked variation in fibre size with internalisation of nuclei and pyknosis, focal necrosis and regeneration, and a lack of inflammatory cells [21]. By contrast, oesophageal smooth muscle appears histologically normal.

Advanced cases of Duchenne muscular dystrophy can result in oesophageal dysmotility and gastric dilatation with evidence of oedema and loss of smooth muscle fibres in the lower oesophagus [22–24]. The fibres that remain are disoriented, variable in size and vacuolated. There is no inflammatory reaction. The changes are less severe than those seen in scleroderma and the myenteric plexus is not involved.

Diffuse oesophageal spasm and other motility disorders of the oesophagus

Diffuse oesophageal spasm [25] is a condition of unknown cause characterised by uncoordinated oesophageal contraction, one of four major patterns of oesophageal manometric abnormalities recognised [7]. It affects males, predominantly, and is usually associated with dysphagia and angina-type chest pain. Radiological studies show segmental spasm (tertiary contractions), giving a corkscrew or curling oesophagus with the appearance of pseudo-diverticula. Manometrically the condition is manifest by uncoordinated ('spastic') activity (simultaneous, retrograde, segmental contractions) in the smooth muscle portion of the oesophagus. In cases that have come to surgery, the oesophagus has been reported to be normal in most with muscular hypertrophy only in a few, although details of the latter are scanty. This condition differs from, and has been confused in the literature with, idiopathic or diffuse muscular hypertrophy, a disorder that is related to, and may coexist with, so-called oesophageal leiomyomatosis (see Chapter 8).

Other patterns of abnormal oesophageal motility include inadequate lower oesophageal sphincter relaxation (classic achalasia, discussed below), nutcracker oesophagus, a term coined by Castell [26] characterised by hypercontraction, and oesophageal hypocontraction, for which the condition scleroderma has long been the paradigm.

Achalasia

In this condition there is obstruction to the onward passage of food at the level of the cardia [27,28]. The annual incidence of new cases in one survey on a stable UK population was 0.5 in 10 000 and the prevalence 8 in 10 000. It is most frequent in patients over the age of 60 [29]. There is evidence of regional variations in its prevalence [30]. Clinically, patients have pain, regurgitation and dyspepsia over a long period, followed by episodes of respiratory infection due to overspill and may die from inhalational pneumonia.

Manometric studies demonstrate failure of relaxation of the lower oesophageal sphincter in response to swallowing, absence of peristalsis in the smooth muscle of the oesophageal body, low-amplitude non-peristaltic contractions, a normal or high resting lower oesophageal sphincter pressure and increased intra-oesophageal pressure [1]. Radiologically, there is a narrow constricted distal segment and gross proximal dilatation, with distal beak-like narrowing being the characteristic feature on barium swallow.

Macroscopically, the characteristic appearance of end-stage achalasia is of an enormously dilated and lengthened oesophagus (mega-oesophagus) that is filled with stagnant fluid and partially digested food and occupies the entire mediastinum, tapering down at the level of the cardio-oesophageal junction. There is considerable hypertrophy of the muscularis propria, particularly the circular layer. Histologically, there is a marked reduction or complete absence of ganglion cells in the myenteric plexus, variable infiltrates of lymphocytes and eosinophils with a patchy distribution in and around the myenteric nerves, and widespread fibrosis involving the myenteric nerves. Inflammatory and reactive epithelial changes are seen in the mucosa, presumably as a response to stasis, and food material, bacteria or *Candida* species may be present on the luminal surface [31].

A study evaluating the changes in deep muscle strips, obtained at oesophago-myotomy from patients with early achalasia, has demonstrated myenteric inflammation, predominantly in the form of CD3-/CD8-positive T lymphocytes expressing activation markers [32], even in patients with normal numbers of ganglion cells, suggesting that achalasia results from a primary inflammatory process, with destruction of myenteric ganglion cells and nerves as a secondary feature [33]. What initiates this inflammatory process remains unknown. Achalasia has occasionally been reported in siblings [34] and there is a significant association with HLA genotype DQA1*0103 and DQB1*0603 alleles [35]. The latter finding raises the possibility of an immunogenetic mechanism in the pathogenesis of achalasia. Viruses, such as measles and neurotrophic viruses with a predilection for squamous epithelium, such as varicella-zoster and herpes simplex 1, have also been implicated as initiating agents [36–38]. Lewy bodies, identical to those seen in Parkinson's disease, have been described in the myenteric plexus neurons as well as the dorsal motor nucleus of the vagus nerve in patients with achalasia [39].

It appears that, in achalasia, nitric oxide-containing neurons are more sensitive than cholinergic nerves to the pathological insult. This is consistent with the findings of a marked reduction in nitric oxide synthase in the region of the sphincter [40], the cholinergic hyper-responsiveness of achalasia smooth muscle [41] and the successful use of botulinum toxin (a potent inhibitor of the release of acetylcholine from nerve endings) locally injected into the region of the lower oesophageal sphincter [42]. More traditional treatments for this condition have been either endoscopic pneumatic dilatation or Heller's myotomy.

The most sinister complication of achalasia is the development of squamous cell carcinoma. A prospective study of patients treated by pneumatic dilatation estimated a 33-fold increased risk compared with an age- and sex-matched population, with an average interval of 17 years from the onset of dysphagia to the diagnosis of malignancy [43]. An occasional case of adenocarcinoma arising in a columnar-lined (Barrett's) oesophagus has been reported in achalasia patients after Heller's myotomy, a procedure often associated with subsequent reflux oesophagitis [44]. Small cell carcinoma has also been reported [45].

A number of conditions may give rise to clinical, radiological and manometric features identical to those of idiopathic achalasia. The term 'secondary achalasia' (pseudo-achalasia) is applied in these cases. The most common cause is tumours at the cardio-oesophageal junction or in close proximity to it. Small cell carcinoma may produce a para-neoplastic syndrome involving neuropathy of the myenteric plexus. Other causes include truncal vagotomy [46], secondary amyloidosis [47], sarcoidosis [48], pancreatic pseudocyst [49] and involvement in multiple endocrine neoplasia type 2B [50]. Chagas' disease is described Chapter 4.

Diverticula, rings and webs

Most oesophageal diverticula are acquired, congenital examples being rare. Diverticula can be categorised as true diverticula (containing all layers of the wall), false diverticula (containing only the mucosa) and intramural, in which mucosal out-pouching occurs within the wall. *Pulsion diverticula* are consequent on raised intraluminal pressure and *traction diverticula* occur when the oesophagus is secondarily involved from without, usually by inflammation and fibrosis, adherent neoplastic or tuberculous lymph nodes. Traction diverticula are more common at or below the tracheal bifurcation.

Pulsion diverticula occur at either end of the oesophagus. They are most common at the upper end (pharyngo-oesophageal or Zenker's diverticulum) [51] where increased hypopharyngeal pressure produces herniation posteriorly between the cricopharynx and the inferior pharyngeal constrictor muscles (Killian's triangle). The primary abnormality appears to be incomplete opening of the upper oesophageal sphincter, whereas neuromuscular pharyngo-sphincteric coordination and sphincter relaxation are normal [52]. Patients are generally middle-aged or elderly and may be asymptomatic or present with dysphagia, regurgitation of undigested food often swallowed hours earlier, aspiration pneumonia and voice changes [53]. Bleeding and perforation can also develop. The diverticula have a narrow neck and all layers of the posterior pharyngeal wall are present, although the muscularis propria is attenuated. Histology of cricopharyngeus has shown marked changes, including fibro-adipose replacement and fibre degeneration [54]. An increased frequency of squamous cell carcinoma has been reported in Zenker's diverticula [55].

Mid-thoracic and epiphrenic diverticula occur within the distal third of the oesophagus and frequently accompany conditions causing functional or structural obstruction such as hiatus hernia, diffuse oesophageal spasm and achalasia [56]. They are usually asymptomatic and discovered during routine radiological examination for unrelated complaints. They are wide-mouthed and can reach a large size. Complications are often due to underlying oesophageal motility disorders and include obstruction, bezoar formation and cardiac dysrhythmias.

Intramural oesophageal diverticulosis, or pseudo-diverticulosis, is an uncommon condition in which there is dilatation of excretory ducts of the submucosal oesophageal glands. If multiple, there is a characteristic radiological picture of numerous small flask- or collar button-shaped out-pouchings projecting perpendicularly from the lumen [57,58]. They may not be visible during endoscopic examination. When only a portion of the oesophagus is involved, it tends to be the proximal third and is characterised by wall thickening. Most cases have occurred in the sixth and seventh decades. The aetiology and pathogenesis are not clear. Similar, but less extensive, changes have been described post mortem where they have been associated with marked chronic inflammation of the submucosal ducts and glands [59]. A non-specific oesophagitis has been present in most clinical cases, often associated with disorders of oesophageal motility and stricture formation. Dilatation of the latter, or treatment of oesophagitis, has reversed the process in some cases [60]. Candida organisms have been present in around 8% of cases [58].

Acquired hiatus hernia

Most diaphragmatic hernias are acquired and many present in late adult life. It is a common condition, being found in 1–3% of adults on routine barium examination and the prevalence rises further when the prone position is adopted or on increasing intra-abdominal pressure [61]. There is wide geographical variation in its prevalence, with the condition being uncommon in Africa [62,63].

There are two main types: 'sliding' or type I hiatus hernia, and 'rolling' hiatus hernia (encompassing types II, III and IV), which in some instances may be combined [64]. The so-called *sliding* hiatus hernia accounts for about 85–95% of the total. The stomach and the lowest 10–20 mm of the oesophagus move through the oesophageal diaphragmatic hiatus, which becomes enlarged, because either the diaphragm muscle has failed or the phreno-oesophageal ligament has stretched. Sliding hernias are thought to relate to increased intra-abdominal pressure associated with chronic cough, kyphosis and obesity, but some may be familial [65]. The main complication of this type of hernia is reflux oesophagitis, although most patients are free of symptoms and have no evidence of reflux, dependent on hernia size [66]. Conversely, in 50% of patients with moderate-to-severe reflux disease the significant pathophysiological factor is hiatus hernia [67].

It is now appreciated that both the intrinsic smooth muscle of the distal oesophagus and the skeletal muscle of the crural diaphragm constitute the sphincter mechanism at the lower end of the oesophagus and contribute to the oesophago-gastric junction pressure which acts as a barrier to reflux. Upward misplacement of the gastro-oesophageal junction will not necessarily therefore result in its malfunction. However the presence of a large and non-reducing hernial sac may impair oesophageal emptying and acid clearance [68,69].

Rolling hiatus hernias are much less common, have a female preponderance and include types II, III and IV, all examples of para-oesophageal hernias. In its pure form (type II) the oesophago-gastric junction remains fixed posteriorly to the peri-aortic fascia in its native position but, due to a widened hiatus and a weakened phreno-oesophageal ligament, the gastric fundus protrudes alongside and anterior to the oesophagus into the posterior mediastinum. However, in practice many examples are mixed hernias with some degree of a 'sliding' element (type III) [70]. Often the herniation is progressive and, in extreme cases, the whole stomach may enter the thorax. Other organs such as the small bowel, colon and spleen may also enter the hernia sac (type IV).

Compared with sliding types of hernia, reflux oesophagitis is uncommon in the pure type of para-oesophageal hernia but bleeding from erosions or ulcer may occur, and ulcers may perforate with mediastinal inflammation and abscess [71]. With giant hernias, obstruction, incarceration and strangulation may result [72–74]. Increase in intra-abdominal pressure, as with sliding hernias, is thought to be important in the pathogenesis and rolling hiatus hernias may occur after previous surgery in the region of the diaphragmatic hiatus. *Traumatic* hernias after a breach of the diaphragm have also been reported [75].

Muscular and connective tissue changes associated with eosinophilic oesophagitis

Eosinophilic oesophagitis is more comprehensively covered in Chapter 4 but a short description of its effects on the musculature and connective tissues of the oesophagus is appropriate here. The disease was first reported only in 1977 but has gained widespread recognition more recently. It is an important and established cause of dysphagia with children and adult patients often presenting with food bolus impaction or signs of gastrointestinal reflux (GORD). The basis for dysphagia is not clearly understood [76]. The chronic inflammatory process may lead to transmural thickening of the oesophageal wall with fibrosis and collagen deposition. Manometry has been shown to be abnormal in half of patients with, most commonly, non-specific peristaltic abnormalities or high-amplitude contractions, spasms, tertiary contractions and aperistalsis. More recently mild asynchrony between circular and longitudinal muscle contraction during peristalsis has been proposed, due specifically to longitudinal muscle dysfunction [77].

References

1. Cohen S. Classification of the esophageal motility disorders. *Gastroenterology* 1983;**84**:1050.
2. Mukhopadhyay A, Graham D. Esophageal motor dysfunction in systemic diseases. *Arch Intern Med* 1976;**136**:583.
3. Castell DO. Oesophageal motility and its disorders. *Curr Opin Gastroenterol* 1986;**2**:504.
4. Ekberg O, Wahlgren L. Dysfunction of pharyngeal swallowing – a cineradiographic investigation in 854 dysphagic patients. *Acta Radiol* 1985;**26**:389.
5. Gelfand MD, Botoman VA. Esophageal motility disorders; a clinical overview. *Am J Gastroenterol* 1987;**82**:181.
6. Mittal RK, Balaban DH. The esophagogastric junction. *N Engl J Med* 1997;**336**:924.
7. Spechler SJ, Castell DO. Classification of oesophageal motility abnormalities. *Gut* 2001;**49**:145.
8. Lock G, Holstege A, Lang B, Schölmerich J. Gastrointestinal manifestations of progressive systemic sclerosis. *Am J Gastroenterol* 1997;**92**:763.
9. McKinley M, Sherlock P. Barrett's esophagus with adenocarcinoma in scleroderma. *Am J Gastroenterol* 1984;**79**:438.
10. Katzka DA, Reynolds JC, Saul SH, et al. Barrett's metaplasia and adenocarcinoma of the esophagus in scleroderma. *Am J Med* 1987;**82**:46.
11. Girsson AJ, Akesson A, Gustafson T, et al. Cineradiography identifies esophageal candidiasis in progressive systemic sclerosis. *Clin Exp Rheumatol* 1989;**7**:43.
12. Treacy WL, Bagenstoss AH, Slocum CH, Code CF. Scleroderma of the esophagus, a correlation of histologic and physiologic findings. *Ann Intern Med* 1963;**59**:351.
13. Atkinson M, Summerling MD. Oesophageal changes in systemic sclerosis. *Gut* 1966;**7**:402.
14. Howe S, Eaker EY, Sallustio JE, et al. Antimyenteric neuronal antibodies in scleroderma. *J Clin Invest* 1994;**94**:761.
15. Roberts CGP, Hummers LK, Ravich WJ, Wigley FM, Hutchins GM. A case–control study of the pathology of oesophageal disease in systemic sclerosis (scleroderma). *Gut* 2006;**55**:1697.
16. Gutierrez F, Valenzuela JE, Ehresmann GR, et al. Esophageal dysfunction in patients with mixed connective tissue diseases and systemic lupus erythematosus. *Dig Dis Sci* 1982;**27**:592.
17. Lapadula G, Muolo P, Semeraro F, et al. Esophageal motility disorders in the rheumatic diseases: a review of 150 patients. *Clin Exp Rheumatol* 1994;**12**:515.
18. Ljubich P, Parkman HP, Fisher RS, Sorokin JJ, Conaway DC. Diffuse gastrointestinal dysmotility in a patient with rheumatoid arthritis. *Am J Gastroenterol* 1993;**88**:1443.
19. Levine JJ, Illowite NT. Scleroderma-like esophageal disease in infants breast fed by mothers with silicone breast implants. *JAMA* 1994;**271**:213.
20. Jaredeh S. Muscle disorders affecting oral and pharyngeal swallowing. *GI Motility online* 2006;doi:10.1038/gimo35.
21. Eckardt VF, Nix W, Kraus W, Bohl J. Esophageal motor function in patients with muscular dystrophy. *Gastroenterology* 1986;**90**:628.
22. Bevans M. Changes in the musculature of the gastrointestinal tract and in the myocardium in progressive muscular dystrophy. *Arch Pathol* 1945;**40**:225.
23. Leon SH, Shuffler MD, Kettler M, et al. Chronic intestinal pseudo-obstruction as a complication of Duchenne's muscular dystrophy. *Gastroenterology* 1986;**90**:455.
24. Barohn RJ, Levine EJ, Olson JO, Mendell JR. Gastric hypomotility in Duchenne muscular dystrophy. *N Engl J Med* 1988;**319**:15.
25. Dalton CB, Castell DO, Hewson EG, et al. Diffuse esophageal spasm. A rare motility disorder not characterized by high-amplitude contractions. *Dig Dis Sci* 1991;**36**:1025.
26. Dalton CB, Castell DO, Richter JE. The changing faces of the nutcracker oesophagus. *Am J Gastroenterol* 1988;**83**:623.
27. Barrett NR. Achalasia of the cardia. Reflections on a clinical study of over 100 cases. *BMJ* 1964;**i**:1135.
28. Walzer N, Hirano I. Achalasia. *Gastroenterol Clin North Am* 2008 **37**:807.
29. Mayberry JF, Atkinson M. Studies of incidence and prevalence of achalasia in the Nottingham area. *Q J Med* 1985;**56**:451.
30. Mayberry JF, Atkinson M. Variations in the presence of achalasia in Great Britain and Ireland; an epidemiological study based on hospital admissions. *Q J Med* 1987;**62**:67.
31. Goldblum JR, White RI, Orringer MB, et al. Achalasia. A morphologic study of forty-two resected specimens. *Am J Surg Pathol* 1994;**18**:327.
32. Clark SB, Rice TW, Tubbs RR, et al. The nature of the myenteric infiltrate in achalasia: an immunohistochemical analysis. *Am J Surg Pathol* 2000;**24**:1153.
33. Goldblum JR, Rice TW, Richter JE. Histopathologic features in esophagomyotomy specimens from patients with achalasia. *Gastroenterology* 1996;**111**:648.
34. Bosher P, Shaw A. Achalasia in siblings. Clinical and genetic aspects. *Am J Dis Child* 1981;**135**:709.
35. Ruis-de-Leon A, Mendoza J, Sevilla-Mantilla C, et al. Myenteric antiplexus antibodies and class II HLA in achalasia. *Dig Dis Sci* 2002;**47**:15.
36. Robertson CS, Martin BAB, Atkinson M. Varicella-zoster virus DNA in the oesophageal myenteric plexus in achalasia. *Gut* 1993;**34**:299.
37. Park W, Vaezi MF. Etiology and pathogenesis of achalasia: the current understanding. *Am J Gastroenterol* 2005;**100**:1404.

38. Castagliuolo I, Brun P, Costantini M, et al. Esophageal achalasia: is the herpes simplex virus really innocent? *J Gastrointest Surg* 2004;**8**:24.

39. Qualman SJ, Haupt HM, Yang P, Hamilton SR. Esophageal Lewy bodies associated with ganglion cell loss in achalasia. Similarity to Parkinson's disease. *Gastroenterology* 1984;**87**:848.

40. Mearin F, Mourelle M, Guarner F, et al. Patients with achalasia lack nitric oxide synthase in the gastro-oesophageal junction. *Eur J Clin Invest* 1993;**23**:724.

41. Holloway RH, Dodds WJ, Helm JF, Hogan WJ, Dent J, Arndorfer RC. Integrity of cholinergic innervation to the lower esophageal sphincter in achalasia. *Gastroenterology* 1986;**90**:924.

42. Pasricha PJ, Rai R, Ravich WJ, Hendrix TR, Kalloo AN. Botulinum toxin for achalasia: long-term outcome and predictors of response. *Gastroenterology* 1996;**110**:1410.

43. Meijssen MAC, Tilanus HW, van Blankenstein M, Hop WCJ, Ong GL. Achalasia complicated by oesophageal squamous cell carcinoma: a prospective study in 195 patients. *Gut* 1992;**33**:155.

44. Gallez JF, Berger F, Moulinier B, Partensky C. Esophageal adenocarcinoma following Heller myotomy for achalasia. *Endoscopy* 1987;**19**:76.

45. Proctor DD, Fraser JL, Mangano MM, Calkins DR, Rosenberg SJ. Small cell carcinoma of the esophagus in a patient with long-standing primary achalasia. *Am J Gastroenterol* 1992;**87**:664.

46. Greatorex RA, Thorpe JAC. Achalasia-like disturbance of oesophageal motility following truncal vagotomy and antrectomy. *Postgrad Med J* 1983;**59**:100.

47. Suris X, Moya F, Panes J, del Olmo JA, Sole M, Munoz-Gomez J. Achalasia of the esophagus in secondary amyloidosis. *Am J Gastroenterol* 1993;**88**:1959.

48. Boruchowicz A, Canva-Delcambre Z, Guillemot F, et al. Sarcoidosis and achalasia: a fortuitous association (letter)? *Am J Gastroenterol* 1996;**91**:413.

49. Woods CA, Foutch PG, Waring JP, Sanowski RA. Pancreatic pseudocyst as a cause for secondary achalasia. *Gastroenterology* 1989;**96**:235.

50. Ghosh P, Linder J, Gallagher TF, Quigley EM. Achalasia of the cardia and multiple endocrine neoplasia 2B. *Am J Gastroenterol* 1994;**89**:1880.

51. Achtar E. Zenker's diverticulum *Dig Dis* 1998;**16**:144.

52. Cook IJ, Gabb M, Panagopoulos V, et al. Pharyngeal (Zenker's) diverticulum is a disorder of upper esophageal sphincter opening. *Gastroenterology* 1992;**103**:1229.

53. Watemberg S, Landau O, Avrahami R. Zenker's diverticulum: reappraisal. *Am J Gastroenterol* 1996;**91**:1494.

54. Cook IJ, Blumbergs P, Cash K, et al. Structural abnormalities of the cricopharyngeus muscle in patients with pharyngeal (Zenker's) diverticulum. *J Gastroenterol Hepatol* 1992;**7**:556.

55. Wychulis AR, Gunnlaugsson GH, Clagett OT. Carcinoma occurring in pharyngo-esophageal diverticulum: report of three cases. *Surgery* 1969;**66**:976.

56. Evander A, Little AG, Ferguson MK, Skinner DB. Diverticula of the mid- and lower esophagus: pathogenesis and surgical management. *World J Surg* 1986;**10**:820.

57. Mendl K, McKay JM, Tanner CH. Intramural diverticulosis of the oesophagus and Rokitansky–Aschoff sinuses in the gallbladder. *Br J Radiol* 1960;**33**:496.

58. Fromkes J, Thomas FB, Mekhjian H et al. Esophageal intramural pseudodiverticulosis. *Dig Dis* 1977;**22**:690.

59. Medeiros LJ, Doos WG, Balogh K. Esophageal intramural pseudodiverticulosis. a report of two cases with analysis of similar, less extensive changes in 'normal' autopsy esophagi. *Hum Pathol* 1988;**19**:928.

60. Dua KS, Stewart E, Arndorfer R, Shaker R. Esophageal intramural pseudodiverticulosis associated with achalasia. *Am J Gastroenterol* 1996;**91**:1859.

61. Atkinson M. The patho-physiology of gastro-oesophageal reflux. In: Truelove SC, Ritchie JA (eds), *Topics in Gastroenterology*, Vol. 4. Oxford: Blackwell Scientific Publications, 1976: 67.

62. Burkitt DP, James PA. Low-residue diets and hiatus hernia. *Lancet* 1973;**i**:128.

63. Bassey OO, Eyo EE, Akinhanmi GA. Incidence of hiatus hernia and gastro-oesophageal reflux in 1030 prospective barium meal examinations in adult Nigerians. *Thorax* 1977;**32**:356.

64. Kahrilas PJ, Pandolfino JE. Hiatus hernia. *GI motility online* 2006 doi:10.1038/gim048.

65. Carré IJ, Johnston BT, Thomas PS, Morrison PJ. Familial hiatus hernia in a large five generation family confirming true autosomal dominant inheritance. *Gut* 1999;**45**:649.

66. Jones MP, Sloan SS, Rabine JC, Ebert CC, Huang CF, Kahrilas PJ. Hiatus hernia size is the dominant determinant of esophagitis presence and severity in gastroesophageal reflux disease. *Am J Gastroenterology* 2001;**96**;1711.

67. Wright RA, Hurwitz AL. Relationship of hiatus hernia to endoscopically proved reflux esophagitis. *Dig Dis Sci* 1979;**24**:311.

68. Mittal RK, Lange RC, McCallum RW. Identification and mechanism of delayed oesophageal acid clearance in subjects with hiatus hernia. *Gastroenterology* 1987;**92**:130.

69. Sloan S, Kahrilas PJ. Impairment of esophageal emptying with hiatus hernia. *Gastroenterology* 1991;**100**:596.

70. Wo JM, Branum GD, Hunter JG, Trus TN, Mauren SJ, Waring JP. Clinical features of type III (mixed) paraesophageal hernia. *Am J Gastroenterol* 1996;**91**:914.

71. Meredith HC, Seymour EQ, Vujic I. Hiatus hernia complicated by gastric ulceration and perforation. *Gastrointest Radiol* 1980;**5**:229.

72. Pearson FG, Cooper JD, Ilves R, et al. Massive hiatus hernia with incarceration: a report of 53 cases. *Ann Thoracic Surg* 1983;**35**:45.

73. Dunn DB, Quick G. Incarcerated paraesophageal hernia. *Am J Emerg Med* 1990;**8**:36.

74. Haas O, Rat P, Christophe M, et al. Surgical results of intrathoracic gastric volvulus complicating hiatus hernia. *Br J Surg* 1990;**77**:1379.

75. Sebayel MI, Qasabi QO, Katugampola W, Ahmed I. Traumatic diaphragmatic hernia: review of 15 cases. *Br J Accident Surg* 1989;**20**:94.

76. Attwood SE. Mechanisms underlying dysphagia in eosinophilic oesophagitis. *Gut* 2009;**58**:1041.

77. Korsapati H, Babaei A, Bhargava V, et al. Dysfunction of the longitudinal muscles of the oesophagus in eosinophilic oesophagitis. *Gut* 2009;**58**:1056.

CHAPTER 4

Inflammatory disorders of the oesophagus

Laura W. Lamps

University of Arkansas for Medical Sciences, Little Rock, AZ, USA

Classification

Inflammation of the oesophagus is very common and can result from numerous causes; in any individual patient it may be multifactorial. The pathological features are frequently non-specific and a careful correlation with clinical factors is often essential in determining the aetiology.

Gastro-oesophageal reflux disease (GORD), also known as peptic oesophagitis, is one of the most common chronic inflammatory conditions, reportedly affecting up to 40% of people in the western world [1]. Oesophageal inflammation may also be a consequence of infection [2], allergy (eosinophilic or allergic oesophagitis), ingestion of injurious medications or corrosive chemicals, and irradiation. It is also frequently seen in the mucosa adjacent to tumours. Rarely the oesophagus may be involved in Crohn's disease, idiopathic eosinophilic gastroenteritis and graft-versus-host disease, and there are rare reports of acute necrotising oesophagitis due to ischaemia [3,4].

Inflammatory disorders of the oesophagus are discussed in the sections that follow. Inflammatory polyps of the oesophagus and related lesions are discussed in Chapter 6. Inflammatory conditions of the gastric cardia, along with the associated causes and controversies, are discussed in Chapter 11.

Reflux oesophagitis

Pathogenesis

The central event in GORD is injury to the oesophageal epithelium by contact with acid. GORD occurs in many clinical settings and its pathogenesis is almost certainly multifactorial, although persistent or transient loss of lower oesophageal sphincter tone is generally accepted as the major underlying cause [5–8]. A sliding hiatus hernia is also a common, although not essential, accompaniment [9]. Other associated clinical conditions include impaired oesophageal peristalsis, delayed gastric emptying [10,11], increased gastric acid production and bile reflux from the duodenum [12,13]: this last mechanism is thought to be particularly important after partial gastrectomy [13]. In addition, there is recent evidence to support an association between high body mass index and reflux [14]. Other risk factors and clinical conditions associated with reflux include alcohol use, tobacco use, advancing age, nasogastric intubation, repeated vomiting, surgery that interferes with the gastro-oesophageal junction (GOJ), diabetes and connective tissue disorders (especially scleroderma), although the significance of some of these factors in the pathogenesis of GORD is not completely clear.

Some degree of GORD is commonplace and occurs, for example, in healthy individuals after meals [15] and during early pregnancy [16]. The prevalence of heartburn and/or acid regurgitation experienced at least weekly has been found to be approximately 20% in individuals aged 25–74 years [17]. The reasons why some people with GORD develop oesophagitis, whereas others do not, are not fully understood. Furthermore, there is poor correlation between symptoms of GORD and histological changes. Whether or not inflammation (see below) results from reflux probably depends on a number of factors, including the volume and nature of the refluxate [18,19], the efficiency of secondary peristalsis in clearing the oesophagus of refluxed material

Morson and Dawson's Gastrointestinal Pathology, Fifth Edition. Edited by Neil A. Shepherd, Bryan F. Warren, Geraint T. Williams, Joel K. Greenson, Gregory Y. Lauwers and Marco R. Novelli.

[20], the resistance of oesophageal epithelium to injury, and the neutralising effects of bicarbonate-rich saliva [21] and secretions from the oesophageal glands, which probably also contain bicarbonate [22,23]. Severe GORD that is associated with erosions, ulcers and/or stricture formation predominantly affects elderly white men [24].

The macroscopic appearances of reflux oesophagitis are observed at endoscopy and several grading systems exist to define and classify macroscopic lesions reproducibly [25]. The earliest changes appear to be diffuse or patchy hyperaemia or erythema of the distal oesophageal mucosa due to a marked widening and irregularity of small blood vessels, which are present in the normal mucosa as fine, parallel, longitudinal red lines [26]. The distinction between squamous and columnar mucosa may become indistinct or effaced. At a more advanced stage, the mucosa is friable and bleeds when touched. Linear erosions, which are surrounded by a red halo and covered by a yellow exudate, initially occur on the longitudinal folds of the posterior wall approximately 10–20 mm proximal to the Z-line. With increasing severity, erosions are multiple and confluent and may involve the whole circumference of the lower oesophagus. Chronic GORD can result in a nodular appearance of the mucosa, decreased distensibility of the oesophageal wall, strictures and ulceration. Inflammatory polyps may also occur (see also Chapter 6) [27], and fibrous septum formation (resulting in a double lumen) and oesophago-gastric fistulae have also been reported as complications of chronic disease [28,29].

Of note, more than half the patients with symptomatic reflux have normal oesophageal mucosa or only mild hyperaemia at endoscopy [30]. Moreover, as mentioned above, histologically inflamed mucosa may appear normal endoscopically and hyperaemia does not necessarily indicate histological inflammation [31–33]. When there are erosions or ulcers at endoscopy, however, there is better correlation with histological evidence of inflammation in directed biopsies. Due to the lack of correlation between histological and endoscopic findings overall, and to exclude the presence of other conditions such as Barrett's oesophagus, infection or neoplasia, biopsies of the oesophagus are usually warranted in symptomatic patients.

Histology

Reflux changes are typically in the distal oesophagus and they may be patchy [31,34,35]. Mild squamous hyperplasia and reactive epithelial changes occur normally in the lowermost 20 mm of the squamous-lined oesophageal mucosa as a result of 'physiological' reflux [31,32], and thus biopsies should be obtained more than 20 mm above the GOJ.

The injury pattern in GORD is non-specific, although characteristic, and typically consists of basal cell hyperplasia [34,36,37], elongation and congestion of the lamina

propria papillae, and increased intraepithelial inflammation consisting of eosinophils, neutrophils and lymphocytes [38] (Figure 4.1). The basal cell layer should comprise more than 15% of the thickness of the oesophageal epithelium and the connective tissue papillae of the lamina propria

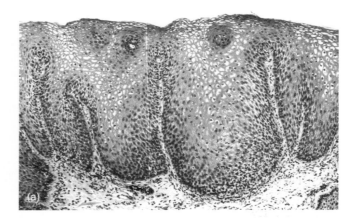

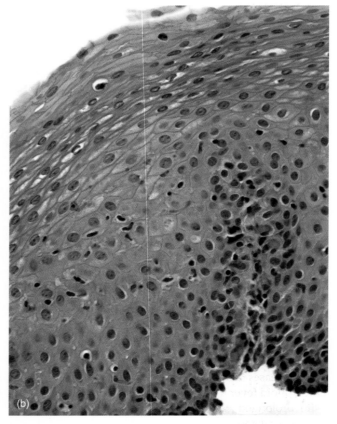

Figure 4.1 Reflux changes: (a) there is thickening of the basal cell layer of the oesophageal epithelium and elongation of connective tissue papillae, which approach the surface. (b) Scattered eosinophils, intraepithelial lymphocytes and nucleated squamous cells at the surface of the epithelium are also frequent findings.

should extend more than two-thirds of the distance to the surface. However, true basal cell hyperplasia may be difficult to appreciate in small, poorly orientated pinch biopsies. Other histological changes in GORD include a lack of surface maturation (as indicated by nucleated keratinocytes at the surface), intercellular oedema, ballooning degeneration of keratinocytes and dilatation of lamina propria capillaries [38,39], although the last may be caused by rough handling of the tissue by biopsy forceps because it is also seen in normal control individuals [40].

The inflammatory cells in reflux include eosinophils, neutrophils and lymphocytes, although none or all of these cells may be present in a single specimen, especially in a patient who has been treated with anti-reflux therapy. Although neutrophils in the oesophageal epithelium always indicate a pathological process, they are neither sensitive nor specific for GORD. Increased eosinophils are often present in patients with GORD [41]. Occasional intra-epithelial eosinophils may be seen in asymptomatic adults in the distal oesophagus, however, and are not diagnostic of GORD if few in number and not associated with other histological changes of reflux [42]. This does not appear to be the case in children, where the presence of even occasional eosinophils is a valuable diagnostic aid [42–44]. The finding of larger numbers of eosinophils, especially with prominent clustering or degranulation, should raise the possibility of other causes of oesophagitis, such as eosinophilic oesophagitis, adverse drug reaction or parasitic infection (see below). Lymphocytes are considered a normal intra-epithelial component of the oesophageal mucosa [38,45–48], both in the lamina propria and between squamous epithelial cells, where they may have an elongated irregular outline and have been termed 'squiggle cells'. Therefore, their presence is not informative. Lymphocytes may be present in increased numbers in patients with GORD but in isolation this finding has no significance because normal control individuals may also have increased numbers of lymphocytes [46–48].

Infective oesophagitis

In immunocompetent individuals, the oesophagus is usually very resistant to infection. Most individuals who have infections of the oesophagus have impaired host responses, although an oesophagitis can occur in the course of infectious diseases such as measles, scarlet fever, diphtheria and typhoid fever in otherwise immunocompetent patients. With prolonged derangements of immunity, a variety of fungal, viral and bacterial agents may cause oesophagitis.

Herpes simplex virus oesophagitis

The oesophagus is the most common site of gastrointestinal herpes infection [49]. Although herpes simplex virus (HSV) infection is most often seen in immunocompromised patients, including those with underlying lymphoma, leukaemia and AIDS, transplant recipients and burns victims, it is not limited to this group [50,51]. Immunocompromised patients with HSV often, however, have disseminated infection at the time of diagnosis, which may be life-threatening [2,52,53]. Other complications include extensive mucosal necrosis, gastrointestinal bleeding [54,55], oesophageal strictures, super-infection by other infective agents and perforation [56].

The middle and distal thirds of the oesophagus are most commonly involved. The earliest changes at endoscopy are small discrete vesicles with an erythematous base. These subsequently give rise to multiple ulcers that are usually shallow (Figure 4.2a) and generally associated with an exudate [52]. Many patients, however, have a non-specific erosive oesophagitis.

Microscopically the characteristic features of herpetic infection occur in squamous epithelium at the margin of ulcers or erosions. Inflammatory changes include focal ulceration, a neutrophilic infiltrate and an inflammatory exudate which often contains sloughed epithelial cells (Figure 4.2b). Prominent aggregates of macrophages in the adjacent tissue have also been proposed as a sensitive and fairly specific marker of HSV infection [57]. There are two types of viral inclusions in HSV infection: homogeneous 'ground glass' or smudge cells (Figure 4.2c) and acidophilic inclusions with a surrounding clear halo and peripheral chromatin margination (Cowdry type A). Multinucleate giant cells are variably present as well [52,53]. Viral inclusions are found only in a minority of biopsy specimens and the best place to find them is within the squamous mucosa at the edges of ulcers and in sloughed cells within the exudate. Immunohistochemical stains are useful in confirming HSV infection and biopsies from the edges of the ulcer can be sent for viral culture when HSV infection is suspected [53].

Cytomegalovirus oesophagitis

Cytomegalovirus (CMV) most commonly presents as an opportunistic pathogen in patients with suppressed immune systems, including those with AIDS and following solid organ or bone marrow transplantation [53,58]. Moreover, CMV is the most common overall pathogen in patients with AIDS. The endoscopic appearances vary from a diffuse oesophagitis to single or multiple ulcers, usually in the distal oesophagus, which may reach a large size [59]. The ulcers may be either superficial or deep [53,59,60].

The histological spectrum of CMV infection is varied as well, ranging from minimal inflammation to ulceration with prominent granulation tissue and necrosis. Characteristic inclusions are usually found in the ulcer base, because CMV infects endothelial cells, pericytes, fibroblasts,

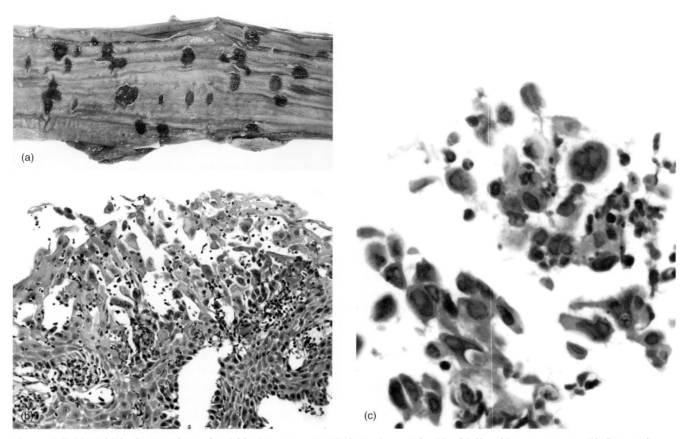

Figure 4.2 (a) Multiple discrete ulcers of variable sizes are present in herpetic oesophagitis. (b) Sloughing squamous epithelium and a neutrophilic infiltrate, as well as viral inclusions typical of herpes simplex virus, are seen at the edge of a herpetic ulcer. (c) Characteristic 'ground-glass' or 'smudge cell' inclusions are seen within squamous cells.

macrophages and smooth muscle cells, but not the squamous epithelium. Characteristic inclusions can be either intracytoplasmic or intranuclear, and infected cells show both nuclear and cytoplasmic enlargement (hence the name 'cytomegalovirus'). Inclusions may have the typical 'owl's-eye' appearance in the nucleus (Figure 4.3), or exist as basophilic granular inclusions in the cytoplasm [53,60]. The diagnosis is easily missed when only rare inclusions are present, so examination of multiple levels, immunohistochemistry, molecular assays and viral culture may be helpful diagnostic aids [53,61].

Chronic HIV-associated oesophageal ulcers

Chronic idiopathic oesophageal ulcers reportedly cause approximately 40–50% of ulcers found in HIV-infected patients [62–64]. Evidence of HIV within the ulcerative lesions has been demonstrated by multiple methods [65], suggesting that the virus is capable of producing ulcers in the absence of other pathogens. However, the ability of

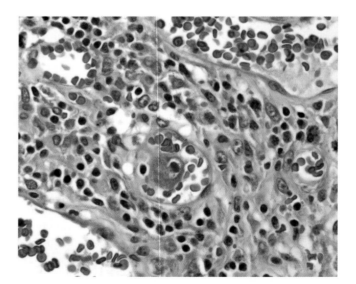

Figure 4.3 Oesophageal cytomegalovirus (CMV) infection: a characteristic 'owl's eye' CMV inclusion is present within an endothelial cell at the base of an ulcer.

HIV to directly cause these ulcers remains controversial. The middle oesophagus is the most common location, followed by the distal oesophagus. Endoscopically, the ulcers consist of one or more well-circumscribed lesions of variable depth [66,67]. They can be quite large, exceeding 30 mm. They often have irregular margins and overhanging, oedematous edges. They are frequently linear and mucosal bridges and sinus tract formation may occur, as well as stricture formation and fatal bleeding if the ulcer erodes into vessels [63]. Histologically, the ulcers contain granulation tissue with a mixed acute and chronic inflammatory infiltrate that often contains eosinophils [62]. By definition, histochemical stains and immunohistochemical stains for identifiable pathogens must be negative and rigorous clinical exclusion of other pathogens is also necessary [53,62].

Other viruses

Epstein–Barr virus (EBV) has been demonstrated by DNA *in situ* hybridisation techniques in biopsy material from oesophageal ulcers of AIDS patients [68] and papovavirus and human herpes virus 6 have also been isolated from the oesophagus in this population [69,70]. The oesophagus may also be involved in herpes zoster infection and the viral inclusions are indistinguishable from HSV by light microscopy alone [71,72]. Immunohistochemistry and viral culture, along with molecular assays, can aid in distinguishing between HSV and herpes zoster/varicella infection.

Candida oesophagitis

This is the most common infective cause of oesophagitis. *Candida albicans* is most frequently the causative agent but other species such as *C. krusei, C. tropicalis, C. stellatoidea* and *C. glabrata* (also known as *Torulopsis glabrata*) may produce similar manifestations [73–75]. *C. albicans* is a normal commensal that colonises the oesophagus in up to 20% of the population [76] but it may become pathogenic under a variety of circumstances including underlying malignancy, diabetes, steroid use, immunosuppressive therapy, radiation and the use of broad-spectrum antibiotics that results in changes in the micro-ecology of the gut flora [77,78]. HIV infection is also a significant risk factor and individuals with a persistently low CD4 count appear at most risk for oesophageal candidiasis [79]. Interference with oesophageal peristalsis, occurring in diseases such as achalasia and scleroderma, and hypochlorhydria due to acid-suppressant therapy or after gastric surgery can also predispose to candida infection [80]. *Candida* spp. may also super-infect ulcers caused by other processes, including HSV or peptic ulcers, or those caused by neoplasms.

Candida oesophagitis may be asymptomatic, particularly in immunocompetent individuals. Complications are more common in immunocompromised patients and with extensive and deeply invasive infection, and include perforation, fistula formation and strictures [81,82]. The last are most frequent in the upper oesophagus where they may complicate intramural oesophageal pseudo-diverticulosis, an inflammatory disorder of unknown cause in which there is dilatation of the excretory ducts of submucosal glands. The gastrointestinal tract is also a common portal of entry for disseminated candidiasis, which is associated with considerable morbidity and mortality, and commonly occurs in the setting of granulocytopaenia [73,83].

Macroscopically, the oesophagus typically contains adherent white or cream plaques in the middle and lower oesophagus which can be scraped away to reveal the ulcerated mucosa underneath (Figure 4.4a). Such features are thought to be almost diagnostic at endoscopy. Confluence of the plaques can produce a pseudo-membrane which may be accompanied by erosion or superficial ulceration. The associated inflammatory response ranges from minimal (especially in immunocompromised patients) to marked with prominent neutrophilic infiltrates, erosions, ulceration and necrosis. When pseudo-membranes are present, they are composed of a mixture of yeasts, necrotic debris and fibrin. Granulomas are seen occasionally. The presence of numerous intra-epithelial neutrophils in the squamous mucosa is a common finding and should provoke a careful search for yeasts (Figure 4.4b) [73,77,84]. *Candida* spp. typically produce a mixture of budding yeasts intermingled with pseudo-hyphae and occasional true hyphae. *Candida* spp. may be appreciated in haematoxylin and eosin (H&E)-stained sections when numerous, but also stain with Grocott's methenamine silver (GMS) stain, and are bright fuchsia in a periodic acid–Schiff (PAS) stain (Figure 4.4c,d). *C. glabrata* features budding yeast forms but does not produce hyphae or pseudo-hyphae [84,85]. In many cases invasion affects only the superficial epithelium but deeper extension with ulceration can occur.

Other fungi

Fungi other than *Candida* spp. that may infect the oesophagus include *Aspergillus* spp. [84,86], zygomycetes [87,88], blastomyces [89], *Cryptococcus neoformans* [90] and *Histoplasma capsulatum* [91,92].

Mycobacterial infection

Most cases of oesophageal *Mycobacterium tuberculosis* (MTb) infection are part of disseminated disease in patients with pulmonary infections [93–95], although rare primary cases have been reported [96]. Infection results from either the swallowing of infected sputum or direct involvement

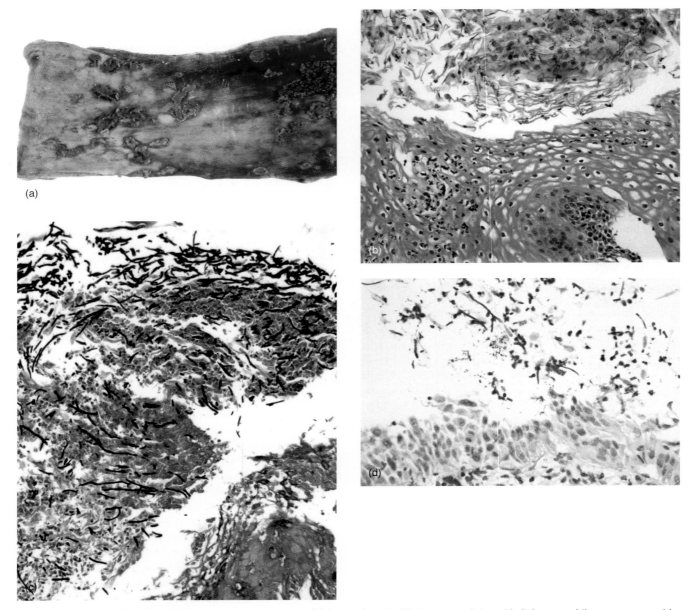

Figure 4.4 (a) Multiple adherent plaques are present in candidal oesophagitis. (b) Numerous intraepithelial neutrophils are present, with an overlying exudate composed of yeast and sloughed squamous cells. Yeast forms stain with (c) Grocott's methenamine silver stain or (d) periodic acid–Schiff stain , showing the characteristic mixture of budding yeast and pseudo-hyphae.

of the oesophagus by a tuberculous hilar lymph node or infected lung. Clinically, oesophageal MTb may mimic oesophageal carcinoma [97]. The characteristic lesions are caseating, often confluent, granulomas, present at any level of the wall of the oesophagus [53,93]. Acid-fast stains may demonstrate organisms within granulomas but culture and/or molecular assays may be required for the diagnosis. *Mycobacterium avium-intracellulare* complex (MAI) occasionally involves the oesophagus in patients with AIDS [98].

Other bacterial infections

Bacterial oesophagitis is rare and usually found in immunocompromised or severely debilitated patients. Strictly defined, this diagnosis requires the histological demonstration of invasive bacteria within the wall of the oesophagus, as well as exclusion of viral, fungal and neoplastic processes, and no history of oesophageal surgery [99]. Implicated bacteria include a wide range of Gram-positive and Gram-negative bacteria such as *Staphylococcus aureus*,

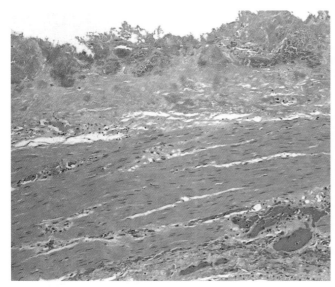

Figure 4.5 Bacterial oesophagitis, featuring clusters of bacteria present within the mucosa and submucosa, along with mucosal necrosis.

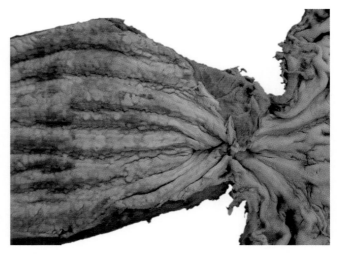

Figure 4.6 Mega-oesophagus due to Chagas' disease. (Photograph courtesy of Dr Dennis Baroni-Cruz.)

streptococci, *Lactobacillus acidophilus* and *Klebsiella pneumoniae* [99,100]. Endoscopy may demonstrate a variety of findings including ulceration, pseudo-membrane formation and haemorrhage, which may mimic other more common pathogens such as *Candida* spp. and HSV. Histological findings include acute inflammation and necrosis, with bacteria demonstrable within the wall of the oesophagus (Figure 4.5) [99–101]. Ultimately, this condition may lead to sepsis.

Bartonella spp. are another rare cause of oesophageal infection and there are rare reports of both ulcerative lesions (sometimes from involved para-oesophageal lymph nodes [102]) and bacillary angiomatosis associated with numerous oesophageal polyps in a patient with AIDS [103].

Chagas' disease

Chagas' disease is one of the most serious public health problems in South America, and it is also found in Central America, Mexico and, rarely, Texas in the USA [104–107]. It is caused by *Trypanosoma cruzi* and the main vector is the cone-nosed triatomine bug. The trypanosomes develop in the bug's faeces, which are deposited on human skin when the bug bites. They then penetrate the skin to enter the bloodstream and invade smooth muscle and myocardium. They multiply as *Leishmania*-like amastigote forms, which are ingested by either histiocytes adjacent to ganglion cells or the muscle and ganglion cells themselves. The resulting pseudo-cysts rupture and liberate the contained parasites. Some of these release neurotoxins leading to inflammatory damage of the myenteric plexus. Others enter the blood-

stream to repeat the cycle. Parasitic involvement of the enteric nervous system is common and an achalasia-like mega-oesophagus is a frequent manifestation (Figure 4.6).

Histological findings include an inflammatory destruction of the myenteric plexus, with loss of neurons. The parasite itself is rarely seen in the myenteric plexus. Chagas' disease also commonly involves the heart and other areas of the gastrointestinal tract, particularly the colon [104, 105,107].

Eosinophilic oesophagitis

Primary eosinophilic oesophagitis (EO) is a relatively recently described entity that has features that may mimic GORD clinically, endoscopically and histologically [108–111]. However, by definition, patients with EO have normal pH monitoring and fail to respond to anti-reflux therapy. EO occurs most often in children and young adults, although it may affect patients of any age. There is a strong male predominance. Most affected patients have an allergic history, especially asthma, and they may have peripheral eosinophilia. The most common clinical findings in EO are dysphagia and food impaction [108–111]. EO is treated by several modalities including dietary elimination, steroids and leukotriene receptor antagonists.

Macroscopically patients often have concentric mucosal rings (hence the 'feline', 'ringed' or 'trachealised' appearance of the oesophagus). Other findings include small punctate white exudates, tears and stenosis. Histologically, patients usually have more prominent intra-epithelial eosinophilia than seen in GORD, often with more than 15–20 (and in some literature up to 40) eosinophils per high power field. However, there is considerable histological overlap between the two entities [110,112]. Histological

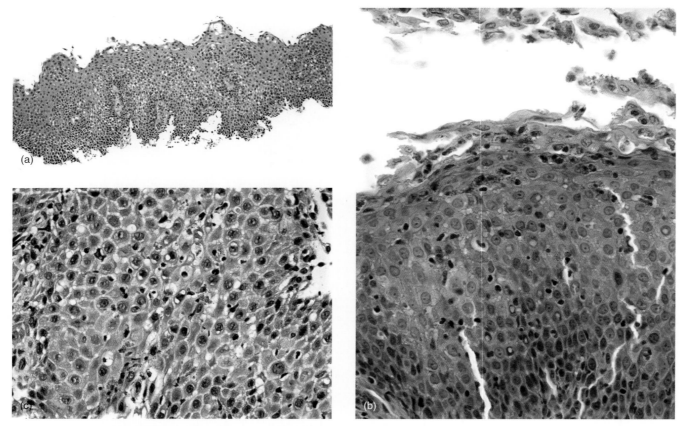

Figure 4.7 Eosinophilic oesophagitis: (a) a low-power view shows spongiosis and numerous eosinophils. (b) A surface predominance of eosinophils, clustering and degranulation of eosinophils and desquamated squamous cells mixed with eosinophils are frequent features. (c) High-power view of spongiosis with numerous eosinophils, some of which are degranulating.

features that favour EO include clustering or micro-abscesses of eosinophils, a predominance of eosinophils within the superficial epithelium, degranulation of eosinophils and abundant eosinophils mixed with desquamated luminal debris (Figure 4.7). Basal cell hyperplasia and oedema are also frequent findings.

It is important to emphasise that the single finding of more than 15–20 eosinophils per high power field is *not* diagnostic of EO, because this can also be seen in severe GORD. The findings favouring EO discussed above, as well as involvement of the mid- and proximal oesophagus (ideally after anti-reflux therapy has already been tried), are helpful in the distinction between these two diseases.

The oesophagus may also be involved in cases of idiopathic eosinophilic gastroenteritis (IEG) [113] and it can be impossible to distinguish EO from IEG if the stomach and duodenum have not been sampled, because most cases of IEG show antral involvement or involvement of other areas of the gastrointestinal tract in addition to the oesophagus. In addition, patients with IEG usually have clinical symptoms of a more generalised disease including nausea, vomiting, diarrhoea and abdominal pain. The presence of full-thickness infiltration of the oesophagus by eosinophil polymorphs has been recently reported in association with oesophageal leiomyomatosis [114].

Other forms of oesophagitis

Many cases of non-infective oesophagitis show non-specific findings including a neutrophilic infiltrate, spongiosis, reactive and degenerative squamous epithelial changes, and erosions or ulcerations. There are many underlying causes (some of which are discussed in more detail below) and careful correlation with clinical findings is often essential to the diagnosis. Carcinomas may also be surrounded by a zone of oesophagitis, so it is important to examine multiple levels of such biopsies to exclude concomitant malignancy.

Pill oesophagitis

Pill oesophagitis is common and is usually caused by prolonged direct mucosal injury from ingested tablets or capsules, particularly large ones [115–118]. Occasionally

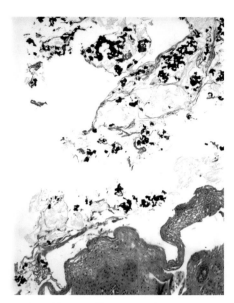

Figure 4.8 Polarisable crystalline material at the luminal surface of the oesophagus, along with sloughing superficial mucosa, in pill oesophagitis.

the contents of the medications themselves may cause the injury. Frequently implicated agents include alendronate sodium [119], antibiotics (particularly tetracyclines) [120], potassium chloride, ferrous sulphate, non-steroidal anti-inflammatory drugs (NSAIDs) and quinidine. Patients often report having taken a pill with little or no fluid before going to bed. Pill oesophagitis occurs more frequently in elderly people and patients with diabetes and/or atrial enlargement are at particular risk for this disorder. Women are affected approximately twice as often as men. Severe cases may lead to perforation.

The most common finding is discrete ulcers, which may be shallow or very deep with extension into the muscularis mucosae [115–118]. Ulcers may be multiple and confluent. The most common location is the junction of the proximal and middle third of the oesophagus where the aortic arch compresses the oesophagus. The mid-oesophagus, adjacent to an enlarged left atrium in elderly patients with or without heart failure, is also a common site. Histological features are non-specific and include an eosinophilic and/or neutrophilic infiltrate, ulceration or erosion, spongiosis and necrosis of squamous epithelium. Stainable crystalline iron may be seen in cases associated with ferrous sulphate. Foreign material may also be present within ulcers and polarisable crystalline material may be associated with cases of alendronate-associated injury (Figure 4.8) [119]. The mucosa surrounding the ulcers is often normal. Pill oesophagitis should be suspected in biopsies that show the above-mentioned histological features in the upper or mid-oesophagus but often the history is necessary to make the diagnosis.

Ingestion of corrosive chemicals may be either accidental or intentional in a suicide attempt. The former occurs mainly in young children and usually involves small quantities, whereas the latter predominantly involves adults who swallow larger amounts. The degree of damage depends on the amount and nature of the ingested substance, as well as the concentration and contact time. After ingestion, the acute phase of necrosis lasts for 4 or 5 days and is associated with oedema and acute inflammation with vascular thrombosis. There may be secondary bacterial infection. A subacute phase follows, with sloughing of superficial necrotic tissue and ulceration, with subsequent repair by granulation tissue and fibrosis. Perforation is most likely during the early part of this phase, in the first 10–12 days after injury [121]. Re-epithelialisation and fibrosis, which may lead to stricture formation, occur in the chronic phase that happens over the next 1–3 months. The strictures that commonly follow lye ingestion may be complicated years later by squamous cell carcinoma [122,123].

Sloughing oesophagitis

Sloughing oesophagitis is defined as superficial mucosal necrosis of the oesophagus that has a characteristic 'sloughing' appearance on endoscopy [124–127]. It is likely to be due to direct contact injury in debilitated people on multiple medications, especially central nervous system depressants or medications known to cause oesophageal injury (see above). It primarily affects middle-aged to older patients, with an equal male:female gender distribution.

At endoscopy, the typical findings are white plaques or sloughing membranes. Non-specific erosions, ulcers and erythema may also be present. Sloughing oesophagitis is most common in the distal and mid-oesophagus but may affect the entire oesophagus.

Histological findings are non-specific and include necrotic, eosinophilic, superficial squamous epithelium, which may be completely or partially detached. The underlying intact mucosa may be very reactive, giving a 'two-toned' appearance to the mucosa. The superficial epithelium may contain flattened dark nuclei, mimicking parakeratosis (Figure 4.9). Vacuolisation and a band of neutrophils may be present at the interface of the necrosis and intact mucosa; however, sometimes there is only minimal inflammation [124–127]. The history of debilitation/multiple medications, the lack of organisms and the unique macroscopic appearance of the oesophagus help to make the diagnosis.

Radiation oesophagitis

Radiation therapy to the chest may be followed by a self-limiting and rarely severe oesophagitis. In some cases,

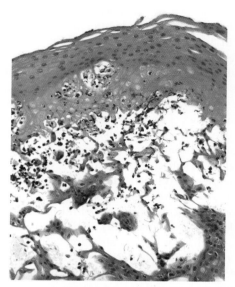

Figure 4.9 Sloughing oesophagitis characterised by separation of the superficial mucosa, neutrophilic inflammation and a 'two-toned' appearance because of the more compact, eosinophilic upper layer of the detached epithelium.

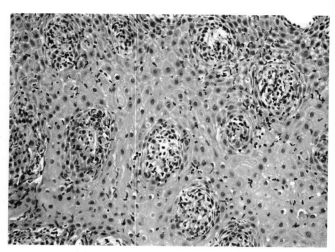

Figure 4.10 The lymphocytic pattern of oesophagitis in a patient with Crohn's disease, showing an exclusively lymphocytic inflammatory infiltrate with a peripapillary distribution.

however, serious complications such as strictures, ulcers and fistula formation occur. These changes are most probably a consequence of ischaemia due to underlying arterial occlusion. Strictures have also been reported at low radiation doses when adjunctive chemotherapy is used [128,129], particularly doxorubicin. Irradiation of squamous cell carcinoma of the oesophagus can result in tracheo-oesophageal fistulae and biopsies performed to detect recurrent carcinoma may show radiation changes with bizarre fibroblasts, oedema and an obliterative vasculitis. Several cases of oesophageal carcinoma that may have been radiation-induced have been reported, with a latent interval ranging from 3 years to 45 years [130,131].

Crohn's disease

Oesophageal involvement by Crohn's disease is well recognised [132–135] and oesophagitis may be the presenting feature of the disease or can occur in the absence of intestinal disease. Its prevalence appears to be higher in children than in adults [136]. The lower third of the oesophagus is the most common site of involvement. Endoscopic appearances are very variable and include erosive oesophagitis, shallow aphthoid ulcers, cobble-stoning and stricture formation [132]. Filiform polyps and fistulae into adjacent viscera have also been reported [137]. Granulomas may be present [137] but biopsies often show non-specific inflammation.

The lymphocytic pattern of oesophagitis

Lymphocytes are a normal component of the squamous epithelium and may be increased in numerous conditions including reflux. 'Lymphocytic oesophagitis' is a recently described entity that remains poorly defined [138,139]. Histologically, the main criterion for this disorder is the presence of increased numbers of lymphocytes in the squamous epithelium, particularly in a peripapillary distribution (Figure 4.10). Granulocytes (including both neutrophils and eosinophils) must be absent or very scanty. Spongiosis is often present. One study [138] has linked lymphocytic oesophagitis with several important entities, including coeliac disease, Crohn's disease and malignancy, particularly in young patients. Other studies [139] have not found the same associations but have found that severe lymphocytic oesophagitis is often a chronic process that is not associated with reflux. Approximately a third of the patients in the latter study had a history of allergy as well. The consensus seems to be that this pattern of inflammation is a non-specific reaction to a variety of insults. However, if a striking lymphocytosis is present in a patient without evidence of reflux, it may be worthwhile considering the possibility that the patient has some other underlying condition.

Oesophagitis and skin diseases

The oesophagus may be involved in a number of skin diseases including pemphigus vulgaris, bullous pemphigoid, benign mucosal pemphigoid, lichen planus, epidermolysis bullosa, toxic epidermal necrolysis (Lyell's disease), Stevens–Johnson syndrome, Darier's disease, tylosis palmaris et plantaris and acanthosis nigricans [140,141]. There are also rare reports of oesophageal involvement in Behçet's disease, featuring discrete, shallow ulcers of the mid-oesophagus with a punched-out appearance and surrounding normal mucosa [142–144]. Loss of peristalsis and lower oesophageal sphincter tone may cause reflux in scleroderma patients and coexistent candidiasis is common [145–147]. Localised epidermolysis bullosa acquisita has also been described in the oesophagus of a patient with intestinal Crohn's disease [148].

Oesophageal graft-versus-host-disease

A desquamative oesophagitis with web formation affecting the upper and mid-oesophagus has been seen in patients with chronic graft-versus-host disease complicating allogeneic bone marrow transplantation [2]. Acute graft-versus-host disease may also involve the oesophageal mucosa in transplanted patients and in non-transplant patients after blood transfusion [149].

References

1. Pettit M: Gastroesophageal reflux disease: Clinical features. *Pharm World Sci* 2005;**27**:417.
2. Baehr PH, McDonald GB. Esophageal infections: risk factors, presentation, diagnosis, and treatment. *Gastroenterology* 1994;**106**:509.
3. Goldenberg SP, Wain SL, Marignani P. Acute necrotizing esophagitis. *Gastroenterology* 1990;**98**:493.
4. Benhaim-Iseni M-C, Petite J-P. Acute necrotizing esophagitis: another case (letter). *Gastroenterology* 1991;**101**:281.
5. Dent J, Holloway RH, Toouli J, Dodds WJ. Mechanisms of lower oesophageal sphincter incompetence in patients with symptomatic gastro-oesophageal reflux. *Gut* 1988;**29**:1020.
6. Dodds WJ, Hogan WJ, Helm JF, Dent J. Pathogenesis of reflux esophagitis. *Gastroenterology* 1981;**81**:376.
7. Timmer R, Breumelhof R, Nadorp JHSM, Smout AJPM. Recent advances in the pathophysiology of gastro-oesophageal reflux disease. *Eur J Gastroenterol Hepatol* 1993;**5**:485.
8. Orlando RC. The pathogenesis of gastroesophageal reflux disease: the relationship between epithelial defense, dysmotility, and acid exposure. *Am J Gastroenterol* 1997;**92**:3S.
9. Gillison EW, Capper WM, Airth GR, et al. Hiatus hernia and heartburn. *Gut* 1969;**10**:609.
10. Baldi F, Corinaldesi R, Ferrarini F, et al. Gastric secretion and emptying of liquids in reflux esophagitis. *Dig Dis Sci* 1981;**26**:886.
11. McCallum RW, Berkowitz DM, Lerner E. Gastric emptying in patients with gastro-esophageal reflux. *Gastroenterology* 1981;**80**:285.
12. Kaye MD, Showalter JP. Pyloric incompetence in patients with symptomatic gastroesophageal reflux. *J Lab Clin Med* 1974;**83**:198.
13. Vaezi MF, Richter JE. Contribution of acid and duodenogastro-oesophageal reflux to oesophageal mucosal injury and symptoms in partial gastrectomy patients. *Gut* 1997;**41**:297.
14. Breckan RK, Paulssen EJ, Asfeldt AM, Mortensen L, Straume B, Florholmen J. The impact of body mass index and *Helicobacter pylori* infection on gastro-oesophageal reflux symptoms: a population-based study in Northern Norway. *Scand J Gastroenterol* 2009;**44**:1060.
15. Kaye MD. Postprandial gastroesophageal reflux in healthy people. *Gut* 1977;**18**:709.
16. Fisher RS, Roberts GS, Grabowski CJ, Cohen S. Altered lower esophageal sphincter function during early pregnancy. *Gastroenterology* 1978;**74**:1233.
17. Locke GR, Talley NJ, Fett SL, Zinsmeister AR, Melton LJ. Prevalence and clinical spectrum of gastroesophageal reflux: a population-based study in Olmsted County, Minnesota. *Gastroenterology* 1997;**112**:1448.
18. Hirschowitz BI. A critical analysis, with appropriate controls, of gastric acid and pepsin secretion in clinical esophagitis. *Gastroenterology* 1991;**101**:1149.
19. Fiorucci S, Santucci L, Chiucchiu S, Morelli A. Gastric acidity and gastroesophageal reflux patterns in patients with esophagitis. *Gastroenterology* 1992;**103**:855.
20. Eriksen CA, Sadek SA, Cranford C, et al. Reflux oesophagitis and oesophageal transit: evidence of a primary oesophageal motor disorder. *Gut* 1988;**29**:448.
21. Helm JF, Dodds WJ, Pelc LR, et al. Effect of esophageal emptying and saliva on clearance of acid from the esophagus. *N Engl J Med* 1984;**310**:284.
22. Meyers RL, Orlando RC. In vivo bicarbonate secretion by human esophagus. *Gastroenterology* 1992;**103**:1174.
23. Brown CM, Rees WDW. Human oesophageal bicarbonate secretion: a phenomenon waiting for a role (commentary). *Gut* 1997;**40**:693.
24. El-Serag HB, Sonnenberg A. Associations between different forms of gastro-oesophageal reflux disease. *Gut* 1997;**41**:594.
25. Lundell LR, Dent J, Bennett JR, et al. Endoscopic assessment of oesophagitis: clinical and functional correlations and further validation of the Los Angeles classification. *Gut* 1999;**45**:172.
26. Hattori K, Winans CS, Archer F, Kirsner JB. Endoscopic diagnosis of esophageal inflammation. *Gastrointest Endosc* 1974;**20**:102.
27. Rabin MS, Bremner CG, Botha JR. The reflux gastroesophageal polyp. *Am J Gastroenterol* 1980;**73**:451.
28. Mihas AA, Slaughter RL, Goldman LN, Hirschowitz BI. Double lumen esophagus due to reflux esophagitis with fibrous septum formation. *Gastroenterology* 1976;**71**:136.
29. Raymond JI, Khan AH, Cain LR, Ramin JE. Multiple esophagogastric fistulas resulting from reflux esophagitis. *Am J Gastroenterol* 1980;**73**:430.
30. Knuff TE, Benjamin SB, Worsham GF, et al. Histologic evaluation of chronic gastroesophageal reflux: an evaluation of biopsy methods and diagnostic criteria. *Dig Dis Sci* 1984;**29**:194.
31. Weinstein WM, Bogoch ER, Bowes KL. The normal human esophageal mucosa: a histological reappraisal. *Gastroenterology* 1975;**68**:40.
32. Schindbleck NE, Wiebecke B, Klauser AG, et al. Diagnostic value of histology in non-erosive gastro-oesophageal reflux disease. *Gut* 1996;**39**:151.
33. Orenstein SR. Gastroesophageal reflux. *Curr Probl Pediatr* 1991;**21**:193.
34. Ismail-Beigi F, Horton PF, Pope CE II. Histological consequences of gastroesophageal reflux in man. *Gastroenterology* 1970;**58**:163.
35. Ismail-Beigi F, Pope CE II. Distribution of the histological changes of gastroesophageal reflux in the distal esophagus of man. *Gastroenterology* 1974;**66**:1109.
36. Johnson LF, DeMeester TR, Haggitt RC. Esophageal epithelial response to gastroesophageal reflux: a quantitative study. *Am J Dig Dis* 1978;**23**:498.
37. Black DD, Haggitt RC, Orenstein SR, et al. Oesophagitis in infants: morphometric histological diagnosis and correlation

with measures of gastroesophageal reflux. *Gastroenterology* 1990;**98**:1408.

38. Haggitt RC. Histopathology of reflux-induced esophageal and supraesophageal injuries. *Am J Med* 2000;**6**(suppl 4a):108.

39. Geboes K, Desmet V, Vantrappen G, et al. Vascular changes in the esophageal mucosa. An early histologic sign of oesophagitis. *Gastrointest Endosc* 1980;**26**:29.

40. Collins BJ, Elliott H, Sloan JM, et al. Esophageal histology in reflux oesophagitis. *J Clin Pathol* 1985;**38**:1265.

41. Brown LF, Goldman H, Antonioli DA. Intraepithelial eosinophils in endoscopic biopsies of adults with reflux esophagitis. *Am J Surg Pathol* 1984;**8**:899.

42. Tummala V, Barwick KW, Sontag SJ, et al. The significance of intraepithelial eosinophils in the histologic diagnosis of gastroesophageal reflux. *Am J Clin Pathol* 1987;**87**:43.

43. Gold BD. Is gastroesophageal reflux disease really a life-long disease: do babies who regurgitate grow up to be adults with GERD complications? *Gastroenterology* 2006;**101**:641.

44. Winter HS, Madara JL, Stafford RJ, et al. Intraepithelial eosinophils: a new diagnostic criterion for reflux oesophagitis. *Gastroenterology* 1982;**83**:818.

45. Mangano MM, Antonioli DA, Schnitt SJ, et al. Nature and significance of cells with irregular nuclear contours in esophageal mucosal biopsies. *Mod Pathol* 1992;**5**:191.

46. Wang HH, Mangano MM, Antonioli DA. Evaluation of T-lymphocytes in esophageal mucosal biopsies. *Mod Pathol* 1994;**7**:55.

47. Jarvis L, Dent J, Whitehead R. Morphometric assessment of reflux esophagitis in fibreoptic biopsy specimens. *J Clin Pathol* 1985;**38**:44.

48. Collins JSA, Watt PCH, Hamilton PW, et al. Assessment of oesophagitis by histology and morphometry. *Histopathology* 1989;**14**:381.

49. Buss DH, Scharyj M. Herpes virus infection of the esophagus and other visceral organs in adults: incidence and clinical significance. *Am J Med* 1979;**66**:457.

50. McKay JS, Day DW. Herpes simplex oesophagitis. *Histopathology* 1983;**7**:409.

51. Deshmukh M, Shah R, McCallum RW. Experience with herpes esophagitis in otherwise healthy patients. *Am J Gastroenterol* 1984;**79**:173.

52. McBane RD, Gross JB. Herpes esophagitis: clinical syndrome, endoscopic appearance, and diagnosis in 23 patients. *Gastrointest Endosc* 1991;**37**:600.

53. Lamps LW. Infectious disorders of the upper gastrointestinal tract (excluding *H. pylori*). *Diagnos Histopathol* 2008;**14**:427.

54. Fishbein PG, Tuthill R, Kressel H, Freidman H, Snape WJ Jr. Herpes simplex esophagitis: a cause of upper gastrointestinal bleeding. *Dig Dis Sci* 1979;**24**:540.

55. Rattner HM, Cooper DJ, Zaman MB. Severe bleeding from herpes esophagitis. *Am J Gastroenterol* 1985;**80**:523.

56. Cronstedt JL, Bouchama A, Hainau B, Halim M, Khouqeer F, Al Darsouny T. Spontaneous esophageal perforation in herpes simplex esophagitis. *Am J Gastroenterol* 1992;**87**:124.

57. Greenson JK, Beschorner WE, Boitnott JK, Yardley JH. Prominent mononuclear cell infiltrate is characteristic of herpes oesophagitis. *Hum Pathol* 1991;**22**:541.

58. Gould B, Kory WP, Raskin JB, Ibe MJ, Redhammer DE. Esophageal biopsy findings in the acquired immunodeficiency syndrome: clinical pathological correlations in **20** patients. *South Med J* 1988;**81**:1395.

59. Wilcox CM, Diehl DL, Cello JP, Margaretten W, Jacobson MA. Cytomegalovirus esophagitis in patients with AIDS. A clinical, endoscopic, and pathologic correlation. *Ann Intern Med* 1990; **113**:589.

60. Chetty R, Roskell DE. Cytomegalovirus infection in the gastrointestinal tract. *J Clin Pathol* 1994;**47**:968.

61. Theise ND, Rotterdam H, Dieterich D. Cytomegalovirus esophagitis in AIDS: diagnosis by endoscopic biopsy. *Am J Gastroenterol* 1991;**86**:1123.

62. Kotler DP, Reka S, Orenstein JM, Fox CH. Chronic idiopathic esophageal ulceration in the acquired immunodeficiency syndrome. *J Clin Gastroenterol* 1992;**15**:284.

63. Pedro-Botet J, Miralles R, Sauleda J, Rubies-Prat J. Idiopathic ulcer of the esophagus in the AIDS syndrome: a potential life-threatening complication. *Gastrointest Endosc* 1989;**35**:470.

64. Wilcox CM. Current concepts of gastrointestinal disease associated with human immunodeficiency virus infection. *Clin Perspect Gastroenterol* 2000;**3**:9.

65. Jalfon IM, Sitton JE, Hammer RA, et al. HIV-1 gp41 antigen demonstration in esophageal ulcers with acquired immunodeficiency syndrome. *J Clin Gastroenterol* 1991;**13**:644.

66. Wilcox CM, Schwartz DA. Endoscopic characterization of idiopathic esophageal ulceration associated with human immunodeficiency virus infection. *J Clin Gastroenterol* 1993;**16**:251.

67. Wilcox CM. Esophageal disease in the acquired immunodeficiency syndrome: etiology, diagnosis, and management. *Am J Med* 1992;**92**:412.

68. Kitchen VS, Helbert M, Francis ND, et al. Epstein–Barr virus associated oesophageal ulcers in AIDS. *Gut* 1990;**31**:1223.

69. Schechter M, Pannain VLN, Viana de Loiveria A. Papova-virus associated esophageal ulceration in a patient with AIDS. *J AIDS* 1991;**5**:238.

70. Corballina M, Lusso P, Gallo RC, et al. Disseminated human herpes-virus 6 infection in AIDS (letter). *Lancet* 1993;**342**:1242.

71. Moretti F, Uberti-Foppa C, Quiros-Roldan E, Fanti L, Lillo F, Lazzarin A. Esophagobronchial fistula caused by varicella zoster virus in a patient with AIDS: a unique case. *J Clin Pathol* 2002;**55**:397.

72. Kroneke K, Cuadrado R. Esophageal stricture following oesophagitis in a patient with herpes zoster: case report. *Mil Med* 1984;**149**:479.

73. Walsh TJ, Mertz WG. Pathologic features in the human alimentary tract associated with invasiveness of *C. tropicalis. Am J Clin Pathol* 1986;**85**:498.

74. Jensen KB, Stenderup A, Thomsen JB, Bichel J. Oesophageal moniliasis in malignant neoplastic disease. *Acta Med Scand* 1964;**175**:455.

75. Tom W, Aaron JS. Esophageal ulcers caused by *Torulopsis glabrata* in a patient with acquired immunodeficiency syndrome. *Am J Gastroenterol* 1987;**82**:766.

76. Anderson LI, Frederiksen JH, Appleyard M. Prevalence of oesophageal *Candida* colonization in a Danish population, with special reference to oesophageal symptoms, benign oesophageal disorders, and pulmonary disease. *J Infect Dis* 1992;**165**:389.

77. Eras P, Goldstein MJ, Sherlock P. Candida infection of the gastrointestinal tract. *Medicine* 1972;**5**:367.

78. Vermeersch B, Rysselaere M, Dekeyser K, et al. Fungal colonization of the oesophagus. *Am J Gastroenterol* 1989;**84**:1079.

79. Lopez-Dupla M, Mora-Sanz P, Pintado-Garcia V, et al. Clinical, endoscopic, immunologic, and therapeutic aspects of oropharyngeal and esophageal candidiasis in HIV-infected patients: a survey of 144 cases. *Am J Gastroenterol* 1992;**87**:1771.

80. Larner AJ, Lendrum R. Oesophageal candidiasis after omeprazole therapy. *Gut* 1992;**33**:860.

81. Gonzalez-Crussi IF, Iung OS. Esophageal moniliasis as a cause of death. *Am J Surg* 1965;**109**:634.

82. Weiss J, Epstein BS. Esophageal moniliasis. *Am J Roentgenol* 1962;**88**:718.

83. Maksymiuk AW, Thongprasert S, Hopfer R, et al. Systemic candidiasis in cancer patients. *Am J Medicine* 1984;**77**(suppl 4D):20.

84. Chandler FW, Watts JC. *Pathologic Diagnosis of Fungal Infections.* Chicago: ASCP Press, 1987.

85. Kodsi BE, Wickremesinghe PC, Kozinn PJ, et al. Candida oesophagitis. A prospective study of 27 cases. *Gastroenterology* 1976;**71**:715.

86. Young RC, Bennett JE, Vogel CL, et al. Aspergillosis: the spectrum of the disease in 98 patients. *Medicine* 1970;**49**:147.

87. Thomson SR, Bade PG, Taams M, Chrystal V. Gastrointestinal mucormycosis. *Br J Surg* 1991;**78**:952.

88. Neame P, Ragner D. Mucormycosis: a report of twenty-two cases. *Arch Pathol* 1960;**70**:261.

89. McKenzie R, Khakoo R. Blastomycosis of the esophagus presenting with gastrointestinal bleeding. *Gastroenterology* 1985;**88**:1271.

90. Jacobs DH, Macher AM, Handler R, et al. Esophageal cryptococcosis in a patient with the hyperimunoglobulin E-recurrent infection (Job's) syndrome. *Gastroenterology* 1984;**87**:201.

91. Lee J-H, Neumann DA, Welsh JD. Disseminated histoplasmosis presenting with esophageal symptomatology. *Dig Dis* 1977;**22**:831.

92. Lamps LW, Molina CP, West AB, Haggitt RC, Scott MA. The pathologic spectrum of gastrointestinal and hepatic histoplasmosis. *Am J Clin Pathol* 2000;**113**:64.

93. Jain SK, Jain S, Jain M, Yaduvanshi A. Esophageal tuberculosis: is it so rare? Report of 12 cases and review of the literature. *Am J Gastroenterol* 2002;**97**:287.

94. Gordon AH, Marshall JB. Esophageal tuberculosis: definitive diagnosis by endoscopy. *Am J Gastroenterol* 1990;**85**:174.

95. Dow CJ. Oesophageal tuberculosis: four cases. *Gut* 1981;**22**:234.

96. Seivewright N, Feehalley J, Wicks ACB. Primary tuberculosis of the esophagus. *Am J Gastroenterol* 1984;**79**:842.

97. Laajam MA. Primary tuberculosis of the esophagus: pseudotumoral presentation. *Am J Gastroenterol* 1984;**79**:839.

98. El-Serag HB, Johnston DE. *Mycobacterium avium* complex esophagitis. *Am J Gastroenterol* 1997;**92**:1561.

99. Walsh TJ, Belitsos NJ, Hamilton SR. Bacterial esophagitis in immunocompromised patients. *Arch Intern Med* 1986;**146**:1345.

100. Miller JT Jr, Slywka SW, Ellis JH. Staphylococcal esophagitis causing giant ulcers. *Abdom Imaging* 1993;**18**:115.

101. Ezzell JH Jr, Bremer J, Adamec TA. Bacterial esophagitis: an often forgotten cause of odynophagia. *Am J Gastroenterol* 1990;**85**:498.

102. Lamps LW, Scott MA. Cat scratch disease: historical, clinical, and pathological perspectives. *Am J Clin Pathol* 2004;**121** (Pathology Patterns Supplement):S71.

103. Chang AD, Drachenberg CI, James SP. Bacillary angiomatosis associated with extensive esophageal polyposis: a new mucocutaneous manifestation of acquired immunodeficiency (AIDS). *Am J Gastroenterol* 1996;**91**:2220.

104. Atias A, Neghme A, Mackay LA, Jarpa S. Megaoesophagus, megacolon, and Chagas' disease in Chile. *Gastroenterology* 1963;**44**:433.

105. Earlam RJ. Gastrointestinal aspects of Chagas' disease. *Am J Dig Dis* 1972;**17**:559.

106. Betarello A, Pinotti HW. Oesophageal involvement in Chagas' disease. *Clin Gastroenterol* 1976;**5**:27.

107. de Oliveira RB, Troncon LEA, Dantas RO, Meneghelli UG. Gastrointestinal manifestations of Chagas disease. *Am J Gastroenterol* 1998;**93**:884.

108. Arora AS, Yamazaki K. Eosinophilic esophagitis: asthma of the esophagus? *Clin Gastroenterol Hepatol* 2004;**2**:523.

109. Liacouras CA, Spergel JM, Ruchelli E, et al. Eosinophilic esophagitis: a 10-year experience in 381 children. *Clin Gastroenterol Hepatol* 2005;**3**:1198.

110. Parfitt JR, Gregor JC, Suskin NG, et al. Eosinophilic esophagitis in adults. Distinguishing features from gastroesophageal reflux disease: a study of 41 patients. *Mod Pathol* 2006;**19**:90.

111. Walsh SV, Antonioli DA, Goldman H, et al. Allergic esophagitis in children: a clinicopathological entity. *Am J Surg Pathol* 1999;**23**:390.

112. Rodrigo S, Abboud G, Oh D, et al. High intraepithelial eosinophil counts in esophageal squamous epithelium are not specific for eosinophilic esophagitis in adults. *Am J Gastroenterol.* 2008;**103**:435.

113. Straumann A. Idiopathic eosinophilic gastrointestinal diseases in adults. *Best Pract Res Clin Gastroenterol* 2008;**22**:481.

114. Nicholson AG, Li D, Pastorino U, Goldstraw P, Jeffery PK. Full thickness eosinophilia in esophageal leiomyomatosis and idiopathic eosinophilic esophagitis. A common allergic inflammatory profile? *J Pathol* 1997;**183**:233.

115. Abid S, Mumtaz K, Jafri W, et al. Pill-induced esophageal injury-endoscopic features and clinical outcomes. *Endoscopy* 2005;**37**:740.

116. Kikendall JW, Friedman AC, Ovewole MA, et al. Pill-induced esophageal injury. Case reports and review of the medical literature. *Dig Dis Sci* 1983;**8**:174.

117. Kikendall JW. Pill esophagitis. *J Clin Gastroenterol* 1999;**28**:298.

118. Teplick JG, Teplick SK, Ominsky SH, Haskin ME. Esophagitis caused by oral medication. *Radiology* 1980;**134**:23.

119. Abraham SC, Cruz-Correa M, Lee LA, et al. Alendronate-associated oesophageal injury: pathologic and endoscopic features. *Mod Pathol* 1999;**12**:1152.

120. Kadayifci A, Gulsen MT, Koruk M, Savas MC. Doxycycline-induced pill esophagitis. *Dis Esophagus* 2004;**17**:168.

121. Butler C, Madden JW, Davis WM. Morphologic aspects of experimental lye strictures. I. Pathogenesis and pathophysiologic correlations. *J Surg Res* 1974;**17**:232.

122. Kiviranta UK. Corrosion carcinoma of the oesophagus: 381 cases of corrosion and 9 cases of corrosion carcinoma. *Acta Otolaryngol* 1952;**42**:89.

123. Appelqvist P, Salmo M. Lye corrosion carcinoma of the oesophagus. A review of 63 cases. *Cancer* 1980;**45**:2655.

124. Moore RJ, et al. Sloughing oesophagitis: a distinct histologic and endoscopic entity. *Mod Pathol* 1999;**12**:81A.

125. Pugh JL, et al. Sloughing oesophagitis: a newly recognized clinicopathologic entity. *Gastroenterology* 2005;**128**:636.

126. Purdy JK, et al. Sloughing esophagitis: a type of contact esophageal injury in debilitated patients? *Mod Pathol* 2008;**21**:133A.

127. Carmack SW, Vemulapalli R, Spechler SJ, Genta RM. Esophagitis dissecans superficialis ('sloughing esophagitis'): a clinicopathologic study of 12 cases. *Am J Surg Pathol* 2009;**33**:1789.

128. Greco FA, Brereton HD, Dent H, et al. Adriamycin and enhanced radiation reaction in normal esophagus and skin. *Ann Intern Med* 1976;**85**:294.

129. Newburger PE, Cassady JR, Jaffe N. Esophagitis due to Adriamycin and radiation therapy for childhood malignancy. *Cancer* 1978;**42**:417.

130. Sherrill DJ, Grishkin BA, Galal FS, et al. Radiation associated malignancies of the esophagus. *Cancer* 1984;**54**:726.

131. Vanagunas A, Jacob P, Olinger E. Radiation-induced esophageal injury: a spectrum from esophagitis to cancer. *Am J Gastroenterol* 1990;**85**:808.

132. Huchzermeyer H, Paul F, Seifert E, et al. Endoscopic results in five patients with Crohn's disease of the esophagus. *Endoscopy* 1976;**8**:75.

133. Degryse HRM, DeSchepper AMAP. Aphthoid oesophageal ulcers in Crohn's disease of the ileum and colon. *Gastrointest Radiol* 1984;**9**:197.

134. Freedman PG, Dieterich DT, Balthazar EJ. Crohn's disease of the esophagus: case report and review of the literature. *Am J Gastroenterol* 1984;**79**:835.

135. Geboes K, Janssens J, Rutgeerts P, Vantrappen C. Crohn's disease of the esophagus. *J Clin Gastroenterol* 1986;**8**:31.

136. Lenaerts C, Roy CC, Vaillancourt M, et al. High incidence of upper gastrointestinal tract involvement in children with Crohn's disease. *Pediatrics* 1989;**83**:777.

137. D'Haens G, Rutgeerts P, Geboes K, et al. The natural history of esophageal Crohn's disease: three patterns of evolution. *Gastrointest Endosc* 1994;**296**:300.

138. Rubio CA, Sjodahl K, Lagergren J. Lymphocytic esophagitis: a histologic subset of chronic esophagitis. *Am J Clin Pathol* 2006;**125**:432.

139. Purdy JK, Appelman HD, Golembeski CP, McKenna BJ. Lymphocytic esophagitis: a chronic or recurring pattern of esophagitis resembling allergic contact dermatitis. *Am J Clin Pathol* 2008;**130**:508.

140. Geboes K, Janssens J. The esophagus in cutaneous diseases. In: Vantrappen GR, Hellemans JJ (eds), *Diseases of the Esophagus*. New York: Springer-Verlag, 1974: 823.

141. Walton S, Bennett JR. Skin and gullet. *Gut* 1991;**32**:694.

142. Lockhart JM, McIntyre W, Caperton EM. Esophageal ulceration in Behçet's syndrome. *Ann Intern Med* 1976;**84**:572.

143. Kaplinsky N, Neumann G, Harzahav Y, Frankl O. Esophageal ulceration in Behçet's syndrome. *Gastrointest Endosc* 1977;**23**:160.

144. Mori S, Yoshihara A, Kawamura H, Takeuchi A, et al. Oesophageal involvement in Behçet's disease. *Am J Gastroenterol* 1983;**78**:548.

145. Atkinson M, Summerling MD. Oesophageal changes in systemic sclerosis. *Gut* 1966;**7**:402.

146. Zamost BJ, Hirschberg J, Ippoliti AF, et al. Esophagitis in scleroderma: prevalence and risk factors. *Gastroenterology* 1987;**92**:421.

147. Cohen S, Laufer I, Snape WJ Jr, et al. The gastrointestinal manifestations of scleroderma: pathogenesis and management. *Gastroenterology* 1980;**79**:155.

148. Schattenkirchner SL, Lemann M, Prost C, et al. Localized epidermolysis bullosa acquisita of the esophagus in a patient with Crohn's disease. *Am J Gastroenterol* 1996;**91**:1657.

149. Iwakuma A, Matsuyoshi T, Arikado T, et al. Two cases of postoperative erythroderma: clinical and pathological investigation. *J Jpn Assoc Thoracic Surg* 1991;**39**:209.

CHAPTER 5

Barrett's oesophagus

Neil A. Shepherd

Gloucestershire Cellular Pathology Laboratory, Cheltenham, UK

Introduction

Barrett's oesophagus (columnar-lined oesophagus or CLO) is defined as the replacement of the lower oesophageal squamous mucosa by metaplastic glandular mucosa as a result of gastro-oesophageal reflux disease (GORD). Over recent decades there has been a rapid rise in the incidence of CLO in the UK and in other western populations [1–4]. Although increased endoscopy and its detection at endoscopy may be in part responsible, there is also a true increase in its prevalence [1]. There has also been a striking increase in the incidence of adenocarcinoma complicating CLO. Until about 20 years ago, in western populations, squamous cell carcinoma was the predominant type of oesophageal cancer but the ratio has been reversed with an eightfold increase in adenocarcinoma over the past 30 years [5]. Overall, oesophageal cancer is now the ninth most common cancer and the fifth most common cause of cancer death in the UK [6].

The increasing incidence of CLO in the west can be ascribed to those risk factors that predispose to gastro-oesophageal reflux disease (GORD) (see 'Reflux oesophagitis' in Chapter 4), such as male sex, middle age, being white, obesity, alcohol, smoking and family history. One retrospective case–control study has demonstrated that an overweight man with a long-term history of reflux disease has an 180-fold increased risk of oesophageal adenocarcinoma compared with a lean individual without a history of reflux disease [7]. The role of acid reflux has long been known but, in the 1990s, it became apparent that the reflux of bile and alkali from the duodenum also had an important part to play, particularly with regard to the development of neoplasia [8–10]. Another factor, believed to be protective against CLO, is *Helicobacter pylori* infection of the stomach. It is thought that the lack of *H. pylori* infection in western populations, especially those subtypes such as cagA-positive *H. pylori*, encourages a higher stomach acid level and so promotes the development of CLO if there are other predisposing factors to reflux disease [11,12].

Despite the advances in our understanding of CLO and the factors that lead to its development, there are many unresolved issues [13]. Its histogenesis remains unproven. Originally described by a London surgeon, Norman Barrett, who mistakenly considered it as a 'congenitally short oesophagus' with an attenuated intrathoracic stomach [14,15], it was subsequently realised that the columnar epithelium lined the true anatomical oesophagus [16] and was an acquired disorder in which there is replacement of the squamous epithelium by columnar epithelium at the lower end of the oesophagus [17,18]. In experimental studies, oesophageal injury has been followed by re-epithelialisation with columnar epithelium under conditions of high acid exposure and when squamous barriers to proximal migration of gastric columnar epithelium had been created [19]. Proximal extension of gastric epithelium to replace the damaged squamous epithelium could not explain the development of CLO and alternative proposed mechanisms are metaplasia of stratified squamous epithelium or migration of columnar cells from native oesophageal glands or their ducts [20]. Candidate cells of origin include multipotential stem cells at the basal aspect of the squamous mucosa of the oesophagus and the cells lining oesophageal gland ducts [21].

Morson and Dawson's Gastrointestinal Pathology, Fifth Edition. Edited by Neil A. Shepherd, Bryan F. Warren, Geraint T. Williams, Joel K. Greenson, Gregory Y. Lauwers and Marco R. Novelli.

The varying terminology and classification of the condition cause substantial consternation [22]. This has led some to propose the dropping of the eponym, Barrett's oesophagus, because of the confusion it generates [23]. As there is a natural variation of up to 20 mm between the true oesophago-gastric junction and the squamo-columnar junction, the disease was initially only said to be present when at least 30 mm of columnar-lined epithelium was demonstrated [24]. 'Short-segment CLO' (SSCLO) was introduced to identify those cases in which there was less than 30 mm of columnar-lined epithelium in the lower oesophagus [24,25]. The term 'ultrashort-segment CLO' (USSCLO) was then conceived for cases where there was intestinal metaplasia at the cardia. Conversely, others have used this term to mean true CLO that is effectively microscopic and not demonstrable at endoscopy [26].

Pathologists in western Europe and North America have seen a huge upsurge in the number of biopsies taken from CLO cases and the number of resections, whether endoscopic mucosal resection or oesophago-gastrectomies, undertaken for the neoplastic complications of CLO. Just like the disease and its neoplastic complications, pathologists in the west have had an epidemic of such specimens, such that Barrett's oesophagus now accounts for a considerable proportion of the workload of a western gastrointestinal pathologist. This is despite continuing uncertainties about the role of pathology in the diagnosis of Barrett's oesophagus. Furthermore, the diagnosis and management of the neoplastic complications of CLO, very much the endeavour of pathologists, are also not without controversy and there are very considerable changes afoot in the identification and treatment of the early neoplastic complications of the disease.

Definition, diagnosis and histological appearances

Classic or long-segment CLO is essentially an endoscopic diagnosis [24,27,28]. There are cases where pathology may be diagnostic (Figure 5.1) and endoscopy is not, especially when there is stricturing or peptic ulceration. So, although the pathologist has an undoubted role in the diagnosis of CLO, it is important that he or she understands the limitations of histopathology and is critically reliant on clinical and endoscopic correlation to make an accurate histological assessment. In this regard, we commend the four category reporting strategy of the British Society of Gastroenterology (BSG) to all pathologists, especially when insufficient clinical and endoscopic information is provided or biopsy sampling is suboptimal (Table 5.1) [24].

The diagnosis of SSCLO requires more pathological corroboration [24,29]. However, USSCLO is an entirely pathological diagnosis and it is emphasised that the latter is essentially a gastric disease rather than part of the spectrum of CLO, and is better termed 'cardia intestinal metaplasia' [24,30,31]. Thus, the role of the pathologist in the diagnosis of classic CLO and SSCLO is to corroborate the endoscopic diagnosis. A definitive diagnosis of CLO can be made on the grounds of histopathology alone when glandular metaplasia is seen associated with native oesophageal structures, such as oesophageal gland ducts or submucosal glands, indicating that the glandular metaplasia is unequivocally in the native oesophagus (Figure 5.1) [24,32]. However, this is only seen in about 15% of biopsy sets, so is not helpful for diagnostic purposes in most cases [32].

Although there is no doubt that intestinal metaplasia is a characteristic feature of CLO (Figure 5.2), and is important

Table 5.1 The pathological reporting strategy for columnar-lined oesophagus (CLO)

Category	Reporting strategy	Pathological features	Observations
1	Biopsies diagnostic for CLO	Native oesophageal structures with juxtaposition to glandular mucosa	–
2	Biopsies corroborative of an endoscopic diagnosis of CLO	Intestinalised metaplastic glandular mucosa with or without non-organised arrangement, villous architecture, patchwork of different glandular types	Could yet represent incomplete IM in the stomach, especially hiatus hernia or USSCLO
3	Biopsies in keeping with, but not specific for, CLO	Gastric type mucosa without intestinal metaplasia, non-organised arrangement, patchwork appearance	Could yet represent the GOJ or the stomach, with or without hiatus hernia
4	Biopsies without evidence of CLO	Oesophageal type squamous epithelium with no evidence of glandular epithelium	–

(Reproduced from Hellier MD, Shepherd NA. Diagnosis of columnar-lined oesophagus. In Watson A, Heading RC, Shepherd NA, eds. Guidelines for the diagnosis and management of Barrett's columnar-lined oesophagus. London: British Society of Gastroenterology, 2005, with permission from the British Society of Gastroenterology).

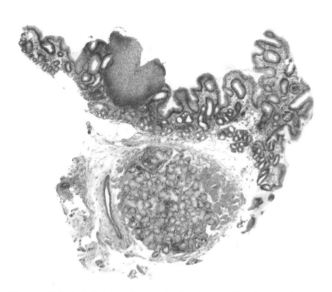

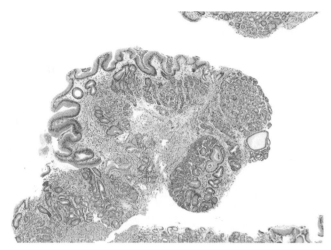

Figure 5.3 This biopsy shows columnar-lined oesophagus with cardiac, fundic and pancreatic epithelial phenotypes all represented.

Figure 5.1 A definitive diagnosis of columnar-lined oesophagus (CLO) can be made from this biopsy specimen. There is glandular mucosa with a squamous island on the surface with juxtaposed native oesophageal structures, a submucosal gland and its duct beneath. In serial sections, the gland duct will lead into, and form, the squamous island.

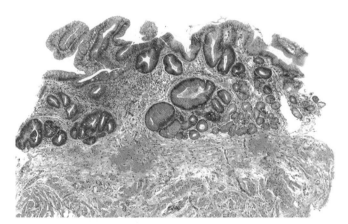

Figure 5.2 Typical columnar-lined oesophagus (CLO) mucosa seen in a biopsy. There is predominant cardiac-type epithelium (right) and intestinalised epithelium (left). Occasional specialised fundic-type glands are also present at right. This is the typical 'patchwork' mucosa of CLO.

in the neoplastic progression of CLO, UK pathological opinion has argued for many years that it should not be used as the defining characteristic of CLO for diagnostic purposes [20,24,33–35], not least because its demonstration depends on the number of biopsies taken [36,37]. This is despite the fact that major reviews of the disease over many years, including the current US management guidelines, have regarded the pathological demonstration of intesti-

nalisation as the defining feature of CLO [38–40]. Now international pathological opinion is undergoing a major rethink concerning the relevance of the demonstration of goblet cells/intestinal metaplasia to the definition and diagnosis of CLO. Recently, two of the world's top gastrointestinal pathologists have argued cogently for the discontinuation of the demonstration of intestinal metaplasia as the defining feature of CLO [31]. Not only do they cite the sampling issue but they also point out that the non-goblet cell population in CLO is biologically intestinalised and shows molecular changes similar to those of the goblet cell population [31,41]. Further, they argue that there is a well-defined risk of neoplasia in those with CLO but without goblet cells, and that it is often difficult to differentiate goblet cells from so-called pseudo-goblet cells histologically [31]. We strongly concur with their views and feel that there are now powerful grounds, internationally, to bring to an end the use of the histological demonstration of intestinal metaplasia/goblet cells as the defining/diagnostic feature of CLO, and resort to defining the disease by endoscopic means with histology becoming corroborative to endoscopy and more of use when the endoscopic features are equivocal (especially in short-segment disease) or when there is extensive ulceration or stricturing [24,31].

Three main types of epithelium are encountered in CLO: cardiac, fundic and intestinal phenotypes [42,43]. The intestinal epithelium is usually of the incomplete type although the complete type is occasionally seen [44,45]. A characteristic histopathological feature of the disease is the presence of a 'patchwork' of these different types (Figure 5.2). Although more commonly seen at the otherwise normal oesophago-gastric junction, a pancreatic phenotype may be also seen within metaplastic glandular mucosa (Figure 5.3). The intestinal metaplasia (IM) in CLO has been termed 'specialised', implying that it is unique to CLO and differs from that seen in the stomach [39,46]. Many attempts have been made to confirm or refute this. Basic mucin histochemical stains have proved unhelpful. Various immunohistochemical stains have also been tried, including cdx2 [47], but again none has been convincingly shown to be specific for IM in CLO. Some encouraging results have been seen with MUC-1 and MUC-6. One study showed that these markers were 90% specific for goblet cells in CLO compared with those in the stomach but their use in routine practice is limited by poor sensitivity of the markers [48].

There has been much debate concerning the value of cytokeratin immunohistochemistry in differentiating true CLO and gastric IM. Some studies have claimed that an exclusive staining pattern is seen in CLO, namely diffuse staining of the glandular epithelium with cytokeratin 7 and staining of the surface epithelium with cytokeratin 20 [49–51]. However, a similar pattern has since been observed in gastric IM, especially immature IM, as well as in biopsies from the gastro-oesophageal junction (GOJ) [52–55]. The use of differential cytokeratin staining in practice is further complicated by evidence that staining patterns may differ because of technical variations in the methods and the types of fixative used: observer variation in the interpretation of staining patterns has also been demonstrated [56,57]. At present, we believe that these methodologies cannot be advocated for the routine pathological differentiation of true intestinal-type glandular metaplasia in the oesophagus from that occurring in the stomach, whether at the cardia or elsewhere.

It has been hypothesised that IM in CLO is preceded by the development of an 'intermediate' or 'transitional' type of epithelium. Multilayered epithelium (ME) has been demonstrated at the squamo-columnar junction and within the columnar mucosa in patients with CLO (Figure 5.4) [58,59]. The morphological, ultrastructural and immunohistochemical features of this epithelium are intermediate between those of squamous epithelium and columnar epithelium, suggesting that MLE represents a precursor stage in the development of CLO [58]. ME has been strongly associated with reflux-associated carditis, when compared with *H. pylori*-induced carditis [60]. However, others have shown that ME is a feature of the 'normal' oesophagogastric junction where it may be seen along with ciliated epithelium, presumably representing a congenital residuum [61]. Similar to Takubo, this author remains to be convinced that ME is specific to CLO and requires further evidence before ME can be regarded as a precursor lesion for CLO, although it may be of some use in the pathological diagnosis of CLO [62].

There are other morphological features that aid the pathologist in the distinction of CLO from cardia IM. These include squamous islands within glandular mucosa, (especially when they are juxtaposed to oesophageal gland ducts), squamous epithelium overlying intestinalised crypts and hybrid glands [21,62,63]. The last are glands with a bimodal composition of intestinalised epithelium in the superficial aspect and cardiac-type epithelium below [62] (Figure 5.5). It has been proposed that these hybrid glands are pathognomonic for CLO [62] and this author has sympathy with this view. Another characteristic feature of Barrett's mucosa is duplication of the muscularis mucosae [64,65]: this causes particular difficulties for pathologists attempting to stage early carcinoma in Barrett's mucosa, especially in endoscopic mucosal resection (EMR) speci-

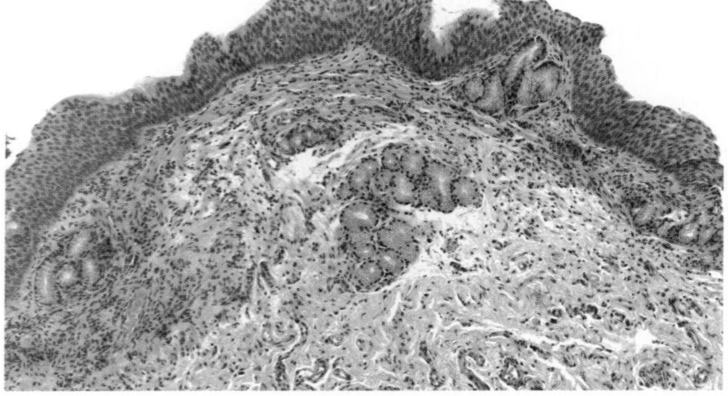

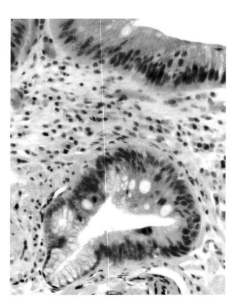

Figure 5.4 Extensive surface multilayered epithelium (ME) overlies cardiac-type mucosa in this columnar-lined oesophagus biopsy.

Figure 5.5 A hybrid gland beneath intestinalised surface mucosa. The gland shows a bimodal composition of intestinalised epithelium superficially and cardiac-type epithelium below.

mens [65]. Many of the aforementioned features do add to the pathologist's armoury in the diagnosis of CLO but it is again stressed that, too often, the pathological features seen on biopsy are not specific and require close correlation with endoscopic features [24,31].

A feature commonly seen in intestinalised CLO mucosa, alongside goblet cells, is the presence of non-goblet columnar cells that also stain positively with Alcian blue. There is evidence to suggest that these 'blue cells' may be more prevalent than goblet cells and may be markers of IM [66]. There is also an apparent association with ME, suggesting that they may represent 'early' goblet cells [67]. Whether such an intermediate phase of IM exists is debatable but it is likely that there are links with the non-goblet cell intestinal differentiation described which has caused us to strongly question the reliance of the demonstration of intestinalisation/goblet cells for the definition and diagnosis of CLO [24,31,41].

The association of hiatus hernia with CLO presents a potential minefield for both pathologists and endoscopists. The two conditions often coexist [68] and distinguishing between the two at endoscopy is frequently difficult. Pathologists, however, know little about the mucosal histological appearances of hiatus hernia, in particular the prevalence of IM, there having been no large-scale standardised studies of the mucosal pathology of the hiatus hernia, an extraordinary state of affairs at the current time. Accurate endoscopico-pathological correlation is therefore essential in these cases [20, 24].

The pathological assessment of CLO depends critically on the endoscopic information provided, especially the site of biopsies and the presence or absence of a hiatus hernia. Adequacy of the size and number of biopsies is also important. To aid the pathologist in the reporting of CLO, the BSG guidelines' four reporting categories are commended and should prevent unhelpful or misleading pathological reports (see Table 5.1) [24]. There also needs to be a major educational exercise of gastroenterologists and other endoscopists to ensure that they understand the role of pathology in the diagnosis of CLO.

SSCLO

This term is used to describe glandular metaplasia in the lower oesophagus measuring less than 30 mm in length, including non-circumferential metaplasia and tongues of columnar epithelium extending from the squamo-columnar junction. SSCLO is much more common, affecting 8–17% of the endoscopic population, compared with 1–2% for classical CLO [5,25,46,69–71]. The disease may be more difficult to diagnose endoscopically, due to its smaller size, particularly when there is associated stricturing, ulceration or a hiatus hernia. Hence corroboration by histology is of more importance than with classical CLO [24]. SSCLO is thought to have significant neoplastic potential but there

is evidence that the length of the segment is directly proportional to the neoplastic risk. There is also evidence to suggest that SSCLO is more likely to regress than classic disease [72]. For these reasons there remains much uncertainty about surveillance strategies for SSCLO [39,70].

USSCLO

This term is one fraught with controversy. Some use this term to imply true glandular metaplasia in the oesophagus that is scarcely or not visible at endoscopy. Most believe that this term refers to IM in the gastric cardia [73,74]. It is now believed that such cardia IM is a gastric disease and is better served by the term 'cardia intestinal metaplasia' (CIM) [30,74]. There is considerable evidence that gastric *H. pylori* infection has a role in its development but reflux disease may also possibly play a part [30]. CIM is a common finding in biopsies from the normal GOJ, being present in 16–35% of an endoscopic population [24,75]. As little is known about its significance or neoplastic potential, current guidelines, including those of the BSG, recommend that the normal GOJ should not be biopsied, and CIM not be diagnosed, in routine practice, mainly because we have no idea how to manage the disease once it has been demonstrated [24,40]. This is not to deny the importance of research into a condition likely to have a considerable bearing on the incidence of junctional adenocarcinoma.

Effects of treatment

Characteristic pathological changes occur as a consequence of the treatment of CLO and these may cause pathological consternation. Acid-suppressive therapy is the mainstay of treatment of reflux disease and many CLO patients are on these drugs [76]. Proton pump inhibitors (PPIs) are widely acclaimed as the agents of choice. They are effective in both providing symptomatic relief and healing erosive GORD. Consequently, there has been much interest in their potential role in inducing regression of CLO. The evidence so far is conflicting. Partial regression can certainly occur [77,78] and one double-blind controlled trial convincingly demonstrated a decrease in both the length and the area of Barrett's segment [79]. Several other studies, however, have shown no regression [76]. Surgical correction of reflux, typically performed laparoscopically and usually using Nissen fundoplication, is aimed at improving the competency of the GOJ through plication of the gastric fundus. The success of acid-suppressive therapy in the management of GORD has lessened the need for surgical intervention [80]. However, studies have indicated that anti-reflux surgery is an effective approach, with overall outcomes equal to and possibly superior to those achieved with medication [81,82].

There is increasing interest in various methods of ablation of CLO, being especially suitable for patients unfit

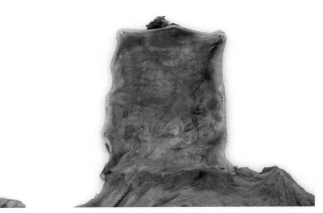

Figure 5.6 A resection specimen of columnar-lined oesophagus (CLO) extensively treated by ablation therapy. There is widespread squamous re-epithelialisation although occasional patches of CLO remain. There was an early cancer in the irregular area, centrally in the oesophageal segment, to the right.

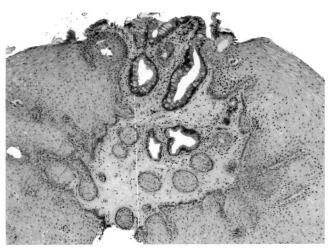

Figure 5.7 Extensive squamous re-epithelialisation as a result of ablation therapy. Not only is there surface squamous re-epithelialisation, but there is also 'metaplasia' of the columnar-lined oesophagus glands themselves to squamous epithelium.

for major surgery. Techniques include laser, photodynamic therapy (PDT), argon beam plasma coagulation (ABC) and radiofrequency ablation (RFA) [83–86]. The pathological response to ablation therapy can be dramatic, with extensive necrosis and florid reactive changes that may be difficult to distinguish from residual dysplasia [87]. The characteristic, and most important, response to treatment is squamous re-epithelialisation of the Barrett's segment (Figures 5.6 and 5.7) [87,88]. This can occur as both endoscopically visible squamous islands and microscopic foci [76,87,88]. Such squamous re-epithelialisation can occur after treatment with PPIs alone or in combination with anti-reflux surgery, laser ablation and PDT [88]. It seems, therefore, that acid-suppressing therapy is necessary for squamous re-epithelialisation to occur. The squamous regeneration occurs in three different ways: the first is encroachment of adjacent squamous epithelium at the squamo-columnar junction; the second, seen particularly after long-term PPI treatment, is extension of squamous epithelium from the superficial portion of the submucosal gland duct, leading to defined squamous islands [88]; and third, squamous metaplasia of Barrett's columnar mucosa itself has been recognised, after laser therapy and PDT, and suggests the existence of multipotential stem cells within Barrett's mucosa [88] (Figure 5.7).

A characteristic feature of ablation therapy is the demonstration of residual CLO glands lying 'hidden' beneath the surface squamous epithelium [88,89]. This causes concerns for the development of concealed neoplasia beneath the squamous mucosa, undetected by routine endoscopic methods [89], although there is some evidence that the buried glandular mucosa may have less neoplastic poten-

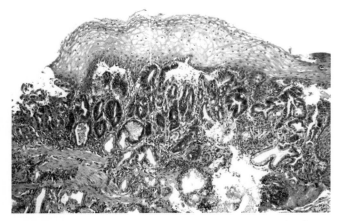

Figure 5.8 Squamous re-epithelialisation in high grade dysplastic columnar-lined oesophagus. The latter diagnosis is clear for the epithelium at the extreme left but the unwary pathologist might regard the isolated glands underneath the surface squamous epithelium as representing invasive adenocarcinoma beneath native oesophageal squamous mucosa.

tial [90,91]. Such glandular epithelium beneath surface squamous re-epithelialisation may also tempt the pathologist into an erroneous diagnosis of dysplasia because the cells of the crypts of intestinalised epithelium appear hyperchromatic and maturation to the surface cannot be seen as a result of the overlying squamous mucosa. When such glands are truly dysplastic, the unwary pathologist may be tempted to interpret this as adenocarcinoma infiltrating beneath native squamous epithelium (Figure 5.8). A feature seen after ablative therapy is that Barrett's glands themselves can undergo squamous re-epithelialisation (see Figure 5.7), suggesting that there is potential for complete squamous re-epithelialisation of Barrett's segment and a plausible reduction in neoplastic potential after ablation therapy [88].

Dysplasia in Barrett's oesophagus

There is consensus that dysplasia in CLO should be categorised according to the Riddell-type classification, originally introduced for dysplasia in ulcerative colitis [40,92–95]. Such a classification has been recommended for use in CLO for 20 years and more [93]. Even so, this author still observes pathologists using the mild, moderate and severe dysplasia classification. As there are well-established guidelines for the management of indefinite for dysplasia, low grade dysplasia and high grade dysplasia [40,95], there can be no excuse for using older and outmoded classifications.

A major problem for pathologists is the lack of definitive criteria for the diagnosis of dysplasia and even more so for the separation of the various categories [93,96,97]. The cytological features of dysplasia have been well described: nuclear enlargement, nuclear pleomorphism, nuclear hyperchromasia, nucleoli, nuclear stratification, increased mitotic activity and atypical mitotic figures are all commonly cited. Although these changes are important, architectural changes are more useful. We believe that a lack of maturation toward the surface is the single most useful criterion for the diagnosis of dysplasia. Villous configuration is also frequently associated with dysplasia, although it is not specific.

It is not possible to define strict criteria for the distinction of low grade dysplasia (Figure 5.9) from high grade dysplasia (Figure 5.10). Tables 5.2 and 5.3 give some guides to help in the differentiation [98,99]. However, there is variation even among experts, and low grade dysplasia and the indefinite category are associated with poorer levels of inter-observer agreement [93,100]. The distinction between dysplasia and carcinoma is also not clear cut, and there are differences in opinion between eastern and western pathologists. In Japan, in particular, emphasis is placed on cytological changes rather than the architecture, and definitive invasion through the basement membrane is not a requirement to diagnose carcinoma. It is mainly these differences that have prompted the introduction of the Vienna system of classification of gastro-intestinal dysplasia, including that in CLO [101,102]. In the system, the term 'non-invasive neoplasia' is used in place of 'low grade' or 'high grade' dysplasia, and an additional subcategory of 'suspicious for invasive carcinoma' is included [101,102]. It has been shown that those cases of high grade dysplasia associated with the 'suspicious' category are much more likely to be associated with coexistent adenocarcinoma, adding credence to the utility of such classification systems [103].

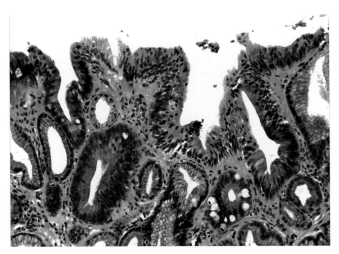

Figure 5.9 Low grade dysplasia in columnar-lined oesophagus. The sharp cut-offs between non-neoplastic foveolar-type epithelium and truly dysplastic epithelium, especially at the surface, are a helpful feature for the diagnosis of true low grade dysplasia.

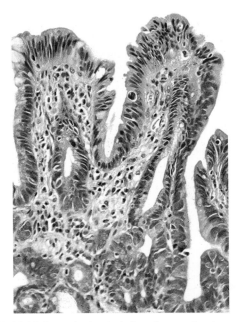

Figure 5.10 High grade dysplasia in columnar-lined oesophagus. There are notable cytological abnormalities with a villiform architecture.

Pathologists are encouraged to use the 'indefinite for dysplasia' category when it is not possible to confidently exclude dysplasia [95,104]. There are many situations, especially those highlighted in Table 5.4, in which a definitive diagnosis of dysplasia cannot and should not be made, and yet it is important to identify the concern for dysplasia

Table 5.2 Useful pathological features for the diagnosis of low and high grade dysplasia in Barrett's oesophagus

Low grade
Cytology approximates to that of mild and moderate adenomatous dysplasia
Nuclei are enlarged, crowded, hyperchromatic and ovoid
Mitotic activity may be substantial and atypical mitoses may be present
Stratification is often present
Architectural change, including villosity, may be present but in the appropriate cytological setting there is loss of the basal–luminal maturation/differentiation axis

High grade
Cytology approximates to that of severe adenomatous dysplasia
Nuclei are enlarged, usually spheroidal and have an open chromatin pattern with nucleoli
Mitotic activity may be substantial and atypical mitoses are usually present
Stratification may be present but there is usually pronounced cellular disorganisation
Architectural change, including villosity, glandular budding and complex glandular structures, is often present
There is loss of the basal–luminal maturation/differentiation axis

(Reproduced from Flejou JF, Svrcek M. Barrett's oesophagus – a pathologist's view. Histopathology, 2007; 50: 3–14).

Table 5.3 Cytological and architectural features of low and high grade dysplasia in columnar-lined oesophagus (CLO)

Feature	Low grade	High grade
Cytology		
Increased N/C ratio	+	++
Loss of cell polarity	–	+
Mitosis	+	++
Atypical mitosis	±	+
Full-thickness nuclear stratification	–	+
Decreased goblet cells (±dystrophic)	+	++
Hyperchromasia	+	++
Multiple nucleoli	±	±
Large irregular (prominent) nucleoli	–	±
Irregular nuclear contour	+	++
Nuclear pleomorphism	–	+
Architecture		
Villiform change	–	±
Crypt budding/branching	±	++
Crowded (back-to-back) crypts	±	++
Irregular crypt shapes	±	+
Intraluminal papilla / ridges	–	±
Lamina propria between glands	+	±

N/C, nuclear/cytoplasmic ratio; –, absent; ±, may be present; +, usually present.
(Reproduced from Diagnosis and grading of dysplasia in Barrett's oesophagus, Odze RD, 59, 1029–1038, 2006 with permission from BMJ Publishing Group Ltd).

Table 5.4 Common causes for error in the pathological diagnosis of dysplasia in columnar-lined oesophagus (CLO)

1. Inflammation and regenerative change
Expansion of proliferative compartment
Hyperproliferation
Nuclear activity
Villous/papillary architecture

2. Polymorphism of cell types
Differences in position of proliferative compartments in different CLO epithelial types
Morphological changes in mucin
Juxtaposition of intestinal mucosa to other blander-appearing cell types

3. Artefact
Biopsy technique, especially crush artefact
Tangential sectioning
Staining variation

4. Squamous re-epithelialisation
Overlying squamous mucosa obscures evidence of maturation
Only prominent intestinal crypt bases seen

to the clinician. Failure to recognise the pathologist's limitations in many of these situations can lead to the dangerous over-calling of dysplasia. One of the most common of these occurs because of the 'patchwork' of the different CLO phenotypes. The intestinal mucosa in CLO has a prominent proliferative zone showing nuclear enlargement and mitotic activity. This can give worrying appearances when seen juxtaposed to relatively bland-appearing cardia-type mucosa. Tangential sectioning can make this assessment even more difficult [95,104].

What are the features that can help one distinguish between true dysplasia and reactive changes? Epithelial changes due to inflammation are usually most prominent in the inflamed foci and there is a gradual reduction in the degree of cytological change towards the non-inflamed areas. In contrast, abrupt transition between normal and abnormal epithelium favours true dysplasia (see Figure 5.9). We believe that the most useful feature, and one that argues against dysplasia, is the presence of surface maturation. However, 'basal crypt dysplasia-like atypia' (BCDA), with surface maturation in a group of patients with long-standing CLO, has been proposed as representing a rare subtype of true dysplasia [105]. We require more evidence before regarding 'basal crypt dysplasia-like atypia' as a form of definite dysplasia, and currently our recommendation is that such cases are categorised as 'indefinite for dysplasia' because this will ensure the correct management for such patients. The assessment of surface maturation can also not be applied to post-treatment specimens where there is squamous re-epithelialisation of the surface: once again categorisation as 'indefinite for dysplasia' is appropriate.

The poorer inter-observer reproducibility of indefinite for dysplasia and low grade dysplasia is well documented [93,100,102,106]. The inter-observer agreement for high grade dysplasia is better [93,100] and this is important because many of these cases will have co-existent adenocarcinoma, especially if ulceration is present [107]. Pathologists should be aware of the implications of the various diagnostic categories for management. Indefinite for dysplasia is managed by early repeat endoscopy and multiple biopsies, often after treatment of inflammation with a course of PPI therapy [40,95]. The management of low grade dysplasia is similar, with close (6-monthly) endoscopic surveillance as long as the disease remains stable [40,95].

In European and North American guidelines that are still current, high grade dysplasia is an indication for oesophagectomy, an operation that carries very significant morbidity and mortality risks, because of the perceived strong association between biopsy-diagnosed high grade dysplasia and (presumed contemporaneous) adenocarcinoma [40,95,103]. However, the treatment of high grade dysplasia and early adenocarcinoma is undergoing major changes at the current time because of the advent of expert endoscopy, especially chromo-endoscopy, narrow band imaging and autofluorescence endoscopy, all of which can accurately identify foci of dysplasia for directed biopsy confirmation [108,109], and the development and wide usage of EMR [110–112]. The last can accurately identify and stage neoplasia complicating CLO (Figures 5.11 and 5.12) [65]. If the neoplasia remains intramucosal, then there is now evidence that the mortality of surgery outweighs the risk of lymph node metastatic disease and thus surgical conservatism, allied to ablative therapy for any remaining neoplastic disease, is an appropriate management strategy

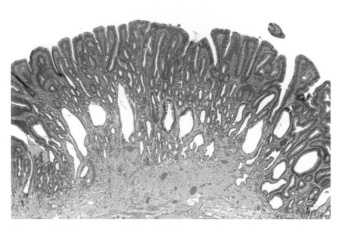

Figure 5.11 Low grade dysplasia in an endoscopic mucosal resection (EMR) specimen. Such specimens generally allow a much fuller assessment, usually with good preservation of architectural and cytological detail, than small biopsies.

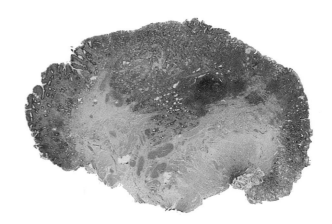

Figure 5.12 A 'whole-mount' slide of an endoscopic mucosal resection undertaken for neoplasia complicating columnar-lined oesophagus. Glandular mucosa is present peripherally with an invasive adenocarcinoma, clear of peripheral and deep margins, present centrally. Duplication of the muscularis mucosae is very evident and, in this section at least, despite the deep invasion, the tumour is not invading the submucosa.

[111,112]. Nevertheless the pathological diagnosis of high grade dysplasia remains one of very considerable import and management guidelines recommend that such a diagnosis be confirmed by a second, preferably expert and specialist, gastrointestinal pathologist [113].

Formerly comprehensive biopsy sampling of Barrett's segment was of paramount importance for the detection of dysplasia. The Seattle biopsy protocol employs quadrantic and segmental (every 20mm) biopsies of the Barrett's segment, preferably using jumbo-type biopsy forceps, in addition to sampling of any visible lesion [39,95,114]. This was developed because endoscopic appearances do not correlate well with the histological diagnosis of dysplasia. High grade dysplasia, and even adenocarcinoma, have been detected in biopsies from macroscopically unremarkable, or minimally abnormal, CLO and dysplasia can also be multifocal and extensive [115]. However, expert endoscopic methods are changing this and it is now generally accepted that most, if not all, significant dysplasia can be detected by these endoscopic methods, allowing directed biopsies rather than the extraordinarily laborious endoscopic and histopathological methodology associated with the Seattle protocol [108,109,114].

It is not surprising, in view of the difficulties encountered in the management of neoplasia complicating CLO, that the search for molecular markers or 'biomarkers' to aid in the diagnosis and grading of dysplasia has been on-going [116–120]. Immunohistochemical detection of p53 protein over-expression and of proliferation markers such as Ki-67 have been extensively assessed [116,121,122]. Although there is no doubt that expression of these markers correlates with increasing grade of dysplasia, it is uncertain whether they add much diagnostic value in practice. We occasionally find p53 immunohistochemistry helpful in confirming recurrent dysplasia, especially when dysplasia has been previously strongly positive, there has been ablative therapy and squamous re-epithelialisation has made the assessment more difficult. Others have found the antibody to α-methylacyl coenzyme A racemase of some use, especially for predicting those cases of 'mucosa indefinite for dysplasia' that may go on to develop high grade dysplasia [123,124]. It is this author's view that most 'biomarkers' should still be regarded as experimental [125] and that their routine use, outside the research setting, cannot be recommended at the current time.

References

1. Prach AT, MacDonald TA, Hopwood DA, Johnston DA. Increasing incidence of Barrett's oesophagus: education, enthusiasm, or epidemiology? *Lancet* 1997;**350**:933.
2. Wild CP, Hardie LJ. Reflux, Barrett's oesophagus and adenocarcinoma: burning questions. *Nat Rev Cancer* 2003;**3**:676.
3. van Soest EM, Dieleman JP, Siersma PD, Sturkenboom MC, Kuipers EJ. Increasing incidence of Barrett's oesophagus in the general population. *Gut* 2005;**54**:1062.
4. Shaheen NJ. Advances in Barrett's esophagus and esophageal adenocarcinoma. *Gastroenterology* 2005;**128**:1554.
5. Watson A. Barrett's oesophagus – 50 years on. *Br J Surg* 2000; **87**:529.
6. Cancer Research UK. *Oesophageal cancer – UK incidence statistics.* Available at: http://info.cancerresearchuk.org/cancerstats/types/oesophagus/incidence/index.htm (accessed 2 February 2010).
7. Lagergren J, Bergstrom R, Lindgren A, Nyren O. Symptomatic gastroesophageal reflux as a risk factor for esophageal adenocarcinoma. *N Engl J Med* 1999;**340**:825.
8. Vaezi MF, Richter JE. Bile reflux in columnar-lined esophagus. *Gastroenterol Clin North Am* 1997;**26**:565.
9. Dixon MF, Neville PM, Mapstone NP, Moayyedi P, Axon AT. Bile reflux gastritis and Barrett's oesophagus: further evidence of a role for duodenogastro-oesophageal reflux? *Gut* 2001;**49**: 359.
10. Owen WJ, Warren BF. Pathogenesis and pathophysiology of columnar-lined oesophagus. In: Watson A, Heading RC, Shepherd NA (eds), *Guidelines for the Diagnosis and Management of Barrett's Columnar-lined Oesophagus.* London: British Society of Gastroenterology, 2005.
11. Blaser MJ. *Helicobacter pylori* and gastric diseases. *BMJ* 1998; **316**:1507.
12. Blaser MJ. Disappearing microbiota: *Helicobacter pylori* protection against esophageal adenocarcinoma. *Cancer Prev Res* 2008; **1**:308.
13. Flejou JF, Svrcek M. Barrett's oesophagus – a pathologist's view. *Histopathology* 2007;**50**:3.
14. Barrett NR. Chronic peptic ulcer of the oesophagus and 'oesophagitis'. *Br J Surg* 1950;**38**:175.
15. Barrett NR. The esophagus lined with gastric mucous membrane. *Surgery* 1957;**41**:881.
16. Allison PR, Johnstone AS. The oesophagus lined with gastric mucous membrane. *Thorax* 1953;**8**:87.
17. Cohen BR, Wolf BS, Som M, Janowitz HD. Correlation of manometric, oesophagoscopic, and radiological findings in the columnar-lined gullet (Barrett syndrome). *Gut* 1963;**4**:406.
18. Goldman MC, Beckman RC. Barrett syndrome. Case report with discussion about concepts of pathogenesis. *Gastroenterology* 1960;**39**:104.
19. Gillen P, Keeling P, Byrne PJ, West AB, Hennessy TPJ. Experimental columnar metaplasia in the canine oesophagus. *Br J Surg* 1988;**75**:113.
20. Coad RA, Shepherd NA. Barrett's oesophagus: definition, diagnosis and pathogenesis. *Curr Diagn Pathol* 2003;**9**:218.
21. Coad RA, Woodman AC, Warner PJ, Barr H, Wright NA, Shepherd NA. On the histogenesis of Barrett's oesophagus and its associated squamous islands: a three-dimensional study of their morphological relationship with native oesophageal gland ducts. *J Pathol* 2005;**206**:388.
22. DeMeester SR, DeMeester TR. Columnar mucosa and intestinal metaplasia of the esophagus: fifty years of controversy. *Ann Surg* 2000;**231**:303.
23. Bani-Hani KE, Bani-Hani BK. Columnar-lined esophagus: time to drop the eponym of 'Barrett': Historical review. *J Gastroenterol Hepatol* 2008;**23**:707.
24. Hellier MD, Shepherd NA. Diagnosis of columnar-lined oesophagus. In: Watson A, Heading RC, Shepherd NA (eds), *Guidelines for the Diagnosis and Management of Barrett's Columnar-lined Oesophagus.* London: British Society of Gastroenterology, 2005.
25. Clark GW, Ireland AP, Peters JH, Chandrasoma P, DeMeester TR, Bremner CG. Short-segment Barrett's esophagus: A prevalent complication of gastroesophageal reflux disease with malignant potential. *J Gastrointest Surg* 1997;**1**:113.
26. Spechler SJ. Barrett's esophagus. *Semin Gastrointest Dis* 1996; **7**:51.
27. Attwood SE, Morris CD. Who defines Barrett's oesophagus: endoscopist or pathologist? *Eur J Gastroenterol Hepatol* 2001; **13**:97.
28. Sharma P, Dent J, Armstrong D, et al. The development and validation of an endoscopic grading system for Barrett's esophagus: the Prague C & M criteria. *Gastroenterology* 2006;**131**:1392.
29. Sampliner RE, Sharma P. Short-segment Barrett's esophagus. *J Clin Gastroenterol* 1998;**26**:357.

30. Goldblum JR. The significance and etiology of intestinal meta-plasia of the esophagogastric junction. *Ann Diagn Pathol* 2002; **6**:67.

31. Riddell RH, Odze RD. Definition of Barrett's esophagus: time for a rethink – is intestinal metaplasia dead? *Am J Gastroenterol* 2009;**104**:2588.

32. Takubo K, Nixon JM, Jass JR. Ducts of esophageal glands proper and Paneth cells in Barrett's esophagus: frequency in biopsy specimens. *Pathology* 1995;**27**:315.

33. Flejou JF. Histological assessment of oesophageal columnar mucosa. *Best Pract Res Clin Gastroenterol* 2008;**22**:671.

34. Gatenby PA, Ramus JR, Caygill CP, Shepherd NA, Watson A. Relevance of the detection of intestinal metaplasia in non-dysplastic columnar-lined oesophagus. *Scand J Gastroenterol* 2008;**43**:524.

35. Takubo K, Vieth M, Aida J, et al. Differences in the definitions used for esophageal and gastric diseases in different countries. Endoscopic definition of the esophagogastric junction, the precursor of Barrett's adenocarcinoma, the definition of Barrett's esophagus, and histologic criteria for mucosal adenocarcinoma or high-grade dysplasia. *Digestion* 2009;**80**:248.

36. Aguirre TV, Sampliner RE. Endoscopic surveillance of columnar-lined esophagus: frequency of intestinal metaplasia detection and impact of antireflux surgery. *Am J Gastroenterol* 2003;**98**:931.

37. Harrison R, Perry I, Haddadin W, et al. Detection of intestinal metaplasia in Barrett's esophagus: an observational comparator study suggests the need for a minimum of eight biopsies. *Am J Gastroenterol* 2007;**102**:1154.

38. Spechler SJ, Goyal RK. The columnar-lined esophagus, intestinal metaplasia, and Norman Barrett. *Gastroenterology* 1996;**110**:614.

39. Sampliner RE. Updated guidelines for the diagnosis, surveillance, and therapy of Barrett's esophagus. *Am J Gastroenterol* 2002;**97**:1888.

40. Wang KK, Sampliner RE. Updated guidelines 2008 for the diagnosis, surveillance and therapy of Barrett's esophagus. *Am J Gastroenterol* 2008;**103**:788.

41. Chaves P, Cardoso P, de Almeida JC, Pereira AD, Leitoa CN, Soares J. Non-goblet cell population of Barrett's esophagus: an immunohistochemical demonstration of intestinal differentiation. *Hum Pathol* 1999;**30**:1291.

42. Paull A, Trier JS, Dalton MD, Camp RC, Loeb P, Goyal RK. The histologic spectrum of Barrett's esophagus. *N Engl J Med* 1976;**295**:476.

43. Chandrasoma PT, Der R, Dalton P, et al. Distribution and significance of epithelial types in columnar-lined esophagus. *Am J Surg Pathol* 2001;**25**:1188.

44. Jass JR. Histopathology of early neoplasia in Barrett's esophagus. In: Imamura M (ed.), *Superficial Esophageal Neoplasm: Pathology, diagnosis and therapy*. Tokyo: Springer-Verlag, 2002: 13.

45. Schreiber DS, Apstein M, Hermos JA. Paneth cells in Barrett's esophagus. *Gastroenterology* 1978;**74**:1302.

46. Spechler SJ. The columnar lined oesophagus: a riddle wrapped in a mystery inside an enigma. *Gut* 1997;**41**:710.

47. Phillips RW, Frierson HF Jr, Moskaluk CA. Cdx2 as a marker of epithelial intestinal differentiation in the esophagus. *Am J Surg Pathol* 2003;**27**:1442.

48. Glickman JN, Shahsafaei A, Odze RD. Mucin core peptide expression can help differentiate Barrett's esophagus from intestinal metaplasia of the stomach. *Am J Surg Pathol* 2003;**27**:1357.

49. Ormsby AH, Goldblum JR, Rice TW et al. Cytokeratin subsets can reliably distinguish Barrett's esophagus from intestinal metaplasia of the stomach. *Hum Pathol* 1999;**30**:288.

50. Ormsby AH, Vaezi MF, Richter JE et al. Cytokeratin immuno-reactivity patterns in the diagnosis of short-segment Barrett's esophagus. *Gastroenterology* 2000;**119**:683.

51. Couvelard A, Cauvin JM, Goldfain D, et al. Cytokeratin immunoreactivity of intestinal metaplasia at normal oesophagogastric junction indicates its aetiology. *Gut* 2001;**49**:761.

52. El-Zimaity HM, Graham DY. Cytokeratin subsets for distinguishing Barrett's esophagus from intestinal metaplasia in the cardia using endoscopic biopsy specimens. *Am J Gastroenterol* 2001;**96**:1378.

53. Glickman JN, Wang H, Das KM, et al. Phenotype of Barrett's esophagus and intestinal metaplasia of the distal esophagus and gastroesophageal junction: an immunohistochemical study of cytokeratins 7 and 20, Das-1 and 45 MI. *Am J Surg Pathol* 2001;**25**:87.

54. DeMeester SR, Wickramasinghe KS, Lord RV, et al. Cytokeratin and DAS-1 immunostaining reveal similarities among cardiac mucosa, CIM, and Barrett's esophagus. *Am J Gastroenterol* 2002; **97**:2514.

55. Mohammed IA, Streutker CJ, Riddell RH. Utilization of cytokeratins 7 and 20 does not differentiate between Barrett's esophagus and gastric cardiac intestinal metaplasia. *Mod Pathol* 2002;**15**:611.

56. Odze R. Cytokeratin 7/20 immunostaining: Barrett's oesophagus or gastric intestinal metaplasia? *Lancet* 2002;**359**:1711.

57. Glickman JN, Ormsby AH, Gramlich TL, Goldblum JR, Odze RD. Interinstitutional variability and effect of tissue fixative on the interpretation of a Barrett cytokeratin 7/20 immunoreactivity pattern in Barrett esophagus. *Hum Pathol* 2005; **36**:58.

58. Glickman JN, Chen YY, Wang HH, Antonioli DA, Odze RD. Phenotypic characteristics of a distinctive multilayered epithelium suggests that it is a precursor in the development of Barrett's esophagus. *Am J Surg Pathol* 2001;**25**:569.

59. Glickman JN, Spechler SJ, Souza RF, Lunsford T, Lee E, Odze RD. Multilayered epithelium in mucosal biopsy specimens from the gastroesophageal junction region is a histologic marker of gastroesophageal reflux disease. *Am J Surg Pathol* 2009;**33**:818.

60. Wieczorek TJ, Wang HH, Antonioli DA, Glickman JN, Odze RD. Pathologic features of reflux and Helicobacter pylori-associated carditis: a comparative study. *Am J Surg Pathol* 2003; **27**:960.

61. Takubo K, Honma N, Arai T. Multilayered epithelium in Barrett's esophagus. *Am J Surg Pathol* 2001;**25**:1460.

62. Srivastava A, Odze RD, Lauwers GY, Redston M, Antonioli DA, Glickman JN. Morphologic features are useful in distinguishing Barrett esophagus from carditis with intestinal metaplasia. *Am J Surg Path* 2007;**31**:1733.

63. Takubo K, Vieth M, Aryal G, et al. Islands of squamous epithelium and their surrounding mucosa in columnar-lined esophagus: A pathognomonic feature of Barrett's esophagus? *Hum Pathol* 2005;**36**:269.

64. Takubo K, Sasajima K, Yamashita K, Tanaka Y, Fujita K. Double muscularis mucosae in Barrett's esophagus. *Hum Pathol* 1991; **22**:1158.

65. Abraham SC, Krasinskas AM, Correa AM, et al. Duplication of the muscularis mucosae in Barrett esophagus: An underrecognized feature and its implication for staging of adenocarcinoma. *Am J Surg Pathol* 2007;**31**:1719.

66. Offner FA, Lewin KJ, Weinstein WM. Metaplastic columnar cells in Barrett's esophagus: a common and neglected cell type. *Hum Pathol* 1996;**27**:885.

67. Chen YY, Wang HH, Antonioli DA, et al. Significance of acid-mucin-positive non-goblet columnar cells in the distal

esophagus and gastroesophageal junction. *Hum Pathol* 1999;**30**: 1488.

68. Cameron AJ. Barrett's esophagus: prevalence and size of hiatus hernia. *Am J Gastroenterol* 1999;**94**:2054.

69. Nandurkar S, Talley NJ, Martin CJ, Ng TH, Adams S. Short segment Barrett's oesophagus: prevalence, diagnosis and associations. *Gut* 1997;**40**:710.

70. Richter JE. Short segment Barrett's esophagus: ignorance may be bliss. *Am J Gastroenterol* 2006;**101**:1183.

71. Gatenby PA, Caygill CP, Ramus JR, Charlett A, Fitzgerald RC, Watson A. Short segment columnar-lined oesophagus: an underestimated cancer risk? A large cohort study of the relationship between Barrett's columnar-lined oesophagus segment length and adenocarcinoma risk. *Eur J Gastroenterol Hepatol* 2007;**19**:969.

72. Weston AP, Badr AS, Hassanein RS. Prospective multivariate analysis of factors predictive of complete regression of Barrett's esophagus. *Am J Gastroenterol* 1999;**94**:3420.

73. Spechler SJ. The role of gastric carditis in metaplasia and neoplasia at the gastroesophageal junction. *Gastroenterology* 1999;**117**:218.

74. Goldblum JR. Ultrashort-segment Barrett's oesophagus, carditis and intestinal metaplasia at the oesophagogastric junction: Pathology, causation and implications. *Curr Diagn Pathol* 2003;**9**:228.

75. Trudgill NJ, Suvarna SK, Kapur KC, Riley SA. Intestinal metaplasia at the squamocolumnar junction in patients attending for diagnostic gastroscopy. *Gut* 1997;**41**:585.

76. Shepherd NA. Barrett's oesophagus and proton pump inhibitors: a pathological perspective. *Gut* 2000;**46**:147.

77. Gore S, Healey CJ, Sutton R, et al. Regression of columnar lined (Barrett's) oesophagus with continuous omeprazole therapy. *Aliment Pharmacol Therap* 1993;**7**:623.

78. Wilkinson SP, Biddlestone L, Gore S, Shepherd NA. Regression of columnar-lined (Barrett's) oesophagus with omeprazole 40 mg daily: results of 5 years of continuous therapy. *Aliment Pharmacol Therap* 1999;**13**:1205.

79. Peters FT, Ganesh S, Kuipers EJ et al. Endoscopic regression of Barrett's oesophagus during omeprazole treatment: a randomised double blind study. *Gut* 1999;**45**:489.

80. Scarpignato C, Pelosini I, Di Mario F. Acid suppression therapy: where do we go from here? *Dig Dis* 2006;**24**:11.

81. O'Riordan JM, Byrne PJ, Ravi N, Keeling PW, Reynolds JV. Long-term clinical and pathologic response of Barrett's esophagus after antireflux surgery. *Am J Surg* 2004;**188**:27.

82. Moayyedi P, Talley NJ. Gastro-oesophageal reflux disease. *Lancet* 2006;**367**:2086.

83. Lovat LB, Jamieson NF, Novelli MR, et al. Photodynamic therapy with *m*-tetrahydroxyphenyl chlorin for high-grade dysplasia and early cancer in Barrett's columnar lined esophagus. *Gastrointestinal Endoscopy* 2005;**62**:617.

84. Ragunath K, Krasner N, Raman VS, et al. Endoscopic ablation of dysplastic Barrett's oesophagus comparing argon plasma coagulation and photodynamic therapy: a randomized prospective trial assessing efficacy and cost-effectiveness. *Scand J Gastroenterol* 2005;**40**:750.

85. Overholt BF, Wang KK, Burdick JS, et al. Five-year efficacy and safety of photodynamic therapy with Photofrin in Barrett's high-grade dysplasia. *Gastrointestinal Endoscopy* 2007;**66**:460.

86. van Visteren FG, Bergmann JJ. Endoscopic therapy using radiofrequency ablation for esophageal dysplasia and carcinoma in Barrett's esophagus. *Gastrointest Endosc Clin N Am* 2010;**20**:55.

87. Odze RD, Lauwers GY. Histopathology of Barrett's esophagus after ablation and endoscopic mucosal resection therapy. *Endoscopy* 2008;**40**:1008.

88. Biddlestone LR, Barham CP, Wilkinson SP, Barr H, Shepherd NA. The histopathology of treated Barrett's esophagus: squamous re-epithelialization after acid suppression and laser and photodynamic therapy. *Am J Surg Pathol* 1998;**22**:239.

89. Sharma P, Morales TG, Bhattacharyya A, Garewal HS, Sampliner RE. Squamous islands in Barrett's esophagus: what lies underneath? *Am J Gastroenterol* 1998;**93**:332.

90. Hornick JL, Mino-Kenudson M, Lauwers GY, Liu W, Goyal R, Odze RD. Buried Barrett's epithelium following photodynamic therapy shows reduced crypt proliferation and absence of DNA content abnormalities. *Am J Gastroenterol* 2007;**103**:38.

91. Bronner MP, Overholt BF, Taylor SL, et al. Squamous overgrowth is not a safety concern for photodynamic therapy for Barrett's esophagus with high-grade dysplasia. *Gastroenterology* 2009;**136**:56.

92. Riddell RH, Goldman H, Ransohoff DF, et al. Dysplasia in inflammatory bowel disease: standardized classification with provisional clinical applications. *Hum Pathol* 1983;**14**:931.

93. Reid BJ, Haggitt RC, Rubin CE, et al. Observer variation in the diagnosis of dysplasia in Barrett's esophagus. *Hum Pathol* 1988;**19**:166.

94. Geboes K, van Eyken P. The diagnosis of dysplasia and malignancy in Barrett's oesophagus. *Histopathology* 2000;**37**:99.

95. Barr H, Shepherd NA. The management of dysplasia. In: Watson A, Heading RC, Shepherd NA (eds), *Guidelines for the Diagnosis and Management of Barrett's Columnar-lined Oesophagus*. British Society of Gastroenterology, 2005.

96. McKenna BJ, Appelman HD. Dysplasia can be a pain in the gut. *Pathology* 2002;**34**:518.

97. Montgomery E. Refining diagnostic criteria for high-grade dysplasia in Barrett esophagus. *Am J Clin Pathol* 2009;**132**:7.

98. Shepherd NA. Dysplasia in Barrett's oesophagus. *Acta Endoscop* 2000;**30**:123.

99. Odze RD. Diagnosis and grading of dysplasia in Barrett's oesophagus. *J Clin Pathol* 2006;**59**:1029.

100. Montgomery E, Bronner MP, Goldblum JR, et al. Reproducibility of the diagnosis of dysplasia in Barrett esophagus: a reaffirmation. *Hum Pathol* 2001;**32**:368.

101. Schlemper RJ, Riddell RH, Kato Y, et al. The Vienna classification of gastrointestinal epithelial neoplasia. *Gut* 2000;**47**:251.

102. Kaye PV, Haider SA, Ilyas M, et al. Barrett's dysplasia and the Vienna classification: reproducibility, prediction of progression and impact of consensus reporting and p53 immunohistochemistry. *Histopathology* 2009;**54**:699.

103. Zhu W, Appelman HD, Greenson JK, et al. A histologically defined subset of high-grade dysplasia in Barrett mucosa is predictive of associated carcinoma. *Am J Clin Pathol* 2009;**132**:94.

104. Yantiss RK, Odze RD. Neoplastic precursor lesions of the upper gastrointestinal tract. *Diagnostic Histopathology* 2008;**14**:437.

105. Lomo LC, Blount PL, Sanchez CA, et al. Crypt dysplasia with surface maturation: a clinical, pathologic and molecular study of a Barrett's esophagus cohort. *Am J Surg Pathol* 2006;**30**:423.

106. Kerkhof M, van Dekken H, Steyerberg EW, et al. Grading of dysplasia in Barrett's oesophagus: substantial interobserver variation between general and gastrointestinal pathologists. *Histopathology* 2007;**50**:920.

107. Montgomery E, Bronner MP, Greenson JK, et al. Are ulcers a marker for invasive carcinoma in Barrett's esophagus? Data from a diagnostic variability study with clinical follow-up. *Am J Gastroenterol* 2002;**97**:27.

108. Curvers WL, Singh R, Song LM, et al. Endoscopic tri-modal imaging for detection of early neoplasia in Barrett's oesopha-

gus: a multi-centre feasibility study using high-resolution endoscopy, autofluorescence imaging and narrow band imaging incorporated in one endoscopy system. *Gut* 2008;**57**:167.

109. Herrero LA, Curvers WL, Bansal A, et al. Zooming in on Barrett oesophagus using narrow-band imaging: an international observer agreement study. *Eur J Gastroenterol Hepatol* 2009;**21**: 1068.

110. Maish MR, DeMeester SR. Endoscopic biomarker as a staging technique to determine the depth of invasion of esophageal adenocarcinoma. *Ann Thoracic Surg* 2004;**78**:1777.

111. Bergman JJGHM. Diagnosis and therapy of early neoplasia in Barrett's esophagus. *Curr Opin Gastroenterol* 2005;**21**:466.

112. Rouw RE, Bergmann JJ. Endoscopic resection of early oesophageal and gastric neoplasia. *Best Pract Res Clin Gastroenterol* 2008;**22**:929.

113. Loft DE, Alderson D, Heading RC. Screening and surveillance in columnar-lined oesophagus. In: Watson A, Heading RC, Shepherd NA (eds), *Guidelines for the Diagnosis and Management of Barrett's Columnar-lined Oesophagus*. British Society of Gastroenterology, 2005.

114. Levine DS, Haggitt RC, Blount PL et al. An endoscopic biopsy protocol can differentiate high-grade dysplasia from early adenocarcinoma in Barrett's esophagus. *Gastroenterology* 1993; **105**:40.

115. Levine DS. Management of dysplasia in the columnar-lined esophagus. *Gastroenterol Clin North Am* 1997;**26**:613.

116. Reid BJ, Blount PL, Rabinovitch PS. Biomarkers in Barrett's esophagus. *Gastrointest Endosc Clin N Am* 2003;**13**:369.

117. Preston SL, Jankowski JA. Drinking from the fountain of promise: biomarkers in the surveillance of Barrett's oesophagus–the glass is half full! *Gut* 2006;**55**:1377.

118. Spechler SJ, Souza RF. Biomarkers and photodynamic therapy for Barrett's esophagus: time to FISH or cut bait? *Gastroenterology* 2008;**135**:354.

119. di Pietro M, Fitzgerald RC. Barrett's oesophagus: an ideal model to study cancer genetics. *Human Genetics* 2009;**126**:233.

120. Jankowski JA, Odze RD. Biomarkers in gastroenterology: between hope and hype comes histopathology. *Am J Gastroenterol* 2009;**104**:1093.

121. Hong MK, Laskin WB, Herman BE, et al. Expansion of the Ki-67 proliferative compartment correlates with degree of dysplasia in Barrett's esophagus. *Cancer* 1995;**75**:423.

122. Whittles CE, Biddlestone LR, Burton A, et al. Apoptotic and proliferative activity in the neoplastic progression of Barrett's oesophagus: a comparative study. *J Pathol* 1999;**187**:535.

123. Dorer R, Odze RD. AMACR immunostaining is useful in detecting dysplastic epithelium in Barrett's esophagus, ulcerative colitis and Crohn's disease. *Am J Surg Pathol* 2006;**7**:871.

124. Sonwalkar S, Rotimi O, Scott N, et al. A study of indefinite for dysplasia in Barrett's oesophagus: reproducibility of diagnosis, clinical outcomes and predicting progression with AMACR (alpha-methylacyl-coA-racemase). *Histopathology* 2010; **66**:900.

125. Riddell RH. The biopsy diagnosis of gastroesophageal reflux disease, 'carditis,' and Barrett's esophagus, and sequelae of therapy. *Am J Surg Pathol* 1996;**20**(suppl 1):S31.

6

Polyps and tumour-like lesions of the oesophagus

Jeremy R. Parfitt and David K. Driman
Western University and London Health Sciences Centre, London, ON, Canada

A number of different types of oesophageal lesions may have a polypoid appearance. These include true neoplasms, both benign and malignant, as well as tumour-like lesions (Table 6.1). Many of the neoplastic lesions are covered in Chapter 7. Consideration is given here to inflammatory/hyperplastic polyps, giant fibrovascular polyps, glycogenic acanthosis and diffuse leiomyomatosis.

Inflammatory/hyperplastic polyp

Inflammatory/hyperplastic polyps are uncommon lesions characterised by hyperplastic epithelium, either gastric foveolar type, squamous, or both, with variable amounts of inflamed stroma [1]. These have a relatively smooth surface and show basal zone hyperplasia with variable erosion of the epithelium, and usually a marked acute inflammatory cell infiltrate of the lamina propria (Figure 6.1a). They are most common around the gastro-oesophageal junction and distal oesophagus and are associated with gastro-oesophageal reflux disease in most cases. They may also be seen with injury due to medication, infection, anastomotic or polypectomy sites, vomiting, photodynamic therapy and eosinophilic oesophagitis [1–4].

Importantly, these lesions can occasionally mimic malignancy when they harbour bizarre stromal cells within areas of granulation tissue or exhibit atypical regenerative hyperplasia of the epithelial component, either squamous or glandular, or both (Figure 6.1b) [5,6]. Stromal cells with marked nuclear enlargement and pleomorphism may mimic melanoma, carcinoma or sarcoma but are immunoreactive for vimentin and sometimes smooth muscle actin,

suggesting that they are of fibroblastic or myofibroblastic origin: these cells are negative for melanocytic, epithelial, histiocytic and endothelial immunohistochemical markers. Further, inflamed, immature-appearing squamous epithelium may show pseudo-epitheliomatous hyperplasia and regenerative cytological atypia, mimicking squamous cell carcinoma. They also have to be differentiated from squamous papillomas, which have an exophytic, papillomatous surface. Rarely atypical inflamed glandular mucosa entrapped within the abnormal stromal cells can also mimic adenocarcinoma.

Giant fibrovascular polyp

These rare and interesting lesions of unknown aetiology can reach an enormous size [7,8]. The majority are attached by a pedicle to the cricopharyngeal area of the upper oesophagus and cases are reported of regurgitation of these polypoid masses into the mouth. They are most frequently seen in middle-aged or elderly men who complain of dysphagia [9]. Although these are benign, they have rarely been reported to cause serious morbidity, including upper airway obstruction, asphyxiation and even death [9,10]. They consist of fibrous tissue, which may be myxomatous, in which there are thin-walled blood vessels. A varying amount of adipose tissue is present and this can be the predominant component. Inflammation is usually insignificant except where ulceration of the overlying epithelium has occurred. Very rarely, malignancy may arise within either the epithelial or stromal components, including squamous cell carcinoma and liposarcoma respectively

Morson and Dawson's Gastrointestinal Pathology, Fifth Edition. Edited by Neil A. Shepherd, Bryan F. Warren,
Geraint T. Williams, Joel K. Greenson, Gregory Y. Lauwers and Marco R. Novelli.
© 2013 Blackwell Publishing Ltd. Published 2013 by Blackwell Publishing Ltd.

[11,12]. Even when large, they may be missed on endoscopic examination because their surface is similar to normal oesophageal mucosa [13]. They should be differentiated from inflammatory fibroid polyps, which do rarely occur in the oesophagus and appear similar to their counterparts elsewhere in the gastrointestinal tract [14–16].

Table 6.1 Classification of polyps of the oesophagus

Tumour-like lesions	
Epithelial	Developmental cysts/duplications
	Heterotopias (gastric, sebaceous)
	Inflammatory/hyperplastic polyp[a]
	Glycogenic acanthosis[a]
Mesenchymal	Giant fibrovascular polyp[a]
	Inflammatory fibroid polyp
	Diffuse leiomyomatosis[a]
Benign neoplasms	
Epithelial	Squamous papilloma
	Polypoid dysplasia in Barrett's oesophagus
Mesenchymal	Granular cell tumour
	Leiomyoma
Malignant neoplasms	
Epithelial	Spindle cell carcinoma
	Conventional squamous cell carcinoma
	Adenocarcinoma
Mesenchymal	Gastrointestinal stromal tumour (GIST)
	Leiomyosarcoma
Other	Endocrine tumours
	Melanoma
	Choriocarcinoma
	Metastases

[a]Covered in this chapter.

Glycogenic acanthosis

This term has been used to describe plaque-like, rarely polypoid, lesions, which occur particularly in the lower oesophagus and usually on the longitudinal folds. They are discrete, white, round or oval, smooth-surfaced lesions, mostly under 5 mm maximum dimension, which have been observed in up to 15% of upper endoscopies [17,18]. At postmortem examination, they are almost invariable in the adult oesophagus [19]. Histologically, there is hyperplasia of the squamous epithelium with elongation of the papillae and hypertrophy of cells, particularly in the superficial layers (Figure 6.2a). These contain abundant glycogen, best demonstrated with a periodic acid–Schiff (PAS) stain, with and without diastase (Figure 6.2b). There is no cellular atypia, keratosis or excess parakeratosis and usually no associated inflammation. Although these lesions have no relationship to malignancy, their pathogenesis and natural history are not known. Very rarely, diffuse involvement of the oesophagus by glycogenic acanthosis may be due to Cowden's disease and *PTEN* mutation has been documented in this instance [20,21].

Diffuse leiomyomatosis

This occurs mainly in adolescents and young adults as a marked, diffuse thickening of the oesophageal wall, with or without nodularity, and extending distally in some cases to involve the proximal stomach [22,23]. Histologically, there is diffuse hypertrophy of smooth muscle, often with a whorled pattern and a considerable amount of intermingled fibrous tissue. Neural and vascular elements may also be prominent and an infiltrate of lymphocytes and plasma cells is common. In rare cases, eosinophilic infiltration may

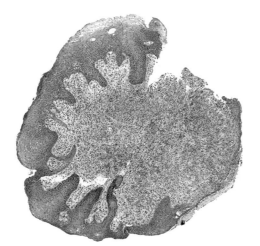

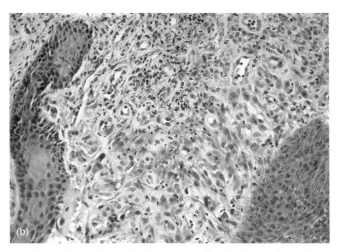

Figure 6.1 (a) Inflammatory/hyperplastic polyp with a smooth surface, basal zone hyperplasia, focal erosion and underlying inflamed, granulation tissue-like stroma. (b) Inflammatory/hyperplastic polyp with bizarre stromal cells lying within granulation tissue with abundant acute inflammation.

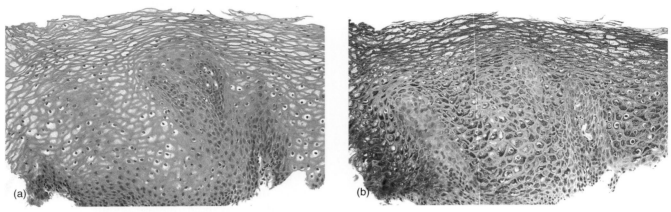

Figure 6.2 (a) Glycogenic acanthosis with hyperplastic squamous epithelium with elongation of the papillae and cells with abundant clear cytoplasm. (b) Glycogenic acanthosis with abundant glycogen within hyperplastic squamous epithelium, demonstrated with a periodic acid–Schiff stain.

be striking [24,25]. In a significant proportion of the reported cases, oesophageal leiomyomatosis has been familial and associated with Alport's syndrome [26–29]. On the other hand, only rare patients with Alport's syndrome, characterised by haematuric nephropathy and sensorial hearing loss, with deafness and/or ocular lesions, will develop oesophageal leiomyomatosis, which arises in those harbouring deletions of the *COL4A5* and *COL4A6* genes [30,31].

Other associations have included uterine and vulval leiomyomas, tracheobronchial leiomyomatosis, pyloric stenosis, and small bowel and anorectal involvement, as well as visceral malignancies occurring at a relatively young age [30,32,33]. Oesophageal leiomyomatosis has been separated by some authors from diffuse or giant muscular hypertrophy of the oesophagus, where nodularity is not a feature. Nevertheless the finding of both patterns in the same patient or in different members of implicated families suggests that they represent differing manifestations of the same condition [34].

References

1. Abraham SC, Singh VK, Yardley JH, Wu TT. Hyperplastic polyps of the esophagus and esophagogastric junction. Histologic and clinicopathologic findings. *Am J Surg Pathol* 2001;**23**:1180.
2. Staples DC, Knodell RG, Johnson LF. Inflammatory pseudotumor of the esophagus. A complication of gastroesophageal reflux. *Gastrointest Endosc* 1978;**24**:175.
3. Rabin MS, Bremner CG, Botha JR. The reflux gastroesophageal polyp. *Am J Gastroenterol* 1980;**73**:451.
4. Mulder DJ, Gander S, Hurlbut DJ, Soboleski DA, Smith RG, Justinich CJ. Multiple squamous hyperplastic-fibrous inflammatory polyps of the oesophagus: a new feature of eosinophilic oesophagitis? *J Clin Pathol* 2009;**62**:845.
5. Gill P, Piris J, Warren BJ. Bizarre stromal cells of the oesophagus. *Histopathology* 2003;**42**:88.
6. Arista-Nasr J, Rivera I, Martinez-Benitez B, Bornstein-Quevedo L, Orozco H, Lugo-Guevara Y. Atypical regenerative hyperplasia of the esophagus in endoscopic biopsy. A mimicker of squamous esophagic carcinoma. *Arch Pathol Lab Med* 2005;**129**:899.
7. Patel J, Kieffer RW, Martin M, Avant GR. Giant fibrovascular polyp of the esophagus. *Gastroenterology* 1984;**87**:953.
8. Penagini R, Ranzi T, Vellio P, et al. Giant fibrovascular polyp of the oesophagus: report of a case and effects on oesophageal function. *Gut* 1989;**30**:1624.
9. Fries MR, Galindo RL, Flint PW, Abraham SC. Giant fibrovascular polyp of the esophagus. A lesion causing upper airway obstruction and syncope. *Arch Pathol Lab Med* 2003;**127**:485.
10. Sargent RL, Hood IC. Asphyxiation caused by giant fibrovascular polyp of the esophagus. *Arch Pathol Lab Med* 2006;**130**:725.
11. Cokelaere K, Geboes K. Squamous cell carcinoma in a giant oesophageal fibrovascular polyp. *Histopathology* 2001;**38**:586.
12. Jakowski JD, Wakely PE. Rhabdomyomatous well-differentiated liposarcoma arising in giant fibrovascular polyp of the esophagus. *Ann Diagnos Pathol* 2009;**13**:263.
13. Burrell M, Toffler R. Fibrovascular polyp of the esophagus. *Dig Dis* 1973;**18**:714.
14. Wolf BC, Khettry U, Leonardi HK, Neptune WB, Bhattacharrya AK, Legg MA. Benign lesions mimicking malignant tumors of the esophagus. *Hum Pathol* 1988;**19**:148.
15. Yamane T, Uchiyama K, Ishi T, et al. Case of inflammatory fibroid polyp of the esophagogastric junction. *Dig Endosc* 2009;**21**:97.
16. Godey SK, Diggory RT. Inflammatory fibroid polyp of the oesophagus. *World J Surg Oncol* 2005;**3**:30.
17. Bender MD, Allison J, Cuartas F, Montgomery C. Glycogenic acanthosis of the esophagus: a form of benign epithelial hyperplasia. *Gastroenterology* 1973;**65**:373.
18. Stern Z, Sharon P, Ligumsky M, et al. Glycogenic acanthosis of the esophagus. A benign but confusing endoscopic lesion. *Am J Gastroenterol* 1980;**74**:261.
19. Rywlin AM, Ortega R. Glycogenic acanthosis of the esophagus. *Arch Pathol* 1970;**90**:439.
20. Kay PS, Soetikno RM, Mindelzun R, Young HS. Diffuse esophageal glycogenic acanthosis: an endoscopic marker of Cowden's disease. *Am J Gastroenterol* 1997;**92**:1038.

21. McGarrity TJ, Wagner Baker MJ, Ruggiero FM, et al. GI polyposis and glycogenic acanthosis of the esophagus associated with PTEN mutation positive Cowden syndrome in the absence of cutaneous manifestations. *Am J Gastroenterol* 2003;**98**:1429.

22. Fernandez JP, Mascarenhas MJ, Da Costa JC, Correia JP. Diffuse leiomyomatosis of the esophagus. A case report and review of the literature. *Am J Dig Dis* 1976;**20**:684.

23. Heald J, Moussalli H, Hasleton PS. Diffuse leiomyomatosis of the oesophagus. *Histopathology* 1986;**10**:755.

24. Morris CD, Wilkinson J, Fox D, Armstrong GR, Attwood SEA. Diffuse esophageal leiomyomatosis with localized dense eosinophilic infiltration. *Dis Esoph* 2002;**15**:85.

25. Nicholson AG, Li D, Pastorino U, Goldstraw P, Jeffery PK. Full thickness eosinophilia in oesophageal leiomyomatosis and idiopathic eosinophilic oesophagitis. A common allergic inflammatory profile? *J Pathol* 1997;**183**:233.

26. Guthrie KJ. Idiopathic muscular hypertrophy of esophagus, pylorus, duodenum and jejunum in a young girl. *Arch Dis Child* 1945;**20**:176.

27. Cochat P, Guiband P, Torres R, Roussel B, Guarner V, Larbre F. Diffuse leiomyomatosis in Alport syndrome. *J Pediatr* 1988;**113**:339.

28. Legius E, Proesmans W, van Damme B, Geboes K, Lerut T, Eggermont E. Muscular hypertrophy of the oesophagus and 'Alport-like' glomerular lesions in a boy. *Eur J Pediatr* 1990;**149**:623.

29. Bloch P, Quijada J. Diffuse leiomyomatosis of the oesophagus. Analysis of a case and review of the literature. *Gastroenterol Clin Biol* 1992;**16**:890.

30. Pujol J, Pares D, Mora L, Sans M, Jaurrieta E. Diagnosis and management of diffuse leiomyomatosis of the oesophagus. *Dis Esoph* 2000;**13**:169.

31. Zheng K, Harvey S, Sado Y, et al. Absence of the α6(IV) chain of collagen type IV in Alport syndrome is related to a failure at the protein assembly level and does not result in diffuse leiomyomatosis. *Am J Pathol* 1999;**154**:1883.

32. Azzie G, Bensoussan A, Spitz L. The association of anorectal leiomyomatosis and diffuse oesophageal leiomyomatosis. *Pediatr Surg Int* 2003;**19**:424.

33. Guillem P, Delcambre F, Cohen-Solal L, et al. Diffuse esophageal leiomyomatosis with perirectal involvement mimicking Hirschsprung disease. *Gastroenterology* 2001;**120**:216.

34. Lonsdale RN, Roberts PF, Vaughan R, Thiru S. Familial oesophageal leiomyomatosis and nephropathy. *Histopathology* 1992;**20**:127.

CHAPTER 7

Tumours of the oesophagus

Amitabh Srivastava[1,2] and Robert D. Odze[1,2]

[1]Harvard Medical School, Boston, MA, USA
[2]Brigham and Women's Hospital, Boston, MA, USA

Benign epithelial tumours

Squamous cell papilloma

Squamous cell papilloma is the most common benign tumour of the oesophagus. These lesions have a multi-lobulated appearance with a granular or warty surface and firm consistency (Figure 7.1). They are usually small in size (15 mm in diameter) and may be multiple in number [1]. The lower third of the oesophagus is the most common site. Histologically, they usually have a papillary architecture and a central core of vascular connective tissue, covered by acanthotic stratified squamous epithelium, with no atypia and good differentiation from the basal to the surface layers. Cytological changes suggestive of human papillomavirus (HPV) effect, such as nuclear hyperchromasia and binucleation, may be present [2,3]. In two recent series, the presence of HPV DNA was demonstrated in squamous cell papillomas using the polymerase chain reaction (PCR) [4,5]. Squamous cell papillomas should be differentiated from inflammatory polyps and verrucous carcinoma [6,7]. Inflammatory polyps have a relatively smooth surface and show basal cell hyperplasia with erosion of the epithelium and acute inflammation in the lamina propria. Rare examples of oesophageal papillomatosis complicated by carcinoma have been reported [8].

Adenoma and polypoid glandular dysplasia

True oesophageal adenomas are rare. Most lesions previously described as oesophageal adenomas represent polypoid dysplasia associated with Barrett's oesophagus [9,10]. Dysplasia in this pre-malignant condition may result in polypoid masses with a tubular or villous configuration. These lesions are best described as polypoid dysplasia arising in Barrett's oesophagus, rather than adenoma, since intervening flat mucosa may also be dysplastic [11]. Dysplasia complicating Barrett's oesophagus is more comprehensively dealt with in Chapter 5.

Miscellaneous lesions

Oesophageal epithelial neoplasms of salivary gland type with a presumptive origin from submucosal glands or ducts are extremely rare (Figure 7.2). Examples of canalicular adenoma, pleomorphic adenoma and sialadenoma papilliferum have all been reported in the oesophagus [12–16].

Malignant epithelial tumours

Oesophageal cancer is the eighth most common type of malignancy worldwide and the sixth most common cause of mortality from cancer. Worldwide, at least 90% of oesophageal carcinomas are squamous cell carcinomas [17]. Adenocarcinoma is the second most common and other types, such as small cell carcinoma and malignant melanoma, are rare. In the USA, the incidence of oesophageal adenocarcinoma has increased from 0.5–0.9/100 000 in the 1970s to 3.2–4.0/100 000 in the 1980s and 1990s. In England and Wales, there has been a similar increase of about 39% every 5 years in men and 37% every 5 years in women. This increase has been seen across all socioeconomic groups [18]

Morson and Dawson's Gastrointestinal Pathology, Fifth Edition. Edited by Neil A. Shepherd, Bryan F. Warren, Geraint T. Williams, Joel K. Greenson, Gregory Y. Lauwers and Marco R. Novelli.
© 2013 Blackwell Publishing Ltd. Published 2013 by Blackwell Publishing Ltd.

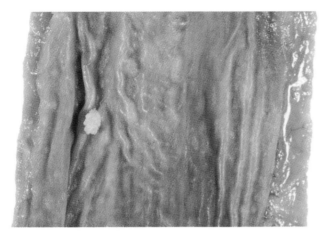

Figure 7.1 Squamous cell papilloma: this small warty lesion was an incidental finding in the middle third of the oesophagus post mortem.

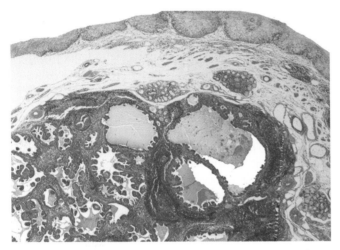

Figure 7.2 Warthin's tumour of the oesophagus: it involves the submucosal glands and shows cysts lined by columnar cells with abundant eosinophilic cytoplasm and a prominent lymphoid stroma.

but has been most pronounced in affluent populations [19–23]. Analyses of cancer incidence data have shown that, in North America and Europe, the incidence of oesophageal adenocarcinoma has been rising steadily since the mid-1970s, when it originally accounted for about 16% of all oesophageal cancers among white men in the USA. In the late 1990s this number approached 50%. The rates of adenocarcinomas of the proximal stomach ('cardia') have also increased, although to a lesser extent than oesophageal adenocarcinoma. Over the same period of time, there has been a decline in the rate of oesophageal squamous cell carcinoma, e.g. the rate of squamous cell carcinoma was reported to have declined by 23% in one study. There has also been a decline in adenocarcinomas involving more distal portions of the stomach [24,25]. A large majority of

adenocarcinomas of the oesophagus and the oesophago-gastric junction are presumed to arise from a columnar-lined (Barrett's) oesophagus.

Squamous cell carcinoma

Clinical features

Squamous cell carcinoma of the oesophagus, although relatively infrequent in most of western Europe and North America, is a major disease for a large proportion of the world's population. About 80% of cases occur within developing countries [26]. In the USA, squamous cell carcinoma continues to represent the most common type of oesophageal cancer in African Americans. Dysphagia and weight loss are the usual presenting symptoms. Hypercalcaemia may be present in a subset of patients. An association with concurrent squamous cell carcinoma of the head and neck region has also been described.

Epidemiology

The highest oesophageal cancer rates are found in the Asian oesophageal cancer belt region, which extends from Turkey to Iran, Iraq and Kazakhstan to northern China. Squamous cell carcinoma is the most prevalent type of oesophageal cancer in this region. However, even within this endemic region, there are striking variations in incidence. In fact, there are sharp gradients of incidence between regions that lie only a few hundred miles apart. Thus, in northern China, there is a 60-fold decrease for men and a 90-fold decrease for women between the north-east region of Henan province and the northern Shansi region, areas that lie only 300 miles apart [27,28]. Similarly, in the Transkei in South Africa and in Uganda, the incidence also varies widely. Clearly defined localities show 10- to 20-fold differences in incidence [29]. Even in Europe, where the incidence of squamous cell carcinoma is low, pockets of high incidence occur, such as in Normandy and Brittany, although there is a marked variation in incidence between the different communes in these respective areas [30]. The increased risk is predominantly among males, where the incidence rate rises to 56 in 100 000, with a male:female ratio of 23:1. The previously reported high rates of cancer in parts of Scandinavia, particularly those that occur in the post-cricoid region and upper oesophagus, which predominantly affected women and were associated with anaemia, dysphagia, hypochlorhydria and other signs of iron and vitamin deficiency (Paterson Brown–Kelly or Plummer–Vinson syndrome) [31,32], have now largely disappeared.

Aetiology and associations

Predisposing factors

The aetiology of squamous cell carcinoma is unknown. However, multiple factors seem to be involved. In fact, epidemiological studies have provided evidence that causative agents may differ between geographical and high-risk versus low-risk areas and may act synergistically.

Alcohol and tobacco Cigarette smoking and alcohol consumption have both been associated with an increased predisposition for oesophageal cancer. Both factors have a stronger association with squamous cell carcinoma than oesophageal adenocarcinoma. Smokers are at three to seven times greater risk of developing squamous cell carcinoma compared with the general population [33–36]. Among combined drinkers and smokers, the risk rises considerably with increased alcohol consumption, compared with increasing tobacco consumption. Consumption of spirits may be more potent rather than beer or wine in promoting carcinogenesis [36]. In the UK, variations in the rate of oesophageal cancer have closely paralleled total alcohol consumption, with only a short lag, suggesting that the effect of alcohol may be on the later stages of carcinogenesis, as a tumour promoter [37]. Interestingly, the occurrence of cancer in high-incidence areas in Africa correlates with the use of maize as the principal ingredient of homemade beer, which has replaced traditional millets and sorghum [38]. Mate is a drink commonly consumed in some parts of South America. These geographical areas, including southern Brazil, north-east Argentina, Uruguay and Paraguay, are also those associated with highest incidence rates of oesophageal cancer in South America.

There is a statistically higher incidence of oesophageal carcinomas among patients who smoke or chew tobacco, and this is equally true for pipe users and cigar and cigarette smokers [39]. Oesophageal carcinomas are not infrequently associated with multiple primary tumours in the mouth, pharynx, stomach or intestine [40,41]. It has been suggested that this finding may be related to ingestion of nicotine and other carcinogenic substances [41]. A postmortem study in American men with a known smoking history showed 'atypical' nuclei in the basal layer of the squamous epithelium of the oesophagus in 6.6% of non-smokers and no cases of carcinoma *in situ*, whereas basal atypia was found in 79.8% and carcinoma *in situ* in 1.9% of smokers [42]. In some high-risk populations in South Africa and India, tobacco appears to play a more important role than alcohol [43,44]. Thus, in South Africa, smoking of pipe tobacco showed a positive association with oesophageal cancer [44]. Tobacco pyrolysis products from the Transkei region have been shown to have mutagenic activity in the Ames test [45]. Measurement of urinary morphine metabolites have indicated that addiction is common in high-incidence areas, occurring in about 50% of men and women aged 35 or more [46]. Mutagens in sukhteh (opium dross) and in morphine and opium pyrolysates have been identified and characterised [47–49] and are thought to be factors involved in the aetiology of oesophageal cancer. There are,

however, exceptions to the finding of a strong association between tobacco use and squamous cell carcinoma. In the Taihang mountain regions of China and in Golestan Province in Iran, cigarette smoking has been shown to be a minor risk factor, with a relative risk of about 1.5, even though both areas are endemic for squamous cell carcinoma [50,51]. The reasons for this discrepancy are unknown. It is possible that other high-risk factors in these regions may dilute the contribution of smoking in the pathogenesis of squamous cell carcinoma.

Diet In northern Iran, detailed dietary surveys have found clear regional associations, e.g. a diet rich in home-baked bread and tea has been linked to geographical regions where there is a high incidence of oesophageal cancer. These populations showed low calorie and total protein intake and low intake of vitamin A, riboflavin and vitamin C [46]. It has been estimated that the risk of oesophageal cancer may be reduced by as much as 20% per 50 g of fruits and vegetables consumed per day. The decrease in risk is most probably related to squamous cell carcinoma only, with little or no impact on oesophageal adenocarcinoma [52,53]. The association between oesophageal cancer and consumption of hot foods and drinks, or of pickled vegetables, remains controversial.

The results of two large chemoprevention trials in China have been disappointing. The Linxian Dysplasia trial, which enrolled 3300 individuals, and the Linxian General Population trial, which included 30 000 people, both found no reduction in risk of oesophageal cancer after 5–6 years of nutritional supplement usage [54,55]. There are some data to suggest that selenium and zinc may play a role in the aetiology of oesophageal squamous cell carcinoma as well [56,57].

Infectious agents Fungal oesophagitis, mostly due to *Candida* spp., is very common in the Linxian province of China. It usually involves the middle third of the oesophagus and has been postulated as a possible aetiological factor in oesophageal carcinogenesis. Recent research has focused on the role of HPV infection in oesophageal carcinogenesis [58–64]. Histological changes in oesophageal squamous cell carcinomas, similar to condylomatous genital lesions, have been observed [65]. There have been multiple studies on the prevalence of HPV in squamous carcinoma of the oesophagus, with detection rates varying from 0% to 71%. This variation may be due to true geographical variation in pathogenesis, variation in techniques used to detect HPV and different thresholds for classifying cases as HPV positive. In some instances, it may simply reflect sample contamination during PCR. The marked differences in the association of oesophageal cancer with HPV infection has led the International Agency for Research on Cancer (IARC) to conclude recently that 'there is inadequate evidence in humans for carcinogenicity of HPV in the oesophagus' [66].

Exogenous factors It has been known for many years that there is an increased risk of oesophageal carcinoma after ingestion of lye (crude sodium hydroxide with sodium carbonate), commonly after a time interval of 40 years [67,68]. The evidence for development of cancer in strictures due to other causes is less convincing [69]. A number of cases of oesophageal cancer have been reported after therapeutic irradiation for neck and spinal diseases [70] and irradiation to the chest for breast carcinoma and, less frequently, for lymphoma [71]. Other postulated exogenous factors, which may play a role in certain populations, include the ingestion of bracken fern [72] and plant irritants in foods [73]. Studies from Linxian and Golestan regions of China and Iran, respectively, also suggest a possible role of polycyclic aromatic hydrocarbons in the pathogenesis of oesophageal cancer [74,75].

Genetic factors

One study from northern Iran showed that 47% of patients in the high-risk region of Turkoman Sahara have a positive family history of oesophageal cancer, compared with only 2% among the low-risk population of non-Turkoman [76]. Cases of oesophageal cancer in families associated with keratosis palmaris and plantaris (tylosis), inherited as an autosomal dominant characteristic, have been described [77–79]. Recently, linkage analysis mapped the tylosis oesophageal cancer (TOC) gene locus to chromosome 17q25 [80] and this locus is commonly deleted in sporadic oesophageal squamous cell carcinomas, suggesting the existence of a tumour suppressor gene for oesophageal squamous cell carcinoma at this site [81].

Acetaldehyde, which is produced during alcohol metabolism, is eliminated from the body by the enzyme aldehyde dehydrogenase, which, in turn, is a product of the gene *ALDH2*. The *1/*2 heterozygous polymorphism of the *ALDH2* gene has been shown to confer an increased risk of oesophageal squamous cell carcinoma and may be a manifestation of gene–environment interaction because the increase in risk observed with this genotype is strongly related to the degree of alcohol consumption [82,83]. In addition, the *2/*2 homozygous genotype of *ALDH2* gene is associated with a lower risk of squamous cell carcinoma [84]. Another example of genetic susceptibility for oesophageal cancer involves the C677 T polymorphism in the gene methylenetetrahydrofolate reductase. The *TT* and *TC* genotypes of this gene have been shown to confer an increased risk of squamous dysplasia, and cancer, compared with the *CC* genotype [85].

Associated conditions

An increased risk of oesophageal cancer has been reported in patients with achalasia [86]. One long-term follow-up cohort study of achalasia patients from Sweden reported a ten-fold increase in risk of both squamous cell carcinoma and adenocarcinoma. Other conditions associated with an increased risk of oesophageal cancer include diverticula [87,88], the Plummer–Vinson syndrome [89] and coeliac disease [90,91]. One report has documented squamous cell carcinoma within a duplication cyst of the oesophagus [92]. Oesophageal carcinoma is also associated with tumours in other organs, particularly the oropharynx and larynx [93,94]. This presumably relates to shared risk factors, particularly heavy smoking and high alcohol intake [95].

Pathology

Precancerous lesions

Oesophagitis Chronic oesophagitis is common in populations where there is a high incidence of oesophageal carcinoma, such as northern China and Iran. It usually involves the middle and lower thirds of the oesophagus. Histologically, acanthosis of the epithelium with swollen clear squamous cells corresponds to the 'white' patches seen at endoscopy. However, one endoscopic study carried out in Linxian province, in a population with a previous diagnosis of dysplasia after screening by oesophageal balloon cytology, has cast doubt on the role of oesophagitis as a precursor lesion. Epithelial atrophy was not observed in any of the patients this study [96].

Squamous dysplasia Squamous dysplasia is a precursor of oesophageal squamous cell carcinoma. Dysplasia may appear endoscopically as areas of friable or erythematous mucosa, erosions, plaques or nodules. Ill-defined irregularities of the mucosal surface, or white patches, may also be present. In a very small proportion of cases, foci of dysplasia or cancer may appear endoscopically normal [97]. Application of Lugol's iodine leads to enhanced visualisation of the dysplastic foci on endoscopy [98]. Most reports of oesophageal squamous dysplasia are from countries with a high incidence of squamous cell carcinoma, particularly China. In one mass survey using the abrasive balloon technique to obtain cytological specimens and carried out over a 9-year period on 21581 inhabitants aged >30 years in Linxian county, 12.7% showed mild dysplasia and 1.2% had severe dysplasia whereas, in 0.9%, the appearances were consistent with invasive squamous cell carcinoma [99]. The age distribution of dysplasia and carcinoma suggested a continuous progression from mild to severe dysplasia and carcinoma *in situ*. Moreover, follow-up studies of patients with severe dysplasia showed progression to cancer in about a quarter of all cases. Another prospective follow-up study from Linxian [100] found that moderate and severe dysplasia and carcinoma *in situ* were the only histological lesions associated with a significantly increased risk of squamous cell carcinoma within 3.5 years of endoscopic biopsy diagnosis. Increasing grades of dysplasia were associated with increasing risk, although severe dysplasia and carcinoma *in situ* were associated with similar degrees of risk. There are also data to suggest that dysplasia may be reversible [101].

Further evidence of the role of dysplasia as a precancerous lesion comes from its frequent occurrence in areas adjacent to, or distant from, invasive squamous cell carcinoma when oesophagectomy specimens have been studied in detail [102–105]. One investigation found that the prevalence of dysplasia at the margins of invasive carcinoma was inversely related to the depth of invasion of the main lesion [106], supporting the view that such changes are not secondary to lateral intraepithelial spread of tumour but represent a primary field transformation from which invasive carcinoma has subsequently arisen. Moreover, multicentric tumours may be present in 15–30% of squamous cell carcinomas, further supporting the idea of a 'field effect' in carcinogenesis [107,108].

The histological criteria for squamous dysplasia include architectural and cytological abnormalities. Two classifications have been used. The original defines dysplasia as mild when <25% of the basal epithelium is involved, moderate when 25–50% of the basal epithelium is involved and severe when >50% of the mucosa is involved. A two-tiered system, in which low grade dysplasia is defined as <50% and high grade dysplasia as >50% involvement of the epithelium with neoplastic cells, is preferred. Cytological features of dysplasia include a high nuclear:cytoplasmic ratio, nuclear hyperchromasia and pleomorphism, and increased mitotic activity. Dysplasia may also spread in a Pagetoid fashion or into underlying oesophageal gland ducts [109, 110]. In some cases, the presence of koilocytotic change may reflect an underlying HPV infection [2,111].

Regenerative changes secondary to inflammation, pseudo-epitheliomatous hyperplasia, or the effects of radiation or chemotherapy may mimic dysplasia. Unlike dysplasia, regenerative epithelium shows surface maturation and does not show significant nuclear crowding; nuclear overlapping and atypical mitoses are typically absent. Vesicular chromatin, with prominent nucleoli, is often present in the nuclei of regenerating epithelium. In the presence of significant inflammation, a diagnosis of dysplasia should be made with caution. In cases of uncertainty, a diagnosis of 'indefinite for dysplasia' is appropriate. Radiation change causes cells to enlarge and develop prominent cytoplasmic vacuolation. Moreover, similar changes may also be present in surrounding stromal fibroblasts and mesenchymal cells.

Macroscopic features

Squamous cell carcinoma is rare in the upper third of the oesophagus, most common in the middle third and less frequent in the lower third. The distribution in one large series from Linxian, China, based on a combination of balloon cytology, oesophagoscopy and radiological examination, found involvement by tumour of the upper third of the oesophagus in 11.7%, the middle third in 63.3% and the lower third in 24.9% [112]. Macroscopically, squamous cell carcinomas may be exophytic, ulcerating or infiltrating or they may show a combination of these features (Figures 7.3–7.5). The tumour often results in a stricture, which is usually irregular, friable and haemorrhagic. True papillary or verrucous squamous cell carcinoma is uncommon and occurs usually as a large, warty, slowly growing neoplasm [113]. Most have occurred in the upper third and, in some, there has been a history of achalasia, a diverticulum or caustic stricture [114–116]. Rarely, a diffuse infiltrative type of growth, resembling a 'leather bottle stomach', may involve the oesophagus. Superficial spreading carcinomas, with extensive intramucosal involvement and a propensity to permeate lymphatics and metastasise to lymph nodes, have also been described [117]. Squamous cell carcinomas situated in the post-cricoid region of the oesophagus do not differ appreciably from those of the middle and lower thirds.

Microscopic features

Oesophageal squamous cell carcinomas show all grades of differentiation. Well differentiated lesions show well-

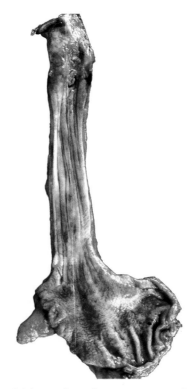

Figure 7.3 Superficial oesophageal cancer: an extensive erosive lesion found incidentally post mortem in middle third of oesophagus.

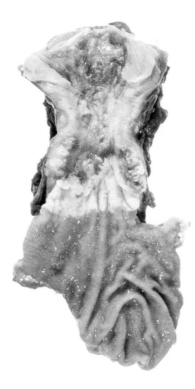

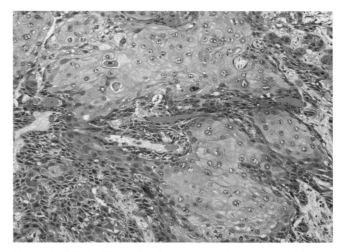

Figure 7.6 Well differentiated squamous cell carcinoma with keratinisation.

Figure 7.4 An extensively ulcerated squamous cell carcinoma of the lower third of the oesophagus resulting in a stricture.

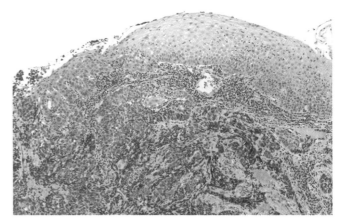

Figure 7.7 Poorly differentiated squamous cell carcinoma. Tumour is seen infiltrating below oesophageal squamous mucosa. There is focal squamous dysplasia (at left) in the surface epithelium, serving to corroborate the squamous nature of the infiltrating tumour.

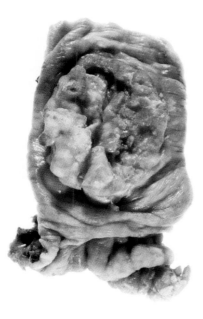

Figure 7.5 A nodular and ulcerated squamous cell carcinoma involving the upper oesophagus. Multifocal squamous carcinoma *in situ* was also present but is not grossly apparent in this case.

defined nests of tumour cells with keratinisation (Figure 7.6) whereas poorly differentiated tumours show sheets of undifferentiated tumour cells without any evidence of keratinisation (Figure 7.7). Some tumours may show a predominance of basaloid tumour cells with peripheral palisading, similar to a basal cell carcinoma in the skin. In most tumours, keratin pearls or intercellular bridges are present. Variation of cellular differentiation in different parts of the tumour is common. Histochemical, immuno-histochemical and ultrastructural studies have confirmed morphological heterogeneity, e.g. approximately 30% of tumours show focal adenocarcinomatous differentiation [118–120].

Natural history and prognosis

Superficial oesophageal cancer

Oesophageal cancer may be confined to the mucosa or spread only into the submucosa, with or without lymph node metastasis. These tumours are referred to as 'superficial cancers'. Most reports of superficial squamous cell carcinoma are from China or Japan [121–123] but series have also been reported from Europe [124–126] and the USA [127]. In China, the majority of cases have been detected in mass surveys involving balloon cytology and radiological examinations in high-incidence areas. However, the prognosis of early oesophageal cancer differs from early gastric cancer, with 5-year survival rates in the 50–60% range in oesophageal cancers with submucosal infiltration. This is largely due to the fact that 30–40% of patients with submucosal invasion also have lymph node metastatic disease [125,128,129]. This has led some authors to suggest that the term 'early' oesophageal cancer should be restricted to cases in which there is carcinoma *in situ* (intraepithelial dysplasia/neoplasia) or intramucosal carcinoma only, cases in which the prognosis approaches 100% [129–131]. In one study, the presence of an elevated component in superficial oesophageal cancer [132] was an important macroscopic feature suggesting submucosal invasion and a high probability of lymph node involvement. Some superficial carcinomas occupy a large area of the oesophagus [133–135]. Endoscopic ultrasonography has been used to assess the depth of invasion and peri-oesophago-gastric lymph node metastatic disease in cases of superficial oesophageal carcinoma [136]. Observations such as these are important because, increasingly, non-surgical interventions such as photodynamic therapy [137] and endoscopic resection [138] are being considered in the treatment of precursor lesions.

Deep oesophageal cancer

Vertical spread through the muscularis propria is common in oesophageal squamous cell carcinomas. Adjacent structures such as the trachea, aorta and pericardium may be involved in locally advanced tumours. The risk of nodal metastasis increases with the depth of invasion and rises dramatically once tumours have penetrated the submucosa. Thus, intramucosal tumours have a less than 5% risk of nodal metastasis compared with tumours that invade the submucosa, where the risk approaches 45% [139,140]. Skip metastases may be present in oesophageal cancers and distant metastases to the lungs and liver have been reported in up to 50% of all squamous cell carcinomas [141]. Overall, the 5-year survival rate in squamous cell carcinoma is about 30–40%. Tumour stage remains the most significant prognostic factor in patients treated by oesophagectomy. Submucosal tumours have a 5-year survival rate of about 70%, which is reduced to 50% for tumours that invade the

Table 7.1 TNM staging of oesophageal carcinoma (7th edn, 2010)

T	Primary tumour	
	pT1	Tumour invades lamina propria, muscularis mucosae or submucosa T1a: invades lamina propria or muscularis mucosae T1b: invades submucosa
	pT2	Tumour invades muscularis propria
	pT3	Tumour invades adventitia
	pT4	Tumour invades adjacent structures T4a: resectable tumour invading pleura, pericardium or diaphragm T4b: unresectable tumour invading other structures (aorta, vertebra, trachea, etc.)
N	Regional lymph nodes	
	pN0	No regional lymph node metastases
	pN1	Regional lymph node metastases involving one to two nodes
	pN2	Three to six positive lymph nodes
	pN3	Seven or more positive lymph nodes
M	Distant metastasis	
	M1	Distant metastasis/metastases present

muscularis propria and to about 25% for tumours that infiltrate the adventitia [142–146].

The TNM (tumour–node–metastasis) staging system proposed by the American Joint Committee on Cancer (AJCC) has been revised recently and is significantly different to previous editions. The staging criteria in this seventh edition are outlined in Table 7.1. The number of lymph nodes examined in oesophagectomy specimens has been shown to be an independent prognostic factor in a number of studies [147–149]. Histopathological examination for extent of residual tumour has also been proposed as a prognostic factor after neoadjuvant therapy for oesophageal squamous cell carcinoma [150].

Histological variants

Verrucous carcinoma

Verrucous squamous cell carcinoma of the oesophagus is extremely rare. These tumours are large, exophytic neoplasms with a papillary or warty appearance, often associated with stricture formation. They can arise at any site in the oesophagus. Similar tumours occur at other sites, notably the oral cavity, larynx, glans penis, vulva and anal canal [151]. The age range of patients is broad but there is

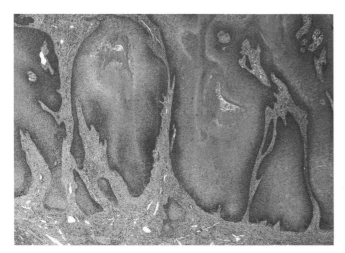

Figure 7.8 Verrucous carcinoma: well differentiated squamous cell carcinoma with surface maturation and broad, pushing margins at the base. Foci of invasion are obvious at the deep aspect in this section.

a male predilection. Most cases occur in the upper third of the oesophagus [114]. In some patients, there is a history of achalasia, diverticulum [114], post-cricoid web [152] or lye-associated stricture [115].

Histologically, verrucous carcinoma consists of papillary projections of well differentiated squamous cells, with parakeratosis and hyperkeratosis most prominent between papillae (Figure 7.8). In biopsies, evidence of invasion is frequently lacking so that a pathologist unaware of the endoscopic appearances may interpret the 'bland' features as a benign process. Multiple biopsy sets often result in the failure of the pathologist to be able to make a definitive diagnosis of malignancy. This is one tumour, in particular, where diagnostic endoscopic mucosal resection (EMR) may be required to make the appropriate diagnosis. Invasion is typically in the form of a broad pushing front and may be difficult to diagnose with certainty even in EMRs and resection specimens. Despite features of low grade malignancy and the fact that metastases are uncommon [113], this tumour has a poor prognosis because of its propensity to invade locally, with fistula formation [153].

Carcinosarcoma (spindle cell carcinoma)

First described by Virchow in 1865, carcinosarcoma of the oesophagus has also been termed 'polypoid carcinoma', 'sarcomatoid carcinoma' and 'spindle cell carcinoma'. These tumours are uncommon and represent about 2% of all oesophageal carcinomas. They predominantly afflict adult men aged between 40 and 90 years, usually as a bulky polypoid growth in the middle or lower oesophagus (Figure 7.9). Microscopically, the tumours show a mixture of 'sarcomatous' elements composed of interlacing bundles of spindle-shaped cells in which bizarre giant cells may

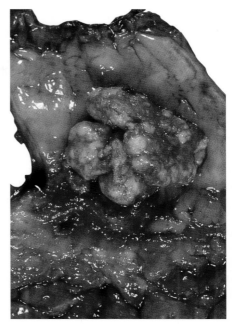

Figure 7.9 Carcinosarcoma: a large lobulated polypoid growth is present at the lower end of the oesophagus.

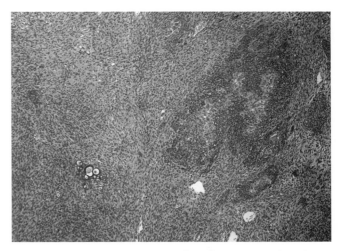

Figure 7.10 Carcinosarcoma (spindle cell carcinoma): foci of poorly differentiated squamous cell carcinoma with broad areas of interlacing spindle cells and focal cartilaginous differentiation.

also be present. Osseous and cartilaginous differentiation may occur (Figure 7.10).

An epithelial component of squamous or undifferentiated carcinoma is typical but may be focal and difficult to detect. Occasionally an adenocarcinomatous [154], adenocystic [155], neuro-endocrine or glandular component may be present [156]. In most tumours, the sarcomatous pattern predominates, with inconspicuous intramucosal or invasive squamous cell carcinoma confined to small areas at the base of the pedicle. Areas of transition from typical squamous cell carcinoma to sarcoma are often present

[155,157]. The demonstration of tonofibrils and well-developed desmosomes in the spindle cells [154,158], together with evidence of collagen production [159] on ultrastructural examination, suggests that the sarcomatous cells are squamous cells in origin. Immunohistochemical studies have demonstrated disparate findings. Some authors have shown immunoreactivity to keratin in the spindle cell component [160,161] whereas others have reported negative reactions to keratin and variable positivity for desmin, smooth muscle actin, vimentin, α_1-anti-chymotrypsin and α_1-anti-trypsin [156,162,163]. Recent studies on clonality of these tumours have also led to disparate results [164,165]. Biopsies of these tumours may suggest a highly malignant undifferentiated sarcoma, although in most of reported cases, squamous cell carcinoma (of varying degrees of differentiation) has been present. Although haematogenous spread is more common in carcinosarcomas than pure squamous cell carcinoma, the overall 5-year survival rate has been shown to be similar in recent studies [154,166].

Basaloid–squamous cell carcinoma

These tumours usually occur in elderly men, involve the mid- or distal oesophagus and typically present at an advanced stage. Tumours with similar histology have been reported in the larynx, pharynx, base of tongue and hard palate [167]. In the oesophagus, basaloid carcinoma comprises about 1.9–11.3% of all squamous cell carcinomas [168,169]. Basaloid carcinomas show a biphasic or multiphasic growth pattern. There is, by definition, a variable amount of undifferentiated basaloid component in the form of solid sheets, anastomosing trabeculae, festoons or microcystic structures, and these areas are usually associated with a high mitotic index, frequent comedo-type necrosis and stromal hyalinisation (Figure 7.11). The neoplastic squamous component, either *in situ* or invasive, may be inconspicuous. Foci of adenocarcinoma, small cell carcinoma or even spindle cell carcinoma have also been described [168]. Most cases in the literature reported as 'adenoid cystic carcinomas' of the oesophagus probably represent basaloid–squamous cell carcinomas. The rare, genuine examples of oesophageal adenoid cystic carcinoma have a less aggressive clinical course (see below) [170,171]. The prognosis of patients with basaloid–squamous cell carcinoma does not differ significantly from conventional squamous cell carcinoma [169].

Adenocarcinoma

Oesophageal adenocarcinoma arises, most commonly, on a background of Barrett's oesophagus. In fact, the first case of malignancy arising in Barrett's oesophagus was reported by one of the original co-authors of this textbook [172]. There has been a very large increase in the incidence of oesophageal adenocarcinoma in recent decades, particu-

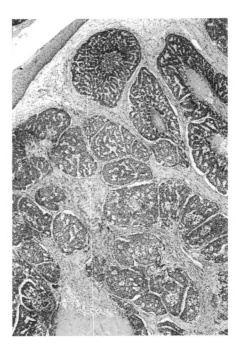

Figure 7.11 Basaloid–squamous carcinoma: lobules of basaloid cells with a festooning appearance peripherally are present deep to oesophageal epithelium. Central necrosis is seen in several of the tumour lobules.

larly in the USA and Europe. The pathogenesis of Barrett's oesophagus and its malignant potential are discussed in detail in Chapter 5. The following discussion focuses on clinical, epidemiological and pathological aspects of oesophageal adenocarcinoma and its variants.

Clinical features

Barrett's oesophagus is a metaplastic pre-cancerous lesion involving the distal oesophagus that occurs in patients with chronic gastro-oesophageal reflux disease and is present in most patients with oesophageal adenocarcinoma. The symptoms of oesophageal adenocarcinoma are non-specific. Early adenocarcinomas detected during surveillance endoscopy for Barrett's oesophagus may be associated with symptoms of the underlying gastro-oesophageal reflux disease. Advanced cancers may present with dysphagia, vomiting, bleeding or anaemia, and manifest as polypoid lesions that bleed easily on contact or as tight stenotic lesions on endoscopy. Most adenocarcinomas involve the distal third of the oesophagus.

Epidemiology

The incidence of oesophageal adenocarcinomas has been rising since the mid-1970s when it accounted for 16% of all oesophageal cancers among white men in the USA. The overall incidence increased from 3.6 per million in 1973 to 25.6 per million in 2006 [18,24,173]. The rates of adenocarcinoma of the gastric cardia have also increased, although to a lesser extent. The incidence has also risen among black men and women during this period but the rates have remained at much lower levels. The increase in incidence is unrelated to diagnostic shifts with reference to location, specificity of cell type or increased use of endoscopy-based diagnosis [174]. Increasing rates of oesophageal adenocarcinoma have also been reported from the UK, Scandinavia, France, Switzerland, Australia and New Zealand [175–180]. A similar increase has been seen in adenocarcinomas involving the gastro-oesophageal junction that also show an association with white male predominance and reflux symptoms, suggesting that they may have a pathogenesis similar to that of distal oesophageal adenocarcinoma. Barrett's oesophagus has been demonstrated in a considerable proportion of tumours centred within 20 mm of the gastro-oesophageal junction [181–183], and the likelihood of finding Barrett's mucosa in junctional cancers is considerably greater in smaller tumours. In larger lesions the metaplastic epithelium may not be identified because it is more likely to be replaced by neoplastic spread of tumour cells [183].

Interestingly, recent incidence trend analysis for oesophageal adenocarcinoma using the SEER (surveillance, epidemiology and end-results) database has shown that the increase in incidence of oesophageal adenocarcinoma may have slowed down and hit a plateau. The rising trend appears to have slowed down from an annual 8.2% increase before 1996 to 1.3% in subsequent years. This may be largely due to changes in incidence of early stage disease, which has changed direction from a 10% annual increase before 1999 to a 1.6% decline subsequently [184].

Aetiology and associations

The underlying risk factors for adenocarcinoma of the distal oesophagus and the gastro-oesophageal junction are significantly different from those of oesophageal squamous cell carcinoma. As mentioned above, oesophageal and gastro-oesophageal adenocarcinomas arise on a background of Barrett's oesophagus and show an association with gastro-oesophageal reflux disease, obesity, dietary factors and smoking, and alcohol consumption, and are inversely associated with gastric colonisation by *Helicobacter pylori*.

Dietary factors

Obesity and being overweight have been consistently shown to be associated with oesophageal adenocarcinoma but not to squamous cell carcinoma [185,186]. This may be related to increased abdominal pressure predisposing to gastro-oesophageal reflux disease and increasing likelihood of developing Barrett's oesophagus [187,188].

Tobacco and alcohol

Smoking is a strong risk factor for oesophageal squamous cell carcinoma but its impact on risk of oesophageal adeno-

carcinoma is comparatively weak. It appears that there is a two- to threefold increased risk in smokers but, unlike squamous cell carcinoma, the risk of oesophageal adenocarcinoma does not decrease substantially after cessation of smoking [189–191]. Changing patterns of smoking may explain the changing incidence of both adenocarcinoma and squamous cell carcinoma of the oesophagus in some countries [174]. Alcohol consumption has not been consistently related to an increased risk for oesophageal adenocarcinoma.

Drugs

The use of aspirin or other non-steroidal anti-inflammatory drugs (NSAIDs) may reduce the risk of oesophageal cancer. A 35% decrease in the risk of oesophageal cancer among NSAID users compared with non-users was shown in a recent meta-analysis [192–196].

Genetic factors

The role of inherited factors in oesophageal adenocarcinoma has been studied recently by a pathway specific evaluation of common genetic variations. Fourteen pathways important in carcinogenesis were explored for genetic variations and single nucleotide polymorphisms (SNPs) of rs3127075 involving *Caspase-7* and rs4661636 involving *Caspase-9* genes were significantly associated with an increased oesophageal adenocarcinoma risk. In the same study, a protective effect was seen for SNP rs572483 in the progesterone receptor gene among women carrying the variant *G* allele but not among men [197]. These initial observations, if confirmed in future larger studies, may provide new screening and surveillance strategies for prevention of oesophageal adenocarcinoma.

Associated conditions

Conditions that predispose to reflux oesophagitis are also associated with an increased risk of adenocarcinoma. They include achalasia [198,199], scleroderma [200,201] and the Zollinger–Ellison syndrome [202]. Unlike oesophageal squamous cell carcinoma, patients with oesophageal adenocarcinoma do not appear to be at an increased risk of extra-oesophageal malignancies [203], apart from a possible modest increased risk of colorectal cancer [204].

Pathological features

Macroscopic appearances

The largest group of oesophageal adenocarcinomas involve the distal third of the oesophagus and present as ulcerating, infiltrative lesions, frequently associated with stenosis of the oesophageal lumen (40–50%) (Figure 7.12). A minority are fungating (20–25%), flat (10–15%) or polypoid (5–10%) in appearance [205,206]. A diffusely infiltrative growth pattern resembling linitis plastica in the stomach is rarely seen [207]. Early cancers detected during surveillance

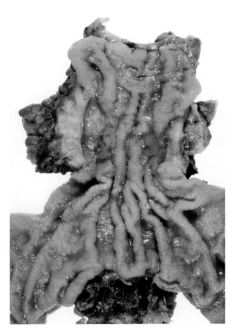

Figure 7.12 Ulcerated adenocarcinoma arising in columnar-lined oesophagus.

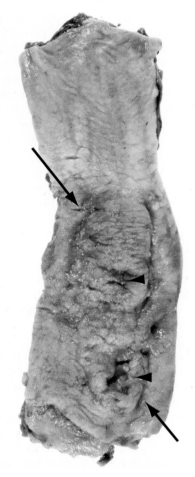

Figure 7.13 This oesophagectomy specimen shows the upper part lined by squamous epithelium and the lower part lined by columnar epithelium, in which there is extensive raised villous dysplasia (arrows) with ulcers (arrowheads) corresponding histologically to multifocal malignant change.

of patients with Barrett's oesophagus may be invisible on endoscopy or appear as small, depressed or elevated lesions [208]. Multicentric tumours have also been described [206,209]. Barrett's oesophagus is often apparent in the background, although in large tumours this may be obliterated completely by the tumour mass. In some of these larger tumours an origin from Barrett's oesophagus can be demonstrated by careful histological examination (Figure 7.13). Patients in whom oesophagectomy is performed after neoadjuvant chemoradiation therapy may not show any residual lesion on gross examination (Figure 7.14). In most cases only a flat ulcerated lesion or an indurated scar is seen at the primary tumour site [210].

Microscopic appearances

Histologically, these tumours show a similar spectrum as adenocarcinomas arising in the stomach. High grade dysplasia is commonly seen in adjacent columnar epithelium [205,211] and may be multifocal (Figure 7.15). Most tumours show a tubular or papillary growth pattern with variable grades of differentiation (Figure 7.16a–d). Well differentiated tumours show more than 95% gland formation, with columnar to cuboidal cells, hyperchromatic or vesicular nuclei, and a variable amount of eosinophilic or clear cytoplasm. Moderately differentiated tumours show gland formation in 50–95% of the tumour and poorly differentiated tumours show less than 50% glandular differentiation. The degree of nuclear pleomorphism parallels the grade of dif-

ferentiation and large, bizarre pleomorphic nuclei are more commonly seen in poorly differentiated tumours. About 5–10% tumours are of the mucinous (colloid) type and show prominent pools of extracellular mucin with floating clusters of tumour cells. Signet ring cell carcinoma phenotype may also be seen in about 5% of cases. Multidirectional differentiation may be present in some tumours and foci of squamous, endocrine cell and Paneth cell differentiation have been described in oesophageal adenocarcinomas [212]. Pagetoid spread into overlying squamous epithelium has been reported and occurs almost always in association with poorly differentiated adenocarcinoma [213].

The presence of duplicated muscularis mucosae in patients with Barrett's oesophagus may lead to errors in staging of early adenocarcinomas. The deep second layer of muscularis mucosae is often thick and may be mistaken

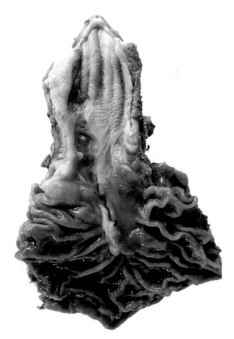

Figure 7.14 Residual tumour may not be grossly visible in resections performed after neoadjuvant chemoradiation therapy. An ulcerated scar is all that remains in the distal oesophagus in this patient with a complete pathological response to treatment. No residual tumour was identified on microscopic examination.

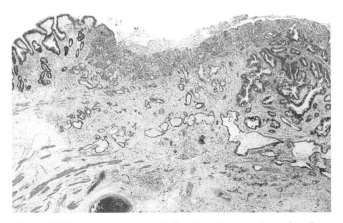

Figure 7.15 Adenocarcinoma infiltrating the oesophageal wall: note high grade epithelial dysplasia at upper left. There is reduplication of the muscularis mucosae.

for muscularis propria [214–216] in an EMR specimen leading to over-staging of invasive carcinomas in about 7% of cases [215]. Carcinomas invading between the two layers of muscularis mucosae are associated with lymphovascular invasion in about 10% of cases [215–216].

In oesophagectomies performed after neoadjuvant therapy, residual tumour is often present in small, isolated clusters in association with dense fibrosis or pools of mucin. Tumour cells may appear more pleomorphic and show endocrine cell differentiation as a consequence of treatment-related changes. Large pools of mucin without any viable tumour cells, with or without calcific deposits, may be present in some cases and should not be reported as residual tumour [217] because these are not associated with increased risk of recurrence or distant metastasis. The amount of residual carcinoma (0%, 1–50% and >50%) seen in resections performed after preoperative chemoradiation has been shown to be a reproducible predictor of survival in some studies [218].

Immunohistochemical studies

Isolated tumour cells in post-neoadjuvant therapy resection specimens may be difficult to distinguish from reactive mesenchymal cells and immunostains for cytokeratins can be helpful in these cases. Cytokeratin stains may also help to determine the deepest extent of tumour invasion for accurate staging when the residual tumour is present predominantly as single cells. In small biopsy specimens, the distinction of primary oesophageal adenocarcinoma from secondary tumours may be an issue. Oesophageal spread from gastric, pulmonary or breast carcinoma is the most common consideration in the differential diagnosis. Immunoreactivity for thyroid transcription factor (TTF-1) and oestrogen receptor is useful in distinguishing oesophageal tumours from pulmonary and breast primaries, respectively. Distinguishing gastric carcinomas with extension into the oesophagus from primary oesophageal adenocarcinoma is virtually impossible using immunohistochemical studies. The presence of Barrett's oesophagus with dysplasia adjacent to the carcinoma is the only convincing and reliable evidence in favour of an oesophageal primary.

Molecular findings

Oesophageal adenocarcinoma arises from Barrett's oesophagus through a progressive, step-wise accumulation of genetic abnormalities. Alterations in DNA content in the form of aneuploidy and tetraploidy are early changes and may occur even before morphological evidence of dysplasia in Barrett's oesophagus [219]. Common alterations in adenocarcinomas include inactivation of p16, p27 and p53, through mutation or transcriptional silencing and overexpression of cyclin D1 [220–222]. Amplification of epidermal growth factor receptor (EGFR) and human epidermal growth factor receptor 2 (HER2) also occur in 15–30% of cases [223,224]. Recent studies have highlighted the importance of micro-RNAs in the pathogenesis of oesophageal adenocarcinoma. Upregulation of miR-196a has been shown in oesophageal adenocarcinoma and is believed to target annexin A1 leading to suppression of apoptosis and enhancement of cell survival [225].

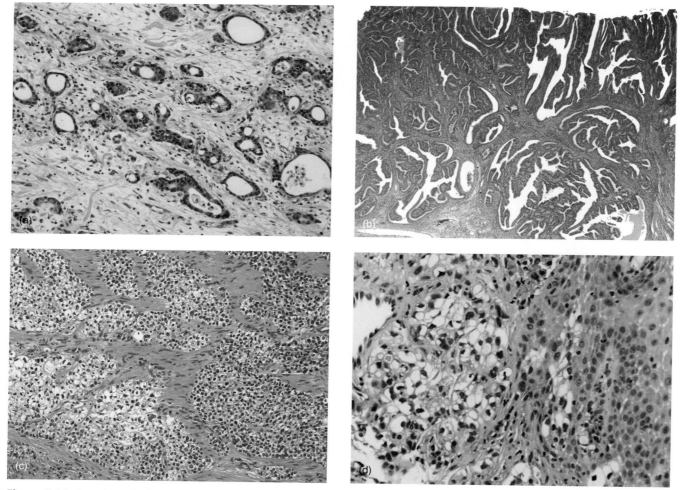

Figure 7.16 Oesophageal adenocarcinomas may show a (a) tubular, (b) papillary or (c) solid architecture on microscopy. (d) Prominent clear cell change, mimicking metastatic renal cell carcinoma, may also be present in some cases.

Natural history and prognosis

Tumour stage remains the best prognostic indicator in oesophageal adenocarcinoma. Survival rates between 80 and 100% are reported for tumours confined to the mucosa or submucosa, but decline significantly to about 10–20% for those that invade deep into the muscularis propria [226–228]. Nodal metastasis to peri-oesophageal and peri-gastric lymph nodes occurs in 50–60% of patients and appears to be closely related to the depth of tumour infiltration. Risk of nodal metastasis is between <5% for intramucosal cancers and >30% for tumours with submucosal invasion. The number of positive lymph nodes is also of prognostic value [229–231] and this is reflected in the recently updated TNM classification, which is summarised in Table 7.1. Distant spread occurs most commonly to the liver and lungs. Histological type is not considered an independent prognostic factor but mucinous and signet ring cell carcinomas have been shown to be associated with poor survival on multi-variate analysis in some studies [232]. Absence of residual tumour (complete pathological response) in resections performed after neoadjuvant therapy is associated with a good outcome whereas persistent nodal disease is a strong adverse prognostic indicator [233–235].

Treatment

Oesophagectomy used to be the standard treatment for high grade dysplasia and early adenocarcinoma. With the realisation that the risk of nodal metastasis in cancer confined to the mucosa is <5%, a figure that is less than the peri-operative mortality for oesophagectomy in many centres, there has been much interest in oesophagus-preserving forms of endoscopic therapy for high grade dysplasia and intramucosal adenocarcinoma. Radiofrequency ablation, EMR and endoscopic submucosal dissection are being increasingly used for treatment instead of oesophagectomy. Patient selection for these procedures is critical and endoscopic forms of therapy are best reserved for well differentiated early cancers with no evidence of lymphovascular invasion. Approximately 10% of patients treated by endoscopy will develop metachronous tumours and, therefore, ablation of background Barrett's oesophagus is often performed after endoscopic resection. Patients with multifocal high grade dysplasia or cancer, those with long-segment Barrett's oesophagus and a large fixed hiatus hernia and severe symptoms, and those with marked oesophageal dysmotility are best treated with vagus-sparing oesophagectomy.

Advanced tumours are treated by neoadjuvant chemoradiation therapy to shrink down the tumour size, followed by complete surgical resection. In a recent meta-analysis of neoadjuvant therapy for oesophageal cancer, data from 3640 patients treated between 2000 and 2008 were analysed. The chemoradiation-related mortality rate was 2.3% and the in-house mortality rate after surgery was 5.2%. A complete resection with negative margins (R0) and complete pathological response (pCR) were reported for 88.4% and 25.8% patients, respectively. The overall 5-year survival rate varied from 16% to 59% for all patients, and from 34% to 62% for patients with pCR [236].

Adenocarcinoma variants

Non-Barrett's oesophagus-associated adenocarcinomas
Occasional reports have described tumours arising in heterotopic gastric mucosa in the cervical oesophagus [237–241] and some have reported tumours with a morphological resemblance to salivary gland tumours in the middle third of the oesophagus, presumably arising from the submucosal gland/ ducts. Proximal adenocarcinomas with no evidence of Barrett's oesophagus between the tumour and the gastro-oesophageal junction may also occur but are extremely rare.

Carcinomas with mixed squamous and glandular differentiation
These are uncommon aggressive tumours in which the tumour shows bidirectional differentiation. They have been described as adenosquamous or mucoepidermoid carcinoma in the literature depending on whether the two components are discrete (adenosquamous) or intimately associated with each other (mucoepidermoid). Adenosquamous carcinomas show a greater degree of nuclear pleomorphism in the squamous component compared with mucoepidermoid carcinoma. A background of Barrett's oesophagus is often present [206,242–244]. The prognosis of these tumours remains uncertain due to their rarity and tumour stage at presentation is the best predictor of survival.

Adenoid cystic carcinoma
Most reported cases of adenoid cystic carcinoma in the past most probably represent examples of basaloid squamous cell carcinoma. True adenoid cystic carcinomas of the oesophagus do occur but are extremely rare [170,171,245]. As in the salivary glands, true examples of this tumour show a biphasic phenotype with predominance of basal/ myoepithelial cells and interspersed ductal structures. The growth pattern is solid, cribriform or tubular and abundant basement membrane-like myxohyaline stroma is present. Marked nuclear pleomorphism, brisk mitotic activity and necrosis are not features of adenoid cystic carcinoma and should alert the pathologist to the possibility of a basaloid squamous cell carcinoma. The ductal cells stain with cytokeratin and the basal/myoepithelial cells with S100 and actin. Typical adenoid cystic carcinomas are slow-growing tumours that rarely metastasise and have a better prognosis than basaloid squamous cell carcinomas, with which they are often confused.

Small cell undifferentiated carcinoma
Since the first description of primary small cell carcinoma of the oesophagus, many more examples of this tumour have been described. Reviews of large series of primary oesophageal carcinomas show a 1–2.4% prevalence of primary small cell carcinoma of the oesophagus [246–249]. In most cases, these tumours are large and protuberant and arise in the middle and lower thirds of the oesophagus. On histological examination, small, fusiform or polygonal cells with little cytoplasm, hyperchromatic nuclei and inconspicuous nucleoli are present, arranged in sheets or anastomosing cords and ribbons. Crush artefact of the tumour cells is common (Figure 7.17), particularly in biopsy material and rosette formation may be present. Squamous differentiation has been described, as well as foci of glandular differentiation, particularly in resection specimens when examined thoroughly [250]. About a third of cases may show areas of squamous cell carcinoma *in situ* [251]. 'Carcinoid'-like areas within an otherwise typical small cell carcinoma have also been reported occasionally [248].

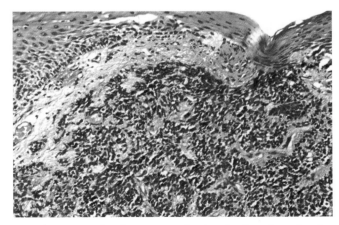

Figure 7.17 Small cell carcinoma showing focal crush artefact is present deep to oesophageal epithelium.

If spread from the lung can be ruled out [252], confirmation that the tumour is a primary small cell carcinoma and not an undifferentiated squamous cell carcinoma depends on the demonstration of endocrine differentiation by chromogranin, CD56 and synaptophysin immunostains or the finding of neurosecretory granules on ultrastructural examination. Poorly differentiated squamous cell carcinomas and adenocarcinomas may stain positively with p63 and cdx-2, respectively, and are helpful in arriving at the correct diagnosis. Primary small cell carcinoma of the oesophagus often expresses TTF-1 so this marker does not distinguish between a primary tumour of the oesophagus and spread from a bronchopulmonary small cell carcinoma.

The prognosis of these tumours is poor with a median survival between 3 and 12 months [247]. Occasional long-term survivors have been reported [253–255]. As with small cell carcinomas of the lung, multi-drug chemotherapy and radiation probably offer the best chance for improvement in survival, with resection reserved for the minority of tumours without evidence of distant metastasis [253].

Choriocarcinoma

Choriocarcinoma of the oesophagus is a rare tumour and has been reported in both men and women [256–259]. They are large, exophytic, fungating tumours with extensive haemorrhage and necrosis. Foci of typical squamous cell carcinoma or Barrett's oesophagus-associated adenocarcinoma are present in many cases. An admixture of syncytiotrophoblast and cytotrophoblast is present on histological examination and one tumour with yolk sac-like differentiation has also been described [258]. The possibility of contiguous spread from a mediastinal germ cell tumour should be excluded in these cases. Most patients have widespread metastatic disease at presentation and the overall prognosis is extremely poor.

Well differentiated endocrine (carcinoid) tumour

Although the designation 'endocrine tumour' or 'neuroendocrine tumour' is now preferred in many quarters, including the World Health Organization (WHO) classifications of 2002 and 2010, most of the small amount of literature on oesophageal tumours uses the alternative nomenclature of 'carcinoid' and this is used here. Oesophageal carcinoids, initially described in 1969, are the rarest of all gastrointestinal carcinoid tumours. In a meta-analysis of 8305 carcinoids of various sites, only three were from the oesophagus, representing only 0.05% of all gastrointestinal carcinoids [260]. The tumours show a striking male predominance (6:1) and present at a variable age. Clinical presentation with carcinoid syndrome is extremely rare [261].

The majority of tumours occur in the distal third of the oesophagus or at the gastro-oesophageal junction. Carcinoids of the oesophagus occur in two clinical scenarios: as a solitary, circumscribed, polypoid lesion or in association with Barrett's oesophagus. Increased numbers of endocrine cells have been described in some cases of Barrett's oesophagus [262,263] and this may contribute to the development of oesophageal carcinoids. These tumours were initially thought to be associated with a poor prognosis [264]. More recent data suggest that cases previously reported as oesophageal carcinoids with an adverse outcome may have been examples of small cell carcinoma due to the presence of high mitotic activity and necrosis [265,266]. Hoang et al. described four new cases in 2002 and reviewed the outcome of other reported cases in literature. All 11 patients with primary oesophageal carcinoids were alive and disease free after 1–23 years of follow-up [267]. This suggests that the prognosis of oesophageal carcinoids is favourable in most instances and that stage at presentation is probably the best prognostic indicator.

Malignant melanoma

It is now well recognised that melanocytes may be identified in normal oesophageal mucosa in 4–8% of normal individuals [268–271]. In a postmortem study of 100 consecutive cases in 1963, basal melanocytes were demonstrated in the oesophagus in four otherwise unremarkable specimens [268]. Benign appearing melanocytosis and atypical junctional lesions, similar to those seen in the skin, have also been described in association with primary oesophageal malignant melanomas. Melanocytosis has been reported in about 25% of primary melanomas of the oesophagus [272].

Metastatic malignant melanoma involves the oesophagus in about 4% of patients with disseminated disease [273]. Therefore, a melanoma presenting in the oesophagus is still much more likely to represent a metastasis rather than a primary tumour. In a recent analysis using the SEER database, the age-adjusted rates of cutaneous, anorectal and oesophageal malignant melanoma were 70.1, 0.27 and 0.03 per million population, respectively [274]. The diagnostic criteria for primary oesophageal melanoma require demonstration of melanocytes in adjacent epithelium with melanocytosis or junctional changes [275]. Most primary oesophageal melanomas are melanotic and show pigmentation on gross and microscopic examination. Examples of primary amelanotic melanoma of the oesophagus have also been described [276].

Primary malignant melanomas have been reported mostly in elderly people in the sixth to seventh decades of life. They are twice as common in men and most often involve the middle or lower third of the oesophagus. Patients present with pain, weight loss or dysphagia. Most lesions appear as polypoid lesions that bulge into the lumen upon endoscopy. The tumours are large, polypoid and

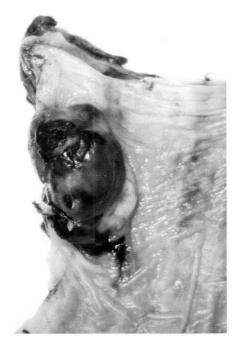

Figure 7.18 Malignant melanoma: a protuberant, superficially ulcerated, pigmented tumour of the middle third of the oesophagus.

friable, with or without obvious pigmentation on gross examination (Figure 7.18). Satellite lesions, melanocytosis or atypical junctional lesions are often present [277–281]. Histologically, spindle and/or epithelioid tumour cells are present which contain melanin pigment demonstrable by conventional stains and are positive for S100, Melan-A and HMB45 immunostains [282]. Both primary and secondary malignant melanomas involving the oesophagus have a poor prognosis. Surgical resection remains the mainstay of therapy for primary tumours, but almost half the patients have disseminated disease at presentation. The mean survival after diagnosis is only about 13 months [283].

Mesenchymal tumours

Gastrointestinal stromal tumours

Gastrointestinal stromal tumours (GISTs) are uncommon in the oesophagus. Dysphagia is the most common symptom in clinically symptomatic cases. However, a significant number of oesophageal GISTs are detected incidentally during examination of oesophagectomies performed for another malignancy. In a series of 150 oesophagectomies performed for oesophageal or oesophago-gastric junction adenocarcinomas, incidental GISTs were detected in 10% of cases [284]. Most tumours occur in the lower third of the oesophagus [285].

The histological and immunophenotypic features of oesophageal GISTs are similar to their much more common counterparts in the stomach (see 'GISTs in the stomach', Chapter 14). Both spindle and epithelioid cell types have been described and the tumour cells stain consistently with KIT and CD34 [286,287]. Desmin positivity, when present, is focal, unlike the diffuse strong positivity seen in leiomyomas. KIT positivity is also seen in melanoma and is a potential pitfall in primary or metastatic amelanotic melanoma involving the oesophagus, which may be mistaken for a GIST [288]. Melanocytic markers Melan A and HMB45 are helpful in arriving at the correct diagnosis. Miettinen et al. reported a series of 17 cases in which 9 patients died of their disease. However, all fatal cases were more than 100 mm in size and one had more than 5 mitoses per 50 high power fields [285]. The incidentally detected tumours in oesophagectomy specimens are invariably associated with an excellent outcome.

Granular cell tumours

Originally reported as a granular cell myoblastoma by Abrikossoff in 1926 [289], granular cell tumours are now regarded as tumours related to Schwann cells. Although skin and subcutaneous soft tissue are the most common site, between 2.7% and 8.1% occur in the gastrointestinal tract [290–293]. About a third of all gastrointestinal granular cell tumours occur in the oesophagus and another 10% in the stomach [294,295]. Examples of multiple tumours involving the oesophagus or stomach or both have also been reported [296]. The majority are found incidentally during upper gastrointestinal endoscopy, where they appear as sessile, yellow, firm nodules, <5 mm in size. Dysphagia, bleeding or abdominal discomfort has been present in symptomatic cases. Most tumours are located in the submucosa (Figure 7.19a) with the overlying squamous epithelium often showing some degree of pseudo-epitheliomatous hyperplasia [297]. The histological appearance is quite uniform from case to case. The tumour cells are oval to spindle in shape with abundant granular eosinophilic cytoplasm and the nuclei are often small and pyknotic (Figure 7.19b). Nucleoli are not prominent and mitoses are seldom present. Diffuse strong S-100 positivity is typical.

Granular cell tumours (GCTs) are usually entirely benign but malignant examples, similar to those in soft tissue, have been reported [298–300]. In a recent report from the Netherlands 52 new cases from 1988–1994 were analysed. Most of the GCTs were solitary (42/44) and localised in the distal oesophagus (33/44). Endoscopic follow-up in 16/17 patients left untreated for 1–60 months showed stable tumour size or regression [301]. The outcome in oesophageal granular cell tumours in almost invariably benign and these patients can be safely followed up endoscopically or alternatively

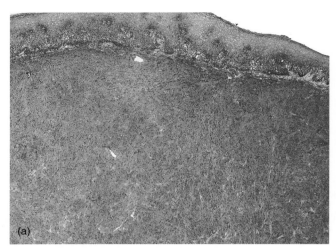 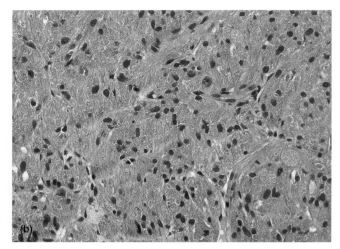

Figure 7.19 Granular cell tumours are located in the submucosa (a) and show large cells with abundant coarsely granular, eosinophilic cytoplasm and pyknotic nuclei (b).

the tumours removed by EMR. Formal oesophageal resection is reserved for patients who are symptomatic, where the tumour is >10 mm in size or cases that show atypical endoscopic, ultrasonographic or histological findings [301,302].

Leiomyomas/smooth muscle tumours

A leiomyoma is the most common benign tumour of the oesophagus [303]. Unlike other parts of the gastrointestinal tract, a large majority of mesenchymal tumours at this site show true smooth muscle differentiation. Leiomyomas are slightly more common in males (1.9:1) and are seen most commonly in the lower oesophagus. Tumours may be single or multiple and careful postmortem studies have identified tiny, subclinical lesions, mostly close to the oesophago-gastric junction, in almost 8% of individuals [304]. A more recent study of oesophagectomies performed after neoadjuvant chemoradiation therapy showed incidental leiomyomas in over 45% of resection specimens [284]. Symptomatic tumours present with dysphagia or pain but nearly half the cases are asymptomatic and detected incidentally on endoscopy performed for an unrelated reason.

These tumours may originate either from the muscularis mucosae or the muscularis propria and present either as a polypoid mass projecting into the lumen or as a lobulated, intramural tumour, occasionally with crater-like ulceration of the mucosal surface [305]. Flat, intramural growths are uncommon. Occasionally, the mass may be mainly extra-oesophageal in position. The cut surface is grey–white and foci of degenerative change or calcification may be seen. Enucleation may be adequate therapy if the tumours are small and oesophagectomy is reserved for patients with large lesions [306,307].

Oesophageal leiomyomatosis is a rare hamartomatous disorder and has been described mostly in children. An association with Alport's syndrome has been reported and a recent report showed partial deletion of smooth muscle-specific genes, *COL4A5* and *COL4A6*, in a patient with Alport's syndrome-associated oesophageal leiomyomatosis [308].

Although most smooth muscle tumours of the oesophagus are benign, the histological distinction between leiomyoma and leiomyosarcoma can be difficult in some cases. Increased cellularity, nuclear atypia, brisk mitotic activity and tumour cell necrosis are the best indicators of malignancy. It is probable that many tumours reported as primary sarcomas of the oesophagus may be examples of spindle cell carcinoma. Immunohistochemical positivity for markers of epithelial differentiation can be helpful in making the distinction.

Neural tumours

All morphological types of peripheral nerve sheath tumours have been described as primary tumours in the oesophagus. Thus, schwannomas, neurofibromas and even rare examples of primary oesophageal perineuriomas have been reported [309–314]. Plexiform schwannoma involving the oesophagus in the setting of neurofibromatosis type 2 has also been described [315].

Other tumours

A whole range of benign and malignant connective tissue tumours of the oesophagus has also been reported. Benign lesions include lipomas [316], rhabdomyomas [317], haemangiomas [318], lymphangiomas [319], glomus tumours [320], inflammatory myofibroblastic tumours [321], chondromas and osteochondromas [322]. Some of these can be considered hamartomas rather than true neoplasms [323]. Primary sarcomas of the oesophagus have also been reported [324–331]. It is important to sample a tumour extensively to exclude the possibility of sarcomatous differentiation in a spindle cell carcinoma before a diagnosis of primary oesophageal sarcoma is made.

Secondary tumours

Secondary tumours in the oesophagus are rare but may cause obstruction and mimic a primary tumour. They may be the result of direct spread from adjacent organs or of spread by the lymphatics or the bloodstream. Direct spread occurs most commonly from carcinoma of the stomach into the lower end of the oesophagus, less commonly from the bronchus/lung or thyroid [332–334]. Immunohistochemical analysis with TTF-1 may be helpful in the latter instances to exclude a primary oesophageal tumour, although primary small cell carcinoma of the oesophagus may be positive for this marker. Lymphatic spread has been described from carcinoma of the breast [332,333,335,336] and bloodstream metastasis from primary tumours in the testis [333], prostate [337,338], kidney [339], endometrium [340] and pancreas [332]. Examples of metastatic disease to the oesophagus from primary pharyngeal tumours are more likely to be examples of multiple primary tumours.

Leukaemia and lymphoma

Leukaemias of all types, particularly acute myeloblastic and acute lymphoblastic forms, commonly involve the gastrointestinal tract, with gut involvement in almost half of all patients with leukaemia shown post mortem [341]. This is either directly by tumour cells or by the various complications of the disease, namely immunodeficiency, coagulation disorders and drug toxicity. In their mildest form, in the oesophagus, they present as subepithelial haemorrhages, which may induce secondary epithelial erosion. Infiltration by leukaemic cells occurs in the submucosa either as microscopic deposits or as macroscopic nodules that undergo necrosis and ulceration [342]. These lesions are often complicated by secondary fungal infections, especially with *Candida* spp., particularly when irradiation or anti-mitotic drugs have been used. Secondary bacterial infection with formation of a pseudo-membrane of debris, fibrin and bacteria also occurs. Chronic graft-versus-host disease not infrequently results in a desquamative oesophagitis in patients after allogeneic bone marrow transplantation [343].

Lymphomatous involvement of the oesophagus is mostly a secondary manifestation in the course of generalised disease. It occurs rarely in Hodgkin lymphoma, either by compression or due to infiltration from affected medias-

tinal lymph nodes and dysphagia can be the presenting symptom [344,345]. It can also occur with non-Hodgkin's lymphomas. A few cases of primary Hodgkin's lymphoma [345,346] and non-Hodgkin's malignant lymphoma of both B- and T-cell phenotype, of the oesophagus, have also been reported [347–350]. Some have occurred in patients with the HIV/AIDS [351–353]. Apparent primary extramedullary plasmacytomas of the oesophagus have been described [354,355]. Rare cases of focal lymphoid hyperplasia [356, 357] and of lymphomatoid granulomatosis in patients with HIV infection, involving the oesophagus, have also been reported [358].

References

1. Parnell SAC, Peppercorn MA, Antonioli DA, Cohen MA, Joffe N. Squamous cell papilloma of the esophagus. Report of a case after peptic esophagitis and repeated bougienage with review of the literature. *Gastroenterology* 1978;**74**:910.
2. Winkler B, Capo V, Reumann W, et al. Human papillomavirus infection of the esophagus. A clinico-pathologic study with demonstration of papillomavirus antigen by the immunoperoxidase technique. *Cancer* 1985;**55**:149.
3. Lavergne D, DeVilliers EM. Papillomavirus in esophageal papillomas and carcinomas. *Int J Cancer* 1999;**80**:680.
4. Odze R, Antonioli D, Shocket D, Noble-Topham S, Goldman H, Upton M. Esophageal squamous papillomas. A clinicopathologic study of 38 lesions and analysis for human papillomavirus by the polymerase chain reaction. *Am J Surg Pathol* 1993; **17**:803.
5. Carr NJ, Bratthauer GL, Lichy JH, Taubenberger JK, Monihan JM, Sobin LH. Squamous cell papillomas of the esophagus: a study of 23 lesions for human papillomavirus by in situ hybridization and the polymerase chain reaction. *Hum Pathol* 1994; **25**:536.
6. Staples DC, Knodell RG, Johnson LF. Inflammatory pseudotumor of the esophagus. A complication of gastroesophageal reflux. *Gastrointest Endosc* 1978;**24**:175.
7. Rabin MS, Bremner CG, Botha JR. The reflux gastroesophageal polyp. *Am J Gastroenterol* 1980;**73**:451.
8. Waluga M, Hartleb M, Sliwinski ZK, et al. Esophageal squamous cell papillomatosis complicated by carcinoma. *Am J Gastroenterol* 2000;**95**:1592.
9. McDonald GB, Brand DL, Thorning DR. Multiple adenomatous neoplasms arising in columnar-lined (Barrett's) esophagus. *Gastroenterology* 1977;**72**:1317.
10. Lee RG. Adenomas arising in Barrett's esophagus. *Am J Clin Pathol* 1986;**85**:629.
11. Thurberg BL, Duray PH, Odze RD. Polypoid dysplasia in Barrett's esophagus: A clinico-pathologic, immunohistochemical and molecular study of five cases. *Hum Pathol* 1999;**30**:745.
12. Banducci D, Rees R, Bluett MK, et al. Pleomorphic adenoma of the cervical esophagus: A rare tumor. *Ann Thorac Surg* 1987; **44**:653.
13. Rouse RV, Soetikno RM, Baker RJ, et al. Esophageal submucosal gland duct adenoma. *Am J Surg Pathol* 1995;**19**:1191.
14. Su J-M, Hsu H-K, Hsu P-I, Wang C-Y, Chang H-C. Sialadenoma papilliferum of the esophagus. *Am J Gastroenterol* 1998;**93**:461.
15. Harada O, Ota H, Katsuyama T, et al. Esophageal gland duct adenoma: Immunohistochemical comparison with the normal esophageal gland and ultrastructural analysis. *Am J Surg Pathol* 2007;**31**:469.

16. Grimm EE, Rulyak SJ, Sekijima JH, Yeh MM. Canalicular adenoma arising in the esophagus. *Arch Pathol Lab Med* 2007; **131**:1595.

17. Kamangar F, Dores GM, Anderson WF. Patterns of cancer incidence, mortality, and prevalence across five continents: defining priorities to reduce cancer disparities in different geographic regions of the world. *J Clin Oncol* 2006;**24**:2137.

18. Jemal A, Siegel R, Xu J, Ward E. Cancer statistics 2010. *CA Cancer J Clin* 2010;**60**:277.

19. Vizcaino AP, Moreno V, Lambert R, Parkin DM. Time trends incidence of both major histologic types of esophageal carcinomas in selected countries 1973–1995. *Int J Cancer* 2002;**99**:860. (Erratum in: *Int J Cancer* 2002;**101**:599.)

20. Botterweck AA, Schouten LJ, Volovics A, Dorant E, van Den Brandt PA. Trends in incidence of adenocarcinoma of the oesophagus and gastric cardia in ten European countries. *Int J Epidemiol* 2000;**29**:645.

21. Wu X, Chen VW, Andrews PA, Ruiz B, Correa P. Incidence of esophageal and gastric cancers among Hispanics, non-Hispanic whites and non-Hispanic blacks in the United States: subsite and histology differences. *Cancer Causes Control* 2007; **18**:585.

22. Trivers KF, Sabatino SA, Stewart SL. Trends in esophageal cancer incidence by histology, United States 1998–2003. *Int J Cancer* 2008;**123**:1422.

23. Baquet CR, Commiskey P, Mack K, Meltzer S, Mishra IS. Esophageal cancer epidemiology in blacks and whites: racial and gender disparities in incidence, mortality, survival rates and histology. *J Natl Med Assoc* 2005;**97**:1471.

24. Blot WJ, Devesa SS, Kneller RW, Fraumeni JF Jr. Rising incidence of adenocarcinoma of the esophagus and gastric cardia. *JAMA* 1991;**265**:1287.

25. Blot WJ, Devesa SS, Fraumeni JF Jr. Continuing climb in rates of esophageal adenocarcinoma: an update (letter). *JAMA* 1993; **270**:1320.

26. Parkin DM, Bray F, Ferlay J, Pisani P. Global Cancer Statistic 2002. *CA Cancer J Clin* 2005;**55**:74.

27. Coordinating group for research on the aetiology of oesophageal cancer of north China. The epidemiology of oesophageal cancer in north China and preliminary results in the investigation of its aetiological factors. *Sci Sin* 1975;**18**:131.

28. Lu JB, Yang WX, Liu JM, Li YS, Qin YM. Trends in morbidity and mortality for oesophageal cancer in Linxian County 1959–1983. *Int J Cancer* 1985;**36**:643.

29. Rose E, McGlashan ND. The spatial distribution of oesophageal carcinoma in the Transkei, South Africa. *Br J Cancer* 1975;**31**:197.

30. Tuyns AJ, Masse LMF. Mortality from cancer of the oesophagus in Brittany. *Int J Epidemiol* 1973;**2**:242.

31. Jacobs A, Cavill IAJ. Pyridoxine and riboflavin status in the Paterson–Kelly syndrome. *Br J Haematol* 1968;**14**:153.

32. Wynder EL. Etiological aspects of squamous cancer of the head and neck. *JAMA* 1971;**215**:452.

33. Morita M, Kumashiro R, Kubo N, et al. Alcohol drinking, cigarette smoking, and the development of squamous cell carcinoma of the esophagus: epidemiology, clinical findings, and prevention. *Int J Clin Oncol* 2010;**15**:126.

34. Islami F, Fedirko V, Tramacere I, et al. Alcohol drinking and esophageal squamous cell carcinoma with focus on light-drinkers and never-smokers: A systematic review and meta-analysis. *Int J Cancer* 2010;**129**:2473.

35. Wang JM, Xu B, Rao JY, Shen HB, Xue HC, Jiang QW. Diet habits, alcohol drinking, tobacco smoking, green tea drinking, and the risk of esophageal squamous cell carcinoma in the Chinese population. *Eur J Gastroenterol Hepatol* 2007; **19**:171.

36. Pandeya N, Williams G, Green AC, Webb PM, Whiteman DC. Australian Cancer Study: Alcohol consumption and the risks of adenocarcinoma and squamous cell carcinoma of the esophagus. *Gastroenterology* 2009;**136**:1215.

37. Chilvers C, Fraser P, Beral V. Alcohol and esophageal cancer: an assessment of the evidence from routinely collected data. *J Epidemiol Commun Health* 1979;**33**:127.

38. Cook P. Cancer of the oesophagus in Africa. *Br J Cancer* 1971; **25**:853.

39. Paymaster JC, Sanghui LD, Gangadharan P. Cancer of the gastrointestinal tract in Western India: epidemiological study. *Cancer* 1968;**21**:279.

40. Epstein SS, Payne PM, Shaw HJ. Multiple primary malignant neoplasms in the air and upper food passages. *Cancer* 1960; **13**:137.

41. Shanta V, Krishnamurthi S. Further study in aetiology of carcinomas of the upper alimentary tract. *Br J Cancer* 1963;**17**:8.

42. Auerbach O, Stout AP, Hammond EC, Garfinkel L. Histologic changes in esophagus in relation to smoking habits. *Arch Environ Health* 1965;**11**:4.

43. Jussawalla DJ, Deshpande VA. Evaluation of cancer risk in tobacco chewers and smokers: an epidemiologic assessment. *Cancer* 1971;**28**:244.

44. Bradshaw E, Schonland M. Smoking, drinking and oesophageal cancer in African males of Johannesburg, South Africa. *Br J Cancer* 1974;**30**:157.

45. Hewer T, Rose E, Ghadirian P, et al. Ingested mutagens from opium and tobacco pyrolysis products and cancer of the oesophagus. *Lancet* 1978;**ii**:494.

46. Iran–IRAC Joint Study Group. Esophageal cancer studies in the Caspian littoral of Iran: results of population studies – a prodrome. *J Natl Cancer Inst* 1977;**59**:1127.

47. Malaveille C, Friesen M, Camus A-M, et al. Mutagens produced by the pyrolysis of opium and its alkaloids as possible risk factors in cancer of the bladder and oesophagus. *Carcinogenesis* 1982;**3**:557.

48. Ghadirian P, Stein GF, Gorodetzky C, et al. Oesophageal cancer studies in the Caspian littoral of Iran: some residual results, including opium use as a risk factor. *Int J Cancer* 1985;**35**:593.

49. Friesen M, O'Neill IK, Malaveille C, et al. Characterization and identification of 6 mutagens in opium pyrolysates implicated in oesophageal cancer in Iran. *Mutat Res* 1985;**150**:177.

50. Tran GD, Sun XD, Abnet CC, et al. Prospective study of risk factors for esophageal and gastric cancers in the Linxian general population trial cohort in China. *Int J Cancer* 2005;**113**:456.

51. Nasrollahzadeh D, Kamangar F, Aghcheli K, et al. Opium, tobacco, and alcohol use in relation to oesophageal squamous cell carcinoma in a high-risk area of Iran. *Br J Cancer* 2008;**98**: 1857.

52. World Cancer Research Fund/American Institute for Cancer Research. *Food, Nutrition, Physical Activity, and the Prevention of Cancer: A global perspective*. Washington, DC: AICR, 2007.

53. Freedman ND, Park Y, Subar AF, et al. Fruit and vegetable intake and esophageal cancer in a large prospective cohort study. *Int J Cancer* 2007;**121**:2753.

54. Li JY, Taylor PR, Li B, et al. Nutrition intervention trials in Linxian, China: multiple vitamin/mineral supplementation, cancer incidence, and disease-specific mortality among adults with esophageal dysplasia. *J Natl Cancer Inst* 1993;**85**:1492.

55. Blot WJ, Li JY, Taylor PR, et al. Nutrition intervention trials in Linxian, China: supplementation with specific vitamin/mineral combinations, cancer incidence, and disease-specific mortality in the general population. *J Natl Cancer Inst* 1993;**85**:1483.

56. Taylor PR, Qiao YL, Dawsey SM, et al. Total and cancer mortality following supplementation with multi-vitamins and min-

erals: Post-intervention follow-up of the general population nutrition intervention trial in Linxian, China. *Cancer Epidemiol Biomarkers Prev* 2004;**13**:1843s.

57. Abnet CC, Lai B, Qiao YL, et al. Zinc concentration in esophageal biopsy specimens measured by x-ray fluorescence and esophageal cancer risk. *J Natl Cancer Inst* 2005;**97**:301.

58. Chen B, Yin H, Dhurandar N. Detection of human papillomavirus DNA in esophageal squamous cell carcinomas by the polymerase chain reaction using general consensus primers. *Hum Pathol* 1994;**25**:920.

59. Suzuk L, Noffsinger AE, Hui YZ, Fenoglio-Preiser CM. Detection of human papillomavirus in esophageal squamous cell carcinoma. *Cancer* 1996;**78**:704.

60. Fidalgo PO, Cravo ML, Chaves PP, Leit'o CN, Mira FC. High prevalence of human papillomavirus in squamous cell carcinoma and matched normal esophageal mucosa. Assessment by polymerase chain reaction. *Cancer* 1995;**76**:1522.

61. Turner JR, Shen LH, Crum CP, et al. Low prevalence of human papillomavirus infection in esophageal squamous cell carcinomas from North America: Analysis by a highly sensitive and specific polymerase chain reaction-based approach. *Hum Pathol* 1997;**28**:174.

62. Poljak M, Cerar A, Seme K. Human papillomavirus infection in esophageal carcinomas: A study of 121 lesions using multiple broad-spectrum polymerase chain reactions and literature review. *Hum Pathol* 1998;**29**:266.

63. Chang F, Syrjanen S, Shen Q, et al. Human papillomavirus involvement in esophageal carcinogenesis in the high-incidence area of China: A study of 700 cases by screening and type-specific in situ hybridization. *Scand J Gastroenterol* 2000;**35**:123.

64. Farhadi M, Tahmasebi Z, Merat S, et al. Human papillomavirus in squamous cell carcinoma of esophagus in a high-risk population. *World J Gastroenterol* 2005;**11**:1200.

65. Syrjänen KJ. Histological changes identical to those of condylomatous lesions found in esophageal squamous cell carcinomas. *Arch Geschwulstforsch* 1982;**52**:283.

66. International Agency for Research on Cancer. Human papillomaviruses. *IARC Monogr Eval Carcinog Risks Hum* 2007; **90**:1.

67. Kiviranta UK. Corrosion carcinoma of the oesophagus: 381 cases of corrosion and 9 cases of corrosion carcinoma. *Acta Otolaryngol* 1953;**42**:89.

68. Appelqvist P, Salmo M. Lye corrosion carcinoma of the esophagus. A review of 63 cases. *Cancer* 1980;**45**:2655.

69. Benedict EB. Carcinoma of the esophagus developing in benign stricture. *N Engl J Med* 1941;**224**:408.

70. Chudecki B. Radiation cancer of the thoracic oesophagus. *Br J Radiol* 1972;**45**:303.

71. Fekete F, Mosnier H, Belghiti J, et al. Esophageal cancer after mediastinal irradiation. *Dysphagia* 1994;**9**:289.

72. Hirayama T. Diet and cancer. *Nutr Cancer* 1979;**1**:67.

73. O'Neill CH, Clarke G, Hodges GM, et al. Silica fragments from millet bran in mucosa surrounding oesophageal tumours in patients in northern China. *Lancet* 1982;**i**:1202.

74. Roth MJ, Guo-Qing W, Lewin KJ, et al. Histopathologic changes seen in esophagectomy specimens from the high-risk region of Linxian, China: potential clues to an etiologic exposure? *Hum Pathol* 1998;**29**:1294.

75. Roth M, QIAO Y, Rothman N, et al. High urine 1-hydroxypyrene glucuronide concentration in Linxian, China, an area of high risk for squamous oesophageal cancer. *Biomarkers* 2001;**6**:381.

76. Ghadirian P. Familial history of esophageal cancer. *Cancer* 1985;**56**:2112.

77. Howel-Evans W, McConnell RB, Clarke CA, Sheppard PM. Carcinoma of the oesophagus with keratosis palmaris et plantaris (tylosis). A study of two families. *Q J Med* 1958; **27**:413.

78. Ashworth MT, Nash JGR, Ellis A, Day DW. Abnormalities of differentiation and maturation in the oesophageal squamous epithelium of patients with tylosis: morphological features. *Histopathology* 1991;**19**:303.

79. Marger RS, Marger D. Carcinoma of the esophagus and tylosis. A lethal genetic combination. *Cancer* 1993;**72**:17.

80. Kelsell DP, Risk JM, Leigh IM, et al. Close mapping of the focal non-epidermolytic palmoplantar keratoderma (PPK) locus associated with oesophageal cancer (TOC). *Hum Mol Genet* 1996;**5**:857.

81. Iwaya T, Maesawa C, Ogasawara S, Tamura G. Tylosis esophageal cancer locus on chromosome 17q25.1 is commonly deleted in sporadic human esophageal cancer. *Gastroenterology* 1998; **114**:1206.

82. Yokoyama A, Kato H, Yokoyama T, et al. Genetic polymorphisms of alcohol and aldehyde dehydrogenases and glutathione S-transferase M1 and drinking, smoking, and diet in Japanese men with esophageal squamous cell carcinoma. *Carcinogenesis* 2003;**23**:1851.

83. Yokoyama A, Muramatsu T, Ohmori T, et al. Alcohol and aldehyde dehydrogenase gene polymorphisms and oropharyngolaryngeal, esophageal and stomach cancers in Japanese alcoholics. *Carcinogenesis* 2001;**22**:433.

84. Lewis SJ, Smith GD. Alcohol, ALDH2, and esophageal cancer: a meta-analysis which illustrates the potentials and limitations of a Mendelian randomization approach. *Cancer Epidemiol Biomarkers Prev* 2005;**14**:1967.

85. Larsson SC, Giovannucci E, Wolk A. Folate intake, *MTHFR* polymorphisms, and risk of esophageal, gastric, and pancreatic cancer: a meta-analysis. *Gastroenterology* 2006;**131**:1271.

86. Pierce WS, MacVaugh H III, Johnson J. Carcinoma of the esophagus arising in patients with achalasia of the cardia. *J Thorac Cardiovasc Surg* 1970;**59**:335.

87. Shin MS. Primary carcinoma arising in the epiphrenic esophageal diverticulum. *South Med J* 1971;**64**:1022.

88. Saldana JG, Cone RO, Hopens TA. Carcinoma arising in an epiphrenic esophageal diverticulum. *Gastrointest Radiol* 1982; **7**:15.

89. Wynder EL, Hultberg S, Jacobsson F, Bross IJ. Environmental factors in cancer of upper alimentary tract: Swedish study with special reference to Plummer–Vinson (Paterson–Kelly) syndrome. *Cancer* 1957;**10**:470.

90. Holmes GKT, Stokes PL, Sorahan TM, Prior P, Waterhouse JAH, Cooke WT. Coeliac disease, gluten-free diet, and malignancy. *Gut* 1976;**17**:612.

91. Cooper BT, Holmes GKT, Ferguson R, Cooke WT. Celiac disease and malignancy. *Medicine* 1980;**59**:249.

92. Tapia RH, White VA. Squamous cell carcinoma arising in a duplication cyst of the esophagus. *Am J Gastroenterol* 1985; **80**:325.

93. Goodner JT, Watson WL. Cancer of the esophagus: its association with other primary cancers. *Cancer* 1956;**9**:1248.

94. Mandard AM, Chasle J, Marnay J, et al. Autopsy findings in 111 cases of esophageal cancer. *Cancer* 1981;**48**:329.

95. Morita M, Kuwano H, Ohno S, et al. Multiple recurrence of carcinoma in the upper aerodigestive tract associated with esophageal cancer. Reference to smoking, drinking and family history. *Int J Cancer* 1994;**58**:207.

96. Dawsey SM, Lewin KJ, Liu F-S, Wang G-Q, Shen Q. Esophageal morphology from Linxian, China. Squamous histologic findings in 754 patients. *Cancer* 1994;**73**:2027.

97. Dawsey SM, Wang G-Q, Weinstein WM, et al. Squamous dysplasia and early esophageal cancer in the Linxian region of

China: distinctive endoscopic lesions. *Gastroenterology* 1993;**105**: 1333.

98. Hashimoto CL, Iriya K, Baba ER, et al. Lugol's dye spray chromoendoscopy establishes early diagnosis of esophageal cancer in patients with primary head and neck cancer. *Am J Gastroenterol* 2005;**100**:275.

99. Coordinating Group for Research on Etiology of Esophageal Cancer in North China. The epidemiology and etiology of esophageal cancer in north China. *Chinese Med J* 1975;**1**:167.

100. Dawsey SM, Lewin KJ, Wang G-Q, et al. Squamous esophageal histology and subsequent risk of squamous cell carcinoma of the esophagus. A prospective follow-up study from Linxian, China. *Cancer* 1994;**74**:1686.

101. Coordinating Groups for the Research of Esophageal Carcinoma. Honan Province and Chinese Academy of Medical Sciences. Studies on relationship between epithelial dysplasia and carcinoma of the esophagus. *Chinese Med J* 1975;**1**:110.

102. Mandard AM, Marnay J, Gignoux M, et al. Cancer of the esophagus and associated lesions: detailed pathologic study of 100 esophagectomy specimens. *Hum Pathol* 1984;**15**:660.

103. Kuwano H, Morita M, Matsuda H, et al. Histopathologic findings of minute foci of squamous cell carcinoma in the human esophagus. *Cancer* 1991;**68**:2617.

104. Nagamatsu M, Mori M, Kuwano H, et al. Serial histologic investigation of squamous epithelial dysplasia associated with carcinoma of the esophagus. *Cancer* 1992;**69**:1094.

105. Morita M, Kuwano H, Yasuda M, et al. The multicentric occurrence of squamous epithelial dysplasia and squamous cell carcinoma in the esophagus. *Cancer* 1994;**74**:2889.

106. Kuwano H, Matsuda H, Matsuoka H, Kai H, Okudaira Y, Sugimachi K. Intra-epithelial carcinoma concomitant with esophageal squamous cell carcinoma. *Cancer* 1987;**59**:783.

107. Kuwano H, Ohno S, Matsuda H, Mori M, Sugimachi K. Serial histologic evaluation of multiple primary squamous cell carcinomas of the esophagus. *Cancer* 1988;**61**:1635.

108. Pesko P, Rakic S, Milicevic M, Bulajic P, Gerzic Z. Prevalence and clinicopathologic features of multiple squamous cell carcinoma of the esophagus. *Cancer* 1994;**73**:2687.

109. Tajima Y, Nakanishi Y, Tachimori Y, et al. Significance of involvement by squamous cell carcinoma of the ducts of esophageal submucosal glands: Analysis of 201 surgically resected superficial squamous cell carcinomas. *Cancer* 2000;**89**:248.

110. Chu P, Stagias J, West AB, Traube M. Diffuse pagetoid squamous cell carcinoma in situ of the esophagus: A case report. *Cancer* 1997;**79**:1865.

111. Hille JJ, Markowitz S, Margolius KA, Isaacson C. Human papillomavirus and carcinoma of the esophagus. *N Engl J Med* 1985; **312**:1707.

112. Liu FS. Pathology of the esophageal cancer. *Cancer Res Prev Treat* 1976;**3**:74.

113. Meyerowitz BR, Shea LT. The natural history of squamous verrucose carcinoma of the esophagus. *J Thorac Cardiovasc Surg* 1971;**61**:646.

114. Minielly JA, Harrison EG Jr, Fontana RS, Payne WS. Verrucous squamous cell carcinoma of the esophagus. *Cancer* 1967;**20**:2078.

115. Parkinson AT, Haidak GL, McInerney RP. Verrucous squamous cell carcinoma of the esophagus following lye stricture. *Chest* 1970;**57**:489.

116. Agha FP, Weatherbee L, Sams JS. Verrucous carcinoma of the esophagus. *Am J Gastroenterol* 1984;**79**:844.

117. Soga J, Tanaka O, Sasaki K, Kawaguchi M, Muto T. Superficial spreading carcinoma of the esophagus. *Cancer* 1982;**50**:1641.

118. Kuwano H, Ueo H, Sugimachi K, et al. Glandular or mucussecreting components in squamous cell carcinoma of the esophagus. *Cancer* 1985;**56**:514.

119. Takubo K, Sasajima K, Yamashita K, et al. Morphological heterogeneity of esophageal carcinoma. *Acta Pathol Jpn* 1989;**39**:180.

120. Newman J, Antonakopoulos GN, Darnton SJ, Matthews HR. The ultrastructure of oesophageal carcinomas: multidirectional differentiation. A transmission electron microscopic study of 43 cases. *J Pathol* 1992;**167**:193.

121. Kato H, Tachimori Y, Watanabe H, et al. Superficial esophageal carcinoma. Surgical treatment and the results. *Cancer* 1990;**66**: 2319.

122. Yoshinaka H, Shimazu H, Fukumoto T, Baba M. Superficial esophageal carcinoma: a clinicopathological review of 59 cases. *Am J Gastroenterol* 1991;**86**:1413.

123. Chinese authors. Pathology of early esophageal squamous cell carcinoma. *Chinese Med J* 1977;**3**:180.

124. Barge J, Molas G, Maillard JN, et al. Superficial oesophageal carcinoma: an oesophageal counterpart of early gastric cancer. *Histopathology* 1981;**5**:499.

125. Bogomoletz VW, Molas G, Gayet B, Potet F. Superficial squamous cell carcinoma of the esophagus. A report of 76 cases and review of the literature. *Am J Surg Pathol* 1989;**13**:535.

126. Hölscher AH, Bollschweiler E, Schneider PM, Siewert JR. Prognosis of early esophageal cancer. Comparison between adeno- and squamous cell carcinoma. *Cancer* 1995;**76**:178.

127. Schmidt LW, Dean PJ, Wilson RT. Superficially invasive squamous cell carcinoma of the esophagus. A study of seven cases in Memphis, Tennessee. *Gastroenterology* 1986;**91**:1456.

128. Watanabe H, Tada T, Iwafuchi M, et al. New definition and macroscopic characteristics of early carcinoma of the esophagus. *Stomach Intest* 1990;**25**:1075.

129. Goseki N, Koike M, Yoshida M. Histopathologic characteristics of early stage esophageal cancer. A comparative study with gastric carcinoma. *Cancer* 1992;**69**:1088.

130. Kitamura K, Ikebe M, Morita M, Matsuda H, Kuwano H, Sugimachi K. The evaluation of submucosal carcinoma of the esophagus as a more advanced carcinoma. *Hepatogastroenterology* 1993;**40**:236.

131. Kumagai Y, Makuuchi H, Mitomi T, Ohmori T. A new classification system for early carcinomas of the esophagus. *Dig Endosc* 1993;**5**:139.

132. Sugimachi K, Ohno S, Matsuda H, Mori M, Kuwano H. Lugolcombined endoscopic detection of minute malignant lesions of the thoracic esophagus. *Ann Surg* 1988;**208**:179.

133. Tsutsui S, Kuwano H, Yasuda M, et al. Extensive spreading carcinoma of the esophagus with invasion restricted to the submucosa. *Am J Gastroenterol* 1995;**90**:1858.

134. Aouad K, Aubertin J-M, Bouillot J-L, Paraf F, Alexandre JH. Extensive spread of squamous cell carcinoma in situ of the esophagus: an unusual case. *Am J Gastroenterol* 1996;**91**:2421.

135. Chu P, Stagias J, West AB, Traube M. Diffuse pagetoid squamous cell carcinoma in situ of the esophagus. A case report. *Cancer* 1997;**79**:1865.

136. Yoshikane H, Tsukamoto Y, Niwa Y, et al. Superficial esophageal carcinoma: evaluation by endoscopic ultrasonography. *Am J Gastroenterol* 1994;**89**:702.

137. Sibille A, Lambert R, Souquet J-C, Sabben G, Descos F. Longterm survival after photodynamic therapy for esophageal cancer. *Gastroenterology* 1995;**108**:337.

138. Kitamura K, Kuwano H, Yasuda M, et al. What is the earliest malignant lesion in the esophagus? *Cancer* 1996;**77**:1614.

139. Ando N, Ozawa S, Kitagawa Y, et al. Improvement in the results of surgical treatment of advanced squamous esophageal carcinoma during 15 consecutive years. *Ann Surg* 2000;**232**: 225.

140. Eguchi T, Nakanishi Y, Shimoda T, et al. Histopathological criteria for additional treatment after endoscopic mucosal resec-

tion for esophageal cancer: Analysis of 464 surgically resected cases. *Mod Pathol* 2006;**19**:475.

141. Mandard AM, Chasle J, Marnay J, et al. Autopsy findings in 111 cases of esophageal cancer. *Cancer* 1981;**48**:329.

142. Wang LS, Chow KC, Chi KH, et al. Prognosis of esophageal squamous cell carcinoma: Analysis of clinicopathological and biological factors. *Am J Gastroenterol* 1999;**94**:1933.

143. Tajima Y, Nakanishi Y, Ochiai A, et al. Histopathologic findings predicting lymph node metastasis and prognosis of patients with superficial esophageal carcinoma: Analysis of 240 surgically resected tumors. *Cancer* 2000;**88**:1285.

144. Sarbia M, Bittinger F, Porschen R, et al. Prognostic value of histopathologic parameters of esophageal squamous cell carcinoma. *Cancer* 1995;**76**:922.

145. Torres CM, Wang HH, Turner JR, et al. Pathologic prognostic factors in esophageal squamous cell carcinoma: A follow-up study of 74 patients with or without preoperative chemoradiation therapy. *Mod Pathol* 1999;**12**:961.

146. Brucher BL, Stein HJ, Werner M, Siewert JR: Lymphatic vessel invasion is an independent prognostic factor in patients with a primary resected tumor with esophageal squamous cell carcinoma. *Cancer* 2001;**92**:2228.

147. Twine CP, Lewis WG, Morgan MA, et al. The assessment of prognosis of surgically resected oesophageal cancer is dependent on the number of lymph nodes examined pathologically. *Histopathology* 2009;**55**:46.

148. Kelty CJ, Kennedy CW, Falk GL. Ratio of metastatic lymph nodes to total number of nodes resected is prognostic for survival in esophageal carcinoma. *J Thorac Oncol* 2010;**5**:1467.

149. Hu Y, Hu C, Zhang H, Ping Y, Chen LQ. How does the number of resected lymph nodes influence TNM staging and prognosis for esophageal carcinoma? *Ann Surg Oncol* 2010;**17**:784.

150. Brucher BL, Becker K, Lordick F, et al. The clinical impact of histopathologic response assessment by residual tumor cell quantification in esophageal squamous cell carcinomas. *Cancer* 2006;**106**:2119.

151. Kraus TK, Perez-Mesa C. Verrucous carcinoma: clinical and pathologic study of 105 cases involving oral cavity, larynx and genitalia. *Cancer* 1966;**19**:26.

152. Jasim KA, Bateson MC. Verrucous carcinoma of the oesophagus – a diagnostic problem. *Histopathology* 1990;**17**:473.

153. Biemond P, ten Kate FJ, van Blankenstein M. Esophageal verrucous carcinoma: histologically a low-grade malignancy but a fatal disease. *J Clin Gastroenterol* 1991;**13**:102.

154. du Boulay CEH, Isaacson P. Carcinoma of the oesophagus with spindle cell features. *Histopathology* 1981;**5**:403.

155. Talbert JL, Cantrell JR. Clinical and pathologic characteristics of carcinosarcoma of the esophagus. *J Thorac Cardiovasc Surg* 1963;**45**:1.

156. Robertson NJ, Rahamim J, Smith MEF. Carcinosarcoma of the oesophagus showing neuroendocrine, squamous and glandular differentiation. *Histopathology* 1997;**31**:263.

157. Guarino M, Reale D, Micoli G, Forloni B. Carcinosarcoma of the oesophagus with rhabdomyoblastic differentiation. *Histopathology* 1993;**22**:493.

158. Osamura RY, Watanabe K, Shimamura K, et al. Polypoid carcinoma of the esophagus. A unifying term for 'carcinosarcoma' and 'pseudosarcoma'. *Am J Surg Pathol* 1978;**2**:201.

159. Battifora H. Spindle cell carcinoma. Ultrastructural evidence of squamous origin and collagen production by the tumor cells. *Cancer* 1976;**37**:2275.

160. Kuhajda FP, Sun T-T, Mendelsohn G. Polypoid squamous carcinoma of the esophagus: a case report with immunostaining for keratin. *Am J Surg Pathol* 1983;**7**:495.

161. Gal AA, Martin SE, Kernen JA, Patterson MJ. Esophageal carcinoma with prominent spindle cells. *Cancer* 1987;**60**:2244.

162. Linder J, Stein RB, Roggli VL, et al. Polypoid tumor of the esophagus. *Hum Pathol* 1987;**18**:692.

163. Kimura N, Tezuka F, Ono I, et al. Myogenic expression in esophageal polypoid tumors. *Arch Pathol Lab Med* 1989;**113**:1159.

164. Thompson L, Chang B, Barsky SH. Monoclonal origins of malignant mixed tumors (carcinosarcomas). Evidence for a divergent histogenesis. *Am J Surg Pathol* 1996;**20**:277.

165. Iwaya T, Maesawa C, Tamura G, et al. Esophageal carcinosarcoma: a genetic analysis. *Gastroenterology* 1997;**113**:973.

166. Iyomasa S, Kato H, Tachimori Y, Watanabe H, Yamaguchi H, Itabashi, M. Carcinosarcoma of the esophagus: A twenty case study. *Jpn J Clin Oncol* 1990;**20**:99.

167. Wain SL, Kier R, Vollmer RT, Bossen EH. Basaloid-squamous carcinoma of the tongue, hypopharynx and larynx. *Hum Pathol* 1986;**17**:1158.

168. Abe K, Sasano H, Itakura Y, Nishihira T, Mori S, Nagura H. Basaloid-squamous carcinoma of the esophagus. A clinicopathologic, DNA ploidy, and immunohistochemical study of seven cases. *Am J Surg Pathol* 1996;**20**:453.

169. Sarbia M, Verreet P, Bittinger F, et al. Basaloid squamous cell carcinoma of the esophagus. Diagnosis and prognosis. *Cancer* 1997;**79**:1871.

170. Kabuto T, Taniguchi K, Iwanaga T, et al. Primary adenoid cystic carcinoma of the esophagus: report of a case. *Cancer* 1979;**43**:2452.

171. Bell-Thomson J, Haggitt RC, Ellis FH. Mucoepidermoid and adenoid cystic carcinoma of the esophagus. *J Thorac Cardiovasc Surg* 1980;**79**:438.

172. Morson BC, Belcher JR. Adenocarcinoma of the oesophagus and ectopic gastric mucosa. *Br J Cancer* 1952;**6**:127.

173. Brown LM, Devesa SS, Chow WH. Incidence of adenocarcinoma of the esophagus among white men by sex, stage and age. *J Natl Cancer Inst* 2008;**100**:1184.

174. Devesa SS, Blot WJ, Fraumeni JF Jr. Changing patterns in the incidence of esophageal and gastric carcinoma in the United States. *Cancer* 1998;**83**:2049.

175. Powell J, McConkey CC. The rising trend in oesophageal adenocarcinoma and gastric cardia. *Eur J Cancer Prev* 1992;**1**:265.

176. Tuyns AJ. Oesophageal cancer in France and Switzerland: recent time trends. *Eur J Cancer Prev* 1992;**1**:275.

177. McKinney PA, Sharp L, MacFarlane GJ, Muir CS. Oesophageal and gastric cancer in Scotland 1960–90. *Br J Cancer* 1995;**71**:411.

178. Armstrong RW, Borman B. Trends in incidence rates of adenocarcinoma of the oesophagus and gastric cardia in New Zealand 1978–92. *Int J Epidemiol* 1996;**25**:941.

179. Thomas RJ, Lade S, Giles GG, Thursfield V. Incidence trends in oesophageal and proximal gastric carcinoma in Victoria. *Aust N Z J Surg* 1996;**66**:271.

180. Hansen S, Wiig JN, Giercksky KE, Tretli S. Esophageal and gastric carcinoma in Norway 1958–92: incidence time trend variability according to morphological subtypes and organ subsites. *Int J Cancer* 1997;**71**:340.

181. Hamilton SR, Smith RRL, Cameron JL. Prevalence and characteristics of Barrett esophagus in patients with adenocarcinoma of the esophagus or esophagogastric junction. *Hum Pathol* 1988;**19**:942.

182. Clark GWB, Smyrk TC, Burdiles P, et al. Is Barrett's metaplasia the source of adenocarcinoma of the cardia? *Arch Surg* 1994;**129**:609.

183. Cameron AJ, Lomboy CT, Pera M, Carpenter HA. Adenocarcinoma of the esophagogastric junction and Barrett's esophagus. *Gastroenterology* 1995;**109**:1541.

184. Pohl H, Sirovich B, Welch HG. Esophageal adenocarcinoma incidence: are we reaching the peak? *Cancer Epidemiol Biomarkers Prev* ;**19**:1468.

185. Hampel H, Abraham NS, El-Serag HB. Meta-analysis: obesity and the risk for gastroesophageal reflux disease and its complications. *Ann Intern Med* 2005;**143**:199.

186. Kubo A, Corley DA. Body mass index and adenocarcinomas of the esophagus or gastric cardia: a systematic review and meta-analysis. *Cancer Epidemiol Biomarkers Prev* 2006;**15**:872.

187. Brown LM, Swanson CA, Gridley G. Adenocarcinoma of the esophagus: role of obesity and diet. *J Natl Cancer Inst* 1995;**87**:104.

188. Chow WH, Blot WJ, Vaughan TL, et al. Body mass index and risk of adenocarcinomas of the esophagus and gastric cardia. *J Natl Cancer Inst* 1998;**90**:150.

189. Kabat GC, Ng SKC, Wynder EL. Tobacco, alcohol intake, and diet in relation to adenocarcinoma of the esophagus and gastric cardia. *Cancer Causes Control* 1993;**4**:123.

190. Brown LM, Silverman DT, Pottern LM, et al. Adenocarcinoma of the esophagus and esophagogastric junction in white men in the United States: alcohol, tobacco, and socioeconomic factors. *Cancer Causes Control* 1994;**5**:333.

191. Gammon MD, Schoenberg JB, Ahsan H, et al. Tobacco, alcohol, and socioeconomic status and adenocarcinomas of the esophagus and gastric cardia. *J Natl Cancer Inst* 1997;**89**:1277.

192. Corley DA, Kerlikowske K, Verma R, et al. Protective association of aspirin/NSAIDs and esophageal cancer: a systematic review and meta-analysis. *Gastroenterology* 2003;**124**:47.

193. Lindblad M, Lagergren J, Garcia Rodriguez LA. Nonsteroidal anti-inflammatory drugs and risk of esophageal and gastric cancer. *Cancer Epidemiol Biomarkers Prev* 2005;**14**:444.

194. Anderson LA, Johnston BT, Watson RG, et al. Nonsteroidal anti-inflammatory drugs and the esophageal inflammation-metaplasia-adenocarcinoma sequence. *Cancer Res* 2006;**66**:4975.

195. Ranka S, Gee JM, Johnson IT, et al. Non-steroidal anti-inflammatory drugs, lower oesophageal sphincter-relaxing drugs and oesophageal cancer. A case-control study. *Digestion* 2006;**74**:109.

196. Fortuny J, Johnson CC, Bohlke K, et al. Use of anti-inflammatory drugs and lower esophageal sphincter-relaxing drugs and risk of esophageal and gastric cancers. *Clin Gastroenterol Hepatol* 2007;**5**:1154.

197. Liu C, Wu MC, Chen F, et al. A large scale genetic association study of esophageal adenocarcinoma risk. *Carcinogenesis* 2010;**31**:1259.

198. Gallez JF, Berger F, Moulinier B, Partensky C. Esophageal adenocarcinoma following Heller myotomy for achalasia. *Endoscopy* 1987;**19**:76.

199. Goodman P, Scott LD, Verani RR, et al. Esophageal adenocarcinoma in a patient with surgically treated achalasia. *Dig Dis Sci* 1990;**35**:1549.

200. McKinley M, Sherlock P. Barrett's esophagus with adenocarcinoma in scleroderma. *Am J Gastroenterol* 1984;**79**:438.

201. Katzka DA, Reynolds JC, Saul SH, et al. Barrett's metaplasia and adenocarcinoma of the esophagus in scleroderma. *Am J Med* 1987;**82**:46.

202. Symonds DA, Ramsey HE. Adenocarcinoma arising in Barrett's esophagus with Zollinger–Ellison syndrome. *Am J Clin Pathol* 1980;**73**:823.

203. Achkar J-P, Post AB, Achkar E, Carey WD. Risk of extraesophageal malignancy in patients with adenocarcinoma arising in Barrett's esophagus. *Am J Gastroenterol* 1995;**90**:39.

204. Logan RFA, Skelly MM. Barrett's oesophagus and colorectal neoplasia: scope for screening? (commentary). *Gut* 1999;**44**:775.

205. Thompson JJ, Zinsser KR, Enterline HT. Barrett's metaplasia in adenocarcinoma of the esophagus and gastroesophageal junction. *Hum Pathol* 1983;**14**:42.

206. Smith RRL, Hamilton SR, Boitnott JK, Rogers EL. The spectrum of carcinoma arising in Barrett's epithelium: a clinicopathologic study of 26 patients. *Am J Surg Pathol* 1984;**8**:563.

207. Chejfec G, Jablokow VR, Gould VE. Linitis plastica carcinoma of the esophagus. *Cancer* 1981;**51**:2139.

208. Reid BJ, Weinstein WM, Lewin KJ, et al. Endoscopic biopsy can detect high-grade dysplasia or early adenocarcinoma in Barrett's esophagus without grossly recognizable neoplastic lesions. *Gastroenterology* 1988;**94**:81.

209. Witt TR, Bains MS, Zaman MB, Martini N. Adenocarcinoma in Barrett's esophagus. *J Thorac Cardiovasc Surg* 1983;**85**:337.

210. Dunne B, Reynolds JV, Mulligan E, et al. A pathological study of tumour regression in oesophageal adenocarcinoma treated with preoperative chemoradiotherapy. *J Clin Pathol* 2001;**54**:841.

211. Hamilton SR, Smith RRL. The relationship between columnar epithelial dysplasia and invasive adenocarcinoma arising in Barrett's esophagus. *Am J Clin Pathol* 1987;**87**:301.

212. Banner BF, Memoli VA, Warren WH, Gould VE. Carcinoma with multi-directional differentiation arising in Barrett's esophagus. *Ultrastruct Pathol* 1983;**4**:205.

213. Abraham SC, Wang H, Wang KK, Wu TT. Paget cells in the esophagus: Assessment of their histologic features and near universal association with underlying esophageal adenocarcinoma. *Am J Surg Pathol* 2008;**32**:1068.

214. Takubo K, Sasajima K, Yamashita K, et al. Double muscularis mucosae in Barrett's esophagus. *Hum Pathol* 1991;**22**:1158.

215. Lewis JT, Wang KK, Abraham SC. Muscularis mucosae duplication and the musculo-fibrous anomaly in endoscopic mucosal resections for Barrett esophagus: implications for staging of adenocarcinoma. *Am J Surg Pathol* 2008;**32**:566.

216. Abraham SC, Krasinskas AM, Correa AM, et al. Duplication of the muscularis mucosae in Barrett esophagus: an underrecognized feature and its implication for staging of adenocarcinoma. *Am J Surg Pathol* 2007;**31**:1719.

217. Hornick JL, Farraye FA, Odze RD. Prevalence and significance of prominent mucin pools in the esophagus post neoadjuvant chemoradiotherapy for Barrett's-associated adenocarcinoma. *Am J Surg Pathol* 2006;**30**:28.

218. Wu TT, Chirieac LR, Abraham SC, et al. Excellent interobserver agreement on grading the extent of residual carcinoma after preoperative chemoradiation in esophageal and esophagogastric junction carcinoma: a reliable predictor for patient outcome. *Am J Surg Pathol* 2007;**31**:58.

219. Rabinovitch PS, Longton G, Blount PL, et al. Predictors of progression in Barrett's esophagus: III. Baseline flow cytometric variables. *Am J Gastroenterol* 2001;**96**:2071.

220. Wongsurawat VJ, Finley JC, Galipeau PC, et al. Genetic mechanisms of p53 LOH in Barrett's esophagus: Implications for biomarker validation. *Cancer Epidemiol Biomarkers Prev* 2006;**15**:509.

221. Lai LA, Paulson TG, Li X, et al. Increasing genomic instability during premalignant neoplastic progression revealed through high resolution array-CGH. *Genes Chromosomes Cancer* 2007;**46**:532.

222. Wong DJ, Paulson TG, Prevo LJ, et al. P16INK4a lesions are common, early abnormalities that undergo clonal expansion in Barrett's metaplastic epithelium. *Cancer Res* 2001;**61**:8284.

223. Thompson SK, Sullivan TR, Davies R, Ruszkiewicz AR. HER-2/neu gene amplification in esophageal adenocarcinoma and its influence on survival. *Ann Surg Oncol* 2011;**18**:2010.

224. Cronin J, McAdam E, Danikas A, et al. Epidermal growth factor receptor (EGFR) is overexpressed in high-grade dysplasia and adenocarcinoma of the esophagus and may represent a biomarker of histological progression in Barrett's esophagus (BE). *Am J Gastroenterol* 2011;**106**:46.

225. Kan T, Meltzer SJ. MicroRNAs in Barrett's esophagus and esophageal adenocarcinoma. *Curr Opin Pharmacol* 2009;**9**:727.

226. Paraf F, Flejou JF, Pignon JP, et al. Surgical pathology of adenocarcinoma arising in Barrett's esophagus: Analysis of 67 cases. *Am J Surg Pathol* 1995;**19**:183.

227. Torres C, Turner JR, Wang HH, et al. Pathologic prognostic factors in Barrett's associated adenocarcinoma: A follow-up study of 96 patients. *Cancer* 1999;**85**:520.

228. van Sandick JW, van Lanschot JJ, ten Kate FJ, et al. Pathology of early invasive adenocarcinoma of the esophagus or esophagogastric junction: Implications for therapeutic decision making. *Cancer* 2000;**88**:2429.

229. Rice TW, Blackstone EH, Rybicki LA, et al. Refining esophageal cancer staging. *J Thorac Cardiovasc Surg* 2003;**125**:1103.

230. Wijnhoven BP, Tran KT, Esterman A, et al. An evaluation of prognostic factors and tumor staging of resected carcinoma of the esophagus. *Ann Surg* 2007;**245**:717.

231. Thompson SK, Ruszkiewicz AR, Jamieson GG, et al. Improving the accuracy of TNM staging in esophageal cancer: a pathological review of resected specimens. *Ann Surg* Oncol 2008;**15**:3447.

232. Chirieac LR, Swisher SG, Correa AM, et al. Signet-ring cell or mucinous histology after preoperative chemoradiation and survival in patients with esophageal or esophagogastric junction adenocarcinoma. Clin *Cancer Res* 2005;**11**:2229.

233. Chirieac LR, Swisher SG, Ajani JA, et al. Posttherapy pathologic stage predicts survival in patients with esophageal carcinoma receiving preoperative chemoradiation. *Cancer* 2005;**103**:1347.

234. Rohatgi P, Swisher SG, Correa AM, et al. Characterization of pathologic complete response after preoperative chemoradiotherapy in carcinoma of the esophagus and outcome after pathologic complete response. *Cancer* 2005;**104**:2365.

235. Gu Y, Swisher SG, Ajani AJ, Correa AM, et al. The number of lymph nodes with metastasis predicts survival in patients with esophageal or esophagogastric junction adenocarcinoma who receive preoperative chemoradiation. *Cancer* 2006;**106**:1017.

236. Courrech Staal EFW, Aleman BMP, Boot H, van Velthuysen M-LF, van Tinteren H. Systematic review of the benefits and risks of neoadjuvant chemoradiation for oesophageal cancer. *Br J Surg* 2010;**97**:1482.

237. Christensen WN, Sternberg SS. Adenocarcinoma of the upper esophagus arising in ectopic gastric mucosa: two case reports and review of the literature. *Am J Surg Pathol* 1987;**11**:397.

238. Ishii K, Ota H, Nakayama J et al. Adenocarcinoma of the cervical oesophagus arising from ectopic gastric mucosa. The histochemical determination of its origin. *Virchows Arch A Pathol Anat* 1991;**419**:159.

239. Takagi A, Ema Y, Horii S, et al. Early adenocarcinoma arising from ectopic gastric mucosa in the cervical esophagus. *Gastrointest Endosc* 1995;**41**:167.

240. Lauwers GY, Scott GV, Vauthey GN. Adenocarcinoma of the upper esophagus arising in cervical ectopic gastric mucosa: Rare evidence of malignant potential of so-called 'inlet patch.' *Dig Dis Sci* 1998;**43**:901.

241. Alrawi SJ, Winston J, Tan D, et al. Primary adenocarcinoma of cervical esophagus. *J Exp Clin Cancer Res* 2005;**24**:325.

242. Bosch A, Frias Z, Caldwell WL. Adenocarcinoma of the esophagus. *Cancer* 1979;**43**:1557.

243. Ter RB, Govil YK, Leite L, et al. Adenosquamous carcinoma in Barrett's esophagus presenting as pseudoachalasia. *Am J Gastroenterol* 1999;**94**:268.

244. Lam KY, Dickens P, Loke SL, et al. Squamous cell carcinoma of the oesophagus with mucin-secreting component (mucoepidermoid carcinoma and adenosquamous carcinoma): A clinicopathologic study and a review of literature. *Eur J Surg Oncol* 1994;**20**:25.

245. Morisaki Y, Yoshizumi Y, Hiroyasu S, et al. Adenoid cystic carcinoma of the esophagus: Report of a case and review of the Japanese literature. *Surg Today* 1996;**26**:1006.

246. McKeown F. Oat-cell carcinoma of the esophagus. *J Pathol Bacteriol* 1952;**64**:889.

247. Casas F, Ferrer F, Farrús B, Casals J, Biete A. Primary small cell carcinoma of the esophagus. A review of the literature with emphasis on therapy and prognosis. *Cancer* 1997;**80**:1366.

248. Briggs JC, Ibrahim NBN. Oat cell carcinoma of the oesophagus: a clinico-pathological study of 23 cases. *Histopathology* 1983;**7**:261.

249. Law SY-K, Fok M, Lam K-Y, Loke S-L, Ma L-T, Wong J. Small cell carcinoma of the esophagus. *Cancer* 1994;**73**:2894.

250. Mori M, Matsukuma A, Adachi Y et al. Small cell carcinoma of the esophagus. *Cancer* 1989;**63**:564.

251. Takubo K, Nakamura K, Sawabe M, et al. Primary undifferentiated small cell carcinoma of the esophagus. *Hum Pathol* 1999;**30**:216.

252. Delpre G, Kadish U, Glanz I, Avidor I. Endoscopic biopsy diagnosis of oat cell carcinoma of the lung penetrating the esophagus. *Gastrointest Endosc* 1980;**26**:104.

253. Nichols GL, Kelsen DP. Small cell carcinoma of the esophagus: the Memorial Hospital experience 1970–87. *Cancer* 1989;**54**:1531.

254. Hussein AM, Feun LG, Sridhar KS, Benedetto P, Waldman S, Otrakji CL. Combination chemotherapy and radiotherapy for small-cell carcinoma of the esophagus. A case report of long-term survival and review of the literature. *Am J Clin Oncol* 1990;**13**:369.

255. McCullen M, Vyas SK, Winwood PJ, Loehry CA, Parham DM, Hamblin T. Long-term survival associated with metastatic small cell carcinoma of the esophagus treated by chemotherapy, autologous bone marrow transplantation, and adjuvant radiation therapy. *Cancer* 1994;**73**:1.

256. Sasano N, Abe S, Satake O. Choriocarcinoma mimicry of an esophageal carcinoma with urinary gonadotropic activities. *Tohoku J Exp Med* 1970;**100**:153.

257. Kikuchi Y, Tsuneta Y, Kawai T, et al. Choriocarcinoma of the esophagus producing chorionic gonadotropin. *Acta Pathol Jpn* 1988;**38**:489.

258. Wasan HS, Schofield JB, Krausz T, Sikora K, Waxman J. Combined choriocarcinoma and yolk sac tumor arising in Barrett's esophagus. *Cancer* 1994;**73**:514.

259. Merimsky O, Jossiphov J, Asna N, et al. Choriocarcinoma arising in a squamous cell carcinoma of the esophagus. *Am J Clin Oncol* 2000;**23**:203.

260. Modlin IM, Sandor A. An analysis of 8305 cases of carcinoid tumors. *Cancer* 1997;**79**:813.

261. Broicher K, Hienz HA. Karzinoid-Syndrom bei im Osophagus lokalisiertem Primartumor. *Z Gastroenterol* 1974;**12** (suppl 0):377.

262. Buchanan AMJ, Grant S, Freeman HJ. Regulatory peptides in Barrett's esophagus. *J Pathol* 1985;**146**:227.

263. Griffin M, Sweeney EC. The relationship of endocrine cells, dysplasia and carcinoembryonic antigen in Barrett's mucosa to adenocarcinoma of the oesophagus. *Histopathology* 1987;**11**:53.

264. Capella C, Solcia E, Sobin LH, et al. Endocrine tumors of the esophagus. In: Hamilton SR, Aaltonen LA (eds), *World Health Organization Classification of Tumors: Pathology and Genetics of Tumors of the Digestive System.* Lyon, France: IARC Press 2000: 26.

265. Oz MC, Ashley PF, Oz M. Atypical gastroesophageal carcinoid: a case report and review of the literature. *Del Med J* 1897; **12**:785.

266. Ready AR, Soul JO, Newman J, et al. Malignant carcinoid tumor of the oesophagus. *Thorax* 1989;**44**:594.

267. Hoang MP, Hobbs CM, Sobin LH, Albores-Saavedra J. Carcinoid tumors of the esophagus. A Clinicopathologic study of four cases. *Am J Surg Pathol* 2002;**26**:517.

268. De la Pava S, Nigogosyan G, Pickren JW, Cabrera A. Melanosis of the esophagus. *Cancer* 1963;**16**:48.

269. Ohashi K, Kato Y, Kanno J, Kasuga T. Melanocytes and melanosis of the oesophagus in Japanese subjects: analysis of factors effecting their increase. *Virchows Arch A Pathol Anat Histopathol* 1990;**417**:137.

270. Sharma SS, Venkateswaran S, Chacko A, Mathan M. Melanosis of the esophagus: an endoscopic, histochemical, and ultrastructural study. *Gastroenterology* 1991;**100**:13.

271. Bogomoletz WV, Lecat M, Amoros F. Melanosis of the oesophagus in a Western patient. *Histopathology* 1997;**30**:498.

272. DiCostanzo DP, Urmacher C. Primary malignant melanoma of the esophagus. *Am J Surg Pathol* 1987;**11**:46.

273. Wysocki W, Komorowski A, Daradz Z. Gastrointestinal metastases from malignant melanoma: report of a case. *Surg Today* 2004;**34**:542.

274. Cote TR, Sobin LH. Primary melanomas of the esophagus and anorectum: epidemiologic comparison with melanoma of the skin. *Melanoma Res* 2009;**19**:58.

275. Raven RW, Dawson I. Malignant melanoma of the oesophagus. *Br J Surg* 1964;**51**:551.

276. Stringa O, Valdez R, Beguerie JR, et al. Primary amelanotic melanoma of the esophagus. *Int J Dermatol* 2006;**45**:1207.

277. Sakornpant P, Barlow D, Bevan CM. Two cases of primary malignant melanoma of the oesophagus. *Br J Surg* 1964;**51**:386.

278. Piccone VA, Klopstock R, Leveen HH, Sika J. Primary malignant melanoma of the esophagus associated with melanosis of the entire esophagus. First case report. *J Thorac Cardiovasc Surg* 1970;**59**:864.

279. Muto M, Saito Y, Koike T, et al. Primary malignant melanoma of the esophagus with diffuse pigmentation resembling superficial spreading melanoma. *Am J Gastroenterol* 1997;**92**:1936.

280. Musher DR, Lindner AE. Primary melanoma of the esophagus. *Dig Dis Sci* 1974;**19**:855.

281. Sabanathan S, Eng J, Pradhan GN. Primary malignant melanoma of the esophagus. *Am J Gastroenterol* 1989;**84**: 1475.

282. Gown AM, Vogel AM, Hoak D, et al. Monoclonal antibodies specific for melanocytic tumors distinguish subpopulations of melanocytes. *Am J Pathol* 1986;**123**:195.

283. Chalkiadakis G, Wihlm JM, Morand G, Weill-Bousson M, Witz JP. Primary malignant melanoma of the esophagus. *Ann Thorac Surg* 1985;**39**:472.

284. Abraham SC, Krasinskas AM, Hofstetter WL, Swisher SG, Wu TT. 'Seedling' mesenchymal tumors (gastrointestinal stromal tumors and leiomyomas) are common incidental tumors of the esophagogastric junction. *Am J Surg Pathol* 2007; **31**:1629.

285. Miettinen M, Sarlomo-Rikala M, Sobin LH, Lasota J. Esophageal stromal tumors: a clinicopathologic, immunohistochemical, and molecular genetic study of 17 cases with comparison

286. Miettinen M, Virolainen M, Rikala MS. Gastrointestinal stromal tumors. Value of CD34 antigen in their identification from true leiomyomas and schwannomas. *Am J Surg Pathol* 1995;**19**:207.

287. Sarlomo-Rikala M, Kovatich A, Barusevicius A, Miettinen M. CD117: a sensitive marker for gastrointestinal stromal tumors that is more specific than CD34. *Mod Pathol* 1998;**11**:728.

288. Wang S, Thamboo TP, Nga M, Zin T, Cheng A, Tan KB. C-kit positive amelanotic melanoma of the oesophagus: a potential diagnostic pitfall. *Pathology* 2008;**40**:527.

289. Abrikossoff AI. Uber Myome, ausgehend van der quergestneiften willkurlichen Muskulatur. *Virchows Arch Pathol Anat* 1926; **260**:214.

290. McSwain G, Colpitts R, Kreutner A, et al. Granular cell myoblastoma. *Surg Gynecol Obstet* 1980;**150**:703.

291. Fisher ER, Wechsler H. Granular cell myoblastoma – a misnomer. Electron microscopic and histochemical evidence concerning its Schwann cell derivation and nature (granular cell schwannoma). *Cancer* 1962;**15**:936.

292. Mittal KR, True LD. Origin of granules in granular cell tumor. Intracellular myelin formation with autodigestion. *Arch Pathol Lab Med* 1988;**112**:302.

293. Miettinen M, Lehtonen E, Lehtola H, Ekblom P, Lehto VP, Virtanen I. Histogenesis of granular cell tumor. An immunohistochemical and ultrastructural study. *J Pathol* 1984;**142**: 221.

294. Lack E, Worsham G, Callihan M. Granular cell tumor: a clinicopathologic study of 110 patients. *J Surg Oncol* 1980; **13**:301.

295. Johnston J, Helwig EB. Granular cell tumors of the gastrointestinal tract and perianal region: a study of 74 cases. *Dig Dis Sci* 1981;**26**:807.

296. Maekawa H, Maekawa T, Yabuki K, et al. Multiple esophagogastric granular cell tumors. *J Gastroenterol* 2003;**38**:776.

297. Gloor F, Clemencon G. Granular cell tumours ('myoblastomas') of the esophagus. *Endoscopy* 1975;**7**:239.

298. Crawford ES, DeBakey ME. Granular cell myoblastoma: two unusual cases. *Cancer* 1953;**6**:786.

299. Obiditsh-Mayer I, Salzer-Kuntschik M. Malignes, 'gekirntzelliges Neurom' soganntes Myoblastemmoym des Oesophagus. *Beitr Pathol Anat* 1961;**125**:357.

300. Ohmori T, Arita N, Uraga N, Tabei R, Tani M, Okamura H. Malignant granular cell tumor of the esophagus: a case report with light and electron microscopic, histochemical and immunohistochemical study. *Acta Pathol Jpn* 1987;**37**:775.

301. Voskuil JH, Van Dijk MM, Wagenaar SC, Van Vliet ACM, Timmer R, Van Hees PAM. Occurrence of esophageal granular cell tumors in The Netherlands between 1988 and 1994. *Dig Dis Sci* 2001;**46**:1610.

302. Goldblum JR, Rice TW, Zuccaro G, Richter JE. Granular cell tumors of the esophagus: a clinical and pathologic study of 13 cases. *Ann Thorac Surg* 1996;**62**:860.

303. Seremetis MC, Lyons WS, De Cuzman VC, Peabody JW Jr. Leiomyomata of the esophagus. Analysis of 838 cases. *Cancer* 1976; **38**:2166.

304. Takubo K, Nakagawa H, Tsuchiya S, Mitomo Y, Sasajima K, Shirota A. Seedling leiomyoma of the esophagus and esophagogastric junction zone. *Hum Pathol* 1981;**12**:1006.

305. Barrett NR. Benign smooth muscle tumours of the oesophagus. *Thorax* 1964;**19**:185.

306. Mutrie CJ, Donahue DM, Wain JC, et al. Esophageal leiomyoma: A 40-year experience. *Ann Thorac Surg* 2005;**79**:1122.

with esophageal leiomyomas and leiomyosarcomas. *Am J Surg Pathol* 2000;**24**:211.

307. Jiang G, Zhao H, Yang F, et al. Thoracoscopic enucleation of esophageal leiomyoma: a retrospective study on 40 cases. *Dis Esoph* 2009;**22**:279.

308. Anker MC, Arnemann J, Neumann K, Ahrens P, Schmidt H, Konig R. Alport syndrome with diffuse leiomyomatosis. *Am J Med Genet* 2003;**119A**:381.

309. Arai T, Sugimura H, Suzuki M, et al. Benign schwannoma of the esophagus: report of two cases with immunohistochemical and ultrastructural studies. *Pathol Int* 1994;**44**:460.

310. Prevot S, Bienvenu L, Vaillant JC, Saint-Maur PP. Benign schwannoma of the digestive tract: a clinicopathologic and immunohistochemical study of five cases, including a case of esophageal tumor. *Am J Surg Pathol* 1999;**23**:431.

311. Saitoh K, Nasu M, Kamiyama R, et al. Solitary neurofibroma of the esophagus. *Acta Pathol Jpn* 1985;**35**:527.

312. Sica GS, Sujendran V, Warren B, Maynard ND. Neurofibromatosis of the esophagus. *Ann Thorac Surg* 2006;**81**:1138.

313. Ganeshan A, Hon LQ, Soonawalla Z, De Costa H. Plexiform neurofibroma of the oesophagus: a mimicker of malignancy. *Br J Radiol* 2005;**78**:1095.

314. Kelesidis T, Tarbox A, Lopez M, Aish L. Perineurioma of esophagus: a first case report. *Am J Med* Sci 2009;**338**:230.

315. Retrosi G, Nanni L, Ricci R, Manzoni C, Pintus C. Plexiform schwannoma of the esophagus in a child with neurofibromatosis type 2. *J Pediatr Surg* 2009;**44**:1458.

316. Zschiedrich M, Neuhaus P. Pedunculated giant lipoma of the esophagus. *Am J Gastroenterol* 1990;**85**:1614.

317. Pai GK, Pai PK, Kamath SM. Adult rhabdomyoma of the esophagus. *J Pediatr Surg* 1987;**22**:991.

318. Gilbert HW, Weston MJ, Thompson MH. Cavernous haemangioma of the oesophagus. *Br J Surg* 1990;**77**:106.

319. Yoshida Y, Okamura T, Ezaki T, et al. Lymphangioma of the oesophagus: a case report and review of the literature. *Thorax* 1994;**49**:1267.

320. Lewin KJ, Appelman HD. Tumors of the esophagus and stomach. In: *Atlas of Tumor Pathology*. Washington: Armed Forces Institute of Pathology, Third Series, Fascicle 18 1996.

321. Chen Y, Tang Y, Li H, et al. Inflammatory myofibroblastic tumor of the esophagus. *Ann Thorac Surg* 2010;**89**:607.

322. Mahour GH, Harrison EG Jr. Osteochondroma (tracheobronchial choristoma) of the esophagus. Report of a case. *Cancer* 1967;**20**:1489.

323. Saitoh Y, Inomata Y, Tadaki N, et al. Pedunculated intraluminal osteochondromatous hamartoma of the esophagus. *J Otolaryngol* 1990;**19**:339.

324. Bloch MJ, Iozzo RV, Edmunds LH Jr, Brooks JJ. Polypoid synovial sarcoma of the esophagus. *Gastroenterology* 1987;**92**:229.

325. Anton-Pacheco J, Cano I, Cuadros J et al. Synovial sarcoma of the esophagus. *J Pediatr Surg* 1996;**31**:1703.

326. Aagaard MT, Kristensen IB, Lund O, et al. Primary malignant non-epithelial tumours of the thoracic oesophagus and cardia in a 25-year surgical material. *Scand J Gastroenterol* 1990;**25**:876.

327. Willen R, Lillo-Gil R, Willen H, et al. Embryonal rhabdomyosarcoma of the oesophagus: case report. *Acta Chir Scand* 1989;**155**:59.

328. Vartio T, Nickels J, Hockerstedt K, Scheinin TM. Rhabdomyosarcoma of the oesophagus. Virchows *Arch Pathol Anat* 1980;**386**:357.

329. Friedman SL, Wright TL, Altman DF. Gastrointestinal Kaposi's sarcoma in patients with acquired immunodeficiency syndrome. Endoscopic and autopsy findings. *Gastroenterology* 1985;**89**:102.

330. Mansour KA, Fritz RC, Jacobs DM, Vellios F. Pedunculated liposarcoma of the esophagus: a first case report. *J Thorac Cardiovasc Surg* 1983;**86**:447.

331. McIntyre M, Webb JN, Browning GCP. Osteosarcoma of the esophagus. *Hum Pathol* 1982;**13**:680.

332. Toreson WE. Secondary carcinoma of the esophagus as a cause of dysphagia. *Arch Pathol* 1944;**38**:82.

333. Gowing NFC. Secondary tumours. In: Tanner NC, Smithers DW, eds. *Tumours of the Oesophagus*. Edinburgh: Churchill Livingstone, 1961.

334. Hale RJ, Merchant W, Hasleton PS. Polypoidal intra-oesophageal thyroid carcinoma: a rare cause of dysphagia. *Histopathology* 1990;**17**:475.

335. Polk HC Jr, Camp FA, Walker AW. Dysphagia and oesophageal stenosis: manifestations of metastatic mammary cancer. *Cancer* 1967;**20**:2002.

336. Varanasi RV, Saltzman JR, Krims P, Crimaldi A, Colby J. Breast carcinoma metastatic to the esophagus: clinicopathological and management features of four cases, and literature review. *Am J Gastroenterol* 1995;**90**:1495.

337. Gross P, Freedman LJ. Obstructing secondary carcinoma of the esophagus. *Arch Pathol* 1942;**33**:361.

338. Gore RM, Sparberg M. Metastatic carcinoma of the prostate to the esophagus. *Am J Gastroenterol* 1982;**77**:358.

339. Nussbaum M, Grossman M. Metastases to the esophagus causing gastrointestinal bleeding. *Am J Gastroenterol* 1976;**66**:467.

340. Zarian LP, Berliner L, Redmond P. Metastatic endometrial carcinoma to the esophagus. *Am J Gastroenterol* 1983;**78**:9.

341. Winton RR, Gwynn AM, Robert JC, et al. Leukemia and the bowel. *Med J Aust* 1975;**4**:89.

342. Kothur R, Marsh F, Posner G, Dosik H. Endoscopic leukemic polyposis. *Am J Gastroenterol* 1990;**85**:884.

343. McDonald GB, Shulman HM, Sullivan KM, Spencer GD. Intestinal and hepatic complications of human bone marrow transplantation. Part II. *Gastroenterology* 1986;**90**:770.

344. Strauch M, Martin TH, Remmele W. Hodgkin's disease of the oesophagus. *Endoscopy* 1971;**4**:207.

345. Stein HA, Murray D, Warner HA. Primary Hodgkin's disease of the esophagus. *Dig Dis Sci* 1981;**26**:457.

346. Loeb DS, Ribeiro A, Menke DM. Hodgkin's disease of the esophagus: report of a case. *Am J Gastroenterol* 1999;**94**:520.

347. Nagrani M, Lavigne BC, Siskind BN, et al. Primary non-Hodgkin's lymphoma of the esophagus. *Arch Intern Med* 1989;**149**:193.

348. Bolondi L, de Giorgio R, Santi V, et al. Primary non-Hodgkin's T-cell lymphoma of the esophagus: a case with peculiar endoscopic ultrasonographic pattern. *Dig Dis Sci* 1990;**35**:1426.

349. Mengoli M, Marchi M, Rota E, Bertolotti M, Gollini C, Signorelli S. Primary non-Hodgkin's lymphoma of the esophagus. *Am J Gastroenterol* 1990;**85**:737.

350. Pearson JM, Borg-Grech A. Primary ki-1 (CD30)-positive, large cell, anaplastic lymphoma of the esophagus. *Cancer* 1991;**68**:418.

351. Bernal A, del Junco GW. Endoscopic and pathologic features of esophageal lymphoma: a report of four cases in patients with acquired immune deficiency syndrome. *Gastrointest Endosc* 1986;**32**:96.

352. Chow DC, Sheikh SH, Eickhoff L, Soloway GN, Saul Z. Primary esophageal lymphoma in AIDS presenting as a nonhealing esophageal ulcer. *Am J Gastroenterol* 1996;**91**:602.

353. Marnejon T, Scoccia V. The coexistence of primary esophageal lymphoma and *Candida glabrata* esophagitis presenting as dysphagia and odynophagia in a patient with acquired immunodeficiency syndrome. *Am J Gastroenterol* 1997;**92**:354.

354. Morris WT, Pead JL. Myeloma of the oesophagus. *J Clin Pathol* 1972;**25**:537.

355. Ahmed M, Ramos S, Sika S, Leveen HH, Piccone VA. Primary extramedullary esophageal plasmacytoma. First case report. *Cancer* 1976;**38**:943.

356. Sheahan DG, West AB. Focal lymphoid hyperplasia (pseudolymphoma) of the esophagus. *Am J Surg Pathol* 1985;**9**:141.

357. Gervaz E, Potet F, Mahé R, Lemasson G. Focal lymphoid hyperplasia of the oesophagus: report of a case. *Histopathology* 1992; **21**:187.

358. Lin-Greenberg A, Villacin A, Moussa G. Lymphomatoid granulomatosis presenting as ulcerodestructive gastrointestinal tract lesions in patients with human immunodeficiency virus infection. *Arch Intern Med* 1990;**150**:2581.

CHAPTER 8

Miscellaneous conditions of the oesophagus

Raymond F.T. McMahon

University of Manchester, Manchester, UK

Trauma

Rupture and perforation

At its upper end, the oesophagus is relatively well protected by surrounding structures in the neck and traumatic lesions virtually always arise from intraluminal causes. An exception is penetrating injuries from gunshot and knife wounds [1]. Most perforations are iatrogenic, following intubation, dilatation or attempted extraction of foreign bodies [2–4]. The risk of perforation with oesophago-gastro-duodenoscopy is estimated at 0.03%, although this can increase up to 17% depending on the underlying oesophageal condition and other co-morbidities [5]. A more recent cause of iatrogenic injury is the insertion of stents used in temporary or permanent palliation of oesophageal strictures [6]. Plastic stents for benign strictures are less prone to causing injury than metal stents used for palliation of malignant strictures. Other injuries are due to swallowed sharp foreign bodies, especially bones, the impaction of foreign bodies with subsequent fistula formation and the ulceration and inflammation that follow the swallowing of corrosive fluids [7–9]. A high index of suspicion is called for when symptoms follow trans-oesophageal echocardiography [10]. Perforation of the oesophagus has a higher mortality than that of other sites in the gastrointestinal tract [11].

Boerhaave's syndrome classically presents with pain, dyspnoea and shock followed by forceful vomiting [12]. It is a form of rupture of the oesophagus caused by a rapid rise in intraluminal pressure and can follow indirect trauma or be spontaneous, often with associated haematoma [13].

It is rare and occurs as an abrupt longitudinal rent, nearly always in the left lateral wall at the lower end of a previously normal oesophagus [14]. The average tear is 20 mm long and 30–60 mm above the diaphragm [8,12]. It is much more common in males and probably results from a sudden rise in intra-oesophageal pressure due to sudden compression or contraction of the stomach after a blow to the abdomen or over-distension with vomiting. A common complication is surgical emphysema at the base of the neck. Less commonly Boerhaave's syndrome may present with more chronic symptoms of dysphagia and upper abdominal pain, as reported in association with an intrathoracic cyst [15].

Rare causes of sudden and unexpected death associated with oesophageal abnormalities include perforation, haemorrhage, rupture, tumours and involvement with vascular catastrophes such as aorto-oesophageal fistulae [16].

Mallory–Weiss syndrome

Risk factors for Mallory–Weiss tears include a history of alcohol use, recent alcohol binges, anticoagulant use and other coagulopathies, non-steroidal anti-inflammatory use and hiatus hernia [16]. The main common risk factor is alcohol use but, in 23% of cases, no specific risk factor can be identified [17]. Less traumatic events, including vomiting, severe retching and, even, snoring [18], can produce linear partial oesophageal tears, usually just above the cardia on the right lateral wall. The tear may extend to involve the lesser curve of the stomach in the presence of a hiatus hernia [13,19]. These usually involve mainly the mucosa and

Morson and Dawson's Gastrointestinal Pathology, Fifth Edition. Edited by Neil A. Shepherd, Bryan F. Warren, Geraint T. Williams, Joel K. Greenson, Gregory Y. Lauwers and Marco R. Novelli.

submucosa and can be associated with severe haemorrhage; they may progress to ulceration with the risk of subsequent perforation. They have been described following upper endoscopy, particularly in association with hiatus hernia [20], and account for 5–10% of all acute upper gastrointestinal bleeds [21]. They are rare, but described, in children [22]. Although most cases pursue a benign course, the bleeding may be significant and recurrent and require therapeutic endoscopy [23, 24] and surgery. The main predictors of poor outcome in Mallory–Weiss tear are a low haematocrit at presentation and active bleeding at first endoscopy [17].

Oesophageal casts

Very rarely the complete squamous lining of the oesophagus can be vomited as a cast. This can follow the ingestion of extremely hot liquids, be spontaneous [25] or be associated with intramural rupture [26] and Mallory–Weiss syndrome [27]. Despite its apparent severity, healing with mucosal regeneration is the rule. An unusual form of oesophageal cast has been described in acrylic glue sclerotherapy used in the treatment of variceal bleeding where the glue cast adopts the shape of the vessels obliterated [28].

Varices

The normal venous drainage of the oesophagus has four components [29–31]. Small intraepithelial venules drain into a rich superficial submucosal venous plexus running longitudinally. This connects with a deeper plexus of fewer, larger veins, still in the submucosa. From it, perforating veins pass through the muscle coats to reach the serosal plexus. These plexuses link with those of the upper part of the stomach and drain partly into the portal, and partly into the systemic, venous system, forming, with the haemorrhoidal and periumbilical veins, an important linkage between the systemic and portal systems.

In portal hypertension these venous plexuses dilate to form oesophageal varices, consisting of enormously distended venous channels which lie immediately beneath the mucosa and are prone to rupture [29–31]. There is evidence that venous stasis and consequent anoxia produce necrosis and ulceration of the overlying epithelium, which increases this risk [32]. At postmortem examination the varices are collapsed and can be difficult to detect but they can be shown if the oesophagus and stomach are removed by everting the oesophagus or by injection techniques (see Chapter 3).

The treatment of varices was formerly by portacaval shunt but many patients are now given endoscopic sclerotherapy or, more recently, rubber band ligation [33,34]. With the former, when such patients come to necropsy at varying times after injection, a sequence of events can be determined. Initially there is venous thrombosis, most extensive in the submucosa, less marked in muscle coats

and subserosa/adventitia; this is accompanied by extensive superficial and less extensive deep tissue necrosis. Ulceration follows, suggesting that some of the sclerosing fluid has leaked into surrounding tissue. In those patients who survive, a degree of fibrosis and eventual re-epithelialisation follow [35,36] with possible fibrosis and ring formation [37]. This can lead to stenosis with dysphagia and there is evidence that the greater the number of treatments and the amount of sclerosant used the greater the risk of stricture formation [38,39]. A study of rabbits suggests that paravenous injection leads to perivenal fibrosis with severe venous compression and may be more effective than intravenous injection as a form of treatment [40].

An alternative treatment is to excise a full-thickness ring of oesophagus and then to staple the two ends together; this technique provides an excised ring of tissue and allows previously untreated varices to be examined histologically [41]. Such specimens show dilated vascular channels within and immediately beneath the squamous epithelium, some of which rupture into the lumen. These channels do not have a surrounding basement membrane or an endothelial cell lining but they are probably not artefactual. They may represent a stage in the development of oesophagitis [42,43], although more probably they result from venous congestion [44]. Some reports suggest that the mucosal changes may reflect differences between bleeders and non-bleeders [45,46] but evidence is confusing.

Webs and rings

Oesophageal webs consist of single, or less commonly multiple, thin mucosal membranes that project into the oesophageal lumen. They may arise at all levels but are most frequent in the post-cricoid region, where they are usually attached anteriorly and laterally and have an eccentric lumen posteriorly. A significant proportion of upper oesophageal webs have occurred in women with glossitis and iron deficiency anaemia, the Plummer–Vinson syndrome, alternatively known in the UK as the Paterson Brown–Kelly syndrome [47,48]. They are also seen in patients with epidermolysis bullosa, benign mucous membrane pemphigoid and pemphigus vulgaris, in which they may be the end-result of scarring [49–53]. Other associations have been with heterotopic gastric mucosa [54], chronic graft-versus-host disease following allogeneic bone marrow transplantation [55], after radiotherapy [56] and in patients with coeliac disease [57].

The histological appearances show normal squamous epithelium or there may be acanthosis and parakeratosis and/or hyperkeratosis. Marked basal cell hyperplasia and elongation of submucosal papillae in biopsies from all levels of the oesophagus have been described in patients with multiple oesophageal webs [58]. There is a significant association between the presence of oesophageal webs

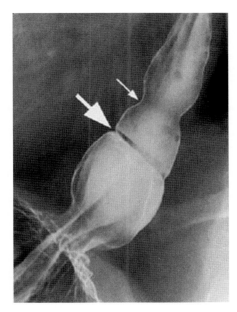

Figure 8.1 Barium swallow of a patient with rings (small and large arrows) of the oesophagus. (Reprinted by permission of Macmillan Publishers Ltd [GI Motility on-line] (doi:10.1038/gim041), 2006.)

and the development of carcinoma of the buccal mucosa or oesophagus and, in one series [47], this occurred in 9 of 58 patients. It has been postulated that the increased cancer risk is related to iron deficiency and anaemia causing oxidative stress and DNA damage [59].

Two types of 'ring' are found in the oesophagus. Mucosal rings (so-called 'B' rings) are found at the lower end of the oesophagus and consist of a symmetrical concentric transverse fold of mucosa projecting into, and completely encircling, the lumen [60] (Figure 8.1). Such rings are not uncommon at postmortem examination [61] or endoscopy [62]. Most patients are asymptomatic but dysphagia may develop with decreasing diameter of the lumen. Histological studies have in general shown that the upper surface of the ring consists of normal squamous epithelium and the lower surface of junctional epithelium. The core of the ring consists of connective tissue, fibres of the muscularis mucosae and blood vessels. A sliding hiatus hernia is a frequent accompaniment.

Muscular rings (so-called 'A' rings or Schatzki's rings) are found somewhat proximal to mucosal rings and consist of a concentric thickening of the main muscle coat corresponding to the lower oesophageal sphincter and covered on both upper and lower surfaces by squamous epithelium [62,63] (Figure 8.1).

The finding of rings endoscopically within the mid- to lower oesophagus is part of the clinical spectrum of eosinophilic oesophagitis producing a corrugated or 'feline' appearance [64,65] (see Chapter 4, 'Eosinophilic oesophagitis').

Barium sulphate in the oesophagus

Barium sulphate is frequently, and on occasions repeatedly, used in the study of oesophageal stenosis and stricture, and barium is sometimes seen in histological sections [66], either as fine greenish non-birefringent granules, often within vessels, or as larger birefringent rhomboid crystals in granulation tissue [67].

References

1. Horwitz B, Krevsky B, Buckman RF Jr, Fisher RS, Dabezies MA. Endoscopic evaluation of penetrating esophageal injuries. *Am J Gastroenterol* 1993;**88**:1249.
2. Ajalat GM, Mulder DG. Esophageal perforations: the need for an individualised approach. *Arch Surg* 1984;**119**:1318.
3. Wesdorp ECE, Bartelsman JFWM, Huitbregbe K, Jager FCAH, Tytgat GN. Treatment of instrumental oesophageal perforation. *Gut* 1984;**25**:398.
4. Panzini L, Burrell MI, Traube M. Instrumental esophageal perforation: chest film findings. *Am J Gastroenterol* 1994;**89**:367.
5. Bhatia NL, Collins JM, Nguyen CC, Jaroszewski DE, Vikram HR, Charles JC. Esophageal perforation as a complication of esophagogastroduodenoscopy. *J Hosp Med* 2008;**3**:256.
6. Karbowski M, Scembre D, Kozarek R, Ayub K, Low D. Polyflex self-expanding, removable plastic stents: assessment of treatment efficacy and safety in variety of benign and malignant conditions of the esophagus. *Surg Endosc* 2008;**22**:1326.
7. Rossoff L Sr, White EJ. Perforation of the esophagus. *Am J Surg* 1974;**128**:207.
8. Michel L, Grills HC, Malt RA. Esophageal perforation. *Ann Thoracic Surg* 1982;**33**:203.
9. Pace F, Antinori S, Repici A. What is new in esophageal injury (infection, drug-induced, caustic, stricture, perforation)? *Curr Opin Gastroenterol* 2009;**25**:372.
10. Elsayed H, Page R, Agarwal S, Chalmers J. Oesophageal perforation complicating intraoperative transoesophageal echocardiography: suspicion can save lives. *Interact Cardiovasc Thorac Surg* 2010;**11**:380.
11. Berry BE, Ochsner JL. Perforation of the esophagus: a 30 year review. *J Thorac Cardiovasc Surg* 1973;**65**:1.
12. de Schipper JP, Pull ter Gunne AF, Oostvogel HJ, van Laarhoven CJ. Spontaneous rupture of the oesophagus: Boerhaave's syndrome in 2008. Literature review and treatment algorithm. *Dig Surg* 2009;**26**:1.
13. Yeoh NTL, McNicholas T, Rothwell-Jackson RL, Goldstraw P. Intramural rupture and intramural haematoma of the oesophagus. *Br J Surg* 1985;**72**:958.
14. Mackler SA. Spontaneous rupture of the esophagus: an experimental and clinical study. *Surg Gynecol Obstet* 1952;**95**:345.
15. Malik UF, Young R, Pham HD, et al. Chronic presentation of Boerhaave's syndrome. *BMC Gastroenterology* 2010;**10**:29.
16. Byard RW. Esophageal causes of sudden and unexpected death. *J Forensic Sci* 2006;**51**:390.
17. Kortas DY, Haas LS, Simpson WG, Nickl NJ, Gates LK. Mallory–Weiss tear: predisposing factors and predictors of a complicated course. *Am J Gastroenterol* 2001;**96**:2836.
18. Merill JR. Snore-induced Mallory–Weiss syndrome. *J Clin Gastroenterol* 1987;**9**:88.
19. Atkinson M, Bottrill MB, Edwards AT, Mitchell WM, Peet BG, Williams RE. Mucosal tears at the oesophago-gastric junction (the Mallory–Weiss syndrome). *Gut* 1961;**2**:1.

20. Baker RW, Spiro AH, Trnka YM. Mallory–Weiss tear complicating upper endoscopy: case reports and review of the literature. *Gastroenterology* 1982;**82**:140.

21. Bharucha AE, Gostout CJ, Balm RK. Clinical and endoscopic risk factors in the Mallory–Weiss syndrome. *Am J Gastroenterol* 1997;**92**:805.

22. Powell TW, Herbst CA, Usher M. Mallory–Weiss syndrome in a 10-month old infant requiring surgery. *J Pediatr Surg* 1984;**19**:596.

23. Harris JM, DiPalma JA. Clinical significance of Mallory–Weiss tears. *Am J Gastroenterol* 1993;**88**:2056.

24. Bataller R, Llach J, Salmeron JL, et al. Endoscopic sclerotherapy in upper gastrointestinal bleeding due to the Mallory–Weiss syndrome. *Am J Gastroenterol* 1994;**89**:2147.

25. Stevens AE, Dove GAW. Oesophageal cast: oesophagitis dissecans superficialis. *Lancet* 1960;**ii**:1279.

26. Marks IN, Keet AD. Intramural rupture of the oesophagus. *BMJ* 1968;**ii**:536.

27. Khan AA, Burkhart CR. Esophageal cast. *J Clin Gastroenterol* 1985;**7**:409.

28. Wang Y, Cheng L, Li N, Wu K, Zhai J, Wang J. Study of glue extrusion after endoscopic N-butyl-2-cyanoacrylate injection on gastric variceal bleeding. *World J Gastroenterol* 2009;**15**:4945.

29. Kitano S, Terblanche J, Kahn D, Bornman PC. Venous anatomy of the lower oesophagus in portal hypertension: practical implications. *Br J Surg* 1986;**73**:525.

30. Helton WS, Johansen K. Portal hypertension and bleeding esophagogastric varices. *Ann Vasc Surg* 1996;**10**:415.

31. Pacquet KJ. Causes and pathomechanisms of oesophageal varices development. *Med Sci Monit* 200;**6**:915.

32. Allison PR. Bleeding from gastro-oesophageal varices. *Ann R Coll Surg* 1959;**25**:298.

33. Laine L, Cook D. Endoscopic ligation compared with sclerotherapy for treatment of esophageal variceal bleeding: a meta-analysis. *Ann Intern Med* 1995;**123**:280.

34. Garcia-Pagan JC, Bosch J. Endoscopic band ligation in the treatment of portal hypertension. *Nature Clin Pract Gastroenterol Hepatol* 2005;**2**:526.

35. Fabiani B, Degott C, Ramond MJ, Valla D, Benhamou JP, Potet F. Endoscopic obliteration of esophagogastric varices with bucrylate II – histopathological study in 12 post-mortem cases. *Gastroenterol Clin Biol* 1986;**10**:580.

36. Matsumoto S. Clinicopathological study of sclerotherapy of esophageal varices. I. A review of 26 autopsy cases. *Gastroenterol Jpn* 1986;**21**:99.

37. Triantos C, Manolakopoulos S, Anastasiou J, et al. Fibrous band formation in cirrhotics treated with band ligation. *Hepatogastroenterology* 2008;**55**:108.

38. Evans DMD, Jones DB, Cleary BK, Smith PM. Oesophageal varices treated by sclerotherapy: a histopathological study. *Gut* 1982;**23**:615.

39. Schellong H, von Maercke PH, Bueb G, Pichlmaeir H. Oesophageal stenosis – a complication of sclerotherapy of oesophageal varices. *Endoscopy* 1986;**18**:223.

40. Jensen LS, Dybdahl H, Juhl C, Nielsen TH. Endoscopic sclerotherapy of esophageal varices in an experimental animal model: a histomorphologic study. *Scand J Gastroenterol* 1986;**21**:725.

41. Sorensen T, Burcharth F, Pedersen ML, Findahl F. Oesophageal stricture and dysphagia after endoscopic sclerotherapy for bleeding varices. *Gut* 1984;**25**:473.

42. Spence RAJ, Sloan JM, Johnston GW, Greenfield A. Oesophageal mucosal changes in patients with varices. *Gut* 1983;**24**:1024.

43. Geboes K, Desmet V, Vantrappen G. Esophageal histology in the early stage of gastroesophageal reflux. *Arch Pathol Lab Med* 1979;**103**:205.

44. Geboes K, Desmet V, Vantrappen G, Mebis J. Vascular changes in the esophageal mucosa. *Gastrointest Endosc* 1980;**26**:29.

45. El-Zayadi A, Montasser MF, Girgis F, El-Okby S, Botros B, Mohran Z. Histological changes of the esophageal mucosa in bleeding versus non-bleeding varices. *Endoscopy* 1989;**21**:205.

46. Hirata M, Kawasaki S, Sanjo K, Idezuki Y. Histopathological study of oesophageal mucosa in patients with varices: a comparison between bleeders and non-bleeders. *Br J Surg* 1991;**78**:1352.

47. Shamma'a MH, Benedict EB. Esophageal webs. A report of 58 cases and an attempt at classification. *N Engl J Med* 1958;**259**:378.

48. Novacek G. Plummer–Vinson syndrome. *Orphanet J Rare Dis* 2006;**1**:36.

49. Benedict EB, Lever WF. Stenosis of esophagus in benign mucous membrane pemphigus. *Ann Otol Rhinol Laryngol* 1952;**61**:1121.

50. Marsden RA, Sambrook-Gower FJ, MacDonald AF, Main RA. Epidermolysis bullosa of the oesophagus with oesophageal web formation. *Thorax* 1974;**29**:287.

51. Johnston DE, Koehler RE, Balfe DM. Clinical manifestations of epidermolysis bullosa dystrophica. *Dig Dis Sci* 1981;**26**:1144.

52. Shields HM, Shaffer K, O'Farrell RP, et al. Gastrointestinal manifestations of dermatologic disorders. *Clin Gastroenterol Hepatol* 2007;**5**:1010.

53. Ntoumazios SK, Voulgari PV, Potsis K, Koutis E, Tsifetaki N, Assimakopoulos DA. Esophageal involvement in scleroderma: gastroesophageal reflux, the common problem. *Semin Arthritis Rheum* 2006;**36**:173.

54. Jerome-Zapadka KM, Clarke MR, Sekas G. Recurrent upper esophageal webs in association with heterotopic gastric mucosa: case report and literature review. *Am J Gastroenterol* 1994;**89**:421.

55. McDonald GB, Shulman HM, Sullivan KM, Spencer GD. Intestinal and hepatic complications of human bone marrow transplantation. Part I. *Gastroenterology* 1986;**90**:460.

56. Papazian A, Capron J-P, Ducroix J-P, Dupas J-L, Quenem C, Besson P. Mucosal bridges of the upper esophagus after radiotherapy for Hodgkin's disease. *Gastroenterology* 1983;**84**:1028.

57. Sinha SK, Nain CK, Udawat HP, et al. Cervical esophageal web and celiac disease. *J Gastroenterol Hepatol* 2008;**23**:1149.

58. Janisch HD, Eckardt VF. Histological abnormalities in patients with multiple esophageal webs. *Dig Dis Sci* 1982;**27**:503.

59. Pra D, Rech Franke SI, Pegas Henriques JA, Fenech M. A possible link between iron deficiency and gastrointestinal carcinogenesis. *Nutr Cancer* 2009;**61**:415.

60. MacMahon HE, Schatski R, Gary JE. Pathology of a lower esophageal ring. *N Engl J Med* 1958;**259**:1.

61. Goyal RK, Bauer JL, Spiro HM. The nature and location of lower esophageal ring. *N Engl J Med* 1971;**284**:1175.

62. Arvanitakis C. Lower esophageal ring: endoscopic and therapeutic aspects. *Gastrointest Endosc* 1977;**24**:17.

63. Jalil S, Castell DO. Schatzki's ring: a benign cause of dysphagia in adults. *J Clin Gastroenterol.* 2002;**35**:295.

64. Yan BM, Shaffer EA. Eosinophilic esophagitis: a newly established cause of dysphagia. *World J Gastroenterol* 2006;**12**:2328.

65. Odze RD. Pathology of eosinophilic esophagitis: what the clinician needs to know. *Am J Gastroenterol* 2009;**104**:485.

66. Womack C. Unusual histological appearances of barium sulphate – a case report with scanning electron microscopy and energy dispersive X-ray analysis. *J Clin Pathol* 1984;**37**:488.

67. Levison DA, Crocker PR, Smith A, Blackshaw AJ, Bartram CI. Varied light and scanning electron microscopic appearances of barium sulphate in smears and histological sections. *J Clin Pathol* 1984;**37**:481.

PART 2

Stomach

The normal stomach: anatomy, specimen dissection and histology relevant to pathological practice

Shinichi Ban

Saiseikai Kawaguchi General Hospital, Saitama, Japan

Anatomy and specimen dissection

Gross anatomy

The stomach plays an important role in the early stages of digestion by controlling onward transmission of food, breaking it down into a semi-fluid consistency (mechanical digestion) and adding secretions (chemical digestion). It also serves as an endocrine and immunological organ.

The stomach, which develops as an unequal dilatation of the foregut, is located in the left upper quadrant of the abdomen. It forms a J-shaped dilated sac that extends from the lower end of the oesophagus (the gastro-oesophageal junction), several centimetres below the level of the diaphragm and to the left of the midline, to end at the gastro-duodenal junction just to the right of the midline. The size and position of the stomach change according to body position and the quantity of contents.

The supero-medial concavity and infero-lateral convexity of the stomach are termed the 'lesser curvature' and 'greater curvature', respectively. The ventral and dorsal aspects are termed the 'anterior wall' and 'posterior wall', respectively. Almost the entire external surface of the stomach is invested in visceral peritoneum, which contributes to the formation of the omentum and the peritoneal ligaments which loosely fix the stomach to the surrounding structures. These are: the gastro-phrenic ligament which connects the upper dome of the stomach (gastric fundus) to the diaphragm; the greater omentum suspended from the greater curvature and attaching to the transverse colon and its mesocolon; the gastro-splenic ligament between the upper left margin of the greater omentum and the spleen; and the lesser omentum (hepato-gastric ligament and hepato-duodenal ligament) between the lesser curvature (and proximal part of the duodenum) and the inferior aspect of the liver.

The stomach is divisible into four zones (Figure 9.1): the cardia, fundus, body (corpus) and antrum (pyloric antrum). The *cardia* is a narrow, macroscopically indistinct zone extending for a few centimetres immediately distal to the gastro-oesophageal junction; it merges distally into the fundus and may be distinguishable only by its histology. The *fundus* is the upper dome-shaped portion which lies above a line drawn horizontally through the gastro-oesophageal junction, whereas the *body (corpus)* comprises about two-thirds of the remainder of the stomach. The *antrum* (pyloric antrum) is an infundibular canal comprising the distal third of the stomach, leading into the *pylorus* (pyloric ring), a circumferentially thickened ridge that separates the stomach from the duodenum. The incisural notch, which is a small bend in the mid-lesser curvature, can be used as a rough macroscopic landmark between the body and the antrum [1]. Practically, the only reliable distinguishing feature between the body and the antrum of the stomach is the difference in histological characteristics of the mucosa. However, even the histological boundary between the body and the antrum can progress proximally as a consequence of either ageing or chronic gastritis [2–4].

The gastric wall comprises four layers: the mucosa delineated below by the muscularis mucosae, submucosa, muscularis propria and subserosa covered by the serosa (Figure 9.2). The gastric mucosal surface, especially in the fundus and the body, displays coarse, longitudinal folds ('rugae'),

Morson and Dawson's Gastrointestinal Pathology, Fifth Edition. Edited by Neil A. Shepherd, Bryan F. Warren, Geraint T. Williams, Joel K. Greenson, Gregory Y. Lauwers and Marco R. Novelli.
© 2013 Blackwell Publishing Ltd. Published 2013 by Blackwell Publishing Ltd.

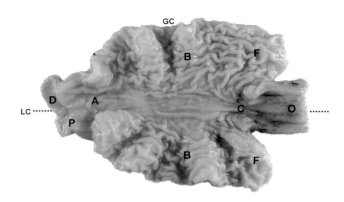

Figure 9.1 Gross appearance of the gastric mucosal surface of a 4-month-old infant (postmortem case), opened along the greater curvature. Gastric folds (rugae) running parallel to the lesser curvature are obvious in a stomach with no mucosal atrophy. LC, lesser curvature; GC, greater curvature; O, oesophagus; C, cardia, F, fundus; B, body (corpus); A, antrum; P, pylorus; D, duodenal mucosal folds.

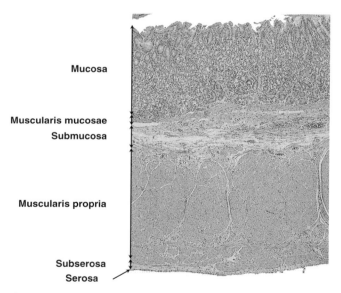

Figure 9.2 View of the layered structure of the gastric wall (same case as Figure 9.1).

which consist of the mucosa and the muscularis mucosae with cores of submucosal tissue (Figure 9.1). The thickness of the gastric rugae is variable, depending on the degree of distension of the stomach. Also, the fundus and body mucosae are freely mobile on the muscle beneath, whereas the antral mucosa is flattened, less rugose and more firmly anchored.

On close examination, the mucosal micro-architecture is composed of polygonal elevations centred on glandular openings (foveolae or pits) and separated by thin narrow grooves (areae gastricae), and can be demonstrated on radiological double-contrast barium as fine reticulation [1]. Under the dissecting microscope, the mucosal surface of the body/fundus differs from that of the antrum, showing a 'Morocco leather' appearance, whereas the antral mucosa has a coarser leaf-like or sulciolar pattern [5,6]. Recognising the semi-microscopic features of the gastric mucosa is important because recent advances in magnifying endoscopy enable their recognition in vivo along with their microvascular architecture [7,8].

Under magnifying endoscopy with narrow band imaging (NBI), the body/fundus mucosa shows a regular honeycomb pattern, each space of which is delineated by fine subepithelial capillary networks and has a central crypt opening, whereas the antral mucosa shows a coarse mesh-like pattern with coiled capillaries (Figure 9.3a,b). These findings serve as a basis for the diagnosis of early gastric neoplasms [9].

The stomach has a generous blood supply derived from branches of the coeliac, hepatic and splenic arteries. The gastric cardia and the lesser curvature are supplied by the left gastric artery, derived from the coeliac axis, and the right gastric artery from the hepatic artery. The proximal greater curvature is vascularised by the left gastro-epiploic artery and the short gastric arteries from the splenic artery, and the distal greater curvature by the right gastro-epiploic artery from the hepatic artery. The arterial branches penetrate the gastric wall with abundant collateral vessels. The major veins parallel the corresponding arteries and venous return is via the portal venous system. Notably, part of the venous return from the lower oesophagus drains into the systemic venous system via the oesophageal veins but also enters the portal system through the left gastric vein, this communication between systemic and portal venous systems explaining the formation of oesophageal and gastric varices in portal hypertension [10].

Numerous lymphatic channels, communicating with the deeper aspect of the mucosa and the submucosa, join with the major lymphatic trunks, generally running along the major arteries and veins. They drain into the lymph nodes near the main arteries. The left gastric nodes are located along the lesser curvature and the right gastric and hepatic nodes along the lesser curvature of the antrum. The pyloric or subpyloric nodes are situated near the head of the pancreas and the paracardial nodes around the gastro-oesophageal junction. The pancreatico-splenic nodes are present along the proximal greater omentum and the right gastro-epiploic nodes along the distal greater curvature [11].

The stomach is extrinsically innervated by the autonomic nervous system (parasympathetic and sympathetic). The parasympathetic supply comes from the terminal branches of the vagus nerve. The anterior vagal trunk is derived from the left vagus nerve which divides into hepatic and anterior gastric branches. The posterior vagal trunk issues from the

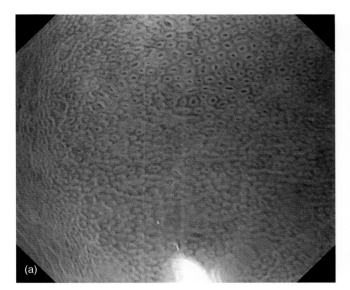 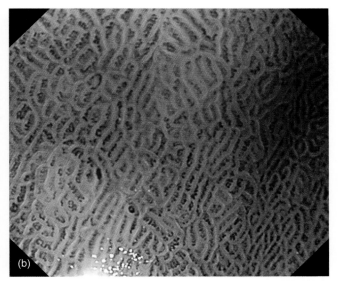

Figure 9.3 Semi-microscopic features of the gastric mucosa visualised by magnifying endoscopy with narrow band imaging (NBI). The body mucosa shows a regular honeycomb pattern delineated by fine subepithelial capillary networks and with central crypt openings (a), whereas the antral mucosa shows a coarse mesh-like pattern with coiled capillaries (b). (Courtesy of Dr K. Nonaka, Department of Gastroenterology, Saitama Medical University International Medical Center, Saitama, Japan.)

right vagus nerve and branches into the coeliac and posterior gastric nerves. This division is (or has been) surgically important because selective vagotomy allows preservation of the hepatic and coeliac branches, which may reduce the incidence of post-vagotomy diarrhoea. Sympathetic innervation derives from the sixth to ninth thoracic segments of the spinal cord, reaching the coeliac ganglion via the greater splanchnic nerves and spreading to the stomach along the gastric and gastro-epiploic arteries [12].

Specimen dissection

Proper and systematic handling and dissection of the resected stomach are cardinal for optimal pathological assessment, especially of tumours. After dissection of the regional lymph nodes, gastrectomy specimens are usually opened along the greater curvature, pinned along the opened edge on a corkboard or hard rubber board, with the mucosal surface uppermost and immersed in formalin solution for fixation. If a lesion is on or near the greater curvature, the specimen can be opened along the lesser curvature line or through a line shifted to the anterior or posterior wall. When pinned, the mucosa should be gently stretched to avoid concealing lesions between mucosal folds. Photography of the specimen is encouraged because it aids reconstruction of the lesions after sampling. The site of the tumour within the stomach should be properly recorded along the length of stomach (greater and lesser curves) and the segments of oesophagus and duodenum present identified and measured.

After suitable fixation (overnight for formalin), the lesions should be systematically sectioned through a line usually parallel to the lesser curvature (Figure 9.4a). Alternatively they can be sectioned in a cruciform fashion (Figure 9.4b). Either way, the extent of spread of neoplastic lesions in both horizontal and vertical directions (depth of invasion), including the relationship to the serosal aspect, should be examined carefully and recorded. The resection margins should also be sampled properly [13]. After careful gross examination for lymph nodes, a clearing solution can be used as this can increase the number of lymph nodes retrieved (Table 9.1). All lymph nodes in the main specimen, and all those submitted separately, should be submitted for histological assessment. Recommendations as to the analysis of subsite distribution of involved lymph nodes vary in different countries and the interested reader should interrogate the appropriate guidelines for specimen dissection such as those of the Japanese Gastric Cancer Association [13], the Royal College of Pathologists of the UK (www.rcpath.org/resources/pdf/G013GastricDataset FINALJan07.pdf) and the College of Pathologists of the USA (www.cap.org/apps/docs/committees/cancer/cancer_ protocols/2011/Stomach_11protocol.pdf).

Appropriate handling and reporting of specimens from endoscopic mucosal resection (EMR) and endoscopic submucosal dissection (ESD) are essential in guiding additional therapeutic options. The specimens should be evenly pinned on a board along the resection edge so as to avoid the edge curling up when immersed in formalin solution. They should be entirely sectioned at 2-mm intervals in a

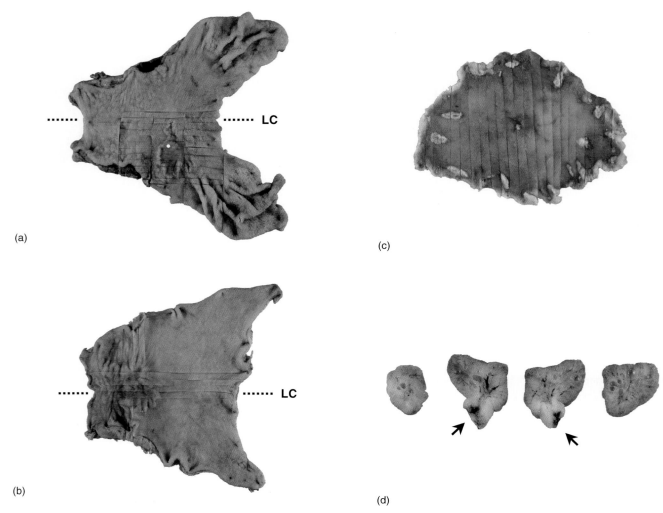

(a)

(b)

(c)

(d)

Figure 9.4 Dissection of gastric specimens: (a) a distal gastrectomy specimen with a depressed type geographic carcinoma on the posterior wall of the lower corpus, sectioned through parallel to the lesser curvature (LC). Although the carcinoma was mostly limited to the mucosa and submucosa, the muscularis propria was focally invaded (white spot), emphasising the importance of thorough examination. (b) Distal gastrectomy with an ulcerative-type carcinoma of the antrum, cut in a cruciform fashion. (c) Endoscopic submucosal dissection (ESD) for a small depressed carcinoma, which was entirely sliced in 2-mm sections. (d) Cut surfaces of a polypectomy specimen divided through the line involving the resection edge of the stalk (arrows).

Table 9.1 Summary of recommended sections of gastric neoplasia

Sections of tumour for assessment of:
  Diagnosis
  Depth of invasion
  Margins – proximal, distal, radial/circumferential (the latter mainly close to the oesophago-gastric junction)
  Relation of tumour to adjacent stomach

Sections to assess background mucosa:
  Atrophy and gastritis
  Dysplasia
  Other lesions

Exhaustive dissection and submission of all lymph nodes

direction that takes into consideration the position of the tumour and where it is near the resection margins [13–15] (Figure 9.4c). The pathological diagnosis, tumour grade, depth of extension, presence or absence of lymphovascular invasion and status of all circumferential and deep margins should all be reported.

After formalin fixation, polypectomy specimens should be cut through the line of the resection edge of the stalk and the submucosa of the polyp head and the stalk, to assess the head and/or stalk for invasion (Figure 9.4d). The quality of the margin should be recorded, if possible.

Once proper sampling has been performed, microscopic analysis will finalise the reporting of an accurate pathological diagnosis, grading and staging. In the 2010 edition of the AJCC/UICC TNM system, the staging for gastric carcinoma has been substantially modified, e.g. T1 has been subdivided so that mucosal and submucosal depth of invasion is delineated. Furthermore, T2a and T2b have been separated into T2 (muscularis propria) and T3 (subserosa), and the former T3 and T4 changed to T4a (penetrates serosa) and T4b (invades adjacent structures) respectively. The divisions of regional lymph node involvement have also been changed [16,17].

Histology

The gastric mucosa

The gastric mucosa consists of the epithelium supported by loose connective tissue, the lamina propria. The epithelial component is composed of two compartments: the gastric pits (foveolae), representing the invagination of the surface epithelial lining, and the deep glandular compartment. The different types of glands (cardiac, fundic and pyloric) define the different zones of the stomach (cardia, fundus and body, and antrum). Endocrine cells are scattered in the glandular compartment throughout the stomach. The mucosal surface is normally covered by a thick mucin gel layer (Figure 9.5).

The surface (foveolar) epithelium

The surface (foveolar) epithelium that covers the surface and lines the pits is the same in all zones of the stomach. It consists of a single layer of tall, columnar, mucus-secreting cells with basal rounded or oval nuclei and supranuclear, mucin-filled cytoplasm that is pale pink with the haematoxylin and eosin (H&E) stain (Figure 9.5) and positive for the periodic acid–Schiff (PAS) reaction. Electron microscopy demonstrates that the individual cells are linked by junctional complexes and that the lateral cell membranes interdigitate. The luminal aspect of each cell is covered by short pleomorphic microvilli which are coated by the glycocalyx. The cytoplasm displays supranuclear

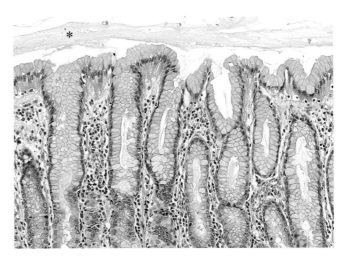

Figure 9.5 Surface (foveolar) epithelium covering the surface and pits of normal gastric body mucosa. The epithelium consists of a single layer of tall columnar mucus-secreting cells with basal rounded or oval nuclei and supranuclear mucin-filled cytoplasm. Part of the mucin gel layer is observed on the mucosal surface (asterisk).

membrane-bound granules of mucin, measuring between 0.1 μm and 1.0 μm in diameter. Most granules are uniformly electron dense but some are mottled, with a denser zone present beneath the limiting membrane. The mucin granules originate from well-developed Golgi complexes [18–20].

The fundic (oxyntic) glands

Body and fundic mucosa is characterised by the fundic (oxyntic) glands. The mucosal thickness varies from 400 μm to 1500 μm with the superficial pits (foveolae) comprising about 25% of the total thickness and the deep glands the remaining 75%. The fundic glands consist of tightly packed straight tubules arranged perpendicularly to the surface (Figure 9.6). They extend from the base of the pits to the muscularis mucosae, where they undergo some coiling, and in cross-section may appear as acini. Several glands open into the bottom of each pit through the neck region of the glands, the upper part of which forms a slight constriction (isthmus). Apart from endocrine cells (described below), the fundic glands contain three types of specialised cells: mucous neck cells, parietal (oxyntic) cells and chief (zymogenic) cells.

Mucous neck cells

Single or forming small groups, these cells mingle with parietal cells in the neck region. A few are also present in the lower part of the glands. They are mucus-secreting cells but differ from surface epithelial cells in being lower columnar and more triangular in shape, with pale cytoplasm and

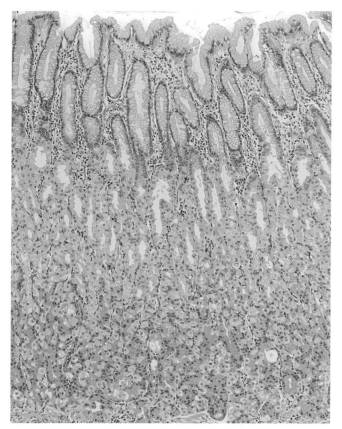

Figure 9.6 Full-thickness view of the body mucosa: the fundic glands consist of tightly packed straight tubules arranged perpendicular to the surface and comprising approximately 75% of the mucosal thickness.

basally located nuclei (Figure 9.7a). They are highlighted by the PAS reaction but are often difficult to recognise on H&E staining. On electron microscopy [20], the mucin granules, which are produced by supranuclear Golgi complexes, are larger than those of the surface epithelial cells. They are coarsely stippled or show variable electron density.

The function of the mucous neck cell is controversial. Some regard these cells as transitional cells in the differentiation of gastric stem cells to zymogenic or chief cells [21,22]. On the basis of these cells' ability to proliferate, which results in pseudo-pyloric gland formation [23], and their secretion of luminally active peptides (such as trefoil peptides, pancreatic secretory trypsin inhibitor and epidermal growth factor), others have concluded that mucous neck cells comprise a distinctive, functional cell lineage with a role of protecting the gastric mucosa from the effects of secreted gastric acid [24].

Parietal (oxyntic) cells

The parietal cells are the source of hydrochloric acid and intrinsic factor. They are located throughout the glands but especially in the upper part. They are large, round or pyramidal in shape, 20–35 μm in diameter, and have central nuclei and eosinophilic, fine granular cytoplasm (Figure 9.7b). The longest side of these cells lies next to the basement membrane and the apical end is wedged between adjoining cells. On ultrastructural examination [20], the cytoplasm reveals numerous mitochondria containing electron-dense granules, to which the cytoplasmic eosinophilia on H&E staining is mainly attributable. The free apical surfaces are invaginated to form branching tubular

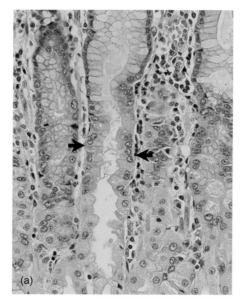
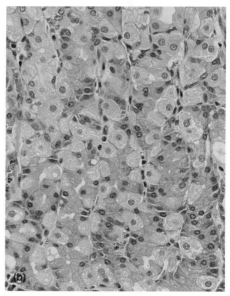

Figure 9.7 Fundic gland mucosa: (a) the neck region composed of mucous neck cells (arrows) and parietal cells. The former are low columnar or triangular cells with pale cytoplasm and basally located nuclei. (b) The deeper glands consist of pyramid-shaped parietal cells with eosinophilic, fine granular cytoplasm and central nuclei, and chief cells with cuboidal or low columnar, granular basophilic cytoplasm and basal nuclei.

structures with numerous microvilli, termed the 'intracellular canalicular system'. Adjacent to it in the cytoplasm are the tubulovesicles, which, when stimulated, fuse to the intracellular canalicular system to secrete acid [25]. Proton pump inhibitor therapy is associated with a decrease in tubulovesicles and microvilli of secretory canaliculi. The changes may possibly be ascribed to the degradation of the membrane in lysosomes because the proton pumps on the membranes bound irreversibly with omeprazole are probably destined to be degraded in lysosomes [26].

Chief (zymogenic) cells

The chief cells secrete pepsinogen (pepsin precursor) and lie mainly in the deeper parts of the glands. They tend to be more numerous towards the cardiac end of the body mucosa, in contrast to parietal cells, which are more numerous distally [27]. They are cuboidal or low columnar cells with coarse granular basophilic cytoplasm and basally situated nuclei (Figure 9.7b). On ultrastructural examination [20], the cytoplasm is full of granular endoplasmic reticulum and free ribosomes, to which light microscopic basophilia is attributed. Zymogen granules, which are membrane-bound homogeneous spheres, 0.5–3.0 μm in diameter, are present in the apical supranuclear region.

Pepsinogen is classified into pepsinogen I (PGI) and pepsinogen II (PGII). Although chief cells are the main source of PGI and PGII, PGI is present in mucous neck cells and also PGII in pyloric and cardiac gland cells as well as mucous neck cells. Pepsinogens can be useful immunohistochemical markers for the identification of cell types [28–30]. In countries with a high incidence of gastric cancer, testing for serum pepsinogen, as a marker for chronic atrophic gastritis (and particularly the PGI : PG II ratio), has

been incorporated, with variable success, into screening programmes to identify those at high risk [31].

The pyloric glands

The mucosa of the antral and pyloric regions contains the pyloric glands. It is from 200 μm to 1100 μm thick and the gastric pits are deeper (about a third to a half of the mucosal thickness) than those of the fundus and the body (Figure 9.8a). The pyloric glands are branched tubules that do not always lie perpendicular to the surface. In cross-section, they appear as clusters separated by abundant intervening stroma, often with thin smooth muscle bundles extending up from the muscularis mucosae (Figure 9.8b). They consist of PAS-positive mucus-secreting cells with faintly granular cytoplasm and basal depressed nuclei on H&E. Occasional parietal cells are present in the pyloric glands, whereas no chief (zymogenic) cells can be demonstrated. On electron microscopy [20], pyloric gland cells have abundant heterogeneous mucin granules and homogeneous granules (similar to the zymogen granules of the chief cells) which are produced by supranuclear Golgi complexes.

The cardiac glands

The cardiac mucosa, also referred to as junctional mucosa because it straddles the anatomical boundary of the oesophagus and stomach, is similar in morphology to the mucosa of the antral and pyloric regions. Cardiac glands are compound or branching tubular glands, and tend to be grouped in lobules separated by connective tissue with prolongations of the smooth muscle bundles from the

Figure 9.8 (a) Full-thickness view of the antral mucosa: the pyloric glands are branched tubules that do not always lie perpendicular to the surface and appear as clusters separated by abundant intervening stroma, comprising approximately half the mucosal thickness. (b) Pyloric glands consisting of mucus-secreting cells with faintly granular cytoplasm and basal depressed nuclei, around which are thin smooth muscle bundles growing up from the muscularis mucosae.

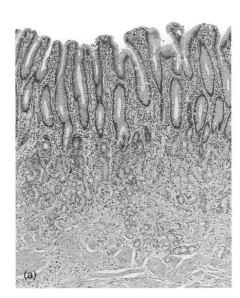 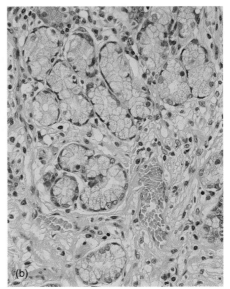

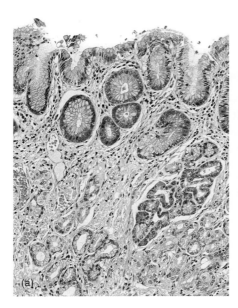 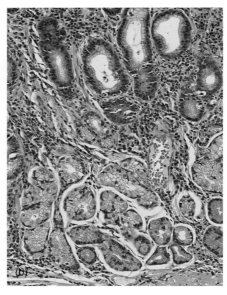

Figure 9.9 (a) Cardiac mucosa similar in morphology to the mucosa of the antral and pyloric regions. (b) Intermediate (transitional) zone mucosa consisting of the pits occupying approximately half the mucosal thickness, with the glandular component comprising mixed fundic and pyloric glands.

muscularis mucosae (Figure 9.9a). They consist of mucus-secreting glands not distinguishable from pyloric glands. Other cells present in smaller numbers include parietal cells and endocrine cells. Chief cells are rare. On electron microscopy [19], cardiac gland cells have electron-dense mucin granules and granules mottled in appearance with developed supranuclear Golgi complexes.

The cardia is defined as the zone between the end of the oesophagus and the fundus/body of the stomach. It usually extends downwards for a few centimetres of the cardio-oesophageal junction. However, there is marked individual variation and there is considerable controversy as to its significance and extent [32–36]. Some authors even deny the existence of the cardiac zone as a normal physiological structure and contend that its presence is always pathological [32,33].

The intermediate (transitional) zone

The junctional area between the fundic gland mucosa and the pyloric gland mucosa is referred to as the intermediate (transitional) zone mucosa. This mucosa usually consists of pits occupying about half the mucosal thickness and glandular compartments comprising mixed fundic and pyloric glands with abundant stroma, similar to the structure of the antral mucosa (Figure 9.9b).

As a consequence of ageing or chronic gastritis, the area of the pyloric glands expands proximally from the antral mucosa far up along the lesser curvature, reaching almost to the cardia and spreading into the body/fundus mucosa of both anterior and posterior walls [2–4]. Atrophic fundic glands are replaced by mucus-secreting glands similar to the pyloric glands, a process that has been termed 'pseudo-pyloric gland metaplasia' (Figure 9.10a) and the intermediate (transitional) zone moves proximally. Pseudo-pyloric glands derived from fundic glands can be identified by their expression of PGI. The original antral mucosa can be distinguished by the presence of clear endocrine gastrin-producing cells in the middle portion of the mucosa (see below) [37].

Intestinal metaplasia, another major type of epithelial metaplasia, is associated with the expansion of pseudo-pyloric gland mucosa due to chronic gastritis. In intestinal metaplasia, the surface and pit epithelia are replaced by epithelium that morphologically and histochemically resembles that of the small and/or large intestine [38,39] (Figure 9.10b). The simplest classification of the intestinal metaplasia is complete or incomplete, the former representing a resemblance of normal small bowel epithelium characterised by enterocytes with a brush border, goblet cells and some Paneth cells and the latter consisting of intestinal-type goblet cells and gastric foveolar-like mucus-secreting cells. It should be noted that the intestinalised mucosa is different from non-intestinalised mucosa, not only in the type of epithelium but also in the types of endocrine cells and stromal cells (see below). Other, less common metaplastic changes of the gastric epithelium are ciliated metaplasia observed in the pyloric glands [40] and at the oesophago-gastric junction (see Chapter 1), and pancreatic acinar metaplasia in the cardiac glands (see Chapter 1) [41].

Endocrine cells

Endocrine cells are widely but patchily distributed in the various epithelia of the stomach and their products are important regulators of gastrointestinal physiology [42,43].

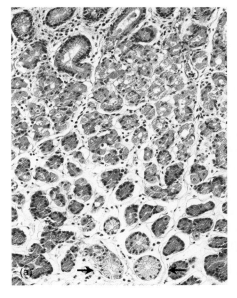
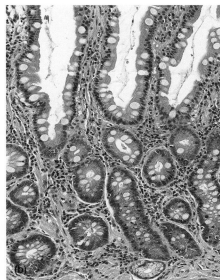

Figure 9.10 Metaplasia of the gastric mucosa: (a) pseudo-pyloric gland metaplasia in the base of the fundic glands (arrows), appearing as mucus-secreting glands. (b) Intestinal metaplasia. The surface and pit epithelia are replaced by epithelium resembling that of the small intestine, including absorptive cells with brush borders, goblet cells and Paneth cells.

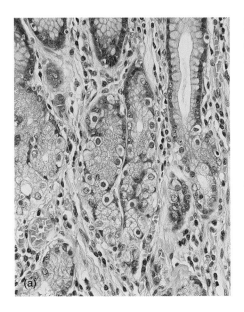
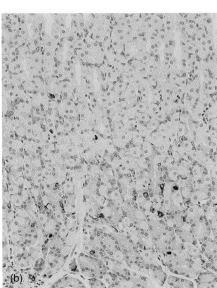

Figure 9.11 Endocrine cells in the gastric mucosa: (a) gastrin-producing G cells in the neck region of the antral mucosa have a clear or pale cytoplasm. (b) Endocrine cells in the body mucosa, as demonstrated by chromogranin A immunostaining, are evident mainly at the base of the fundic glands.

They can sometimes be recognised on H&E-stained preparations as rounded clear or pale cells, or pyramid-shaped eosinophilic cells in the glandular compartment, often wedged between the basement membrane and the other epithelial cells. The cytoplasm of the endocrine cells contains granules that are smaller than those of Paneth cells. These granules are either dispersed in the cytoplasm or concentrated beneath the nucleus. In the pyloric gland mucosa, endocrine cells often have a narrow apex that reaches the gland lumen (open type) whereas it does not in the fundic gland mucosa (closed type) [20]. A few endo-

crine cells are also scattered in the lamina propria near the glandular base.

Endocrine cell types in the gastric mucosa are site-dependent [42,43]. In the antrum, the predominant endocrine cells are gastrin-producing G cells. They are common in the neck and upper gland regions, showing clear or pale cytoplasm (Figure 9.11a). Enterochromaffin-like (ECL) cells, a source of histamine, are confined to the body/fundus and are the most common endocrine cells there. They are evident mostly in the basal third of the mucosa (Figure 9.11b) and are particularly associated with chief cell-rich areas. ECL cells are often hard to discern in routine H&E stained preparations.

Gastrin released from the G cells stimulates ECL cells to produce histamine, which triggers acid secretion from the parietal cells. Enterochromaffin (EC) cells containing serotonin (5-hydroxytryptamine) and somatostatin-producing D cells are scattered throughout the stomach. A minority of other endocrine cell types is also present. In intestinal metaplasia, intestinalised epithelium contains an increased number of intestinal-type endocrine cells such as glicentin-containing cells and a decreased number of other endocrine cells [44,45].

In formalin-fixed material, endocrine cells can be highlighted by classic silver impregnation. EC cells and some ECL cells are argentaffin using the Fontana–Masson technique, whereas most other gastric endocrine cells are argyrophilic using the Grimelius technique. Some endocrine cells, however, fail to stain with either method. Nowadays, immunohistochemistry using either antibodies against general endocrine markers specific to each endocrine cell type, such as the chromogranins, synaptophysin and CD56 (NCAM), or antibodies against amines or polypeptide products, such as gastrin and somatostatin, are more widely utilised to demonstrate endocrine cells (Figure 9.11b).

Ultrastructurally, each type of endocrine cell contains distinctive granules. The granules of gastrin-producing G cells are spherical and membrane bound, and have a variably electron-dense core and an average diameter of 150–250 nm [42].

Renewal of gastric epithelial cells

There is a constant renewal of gastric epithelial cells originating from stem cells. The stem cells are believed to lie in the compartment between the pits and the glands (the neck region). Proliferating cells, which can be demonstrated by MIB1 (Ki-67 antigen) immunohistochemistry, are distributed there in the so-called regenerative or proliferative zone (Figure 9.12a). The surface epithelial cells migrate upward with maturation and detach from the mucosal surface within several days, whereas glandular cells, including endocrine cells, migrate downward with maturation and persist for several weeks (pyloric gland cells and endocrine cells) or several hundred days (chief cells and parietal cells) [46–49]. As described above, mucous neck cells may be immature zymogenic cells. In intestinal metaplasia, the regenerative zone shifts more deeply into the mucosa [50] (Figure 9.12b).

Mucin of the gastric mucosa

Mucin is a glycoprotein composed of a central protein core and carbohydrate side chains. In the normal stomach, the mucin produced by the foveolar epithelium, mucous neck cells and pyloric/cardiac glands is mostly neutral, i.e. PAS positive and Alcian blue pH 2.5 negative. However, mucous neck cells may contain a small amount of acidic mucin (sialomucin and sulphomucin) and be faintly stained by Alcian blue pH 2.5. Other techniques can demonstrate unique mucin phenotypes for each cell type, e.g. the surface foveolar epithelium stains with galactose oxidase–Schiff (GOS), whereas the pyloric glands and mucous neck cells show paradoxical concanavalin A staining (PCS) (class III reactivity) [51]. The mucin gel secreted by the epithelial cells forms a stable layer 100 μm in thickness on the mucosal surface [52], in which bicarbonate ions produced by the lining epithelium are trapped and neutralise luminal hydrochloric acid to maintain the mucosal surface pH at 7.

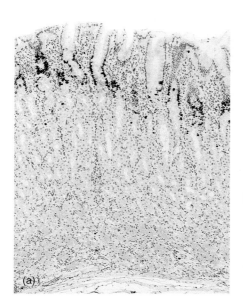

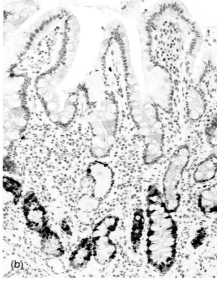

Figure 9.12 Proliferating cells in the gastric mucosa demonstrated by MIB1 immunostaining: (a) MIB1-positive proliferating cells are located in the neck region of the fundic gland mucosa (the proliferative zone). (b) In intestinalised mucosa, the proliferative zone shifts toward the deeper portion of the mucosa.

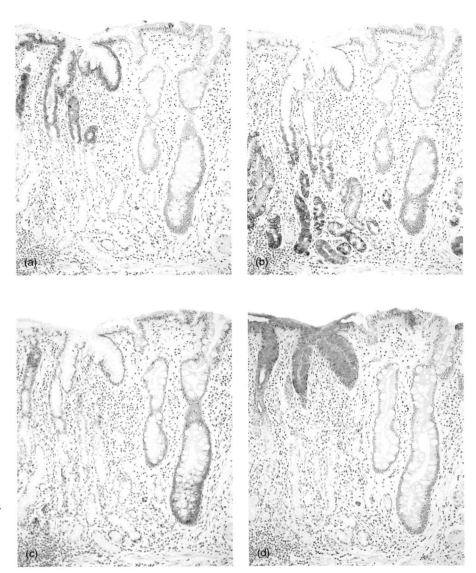

Figure 9.13 Mucin immunohistochemistry of pyloric mucosa with focal intestinal metaplasia. (a) MUC5AC and (d) human gastric mucin (HGM) is expressed in the surface foveolar epithelium, whereas (b) MUC6 is expressed in the pyloric glands. (c) Goblet cells of the intestinalised epithelium (right) are immunoreactive to MUC2.

Recently, monoclonal antibodies against mucin core proteins have become widely used to detect various types of mucins [53,54]; MUC5AC is expressed in the surface foveolar epithelium (Figure 9.13a) and MUC6 in pyloric/cardiac glands and mucous neck cells (Figure 9.13b). MUC2 is not expressed in the normal stomach but is positive in the goblet cells of intestinal metaplasia (Figure 9.13c). Other monoclonal antibodies for mucin identification are human gastric mucin (HGM) for surface foveolar epithelium mucin (recognising the side sugar chains of the MUC5AC mucin) (Figure 9.13d) [55] and M-GGMC-1 for pyloric gland mucin stained by PCS [56]. These mucin phenotypes, as well as PGI/-II expression, are useful for the identification of cell lineages. In practice, incomplete intestinal metaplasia is characterised by the co-expression of 'gastric' mucins and MUC2 'intestinal' mucin, reflecting aberrant cellular differentiation [57]. Similarly, gastric carcinomas commonly express a combination of various mucins [53,54].

The lamina propria

The epithelial component of the gastric mucosa is supported by the lamina propria, a fine network of connective tissue fibres (reticulin fibres with collagen and elastic fibres) in which lie fibroblasts, inflammatory cells, blood vessels, lymphatics and nerve fibres. The lamina propria is scant around the tightly packed fundic glands and abundant in the pyloric/cardiac glands. A spray of smooth muscle fibres extending from the muscularis mucosae into the lamina propria is observed, especially in the antrum. In contrast to the small and large intestinal mucosae, the normal gastric mucosa has scant pericryptal myofibroblasts, although they are seen around the glands in intestinal metaplasia [58].

Even in normal-appearing stomach, some inflammatory cells usually exist in the lamina propria, mainly around the gastric pits. The inflammatory cells include lymphocytes, plasma cells, macrophages, mast cells, eosinophils and rare isolated neutrophils. Lymphoid aggregates or follicles with no germinal centre may also be observed but whether lymphoid aggregates or follicles are ever seen in the absence of gastritis, especially *Helicobacter pylori*-related gastritis, is controversial [37]. B lymphocytes and plasma cells are the predominant inflammatory cells. The number of plasma cells varies but the ratio of IgA, IgG and IgM detected in plasma cells seems to be fairly constant: plasma cells containing IgA predominate [59,60]. These plasma cells containing IgA are scattered in the lamina propria of body mucosa but are more numerous in the antral region [61]. The concentration of IgA plasma cells is higher in the superficial aspect of the mucosa compared with its mid-portion which is richer in IgG plasma cells [60]. When intestinal metaplasia is present, IgG-containing plasma cells decrease in number and the expression of secretory components in intestinalised epithelium becomes obvious, suggesting changes in mucosal immune responses [60]. The lamina propria also has small numbers of T lymphocytes and intra-epithelial lymphocytes, over 95% of which are of T-cell type, may also be identified, although far less frequently than in the small bowel mucosa [60,62].

The microvasculature of the mucosa in the body/fundus differs from that in the antrum. Within the body mucosa, capillaries extend at right angles to the surface and form a network beneath the surface epithelial layer surrounding the gastric pits, which is drained by sparse collecting venules. There are no arteriovenous anastomoses and blood must reach the mucosal surface before it can enter the venous return. In the antral mucosa, there are two distinct capillary beds: a basal capillary system branching out from short arterioles and a superficial capillary network originating from long arterioles ascending into the mucosa [10]. These two different systems are identified by different patterns on magnifying endoscopy [7,8] (Figure 9.3a,b).

The lymphatics are limited to the deep portion above the muscularis mucosae (Figure 9.14) [10,63,64]. Their absence from the superficial mucosa correlates with the low prevalence of lymph nodal metastases in intramucosal gastric cancer [63,64].

Muscularis mucosae

Underlying the mucosa is the muscularis mucosae, a thin double layer of smooth muscle tissue that varies in thickness from 30 μm to 200 μm and is thicker in the antrum than

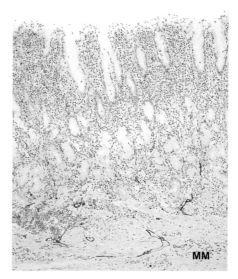

Figure 9.14 Mucosal lymphatics revealed by D2-40 (podoplanin) immunostaining. The small lymphatic channels are distributed in and just above the muscularis mucosae (MM) but not in the upper half of the mucosa.

in the fundus [65]. The muscularis mucosae consists of the inner circular layer and outer longitudinal layer, and contains some elastic fibres. It does not normally show fragmentation or infiltration by inflammatory cells. In the antrum, vertical thin fascicles extend up into the mucosa and separate pyloric glands.

Submucosa

The submucosa is a thick layer of loose connective tissue beneath the muscularis mucosae, with relatively thick arteries, veins and lymphatics forming major plexuses, as well as nerves and the submucosal nerve plexus of Meissner. The submucosa is rich in elastic fibres and also contains fibroblasts, adipocytes, smooth muscle cells and mast cells.

Muscularis propria

The stomach has three muscle coats. The *inner circular* coat surrounds the whole stomach and is continuous with that of the oesophagus. The *outer longitudinal* coat runs from the oesophagus to the duodenum and is continuous with their longitudinal fibres. Internal to the circular coat, additional *inner oblique fibres* run down from the cardia more or less parallel to the lesser curvature and blend with the circular coat on the greater curvature (Figure 9.15). At the pylorus, the inner circular muscle thickens and forms distinct proximal and distal loops which unite in a torus along the lesser curvature, forming the pyloric sphincter. The nerves and

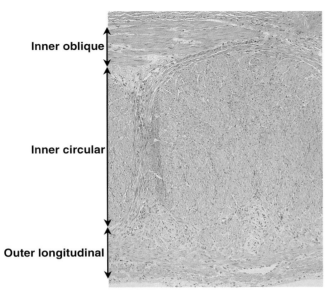

Figure 9.15 Illustration of the three-layer muscle coat of the stomach (the same case as Figure 9.1).

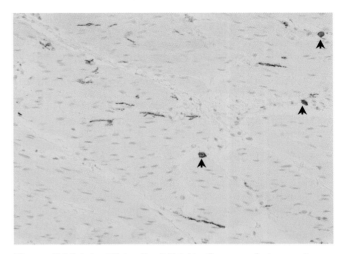

Figure 9.16 Interstitial cells of Cajal in the muscularis propria revealed by Kit immunostaining. Kit-positive spindle-shaped cells are scattered in the smooth muscle tissue. Scattered mast cells are also positive for Kit (arrows).

ganglion cells of the myenteric plexus of Auerbach are found between the inner circular and outer longitudinal coats.

Neural networks of the gastric wall and interstitial cells of Cajal

The stomach is richly innervated by both extrinsic and intrinsic nervous systems [66]. The extrinsic system includes the parasympathetic and sympathetic autonomic nerve supplies mentioned above, which include parasympathetic and sympathetic motor neurons and accompanying sensory neurons. The intrinsic system forms proper nerve plexuses (submucosal plexuses of Meissner and myenteric plexuses of Auerbach). Integration of these two elements enables the stomach to respond to both local and external stimuli by regulating motility, local blood flow, secretion, endocrine functions and mucosal defence mechanisms. In the wall, rich networks of cholinergic nerves are observed and a similar network is present for gastric glands in the mucosa, whereas adrenergic neurons are scantier [67]. Other types of neurons are also present in the gastric mucosa, such as peptidergic (peptide-containing) and nitrergic (nitric oxide synthetase-containing) neurons [66].

In the muscle coat, interstitial cells of Cajal are interposed between smooth muscle cells and neurons. They are pacemaker cells that regulate autonomous motility of the smooth muscle cells, also playing a role in mediating neurotransmission [68,69]. They are spindle-shaped or stellate and most are immunoreactive with c-kit (CD117) antibodies [70] (Figure 9.16).

Subserosa and serosa

The subserosa is a thin layer of loose areolar tissue containing blood vessels, lymphatics and nerve fibres. It is enclosed by the serosa, composed of a sheet of flattened mesothelial cells continuous with the serosal lining of the peritoneal cavity. When inflamed, the mesothelial cells easily show reactive swelling and nuclear atypia, which must not be misinterpreted as malignant cells, particularly in peritoneal cytology [13].

References

1. Rubesin SE, Levine MS, Laufer I. Double-contrast upper gastrointestinal radiography: a pattern approach for diseases of the stomach. *Radiology* 2008;**246**:33.
2. Kimura K. Chronological transition of the fundic-pyloric border determined by stepwise biopsy of the lesser and greater curvatures of the stomach. *Gastroenterology* 1972;**63**:584.
3. Sugano H, Nakamura K, Kato Y. Pathological studies of human gastric cancer. *Acta Pathol Jpn* 1982;**32**(suppl 2):329.
4. El-Zimaity HM. Gastric atrophy, diagnosing and staging. *World J Gastroenterol* 2006;**12**:5757.
5. Salem SN, Truelove SC. Dissecting microscope appearances of the gastric mucosa. *BMJ* 1964;**2**:1503.
6. Yoshii T. Comparative study on chronic gastritis with dissecting microscopic findings of stained stomach and histological findings: application to endoscopic diagnosis. *Progress of Digestive Endoscopy* 1976;**9**:49 (in Japanese).
7. Yao K, Oishi T. Microgastroscopic findings of mucosal microvascular architecture as visualized by magnifying endoscopy. *Dig Endosc* 2001;**13** (Suppl):S27.
8. Yao K. Gastric microvascular architecture as visualized by magnifying endoscopy: body and antral mucosa without pathologic change demonstrate two different patterns of microvascular architecture. *Gastrointest Endosc* 2004;**59**:596.

9. Yao K, Takaki Y, Matsui T, et al. Clinical application of magnification endoscopy and narrow-band imaging in the upper gastrointestinal tract: new imaging techniques for detecting and characterizing gastrointestinal neoplasia. *Gastrointest Endosc Clin N Am* 2008;**18**:415.

10. Gannon G. The vascular and lymphatic drainage. In: Whitehead R (ed.), *Gastrointestinal and Oesophageal Pathology*. Edinburgh: Churchill Livingstone, 1995: 129.

11. Levin KJ, Appelman HD. The stomach: embryology, normal anatomy, and tumor derivation. In: *Atlas of Tumor Pathology*, 3rd series. Fascicle 18 *Tumors of the Esophagus and Stomach*. Washington DC: AFIP, 1996: 175.

12. Moore KL, Dalley AF. *Clinically Oriented Anatomy*. Philadelphia, PA: Lippincott Williams & Wilkins, 2005.

13. Japanese Gastric Cancer Association. Japanese Classification of Gastric Carcinoma – 2nd English Edition. *Gastric Cancer* 1998; **1**:10.

14. Lauwers GY, Ban S, Mino M, et al. Endoscopic mucosal resection for gastric epithelial neoplasms: a study of 39 cases with emphasis on the evaluation of specimens and recommendations for optimal pathologic analysis. *Mod Pathol* 2004;**17**:2.

15. Ono H. Early gastric cancer: diagnosis, pathology, treatment techniques and treatment outcomes. *Eur J Gastroenterol Hepatol* 2006;**18**:863.

16. Edge SB, Byrd DR, Carducci MA, Compton CC, eds. *American Joint Committee on Cancer (AJCC) Cancer Staging Manual*, 7th edn. New York: Springer, 2009.

17. Sobin LH, Gospodarowicz MK, Wittekind CH, eds. *International Union against Cancer (UICC): TNM classification of malignant tumors*, 7th edn. Oxford: Wiley-Blackwell, 2009

18. Stockton M, McColl I. Comparative electron microscopic features of normal, intermediate and metaplastic pyloric epithelium. *Histopathology* 1983;**7**:859.

19. Krause WJ, Ivey KJ, Baskin WM, Mackercher PA. Morphological observations on the normal human cardiac glands. *Anat Rec* 1978;**192**:59.

20. Toner PG, Cameron CHS. The gastric mucosa. In: Whitehead R (ed.), *Gastrointestinal and Oesophageal Pathology*. Edinburgh: Churchill Livingstone, 1995: 15.

21. Karam SM, Leblond CP. Dynamics of epithelial cells in the corpus of the mouse stomach. III. Inward migration of neck cells followed by progressive transformation into zymogenic cells. *Anat Rec* 1993;**236**:297.

22. Bockman DE, Sharp R, Merlino G. Regulation of terminal differentiation of zymogenic cells by transforming growth factor α in transgenic mice. *Gastroenterology* 1995;**108**:447.

23. Hattori T, Helpap B, Gedigk P. The morphology and cell kinetics of pseudopyloric glands. *Virchows Arch B Cell Pathol Incl Mol Pathol* 1982;**39**:31.

24. Hanby AM, Poulsom R, Playford RJ, Wright NA. The mucous neck cell in the human gastric corpus: a distinctive, functional cell lineage. *J Pathol* 1999;**187**:331.

25. Forte JG, Forte TM, Black JA, Okamoto C, Wolosin JM. Correlation of parietal cell structure and function. *J Clin Gastroenterol* 1983;**5** Suppl 1:17.

26. Furuhashi M, Nakahara A, Fukutomi H, Kominami E, Uchiyama Y. Changes in subcellular structures of parietal cells in the rat gastric gland after omeprazole. *Arch Histol Cytol* 1992;**55**:191.

27. Hogben CAM, Kent TH, Woodward PA, Sill AJ. Quantitative histology of the gastric mucosa: man, dog, cat, guinea pig, and frog. *Gastroenterology* 1974;**67**:1143.

28. Samloff IM. Cellular localization of group 1 pepsinogens in human gastric mucosa by immunofluorescence. *Gastroenterology* 1971;**61**:185.

29. Cornaggia M, Riva C, Capella C, Solcia E, Samloff IM. Subcellular localization of pepsinogen II in stomach and duodenum by the immunogold technique. *Gastroenterology* 1987;**92**:585.

30. Sano J, Miki K, Ichinose M, et al. In situ localization of pepsinogens I and II mRNA in human gastric mucosa. *Acta Pathol Jpn* 1989;**39**:765.

31. Kim HY, Kim N, Kang JM, et al. Clinical meaning of pepsinogen test and *Helicobacter pylori* serology in the health check-up population in Korea. *Eur J Gastroenterol Hepatol* 2009;**21**:606.

32. Chandrasoma PT, Der R, Ma Y, Dalton P, Taira M. Histology of the gastro-oesophageal junction: an autopsy study. *Am J Surg Pathol* 2000;**24**:402.

33. Sarbia M, Donner A, Gabbert HE. Histopathology of the gastro-oesophageal junction: a study on 36 operation specimens. *Am J Surg Pathol* 2002;**26**:1207.

34. Glickman JN, Fox V, Antonioli DA, Wang HH, Odze RD. Morphology of the cardia and significance of carditis in pediatric patients. *Am J Surg Pathol* 2002;**26**:1032.

35. De Hertogh G, Van Eyken P, Ectors N, Tack J, Geboes K. On the existence and location of cardiac mucosa: an autopsy study in embryos, fetuses, and infants. *Gut* 2003;**52**:791.

36. Nakanishi Y, Saka M, Eguchi T, Sekine S, Taniguchi H, Shimoda T. Distribution and significance of the oesophageal and gastric cardiac mucosae: a study of 131 operation specimens. *Histopathology* 2007;**51**:515.

37. El-Zimaity H. How to interpret biopsies for 'gastritis'. *Pathol Case Reviews* 2008;**13**:157.

38. Jass JR, Filipe MI. The mucin profiles of normal gastric mucosa, intestinal metaplasia and its variants and gastric carcinoma. *Histochem J* 1981;**13**:931.

39. Inada K, Nakanishi H, Fujimitsu Y, et al. Gastric and intestinal mixed and solely intestinal types of intestinal metaplasia in the human stomach. *Pathol Int* 1997;**47**:831.

40. Rubio CA, Nesi G, Zampi GC, et al. Gastric ciliated metaplasia. A study of 3406 gastrectomy specimens from dwellers of the Atlantic and the Pacific basins. *J Clin Pathol* 2005;**58**:605.

41. Doglioni C, Laurino L, Dei Tos AP, et al. Pancreatic (acinar) metaplasia of the gastric mucosa. Histology, ultrastructure, immunocytochemistry, and clinicopathologic correlations of 101 cases. *Am J Surg Pathol* 1993;**17**:1134.

42. Falkmer S, Wilander E. The endocrine cell population. In: Whitehead R (ed.) *Gastrointestinal and Oesophageal Pathology*. Edinburgh: Churchill Livingstone, 1995: 63.

43. Fenoglio-Preiser CM. Gastrointestinal neuroendocrine lesions. In: *Gastrointestinal Pathology. An Atlas and Test*, 3rd edn. Philadelphia, PA: Lippincott Williams & Wilkins. 2008: 1099.

44. Tsutsumi Y, Nagura H, Watanabe K, Yanaihara N. A novel subtyping of intestinal metaplasia of the stomach, with special reference to the histochemical characterizations of endocrine cells. *Virchows Arch A Pathol Anat Histopathol* 1983;**401**:73.

45. Otsuka T, Tsukamoto T, Mizoshita T, et al. Coexistence of gastric- and intestinal-type endocrine cells in gastric and intestinal mixed intestinal metaplasia of the human stomach. *Pathol Int* 2005;**55**:170.

46. Hattori T. On cell proliferation and differentiation of the fundic mucosa of the golden hamster. Fractographic study combined with microscopy and 3H-thymidine autoradiography. *Cell Tissue Res* 1974;**148**:213.

47. Hattori T, Fujita S. Tritiated thymidine autoradiographic study of cell migration and renewal in the pyloric mucosa of golden hamsters. *Cell Tissue Res* 1976;**175**:49.

48. Hattori T, Niki H, Fujita S. Tritiated thymidine autoradiographic study on the origin and renewal of argentaffin cells in the pyloric gland of hamsters. *Cell Tissue Res* 1977;**181**:15.

49. Fujimoto S, Hattori T, Kimoto K, Yamashita S, Fujita S, Kawai K. Tritiated thymidine autoradiographic study on origin and renewal of gastrin cells in antral area of hamsters. *Gastroenterology* 1980;**79**:785.

50. Hattori T, Fujita S. Tritiated thymidine autoradiographic study on histogenesis and spreading of intestinal metaplasia in human stomach. *Pathol Res Pract* 1979;**164**:224.

51. Ota H, Katsuyama T, Akamatsu T, et al. Application of mucin histochemistry for pathological diagnosis-expression of gastric phenotypes in metaplastic and neoplastic lesions and its relation to the organoid differentiation. *Acta Histochem Cytochem* 1995; **28**:43.

52. Ota H, Katsuyama T, Ishii K, Nakayama J, Shiozawa T, Tsukahara Y. A dual staining method for identifying mucins of different gastric epithelial mucous cells. *Histochem J* 1991;**23**:22.

53. Jass JR. Mucin core proteins as differentiation markers in the gastrointestinal tract. *Histopathology* 2000;**37**:561.

54. Corfield AP, Myerscough N, Longman R, Sylvester P, Arul S, Pignatelli M. Mucins and mucosal protection in the gastrointestinal tract: new prospects for mucins in the pathology of gastrointestinal disease. *Gut* 2000;**47**:589.

55. Nordman H, Davies JR, Lindell G, de Bolós C, Real F, Carlstedt I. Gastric MUC5AC and MUC6 are large oligomeric mucins that differ in size, glycosylation and tissue distribution. *Biochem J* 2002;**364** (Pt 1):191.

56. Nakamura N, Ota H, Katsuyama T, et al. Histochemical reactivity of normal, metaplastic, and neoplastic tissues to alpha-linked *N*-acetylglucosamine residue-specific monoclonal antibody HIK1083. *J Histochem Cytochem* 1998;**46**:793.

57. Reis CA, David L, Correa P, et al. Intestinal metaplasia of human stomach displays distinct patterns of mucin (MUC1, MUC2, MUC5AC, and MUC6) expression. *Cancer Res* 1999;**59**:1003.

58. Mutoh H, Sakurai S, Satoh K, et al. Pericryptal fibroblast sheath in intestinal metaplasia and gastric carcinoma. *Gut* 2005;**54**:33.

59. Kreuning P, Bosman FT, Kuiper G, van der Wal AM, Lindeman J. Gastric and duodenal mucosa in 'healthy' individuals. An endoscopic and histopathological study of 50 volunteers. *J Clin Pathol* 1978;**31**:69.

60. Tsutsumi Y, Nagura H, Watanabe K. Immune aspects of intestinal metaplasia of the stomach: an immunohistochemical study. *Virchows Arch A Pathol Anat Histopathol* 1984;**403**:345.

61. Isaacson P. Immunoperoxidase study of the secretory immunoglobulin system and lysozyme in normal and diseased gastric mucosa. *Gut* 1982;**23**:578.

62. Selby WS, Janossy G, Jewell DP. Immunohistological characterisation of intraepithelial lymphocytes of the human gastrointestinal tract. *Gut* 1981;**22**:169.

63. Lehnert T, Erlandson RA, DeCosse JJ. Lymph and blood capillaries of the human gastric mucosa. A morphologic basis for metastasis in early gastric carcinoma. *Gastroenterology* 1985;**89**:939.

64. Listrom MB, Fenoglio-Preiser CM. Lymphatic distribution of the stomach in normal, inflammatory, hyperplastic, and neoplastic tissue. *Gastroenterology* 1987;**93**:506.

65. Yamada Y, Kato Y, Sugano H. Significance of the lamina muscularis mucosae of the stomach in invasiveness of gastric cancer. *Gan No Rinsho* 1984;**30**:1657 (in Japanese with English abstract).

66. Ekblad E, Mei Q, Sundler F. Innervation of the gastric mucosa. *Microsc Res Tech* 2000;**48**:241.

67. Kyosala K, Rechardt L, Veijola L, Waris T, Penttila O. Innervation of the human gastric wall. *J Anat* 1980;**131**:453.

68. Takayama I, Horiguchi K, Daigo Y, Mine T, Fujino MA, Ohno S. The interstitial cells of Cajal and a gastroenteric pacemaker system. *Arch Histol Cytol* 2002;**65**:1.

69. Sanders KM, Ward SM. Kit mutants and gastrointestinal physiology. *J Physiol* 2007;**578** (Pt 1):33.

70. Torihashi S, Horisawa M, Watanabe Y. c-Kit immunoreactive interstitial cells in the human gastrointestinal tract. *J Auton Nerv Syst* 1999;**75**:38.

10

Congenital abnormalities of the stomach

Michio Shimizu[1] and Do-Youn Park[2]

[1]Saitama Medical University, Saitama International Medical Center, Saitama, Japan
[2]Pusan National University College of Medicine, Pusan National University Hospital, Busan, Republic of Korea

Normal development

The gastrointestinal tract is derived largely from the endodermal germ layer, which gives rise to the epithelium, while the mesoderm is responsible for the development of the smooth muscle layer, the mesenchyme and numerous cell types [1]. The stomach develops from the embryonic foregut. The fusiform dilatation that will form the future stomach appears during weeks 4–5 of gestation, when the embryo is 4mm long. During the next 8 weeks, the stomach, which originates in the neck at the level of the third to fifth cervical segments, will descend into the abdomen at the level of the tenth thoracic to third lumbar segments. The greater and lesser curvatures develop during weeks 6 and 7. Eventually, the distal end of the stomach moves to the right and becomes the pylorus, whereas the proximal end moves to the left and evolves into the oesophago-gastric junction. During this period, gastric rugae appear and gastric pits develop in weeks 7–10. By week 14, the characteristic anatomical features can be identified, namely the greater curvature, lesser curvature, fundus, body, antrum and pylorus [2].

Gastric glands develop by the end of the third month [3]. Parietal cells and enterochromaffin cells appear in weeks 9–11 [4]. Later, chief cells can be identified and mucous neck cells can be observed by week 16 [5]. The circular muscle layer forms in about weeks 7–8 of embryonic life, followed by the longitudinal layer in weeks 11–12. The muscularis mucosae develops much later, in week 20.

At the molecular level, the structuring of the developing stomach involves cross-talk between the endoderm and the mesoderm through the action of morphogenism which belongs to the Hedgehog signalling pathway. Accordingly, defective Hedgehog signalling may play a role in the development of congenital malformations [6].

Developmental abnormalities

Congenital agastria

A single case of congenital agastria in a viable fetus has been reported [7]. In this patient, the oesophagus joined the first part of the duodenum. However, there was microscopic evidence of fundic-type gastric mucosa at the oesophago-duodenal junction. The patient also presented with micrognathia and a cleft soft palate. A jejunal pouch allowed the boy to grow and develop well for several years, although he ultimately died after repeated episodes of acute enteritis [7].

Congenital microgastria

This is a rare congenital anomaly, with fewer than 100 cases reported in the English literature [8]. In microgastria, the stomach is not only small but also tubular and often non-rotated, with no clear identification of cardia, body or antrum [9]. This may be caused by a failure of development of the dorsal mesogastrium. Symptoms include failure to thrive, vomiting and recurrent aspiration pneumonia. Microscopically, the gastric wall shows hypoplasia [10,11]. Cases of isolated congenital microgastria are exceptional and microgastria is often associated with other anomalies, such as: asplenia, intestinal malrotations and duodenal atresia; cardiopulmonary, renal and central nervous system (CNS) anomalies; laryngo-tracheobronchial clefts; and limb reduction defects [8,9,12–14]. It has been suggested that microgastria in association with limb reduction defects and CNS anomalies has a genetic basis, with an autosomal recessive pattern of inheritance [15].

Atresia, webs and diaphragms

Gastric atresia, webs and diaphragms, and infantile hypertrophic pyloric stenosis, represent common aetiologies of gastric outlet obstruction in infancy and childhood. Others include heterotrophic pancreas and acquired causes (peptic ulcer, caustic ingestion, tumour, chronic granulomatous disease and eosinophilic gastroenteritis) [16].

Atresia of the stomach, defined as a complete segmental defect (with or without a remnant fibrous cord), is an extremely rare condition. Related anomalies include webs and diaphragms. Antral diaphragm or web is a simple submucosal web covered by gastric mucosa, which lacks abnormal musculature. These anomalies share the same pathogenesis, namely abnormal fusion of redundant endoderm around 8 weeks' gestation with failure to develop a patent gastric lumen [17]. Gastric atresia may be associated with duodenal atresia, trisomy 21 and epidermolysis bullosa [18,19]. In many cases, polyhydramnios will be noted during pregnancy [20]. Deficient integrin $\alpha6\beta4$ complex located in hemi-desmosomes may represent a common mechanism [21]. Gastric atresia and complete web will manifest themselves shortly after birth with persistent non-bilious vomiting. An incomplete web may be associated instead with abdominal distension, intermittent vomiting, epigastric pain or failure to thrive. Successful treatments can either be surgical (excision with pyloroplasty) or endoscopic (balloon dilatation or transection) [16].

Congenital pyloric stenosis

Infantile hypertrophic pyloric stenosis occurs in about 3 of every 1000 live births [22]. It is five times more common in boys than in girls and is more often than not familial. Congenital pyloric stenosis arises in an otherwise healthy infant, usually manifesting itself between 3 and 12 weeks of age, making it the most common indication for surgical intervention in infancy. Failure to diagnose the condition often results in weight loss, dehydration and metabolic abnormalities. The typical presentation is the development of projectile, non-bilious vomiting. Gastric peristaltic waves can be observed externally and abdominal palpation can reveal a thickened pylorus, or 'olive', in the right upper quadrant. Abdominal sonographic examination will secure the diagnosis by demonstrating the hypertrophied pylorus (muscle thickness of at least 3 mm) [23] (Figure 10.1).

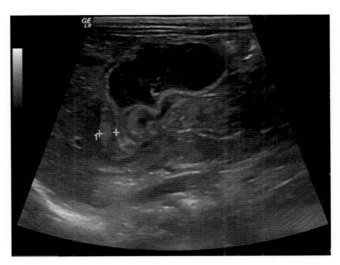

Figure 10.1 Abdominal sonographic examination demonstrating a thickened hypertrophic pylorus (white crosses). (Courtesy of Michael S. Gee, MD, PhD, Massachusetts General Hospital, Boston, USA.)

Microscopically, hypertrophic pyloric stenosis is characterised by concentric hypertrophy and thickening of the circular and longitudinal muscle of the pylorus with fibrosis [24]. There are, however, documented cases of early onset (including presentation at birth) hypertrophic pyloric stenosis, in which there is a notable family history of pyloric stenosis [25]. The aetiology of pyloric stenosis is unclear but may include genetic and environmental components. The role of breast milk feeding has been implicated in early onset cases [26].

Duplication

Gastric duplication accounts for between 3% and 20% of gastrointestinal duplications and affects females more often than males [27]. Controversy exists over the embryological origin of this anomaly. The description of cases with respiratory-type mucosa and seromucinous glands, along with the presence of pulmonary sequestration, has been used to support the theory of an origin from supernumerary foregut buds [27]. Gastric duplications can be tubular or cystic [28]. The cystic type does not communicate with the gastric lumen and is mostly located on the greater curvature or at the pylorus (Figure 10.2). It may present with ulceration, bleeding, rupture or carcinoma, and can mimic pancreatic pseudocyst or mucinous cystadenoma [29,30].

Microscopically, all layers of the stomach are identified and the mucosa resembles normal gastric mucosa. Small intestinal mucosa can also be seen. Gastric duplication can be associated with other anomalies, such as double oesophagus, gastrointestinal malrotations, multi-cystic kidney and pulmonary sequestration [31,32]. Although it

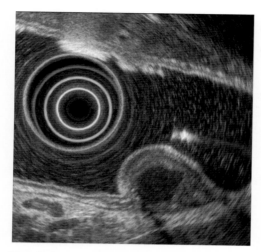

Figure 10.2 Endoscopic ultrasound appearance of cystic-type gastric duplication. The cyst does not communicate with the lumen. (Courtesy of Gwang Ha Kim, MD, PhD, Pusan National University Hospital, Busan, Republic of Korea.)

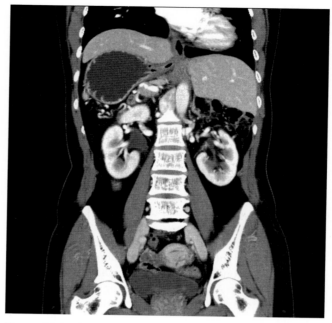

Figure 10.3 Abdominal CT scan of a patient with dextrogastria. The stomach is located on the right side and is compressed by the liver. (Courtesy of Gwang Ha Kim, MD, PhD, Pusan National University Hospital, Busan, Republic of Korea.)

is usually diagnosed during the first year of life, it may be discovered in adults, in whom the diagnosis can be challenging. Due to the risk of gastric cancer, surgical excision of the duplication is considered optimal treatment [33].

Diverticula

Gastric diverticula are an uncommon form of diverticular disease, accounting for much less than 5% of all gastrointestinal diverticula [34]. Congenital and acquired forms are recognised. Congenital diverticula comprise around 70% of all gastric diverticula [35]. Typically, they are located on the posterior wall of the stomach just below the gastro-oesophageal junction and may contain ectopic pancreatic tissue [36]. In contrast, acquired diverticula, typically seen in adults, are pseudo-diverticula (lacking muscular layers), usually distally located at or near the gastric antrum [35]. They are often associated with gastric tumours, peptic ulcer disease, pancreatitis or prior surgery [37].

Gastric diverticula usually remain asymptomatic. When symptomatic, upper abdominal pain, nausea and vomiting are the most common complaints [35,38]. Massive bleeding or perforation is uncommon. Not unexpectedly, given the posterior location, physical examination of most children with this disorder is unremarkable. The ability to definitively diagnose a gastric diverticulum can be difficult. Large diverticula may be difficult to distinguish from a communicating gastric duplication. Ultrasonography or CT is commonly the first radiographic study performed to evaluate abdominal symptoms in children; either can suggest the diagnosis of a gastric diverticulum but the findings may not be specific. Orally administered contrast should be given to

facilitate the diagnosis of gastric diverticula during CT. Surgical treatment is recommended only in complicated or symptomatic cases.

Dextrogastria

Dextrogastria occurs in 1 of every 6000–8000 births [39]. The stomach is displaced to the right of the midline and lies completely behind the liver or above it. It is commonly associated with situs inversus. Despite misplacement, the structure and function of the stomach are usually entirely normal (Figure 10.3).

Heterotopias

Heterotopic pancreas, observed in up to 1 in 500 laparotomies, is the most common form of heterotopia diagnosed in the stomach. It is also the second most common pancreatic congenital abnormality after pancreas divisum [40]. Heterotopic pancreas tends to be more frequent in males than in females. Its pathogenesis is controversial but it may be secondary to the abnormal location of developing pancreatic buds during embryogenesis. Usually asymptomatic, gastric heterotopia is commonly an incidental finding on imaging studies, at endoscopy or post mortem. Only a few cases are clinically significant, particularly larger lesions, which can be associated with abdominal pain, vomiting,

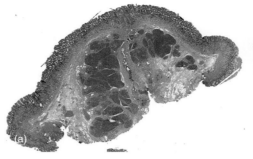
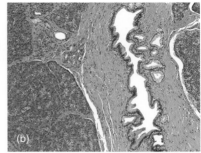

Figure 10.4 Heterotopic pancreas: (a) this gastric endoscopic mucosal resection specimen shows well-organised submucosal pancreatic lobules centred around a mid-size duct. (b) Higher magnification reveals benign pancreatic acini and duct.

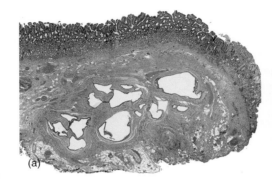
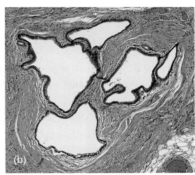

Figure 10.5 Heterotopic pancreas, 'adenomyoma' variant: (a) this lesion is composed of only dilated pancreatic ducts. (b) This benign condition should not be confused with a neoplastic lesion.

gastric outlet obstruction and even dysphagia in the very rare cases located near the gastro-oesophageal junction [41–44]. Gastric heterotopic pancreas is commonly situated in the submucosa of the distal stomach, most often within 50 mm of the pylorus. It is usually seen at endoscopy as a solitary, umbilicated submucosal lesion with occasional erosions of the overlying mucosa. The submucosal location of pancreatic heterotopia lends itself to endoscopic ultrasound evaluation with recognition of features distinguishing it from gastrointestinal stromal tumour (GIST) and leiomyoma, the major clinical and endoscopic differential diagnoses (by its hypoechoic nature) [45,46].

Heterotopic pancreas is variably composed of pancreatic acini, ducts or islets. Some cases contain all components of the pancreas, including ducts, acini and endocrine islets, whereas others consist of pancreatic ducts only (Figure 10.4). These are usually characterised by only dilated pancreatic ducts and are surrounded by prominent smooth muscle proliferation. They have also been termed 'adenomyomas' or 'myoepithelial hamartomas' (Figure 10.5). Other cases consist of only acinar tissue (exocrine pancreas), whereas some consist of only islet cells (endocrine pancreas) [47]. Ectopic pancreatic tissue can undergo secondary changes and complications, such as acute pancreatitis, pseudocyst formation, development of mucinous cysts and pancreatic intraepithelial neoplasia [48–55]. Rare cases of ectopic pancreatic tissue complicated by adenocarcinoma or even endocrine tumour have been described [54,56–58]. In symptomatic lesions, if a preoperative diagnosis can be secured, minimally invasive techniques should be the treatment of choice, including endoscopic resection and laparoscopic surgery [46].

Submucosal heterotopic glands of the stomach occur in 11% of resected stomachs. They are usually found in the distal half of the stomach and may be diffuse or localised [59] (Figure 10.6). Heterotopic gastric glands have also been reported as diffuse submucosal cysts or gastritis cystica profunda [60–62] and they may be a risk factor for multiple gastric cancers [63].

Volvulus

Gastric volvulus is a rare condition, defined as an abnormal rotation of the stomach leading to partial or total obstruction. Gastric volvulus usually, but not always, occurs with various causes of diaphragmatic defects, including para-oesophageal hernia [64]. Gastric volvulus can be categorised anatomically. Approximately two-thirds of cases are organo-axial volvulus, in which there is volvulus around the long axis of the lesser curve of the stomach, commonly associated with diaphragmatic defects. The stomach effectively turns upside down, so there is obstruction at both the proximal and distal ends. In these cases, rotation is more commonly anterior. The second type is mesenterico-axial volvulus, in which the stomach twists around a line from the middle of the greater curve to the porta hepatis. In some instances, the stomach may also twist around the gastro-hepatic omentum, resulting in torsion rather than volvulus.

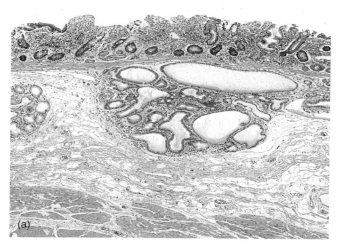
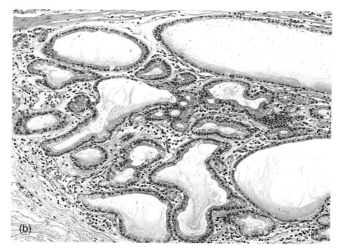

Figure 10.6 Submucosal heterotopic gastric glands: (a) as in this example, the glands are commonly distended and lined by bland mucin-secreting epithelium; (b) no atypia present.

Gastric volvulus is also classified as primary when anchoring structures, such as the gastro-hepatic, gastro-colic, gastro-phrenic and gastro-splenic ligaments, are weak or absent. It can also be secondary to anomalies such as congenital diaphragmatic hernia, hiatus hernia, diaphragmatic eventration, para-oesophageal hernia and wandering spleen. It can also develop after Nissen's fundoplication.

Gastric volvulus may manifest itself acutely or with chronic symptomatology [65,66]. Chronic gastric volvulus is difficult to diagnose because the signs are not specific. Most cases are diagnosed in elderly people, who may complain of recurrent pain and vomiting, and sometimes present with haematemesis. The symptoms in infants and children include non-bilious emesis, epigastric distension and abdominal pain. Failure to thrive due to recurrent foul eructations has also been reported [67]. Acute volvulus is a surgical emergency that presents with haemorrhage, ischaemia and infarction and carries significant mortality if not managed in a timely manner [68]. Surgical treatment is usually recommended and includes reduction, correction of predisposing factors and gastropexy [69].

References

1. McLin VA, Henning SJ, Jamrich M. The role of the visceral mesoderm in the development of the gastrointestinal tract. *Gastroenterology* 2009;**136**:2074.
2. Montgomery RK, Mulberg AE, Grand RJ. Development of the human gastrointestinal tract: twenty years of progress. *Gastroenterology* 1999;**116**:702.
3. Salenius P. On the ontogenesis of the human gastric epithelial cells. A histologic and histochemical study. *Acta Anat Suppl* 1962; **50**:1.
4. Russo P, Ruchelli ED, Piccoli DA. *Pathology of Pediatric Gastrointestinal and Liver Disease*. New York: Springer-Verlag, 2004: 47.
5. Grand RJ, Watkins JB, Torti FM. Development of the human gastrointestinal tract. A review. *Gastroenterology* 1976;**70**:790.
6. van den Brink GR. Hedgehog signaling in development and homeostasis of the gastrointestinal tract. *Physiol Rev* 2007;**87**:1343.
7. Dorney SF, Middleton AW, Kozlowski K, Benjamin BN, Kan AE, Kamath KR. Congenital agastria. *J Pediatr Gastroenterol Nutr* 1987;**6**:307.
8. Jones VS, Cohen RC. An eighteen year follow-up after surgery for congenital microgastria-case report and review of literature. *J Pediatr Surg* 2007;**42**:1957.
9. Tanaka K, Tsuchida Y, Hashizume K, Kawarasaki H, Sugiyama M. Microgastria: case report and a review of the literature. *Eur J Pediatr Surg* 1993;**3**:290.
10. Neifeld JP, Berman WF, Lawrence W Jr, Kodroff MB, Salzberg AM. Management of congenital microgastria with a jejunal reservoir pouch. *J Pediatr Surg* 1980;**15**:882.
11. Kroes EJ, Festen C. Congenital microgastria: a case report and review of literature. *Pediatr Surg Int* 1998;**13**:416.
12. Kawaguchi AL, Donahoe PK, Ryan DP. Management and long-term follow-up of patients with type III and IV laryngotracheoesophageal clefts. *J Pediatr Surg* 2005;**40**:158.
13. Siebert JR, Schoenecker KA, Resta RG, Kapur RP. Holoprosencephaly and limb reduction defects: a consideration of Steinfeld syndrome and related condition. *Am J Med Genet A* 2005;**134**:381.
14. Menon P, Rao KL, Cutinha HP, Thapa BR, Nagi B. Gastric augmentation in isolated congenital microgastria. *J Pediatr Surg* 2003;**38**:E4.
15. Al-Gazali LI, Bakir M, Dawodu A, Nath R, Al-Tatari HM, Gerami M. Recurrence of the severe form of microgastria-limb reduction defect in a consanguineous family. *Clin Dysmorphol* 1999;**8**:253.
16. Feng J, Gu W, Li M, et al. Rare causes of gastric outlet obstruction in children. *Pediatr Surg Int* 2005;**21**:635.
17. Mitchell KG, McGowan A, Smith DC, Gillespie G. Pyloric diaphragm, antral web, congenital antral membrane: a surgery rarity? *Br J Surg* 1979;**66**:572.
18. Achiron R, Hamiel-Pinchas O, Engelberg O, et al. Aplasia cutis congenita associated with epidermolysis bullosa and pyloric atresia: the diagnostic role of prenatal ultrasonography. *Prenat Diagn* 1992;**12**:765.
19. Sarin YK. Pyloric atresia associated with intestinal atresia. *Indian Pediatr* 2000;**37**:206.
20. Ferguson C, Morabito A, Bianchi A. Duodenal atresia and gastric antral web. A significant lesson to learn. *Eur J Pediatr Surg* 2004; **14**:120.

21. Lachaux A, Bouvier R, Loras-Duclaux I, Chappuis JP, Meneguzzi G, Ortonne JP. Isolated deficient alpha6beta4 integrin expression in the gut associated with intractable diarrhea. *J Pediatr Gastroenterol Nutr* 1999;**29**:395.

22. Schechter R, Torfs CP, Bateson TF. The epidemiology of infantile hypertrophic pyloric stenosis. *Paediatr Perinatol Epidemiol* 1997;**11**:407.

23. Hernanz-Schulman M. Infantile hypertrophic pyloric stenosis. *Radiology* 2003;**227**:319.

24. Solowiejczyk M, Holtzman M, Michowitz M. Congenital hypertrophic pyloric stenosis: a long-term follow-up of 41 cases. *Am Surg* 1980;**46**:567.

25. Demian M, Nguyen S, Emil S. Early pyloric stenosis: a case control study. *Pediatr Surg Int* 2009;**25**:1053.

26. Davanzo R, Perini R, Ventura A, Guastalla P. Infantile hypertrophic pyloric stenosis and cow's milk intolerance. *Pediatr Med Chir* 1987;**9**:77.

27. Theodosopoulos T, Marinis A, Karapanos K, et al. Foregut duplication cysts of the stomach with respiratory epithelium. *World J Gastroenterol* 2007;**13**:1297.

28. Perek A, Perek S, Kapan M, Göksoy E. Gastric duplication cyst. *Dig Surg* 2000;**17**:634.

29. D'Journo XB, Moutardier V, Turrini O, et al. Gastric duplication in an adult mimicking mucinous cystadenoma of the pancreas. *J Clin Pathol* 2004;**57**:1215.

30. Wieczorek RL, Seidman I, Ranson JH, Ruoff M. Congenital duplication of the stomach: case report and review of the English literature. *Am J Gastroenterol* 1984;**79**:597.

31. Knight J, Garvin PJ, Lewin E Jr, Gastric duplication presenting as a double oesophagus. *J Pediatr Surg* 1983;**18**:300.

32. Thornhill BA, Cho KC, Morehouse HT. Gastric duplication associated with pulmonary sequestration. CT manifestations. *Am J Roentgenol* 1982;**138**:1168.

33. Kuraoka K, Nakayama H, Kagawa T, Ichikawa T, Yasui W, Adenocarcinoma arising from a gastric duplication cyst with invasion to the stomach: a case report with literature review. *J Clin Pathol* 2004;**57**:428.

34. Simstein NL. Congenital gastric anomalies. *Am Surg* 1986;**52**:264.

35. Rodeberg DA, Zaheer S, Moir CR, Ishitani MB. Gastric diverticulum: a series of four pediatric patients. *J Pediatr Gastroenterol Nutr* 2002;**34**:564.

36. Elliott S, Sandler AD, Meehan JJ, Lawrence JP. Surgical treatment of a gastric diverticulum in an adolescent. *J Pediatr Surg* 2006;**41**:1467.

37. Eras P, Beranbaum SL. Gastric diverticula: congenital and acquired. *Am J Gastroenterol* 1972;**57**:120.

38. Velanovich V. Gastric diverticulum. Endoscopic and radiologic appearance. *Surg Endosc* 1994;**8**:1338

39. Hewlett PW. Isolated dextrogastria. *Br J Radiol* 1982;**55**:678.

40. Lai EC, Tompkins RK. Heterotopic pancreas. Review of a 26 year experience. *Am J Surg* 1986;**15**:697.

41. Rodriguez FJ, Abraham SC, Allen MS, Sebo TJ. Fine-needle aspiration cytology findings from a case of pancreatic heterotopias at the gastroesophageal junction. *Diagn Cytopathol* 2004;**31**:175.

42. Shalaby M, Kochman ML, Lichtenstein GR. Heterotopic pancreas presenting as dysphagia. *Am J Gastroenterol* 2002;**97**:1046.

43. Ogata H, Oshio T, Ishibashi H, Takano S, Yagi M. Heterotopic pancreas in children: review of the literature and report of 12 cases. *Pediatr Surg Int* 2008;**24**:271.

44. Ormarsson OT, Haugen SE, Juul I. Gastric outlet obstruction caused by heterotopic pancreas. *Eur J Pediatr Surg* 2003;**13**:410.

45. Kim JH, Lim JS, Lee YC, et al. Endosonographic features of gastric ectopic pancreases distinguishable from mesenchymal tumors. *J Gastroenterol Hepatol* 2008;**23**:e301.

46. Ormarsson OT, Gudmundsdottir I, Mårvik R. Diagnosis and treatment of gastric heterotopic pancreas. *World J Surg* 2006;**30**:1682.

47. Hammock L, Jorda M. Gastric endocrine pancreatic heterotopia. *Arch Pathol Lab Med* 2002;**126**:464.

48. Hirasaki S, Tanimizu M, Moriwaki T, Nasu J. Acute pancreatitis occurring in gastric aberrant pancreas treated with surgery and proved by histological examination. *Intern Med* 2005;**44**:1169.

49. Mulholland KC, Wallace WD, Epanomeritakis E, Hall SR. Pseudocyst formation in gastric ectopic pancreas. *JOP* 2004;**10**:498.

50. Kaufman A, Storey D, Lee CS, Murali R. Mucinous cyst exhibiting severe dysplasia in gastric heterotopic pancreas associated with gastrointestinal stromal tumour. *World J Gastroenterol* 2007;**21**:5781.

51. Rimal D, Thapa SR, Munashighe N, Chitre VV. Symptomatic gastric heterotopic pancreas: clinical presentation and review of the literature. *Int J Surg* 2008;**6**:e52.

52. Burke GW, Binder SC, Barron AM, Dratch PL, Umlas J. Heterotopic pancreas: gastric outlet obstruction secondary to pancreatitis and pancreatic pseudocyst. *Am J Gastroenterol* 1989;**84**:52.

53. Wilde GE, Gakhal M, Sartip KA, Corso MJ, Butt WG. Pancreatitis in initially occult gastric heterotopic pancreas. *Clin Imaging* 2007;**31**:356.

54. Osanai M, Miyokawa N, Tamaki T, Yonekawa M, Kawamura A, Sawada N. Adenocarcinoma arising in gastric heterotopic pancreas: clinicopathological and immunohistochemical study with genetic analysis of a case. *Pathol Int* 2001;**51**:549.

55. Emerson L, Layfield LJ, Rohr LR, Dayton MT. Adenocarcinoma arising in association with gastric heterotopic pancreas: A case report and review of the literature. *J Surg Oncol* 2004;**87**:53.

56. Song DE, Kwon Y, Kim KR, Oh ST, Kim JS. Adenocarcinoma arising in gastric heterotopic pancreas: a case report. *J Korean Med Sci* 2004;**19**:145.

57. Chetty R, Weinreb I. Gastric neuroendocrine carcinoma arising from heterotopic pancreatic tissue. *J Clin Pathol* 2004;**57**:314.

58. Guillou L, Nordback P, Gerber C, Schneider RP. Ductal adenocarcinoma arising in a heterotopic pancreas situated in a hiatus hernia. *Arch Pathol Lab Med* 1994;**118**:568.

59. Yamagiwa H, Matsuzaki O, Ishihara A, Yoshimura H. Heterotopic gastric glands in the submucosa of the stomach. *Acta Pathol Jpn* 1979;**29**:347.

60. Iwanaga T, Koyama H, Takahashi Y, Taniguchi H, Wada A. Diffuse submucosal cysts and carcinoma of the stomach. *Cancer* 1975;**36**:606.

61. Franzin G, Novelli P. Gastric cystica profunda. *Histopathology* 1981;**5**:535.

62. Fonde EC, Rodning CB. Gastritis cystica profunda. *Am J Gastroenterol* 1986;**81**:459.

63. Tsuji T, Iwahashi M, Nakamori M, et al. Multiple early gastric cancer with gastritis cystica profunda showing various histological types. *Hepatogastroenterology* 2008;**55**:1150.

64. Godshall D, Mossallam U, Rosenbaum R. Gastric volvulus: case report and review of the literature. *J Emerg Med* 1999;**17**:837.

65. Miller DL, Pasquale MD, Seneca RP, Hodin E. Gastric volvulus in the pediatric population. *Arch Surg* 1991;**126**:1146.

66. Patel NM. Chronic gastric volvulus: report of a case and review of literature. *Am J Gastroenterol* 1985;**80**:170.

67. Cribbs RK, Gow KW, Wulkan ML. Gastric volvulus in infants and children. *Pediatrics* 2008;**122**:e752.

68. Rashid F, Thangarajah T, Mulvey D, Larvin M, Iftikhar SY. A review article on gastric volvulus: A challenge to diagnosis and management. *Int J Surg* 2010;**8**:18.

69. Joshi M, Parelkar S, Sanghvi B, Agrawal A, Mishra P, Pradeep SH. Gastric volvulus in children: experience of 6 years at a tertiary care centre. *Afr J Paediatr Surg* 2010;**7**:2.

CHAPTER 11

Inflammatory disorders of the stomach

Hala El-Zimaity[1] and Robert H. Riddell[2]

[1]University of Toronto, Toronto, ON, Canada
[2]Mount Sinai Hospital, Toronto, ON, Canada

The term 'gastritis' is often used loosely by clinicians to describe any condition in which upper central abdominal discomfort or pain, heartburn and nausea or vomiting is a conspicuous symptom, although clinical signs and radiological examinations are negative. Further, endoscopists blithely make the diagnosis when they see redness of the gastric mucosa, a situation most often caused not by inflammation but by a failure to fully inflate the stomach at endoscopy. There is also frequently poor correlation of symptoms, endoscopic appearance of the stomach and histology of the mucosa, underscoring that biopsy and subsequent histological examination are essential. It is usually possible to subdivide gastric pathology into 'gastritis' for mucosal changes associated with inflammation and 'gastropathy' for non-inflammatory conditions. Nevertheless, their aetiologies and pathogenic mechanisms frequently overlap, and, for example, inflammation can be seen in gastropathies associated with erosions.

Classification of 'gastritis' and 'gastropathies'

Although no classification satisfies everyone, most lesions can be classified into 'gastropathies', 'gastritides' and 'endoscopic gastropathies'. In practical terms, a pathology report should have an indication of the aetiology (or a differential diagnosis) rather than a microscopic description.

Gastropathies

Gastropathies are conditions in which non-inflammatory changes predominate. This group includes pathology demonstrating primary epithelial reactive changes (e.g. chemical/reflux gastropathy) and a smaller subset of conditions with a predominance of vascular pathology (e.g. portal hypertensive gastropathy and gastric antral vascular ectasia [GAVE]) (Table 11.1).

Gastropathies with predominant epithelial changes

Reactive gastropathy

Dixon and his colleagues first described this condition in a series of patients who had undergone previous gastric surgery for peptic ulcer and presented with reflux of bile into the stomach [1]. Similar changes were later recognised in association with long-term ingestion of non-steroidal anti-inflammatory drugs (NSAIDs) [2,3]. In the absence of inflammation (which is the case in the absence of erosions), the term 'gastropathy' is commonly used. Synonyms include reflux, NSAID and chemical gastropathy.

The condition is seen in its most severe form in biopsies taken from gastric mucosa proximal to a previously performed gastro-enteric anastomosis. In most instances, however, the changes are subtle. In the absence of previous surgery, a history of NSAID ingestion may be present and, if not, should be suggested in the report. However, reactive gastropathy may occur in association with a variety of other conditions. It is found in some cases of heavy alcohol ingestion [4] and in almost 10% of healthy volunteers with no history of drug ingestion [5].

The histological features are primarily foveolar hyperplasia, marked mucin depletion, epithelial nuclear enlargement, prominence of (the normal) smooth muscle within

Morson and Dawson's Gastrointestinal Pathology, Fifth Edition. Edited by Neil A. Shepherd, Bryan F. Warren,
Geraint T. Williams, Joel K. Greenson, Gregory Y. Lauwers and Marco R. Novelli.
© 2013 Blackwell Publishing Ltd. Published 2013 by Blackwell Publishing Ltd.

Table 11.1 Classification of gastropathies

Category	Subcategory	
Gastropathy	Predominant epithelial changes	Chemical/reflux gastropathy Alcoholic gastropathy Drug- and caustic-induced injury Graft-versus-host disease Radiation/chemotherapy Ischaemia
	Predominant vascular pathology	Gastric antral vascular ectasia Portal hypertension Haemorrhagic/shock gastropathy

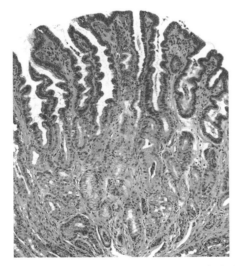

Figure 11.1 Reactive gastropathy: the changes include foveolar hyperplasia and tortuosity with hyperchromasia of surface epithelial cells. The lamina propria contains occasional elongated spindle-shaped smooth muscle cells.

the lamina propria and a reduction in the number of inflammatory cells [1]. Indeed the last is exemplified by the original Dixon scoring system, in which a diminution of inflammatory cells scores positively and is more likely to result in a diagnosis of reactive gastropathy. Other features include vascular congestion and oedema of the lamina propria. With foveolar hyperplasia, there is elongation and increased tortuosity of the foveolae (gastric pits), especially in the antrum. In addition, there may be hyperchromatism and enlargement of the nuclei of the mucosa-lining cells, features that sometimes may be sufficiently marked to be confused with dysplasia (Figure 11.1). The mucosa having mucin depletion causes it to appear red endoscopically.

It is possible that oedema contributes to making the normal smooth muscle cells more prominent but it has been postulated that real smooth muscle proliferation could be due to platelet-derived growth factor released by repeated leakage from vessels as a result of damage induced by bile or repeated surface erosions caused by NSAIDs [6]. Reduction in the number of inflammatory cells within the lamina propria may also be more apparent than real, again resulting from the accompanying oedema. Moreover, it has been noted that biopsies taken adjacent to mucosal ulcers caused by chronic salicylate use also show surprisingly little inflammation of the mucosa [7]. Although many of the histological features of reactive gastropathy are subjective, there is good correlation with biochemical evidence of bile reflux when formal scoring systems are used [3]. Nevertheless, it is sometimes difficult to distinguish mild changes from normality.

When concomitant *Helicbacter pylori* infection is present, it increases the likelihood of NSAID-induced mucosal damage. In such cases the oedema and smooth muscle may be obscured and the paucity of inflammatory cells completely reversed [8]. In contrast, reactive gastropathy in the postoperative stomach due to significant bile reflux is seldom colonised by *H. pylori* [9].

Although the association between reactive gastropathy and NSAID ingestion is established [10–13], sensitivity is low. Using a semi-quantitative technique based on severity of each of the histological features [1], a diagnosis of reactive gastropathy was possible in only a third of NSAID users [5], with the most consistent abnormalities being foveolar hyperplasia and prominent smooth muscle fibres in the lamina propria.

Reactive gastropathy and other mucosal changes in the operated stomach

Reactive gastropathy is seen in its most florid form in the operated stomach. It has been suggested that duodeno-gastric reflux is the cause and the presence of an excess of bile acids and activated pancreatic juice with enteric organisms is a potent combination. Cystic change proximal to the stoma is also well recognised and may be florid such that cystically dilated glands become displaced into the submucosa or even the external muscle coat. This may result in the formation of a polyp or tumour that should be distinguished carefully from adenocarcinoma. The condition has been described as gastritis cystica polyposa or profunda [14]. Of note, there are some similarities with the changes seen in solitary ulcer syndrome of the rectum and some of the changes may be secondary to mucosal prolapse in the vicinity of the stoma. Peristomal typical hyperplastic polyps, either single or multiple, have been reported in about 10% of patients at long-term follow-up [15,16].

There is an increased relative risk of carcinoma developing in the gastric stump, particularly when more than 20 years have elapsed following partial gastrectomy. Epithelial dysplasia, either flat or polypoid, may help to identify patients at increased risk [17,18]. The distinction between genuine dysplasia and the much more common reactive 'atypia' in foveolar hyperplasia can be difficult, and is almost certainly responsible for some reports claiming a high prevalence (up to 40%) of post-gastrectomy low grade dysplasia. Such over-diagnosis is supported by the observation that the lesions were not observed to progress to malignancy; rather they tend to regress [19,20]. By contrast, in one large prospective series, unequivocal severe dysplasia was a rare diagnosis that progressed to intramucosal carcinoma [21].

Chronic atrophic gastritis is also common after gastroenterostomy, developing in 54% of patients within 2 years of surgery [22]. This is mainly limited to the mucosa around the stoma. A selective loss of parietal cells leaving glands composed of mucus and chief cells has been noted [23]. Glands frequently become irregular and cystic. Pyloric/pseudo-pyloric metaplasia (also known as ulcer-associated cell lineage) and intestinal metaplasia are both common in this situation.

Gastropathies with predominant vascular changes

Portal hypertensive gastropathy or congestive gastropathy

Portal hypertensive gastropathy (PHG) [24] affects over 60% of patients with cirrhosis, although less than 25% have severe lesions [25,26]. Although minor lesions appear to be of little significance, severe cases of PHG are of clinical importance due to the associated bleeding. This may be insidious, resulting in iron-deficiency anaemia, or severe enough to warrant emergency endoscopy and blood transfusion. Of note, bleeding from congestive gastropathy may be more common after sclerotherapy of oesophageal varices [27]. Endoscopically, the mucosal appearance varies from mild hyperaemia to severe haemorrhages with 'cherry-red' spots similar to those of oesophageal varices. Histologically, mucosal capillary dilatation and congestion are the principal features, whereas inflammation is frequently absent. Of note, the diagnosis of PHG may not always be apparent on biopsy if using only routine haematoxylin and eosin (H&E) staining and immunocytochemistry may be required to highlight mucosal capillaries [28].

Histology reveals focal ectasia of capillaries immediately beneath the surface, with an increase in the number and diameter of both mucosal and submucosal blood vessels. The vascular congestion and dilatation are out of proportion to any concomitant inflammatory cell infiltrate [27–29]. The vascular ectasia is present in both the proximal and distal stomach. In cases where the whole stomach has been available for examination, there is marked dilatation and tortuosity of submucosal veins, especially in the corpus and cardia, possibly corresponding to gastric varices [27].

Gastric antral vascular ectasia ('watermelon' stomach)

This condition is characterised by similar histological and endoscopic changes to those of congestive gastropathy. Although the condition is sometimes associated with portal hypertension, in many cases this is absent. The entity is rare and was described in a series of just three patients with severe iron deficiency anaemia due to bleeding from the lesion: this communication applied the term 'watermelon stomach' on account of the characteristic findings at endoscopy [30]. The condition affects middle-aged and elderly individuals with a marked female predominance. Iron deficiency anaemia is the most common presenting symptom. Endoscopy shows characteristic longitudinal, almost parallel, mucosal folds within the antrum with prominent congested vessels in the apices of the folds giving a striped appearance [30–32]. Histology of the antral mucosa shows prominent dilated, congested, mucosal capillaries beneath the epithelial surface. In addition, microthrombi are present within some vessels and there is fibromuscular hyperplasia in the lamina propria, with prominent smooth muscle cells extending upwards perpendicular to the muscularis mucosae [31,32] (Figure 11.2). Active inflammation is absent. The antral mucosa may be hypertrophic but atrophic gastritis of the corpus and hypergastrinaemia were reported to be common in one series [33]. In antral biopsies, the combination of capillary ectasia, fibrin thrombi and fibromuscular spindle cell proliferation in the lamina propria

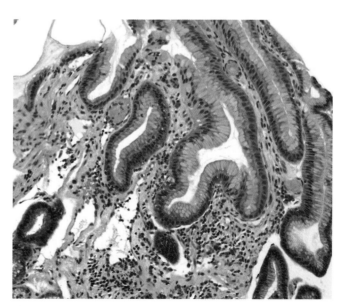

Figure 11.2 Gastric antral vascular ectasia (GAVE): the lesion is characterised by dilated capillaries in the superficial mucosa with occasional thrombi. Fibromuscular spindle cells are noted. (Courtesy of Lisa A. Cerilli, MD, University of Michigan, USA.)

should alert the pathologist to the diagnosis [34]. The condition is important, because it is increasingly recognised as a cause of gastrointestinal bleeding. Extension of lesions beyond the antrum to the proximal stomach may occur, especially in association with diaphragmatic hernia [35].

Vasculitis

Within the gastrointestinal tract, the small intestine and gallbladder are the sites most frequently involved by vasculitis, whereas the stomach is seldom affected [36]. Occasional cases presenting with gastrointestinal haemorrhage [37] or refractory gastric ulcer [26] have been reported. Depending on the condition, the blood vessels may show characteristic changes, often with an eosinophilic fibrinoid infiltrate and occasional giant cells. Henoch–Schönlein purpura may affect small vessels of the gastric mucosa. There is focal intramucosal haemorrhage accompanied by an intense acute inflammation. Leukocytoclasis is often present. These changes often obscure the underlying eosinophilic fibrinoid degeneration in affected capillaries, making biopsy diagnosis difficult without relevant clinical information (Figure 11.3). Extensive necrotising granulomatous infiltration of the submucosa, muscularis propria and serosa of the stomach, with a heavy eosinophilic infiltrate, has been reported in the stomach in association with allergic granulomatosis (Churg–Strauss syndrome) [38].

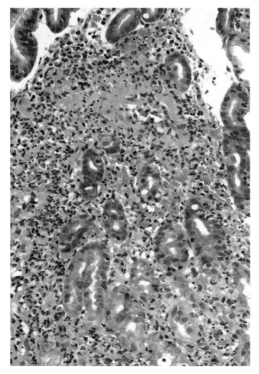

Figure 11.3 Gastric mucosa in Henoch–Schönlein purpura: there is intense acute inflammation and leukocytosis with haemorrhage around affected capillary vessels, which show eosinophilic fibrinoid degeneration.

Gastritides

As acute gastritis is not biopsied on a regular basis, we first address its chronic phase, a stage that is more commonly encountered in practice. We should not forget that chronic gastritis is essentially a histological diagnosis and that the correlation between clinical symptoms, endoscopic appearance and histology is notoriously poor [39]. Thus, gastric biopsy is an essential part of endoscopic examination even if no specific lesion such as an ulcer is seen [4]. It is incumbent on the pathologist to provide all information relevant to the correct diagnosis and subsequent treatment, if at all possible.

The classification of chronic gastritis

Many classifications have been designed over the years. Whitehead and his colleagues advocated classifying chronic gastritis according to mucosal type, the grade of gastritis, whether it is superficial or atrophic, and the type of associated metaplasia [40]. Strickland and Mackay classified chronic gastritis into type A and type B based on topography. Type A refers to gastritis involving the corpus and often associated with parietal cell autoantibodies and minimal antral involvement. Type B gastritis involves the distal stomach predominantly with only patchy involvement of the corpus [41]. Wyatt and Dixon proposed a classification based on histological features and pathogenesis. This consisted of type A (autoimmune), type B (bacterial) and type C (chemical or reflux gastritis) [42].

The most recent and now perhaps most widely used classification of chronic gastritis is the Sydney system, which was devised by an international working party and attempted to draw many previous classifications together and to combine histological and endoscopic assessment [43,44]. This system, combining aetiology, topography and morphology, relies on obtaining at least two mucosal biopsies from both the antrum and the corpus, in addition, of course, to biopsies of any specific lesions. These multiple mucosal biopsies are said to be essential for the proper assessment of the extent and severity of gastritis. As endoscopy is neither a sensitive nor a specific method for diagnosing gastritis [45], the discussion here is limited to histology.

The Sydney classification was introduced in an attempt to produce standardised interpretation of gastric biopsies and to allow semi-quantitative assessment of progression or regression of histological abnormalities. Five histological variables – chronic inflammation, activity (neutrophil infiltration), atrophy, intestinal metaplasia and *H. pylori* density – are graded as mild, moderate or severe. The system is easy to apply but inter-observer variation remains an issue, especially with regard to grading [46,47]. Although widely used, the system has not met with universal approval and an alternative classification based on morphological and probable aetiological considerations has been proposed [48,49].

In the revised 1994 version of the Sydney classification, the necessity for multiple biopsies (at least five) from antrum, corpus and incisura angularis was emphasised in order to permit assessment of the distribution of gastritis, atrophy and intestinal metaplasia. In addition, the value of grading these variables as a means of monitoring progression of disease or response to treatment was emphasised, as was the use of visual analogue scales as a template for grading inflammation and atrophy, a method previously shown to be convenient and reasonably accurate [49,50].

In practical terms, we seldom see Sydney-type biopsies undertaken for the routine histological assessment of the stomach. Some have argued that the system is more appropriate for research and provides little evidence for the routine management of the individual patient. In that regard, the system was established mainly by pathologists and there has been little correlation with clinical features and, in particular, the utility of the Sydney system for the subsequent management of the individual patient.

Distinctive types of gastritis

The designation 'distinctive' or 'specific' refers to histological features that markedly narrow the differential diagnosis or are, occasionally, pathognomonic. For simplicity, gastritis is subclassified into infectious and non-infectious gastritides and those seen as part of a systemic involvement (Table 11.2).

Chronic gastritis associated with *H. pylori* infection
Since the association between *H. pylori* infection and chronic gastritis was 're-discovered' by Warren and Marshall [51]

it is now clear that the organism is the principal cause of chronic gastritis. *H. pylori* has undergone various name changes since its identification. It was first known as *Campylobacter pyloridis*, then *Campylobacter pylori*. It is not, however, a member of the Campylobacter genus [52]. The organism is now universally known as *Helicobacter pylori* [53].

H. pylori is aetiologically linked to histological gastritis, peptic ulcer disease, marginal zone lymphoma and gastric carcinoma, in addition to other conditions (Table 11.3). The vast majority of cases of *H. pylori* gastritis present to clinicians and pathologists alike as chronic gastritis. There is, however, evidence, albeit scanty, that, in the initial stages of infection, there is an acute gastritis, a transient condition followed by either resolution within 11–14 days after infection or the onset of chronic gastritis [54,55]. Volunteer studies have shown neutrophil polymorph infiltration of the superficial gastric mucosa with mild degenerative changes in the superficial epithelium.

H. pylori infection is present in approximately 60% of the world population and is, in many communities, acquired before the age of 10 [56]. The prevalence of *H. pylori* infection varies both between and within countries [57–59]. This relates to the known determinants of infection, particularly socioeconomic standards [60]. Differences in prevalence among ethnic groups of similar socioeconomic status reflect differences in the environment and possible host and bacterial genetics. In countries where there has been rapid economic development with associated improvements in standards of living, there is some evidence that the prevalence of infection is declining. In developed countries, it is currently uncommon to find infected children but there is a cohort effect, so that the percentage of infected people increases with age, with about 50% infected in those aged >60

Table 11.2 Classification of gastritis

Category	Subcategory
Infectious	**Bacterial**: *Helicobacter pylori* bacterial infection Non-*H. pylori* bacterial infections – *H. heilmannii*, tuberculosis, syphilis, phlegmonous and emphysematous gastritis **Viral**: cytomegalovirus, herpes **Fungal**: *Candida* spp., *Histoplasma* spp., mucormycosis, aspergillosis **Parasitic**: cryptosporidia, *Anisakis* spp., other protozoa and nematodes
Non-infectious	Inflammatory bowel disease Eosinophilic gastro-enteritis Lymphocytic gastritis Collagenous gastritis
Part of systemic involvement	Graft-versus-host disease Vasculitis (e.g. Churg–Strauss syndrome)

Table 11.3 Gastric conditions associated with *Helicobacter pylori* infection

Acute gastritis
Chronic active gastritis
Duodenal ulceration
Gastric ulceration
Gastric carcinoma
Gastric lymphoma

Extra-gastric conditions that have been associated with *H. pylori* infection
Iron deficiency anaemia[a,b]
Vitamin B$_{12}$ deficiency
Pernicious anaemia
Coronary artery disease
Cerebrovascular disease
Hypertension
Raynaud's phenomenon
Migraine headaches
Hyperemesis gravidarum[c]
Immune (idiopathic) thrombocytopaenic purpura
Hyperammonaemia
Sudden infant death syndrome
Growth retardation 'short stature'[d]
Anorexia of ageing
Rosacea

[a]Baggett HC, Parkinson AJ, Muth PT, Gold BD, Gessner BD. Endemic iron deficiency associated with *Helicobacter pylori* infection among school-aged children in Alaska. *Pediatrics* 2006;**117**:e396–404.
[b]Yokota S, Konno M, Mino E, Sato K, Takahashi M, Fujii N. Enhanced Fe ion-uptake activity in *Helicobacter pylori* strains isolated from patients with iron-deficiency anaemia. *Clin Infect Dis* 2008;**46**:e31–3.
[c]Sandven I, Abdelnoor M, Nesheim BI, Melby KK. *Helicobacter pylori* infection and hyperemesis gravidarum: a systematic review and meta-analysis of case-control studies. *Acta Obstet Gynecol Scand* 2009;**88**:1190–200.
[d]Vilchis J, Duque X, Mera R, et al. Association of *Helicobacter pylori* infection and height of Mexican children of low socioeconomic level attending boarding schools. *Am J Trop Med Hyg* 2009;**81**:1091–6.

[60]. The higher prevalence among elderly people reflects higher infection rates when they were children rather than infection at later ages. Nevertheless, *H. pylori* infection remains common among the socially disadvantaged and in the immigrant population in developed countries.

Although the exact route of transmission is not known, person-to-person transmission is most likely, by oral–oral or faecal–oral routes, as exemplified by data on intrafamilial clustering. The role of external reservoirs in *H. pylori* transmission has not been ruled out, particularly in rural and developing areas [61]. Nevertheless, studies on water yielded inconsistent results that may reflect different water treatment modalities and/or variations in detection procedures.

H. pylori is a curved or spiral shaped bacterium 2–4 μm in length with sheathed flagella at one or occasionally both ends [51]. The organism possesses powerful urease activity, which is the basis for a number of biochemical tests for infection. There is considerable genomic diversity but pathogenicity depends to some extent on the production of various potent proteins, especially vacuolating toxin (vac-A) and cytotoxin-associated protein (cag-A). Strains possessing these cytotoxins are associated with increased inflammation and mucosal damage [62]. Western patients infected with strains carrying the cag-A pathogenicity island (PAI) have a stronger inflammatory response than those infected with strains lacking the island and are at a greater risk of developing peptic ulcers and/or gastric cancer [63,64].

Despite the marked improvement in histological gastritis after eradication, this is not necessarily paralleled by symptomatic improvement. A comprehensive review of publications relating to the effect of *H. pylori* eradication on dyspeptic symptoms indicated that over 25% of patients in whom the organism has been eradicated noted no improvement in symptoms [65]. Further studies on non-ulcer dyspepsia patients with *H. pylori* infection indicate that eradication leads to symptomatic improvement in only approximately 20% of cases [66], and that the placebo effect in untreated patients leads to symptomatic relief as often [67].

Histology

The principal and most obvious histological feature of *H. pylori* gastritis is the infiltration of the lamina propria of the superficial mucosa by plasma cells, lymphocytes and small numbers of eosinophils (Figure 11.4a). However, the intensity of this infiltration varies considerably [68]. In addition, variable numbers of neutrophils are present, characteristically found in and around the epithelium lining the base of gastric pits. In cases of severe inflammation, neutrophils are also present between and adjacent to the surface epithelial cells. The term 'active' chronic superficial gastritis indicates the presence of neutrophils in addition to chronic inflammatory cells (Figure 11.4a). Active inflammation in association with generalised diffuse gastritis is almost invariably associated with the presence of *H. pylori* on the surface of the epithelium and should stimulate a search for the organisms. Although, in many cases of *H. pylori* gastritis, the surface epithelium may show little abnormality, detailed examination indicates that degenerative changes are common. These changes include loss of apical mucus formation within epithelial cells and, less often, micro-erosions and ulcerations [69] (Figure 11.5).

Examination of semi-thin resin-embedded sections demonstrates that the epithelium shows cellular oedema, micropapillae, mucin loss and epithelial denudation. This is

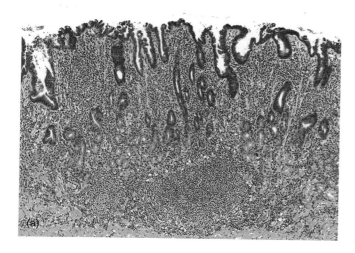

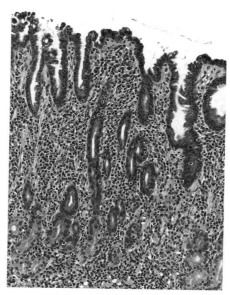

Figure 11.5 Active antral chronic superficial gastritis in *Helicobacter pylori* infection showing intense infiltration of the lamina propria by neutrophils, lymphocytes and plasma cells. Inflammatory cells also infiltrate the surface and glandular epithelial cells.

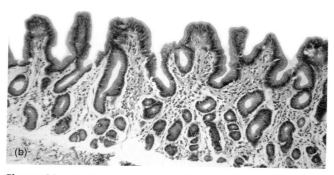

Figure 11.4 (a) Active chronic superficial gastritis affecting the antrum in *Helicobacter pylori* infection. (b) Antral biopsy of a patient with previously detected *H. pylori* infection. The biopsy was taken 11 months after eradication of the organisms. Neutrophils have disappeared but some chronic inflammation remains.

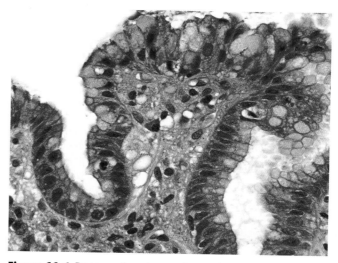

Figure 11.6 Degenerative changes in gastric surface epithelial cells in *Helicobacter pylori* gastritis. Some cells are swollen with loss of apical mucin. Tufting of the surface epithelial cells and micro-erosions are also present.

especially prominent in cells lining the upper foveolae and surface (Figure 11.6). The increased permeability of damaged surface epithelium may permit permeation of bacterial antigens and toxins and increase underlying mucosal inflammatory response and damage [70].

Lymphoid follicles are a common feature of helicobacter gastritis [71], particularly in the antral mucosa and in cases of severe active gastritis in comparison with mild or relatively inactive cases [72,73]. Eradication of the organism leads to a slow decrease in the number of lymphoid follicles and they tend to lose their germinal centres and evidence of lymphoid activation [74]. Marked histological lymphoid hyperplasia, sometimes resulting in antral nodularity on endoscopy, is also a feature of *H. pylori* gastritis in children [75].

After eradication of the organism, there is rapid improvement in the gastritis (see Figure 11.4b). Neutrophils disappear and epithelial cell damage heals within a matter of weeks [76–79]. The chronic inflammatory cell infiltrate, however, regresses more slowly, especially in the antrum. After eradication of *H. pylori*, the antral mucosa was normal in just over half of a series of patients studied 1 year later, although the corpus mucosa was normal in all cases [79]. Other workers have noted a slower disappearance of the mononuclear cell infiltrate stretching over a period of 4 years [78]. Eradication of the organism also leads to a slow decrease in the number of lymphoid follicles [74].

Variation in *H. pylori*-related gastritis

The histological spectrum of *H. pylori* associated gastritis ranges from antral predominant to pangastritis (with and without atrophy) to a corpus predominant pattern. Although host and environmental factors play critical roles in disease outcome, it is well known that the development of a specific disease is associated with a specific gastritis pattern. Duodenal ulcer is typically associated with antral predominant gastritis, little or no oxyntic gland (corpus and fundus) atrophy, and normal or increased acid secretion. Conversely, gastric ulcer and the intestinal type of gastric cancer are typically associated with pangastritis, widespread oxyntic atrophy with varying degrees of intestinal metaplasia, and hypo- or achlorhydria.

The distribution and severity of *H. pylori*-related gastritis (and thus disease risk) is related to the distribution and density of *H. pylori* within the stomach. In turn, the distribution of *H. pylori* is influenced by a person's acid secretory status. *H. pylori* is adapted to the human stomach with its hostile acidic environment by producing large amounts of the enzyme urease. Urease catalyses hydrolysis of urea to yield NH_3 and CO_2 in a thin neutral layer around the outer surface of the bacterium. This increases the pH in its surrounding environment to neutral and allows the bacterium's survival [80]. *H. pylori* further protects itself by swimming through the protective layer of gastric mucus away from the acidic contents of the lumen towards the more neutral pH environment [81]. Nevertheless, *H. pylori* flourishes best at a pH range of 3.5–5 [82] where, in the presence of urea, it can maintain a proton motive force (PMF) across its periplasmic membrane, ensuring a continued supply of energy through ATP synthesis [82].

Regional acidity explains why early *H. pylori* gastritis is typically antrum predominant where gastric acidity is reduced by antral mucin. Concomitantly, inflammation in the corpus is mild, superficial or even absent. Chronic inflammatory sequelae, such as intestinal metaplasia, are for the most part (initially) confined to the antrum. Early *H. pylori* gastritis is often characterised by an exaggerated gastrin response to meals and other stimuli [83], which precipitates an increased acid secretion that may cause duodenal ulcer disease. A consistent finding, associated with marked duodenitis, occurring in patients with early *H. pylori* gastritis, is surface gastric metaplasia interspersed between the absorptive and goblet cells of the duodenal epithelium. *H. pylori*, when present in the duodenum,

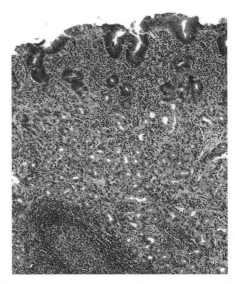

Figure 11.7 *Helicobacter pylori* gastritis in gastric body fundic mucosa. The biopsy displays a dense superficial inflammation of the lamina propria. A large expansive lymphoid nodule is also present.

can be identified only in areas with gastric metaplasia. It is hypothesised that, as with the gastric mucosa proper, *H. pylori* induces inflammation and erosions of gastric metaplasia (and heterotopia) patches [84]. As such, the prevalence of duodenal gastric metaplasia is much lower in 'healthy' volunteers [84].

Over time, there is a gradual reduction in acid-producing mucosa. In turn, the development of hypochlorhydria and achlorhydria facilitates proximal migration of the bacteria and allows the development of corpus gastritis (Figure 11.7) and, eventually, corpus atrophy. This is the setting in which gastric ulcer and later gastric carcinoma develops.

The natural history of *H. pylori* gastritis is for the inflammation to progress from the antrum into the adjacent corpus, resulting in an atrophic advancing front (which may be visible endoscopically), leading to a reduction in acid secretion and, eventually, loss of parietal cells and development of corpus atrophy. The front progresses uniformly and so appears to advance faster on the lesser curve. This scenario is accelerated in the setting of low acid secretion such as with chronic therapy with proton pump inhibitors (PPIs) [85]. Thus, antral predominant gastritis may in some instances represent an earlier stage of atrophic pangastritis, these patterns representing two ends of the spectrum of *H. pylori* infection rather than mutually exclusive diseases.

It is important to remember that, when the microenvironment pH rises above about 5, the bacteria produce ammonia in excess of what is needed to neutralise the much-diminished influx of hydrogen ion. As the micro-environment becomes increasingly alkaline, it is detrimental to the bacteria, which cannot survive at a pH level >8. This explains why *H. pylori* may not be identified in achlorhydric states (gastric atrophy and with continued PPI use) when the inflammatory pattern is clearly that associated with low *H. pylori* density. Further, in patients on PPIs, the organism may migrate to the oxyntic mucosa to find enough acid to survive, explaining the proximal migration of *H. pylori* with both increasing atrophy and PPI use. Not only that, but the organisms seem to migrate deeper into the oxyntic glands, as opposed to their usual superficial location.

The diagnosis of *H. pylori*

Diagnostic testing for *H. pylori* can be divided into invasive and non-invasive methods [86]. Non-invasive methods include serology and the urea breath test. Invasive tests require endoscopy and tests for urease, histology and culture. The choice of test depends on the clinical situation (e.g. if the patient requires evaluation with upper endoscopy anyway) and on other issues such as cost, availability, prevalence of infection, probability of infection, and factors such as the use of PPIs and antibiotics, which may influence certain test results.

Histology is still considered the gold standard for detecting the infection both for untreated individuals and after therapy. The advantages of histology include the ability to document *H. pylori* infection, the degree of inflammation and any associated pathology, e.g. intestinal metaplasia, cancer or lymphoma. However, histology is expensive, certainly compared with simple tests available at the time of endoscopy, and some have doubted whether the additional information provided by histological assessment, apart from confirming the presence of *H pylori* infection, is valuable for the routine management of individual patients in the absence of an endoscopically detected lesion or lesions.

H. pylori are often easily recognised on routine H&E staining. Identifying the bacteria by histology depends on the intra-gastric distribution of *H. pylori* and the number and sites of biopsies taken. Indeed, it is rare to find helicobacter organisms when intestinal metaplasia is present. *H. pylori* may also be present in small numbers of biopsy specimens that are histologically normal, usually 10% or less, especially in the gastric body. Finally, patchy distribution of the organisms may be one of the reasons that a minority of cases of chronic active gastritis lack *H. pylori* [87].

Most pathologists use a special stain for *H. pylori* visualisation. The appearance of the organism varies with the staining technique used. Commonly used special stains can be divided arbitrarily into (1) silver-based stains, (2) non-silver-based stains and (3) immunohistochemistry. The last is particularly useful in patients on PPIs, where bacteria are fewer in number and generally smaller in size. Silver stains include the Warthin–Starry stain, the modified Steiner stain, the El-Zimaity dual stain [88] and the Genta stains [89].

In non-silver-based stains, visualising the bacteria depends on the contrast between the bacteria and tissue sections. In our experience, Diff-Quik has the better sensitivity and specificity whereas the Giemsa stain has suboptimal accuracy, especially with less experienced pathologists. With Leung's alcian yellow stain [90], it is easier to spot blue bacteria against yellow gastric mucin. In equivocal situations (common with chronic PPI use), pathologists may err on the side of overcalling the presence of the bacteria. This might seem unimportant. However, *H. pylori* infection is absent in up to 27% of patients with endoscopically proven duodenal ulcers [91]. Such patients appear to have a significantly worse outcome when treated empirically for the infection [92], almost certainly because they were also ingesting NSAIDs.

Immunohistochemistry is an alternative to silver stains, primarily because the organisms are readily identifiable. It has the potential advantage of not picking up other organisms that may be present in the stomach (enteric, oral) and can proliferate in patients with atrophy or who are taking PPIs. Immunohistochemistry also reduces the false-positive rate, providing greater accuracy [93]. However, we have seen other *Helicobacter* spp. (e.g. *H. heilmannii*) stain positively with antibodies (especially polyclonal) for *H. pylori*. Notably, morphological differences in their spiral morphology are difficult to detect on immunostains. Importantly, anti-*H. pylori* antibodies also stain the coccoid forms of the bacteria. These forms are non-culturable and less virulent, and less likely to colonise and induce inflammation [94]. Indeed they are probably dead. Notably, coccoid forms have never (yet) been shown to be viable, so basing a diagnosis of helicobacter gastritis only on coccoid forms of organisms should arguably never be done or at least should be stated clearly in the report.

In conclusion, no stain is perfect and the best stain is the one that works in the pathologist's own laboratory, bearing in mind that an H&E stain interpreted by inexperienced pathology staff is the least sensitive and the least specific. The sensitivity of the histological diagnosis may be affected by prior treatment with PPIs. As these drugs cause a shift of organisms proximally from antrum to corpus [95], the examination of a single antral biopsy may give false-negative results. Then, as many patients may have received PPI therapy before coming to endoscopy, the recommendation should be reinforced that at least two biopsies taken from both antrum and corpus [43].

Consequences of long-term helicobacter infection

Spontaneous disappearance of the organism and subsequent regression of the chronic gastritis has been reported in about 10% of cases followed over several years [96–98]. It is uncertain if this is genuinely due to successful host defence mechanisms or to antibiotic therapy given for unrelated conditions. Overall, most patients are asymptomatic and do not present for treatment. Thus, the infection lasts for many years in large numbers of people. Consequences of chronic infection include peptic ulceration, atrophic gastritis, autoimmune gastritis and lymphocytic gastritis. Gastric carcinoma and lymphoma are discussed in Chapters 13 and 15, respectively, whereas other outcomes, especially peptic ulceration, are dealt with in the following sections.

Peptic ulcer disease

Inflammation and ulceration of the gastric mucosa occur when noxious factors overwhelm the mucosal defence system. The fact that the stomach secretes hydrochloric acid and pepsinogen (important final mediators of gastric damage) would render this balance precarious if there were not a formidable set of defences against the continuous threat of autodigestion. Thus, before detailed consideration of peptic ulcers and their sequelae is undertaken, it seems reasonable to briefly consider gastric mucosal defence and ulcer pathogenic mechanisms.

Peptic ulcer disease is a heterogeneous group of disorders, having in common mucosal erosion or ulceration. Peptic ulcer disease results when aggressive factors (acid, pepsin, bile, activated pancreatic enzymes, medications, chemicals, ischaemia, radiation, etc.) overwhelm intrinsic defence mechanisms and protective factors. Peptic ulcers are most common in the antral and pre-pyloric regions, at the pylorus itself, and on the anterior and posterior walls of the first part of the duodenum. Peptic ulcers may also be seen after gastroenterostomy, either at the line of anastomosis or in the small bowel immediately distal, or in the second, third or fourth parts of the duodenum or upper jejunum in Zollinger–Ellison syndrome; they can occur within or immediately distal to Meckel's diverticulum if the lining heterotopic mucosa is acid-secreting.

Mucosal defence mechanisms

These can be divided into several components.

The surface mucus layer and gastric mucosal barrier
The surface mucus layer constitutes the first line of defence and is composed of a thin layer of mucus adherent to the mucosal surface. Estimates vary but the layer is thought to be around 180 μm thick [99]. The structure of the mucus layer is not affected by short exposure to bile, ethanol and very low pH, thus limiting the potential damage due to such agents [100] but experimental removal of this layer leads to mucosal erosion [101]. The efficacy of the protective surface mucus layer is enhanced by secretion of bicarbonate by the gastric mucosa, resulting in alkalinisation of the overlying mucus layer [102]. The efficiency of the protection given by the mucus bicarbonate layer is illustrated by a significant pH gradient across the layer, resulting in almost neutral pH on the mucosal side, in contrast to the very acidic levels on the luminal side [103].

The mucus layer is also hydrophobic – a property, conferred by surface-active phospholipid substances produced from the lamellar bodies in parietal cells and mucous neck cells, thought to contribute to protection of the mucosa against autodigestion. The protection is severely compromised by substances such as luminal aspirin with resultant damage to underlying surface mucosal cells. On the contrary, prostaglandins provide protection against such damage and promote healing [104,105].

The next line of defence is a gastric mucosal barrier with surface cell membranes and tight junctions between surface epithelial cells [106]. This barrier restricts the back diffusion of hydrogen ions from acid luminal contents into mucosa and also provides a transmucosal potential difference of around 50 mV [107]. It thus provides mucosal protection against low luminal pH levels. The surface-active phospholipid layer is also a component of the gastric mucosal barrier [108].

Epithelial renewal
The gastric mucosa has the ability to proliferate and replace damaged surface epithelial cells rapidly. The gastric proliferative zone lies at the junction of the base of the surface pits and the tip of the glands [109]. Various experimental studies indicate that, after various types of damage, complete restitution of gastric mucosal integrity can occur between 15 min and 6 h [102,110]. Mucosal injury is rapidly followed by upregulation of numerous genes and expression of peptides and growth factors, a local sequence designed to repair injury and restore the epithelial surface [111]. These include epidermal growth factor (EGF) synthesised in salivary glands and Brunner's glands and in small amounts in gastric mucosa, transforming growth factor α (TGF-α), synthesised in the gastrointestinal mucosa, and gastrin [102,112,113].

Mucosal blood flow
Adequate blood flow is fundamental to epithelial protection, because it enables the mucosa to dispose of hydrogen ions diffusing in from the gastric lumen [113]. Experimental studies indicate that increased hydrogen ion concentration in the lumen causes increased gastric mucosal blood flow, which within limits maintains physiological levels intramucosally pH [114]. Consequently, hypovolaemic shock frequently results in focal ulceration similar to that seen in

acute erosive gastritis [115]. Notably, the duodenal mucosa appears more sensitive to minor degrees of ischaemia than the gastric mucosa [116].

Cytoprotection

Continuous generation of endogenous prostaglandins (PGG_2, prostacyclin or PGI_2] provides mucosal protection and increase in mucosal blood flow via stimulation of mucus secretion, bicarbonate production and phospholipid secretion [117–122]. Prostaglandins also modulate gastric mucosal inflammatory response by inhibiting release of tumour necrosis factor (TNF) from macrophages [123], and TNF and other potentially ulcerogenic inflammatory mediators from mast cells [124,125]. There is evidence that NSAID-induced gastric mucosal damage is related to a reduction in endogenous prostaglandin secretion [126–128].

Mucosal pathogenic mechanisms

The two main factors that may predispose to ulcer formation are NSAIDS, including aspirin, and *H. pylori* infection [129]. Today, with the decline in *H. pylori* prevalence, other aetiological factors, including NSAIDs, play an important role, even in less developed countries [130].

Acid and pepsin

Before *H. pylori* was re-discovered in 1984 [131], it was generally accepted that a duodenal ulcer was due to high acid secretion. Effective measures to reduce acid output, surgical or medical, led to long-term healing.

Helicobacter pylori

H. pylori infection, especially cag-A-positive strains, is highly associated with the occurrence of peptic ulcers. In patients with duodenal ulcers, *H. pylori* infection induces antral gastritis, which leads to hypergastrinaemia and acid hypersecretion. Excess acid entering the duodenal bulb causes duodenal gastric metaplasia, allowing *H. pylori* colonisation. This in turn induces an inflammatory response and, potentially, focal erosions or ulceration [132]. Recently the incidence of duodenal ulcers has decreased substantially in the western world [133], mirroring the fall in *H. pylori* infection [134] and possibly the replacement of aspirin by paracetamol (acetaminophen) as the analgesic of choice. In some western countries, smoking, alcohol and NSAIDs, but not *H. pylori* infection, remain the leading risk factors for duodenal or pre-pyloric ulcer [135].

Drugs

Approximately 30 million people throughout the world take NSAIDs regularly [136]. During a course of NSAID therapy, approximately 15% of patients will develop gastric ulcers and 5% will develop duodenal ulcers. The risk of NSAID-associated ulcer bleeding is higher in elderly women, probably because of the increased consumption of NSAIDs by this group. Although NSAIDs may only slightly increase the risk of duodenal ulcer, they appear to significantly increase the bleeding risk in those with a duodenal ulcer. Aspirin, with its anticoagulant effect, may potentiate this. The contribution of corticosteroids, chemotherapeutic drugs and/or immunosuppressive agents, and ischaemia to the pathogenesis of erosions and ulcers, and their effects on healing of peptic ulcer disease, remain unclear.

Duodeno-gastric reflux

Duodeno-gastric reflux and gastro-oesophageal reflux represent physiological phenomena occurring in the postprandial period and sporadically in the inter-digestive state [78]. Duodenal contents contain not only bile but activated pancreatic enzymes, so are potentially quite injurious. Bile reflux gastropathy is present in a significant proportion of patients with gastro-oesophageal reflux disease (GORD), including Barrett's oesophagus, and is associated with disease severity [137]. Duodeno-gastric reflux is greater in some gastric ulcer patients than in normal individuals.

Environmental factors

Smoking is a risk factor for peptic ulcer disease, associated with the initiation, prolongation and recurrence of gastric ulcer, the risk being directly proportional to the number of cigarettes smoked.

Psychological stress

Emotional factors or disturbances have long been suspected to play a role in the pathogenesis of peptic ulcer disease, e.g. the type A 'hard-driving executive' stereotype in duodenal ulcer disease. Case–control studies have shown a strong association between psychological factors and ulcer disease. Although stressful life events occur with equal frequency in ulcer and control patients, the way in which these events are perceived and responded to differ between the two groups. As a group, peptic ulcer patients have significantly more personality disturbances [138].

Heredity

Genetic heterogeneity was proposed to explain the familial aggregation and the lack of a simple mendelian pattern of inheritance in peptic ulcer disease. Nevertheless, individuals who live in the same household carry the same *H. pylori* strains, independent of kinship, and, in some cases, there is autosomal dominant hyperpepsinogenaemia I [139]. Other rare genetic syndromes accompanied by ulcer disease include systemic mastocytosis, ulcer–tremor–nystagmus syndrome, type IV amyloidosis and multiple lentigines–ulcer syndrome.

Associated diseases

Several diseases appear to be associated with peptic ulcer disease, such as multiple endocrine neoplasia type 1 (MEN 1 with either gastrinoma or possibly hypercalcaemia that may mediate a degree of acid secretion), chronic pulmonary disease, cirrhosis of the liver, systemic mastocytosis and basophilic leukaemia. The pathogenic mechanisms underlying ulcer formation in these disorders are not always clear.

Peptic ulcer epidemiology

The mean age of presentation is about 20 in duodenal ulcers and about 40 in gastric ulcers. In both conditions the incidence rises with age, peaking at around 40 for duodenal ulcers and in the late 50s and early 60s for gastric ulcers. However, no age group is exempt and ulcer disease is well recognised in childhood [140]. Although the incidence of peptic ulcers varies among different groups in the same country, and also among countries, these differences are most likely due to environmental and not racial factors.

From 1980 onward, there has been a decreasing incidence of both gastric and duodenal ulcers, with only a slight decline for gastric ulcer incidence [141]. The overall decline is likely to be due to a combination of factors, including the introduction of acid-suppressive medication, a decreasing prevalence of *H. pylori* in subsequent birth cohorts and the development of eradication treatment for *H. pylori*-positive ulcer patients, which prevents chronic relapsing ulcer disease. However, peptic ulcer disease remains an important clinical problem, with a rise in the proportion of complicated ulcers. This rise has been shown to correlate with oral anticoagulants, NSAIDs and oral corticosteroid intake.

Macroscopic pathology of peptic ulcer disease

Peptic ulcers are usually classified as acute or chronic on the basis of the depth of penetration or degree of healing, rather than their duration. Erosions are defined as shallower defects (above the muscularis mucosae) that involve less than the full thickness of the mucosa, so that some basal gland elements remain. Acute ulcers and erosions tend to heal rapidly and seldom recur if the underlying cause is treated. Erosions tend to be oval or circular in shape, with sharply defined edges, and fresh or altered

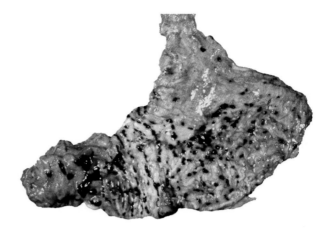

Figure 11.8 Acute erosive gastritis: multiple erosions with bleeding on the mucosal surface, especially in the fundus of the stomach.

blood in the base. They are almost invariably multiple in the gastric mucosa and most measure 1–3 mm in diameter, although some extend up to several centimetres (Figure 11.8). The intervening mucosa appears congested and contains petechial haemorrhages. The distribution of erosions differs with the clinical circumstances. After trauma or sepsis, they are first observed in the fundus near the greater curve and, with time, develop distally, only involving the antrum when the lesions in the body are widespread and severe. This contrasts with erosions caused by NSAIDs and alcohol which, although most frequent in the antrum, can affect all segments of the stomach and duodenum, and do not have a proximal to distal progression. The latter lesions also tend to be smaller and to heal more quickly [142,143].

An acute ulcer is simply an extension of an erosion through the full thickness of the mucosa into the submucosa or deeper into underlying tissues. They tend to be larger than erosions and frequently occur in areas of intense erosion and mucosal congestion, especially on the greater curvature of the stomach. Similar to erosions, they are often multiple. The ulcer bed is similar to that of an erosion and fibrous scar tissue is not prominent in the base. Acute ulcers are considerably less common in the duodenum but in that site they tend to be single. Haemorrhage is a frequent complication of acute ulcer due to ulceration of submucosal vessel walls.

Chronic peptic ulcers, by contrast, are long standing, by definition, and characterised histologically by loss of the full thickness of the mucosa with a variable degree of penetration into the underlying coats and the presence of fibrous tissue in the ulcer base. An ulcer may be regarded as chronic, clinically, when it has failed to heal over a reasonable period of time and, pathologically, when attempts at repair have led to the formation of collagenous fibrohyaline basal scar to such a degree that restoration of the submucosa and muscularis propria is no longer possible; there is often concomitant failure of the mucosa to regenerate satisfactorily. It is generally assumed that all chronic ulcers originate in an acute ulcer that failed to heal. Involvement of the submucosa and muscular coats may produce distortion in the form of pyloric stenosis or an 'hour-glass' constriction. The overlying serosa is often thickened and opaque, and the ulcer base adheres to underlying or overlying strictures, particularly the pancreas. The surrounding mucosa often appears flat and atrophic [144]. The presence of gastritis, either local or more generalised, can be confirmed on microscopy. Occasionally, simple gastric ulcers reach extreme sizes. Lesser curve ulcers tend to enlarge in a saddle-shaped manner and may reach 100 mm or more in diameter [145]. They can also extend longitudinally as 'trench ulcers' along the lesser curve from cardia to incisura [146]. This type shows less fibrosis and the ulceration appears more acute.

Chronic gastric ulcers are comparatively rare in the body mucosa [147,148]. Many arise at the junction of antral and corpus mucosa surrounded by pyloric-type mucosa or metaplastic mucosa of intestinal type, whereas others arise entirely in antral mucosa [147,149]. They are usually single, although multiple ulcers can occur in 6–13% of cases [147,150]. They are usually <20 mm in diameter, often <10 mm, and are round or oval. Smaller ulcers tend to occur near the pylorus [151]. They occur predominantly on the lesser curvature and less often on the posterior wall. The anterior wall and greater curvature are seldom involved [152]. They may lie across the lesser curve in a saddle-shaped form (Figure 11.9) and are commonly found higher up on the lesser curve [153]. The edges are clear cut but not raised or rolled and overhang, producing a flask-like appearance. The base is grey and either blood clot or an eroded vessel can occasionally be seen within the crater.

All large ulcers have to be distinguished from carcinomas and examined closely; distinction can usually be made by the clear-cut overhanging edges and absence of thickening in adjacent mucosa, but multiple biopsies should be taken from the base and circumference to exclude malignancy.

Microscopic pathology of peptic ulcers

Erosions show necrosis of a small area of mucosa of variable depth but not extending down to the muscularis mucosae. The crater of the erosion contains necrotic slough, polymorphs and red blood cells. There is a variable, usually minor, degree of acute inflammation in the adjacent lamina propria with dilatation and congestion of nearby capillar-

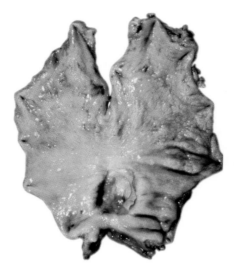

Figure 11.9 A peptic ulcer in a characteristic site, the lower part of the lesser curvature. The edges are clean cut but not raised or rolled. Note the flat, featureless, atrophic-appearing background mucosa.

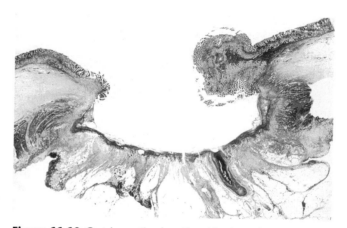

Figure 11.10 Gastric peptic ulceration: histology shows interruption of the muscle coat by fibrous tissue and extensive fibrosis of the ulcer base. An eroded blood vessel is present in the ulcer base. Masson trichrome stain.

ies. On healing most erosions show complete mucosal regeneration and there is no visible residual scarring.

Microscopically, all chronic peptic ulcers have a characteristic structure. In the stage of active necrosis, the base has four recognisable layers. On the luminal aspect there is a narrow zone of fibrinopurulent exudate. Underlying this, there is a layer of acidophilic necrotic tissue. Then there is a zone of granulation tissue of variable vascularity containing young fibroblasts and mononuclear inflammatory cells. This blends with the deepest layer of more dense scar tissue that interrupts and replaces the muscularis propria (Figure 11.10). The granulation tissue in the ulcer base is important

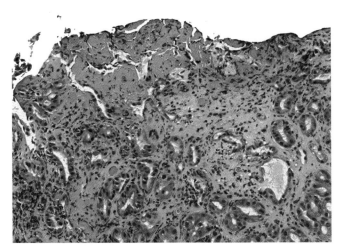

Figure 11.11 Histology of a gastric erosion: necrotic slough is present (top) with underlying stromal fibrosis and atypical regenerative epithelial elements that may simulate dysplasia.

in relation to subsequent healing and experimental studies indicate that stimulation of angiogenesis in this area results in acceleration of ulcer repair [154]. In deep ulcers, the interrupted circular, longitudinal and oblique muscle coats tend to curl upwards at the edges of the ulcer to fuse with the muscularis mucosae [155]. Small veins may show organising or organised thrombus, and arteries in the base of the ulcer may be eroded or show organising thrombus or endarteritis obliterans.

Care must be taken not to mistake granulation tissue in the base of an erosion or acute ulcer for infiltrating carcinoma. This may cause considerable diagnostic difficulty in biopsy material, as prominent and sometimes bizarre endothelial cells and fibroblasts may simulate poorly differentiated infiltrating carcinoma [156] (Figure 11.11). At the ulcer margin, marked regenerative atypia of the adjacent epithelium, which may grow downwards or give rise to islands of mucosa trapped in granulation or fibrous tissue [156], can similarly cause confusion with adenocarcinoma. To avoid a misdiagnosis of carcinoma, good communication with the endoscopist, knowledge of the endoscopic appearances and awareness of this difficult diagnostic problem are important. Mucosal replacement begins from the edges initially as a single layer of cells; in ulcers of 20 mm diameter or less, this ingrowth can extend to cover the whole ulcerated surface with a single layer of epithelium.

Complications of peptic ulceration

Perforation

Acute and chronic gastric and duodenal ulcers, particularly those on the anterior wall, which are not readily walled off by surrounding structures, are liable to perforate. In reported series, duodenal and pyloro-duodenal ulcer perforation is much more common than perforation of gastric ulcers [157,158]. The risk of upper GI bleeding/perforation varies with the development of selective cyclo-oxygenase 2 (COX-2] inhibitors. Drugs that have a long half-life or slow-release formulation and/or are associated with profound and coincident inhibition of both COX isoenzymes are associated with a greater risk of upper gastrointestinal (GI) bleeding/perforation [159]. Cigarette smoking is also a significant risk factor [160].

Perforated peptic ulcers present as a neat, round hole in the floor of the ulcer and the surrounding serosa is hyperaemic, lustreless and partly covered by white flakes of fibrinous exudate. Fine fibrinous adhesions are commonly observed between the lesion and neighbouring organs and, frequently, the hole is plugged by the greater omentum. Any delay in surgical treatment will lead to diffuse peritonitis, at first the result of chemical irritation but, from an early stage, associated with secondary infection from bacterial contamination. Later complications include the formation of local abscesses, sometimes pelvic or subdiaphragmatic.

Haemorrhage

This is the most frequent complication of chronic peptic ulcers (Figure 11.12 and also see Figure 11.10). A 15-year study carried out in general practice before the advent of efficient acid suppression therapy indicated that haemorrhage occurred in 16% of peptic ulcer patients. Post-bulbar duodenal ulcers and stomal ulcers are particularly prone. Risk factors include old age, ingestion of NSAIDs within the preceding 4 weeks, a previous ulcer complication and an ulcer diameter >20 mm. NSAID ingestion has been reported to increase the risk of bleeding two to three times compared with controls and it is probably related to the anti-haemostatic effect of aspirin, in addition to its ulcerogenic effect [161]. Non-aspirin NSAIDs are also associated with increased risk and the combination of a NSAID and paracetamol may be a particular risk [162].

Erosions and acute ulcers are also liable to be associated with acute haemorrhage, because the lamina propria is extremely vascular, and gastric and duodenal submucosal vessels are thin walled and numerous. Peptic ulceration is found in only about 50% of cases admitted for acute upper GI bleeding [163]. A further large study reported similar findings and indicates that bleeding is more commonly associated with chronic duodenal ulcer than gastric ulcer. The incidence of upper GI bleeding increases markedly with age and is more common in men. The overall mortality rate in one study was 14% [164]. Other conditions associated with increased risk of bleeding from peptic ulcers include oral anticoagulant therapy, previous history of

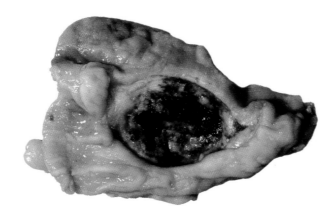

Figure 11.12 Bleeding in a gastric ulcer resected after severe haemorrhage. An eroded artery with fresh blood clot is visible in the ulcer base.

peptic ulcer, heart failure. and/or diabetes and oral corti-costeroid therapy [165].

Pathological examination shows that, in the majority of cases, bleeding results from erosion of a single artery in the floor of an ulcer (see Figure 11.12). More than half of bleeding ulcers are acute in nature, with penetration only as far as the submucosa. Aneurysmal dilatation of the artery at the bleeding point is very common and an intense arteri-tis is present in the wall of the vessel adjacent to the floor of the ulcer in most. Recanalised thrombus, loose intimal proliferation and endarteritis obliterans are observed rarely [163].

Fibrosis and stenosis

Peptic ulceration in the region of the pyloric sphincter or cardia will lead to local fibrosis and possibly stenosis, with signs of obstruction. In pre-modern therapy, there were reports of hour-glass deformities related to dense submu-cosal fibrosis radiating from the lesser curvature. Nowa-days this complication is extremely rare.

Involvement of adjacent organs

A peptic ulcer in the stomach or duodenum is liable to adhere and erode into the pancreas or spleen. Localised pan-creatitis develops at the site of the penetration but impor-tant complications, such as haemorrhage from erosion of the splenic artery and acute haemorrhagic pancreatic necrosis, are very rare. Perforation into the stomach or duo-denum and the transverse colon may lead to a gastrocolic or duodenocolic fistula. Occasionally, a peptic ulcer results in adherence of the stomach or duodenum to the liver with no undue complications, although we have seen occasional cases where biopsy and/or brush cytology have resulted in considerable consternation for the pathologist when

viewing hepatocytes, considerably distorted by the effects of the ulceration and the contents of the stomach/duodenum. Rarely, benign peptic ulcers penetrate to the heart and pericardium [166,167].

Acquired diverticula

Occasionally, a diverticulum develops in association with pyloric stenosis or a peptic ulcer that has penetrated the muscle coats but excited little fibrosis. These are usually single and arise from the posterior wall of the stomach just below the cardia and presenting as an outpouching, in which all coats of the stomach are intact [168].

Clinical variants of peptic ulcer

Practically, there are three major causes of peptic erosions or ulcers: *H. pylori*, medications and, less commonly, Crohn's disease. We focus here only on *H. pylori*-related ulcers.

H. pylori-related ulcers

These ulcers are invariably associated with a pangastritis. In the rare ulcer lying wholly in body mucosa, there is some degree of preceding gastritis [169] but without total destruc-tion of cells that secrete acid or pepsinogen. In the much more common antral and lesser curve ulceration, there is usually local gastritis surrounding the ulcer or, more com-monly, regional gastritis involving the whole antral-type mucosa. This is active chronic gastritis with or without atrophic gastritis. *H. pylori* infection is identified in 60–70% of gastric ulcers, because the organisms are frequently present on the surface of intact mucosa adjacent to the ulcer. Intestinal metaplasia of mucosa surrounding ulcers is common, especially in the antrum, and ulcers often arise in metaplastic epithelium at the junction of corpus and antrum, often at the incisura [170]. Congestion of sur-rounding mucosal capillaries is common and, occasionally, inflammatory polypoid proliferation takes place at an ulcer edge during healing [171]. In contrast, chronic gastric ulcers associated with NSAID ingestion and without con-comitant *H. pylori* infection often have little or no inflam-mation in the adjacent mucosa [7,172].

Duodenal ulceration is typically associated with antral predominant gastritis, little or no oxyntic gland (corpus and fundus) atrophy, and normal or increased acid secre-tion [173,174]. Most chronic duodenal ulcers occur in the first part of the duodenum, usually immediately distal to the pylorus, with approximately 2% of ulcers being post-bulbar [175] (Figure 11.13). The anterior wall is a more common site than the posterior wall. In 10–15% of cases, the ulcers are multiple [176,177] and, not uncommonly, paired on the anterior and posterior walls. Duodenal ulcers are punched out in appearance and scarring often

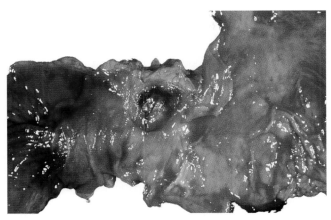

Figure 11.13 A chronic duodenal ulcer: a large ulcer is seen immediately distal to the pylorus.

produces considerable distortion. However, unlike their gastric counterparts, these ulcers do not have show a fusion of muscularis propria with muscularis mucosae at the ulcer edge.

The mucosa adjacent to the ulcer crater shows increased inflammation by polymorphs and mononuclear inflammatory cells with shortening and thickening of villi. Active mucosal inflammation can be observed some distance from the ulcer, even though the mucosa in this area may appear endoscopically normal [178]. Either way, when the ulcer heals, the 'healed' mucosa is often histologically very abnormal [179].

Patchy areas of surface gastric metaplasia are commonly present and occur almost exclusively in the first part of the duodenum [180]. When *H. pylori* is present in the areas of gastric metaplasia, the relative risk of duodenal ulcer increases, possibly by a factor of 50 [181]. Gastric metaplasia, frequently found at the edge of a duodenal ulcer, and the patches of metaplasia are frequently colonised by *H. pylori* [180]. The metaplasia is most often seen at the tips of duodenal villi and is often associated with some blunting of the villi [180]. Duodenal gastric metaplasia is thought to develop as a result of high levels of acidity within the duodenum. It is more extensive in patients with low pH values in gastric juice [182] and both the prevalence and the extent of metaplasia correlate with gastric acid output [183]. *H. pylori* infection of the stomach itself does not appear to correlate with duodenal gastric metaplasia [183,184], but infection may indirectly increase the extent and prevalence of metaplasia via the increased acid secretion that it stimulates. In the absence of duodenal Crohn's disease or other relatively rare conditions, inflammation of the duodenal mucosa is seldom seen unless gastric metaplasia is present and the extent of gastric metaplasia correlates with the degree of inflammation [180]. This lends

support to the proposal that colonisation of islands of gastric metaplasia by *H. pylori* may lead to inflammation of these islands and the surrounding duodenal mucosa, which in turn renders the mucosa more susceptible to acid attack and ulceration. The likely sequence of *H. pylori* infection of the stomach, hyperacidity, gastric metaplasia in the duodenum, colonisation of foci of metaplasia by *H. pylori*, duodenitis and, ultimately, duodenal ulceration has been termed the 'leaking roof' concept [185].

Of note, metaplasia is likely to be a non-specific response to a variety of mucosal insults and chronic inflammation is probably another of these factors [186], e.g. small foci of surface gastric metaplasia (without accompanying inflammation) have been documented in up to two-thirds of normal individuals and also in renal failure. In addition, it occurs in the distal duodenum in the Zollinger–Ellison syndrome [187,188]. Studies indicate that foci of gastric metaplasia in the duodenum are the result of expansion of the surface component of Brunner's glands [189,190]. Although islands of heterotopic oxyntic mucosa are quite common in the duodenum, their role in the genesis of duodenal ulcers has been largely ignored. Carrick et al. [191] have demonstrated that intravenous pentagastrin induces acid production in these islands, suggesting the role of intrinsic duodenal acid secretion and *H. pylori* in the development of duodenal ulceration [191].

NSAIDs, drugs and alcohol-related erosions and acute ulcers

Non-steroidal anti-inflammatory drugs

NSAID ingestion is regarded as the most common cause of acute erosive gastropathy [10]. Mucosal haemorrhage and erosions are extremely common but, in most cases, there are no significant clinical manifestations. However, acute gastric ulceration has been reported in almost 7% of healthy volunteers taking therapeutic doses of aspirin for 1 week [11]. In this study, non-aspirin NSAIDs caused lesser degrees of mucosal damage. A similar endoscopic study showed that gastric and duodenal mucosal haemorrhage is reduced with enteric-coated tablets [12]. It is likely that with long-term therapy mucosal adaptation occurs and the damage may diminish. In contrast to stress-induced lesions that show a predilection for the proximal stomach, the erosions caused by NSAIDs tend to be less florid, and are relatively more common in the antrum [13].

There is little doubt that NSAID ingestion plays an important role in chronic peptic ulceration. Although aspirin has been supplemented or replaced by a large number of newer NSAIDs, all of these, although less damaging to the gastric mucosa, are nevertheless gastric irritants [127,128,192]. Adverse reactions to NSAIDs are one of the most commonly reported drug side effects and, of these, problems related to the GI tract are the most common [193]. The use of aspirin (albeit in low doses) for prophylaxis of cardiovascular disease is now widespread and, in addition, very large amounts of NSAIDs are bought 'over the counter', without prescription for self-medication. Thus, to keep the problem in perspective, in view of the vast quantities of aspirin and other NSAIDs consumed, the increased risk of serious upper GI complications is relatively modest at three- to fourfold [161]. The incidence of peptic ulcers and/or GI bleeding associated with non-aspirin NSAIDs is around 1% [194]. The overall risk of serious GI events in NSAID users is about three times greater than in non-users and the risk is increased in elderly patients with concomitant corticosteroid use. It is highest during the first 3 months of drug therapy [195].

Aspirin and non-aspirin NSAID ingestion appears to be more strongly associated with gastric ulcers rather than duodenal ulcers [196–198] and there is also an increased risk of upper GI bleeding. It is unclear whether this is due to drug-induced mucosal damage or bleeding from a pre-existing ulcer. There is about a threefold increase in the risk of gastric ulceration and upper GI bleeding associated with aspirin consumption [161]. Patients at greatest risk from upper GI complications of NSAIDs are elderly people, especially women [199], and those who have had previous upper abdominal pain, peptic ulcer disease or side effects with NSAID use [200]. Studies on the comparative safety of individual drugs have produced rather confusing conclusions but a recent meta-analysis indicates that ibuprofen carries a relatively low risk, although this may be because it is normally used in comparatively low doses [201]. Indeed, among patients with NSAID-associated GI complications, only a small minority report preceding GI symptoms [202]. In addition to advanced age and previous peptic ulceration, other risk factors for NSAID-induced peptic ulceration include concomitant use of steroids or anticoagulants, high dosage of NSAIDs and serious systemic disease [203].

Detailed discussion of the mechanisms of NSAID-induced gastro-duodenal mucosal damage is beyond the scope of this chapter and only an overview is presented. At low pH, aspirin is in a lipid-soluble, non-ionised form that can be transported across cell membranes. After absorption it can lead to increased cell membrane permeability with resulting influx of sodium, calcium and water, resulting in cell swelling and death [204]. Death of surface epithelial cells allows back diffusion of acid, pepsin and aspirin into the mucosa [106]. The resulting injury to mast cells, endothelial cells and neutrophils may result in release of inflammatory mediators leading to capillary leakage, neutrophil adherence to endothelial cells, vasoconstriction and subsequent local mucosal ischaemia and cellular necrosis [205].

The protective effect of prostaglandins on gastric mucosa is relevant to NSAID-induced gastrotoxicity. Prostaglandins are synthesised by the gastric mucosa from the precursor arachidonic acid. They have a variety of protective actions, including stimulation of mucus secretion, increasing gastric mucosal blood flow [119], and stimulation of both gastric and duodenal bicarbonate secretion [206,207]. Endogenous prostaglandin synthesis by gastric mucosa is inhibited by NSAIDs [126] and subsequent reduction in the protection afforded is likely to leave the mucosa more susceptible to damage. This is supported by the finding that co-treatment with a synthetic prostaglandin analogue, misoprostol, markedly reduces the development of gastric ulcers in patients receiving long-term NSAID therapy [208].

Cyclo-oxygenase is an important enzyme in the production of prostaglandins and is inhibited by aspirin and other commonly used NSAIDs. There are at least two forms of this enzyme: COX-1 and COX-2. The theory that COX-1 is expressed predominantly in the stomach and plays an important part in the production of protective prostaglandins whereas COX-2 is induced at sites of inflammation has led to the possibility that specific COX-2 inhibitors may exhibit an anti-inflammatory effect without concomitant gastrotoxicity [209]. So COX-2-selective NSAIDs were developed to diminish the GI adverse events caused by non-selective NSAIDs (nsNSAIDs) [209]. Nevertheless, COX-2-selective NSAIDs can be associated with increased cardiovascular risk [210]. All NSAIDs are also associated with other side effects, including hypertension, water retention, heart failure and renal insufficiency [211]. Based on these findings, the US Food and Drug Administration (FDA), the European Medicines Agency (EMA) and other scientific societies agree that the medical management of patients who require NSAIDs must be based on the previous assessment of GI and cardiovascular risk factors in the individual patient [212]. Guidelines recommend the use of nsNSAIDs and a gastro-protectant or COX-2-selective NSAID alone in patients with one or more GI risk factors [213]. A COX-2-selective agent plus a PPI is recommended in those with the highest GI risk, whereas nsNSAIDs and COX-2-selective inhibitors should be avoided in patients with high GI and cardiovascular risks [214]. The EMA contraindicates the use of the COX-2 selective agents in patients with previous cardiovascular events, and establishes that adverse cardiovascular events with the use of nsNSAIDs cannot be excluded.

NSAIDs play a significant role in *H. pylori*-negative duodenal and gastric ulcers. NSAID ingestion is regarded as the most common cause of acute erosive gastritis. Mucosal haemorrhages and erosions are extremely common in individuals taking these drugs but, in most cases, there are no significant clinical manifestations. However, acute gastric ulcers have been reported in almost 7% of healthy volunteers taking therapeutic doses of aspirin for 1 week [11]. In the same study, non-aspirin NSAIDs caused lesser degrees of mucosal damage. A similar endoscopic study showed that variable degrees of gastric and duodenal mucosal haemorrhage are common after aspirin therapy, but that enteric-coated tablets reduced the damage [12]. It is likely that, with long-term therapy, mucosal adaptation occurs and the mucosal damage may diminish. The distribution of erosions caused by NSAIDs differs from that of stress-induced lesions, in that they do not show a predilection for the proximal stomach, they tend to be less florid and they are relatively more common in the antrum [13]. A high percentage of the NSAID/aspirin-induced ulcers of the stomach can be correctly diagnosed on the basis of ischaemic necrosis [215].

In view of the widespread prevalence of *H. pylori* infection, especially in the middle-aged and elderly population, it seems reasonable to consider any synergistic association between *H. pylori* and NSAID ingestion. *H. pylori* infection and low-dose aspirin are not only independent causal factors of peptic ulceration and GI bleeding, but also have synergistic and additive effects [216]. Testing for, and cure of, *H. pylori* infection is recommended in patients before the initiation of NSAID therapy, and in those who are currently receiving NSAIDs and have a history of dyspepsia, peptic ulceration or ulcer complications [216,217]. Nevertheless, *H. pylori* eradication is less effective than PPI treatment in preventing ulcer recurrence in long-term NSAID users [217]. In patients receiving long-term NSAIDs, a PPI is more effective in the prevention of ulcer recurrence and bleeding. However, *H. pylori* should be eradicated in patients receiving long-term PPI maintenance treatment to prevent the development of corpus gastritis and gastric atrophy [215–218].

Alcohol-induced gastropathy

Heavy alcohol ingestion is associated with haemorrhagic gastritis. Mucosal petechial haemorrhages are predominantly seen in the proximal stomach in a distribution similar to that of stress-related lesions. Also, after short-term ingestion of large quantities of alcohol, mucosal erosions are commonly found. Although haemorrhagic gastritis is the descriptive term frequently used to describe the end-result of acute and chronic alcohol ingestion, there is little inflammation. The principal feature is intramucosal subepithelial haemorrhages, which impart a congested mucosal appearance on endoscopy [219]. Thus, the term 'acute erosive gastropathy' is more appropriate [4].

Mucosal haemorrhage occurs in 15% of heavy drinkers and can be induced in healthy volunteers after acute alcohol ingestion, even after a single dose. In a detailed histological study, extensive mucosal lesions were observed in <20% of patients studied and resolved rapidly [220]. There is evidence that high concentrations of alcohol lead to exfoliation and necrosis of the superficial gastric mucosa, and

that the damage may be mediated by neutrophils [221]. Exposure to high concentrations of ethanol also leads to reduction in gastric mucosal blood flow [222]. Conversely, nitric oxide released from vascular endothelial cells after alcohol ingestion may exert a protective vasodilator effect [223].

The principal histological feature of alcohol-induced gastric mucosal damage is focal haemorrhage just beneath the surface epithelium [224]. Biopsies also may show patchy 'necrobiosis' of the foveolar region with focal neutrophil infiltration. Mild epithelial cell degeneration in the form of mucus depletion and loss of nuclear polarity is seen particularly in epithelial cells overlying the haemorrhages. Vascular congestion is seen in a minority of cases and inflammation is not intense. Biopsies from adjacent non-haemorrhagic mucosa show oedema, which may involve the full thickness of the mucosa and extend into the submucosa. The risk of major upper GI bleeding increases in proportion to the amount of alcohol consumed [225].

Stress-related erosions

After severe trauma or sepsis, endoscopic studies indicate that mucosal petechiae and erosions appear in the corpus of the stomach within 24h. They may spread distally and involve the antral mucosa [226]. The incidence of such lesions is very high and approaches 100% in seriously ill patients [226,227]. Clinical manifestations are much less common and usually occur 3–10 days after the stressful event. Significant bleeding occurs in 5–20% of cases, although this can be significantly reduced by prophylactic antacids or acid-suppression therapy [228]. With modern intensive care treatment, the risk of significant bleeding, although associated with high mortality, has decreased and is lower than previously thought, except in patients with coagulopathy or respiratory failure [140].

The pathogenesis of stress-related erosive gastritis is not fully understood and is probably due to a variety of factors related to the mucosal defence mechanisms. The importance of gastric acid is indicated by a significant reduction in clinical manifestations of erosive gastritis after prophylactic antacid or acid-suppression therapy [228]. Hypovolaemia has been implicated [229,230]. The mucosa of the gastric corpus has a high energy requirement and it is suggested that hypovolaemic shock causes an energy deficit, leading to depletion of adenosine triphosphate (ATP) levels, which particularly affects the proximal stomach [231]. A further consequence of haemorrhagic shock is to alter the intramucosal acid–base balance and to impair the capacity to buffer luminal acid [115]. Other aetiological factors include oxygen-derived free radicals, with related damage occurring during reperfusion after ischaemia; this damage is reduced by agents that inhibit and scavenge free radicals [232].

Curling's ulcer

Curling's ulcer is the term applied to acute gastroduodenal ulceration after extensive burns. It develops within 24–72 h, predominantly within the proximal stomach as in other cases of stress gastritis, but the antrum and duodenum are also frequently involved [233]. In areas of intense mucosal erosion, there may be progression to gastric ulcer, especially in burns cases complicated by sepsis or haemoconcentration, despite prophylactic antacid therapy [234]. Duodenal ulceration occurs with approximately the same frequency as gastric ulcer [233,234], and is particularly common in children [235].

Cushing's ulcer

The term Cushing's ulcer is used to describe acute gastroduodenal ulceration associated with disease or injury of the central nervous system [236]. Endoscopic studies indicate a high incidence of visible lesions soon after severe head injury [237], although clinically significant complications are considerably less common. In contrast to other forms of stress-associated gastroduodenal disease, Cushing's ulcer is relatively more common in the duodenum and tends to be solitary and deep. Accordingly, perforation is more common [238].

Ulceration and the Zollinger–Ellison syndrome

Zollinger–Ellison syndrome is a rare cause of severe, recurrent and often multiple peptic ulcers. It appears that the marked increase in gastric acid output secondary to hypergastrinaemia alone is sufficient to cause the extensive ulceration, and the prevalence of infection is diminished in these patients compared with the general population [239], probably because the sustained hyperacidity restricts bacterial colonisation and growth. Most patients who develop the syndrome [240] have a primary gastrin-secreting tumour (gastrinoma) in the pancreas that stimulates the acid-secreting cells of the corpus to maximal activity, with consequent liability to duodenal or even jejunal ulceration. The syndrome is characterised by severe and refractory peptic ulceration, which may be multiple and occur in atypical sites such as the distal duodenum and jejunum. The oesophagus also may be involved. In approximately 10% of cases, the tumours arise in the duodenum, most commonly in the second part [241,242]. The most useful diagnostic feature is marked elevation of fasting serum gastrin levels [243].

The incidence of the syndrome is very low [244]. Although most cases are sporadic, in about 20–30% of cases the syndrome is associated with the autosomal dominant syndrome of MEN 1, in which case there are often multiple small gastrinomas in the duodenum and primary tumours in other endocrine organs, notably the parathyroids and the pituitary [243,245]. In such cases, the trophic effects of prolonged hypergastrinaemia on fundal enterochromaffin-like (ECL) cells induce multiple small gastric endocrine (carcinoid) tumours (gastric carcinoidosis) [246]. In a few patients, no tumour is detectable and there is localised hyperplasia of antral G cells, which results in a similar clinical picture [247,248]. Such primary G-cell hyperplasia must be distinguished from secondary forms, which represent a physiological response to hypochlorhydria due to autoimmune atrophic gastritis, truncal vagotomy or, occasionally, prolonged treatment with H2-receptor antagonists or PPIs [249]. In such cases, hyperacidity, peptic ulceration and the Zollinger–Ellison syndrome are absent.

Grossly, the stomach in Zollinger-Ellison syndrome shows very prominent folds in the body, not unlike the appearance in Ménétrier's disease. The body mucosa is thickened due to marked expansion of the specialised glands as a result of proliferation of hypertrophic parietal cells (Figure 11.14). The shrewd observer may also detect ECL hyperplasia which is better demonstrated by immunohistochemistry. Foveolae usually have no associated inflammation. The duodenal mucosa shows features of duodenitis in which gastric metaplasia of the surface epithelium is a prominent feature [187] and villi may be markedly reduced in height or absent. When the Zollinger–Ellison syndrome is due to apparent primary antral G-cell hyperplasia (it is always difficult to know that this is present and that it is primary), the antral endocrine cells are signifi-

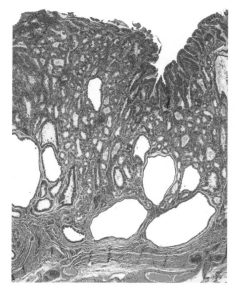

Figure 11.14 Zollinger–Ellison syndrome: the fundic mucosa is markedly thickened. Intramucosal cysts and hyperplastic parietal lining cells are characteristic features as well.

cantly increased in number, sometimes forming small clusters or microcarcinoids [250,251]. Conversely, when the cause is a discrete gastrinoma, the antral G cells become suppressed and their numbers may be either normal or decreased [252].

Atrophic gastritis and gastric atrophy

Atrophic gastritis refers to the finding of variable gland loss associated with or without metaplasia. In the antrum, atrophic gastritis is usually associated with intestinal metaplasia that occupies the full thickness of the mucosa in all or part of a biopsy. Complete or almost complete replacement of the antrum with intestinal metaplasia is associated with a higher cancer risk (even in the absence of corpus atrophy) [253]. In the corpus, atrophy begins at the junction between fundic and antral mucosa [153,253,254]. This usually takes the form of loss of oxyntic glands with extension of mucous neck cells into the pits, replacing them with pseudopyloric (alternatively known as ulcer-associated cell lineage), intestinal, and/or pancreatic metaplasia [253–255]. Corpus atrophy shifts proximally to variable-sized areas on the lesser and greater curves and neighbouring anterior and posterior walls [153,253], such that the antrum appears to expand with advancing atrophic gastritis [153,256]. The rate of progression of *H. pylori* gastritis depends on the acid milieu [254]. On occasion, isolated intestinal metaplasia may happen without adjacent pseudo-pyloric metaplasia. Presumably this is the result of focal injury, possibly related to NSAIDs or aspirin use.

To increase the likelihood of identifying corpus atrophy, when present, it is important to remember several principles:

1. Atrophy begins at the antrum–corpus junction such that, in the early stages of atrophic gastritis, especially in children [257], the location of the histological antral–corpus border would be expected to be nearer to the normal anatomical border [173].

2. Atrophy is gland loss with or without its replacement with fibrosis or metaplastic epithelium [153,253] (Figure 11.15).

3. The atrophic border extends proximally at a similar rate on both curvatures. However, because the lesser curve is much shorter than the greater curve, locations high on the greater curvature are among the last to undergo atrophy [147,253].

Pseudo-pyloric metaplasia

With continuous inflammation and progressive atrophy, there is a progressive loss of specialised cells. Eventually, with the progressive replacement of oxyntic glands by mucous cells, biopsies from the body will resemble antral (pyloric) glands, hence the term 'pseudo-pyloric metapla-

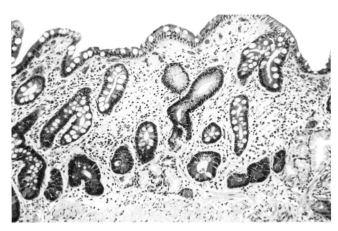

Figure 11.15 Gastric atrophy with extensive intestinal metaplasia, including the complete type with demonstrable Paneth cells at the crypt bases.

sia' (Figure 11.16), which may be misinterpreted as antral mucosa. Pseudo-pyloric metaplasia has also been termed 'ulcer-associated cell lineage'. The differentiation of true antral mucosa from pseudo-pyloric metaplasia can be facilitated by several methods. As G cells are never seen in the body [257], the absence of G cells is particularly useful in recognising pseudo-pyloric metaplasia or, conversely, the presence of G cells indicates that the mucosa is antral. Alternatively, pseudo-pyloric metaplasia stains for pepsinogen I (PG I), which is naturally localised in chief cells, mucous neck cells and transitional mucous neck/chief cells of the oxyntic mucosa, but is not localised in antral gland cells [253,255,258].

Pseudo-pyloric metaplasia has been observed adjacent to benign gastric ulcers proximal to the normal border zone (antrum–corpus junction) [147]. In fact, before the rediscovery of *H. pylori*, a proximally advancing atrophic front with pseudo-pyloric metaplasia was considered part of the normal ageing process [153]. Later, an association was demonstrated between the presence of mucous glands in corpus biopsies and the age of *H. pylori*-infected patients. Pseudo-pyloric metaplasia is considered regenerative in nature [259,260] and is also observed in gastric remnants after distal gastrectomy with gastro-enteric anastomosis, forming a 'neo-antrum' [16].

Intestinal metaplasia

Intestinal metaplasia has two major forms that often coexist. The complete form essentially resembles the colon, with absorptive, goblet, Paneth and endocrine cells but, when well developed, may resemble small intestine with villi. Incomplete intestinal metaplasia consists of gastric mucus-producing cells with goblet cells interspersed

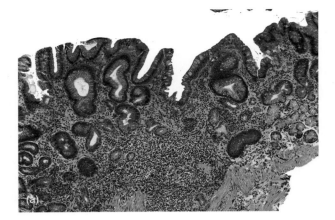

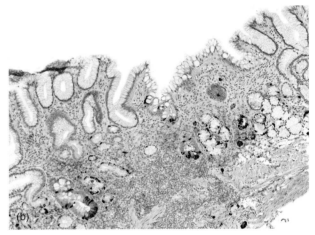

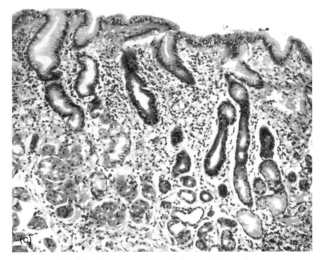

Figure 11.16 (a) Gastric corpus of stomach in autoimmune atrophic gastritis: there is severe atrophy with total loss of parietal cells and replacement by pyloric-type mucosa. A basal lymphocytic infiltrate is noted. Intestinal metaplasia is also focally present. (b) Synaptophysin immunohistochemistry shows linear and nodular hyperplasia of enterochromaffin-like cells in the same case. (c) Another example of autoimmune gastritis with atrophy and pyloric metaplasia with replacement of parietal cells by antral-type mucosa.

among them. As the development of gastric carcinoma is a slow and unpredictable process, and intestinal metaplasia is an easily recognisable marker for atrophy, subtyping intestinal metaplasia using high iron diamine staining might identify subgroups of patients with different risk potentials. Intestinal metaplasia subtyped as III (black-staining sulphomucin in goblet cells of incomplete intestinal metaplasia) (Figure 11.17) is often considered the highest risk precursor lesion for the intestinal form of gastric cancer [261–264], but this is not uniformly accepted. In addition, approximately equal numbers of studies have suggested that intestinal metaplasia either regresses or does not regress after *H. pylori* treatment [97,254,265–271]. Sampling error is the factor probably responsible for this discrepancy. Prior studies suggesting an association of type III intestinal metaplasia with the development of gastric cancer [261–264] did not take into account the higher prevalence of incomplete intestinal metaplasia (type III) in the gastric antrum [253,261–264,272,273]. In practice, areas of intestinal metaplasia (or a certain subtype) are generally small and can easily be missed at follow-up [251,252].

A small percentage of cancer patients show complete replacement of the antral mucosa with intestinal metaplasia and have normal appearing oxyntic mucosa [253]. It is unknown if these individuals lose their G cells and have normal or reduced acid secretion. Continued inflammation with antral atrophy could possibly lead to sufficient destruction of G cells [274], which can result in a fall in acid secretion [275,276]. Alternatively, contiguous sheets of intestinal metaplasia may be an unstable epithelium.

Overall, it is not possible to make recommendations or prognoses based on biopsies (single or multiple) showing sulphomucin expression in areas with intestinal metaplasia [254,277,278]. All data suggest that, in the development of intestinal type of gastric cancer, the extent of mucosal atrophy within a region of the stomach is more important than the type of intestinal metaplasia. Although intestinal metaplasia is a form of atrophy that is easy for pathologists to recognise, it is also important to determine whether intestinal metaplasia is present as an isolated patch within non-atrophic mucosa or amidst an atrophic lawn [173,253]. Thus a patch of intestinal metaplasia in non-atrophic mucosa is a reparative phenomenon and there are no data to suggest that it is associated with an increased risk of carcinoma, and thus there is no perceived benefit in using intestinal metaplasia, demonstrated in gastric biopsies, as a marker for those at increased risk of gastric cancer in practical terms.

Pancreatic metaplasia

In addition to pyloric and intestinal metaplasia, foci of pancreatic acinar metaplasia within the stomach have been

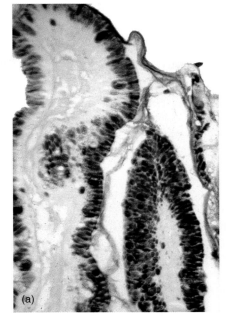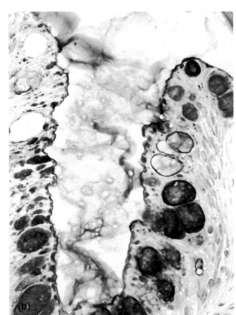

(a)   (b)

Figure 11.17 Type III intestinal metaplasia with (a) sulphomucin (brown) mainly in columnar cells and some goblet cells. Most goblet cells contain sialomucin (blue). (b) Type III intestinal metaplasia stained by Gomori's aldehyde fuchsin showing sulphomucins (purple) in columnar cells and in some goblet cells. Other goblet cells contain sialomucin (blue).

described in association with chronic gastritis [279]. These cells, showing characteristic features of pancreatic acinar cells on light and electron microscopy, and immunoreactivity for pancreatic lipase trypsinogen, occur most frequently within pyloric mucosa affected by active chronic gastritis and atrophic gastritis. Such foci have also been noted in the cardia [280] and fundus. The most frequent association is with *H. pylori* infection but pancreatic metaplasia has also been reported in the fundus in autoimmune gastritis.

PPIs and corpus atrophy

PPIs are potent inhibitors of gastric acid secretion, widely used in the treatment of peptic diseases, and effectively alleviate symptoms and facilitate healing of inflamed or ulcerated mucosa. Frequently, PPIs are also prescribed for a lifetime, in patients with GORD, and in NSAID or aspirin users, such as patients with rheumatoid arthritis or osteoarthritis [281].

However, 20–50% of patients on long-term PPIs may be infected with *H. pylori* unknowingly. As a result, *H. pylori* corpus gastritis is accelerated by low acid secretion secondary to chronic therapy [85,282–292], which in turn affects both the distribution and severity of *H. pylori*-related gastritis [81,283,291]. It facilitates proximal migration of the bacteria [85,285,293,294], and allows the development of a corpus-predominant gastritis rather than a pangastritis [295]. Omeprazole therapy is associated with a reduction in bacterial load, both in the antrum and in the corpus, and a tendency for antral histology to improve; corpus gastritis either does not change or worsens. With omeprazole therapy, not only does the corpus mucosa fail to show

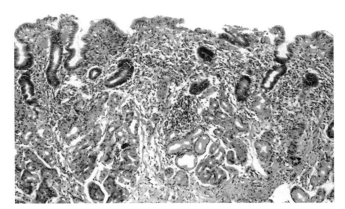

Figure 11.18 Moderate atrophic gastritis of gastric corpus mucosa in chronic Helicobacter pylori infection showing loss of parietal cells in association with active inflammation. Connective tissue has replaced the lost cells.

histological improvement but, rather, there is a significant progression of the inflammatory reaction deeper within the pit to involve the proliferative zone [294].

Prolonged PPI use in *H. pylori*-negative patients shows no difference in gastric inflammation or atrophy over a 7-year period in one study [294]. In contrast, *H. pylori*-positive patients followed over the same period showed increased inflammation and gastric atrophy [296] (Figure 11.18). These studies highlight the importance of considering *H. pylori* eradication in infected, long-term PPI users. As PPI therapy reduces gastric acidity, it also reduces *H. pylori* density, which then may not be identified in gastric biopsies [294,297,298]. One has to rely on the pattern of inflammation to diagnose the infection. Histopathological features suggestive of long-term PPI use include parietal cell hypertrophy and G-cell hyperplasia.

Other adverse effects associated with long-term and/or high-dose PPI therapy include vitamin B_{12} deficiency irrespective of *H. pylori* status [299,300–302], enteric infections (e.g. *Clostridium difficile*), community-acquired pneumonia, osteopaenia and hip fractures, and small intestinal bacterial overgrowth. The proposed mechanism is that reduced acidity impairs cobalamin release from dietary protein and bacterial overgrowth increases competitive consumption [299,301,302]. It is not uncommon to see a variety of cocci and bacilli in gastric mucosa of patients on high-dose long-term PPIs. These should not be mistaken for *H. pylori* or its coccoid forms. although these colonies can be associated with inflammation, it is often difficult to be sure that the patient does not have helicobacter infection that is being suppressed by the PPIs.

Autoimmune gastritis

Classic autoimmune gastritis (AIG) results from immune-mediated progressive destruction of parietal cells, leading to reduced acid production and reduced or absent intrinsic factor necessary for vitamin B_{12} absorption. In later stages of the disease, vitamin B_{12} deficiency may result in pernicious anaemia. Approximately 90% of patients have antibodies to parietal cells, and 50–70% of patients have antibodies to proton pump H^+/K^+ ATPase and intrinsic factor (IF) [303–305]. The latter autoantibodies are considered by many to be diagnostic of pernicious anaemia [303]. The specificity of the intrinsic factor autoantibody test is high, because false positives in healthy controls have not been reported so far [306–308].

Of note, there are limited longitudinal studies of autoantibodies in patients with AIG [303]. In a contested large study of white patients with pernicious anaemia [303], a trend was showed for gradual disappearance of parietal cell autoantibodies while intrinsic factor autoantibodies became more prevalent [303,309]. Interestingly, the relative prevalence of antibodies to gastric parietal cell and IF was originally described in predominantly elderly white patients of European origin and did not apply in a more diverse patient population, in which anti-parietal cell autoantibodies may be less frequent than IF autoantibodies [310]. Thus anti-parietal cell autoantibody is not only not so specific for AIG but also of limited sensitivity [310].

AIG is far more common in white people [311,312], especially those of Scandinavian descent, and family studies suggest an autosomal recessive trait [313,314]. Affected patients also tend to suffer from other autoimmune diseases such as psoriasis, rosacea, autoimmune thyroid dis-

orders, type 1 diabetes, Sjögren's syndrome and coeliac disease [315,316–320]. This is particularly true in younger individuals, with isolated AIG being rarely recognised before age 30. Clinical symptoms in early stages are non-specific and no different from other forms of chronic gastritides. Once anaemia develops, symptoms resemble those seen in other anaemias (namely fatigue, pallor and shortness of breath). Late complications of vitamin B12 deficiency include neurological abnormalities such as peripheral neuropathy and subacute combined degeneration of the spinal cord [321,322]. The 'cure' for pernicious anaemia centres on replacing vitamin B_{12} for life. Of note, in the presence of hypochlorhydria or achlorhydria, the absorption of non-haem iron is decreased, leading to concomitant iron deficiency anaemia.

Autoimmune gastritis is a corpus-predominant gastritis with severe atrophy of the oxyntic mucosa (see Figure 11.16). Although most believe that the antrum is uninvolved, there is invariably some antral involvement [323], and this may represent an immune response aimed at the scattered parietal cells located within the junctional mucosa. The histopathological diagnosis in the early stages can be challenging, because biopsies reveal chronic inflammation only primarily in the gastric corpus with minimal atrophy and no metaplasia or endocrine cell hyperplasia [324]. In advanced cases, the degree of inflammation may decrease, with loss of virtually all specialised glands of the upper stomach along with pseudo-pyloric, intestinal and/or pancreatic metaplasia [253,324,325].

Immunohistochemical studies have demonstrated an absolute increase in T cells and, more notably, B lymphocytes and an increased IgG:IgA ratio of secreting plasma cells [326]. Although *H. pylori* gastritis may precede AIG, a distinguishing feature between them is usually the presence of ECL and G-cell hyperplasia in AIG secondary to the profound achlorhydria and the high serum gastrin levels [325,327–330] (see Figure 11.16).

Autoimmunity and the role of *H. pylori* gastritis

It is now recognised that the clinical presentation commonly associated with AIG is not specific and can be seen with *H. pylori*-induced gastric atrophy. Interestingly, it has been noted that cross-reacting autoantibodies initiated by *H. pylori* may target parietal cells, hence the implication of *H. pylori* in the genesis of autoimmune gastritis, possibly playing an initiating role [331,332]. It is worth emphasising that parietal cell loss can be widespread in *H. pylori*-induced gastric atrophy and may be associated with a significant increase in autoantibodies [333,334]. Notably, the prevalence of anti-canalicular and parietal cell antibodies increases significantly with the duration of *H. pylori* gastritis, particularly with the development of atrophy of the corpus mucosa [335]. Nevertheless, pernicious anaemia after *H. pylori* infection is still rare and typically occurs in an elderly patient who may have been improperly managed for many years [299]. Interestingly, a decrease of gastric autoantibodies after eradication of *H. pylori* infection has been reported by some [336]. Furthermore, *H. pylori* infection alone cannot explain AIG (latent or active) in children [406–408], or the familial aggregation in the absence of *H. pylori* infection [337].

Alternatively, the prevalence of AIG and pernicious anaemia is three- to fivefold higher in patients with type 1 diabetes mellitus, an autoimmune disease, with respective frequencies of 5–10% and 2–4% compared with 2% and 0.5–1.0% in the general population [338,339]. In another study, 2 of 18 children with juvenile autoimmune thyroid disease had elevated parietal cell antibodies, hypergastrinaemia, and negative histology and serology for *H. pylori* infection [340]. There is a report of a young woman with systemic lupus erythematosus and pernicious anaemia. In this case, parietal cell autoantibodies were absent but high IF autoantibodies were noted. Of note, her anaemia resolved on steroid therapy, whereas IF autoantibodies remained steadily positive [341]. Finally, one patient has been reported with elevated parietal cell antibodies and slightly elevated IF antibodies with mild atrophic gastritis, but no evidence of ongoing or previous *H. pylori* infection [342]. Thus, it can be inferred that individuals with autoimmunity predisposition may develop spontaneous autoantibodies without *H. pylori* infection, suggesting the existence of different pathogenic pathways [341,342]. Corpuspredominant gastritis is classically associated with AIG [313]. However, it has also been described in *H. pylori*-associated atrophic gastritis [343] and particularly in long-term PPI users [295].

Endoscopy and surveillance

Severe gastric atrophy may be evident as thinning of the mucosa, with a paucity of the gastric folds at the greater curvature and prominent vessels [344]. If there is extensive intestinal metaplasia, the mucosa may acquire a silvery sheen. However, none of the endoscopic features is sufficiently specific to render the diagnosis without histological confirmation. The best area to sample for this purpose is the mid-body region on the greater curve, because the mucosa of the lesser curve and transition zones (antral–body, cardiac–body) is commonly thinner than on the greater curve, and could be erroneously interpreted as atrophic.

Gastrin, which is elevated in AIG, has a well-known trophic effect and, in up to 10% of patients, there is an increased risk for gastric endocrine (carcinoid) tumours or adenocarcinomas [345–347]. Patients who develop pernicious anaemia also have a three- to fivefold increased risk for gastric cancer [348,349].

Thus the question of endoscopic surveillance, for potential neoplasia, of patients with AIG is frequently raised. We agree with the recommendation that all patients with AIG should undergo endoscopy with biopsies at least once, at or after the initial diagnosis [350]. We recommend taking four biopsies from the antrum and at least six from the body and fundus; these should be spaced equidistantly along the lesser and greater curvatures. If no endocrine tumours (carcinoids) or dysplastic lesions are discovered, screening at periodic intervals is not likely to be required [351]. One exception concerns patients with a history of gastric cancer in a first-degree relative; here we would be inclined to repeat the examinations, as above, every 5 years. In the rare event that a patient is found to have dysplasia, particularly high grade dysplasia, a second endoscopy and more biopsies should be performed to rule out coexisting carcinoma while, ideally, the lesion should be treated with endoscopic mucosal resection. With regard to microcarcinoidosis, follow-up studies of patients show that they tend not to grow, so that, at best, occasional endoscopy is required. The frequency of such follow-up has not been established.

Juvenile forms of pernicious anaemia

These rare conditions present in three forms [352]. One, occurring in later childhood and adolescence, is associated with gastric atrophy and appears to correspond to the adult type with an unusually early age of onset. In the second, sometimes called 'true' juvenile pernicious anaemia, intrinsic factor is not secreted by parietal cells but the mucosa is histologically normal. The failure to secrete IF is not explained by the presence of an autoantibody. Acid secretion is normal when vitamin B12 is given, although it may be reduced without it. Vitamin B12 is absorbed from the small intestine if IF is added to the diet [353,354]. Finally, the third type results from the failure to absorb vitamin B12–IF complex [355].

The stomach in other types of megaloblastic anaemia

Infestation with *Diphyllobothrium latum* occurs in Scandinavian countries, producing a megaloblastic anaemia. The gastric mucosa shows varying degrees of atrophic gastritis with superficial inflammation and zones of intestinal metaplasia [356]. The condition closely resembles pernicious anaemia.

Immune-mediated pan-gastritis

Cases of pangastritis, involving the entire gastric mucosa, including the whole body and the antrum, unlike in classic AIG, can be seen among *H. pylori*-negative patients

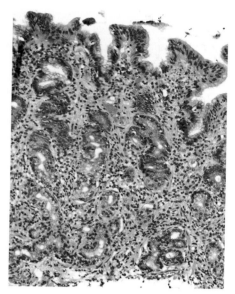

Figure 11.19 Gastritis in a patient with autoimmune enteropathy: the non-specific histological features include lymphocytic exocytosis, increased apoptosis and mild expansion of the lamina propria by chronic inflammatory cells.

[357,358]. Most cases have occurred in the setting of autoimmune enteropathy, other autoimmune disorders or immunodeficiency syndromes (congenital or acquired). The underlying mechanisms are various and not fully understood. Anti-parietal cell and/or anti-IF antibodies have been detected in some patients, whereas others have different autoantibodies, such as anti-enterocyte antibodies or anti-nuclear antibodies. The morphology is variable. In some, a dense mixed inflammatory infiltrate is seen, composed of polyclonal plasma cells and numerous CD3+ T lymphocytes, with variable numbers of CD4-positive and CD8-positive T cells (Figure 11.19). Secondary endocrine cell hyperplasia is absent, suggesting that all types of gastric cells are equally damaged. The development of dysplasia has been seen rarely, suggesting a possible risk of adenocarcinoma.

Acute gastritis

Acute gastritis is an ill-defined term that has been used to cover a wide variety of conditions ranging from life-threatening acute haemorrhagic gastritis (also known as acute stress ulceration or acute erosive gastritis) to transient mild acute inflammation of the gastric mucosa. It commonly presents with a sudden onset and develops when there is an acute imbalance between injury and mucosal repair mechanisms. Biopsy studies are few. Acute gastritis can be broadly divided into three groups: (1) infectious; (2) haemorrhagic (see Stress-related erosions, above); and (3) secondary to drugs, chemotherapy and caustic

injury. Acute haemorrhagic gastritis is associated with multiple mucosal petechiae, acute erosions and ulcers. Acute gastritis may result from the ingestion of corrosives or drugs such as ferrous sulphate; milder forms are seen in patients with uraemia and in the early stages of *H. pylori* infection. The gastritis associated with chronic alcohol abuse is often termed 'haemorrhagic gastritis' on account of the congested inflammation of the mucosa at endoscopy and is thus discussed in the section above. Acute phlegmonous gastritis is a rare disease in which there is suppurative inflammation of the full thickness of the gastric wall.

Phlegmonous and emphysematous gastritis

Phlegmonous gastritis is an uncommon condition characterised by suppurative bacterial infection of the gastric wall. It primarily affects the submucosa but may spread to all layers of the stomach, resulting in necrosis and gangrene. The latter complication, when unassociated with thrombosis of the major vessels, has sometimes been designated *acute necrotising gastritis* [359]. Emphysematous gastritis is probably the same disease but associated with gas-forming bacterial organisms [360]. Both phlegmonous and emphysematous gastritis are rare and potentially life threatening [361].

Phlegmonous gastritis was more common in the pre-antibiotic era [362] but sporadic cases continue to occur and appear to be increasing. Immunosuppression may be involved with cases occurring in association with HIV infection with some cases reported with HIV seroconversion [363,364] particularly during ACTH treatment [365]. Other predisposing factors include disability, gastritis and chronic alcoholism. The route of entry of the infection is often uncertain. Sometimes there is septicaemia, endocarditis [366] or pharyngitis [367]. Very rarely, phlegmonous gastritis may follow endoscopic biopsy [368]. Most cases occur in patients aged 30–70 years. The presentation is usually with nausea, vomiting, and upper abdominal pain and tenderness. Polymorphonuclear leukocytosis is usually present and pyrexia is common but not invariable. Positive blood culture may be detected [369]. In fact, the clinical diagnosis is difficult and many cases may be identified post mortem.

On examination, the gastric wall is thickened, especially the submucosa. Inflammation may involve the whole stomach or be localised, usually to the pyloric canal [367]. The mucosa is often intact, although the folds may be lost. Ulceration may be noted. The serosa is usually covered by a fibrinous exudate. Usually the inflammation and thickening of the wall do not extend proximally or distally, beyond the cardia or pylorus (Figure 11.20). On microscopic examination, there is an intense acute inflammation with abscess formation and oedema, usually centred on the submucosa but also extending into the muscularis propria and subserosa [367]. The most common infective organisms are strep-

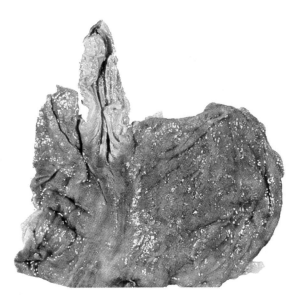

Figure 11.20 A postmortem specimen of acute phlegmonous gastritis: there is loss of the mucosal folds of the proximal stomach due to massive submucosal oedema. Note that there is a sharp demarcation at the oesophago-gastric junction, the distal oesophagus being unaffected.

tococci [362], but staphylococci, *Haemophila influenzae*, *Escherichia coli* and *Proteus spp.* have also been implicated. The condition is frequently fatal, although patients treated surgically have a much better chance of survival [370].

Effects of corrosive poisons

A wide variety of poisons severely affects the stomach, including mineral acids, carbolic acid, Lysol, sodium and potassium hydroxide, sodium hypochlorite (bleach) and sodium acid sulphate. These may be ingested accidentally or with suicidal intent. Such substances are widely used as cleaning agents, descalers and metal polish. They are freely available. Ingestion causes rapid and widespread necrosis of the gastric mucosa, which becomes haemorrhagic and oedematous. The antral mucosa may not be affected, depending on the amount ingested. The mucosal surface is often black due to altered blood and necrosis frequently extends into the muscle coat, resulting in friability of the wall and the likelihood of perforation. Corrosive burns also affect the mouth and surrounding skin and the oesophagus.

Uraemic gastropathy

Small petechial haemorrhages may develop secondary to uraemia and, in severe untreated cases, this may give the appearance of an acute haemorrhagic gastropathy [371].

In fact, superficial gastritis is common, and gastric and duodenal erosions may be seen in patients with chronic renal failure undergoing dialysis treatment [371–374]. When present, erosions and ulcers are important causes of upper GI bleeding. However, the concomitant use of ulcerogenic drugs, such as NSAIDs, may have a compounding effect [375]. Another significant factor is hypersecretion of acid, which frequently occurs during dialysis treatment [376,377]. Severe atrophic gastritis and chronic duodenitis with gastric metaplasia may also be seen [378]. Of note, *H. pylori* infection does not appear to be common in patients undergoing treatment for chronic renal failure [379].

Successful kidney transplantation is frequently associated with hypertrophic mucosal folds in the corpus. Histology shows foveolar hyperplasia, multinucleated parietal cells, and extension of parietal cells into the antrum and even the duodenum. This may be related to long-term steroid therapy and the trophic effects of hypergastrinaemia. In addition, heterotopic calcification may occur and the increased incidence of cytomegalovirus (CMV) infection should be considered in these patients receiving immunosuppression therapy [372].

Other forms of gastritis

Lymphocytic gastritis

Lymphocytic gastritis is the descriptive diagnosis of an uncommon condition characterised by a striking increase in intra-epithelial lymphocytes (IELs) infiltrating the mucosal surface and the foveolae of the stomach. It has numerous aetiologies, so the key is in identifying the associated conditions. Irrespective of the cause, it is usually a chronic condition that appears to persist over many years. Although the number of IELs may diminish with time and fall below the diagnostic threshold, it remains higher than normal [380].

The diagnosis of lymphocytic gastritis can be made only on histology but some cases present the endoscopic features of 'varioliform gastritis', in which there are persistent shallow chronic erosions, often in clusters, set on the surface of prominent rugal mucosal folds of the corpus, but occasionally extending into the antrum. As the erosions may have a volcano-like appearance that resembles the rash of smallpox (or variola), the term 'varioliform gastritis' was coined [381,382]. This condition is recognised on endoscopy and double-contrast radiology [383,384]. Patients present with anorexia, weight loss, epigastric pain and, sometimes, a protein-losing gastro-enteropathy.

Severe forms of lymphocytic gastritis may also be associated with large mucosal folds resembling Ménétrier's disease, both endoscopically and clinically, with protein loss noted in 20% of the patients [385,386]. In one series of cases showing giant gastric mucosal folds and foveolar

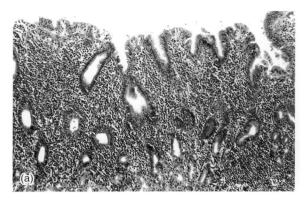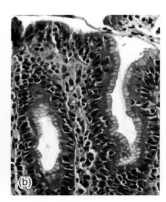

Figure 11.21 Lymphocytic gastritis: (a) low-power view to show dense chronic inflammatory cell infiltrate in the lamina propria and lining foveolar epithelium. (b) High magnification showing increased numbers of intra-epithelial lymphocytes among surface and foveolar epithelial cells.

hyperplasia, over 50% showed lymphocytic gastritis [387]. However, it should be noted that some cases of lymphocytic gastritis show no distinctive endoscopic features [388].

The clinical presentation is variable and depends on the underlying cause. Some reports have attributed a protein-losing gastro-enteropathy to lymphocytic gastritis [389]. Symptoms include abdominal pain, nausea, vomiting, anorexia, weight loss and iron deficiency anaemia [390,391]. Gastrointestinal bleeding [392] has been variably reported. The natural history of patients with lymphocytic gastritis is unclear. Healing after therapy with H_2-receptor blockers or PPIs, as well as without any specific therapy, has been described.

Lymphocytic gastritis has an excess of IELs) defined as >25 IELs/100 epithelial cells [380,381], this being considered the upper limit of normal (Figure 11.21). Typically infiltrating lymphocytes appear morphologically normal and involve both surface and foveolar epithelium but are usually maximal at the surface. These IELs are predominantly T lymphocytes of the cytotoxic/suppressor type (CD3+, CD8+) [380]. A variable increase of chronic inflammatory cells in the lamina propria (Figure 11.21) and/or oedema can be detected. Neutrophils, in close proximity to erosions, as well as epithelial nuclear stratification, may also be present [393]. Although the entire stomach may be involved, the number of IELs varies [381]. Cases limited to the body (about a fifth of total case numbers) or antrum (about a tenth of total case numbers) have been reported. Thus, the condition may not be obvious in all biopsies taken from the same patient and certainly may be missed if only a single biopsy is taken.

The aetiology of lymphocytic gastritis remains uncertain but it is associated with a variety of other pathological entities. The two most common associations are with *H. pylori* infection and coeliac disease in about one-fifth and two-fifths of cases, respectively [394]. However, lymphocytic gastritis can also be seen in the setting of lymphocytic enterocolitis, Crohn's disease, common variable immuno-deficiency, lymphoma, adenocarcinoma, HIV infection and medications such as ticlopidine [395]. In 20% of the cases, a specific aetiology is not recognised.

With regard to the two most common associations, about 4% of *H. pylori*-infected patients have lymphocytic gastritis [380] and, in these, intra-epithelial lymphocytosis tends to be greater in the gastric body [396]. Yet, irrespective of the endoscopic appearance or the distribution of the disease, in the presence of severe lymphocytic gastritis one needs to look carefully for evidence of *H. pylori* infection. The effect of *H. pylori* eradication on the severity of the histological abnormalities is controversial but it does seem to be beneficial.

About 10–30% of patients with coeliac disease have lymphocytic gastritis and the intra-epithelial lymphocytosis associated with coeliac disease tends to be more pronounced in the antrum [397]. The gastric pathology also resolves with a gluten-free diet. Similar HLA associations have been demonstrated in both coeliac disease and lymphocytic gastritis [398], and it is possible that lymphocytic gastritis is part of a spectrum of diffuse lymphocytic gastroenteropathy representing an abnormal immunological reaction to a single or to different antigens [380].

Eosinophilic gastritis

Eosinophilic gastritis refers to a selective predominance of eosinophil neutrophil infiltrates in the gastric mucosa. It could be an isolated involvement of the stomach or part of a generalised eosinophilic gastroenterocolitis. The stomach, especially the antrum, is often involved in the latter process but any part of the gut may be affected and multiple areas of involvement are common. Endoscopic examination reveals thickening and deformity of the antrum with narrowing of the pylorus and diminished peristalsis. The mucosa may appear swollen and reddened with surface erosions.

In adults, eosinophilic gastroenteritis affects mainly patients in the 30- to 40-year age group. The aetiology of eosinophilic gastritis remains obscure in many cases. A history of systemic allergy or asthma is present in about 25% of cases [399]. There may also be a family history; IgE levels are often elevated and food-specific IgE antibodies may be present, becoming apparent on skin testing [397–402]. There is usually a peripheral blood eosinophilia and IgE levels may be raised [403–405]. The clinical manifestations vary depending on the layers of the wall of the gut affected. Patients presenting with vomiting, abdominal pain, diarrhoea, bloody stools, failure to thrive and iron deficiency anaemia usually have mucosal involvement. Obstructive symptoms and dysphagia tend to be associated with muscularis involvement, whereas patients with serosal involvement present with eosinophilic ascites. Protein-losing gastro-enteropathy, ascites and malabsorption are seen in severe cases [406].

Histological examination shows a striking eosinophil polymorph infiltration of the gastric wall accompanied by oedema (Figure 11.22) [399,407]. The submucosa is affected principally but, as suggested by the presenting features outlined above, no layer is exempt. Eosinophils may infiltrate the lamina propria and invade the epithelium of the crypts and mucosal surface. Focal mucosal necrosis and epithelial regenerative changes may be seen.

Although the criteria defining what constitutes an increase of eosinophils are debated, a definitive diagnosis of eosinophilic gastroenteritis requires an eosinophilic infiltration, usually more than 20 eosinophils per high-power field, in one or more areas of the GI tract [408], an absence of alternative causes of eosinophilia (drug reactions, parasitic infections, malignancies) [408] and no involvement outside the GI tract (no systemic eosinophilic pathology).

Histological subclassification of eosinophilic gastroenteritis is determined according to the layer of the GI tract involved (mucosa, submucosa, muscularis propria and subserosa/serosa). The diagnosis is challenging, because eosinophilic infiltration can be patchy [408]. However, diffuse involvement of the gastric antrum is the rule, unlike the patchy involvement of the small intestinal mucosa. Sampling error is thus less likely to occur in the stomach. Yet, as the infiltrate may predominantly affect different mural layers, a full-thickness surgical biopsy may be required to confirm the diagnosis.

Tissue eosinophilia is not specific for eosinophilic gastritis. In practice, increased eosinophils are most commonly associated with other specific inflammatory disorders, the most common being *H. pylori* infection, although eosinophil polymorphs do not usually predominate and eosinophilic pit abscesses are not found. When eosinophilic infiltration is focal and in association with a severe reactive gastropathy, a common association is medications such as NSAIDs. Various diagnoses that should also be considered include inflammatory fibroid polyp, malignant lymphoma, parasitic infection, Langerhans' cell histiocytosis, Crohn's disease, tropical sprue, systemic mastocytosis and chronic granulomatous disease of childhood [408,409,410]. Hypersensitivity to a specific food or protein is another scenario where eosinophils may be increased in the stomach. This happens more frequently in children in whom modest numbers of eosinophils can be seen as a reaction to cows' milk, soy protein or other allergens. Occasionally food allergy changes may also be seen in adults. Although spontaneous cure is common, appropriate modification of the diet may ameliorate the condition. Other patients will require steroid therapy, whereas some may require surgery because of persistent gastric outlet obstruction.

Collagenous gastritis

Collagenous gastritis, first described in 1989, is a rare disorder that can occur in either the antrum or the body or both [411]. A characteristic, but not universal, endoscopic appearance is that of diffuse mucosal nodularity. Other patients may display a diffuse erythematous mucosa [412]. The pathology is similar to that of collagenous colitis, with a thickened band of subepithelial collagen, which ranges from 15 μm to 120 μm, averaging 30–40 μm, in thickness, and lies immediately beneath the surface of the gastric superficial epithelium (Figure 11.23). The thickened subepithelial collagen band is accompanied by dilated capillaries entrapped within the collagen band. This band is, however, discontinuous. In addition, there is a lymphocytic infiltrate of the lamina propria and scattered eosinophils.

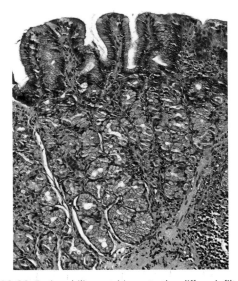

Figure 11.22 Eosinophilic gastritis: note the diffuse infiltration of the lamina propria by chronic inflammatory cells especially eosinophil polymorphs.

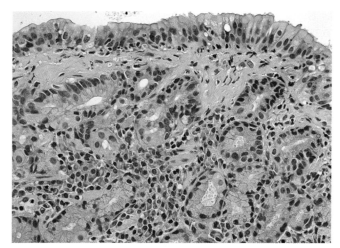

Figure 11.23 Collagenous gastritis: the diagnostic increased subepithelial collagen is easily identified underneath intact epithelial cells. Chronic inflammation of the lamina propria is present as well.

The overlying surface epithelial cells often show degenerative change with flattening and focal detachment of the epithelium. Glandular atrophy is rarely seen and intestinal metaplasia is usually absent [412,413].

The literature divides collagenous gastritis into two phenotypes: childhood and adult onset [413]. The adult-onset subset is associated with a spectrum of conditions, including collagenous colitis, coeliac disease, collagenous sprue and various autoimmune conditions. This condition is more commonly diagnosed in women. In children, collagenous gastritis is often isolated, characterised by anaemia and abdominal pain. The anaemia is believed to result from haemorrhage from dilated capillaries entrapped in the abnormal collagenous matrix [414]. Nevertheless, this subdivision may be arbitrary because the adult-onset phenotype has been described in children, with a case report of collagenous gastritis progressing to collagenous gastroenterocolitis in the adult years [415].

The natural history of collagenous gastritis is variable and uncertain. Most adult patients have a chronic intermittent course [416] with no significant mortality risk or periods of severe deterioration. A more refractory disease seems to characterise cases presenting in young children and early adults, and also when part of a diffuse collagenous gastroenterocolitis. This subtype can be life threatening and responds poorly to steroids and other anti-inflammatory agents.

In adult-onset disease, autoimmune disease, infectious factors and medications have been regarded as possible triggers [417]. Although a genetic predisposition to childhood-onset collagenous gastritis has not been established, familial examples of collagenous colitis have been observed [417].

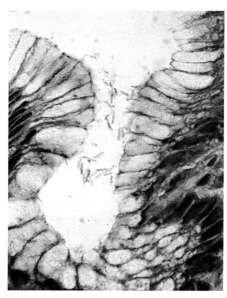

Figure 11.24 *Helicobacter heilmannii* on the gastric mucosal surface. The organisms are larger than *H. pylori* and have several prominent spirals.

Other helicobacter infections of the stomach

At least five different *Helicobacter* spp. (all known to colonise the stomach of animals) comprise this group of organisms. Because of difficulties in isolation and identification, the epidemiology remains poorly understood. Nonetheless, current data suggest that many animals, especially pigs, dogs and cats, constitute reservoir hosts for gastric *Helicobacter* species with zoonotic potential [418].

In a minority of patients (between 0.1% and 2%) with upper GI symptoms, long, tightly coiled spiral bacteria (Figure 11.24), clearly distinct from the smaller gull's wing, S-shaped or comma-shaped *H. pylori*, are observed in gastric biopsies. These bacteria were originally called *Gastrospirillum hominis* [419] but they were subsequently designated *H. heilmannii*, named after the German pathologist, Konrad Heilmann, who first studied the pathology associated with these micro-organisms [420]. *H. heilmannii* is larger than *H. pylori*, measuring up to 7.5 μm in length, with five to eight prominent tight spirals. On this basis, they are usually easily distinguishable from *H. pylori* on light microscopy. The spirals are especially well displayed on scanning electron microscopy [421], whereas transmission electron microscopy shows that, similar to *H. pylori*, the organism possesses sheathed flagellae [421,422,423].

Infection with *H. heilmannii* is associated with chronic or chronic active gastritis [420,421], usually confined to the antrum. This gastritis is usually milder than *H. pylori*-associated gastritis. Features of reactive gastritis with foveolar hyperplasia, vasodilatation and oedema of the lamina propria have been reported in most cases [420]. The organisms are less numerous but longer than *H. pylori*, and occur in small groups or as isolated single organisms within the mucus layer on the mucosal surface or, more often, within foveolae. Touch cytology with smearing of biopsies onto a slide, and subsequent rapid fixation and staining, has resulted in a much higher rate of diagnosis than histological examination of the biopsy alone [422]. The organisms are most easily seen with silver stains. Polymerase chain reaction (PCR) and/or sequencing remain the gold standard for the detection of this genus. The infection may persist for years, and be asymptomatic, or may be associated with symptoms including epigastric pain, vomiting and heartburn [420]. *H. heilmannii* has been implicated in the pathogenesis of gastric ulcers [424] and gastric cancer [425]. In fact, MALT (mucosa-associated lymphoid tissue) lymphoma seems more frequent among patients infected with *H. heilmannii*, although lymphoid aggregates are rare and concomitant infection with *H. pylori* is seldom seen [421,426,427].

Treatment regimens are identical to those used for *H. pylori,* namely triple therapy using combinations of a PPI and two antimicrobial agents. As a result of the low number of in vitro isolates available, very few data exist on the antimicrobial susceptibility and acquired resistance of gastric non-*H. pylori Helicobacter* spp. Nevertheless, acquired resistance to metronidazole may occur with *H. bizzozeronii* and *H. felis* strains of animal origin.

Other bacterial infections in the stomach

A variety of bacterial species colonises the stomach of patients with hypochlorhydria due to chronic atrophic gastritis. There are rare reports of gastric anthrax [428]. Infection with tuberculosis (TB) and syphilis is described below (see 'Granulomatous gastritis'). There is a report of an enterococcus-associated gastritis in a 59-year-old man with diabetes detected 9 months after treatment for *H. pylori*-associated gastritis and ulcers. Mucosal biopsy revealed severe active but focal gastritis adjacent to Gram-positive coccobacilli in short to long chains. Culture grew an enterococcus similar to *Enterococcus hirae* and *E. durans*. No treatment was given and endoscopy 2 months later showed complete resolution of the gastritis and absence of *H. pylori* or enterococci. The presence of NSAID-induced gastric mucosal injury and diabetes mellitus may have been predisposing factors [429].

Opportunistic infections of the stomach

Apart from helicobacter infections, the stomach had been a rare site for microbial infection in the gut. In the early years of HIV/AIDS, such infections were more often seen in the stomach. However, the prevalence of opportunistic gastric infections in HIV-infected patients has declined because of effective antiretroviral therapy. The risk remains for those in whom such therapy is not available and those who are immunocompromised for other reasons (e.g. in cancer patients). Nevertheless, the stomach is relatively rarely affected by such infections compared with the rest of the gut.

Fungal infections of the stomach

In western countries, whether in patients with severe immunocompromise or otherwise, the stomach is an unusual site for fungal infection. The infection may be localised to the stomach or part of a systemic infection.

Candidiasis

Gastric candidiasis may occur as an opportunistic infection in immunosuppressed patients, in those with cancer, and/or after cytotoxic therapy and antibiotic therapy. Patients with alcohol problems and those who ingest corrosive chemicals are also at risk. Two endoscopic patterns are observed. The first and more common is white or yellow plaques, which can be easily abraded to reveal a reddened underlying mucosa. Such plaques are not specific for fungal infection but are very characteristic. Less commonly, chronic infection leads to the formation of warty, umbilicated nodules. Treatment is required, the rationale being to minimise the risk of dissemination or vascular invasion in the bed of the ulcer, especially in the neutropaenic patient.

Candida albicans and, to a lesser extent, *C. tropicalis* and *C. glabrata* (formerly known as *Torulopsis glabrata*) [430,431] may be commonly found in the biopsies from gastric ulcers and erosions in immunocompetent and immunocompromised hosts. In the former situation, the yeast is more likely to be a secondary contaminant rather than a primary infective pathology.

Smears of exudates combined with cultures and examination of biopsy specimens from ulcer edges will establish the diagnosis. Identification of the yeast forms and hyphae is difficult in H&E sections and PAS (periodic acid–Schiff) and/or Grocott's stains are often required. In immunocompetent patients, who probably have biopsies taken to rule out cancer in gastric ulcers, special stains are not usually required to detect fungi, because the organisms are usually secondary contaminants and no specific therapy is then required.

Phycomycosis (mucormycosis)

Gastrointestinal phycomycosis is rare and the organism more often involves the terminal ileum and proximal colon. However, reports of gastric infection have been documented, in adults and in infants and children [432] (Figure 11.25). The organism is usually saprophytic and, invariably, patients with systemic involvement have underlying serious debilitating disease, such as poorly controlled

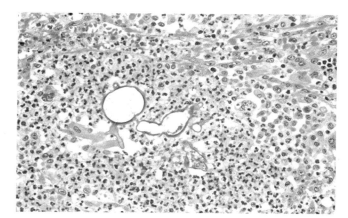

Figure 11.25 Phycomycosis in a gastric ulcer: the fungi are branching and non-septate. Vascular invasion by fungi with subsequent thrombosis occurs frequently. Periodic acid–Schiff stain.

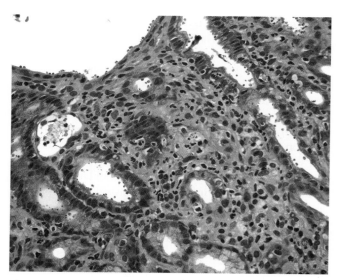

Figure 11.26 Cryptosporidiosis in the stomach: small basophilic parasites are easily identified on the epithelial luminal surface. (Courtesy of Dr Tomas Slavik, Ampath Pathology Laboratories, Pretoria, South Africa.)

diabetes with acidosis, haematological or other malignancies, malnutrition and immunosuppression. Gastric infection results in ulceration and invasion of blood vessels by the fungus, with subsequent thrombosis, and it is often fatal.

Histoplasmosis

Gastrointestinal histoplasmosis is reported primarily in association with HIV/AIDS. Disseminated histoplasmosis rarely involves the stomach and, when it does, the usual feature is bleeding from ulcers or erosions of giant mucosal folds that are infiltrated with numerous histiocytes, usually including demonstrable forms of *Histoplasma capsulatum* [433]. However, histological demonstration of the organisms in tissue does not necessarily imply that they are viable or that the infection is active. Active infection must be proven by culture of the organism from biopsy or resection specimens [434]. *H. duboisii* much more rarely involves the GI tract but this has been reported in a case from Africa, when the clinical and endoscopic features mimicked gastric cancer [435].

Other fungal infections

Gastric involvement by *Cryptococcus neoformans* is rare and is seen together with disseminated disease in immunosuppressed patients [436]. There have also been occasional reports of gastric involvement by *Pneumocystis jiroveci* (formerly *Pneumocystis carinii*) in HIV-positive patients with widespread extrapulmonary pneumocystosis [437,438]. Gastroduodenal pneumocystosis is manifest by small mucosal nodules and erosions. Histology shows a foamy granular exudate within the lamina propria.

Gomori's methenamine silver stain and immunohistochemistry greatly serve to confirm the diagnosis.

Protozoal and nematodal involvement of the stomach

Cryptosporidiosis

This protozoon frequently infects the small and large intestine in immunocompromised patients [439], but detailed evaluation of AIDS patients indicates that gastric infection is more common than previously suspected [440]. Endoscopic examination frequently shows no abnormality, although mucosal oedema and erosions may occur. Histological studies demonstrate that involvement of the antrum is more common than the corpus. The organisms are most frequently found on the luminal border of epithelial cells of gastric pits and accompanied by non-specific active chronic inflammation (Figure 11.26). Colonisation of the mucosa is patchy and examination of multiple biopsies may be advisable [440].

Giardiasis

Giardiasis is a common infection in which *Giardia lamblia* protozoa colonise the gut. It is usually diagnosed, histologically, in duodenal biopsies. However, gastric antral involvement is reported to occur in about 9% of cases [441,442]. In many instances, the underlying mucosal histology is normal and the diagnosis is dependent on the identification of the trophozoite in the mucus close to the mucosal surface [442]. The possible mechanisms for its

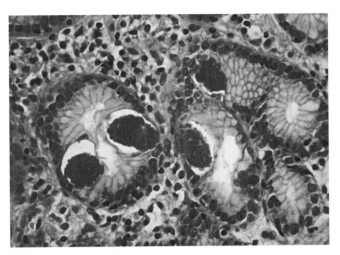

Figure 11.27 Toxoplasmosis infection in the stomach: intraluminal bradyzoites are readily identified. (Courtesy of Dr Tomas Slavik, Ampath Pathology Laboratories, Pretoria, South Africa.)

presence and survival, in the stomach, include intestinal metaplasia, hypochlorhydria or achlorhydria (pathological or iatrogenic) and/or duodenogastric reflux [442].

Toxoplasmosis

Toxoplasmosis is a common opportunistic infection in advanced HIV/AIDS. Gastric infection by *Toxoplasma gondii*, although very rare, has been reported in association with widely disseminated disease [443]. Thickening of the gastric wall and mucosal folds, which may result in gastric outlet obstruction and mucosal ulceration, has been described but, in some cases, endoscopy is normal [443]. Examination of biopsy material shows a corresponding spectrum of abnormalities from full-thickness mucosal necrosis to just oedema and non-specific inflammation. *T. gondii* cysts and tachyzoites can be found within the mucosa (Figure 11.27), and trophozoites can be identified in gastric epithelial cells, endothelial cells, smooth muscle cells and macrophages.

Strongyloidiasis

Strongyloides infection, by the small nematode *Strongyloides stercoralis*, is common in many parts of the world but its primary site of involvement, in the gut, is the upper small intestine. In a healthy host, the parasite does not usually cause symptoms but, in immunocompromised patients, it may lead to overwhelming dissemination and this may include the stomach [444]. Although the adult worms are easy to observe in biopsy material [445], the larvae can be extremely difficult to detect. Thus, critical evaluation is required, of gastric biopsies in patients, in the appropriate clinical setting, showing heavy tissue eosinophilia.

Viral involvement of the stomach

Human herpesviridae (HHV) infections

There are eight distinct viruses in this family known to cause disease in humans (HHV-1, herpes simplex virus 1; HHV-2, herpes simplex virus 2; HHV-3, varicella-zoster virus; HHV-4, Epstein–Barr virus (EBV); HHV-5, cytomegalovirus (CMV); HHV-6, herpes lymphotrophic virus; HHV-7, roseolovirus; and HHV-8, Kaposi's sarcoma-associated herpesvirus [446–8]. In the following section, we discuss herpesviridae infections that have been reported in the gastric mucosa, in descending order of importance or frequency.

Cytomegalovirus infection

Cytomegalovirus infection of the gut occurs in neonates, immunologically deficient adults and, occasionally, in apparently healthy individuals [449–453]. Childhood gastric CMV infection has attracted considerable attention because it causes a Ménétrier-like picture and occurs in apparently immunocompetent patients [454]. It is likely that CMV-infected endothelium narrows vascular channels, inducing local ischaemia [455], and eventually resulting in erosions and mucosal oedematous expansion. Irregular erosions and fold thickening, although considered common manifestations of CMV in terms of the distinctive macroscopic appearance, are not observed in all patients [456]. When present, mucosal thickening can mimic lymphoma or 'linitis plastica', and can cause gastric outlet obstruction [457].

CMV infection has been identified in 13% of HIV-infected patients [451] and is responsible for about 50% of cases of gastro-duodenal ulceration in HIV-positive patients [458]. In the transplant group, the use of azathioprine is regarded as a major risk factor [452,459].

Gastric CMV infection takes two forms. In one, typical intranuclear inclusions are seen in cells of the glandular epithelium without any associated tissue reaction (Figure 11.28). In this form of the disease, the patient is frequently asymptomatic and endoscopy normal. In the second type of infection, there is gastric ulceration and erosions, causing epigastric pain and, on occasion, haemorrhage [453,459]. The ulcers are typically shallow but may be up to 50 mm in diameter, and perforation and fistula formation may occur occasionally as well [460]. CMV intranuclear inclusions may be found in swollen endothelial and stromal cells in the vicinity of the ulcers, in highly vascularised granulation tissue and in intact mucosa. Intra-epithelial inclusions are much less conspicuous in this form of the disease. Infected cells are enlarged and contain large eosinophilic intranuclear inclusions, often, but not always, surrounded by a clear halo. More basophilic intracytoplasmic inclusions are usually present but the former are much more conspicuous. In AIDS patients, who are severely

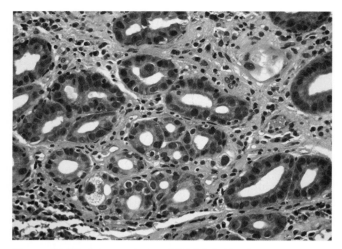

Figure 11.28 Cytomegalovirus (CMV) infection in an immunocompromised HIV-positive patient: characteristic inclusion bodies are easily identified within epithelial cells and stromal cells in the gastric mucosa. (Courtesy of Dr Tomas Slavik, Ampath Pathology Laboratories, Pretoria, South Africa.)

immunocompromised, the histological evidence of CMV infection may be difficult to find in small biopsies and in the absence of a normal antibody response [461]. Immunohistochemistry, using anti-CMV antibody, is useful in this setting. Brush cytology that allows wider sampling of cells can be helpful.

Herpes infection

Gastrointestinal herpes simplex virus (HSV-1 and HSV-2) infection most commonly involves the oesophagus [462]. HSV infection can be recognised in the stomach in association with gastric erosions in the immunocompromised host (especially after radiotherapy and/or chemotherapy and in malignancies) [463]. Endoscopy varies from shallow superficial ulcers that may coalesce in later stages [464] to raised erythematous nodules [465] and the very occasional case of a Ménétrier-like disease associated with HSV. Of note, herpetic gastritis is not necessarily accompanied with concomitant stomatitis or oesophagitis and may be more common than once believed.

Histological findings include acute and chronic inflammation with regenerative epithelial hyperplasia, areas of necrosis and ulceration with fibrinopurulent exudates. Herpetic inclusions are rarely detected in routine staining in the gastric mucosa but can be demonstrated by tissue culture of gastric biopsies or immunohistochemistry. Prophylactic antiviral treatment, often given to prevent CMV infection, may also prevent HSV infection.

Interestingly, the detection of the DNA of HSV-1 in human vagal [466] and/or coeliac ganglia [467], which provide the neural network to gastric tissue, has led some investigators to hypothesise that HSV migrating from the vagal and coeliac ganglia plays a role in recurrent ulceration after vagotomy.

Infection of the stomach with herpes zoster varicella virus is exceedingly rare [468].

Epstein–Barr virus

Rarely, EBV can affect the gut, including the stomach, leading to ulcerative and haemorrhagic lesions [469]. Patients can present with nausea, early satiety, bloating and epigastric pain [469]. The endoscopic differential diagnosis includes NSAID-induced injury, *H. pylori* infection, marginal zone lymphoma and malignancy [469]. Biopsies show epithelial ulceration and a marked expansion of the lamina propria with a diffuse lymphoid infiltrate, which can simulate primary gastric lymphoma. Despite the presence of surface erosions and necrosis, neutrophils are not prominent and only a few foci of active inflammation in crypts and 'pit abscesses' are seen.

The presence of EBV is most frequently demonstrated by *in situ* hybridisation (ISH) for EBV-encoded small RNA-1 (EBER-1) [470]. Importantly, expression of EBER-1 should not be considered a definitive result unless there is diffuse staining [469]. Of particular importance is the recognition of an ulcerative gastritis, secondary to EBV infection, effectively a self-limiting condition, which potentially can be mistaken for gastric lymphoma. EBV infection should be considered in a clinical scenario with severe active gastritis, inexplicably negative for *H. pylori*, and/or when there is rapid resolution without treatment, particularly when the clinical features suggest infectious mononucleosis.

Granulomatous gastritis

Microscopically, a compact, organised collection of mature mononuclear macrophages/histiocytes is the minimum requirement for the diagnosis of a granuloma, regardless of whether the lesion also shows necrosis, lymphocytes, plasma cells or multinucleated giant cells. Gastric mucosal granulomas, reportedly, are found much more frequently in the antrum than in the corpus. However, in common with all granulomatous conditions, sampling error limits the biopsy diagnosis, because granulomas may be scarce.

As the underlying aetiology differs geographically throughout the world, the incidence of granulomatous gastritis varies from 0.08% to 0.35% of all gastric biopsies. A comprehensive survey carried out in Belgium and the UK indicates that Crohn's disease is by far the most common cause of granulomatous gastritis in these countries, followed by idiopathic cases [471]. Less common causes were foreign body granulomas, tumour-associated granulomas and occasional cases of sarcoidosis, Whipple's disease and granulomatous vasculitis. In a study from the USA, Crohn's disease was the most common cause, representing almost half the patients, followed by sarcoidosis [472]. In other series of granulomatous gastritis, especially from Asia,

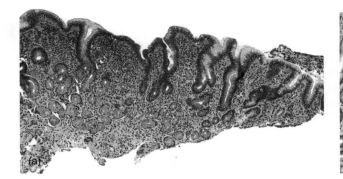

Figure 11.29 Gastric manifestations of Crohn's disease: (a) patchy superficial focally enhanced gastritis in a patient with small intestinal Crohn's disease. (b) Intramucosal, non-necrotising granulomas in a patient with small intestinal Crohn's disease.

Helicobacter sp. was said to be one of the more common causes of granulomatous gastritis [473]. However, that appears not to be the case in North America and Europe, and many informed workers question this association, especially as few studies have shown complete or partial remission after *H. pylori* eradication, and it is generally believed that concurrent helicobacter infection is incidental to the diagnosis of granulomatous gastritis.

Crohn's disease in the stomach

Recognising its importance, the Montreal 2005 system classifies upper GI involvement in Crohn's disease, independent of other locations [474]. However, this classification does not specify a definition of upper tract 'involvement'. Obvious stenosis or ulcerations should prompt a diagnosis; however, aphthous ulcerations are recognised as reappearing sporadically. The North American Inflammatory Bowel Disease Genetics Consortium arbitrarily allows up to 10 minor lesions without indicating significant disease in a given location. Overall, the presence of an abnormal histology, including focally enhanced gastritis and granulomatous inflammation in otherwise normal appearing mucosa, should not be considered sufficient to be classified as gastro-duodenal Crohn's disease, just as such findings in the colon would not alone indicate colonic Crohn's disease.

Gastric manifestations of Crohn's disease are usually seen in younger populations, with patients commonly aged <45 years. The common presenting symptoms are upper GI pain and, less often, vomiting. However, a substantial minority of patients have no gastric symptoms [475]. Notably, there may be clinical and pathological evidence of coexisting disease in the duodenum or the small or large intestine [476,477]. Macroscopically, there can be cobblestoning of the mucosa with thickening of the pyloric region, but, most commonly, endoscopy shows erosions and redness of the mucosa. One feature of advanced involvement of the stomach by Crohn's disease, representing relatively consistent mucosal cobblestoning over a substantial portion of the stomach, is an appearance that has been likened to 'baked beans' with nodules of hyperaemic polypoid mucosa alternating with clefts of ulceration around them.

The proximal stomach is involved only rarely [476]. Abnormal gastric biopsies, if taken, are found in up to 75% of patients with intestinal Crohn's disease. The characteristic feature is focal inflammation, reported by some as 'focally enhanced gastritis', composed of lymphocytes and histiocytes, usually with associated neutrophils in a background of minimally inflamed mucosa (Figure 11.29a) [476,477]. Although these focal lesions frequently occur deep in the mucosa, they may be associated with erosions or degenerative changes in the overlying surface epithelium [475,479]. Concomitant *H. pylori* infection occurs in 10–33% of cases and the associated generalised active gastritis tends to obscure the focal inflammation of Crohn's disease, making diagnosis difficult. Granulomas are seen in less than 15% of gastric biopsies in Crohn's disease, and while obviously important, they are neither a sensitive diagnostic nor pathognomonic feature [476] (Figure 11.29b).

In children, histological evidence suggestive of mucosal involvement of the stomach and duodenum is found in a third of cases with Crohn's ileocolitis [478,479]. Importantly, the notion that any inflammation in the upper GI tract precludes the diagnosis of ulcerative colitis (UC) is no longer accepted, because about two-thirds of Crohn's disease patients and about 50% of UC patients have microscopic abnormalities in the upper GI tract, irrespective of the presence of symptoms, in both adults and children. However, mucosal changes in UC are typically mild and obvious ulcerations are more characteristic of Crohn's disease. Detecting granulomas at upper endoscopy (namely in the oesophagus, stomach and duodenum) appears to be the only pathological abnormality that is useful in the discrimination between Crohn's disease and UC: in 40% versus 0%, respectively [479].

Sarcoidosis

Involvement of the stomach by sarcoidosis represents between 1 and 21% of all cases of granulomatous gastritis [471,473,480–482]. Yet involvement of the gut is rare in sarcoidosis, as a whole, even if the stomach is the most commonly affected site [482,483]. In fact, in patients with sarcoidosis but no GI symptoms, granulomas have been found in biopsies from the stomach, in one series in 10% of cases [480]. Symptoms of GI involvement include haematemesis, epigastric pain, nausea, colicky abdominal pain and diarrhoea. Endoscopy is usually normal but it may show changes ranging from a distal gastritis with or without nodularity, mainly affecting the greater curvature, to ulceration and pyloric stenosis.

Histologically the granulomas are usually well circumscribed and compact, and surrounding non-specific mucosal inflammation is absent or less marked than in Crohn's disease or tuberculosis. Gastric sarcoidosis should never be diagnosed in the absence of evidence of the disease in other sites, and then only when overt aetiologies have been satisfactorily excluded. Elevated angiotensin-converting enzyme levels are helpful in establishing the diagnosis.

Tuberculosis and other mycobacterial infections

The re-upsurge in cases of tuberculosis (TB) over the past two decades in western countries is now well recognised. Those most susceptible are the urban poor, many of whom are immigrants from endemic areas and/or elderly, and severely immunocompromised patients. Extra-pulmonary TB is much more common in HIV-infected patients [484,485] and the possibility of GI infection, particularly in the ileocaecal region and jejunum and ileum, should always be considered in such patients. Gastric TB is rarely present as an isolated infection and is virtually never primary in the stomach. Thus, similar to sarcoidosis, it is unwise to make the diagnosis in the absence of disease elsewhere.

The antrum is the most common site of involvement by gastric TB. Symptoms include epigastric pain, vomiting and haematemesis, and there may be evidence of pyloric obstruction [486–489]. At endoscopy, ulceration of the pyloric region is a common manifestation, often on the lesser curvature. In some cases, there may be a nodular mass, which may simulate carcinoma. A narrowed, deformed antrum can also be observed.

The diagnosis may be made on histological examination of endoscopic biopsies but more often it is made after surgery. The granulomatous inflammation may involve the mucosa, submucosa or subserosa (Figure 11.30). The granulomas may be confluent and, although typically caseating, this is by no means always the rule [486–489]. Regional lymph nodes are frequently enlarged and should be carefully examined, because they frequently contain granulomas, which may not be readily apparent in the gastric wall itself. Demonstration of acid- and alcohol-fast bacilli is pathognomonic and should always be attempted, although frequently unsuccessful. PCR of a biopsy specimen provides a faster, alternative route for the diagnosis, while excluding Crohn's disease with 100% specificity and sensitivity between 27% and 75% [490].

Although much more common in the intestines in HIV/AIDS patients, gastric involvement by *Mycobacterium*

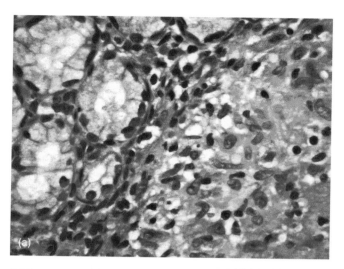

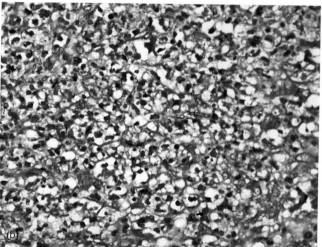

Figure 11.30 Gastric tuberculosis: (a) adjacent to the antral-type glands are large non-necrotising granulomas. (b) In another patient, an acid-fast bacilli stain highlights the presence of numerous mycobacteria. (Courtesy of Dr Tomas Slavik, Ampath Pathology Laboratories, Pretoria, South Africa.)

avium complex is rare in those patients. Microscopically, the lamina propria is expanded by numerous foamy histiocytes and ill-formed granulomas without necrosis. Acid fast bacilli are diagnostic.

Syphilis

Although syphilis is often listed as one of the bacterial infections that does involve the stomach, it has to be admitted that gastric involvement is particularly unusual with many card-carrying GI pathologists having never seen a case in their careers. It may present with diffuse enlargement of the gastric folds and multiple shallow ulcers or erosions [491,492]. Less often, there is a single large ulcer, usually in the antrum. Perforation has been reported [492]. Even though, initially, gastric syphilis had been viewed as a complication of tertiary syphilis, subsequent reports have indicated that the stomach is affected in early syphilis [493]. Of affected patients, only 13% have a prior history of a syphilis diagnosis and 46% had prior (13%) or concurrent (33%) clinical manifestations of the disease [493].

The histological appearances of the gastric mucosa in secondary syphilis are protean. Ill-formed granulomas may be present but the usual finding is a dense intramucosal infiltrate of plasma cells, neutrophils and lymphocytes, often with lymphoid follicle formation. There may be destruction of mucosal glands and lympho-epithelial-like lesions, more usually associated with primary malignant lymphoma. The endarteritis often seen in syphilitic lesions elsewhere may not be present in gastric lesions, especially in biopsies, and the gummas that occur in the tertiary stage or in congenital syphilis [494] are seldom seen in the adult stomach. Thus, the diagnosis should be considered whenever a gastric biopsy shows unusually severe chronic active gastritis, in which plasma cells are especially prominent, with glandular destruction in the absence of *H. pylori*. These features can, however, only hint at an unusual infectious or inflammatory condition and are by no means diagnostic for syphilitic gastritis. The key lies in thinking of the diagnosis and looking for the organism in the sections and/or requesting serological evaluation.

Demonstration of *Treponema pallidum*, a Gram-negative spirochaete bacterium measuring 8–15 μm in length and 0.1– 0.2 μm in diameter [495], is challenging in mucosal biopsies. It can be achieved using silver stains such as Warthin–Starry, Dieterle and/or the modified Steiner silver stain [496], but identification is difficult, especially with a background of elastic or reticulin fibres. Practically, the use of specific immunohistochemistry, immunofluorescence or the PCR to detect bacterial DNA is advisable when the diagnosis is suspected [497].

Food and foreign body granulomas
These foreign body-type, non-epithelioid granulomas are usually easily distinguishable from other forms of granulomatous gastritis. Some are obviously related to visible food particles, such as vegetable matter or the insoluble coatings of cereals, in the mucosa or more deeply if there is an associated active or healed peptic ulcer. Other causes include kaolin, talc and suture material. Granulomas may be the result of small breaches in the gastric mucosa that allow gastric juice to digest the muscularis mucosae, producing partial necrosis and inciting a granulomatous response [498]. Finally, crystalline iron material may also be found in gastric mucosa in patients taking therapeutic oral iron medication [499] (see below).

Idiopathic granulomatous gastritis
This is a diagnosis of exclusion. It refers to the histological finding of isolated mucosal granulomas with no known association or cause. It has been reported in 25–41% of all granulomatous gastritis cases. However, the concept of a distinct clinicopathological entity has been questioned, due to lack of adequate clinical information and follow-up in many studies [500]. In some cases it may be the initial presentation of Crohn's disease or sarcoidosis but only long-term follow-up can truly clarify the ultimate diagnosis. In Japan, idiopathic granulomatous gastritis is also reported as 'isolated gastric sarcoidosis' [501].

Similar to other granulomatous gastritides, idiopathic granulomatous gastritis has been associated with marked gross structural changes, especially in the gastric antrum. There may be stricturing or mass lesions, which may simulate carcinoma, and ulcerative lesions, which may perforate. The findings are said to be related to the depth of involvement by granulomas in the gastric wall. In practice, we would strongly discourage the use of the term 'idiopathic granulomatous gastritis' as a pathological diagnosis, because the aetiology may become obvious only after many years of follow-up. Furthermore, in some of these patients, the granulomas have been shown to disappear on follow-up biopsies without any treatment. Thus, we would recommend a descriptive designation of 'granulomatous gastritis of uncertain aetiology'.

Anisakiasis
Gastric anisakiasis occurs mainly in Japan but cases are reported from elsewhere, such as the western USA [502]. The condition is caused by penetration of the gastric mucosa by anisakis larvae. *Phocanema decipiens* larvae may also be involved. Ingestion of uncooked infected fish may result in the larvae being coughed up or vomited but larval attachment to the gastric wall usually results in acute or chronic anisakiasis. The former is characterised by epigastric pain, nausea and vomiting with oedema of the gastric mucosa around the larvae. The larvae can be removed by forceps at the time of endoscopy [503]. Chronic disease may ensue, during which the larvae die and the oedematous mucosa becomes infiltrated by eosinophils and epithelioid cell granulomas. Hence anisakiasis is not only a potential cause of 'granulomatous gastritis', but also a potent cause of 'eosinophilic gastritis'. Ultimately, the larvae may disappear, leaving only unidentifiable fragments and the chronic inflammatory residua [504].

Other causes of granulomatous gastritis
Rare causes of granulomatous gastritis include Whipple's disease, Langerhans' cell histiocytosis and vasculitis. Involvement of the stomach in Whipple's disease is exceedingly rare. Granulomatous gastritis with non-caseating granulomas containing macrophages with PAS-positive particles has been reported in a patient with duodenal involvement [505].

Langerhans' cell histiocytosis (formerly known as histiocytosis X) occasionally involves the GI tract. Gastric involvement may manifest as multiple mucosal polyps [506]. In some cases the mucosal infiltrate of histiocytes, eosinophils and lymphocytes may take the form of distinct non-caseating giant cell granulomas [507]. Gastric manifestation in patients with common variable immunodeficiency and X-linked agammaglobulinaemia has also been documented with occasional ill-defined granulomas [508]. A variety of accompanying abnormalities include single cell necrosis within glands and increased numbers of mononuclear cells within the lamina propria, together with a lymphocytic infiltration of the foveolae areas.

Other causes of granulomatous gastritis include chronic granulomatous disease, amyloidosis, rheumatoid nodules and/or rheumatoid arthritis, a reaction to nearby malignancy and vasculitis.

Iatrogenic gastritis/gastropathy

In addition to NSAID-related mucosal injury, a wide and ever-growing spectrum of iatrogenic gastric mucosal pathology is being detected. The distribution, severity and mechanisms vary depending on the causative agents.

Gastric mucosal calcinosis

This term is used when partially calcified refractile crystals are found beneath the surface epithelium, frequently associated include foveolar hyperplasia and mucosal oedema (Figure 11.31). The small, purple crystals are more commonly seen in orthotopic transplant recipients and chronic renal failure patients receiving either aluminium-containing antacids or sucralfate [509].

Iron therapy

Patients prescribed iron therapy frequently develop mucosal erythema and erosions. Microscopically, diagnostic golden brown iron crystals can be embedded in the lamina propria, present in stromal cells, encrusting the damaged epithelium or even in vessel walls (Figure 11.32) [510]. The mucosa is characterised by regenerative foveolar hyperplasia but infarct-like necrosis can be observed as well. The differential diagnosis includes glandular siderosis, which may be associated with systemic iron overload or haemochromatosis. In these circumstances the accumu-

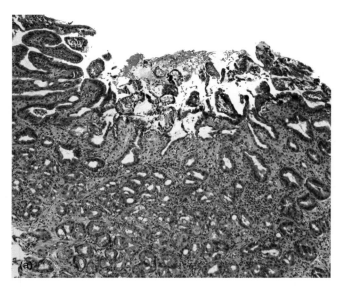

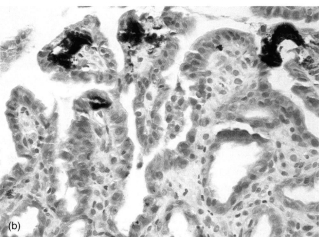

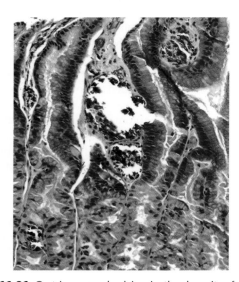

Figure 11.31 Gastric mucosal calcinosis: the deposits of cyanophilic crystals encrusted within the lamina propria are diagnostic.

Figure 11.32 Iron-induced gastropathy: (a) crystalline iron in the gastric lamina propria of a patient taking oral iron medication. The marked regenerative atypia should not be mistaken for dysplasia. (b) An iron histochemical stain highlights the iron crystals encrusting the mucosal surface.

lation of iron is deep in the mucosa and not associated with features of acute mucosal damage [510,511].

Colchicine

Patients prescribed colchicine, and with altered renal or hepatic function, may develop mucosal changes reflecting the inhibition of tubulin polymerisation if the alkaloid reaches toxic levels. The epithelium shows loss of polarity, nuclear pseudo-stratification and increased apoptosis. Characteristic mitotic figures, arrested in metaphase, with the chromosomes often arranged as 'ring' mitoses, can be observed [512].

Chemoradiation-related gastritis/gastropathy

Chemotherapeutic agents can produce various mucosal changes including ulceration and epithelial abnormalities with eosinophilia, vacuolation and pleomorphic nuclei. Sometimes the changes are less pronounced, although enhanced apoptosis is often a prominent feature (Figure 11.33). Reactive changes of stromal endothelial cells and fibroblasts are common as well. These changes can result in appearances that themselves may mimic neoplasia and are especially seen after hepatic arterial infusion of such chemotherapeutic agents [513–515].

Radiation gastritis

Gastric lesions associated with irradiation

Radiation therapy, either external beam radiotherapy or brachytherapy for upper abdominal neoplasia or in bone marrow transplant recipients, results in three different forms of pathology [516–519]:

1. *Radiation gastritis*: radiation gastritis may develop a few days to a few months after exposure. The changes can be noted as early as 8–10 days after irradiation, including nuclear karyorrhexis and cytoplasmic eosinophilia of the gastric pit epithelium. Mucosal oedema and congestion develop at a later stage, usually accompanied by submucosal collagen bundle swelling, fibrin deposition and telangiectasia. Inflammation is not a prominent feature. Glandular necrosis with characteristic radiation-induced nuclear atypia usually follows. There may be extensive mucosal necrosis and surface ulceration. The vessel walls become swollen and their lumina reduced in size. The mucosa usually regenerates but varying degrees of atrophy with submucosal fibrosis, mucosal and submucosal oedema, and endarteritis of small arteries often persist (Figure 11.34). Fibroblasts with bizarre, hyperchromatic nuclei are characteristic of radiation injury. In severe cases, mucosal ulceration and haemorrhage, with possible late radiation effects such as endothelial proliferation and fibrinoid necrosis of the vessel walls, can be seen. Mucosal recovery is usually complete within 2–3 months [520,521].

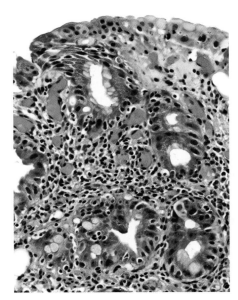

Figure 11.33 Chemotherapy-induced gastritis in a patient who received a multi-drug protocol for pulmonary adenocarcinoma. The non-specific changes include lymphocytic exocytosis, apoptosis, regenerative epithelial changes and increased lamina propria cellularity.

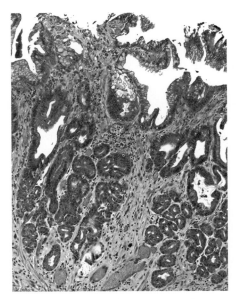

Figure 11.34 Radiation-induced gastritis in patient treated for gastro-oesophageal adenocarcinoma. Characteristic features include oedematous and partially hyalinised stroma with telangiectatic blood vessels. Architectural glandular disarray is marked as well as degenerative and regenerative epithelial change.

2. *Acute ulceration*: acute gastric ulceration may occur 1–2 months after irradiation. The ulcer is usually deep and penetrating and is often accompanied by pain and bleeding. Perforation, however, is rare, because the ulcer usually becomes walled off by surrounding structures. Other histological features characteristic of radiation damage are usually present as well.

3. *Chronic ulceration:* chronic ulcers may develop from a few months to several years after irradiation. They are usually solitary and occur principally in the antrum. The histology is similar to that of the 'usual' gastric ulcer, except that there are atypical fibroblasts in the ulcer base. Furthermore, the endothelial cells lining capillaries may also appear bizarre and unusually prominent [522]. In addition, there may be an excessive amount of antral fibrosis, which frequently appears hyalinised appearance and is accompanied by hyalinisation of blood vessel walls.

Emphasis has recently been drawn to the effects of selective intra-arterial radiation therapy (SIRT), which is used to manage selected patients with hepatocellular carcinoma, unresectable hepatic metastatic endocrine tumours and colorectal liver metastases. Inappropriate high levels of delivery of yttrium-90-coated spheres to arteries supplying the stomach, duodenum or pancreas, as well as other organs, causes serious complications. In the stomach, the mucosal changes range from apoptosis, epithelial flattening and glandular cystic dilatation to nuclear atypia, capillary ectasia and prominent endothelial cells. These adverse effects have been reported with an incidence of up to 30%, generally within the first 2 months after the procedure [523].

Hypertrophic gastritis and hypertrophic gastropathy

Hypertrophic gastropathy refers simply to thickened gastric folds, irrespective of associated symptoms or the underlying pathology. There are numerous causes of giant gastric folds, which can be focal or diffuse. They include primary epithelial hyperplasia of the mucosa ('classic' Ménétrier's disease) and Zollinger–Ellison syndrome and secondary disorders such as tumour infiltration (especially lymphoma), infections (CMV, histoplasmosis, syphilis) and granulomatous diseases.

There is debate and confusion as to whether Ménétrier's disease should be used as an overall term to describe hypertrophy of the gastric mucosa or whether it should be confined to cases without significant inflammation. Some authorities consider that Ménétrier's disease should be restricted to cases of idiopathic gastric mucosal hypertrophy with massive foveolar hyperplasia without gastritis [396]. Others define Ménétrier's disease as hypertrophic gastropathy with hypoproteinaemia, regardless of the histology. Ménétrier's disease is further considered in Chapter 12 but is also included for discussion here because of its potential association with inflammatory pathology of the stomach.

Without getting too deeply involved in semantics, hypertrophy of the gastric mucosa may be due to a variety of causes and different aetiologies should be considered in such cases. These include lymphocytic gastritis [380], gastric syphilis [492], CMV infection, histoplasmosis, Canada–Cronkhite syndrome, Zollinger–Ellison syndrome, carcinoma and lymphoma. An association between hypertrophic gastritis and *H. pylori* infection has been identified and may represent an unusual form of *H. pylori* gastritis [524]. In some instances *H. pylori*-associated hypertrophic gastritis is accompanied by protein-losing enteropathy [524]. The histology in this condition differs from classic Ménétrier's disease in that both mucosal thickening and foveolar hyperplasia are less marked and inflammation more intense [525]. Such cases have been called 'enlarged fold gastritis'. The mucosa in *H. pylori*-associated hypertrophic gastritis reverts to normal after eradication of the infection [525]. In the Zollinger–Ellison syndrome, thickening of the gastric corpus mucosa is due to hyperplasia and hypertrophy of acid-producing parietal cells as a result of the gastrin drive. However, sometimes there is no foveolar hyperplasia [526].

Thus, it is important to be aware of the variety of different conditions that may give rise to clinical or radiological enlargement of gastric mucosal folds. If histology supports a diagnosis of hypertrophic change, and for obvious reasons a large biopsy is necessary, pathologists should assess the degree of concomitant inflammation and seek the presence of lymphocytic gastritis and/or *H. pylori*-associated gastritis, before concluding that the appropriate diagnosis is one of Ménétrier's disease. Indeed, there is frequently a poor correlation between endoscopic and/or radiological findings and the histological features. In one series, most patients with large gastric folds identified radiologically or endoscopically did not have clinical or laboratory features of hypertrophic gastropathy. Most of these patients had active chronic gastritis with increased mucosal thickness due to oedema but no foveolar hyperplasia. It may be actually better to refer to these cases as hypertrophic gastropathies and qualify them further as localised or diffuse, with and without protein-losing state, and idiopathic or with a known underlying aetiology. Idiopathic hypertrophic gastropathy may be labelled as true Ménétrier's disease. However, it should be recognised that this condition is very rare and also, curiously, seems to be decreasing in prevalence, with many GI pathologists having not seen a single case, in their own practices, in the last 5 years. This underpins the evidence that most cases of 'hypertrophic gastropathy' have a clear cause once full investigation of the patient has been concluded.

References

1. Dixon MF, O'Connor HJ, Axon AT, King RF, Johnston D. Reflux gastritis: distinct histopathological entity? *J Clin Pathol* 1986; **39**:524.

2. Quinn CM, Bjarnason I, Price AB. Gastritis in patients on non-steroidal anti-inflammatory drugs. *Histopathology* 1993; **23**:341.

3. Sobala GM, King RF, Axon AT, Dixon MF. Reflux gastritis in the intact stomach. *J Clin Pathol* 1990;**43**:303.

4. Carpenter HA, Talley NJ. Gastroscopy is incomplete without biopsy: clinical relevance of distinguishing gastropathy from gastritis. *Gastroenterology* 1995;**108**:917.

5. El-Zimaity HM, Genta RM, Graham DY. Histological features do not define NSAID-induced gastritis. *Hum Pathol* 1996;**27**: 1348.

6. Dixon MF. Recent advances in gastritis. *Curr Diagnos Pathol* 1994;1.

7. Hamilton SR, Yardley JH. Endoscopic biopsy of aspirin-associated chronic gastric ulcers. *Gastroenterology* 1980;**78**:1178.

8. Huang JQ, Sridhar S, Hunt RH. Role of *Helicobacter pylori* infection and non-steroidal anti-inflammatory drugs in peptic-ulcer disease: a meta-analysis. *Lancet* 2002;**359**:14.

9. O'Connor HJ, Wyatt JI, Dixon MF, Axon AT. *Campylobacter* like organisms and reflux gastritis. *J Clin Pathol* 1986;**39**:531.

10. Chamberlain CE. Acute hemorrhagic gastritis. *Gastroenterol Clin North Am* 1993;**22**:843.

11. Lanza FL. A review of gastric ulcer and gastroduodenal injury in normal volunteers receiving aspirin and other non-steroidal anti-inflammatory drugs. *Scand J Gastroenterol Suppl* 1989; **163**:24.

12. Petroski D. A comparison of enteric-coated aspirin granules with plain and buffered aspirin: a report of two studies. *Am J Gastroenterol* 1986;**81**:26.

13. Silvoso GR, Ivey KJ, Butt JH, et al. Incidence of gastric lesions in patients with rheumatic disease on chronic aspirin therapy. *Ann Intern Med* 1979;**91**:517.

14. Franzin G, elli P. Gastritis cystica profunda. *Histopathology* 1981;**5**:535.

15. Janunger KG, Domellof L. Gastric polyps and precancerous mucosal changes after partial gastrectomy. *Acta Chir Scand* 1978;**144**:293.

16. Savage A, Jones S. Histological appearances of the gastric mucosa 15–27 years after partial gastrectomy. *J Clin Pathol* 1979; **32**:179.

17. Domellof L, Eriksson S, unger KG. Carcinoma and possible precancerous changes of the gastric stump after billroth II resection. *Gastroenterology* 1977;**73**:462.

18. Schrumpf E, Serck-Hanssen A, Stadaas J, Aune S, Myren J, Osnes M. Mucosal changes in the gastric stump 20–25 years after partial gastrectomy. *Lancet* 1977;**2**:467.

19. Farrands PA, Blake JR, Ansell ID, Cotton RE, Hardcastle JD. Endoscopic review of patients who have had gastric surgery. *BMJ (Clin Res Ed)* 1983;**286**:755.

20. Watt PC, Sloan JM, Kennedy TL. Changes in gastric mucosa after vagotomy and gastrojejunostomy for duodenal ulcer. *BMJ (Clin Res Ed)* 1983;**287**:1407.

21. Offerhaus GJ, Huibregtse K, de Boer J, et al. The operated stomach: a premalignant condition? A prospective endoscopic follow-up study. *Scand J Gastroenterol* 1984;**19**:521.

22. Pulimood BM, Knudsen A, Coghill NF. Gastric mucosa after partial gastrectomy. *Gut* 1976;**17**:463.

23. Sipponen P, Hakkiluoto A, Kalima TV, Siurala M. Selective loss of parietal cells in the gastric remnant following antral resection. *Scand J Gastroenterol* 1976;**11**:813.

24. Perez-Ayuso RM, Pique JM, Bosch J, et al. Propranolol in prevention of recurrent bleeding from severe portal hypertensive gastropathy in cirrhosis. *Lancet* 1991;**337**:1431.

25. Pique JM. Portal Hypertensive gastropathy. *Baillière's Clin Gastroenterol* 1997;**11**:257.

26. Zaman A, Hapke R, Flora K, Rosen H, Benner K. Prevalence of upper and lower gastrointestinal tract findings in liver transplant candidates undergoing screening endoscopic evaluation. *Am J Gastroenterol* 1999;**94**:895.

27. McCormack TT, Sims J, Eyre-Brook I, et al. Gastric lesions in portal hypertension: inflammatory gastritis or congestive gastropathy? *Gut* 1985;**26**:1226.

28. Foster PN, Wyatt JI, Bullimore DW, Losowsky MS. Gastric mucosa in patients with portal hypertension: prevalence of capillary dilatation and *Campylobacter pylori*. *J Clin Pathol* 1989;**42**:919.

29. Quintero E, Pique JM, Bombi JA, et al. Gastric mucosal vascular ectasias causing bleeding in cirrhosis. A distinct entity associated with hypergastrinemia and low serum levels of pepsinogen I. *Gastroenterology* 1987;**93**:1054.

30. Jabbari M, Cherry R, Lough JO, Daly DS, Kinnear DG, Goresky CA. Gastric antral vascular ectasia: the watermelon stomach. *Gastroenterology* 1984;**87**:1165.

31. Gardiner GW, Murray D, Prokipchuk EJ. Watermelon stomach, or antral gastritis. *J Clin Pathol* 1985;**38**:1317.

32. Suit PF, Petras RE, Bauer TW, Petrini JL, Jr. Gastric antral vascular ectasia. A histologic and morphometric study of 'the watermelon stomach'. *Am J Surg Pathol* 1987;**11**:750.

33. Gostout CJ, Viggiano TR, Ahlquist DA, Wang KK, Larson MV, Balm R. The clinical and endoscopic spectrum of the watermelon stomach. *J Clin Gastroenterol* 1992;**15**:256.

34. Gilliam JH, 3rd, Geisinger KR, Wu WC, Weidner N, Richter JE. Endoscopic biopsy is diagnostic in gastric antral vascular ectasia. The 'watermelon stomach'. *Dig Dis Sci* 1989;**34**:885.

35. Gretz JE, Achem SR. The watermelon stomach: clinical presentation, diagnosis, and treatment. *Am J Gastroenterol* 1998;**93**: 890.

36. Burke AP, Sobin LH, Virmani R. Localized vasculitis of the gastrointestinal tract. *Am J Surg Pathol* 1995;**19**:338.

37. Lee HC, Kay S. Primary polyarteritis nodosa of the stomach and small intestine as a cause of gastro-intestinal hemorrhage. *Ann Surg* 1958;**147**:714; discussion 26.

38. Abell MR, Limond RV, Blamey WE, tel W. Allergic granulomatosis with massive gastric involvement. *N Engl J Med* 1970; **282**:665.

39. Gear MW, Truelove SC, Whitehead R. Gastric ulcer and gastritis. *Gut* 1971;**12**:639.

40. Whitehead R, Truelove SC, Gear MW. The histological diagnosis of chronic gastritis in fibreoptic gastroscope biopsy specimens. *J Clin Pathol* 1972;**25**:1.

41. Strickland RG, Mackay IR. A reappraisal of the nature and significance of chronic atrophic gastritis. *Am J Dig Dis* 1973; **18**:426.

42. Wyatt JI, Dixon MF. Chronic gastritis – a pathogenetic approach. *J Pathol* 1988;**154**:113.

43. Price AB. The Sydney System: histological division. *J Gastroenterol Hepatol* 1991;**6**:209.

44. Misiewicz JJ. The Sydney System: a new classification of gastritis. Introduction. *J Gastroenterol Hepatol* 1991;**6**:207.

45. Khakoo SI, Lobo AJ, Shepherd NA, Wilkinson SP. Histological assessment of the Sydney classification of endoscopic gastritis. *Gut* 1994;**35**:1172.

46. Andrew A, Wyatt JI, Dixon MF. Observer variation in the assessment of chronic gastritis according to the Sydney system. *Histopathology* 1994;**25**:317.

47. Genta RM, Dixon MF. The Sydney System revisited: the Houston International Gastritis Workshop. *Am J Gastroenterol* 1995;**90**:1039.

48. Correa P. Chronic gastritis. In: Whitehead R (ed.), *Gatrointestinal and Oesophageal Pathology*. Edinburgh: Churchill Livingstone, 1995: 485.

49. Dixon MF, Genta RM, Yardley JH, Correa P. Classification and grading of gastritis. The updated Sydney System. International Workshop on the Histopathology of Gastritis, Houston 1994. *Am J Surg Pathol* 1996;**20**:1161.

50. Collins JS, Watt PC, Hamilton PW, Sloan JM, Love AH. Grading of superficial antral gastritis: comparison of cell-counting and photographic-based methods. *J Pathol* 1991;**163**:251.

51. Warren RJ, Marshall B. Unidentified curved bacilli gastric epithelium in active chronic gastritis. *Lancet* 1983;**321**: 1273.

52. Anonymous. *Campylobacter pylori* becomes *Helicobacter pylori*. *Lancet* 1989;**ii**:1019.

53. Goodwin C, Armstrong J, Chilvers T, et al. Transfer of *Campylobacter pylori* and *Campylobacter mustelae* to *Helicobacter* genus as *Helicobacter pylori* comb. and *Helicobacter mustelae* comb., respectively. *Int J Syst Bacteriol* 1989;**39**:397.

54. Marshall BJ, Armstrong JA, McGechie DB, Glancy RJ. Attempt to fulfil Koch's postulates for pyloric Campylobacter. *Med J Aust* 1985;**142**:436.

55. Graham DY, Opekun AR, Osato MS, et al. Challenge model for *Helicobacter pylori* infection in human volunteers. *Gut* 2004; **53**:1235.

56. Menon R, Riera A, Ahmad A. A global perspective on gastrointestinal diseases. *Gastroenterol Clin North Am* 2011;**40**:427.

57. Lam SK, Talley NJ. Report of the 1997 Asia Pacific Consensus Conference on the management of *Helicobacter pylori* infection. *J Gastroenterol Hepatol* 1998;**13**:1.

58. Torres J, Perez-Perez G, Goodman KJ, et al. A comprehensive review of the natural history of *Helicobacter pylori* infection in children. *Arch Med Res* 2000;**31**:431.

59. Malaty HM, El-Kasabany A, Graham DY, et al. Age at acquisition of *Helicobacter pylori* infection: a follow-up study from infancy to adulthood. *Lancet* 2002;**359**:931.

60. Pounder RE, Ng D. The prevalence of *Helicobacter pylori* infection in different countries. *Aliment Pharmacol Ther* 1995; **9**(suppl 2):33.

61. Azevedo NF, Guimaraes N, Figueiredo C, Keevil CW, Vieira MJ. A new model for the transmission of *Helicobacter pylori*: role of environmental reservoirs as gene pools to increase strain diversity. *Crit Rev Microbiol* 2007;**33**:157.

62. Crabtree JE. Gastric mucosal inflammatory responses to *Helicobacter pylori*. *Aliment Pharmacol Ther* 1996;**10** Suppl 1:29.

63. Kusters JG, van Vliet AH, Kuipers EJ. Pathogenesis of *Helicobacter pylori* infection. *Clin Microbiol Rev* 2006;**19**:449.

64. Yamaoka Y. Mechanisms of disease: *Helicobacter pylori* virulence factors. *Nat Rev Gastroenterol Hepatol* 2010;**7**:629.

65. Laheij RJ,sen JB, van de Lisdonk EH, Severens JL, Verbeek AL. Review article: symptom improvement through eradication of *Helicobacter pylori* in patients with non-ulcer dyspepsia. *Aliment Pharmacol Ther* 1996;**10**:843.

66. McColl K, Murray L, El-Omar E, et al. Symptomatic benefit from eradicating *Helicobacter pylori* infection in patients with nonulcer dyspepsia. *N Engl J Med* 1998;**339**:1869.

67. Talley NJ, Janssens J, Lauritsen K, Racz I, Bolling-Sternevald E. Eradication of *Helicobacter pylori* in functional dyspepsia: randomised double blind placebo controlled trial with 12 months' follow up. The Optimal Regimen Cures Helicobacter Induced Dyspepsia (ORCHID) Study Group. *BMJ* 1999;**318**:833.

68. Collins JS, Hamilton PW, Watt PC, Sloan JM, Love AH. Superficial gastritis and *Campylobacter pylori* in dyspeptic patients – a quantitative study using computer-linked image analysis. *J Pathol* 1989;**158**:303.

69. Hui PK, Chan WY, Cheung PS, Chan JK, Ng CS. Pathologic changes of gastric mucosa colonized by *Helicobacter pylori*. *Hum Pathol* 1992;**23**:548.

70. Fiocca R, Luinetti O, Villani L, Chiaravalli AM, Capella C, Solcia E. Epithelial cytotoxicity, immune responses, and inflammatory components of *Helicobacter pylori* gastritis. *Scand J Gastroenterol Suppl* 1994;**205**:11.

71. Wyatt JI, Rathbone BJ. Immune response of the gastric mucosa to *Campylobacter pylori*. *Scand J Gastroenterol Suppl* 1988;**142**: 44.

72. Eidt S, Stolte M. Prevalence of lymphoid follicles and aggregates in *Helicobacter pylori* gastritis in antral and body mucosa. *J Clin Pathol* 1993;**46**:832.

73. Zaitoun AM. The prevalence of lymphoid follicles in *Helicobacter pylori* associated gastritis in patients with ulcers and non-ulcer dyspepsia. *J Clin Pathol* 1995;**48**:325.

74. Genta RM, Hamner HW, Graham DY. Gastric lymphoid follicles in *Helicobacter pylori* infection: frequency, distribution, and response to triple therapy. *Hum Pathol* 1993;**24**:577.

75. Hassall E, Dimmick JE. Unique features of *Helicobacter pylori* disease in children. *Dig Dis Sci* 1991;**36**:417.

76. Rauws EA, Langenberg W, Houthoff HJ, Zanen HC, Tytgat GN. *Campylobacter pyloridis*-associated chronic active antral gastritis. A prospective study of its prevalence and the effects of antibacterial and antiulcer treatment. *Gastroenterology* 1988; **94**:33.

77. Witteman EM, Mravunac M, Becx MJ, et al. Improvement of gastric inflammation and resolution of epithelial damage one year after eradication of *Helicobacter pylori*. *J Clin Pathol* 1995; **48**:250.

78. Tepes B, Kavcic B, Zaletel LK, et al. Two- to four-year histological follow-up of gastric mucosa after *Helicobacter pylori* eradication. *J Pathol* 1999;**188**:24.

79. Valle J, pala K, Sipponen P, Kosunen T. Disappearance of gastritis after eradication of *Helicobacter pylori*. A morphometric study. *Scand J Gastroenterol* 1991;**26**:1057.

80. Mobley HL, Cortesia MJ, Rosenthal LE, Jones BD. Characterization of urease from *Campylobacter pylori*. *J Clin Microbiol* 1988; **26**:831.

81. Schreiber S, Konradt M, Groll C, et al. The spatial orientation of *Helicobacter pylori* in the gastric mucus. *Proc Natl Acad Sci USA* 2004;**101**:5024.

82. Meyer-Rosberg K, Scott DR, Rex D, Melchers K, Sachs G. The effect of environmental pH on the proton motive force of *Helicobacter pylori*. *Gastroenterology* 1996;**111**:886.

83. Graham DY, Opekun A, Lew GM, Klein PD, Walsh JH. *Helicobacter pylori*-associated exaggerated gastrin release in duodenal ulcer patients. The effect of bombesin infusion and urea ingestion. *Gastroenterology* 1991;**100**:1571.

84. Fitzgibbons PL, Dooley CP, Cohen H, Appleman MD. Prevalence of gastric metaplasia, inflammation, and *Campylobacter pylori* in the duodenum of members of a normal population. *Am J Clin Pathol* 1988;**90**:711.

85. Lamberts R, Creutzfeldt W, Struber HG, Brunner G, Solcia E. Long-term omeprazole therapy in peptic ulcer disease: gastrin, endocrine cell growth, and gastritis. *Gastroenterology* 1993;**104**: 1356.

86. Ricci C, Holton J, Vaira D. Diagnosis of *Helicobacter pylori*: invasive and non-invasive tests. *Best Pract Res Clin Gastroenterol* 2007;**21**:299.

87. el-Zimaity HM, al-Assi MT, Genta RM, Graham DY. Confirmation of successful therapy of *Helicobacter pylori* infection: number and site of biopsies or a rapid urease test. *Am J Gastroenterol* 1995;**90**:1962.

88. el-Zimaity HM, Wu J, Akamatsu T, Graham DY. A reliable method for the simultaneous identification of H pylori and gastric metaplasia in the duodenum. *J Clin Pathol* 1999;**52**: 914.

89. Genta RM, Robason GO, Graham DY. Simultaneous visualization of *Helicobacter pylori* and gastric morphology: a new stain. *Hum Pathol* 1994;**25**:221.

90. Vartanian RK, Leung JK, Davis JE, Kim YB, Owen DA. Ael Alcian yellow-toluidine blue (Leung) stain for *Helicobacter* species: comparison with standard stains, a cost-effectiveness analysis, and supplemental utilities. *Mod Pathol* 1998;**11**:72.

91. Chey WD, Wong BC. American College of Gastroenterology guideline on the management of *Helicobacter pylori* infection. *Am J Gastroenterol* 2007;**102**:1808.

92. Bytzer P, Teglbjaerg PS. *Helicobacter pylori*-negative duodenal ulcers: prevalence, clinical characteristics, and prognosis – results from a randomized trial with 2-year follow-up. *Am J Gastroenterol* 2001;**96**:1409.

93. Jonkers D, Stobberingh E, de Bruine A, Arends JW, Stockbrugger R. Evaluation of immunohistochemistry for the detection of *Helicobacter pylori* in gastric mucosal biopsies. *J Infect* 1997;**35**:149.

94. Andersen LP, Rasmussen L. *Helicobacter pylori*-coccoid forms and biofilm formation. *FEMS Immunol Med Microbiol* 2009;**56**:112.

95. Dickey W, Kenny BD, McConnell JB. Effect of proton pump inhibitors on the detection of *Helicobacter pylori* in gastric biopsies. *Aliment Pharmacol Ther* 1996;**10**:289.

96. Tham T, Collins JS, Sloan JM. Long-term effects of *Helicobacter pylori* on gastric mucosa: an 8 year follow-up. *Gastroenterology* 1994;**89**:1355.

97. Niemela S, Karttunen T, Kerola T. *Helicobacter pylori*-associated gastritis. Evolution of histologic changes over 10 years. *Scand J Gastroenterol* 1995;**30**:542.

98. Villako K, Kekki M, Maaroos HI, et al. A 12-year follow-up study of chronic gastritis and *Helicobacter pylori* in a population-based random sample. *Scand J Gastroenterol* 1995;**30**:964.

99. Allen A, Cunliffe WJ, Pearson JP, Venables CW. The adherent gastric mucus gel barrier in man and changes in peptic ulceration. *J Intern Med Suppl* 1990;**732**:83.

100. Bell AE, Sellers LA, Allen A, Cunliffe WJ, Morris ER, Ross-Murphy SB. Properties of gastric and duodenal mucus: effect of proteolysis, disulfide reduction, bile, acid, ethanol, and hypertonicity on mucus gel structure. *Gastroenterology* 1985;**88**(1 Pt 2):269.

101. Turnberg LA. Gastric mucosal defence mechanisms. *Scand J Gastroenterol Suppl* 1985;**110**:37.

102. Allen A, Flemstrom G, Garner A, Kivilaakso E. Gastroduodenal mucosal protection. *Physiol Rev* 1993;**73**:823.

103. Williams SE, Turnberg LA. Demonstration of a pH gradient across mucus adherent to rabbit gastric mucosa: evidence for a 'mucus-bicarbonate' barrier. *Gut* 1981;**22**:94.

104. Goddard PJ, Kao YC, Lichtenberger LM. Luminal surface hydrophobicity of canine gastric mucosa is dependent on a surface mucous gel. *Gastroenterology* 1990;**98**:361.

105. Hills BA. A physical identity for the gastric mucosal barrier. *Med J Aust* 1990;**153**:76.

106. Davenport HW. Salicylate damage to the gastric mucosal barrier. *N Engl J Med* 1967;**276**:1307.

107. Kauffman GL, Jr. The gastric mucosal barrier. Component control. *Dig Dis Sci* 1985;**30**(11 suppl):69S.

108. Hills BA. Gastric surfactant and the hydrophobic mucosal barrier. *Gut* 1996;**39**:621.

109. Eastwood GL. Gastrointestinal epithelial renewal. *Gastroenterology* 1977;**72**(5 Pt 1):962.

110. Svanes K, Ito S, Takeuchi K, Silen W. Restitution of the surface epithelium of the in vitro frog gastric mucosa after damage with hyperosmolar sodium chloride. Morphologic and physiologic characteristics. *Gastroenterology* 1982;**82**:1409.

111. Wong WM, Playford RJ, Wright NA. Peptide gene expression in gastrointestinal mucosal ulceration: ordered sequence or redundancy? *Gut* 2000;**46**:286.

112. Gottfried EB, Korsten MA, Lieber CS. Alcohol-induced gastric and duodenal lesions in man. *Am J Gastroenterol* 1978;**70**:587.

113. Kauffman GL Jr. Mucosal damage to the stomach: how, when and why? *Scand J Gastroenterol Suppl* 1984;**105**:19.

114. Starlinger M, Schiessel R, Hung CR, Silen W. H+ back diffusion stimulating gastric mucosal blood flow in the rabbit fundus. *Surgery* 1981;**89**:232.

115. Kivilaakso E, Fromm D, Silen W. Relationship between ulceration and intramural pH of gastric mucosa during hemorrhagic shock. *Surgery* 1978;**84**:70.

116. Leung FW, Itoh M, Hirabayashi K, Guth PH. Role of blood flow in gastric and duodenal mucosal injury in the rat. *Gastroenterology* 1985;**88**(1 Pt 2):281.

117. Robert A. Cytoprotection by prostaglandins. *Gastroenterology* 1979;**77**(4 Pt 1):761.

118. Bickel M, Kauffman GL Jr. Gastric gel mucus thickness: effect of distension, 16,16-dimethyl prostaglandin E2, and carbenoxolone. *Gastroenterology* 1981;**80**:770.

119. Konturek SJ, Robert A. Cytoprotection of canine gastric mucosa by prostacyclin: possible 115 by increased mucosal blood flow. *Digestion* 1982;**25**:155.

120. Konturek SJ, Tasler J, Bilski J, Kaminska A, Laskiewicz J. Role of prostaglandins in alkaline secretion from the gastroduodenal mucosa exposed to acid and taurocholate. *Scand J Gastroenterol Suppl* 1984;**92**:69.

121. Lichtenberger LM, Richards JE, Hills BA. Effect of 16,16-dimethyl prostaglandin E_2 on the surface hydrophobicity of aspirin-treated canine gastric mucosa. *Gastroenterology* 1985;**88**(1 Pt 2):308.

122. Konturek SJ. Gastric cytoprotection. *Scand J Gastroenterol* 1985;**20**:543.

123. Kunkel SL, Wiggins RC, Chensue SW, Larrick J. Regulation of macrophage tumour necrosis factor production by prostaglandin E2. *Biochem Biophys Res Commun* 1986;**137**:404.

124. Raud J. Vasodilatation and inhibition of mediator release represent two distinct mechanisms for prostaglandin modulation of acute mast cell-dependent inflammation. *Br J Pharmacol* 1990;**99**:449.

125. Hogaboam CM, Bissonnette EY, Chin BC, Befus AD, Wallace JL. Prostaglandins inhibit inflammatory mediator release from rat mast cells. *Gastroenterology* 1993;**104**:122.

126. Konturek SJ, Obtulowicz W, Sito E, Oleksy J, Wilkon S, Kiec-Dembinska A. Distribution of prostaglandins in gastric and duodenal mucosa of healthy subjects and duodenal ulcer patients: effects of aspirin and paracetamol. *Gut* 1981;**22**:283.

127. Simon LS, Mills JA. Nonsteroidal antiinflammatory drugs [second of two parts]. *N Engl J Med* 1980;**302**:1237.

128. Simon LS, Mills JA. Drug therapy: nonsteroidal antiinflammatory drugs [first of two parts]. *N Engl J Med* 1980;**302**:1179.

129. Graham DY. *Campylobacter pylori* and peptic ulcer disease. *Gastroenterology* 1989;**96**(2 Pt 2 suppl):615.

130. Gisbert JP, Calvet X. Review article: *Helicobacter pylori*-negative duodenal ulcer disease. *Aliment Pharmacol Ther* 2009;**30**:791.

131. Marshall BJ, Warren JR. Unidentified curved bacilli in the stomach of patients with gastritis and peptic ulceration. *Lancet* 1984;**i**:1311.

132. Ohkusa T, Okayasu I, Miwa H, Ohtaka K, Endo S, Sato N. *Helicobacter pylori* infection induces duodenitis and superficial duodenal ulcer in Mongolian gerbils. *Gut* 2003;**52**:797.

133. el-Serag HB, Sonnenberg A. Opposing time trends of peptic ulcer and reflux disease. *Gut* 1998;**43**:327.

134. Banatvala N, Mayo K, Megraud F, Jennings R, Deeks JJ, Feldman RA. The cohort effect and *Helicobacter pylori*. *J Infect Dis* 1993;**168**:219.

135. Redeen S, Petersson F, Kechagias S, dh E, Borch K. Natural history of chronic gastritis in a population-based cohort. *Scand J Gastroenterol* 2010;**45**:450.

136. Gibson T. Nonsteroidal anti-inflammatory drugs – another look. *Br J Rheumatol* 1988;**27**:87.

137. Nakos A, Zezos P, Liratzopoulos N, et al. The significance of histological evidence of bile reflux gastropathy in patients with gastro-esophageal reflux disease. *Med Sci Monit* 2009; **15**:CR313.

138. Feldman M, Walker P, Green JL, Weingarden K. Life events stress and psychosocial factors in men with peptic ulcer disease. A multidimensional case-controlled study. *Gastroenterology* 1986;**91**:1370.

139. Rotter JI, Sones JQ, Samloff IM, et al. Duodenal-ulcer disease associated with elevated serum pepsinogen I: an inherited autosomal dominant disorder. *N Engl J Med* 1979;**300**:63.

140. Cook DJ, Fuller HD, Guyatt GH, et al. Risk factors for gastrointestinal bleeding in critically ill patients. Canadian Critical Care Trials Group. *N Engl J Med* 1994;**330**:377.

141. Post PN, Kuipers EJ, Meijer GA. Declining incidence of peptic ulcer but not of its complications: a nation-wide study in The Netherlands. *Aliment Pharmacol Ther* 2006;**23**:1587.

142. Sugawa C, Lucas CE, Rosenberg BF, Riddle JM, Walt AJ. Differential topography of acute erosive gastritis due to trauma or sepsis, ethanol and aspirin. *Gastrointest Endosc* 1973;**19**: 127.

143. Hoftiezer JW, O'Laughlin JC, Ivey KJ. Effects of 24 hours of aspirin, Bufferin, paracetamol and placebo on normal human gastroduodenal mucosa. *Gut* 1982;**23**:692.

144. Tanner NC. Surgery of peptic ulceration and its complications. *Postgrad Med J* 1954;**30**:577.

145. Jennings D, Richardson JE. Giant lesser-curve gastric ulcers. *Lancet* 1954;**267**:343.

146. Kamada T, Fusamoto H, Masuzawa M, Hiramatsu K, Fukui O. 'Trench ulcer' of the stomach. *Am J Gastroenterol* 1975;**63**: 486.

147. Oi M, Oshida K, Sugimura S. The location of gastric ulcer. *Gastroenterology* 1959;**36**:45.

148. Findley JW, Jr. Ulcers of the greater curvature of the stomach. *Gastroenterology* 1961;**40**:183.

149. Stadelmann O, Elster K, Stolte M, et al. The peptic gastric ulcer – histotopographic and functional investigations. *Scand J Gastroenterol* 1971;**6**:613.

150. Magnus HA. The pathology of peptic ulceration. *Postgrad Med J* 1954;**30**:131.

151. Sun DC, Stempien SJ. The Veterans Administration Cooperative Study on Gastric Ulcer. 3. Site and size of the ulcer as determinants of outcome. *Gastroenterology* 1971;**61**(suppl 2): 576.

152. Thomas J, Greig M, McIntosh J, Hunt J, McNeil D, Piper DW. The location of chronic gastric ulcer: a study of the relevance of ulcer size, age, sex, alcohol, analgesic intake and smoking. *Digestion* 1980;**20**:79.

153. Kimura K. Chronological transition of the fundic-pyloric border determined by stepwise biopsy of the lesser and greater curvatures of the stomach. *Gastroenterology* 1972;**63**:584.

154. Szabo S, Folkman J, Vattay P, Morales RE, Pinkus GS, Kato K. Accelerated healing of duodenal ulcers by oral administration of a mutein of basic fibroblast growth factor in rats. *Gastroenterology* 1994;**106**:1106.

155. Newcomb WD. The relationship between peptic ulceration and gastric carcinoma. *Br J Surg* 1932;**20**:279.

156. Isaacson P. Biopsy appearances easily mistaken for malignancy in gastrointestinal endoscopy. *Histopathology* 1982;**6**:377.

157. Dean AC, Clark CG, Sinclair-Gieben AH. The late prognosis of perforated duodenal ulcer. *Gut* 1962;**3**:60.

158. Cohen MM. Treatment and mortality of perforated peptic ulcer: a survey of 852 cases. *Can Med Assoc J* 1971;**105**:263.

159. Masso Gonzalez EL, Patrignani P, Tacconelli S, Garcia Rodriguez LA. Variability among nonsteroidal antiinflammatory drugs in risk of upper gastrointestinal bleeding. *Arthrit Rheum* 2010;**62**:1592.

160. Svanes C, Soreide JA, Skarstein A, et al. Smoking and ulcer perforation. *Gut* 1997;**41**:177.

161. Hawkey CJ. Review article: aspirin and gastrointestinal bleeding. *Aliment Pharmacol Ther* 1994;**8**:141.

162. Rahme E, Barkun A, Nedjar H, Gaugris S, Watson D. Hospitalizations for upper and lower GI events associated with traditional NSAIDs and acetaminophen among the elderly in Quebec, Canada. *Am J Gastroenterol* 2008;**103**:872.

163. Swain CP, Storey DW, Bown SG, et al. Nature of the bleeding vessel in recurrently bleeding gastric ulcers. *Gastroenterology* 1986;**90**:595.

164. Rockall TA, Logan RF, Devlin HB, Northfield TC. Incidence of and mortality from acute upper gastrointestinal haemorrhage in the United Kingdom. Steering Committee and members of the National Audit of Acute Upper Gastrointestinal Haemorrhage. *BMJ* 1995;**311**:222.

165. Weil J, Langman MJ, Wainwright P, et al. Peptic ulcer bleeding: accessory risk factors and interactions with non-steroidal anti-inflammatory drugs. *Gut* 2000;**46**:27.

166. Porteous C, Williams D, Foulis A, Sugden BA. Penetration of the left ventricular myocardium by benign peptic ulceration: two cases and a review of the published work. *J Clin Pathol* 1984;**37**:1239.

167. West AB, Nolan N, O'Briain DS. Benign peptic ulcers penetrating pericardium and heart: clinicopathological features and factors favoring survival. *Gastroenterology* 1988;**94**:1478.

168. Palmer ED. Gastric diverticula. *Int Abstr Surg* 1951;**92**:417.

169. Tatsuta M, Okuda S. Location, healing, and recurrence of gastric ulcers in relation to fundal gastritis. *Gastroenterology* 1975;**69**:897.

170. Stemmermann GN. Intestinal metaplasia of the stomach. A status report. *Cancer* 1994;**74**:556.

171. Mori K, Shinya H, Wolff WI. Polypoid reparative mucosal proliferation at the site of a healed gastric ulcer: sequential gastroscopic, radiological, and histological observations. *Gastroenterology* 1971;**61**:523.

172. MacDonald WC. Correlation of mucosal histology and aspirin intake in chronic gastric ulcer. *Gastroenterology* 1973;**65**:381.

173. El-Zimaity HMT, Gutierrez O, Kim JG, et al. Geographic differences in the distribution of intestinal metaplasia in duodenal ulcer patients. *Am J Gastroenterol* 2001;**96**:666.

174. El-Zimaity H. Gastritis and gastric atrophy. *Curr Opin Gastroenterol* 2008;**24**:682.

175. Kirk RM. Site and localization of duodenal ulcers: a study at operation. *Gut* 1968;**9**:414.

176. Kang JY, Nasiry R, Guan R, et al. Influence of the site of a duodenal ulcer on its mode of presentation. *Gastroenterology* 1986; **90**:1874.

177. Classen M. Endoscopy in benign peptic ucer. *Clin Gastroenterol* 1973;**2**:315.

178. Collins JS, Hamilton PW, Watt PC, Sloan JM, Love AH. Quantitative histological study of mucosal inflammatory cell densities in endoscopic duodenal biopsy specimens from dyspeptic

patients using computer linked image analysis. *Gut* 1990;**31**: 858.

179. Zukerman GR, Mills BA, Koehler RE, Siegel A, Harter HR, DeSchryver-Kecskemeti K. Nodular duodenitis. Pathologic and clinical characteristics in patients with end-stage renal disease. *Dig Dis Sci* 1983;**28**:1018.

180. Wyatt JI, Rathbone BJ, Sobala GM, et al. Gastric epithelium in the duodenum: its association with *Helicobacter pylori* and inflammation. *J Clin Pathol* 1990;**43**:981.

181. Marshall BJ, Goodwin CS, Warren JR, et al. Prospective double-blind trial of duodenal ulcer relapse after eradication of *Campylobacter pylori*. *Lancet* 1988;**ii**:1437.

182. Wyatt JI, Rathbone BJ, Dixon MF, Heatley RV, Axon AT. *Campylobacter pylori* and development of duodenal ulcer. *Lancet* 1988;**1**:118.

183. Harris AW, Gummett PA, Walker MM, Misiewicz JJ, Baron JH. Relation between gastric acid output, *Helicobacter pylori*, and gastric metaplasia in the duodenal bulb. *Gut* 1996;**39**:513.

184. Noach LA, Rolf TM, Bosma NB, et al. Gastric metaplasia and *Helicobacter pylori* infection. *Gut* 1993;**34**:1510.

185. Goodwin CS. Duodenal ulcer, *Campylobacter pylori*, and the 'leaking roof' concept. *Lancet* 1988;**ii**:1467.

186. Savarino V, Mela GS, Zentilin P, et al. Circadian gastric acidity in *Helicobacter pylori* positive ulcer patients with and without gastric metaplasia in the duodenum. *Gut* 1996;**39**:508.

187. James AH. Gastric epithelium in the duodenum. *Gut* 1964;**5**: 285.

188. Parrish JA, Rawlins DC. Intestinal mucosa in the Zollinger–Ellison syndrome. *Gut* 1965;**6**:286.

189. Hanby AM, Poulsom R, Elia G, Singh S, Longcroft JM, Wright NA. The expression of the trefoil peptides pS2 and human spasmolytic polypeptide (hSP) in 'gastric metaplasia' of the proximal duodenum: implications for the nature of 'gastric metaplasia'. *J Pathol* 1993;**169**:355.

190. Kushima R, Manabe R, Hattori T, Borchard F. Histogenesis of gastric foveolar metaplasia following duodenal ulcer: a definite reparative lineage of Brunner's gland. *Histopathology* 1999; **35**:38.

191. Carrick J, Lee A, Hazell S, Ralston M, Daskalopoulos G. *Campylobacter pylori*, duodenal ulcer, and gastric metaplasia: possible role of functional heterotopic tissue in ulcerogenesis. *Gut* 1989; **30**:790.

192. Roth SH. Nonsteroidal anti-inflammatory drug gastropathy. We started it – can we stop it? *Arch Intern Med* 1986;**146**:1075.

193. Brooks PM. Clinical management of rheumatoid arthritis. *Lancet* 1993;**341**:286.

194. Meisel AD. Clinical benefits and comparative safety of piroxicam. Analysis of worldwide clinical trials data. *Am J Med* 1986;**81**(5B):15.

195. Gabriel SE, Jaakkimainen L, Bombardier C. Risk for serious gastrointestinal complications related to use of nonsteroidal anti-inflammatory drugs. A meta-analysis. *Ann Intern Med* 1991;**115**:787.

196. Hawkey CJ. Non-steroidal anti-inflammatory drugs and peptic ulcers. *BMJ* 1990;**300**:278.

197. Taha AS, Dahill S, Sturrock RD, Lee FD, Russell RI. Predicting NSAID related ulcers – assessment of clinical and pathological risk factors and importance of differences in NSAID. *Gut* 1994;**35**:891.

198. Skander MP, Ryan FP. Non-steroidal anti-inflammatory drugs and pain free peptic ulceration in the elderly. *BMJ* 1988;**297**: 833.

199. Clinch D, Banerjee AK, Ostick G, Levy DW. Non-steroidal anti-inflammatory drugs and gastrointestinal adverse effects. *J R Coll Physicians Lond* 1983;**17**:228.

200. Fries JF, Miller SR, Spitz PW, Williams CA, Hubert HB, Bloch DA. Identification of patients at risk for gastropathy associated with NSAID use. *J Rheumatol Suppl* 1990;**20**:12.

201. Henry D, Lim LL, Garcia Rodriguez LA, et al. Variability in risk of gastrointestinal complications with individual non-steroidal anti-inflammatory drugs: results of a collaborative meta-analysis. *BMJ* 1996;**312**:1563.

202. Singh G, Ramey DR, Morfeld D, Shi H, Hatoum HT, Fries JF. Gastrointestinal tract complications of nonsteroidal anti-inflammatory drug treatment in rheumatoid arthritis. A prospective observational cohort study. *Arch Intern Med* 1996; **156**:1530.

203. Wolfe MM, Lichtenstein DR, Singh G. Gastrointestinal toxicity of nonsteroidal antiinflammatory drugs. *N Engl J Med* 1999; **340**:1888.

204. Szabo S, Goldberg I. Experimental pathogenesis: drugs and chemical lesions in the gastric mucosa. *Scand J Gastroenterol Suppl* 1990;**174**:1.

205. Jacobson ED. Circulatory mechanisms of gastric mucosal damage and protection. *Gastroenterology* 1992;**102**:1788.

206. Hogan DL, Ainsworth MA, Isenberg JI. Review article: gastroduodenal bicarbonate secretion. *Aliment Pharmacol Ther* 1994;**8**:475.

207. Forssell H, Olbe L. Continuous computerized determination of gastric bicarbonate secretion in man. *Scand J Gastroenterol* 1985;**20**:767.

208. Graham DY, Agrawal NM, Roth SH. Prevention of NSAID-induced gastric ulcer with misoprostol: multicentre, double-blind, placebo-controlled trial. *Lancet* 1988;**ii**:1277.

209. Rostom A, Muir K, Dube C, et al. Gastrointestinal safety of cyclooxygenase-2 inhibitors: a Cochrane Collaboration systematic review. *Clin Gastroenterol Hepatol* 2007;**5**:818, 28 e1; quiz 768.

210. McGettigan P, Henry D. Cardiovascular risk and inhibition of cyclooxygenase: a systematic review of the observational studies of selective and nonselective inhibitors of cyclooxygenase 2. *JAMA* 2006;**296**:1633.

211. Harirforoosh S, Jamali F. Renal adverse effects of nonsteroidal anti-inflammatory drugs. Expert *Opin Drug Saf* 2009;**8**: 669.

212. Lanas A, Garcia-Tell G, Armada B, Oteo-Alvaro A. Prescription patterns and appropriateness of NSAID therapy according to gastrointestinal risk and cardiovascular history in patients with diagnoses of osteoarthritis. *BMC Med* 2011;**9**:38.

213. Chan FK, Abraham NS, Scheiman JM, Laine L. Management of patients on nonsteroidal anti-inflammatory drugs: a clinical practice recommendation from the First International Working Party on Gastrointestinal and Cardiovascular Effects of Nonsteroidal Anti-inflammatory Drugs and Anti-platelet Agents. *Am J Gastroenterol* 2008;**103**:2908.

214. Burmester G, Lanas A, Biasucci L, et al. The appropriate use of non-steroidal anti-inflammatory drugs in rheumatic disease: opinions of a multidisciplinary European expert panel. *Ann Rheum Dis* 2011;**70**:818.

215. Vieth M, Muller H, Stolte M. Can the diagnosis of NSAID-induced or HP-associated gastric ulceration be predicted from histology? *Z Gastroenterol* 2002;**40**:783.

216. Hunt RH, Bazzoli F. Review article: should NSAID/low-dose aspirin takers be tested routinely for H. pylori infection and treated if positive? Implications for primary risk of ulcer and ulcer relapse after initial healing. *Aliment Pharmacol Ther* 2004;**19**(suppl 1):9.

217. Malfertheiner P, Megraud F, O'Morain C, et al. Current concepts in the management of *Helicobacter pylori* infection: the Maastricht III Consensus Report. *Gut* 2007;**56**:772.

218. El-Zimaity HM. Gastric atrophy, diagnosing and staging. *World J Gastroenterol* 2006;**12**:5757.

219. Palmer ED. Gastritis: a revaluation. *Medicine (Baltimore)* 1954; **33**:199.

220. Laine L, Weinstein WM. Histology of alcoholic hemorrhagic 'gastritis': a prospective evaluation. *Gastroenterology* 1988;**94**: 1254.

221. Kvietys PR, Twohig B, Danzell J, Specian RD. Ethanol-induced injury to the rat gastric mucosa. Role of neutrophils and xanthine oxidase-derived radicals. *Gastroenterology* 1990;**98**: 909.

222. Bou-Abboud CF, Wayland H, Paulsen G, Guth PH. Microcirculatory stasis precedes tissue necrosis in ethanol-induced gastric mucosal injury in the rat. *Dig Dis Sci* 1988;**33**:872.

223. Masuda E, Kawano S, Nagano K, et al. Endogenous nitric oxide modulates ethanol-induced gastric mucosal injury in rats. *Gastroenterology* 1995;**108**:58.

224. Laine L, Weinstein WM. Subepithelial hemorrhages and erosions of human stomach. *Dig Dis Sci* 1988;**33**:490.

225. Kelly JP, Kaufman DW, Koff RS, Laszlo A, Wiholm BE, Shapiro S. Alcohol consumption and the risk of major upper gastrointestinal bleeding. *Am J Gastroenterol* 1995;**90**:1058.

226. Lucas CE, Sugawa C, Riddle J, Rector F, Rosenberg B, Walt AJ. Natural history and surgical dilemma of 'stress' gastric bleeding. *Arch Surg* 1971;**102**:266.

227. Bank S, Misra P, Mausner D, et al. The incidence, distribution and evolution of stress ulcers in surgical intensive care units. *Am J Gastroenetrol* 1980;**74**:76.

228. Shuman RB, Schuster DP, Zuckerman GR. Prophylactic therapy for stress ulcer bleeding: a reappraisal. *Ann Intern Med* 1987; **106**:562.

229. Harjola PT, Sivula A. Gastric ulceration following experimentally induced hypoxia and hemorrhagic shock: in vivo study of pathogenesis in rabbits. *Ann Surg* 1966;**163**:21.

230. Shirazi S, Mueller TM, Hardy BM. Canine gastric acid secretion and blood flow measurement in hemorrhagic shock. *Gastroenterology* 1977;**73**:75.

231. Menguy R, Masters YF. Mechanism of stress ulcer. II. Differences between the antrum, corpus, and fundus with respect to the effects of complete ischemia on gastric mucosal energy metabolism. *Gastroenterology* 1974;**66**:509.

232. Perry MA, Wadhwa S, Parks DA, Pickard W, Granger DN. Role of oxygen radicals in ischemia-induced lesions in the cat stomach. *Gastroenterology* 1986;**90**:362.

233. Czaja AJ, McAlhany JC, Pruitt BA Jr. Acute gastroduodenal disease after thermal injury. An endoscopic evaluation of incidence and natural history. *N Engl J Med* 1974;**291**:925.

234. Nordstrom H, Nettelblad H. Curling's ulcer – a serious complication of the burned patient. *Scand J Gastroenterol Suppl* 1984;**105**:14.

235. Sevitt S. Duodenal and gastric ulceration after burning. *Br J Surg* 1967;**54**:32.

236. Cushing H. Peptic ulcers and the interbrain. *Surg Gynecol Obstet* 1932;**55**:1.

237. Brown TH, Davidson PF, Larson GM. Acute gastritis occurring within 24 hours of severe head injury. *Gastrointest Endosc* 1989;**35**:37.

238. Cheung LY. Thomas G Orr Memorial Lecture. Pathogenesis, prophylaxis, and treatment of stress gastritis. *Am J Surg* 1988; **156**:437.

239. Weber HC, Venzon DJ, Jensen RT, Metz DC. Studies on the interrelation between Zollinger–Ellison syndrome, *Helicobacter pylori*, and proton pump inhibitor therapy. *Gastroenterology* 1997;**112**:84.

240. Zollinger RM, Ellison EH. Primary peptic ulcerations of the jejunum associated with islet cell tumours of the pancreas. *Ann Surg* 1955;**142**:709; discussion, 24.

241. Oberhelman HA Jr. Excisional therapy for ulcerogenic tumours of the duodenum: long-term results. *Arch Surg* 1972;**104**: 447.

242. Stamm B, Hedinger CE, Saremaslani P. Duodenal and ampullary carcinoid tumours. A report of 12 cases with pathological characteristics, polypeptide content and relation to the MEN I syndrome and von Recklinghausen's disease (neurofibromatosis). *Virchows Arch A Pathol Anat Histopathol* 1986; **408**:475.

243. Buchanan KD, Sloan JM, O'Hare MM, Kennedy TL. Zollinger–Ellison syndrome. In: Bouchier IA (ed.), *Textbook of Gastroenterology*. London: Baillière Tindall, 1984: 1339.

244. Watson RG, Johnston CF, O'Hare MM, et al. The frequency of gastrointestinal endocrine tumours in a well-defined population – Northern Ireland 1970–1985. *Q J Med* 1989;**72**:647.

245. Newsome HH. Multiple endocrine adenomatosis. *Surg Clin North Am* 1974;**54**:387.

246. Solcia E, Capella C, Fiocca R, Rindi G, Rosai J. Gastric argyrophil carcinoidosis in patients with Zollinger–Ellison syndrome due to type 1 multiple endocrine neoplasia. A newly recognized association. *Am J Surg Pathol* 1990;**14**:503.

247. Friesen SR, Tomita T. Pseudo-Zollinger–Ellison syndrome: hypergastrinemia, hyperchlorhydria without tumour. *Ann Surg* 1981;**194**:481.

248. Bordi C, Cocconi G, Togni R, Vezzadini P, Missale G. Gastric endocrine cell proliferation. Association with Zollinger–Ellison syndrome. *Arch Pathol* 1974;**98**:274.

249. Lechago J. Gastrointestinal neuroendocrine cell proliferations. *Hum Pathol* 1994;**25**:1114.

250. Lewin KJ, Yang K, Ulich T, Elashoff JD, Walsh J. Primary gastrin cell hyperplasia. Report of five cases and a review of the literature. *Am J Surg Pathol* 1984;**8**:821.

251. Polak JM, Stagg B, Pearse AG. Two types of Zollinger–Ellison syndrome: immunofluorescent, cytochemical and ultrastructural studies of the antral and pancreatic gastrin cells in different clinical states. *Gut* 1972;**13**:501.

252. Arnold R, Hulst MV, Neuhof CH, Schwarting H, Becker HD, Creutzfeldt W. Antral gastrin-producing G-cells and somatostatin-producing D-cells in different states of gastric acid secretion. *Gut* 1982;**23**:285.

253. El-Zimaity HM, Ota H, Graham DY, Akamatsu T, Katsuyama T. Patterns of gastric atrophy in intestinal type gastric carcinoma. *Cancer* 2002;**94**:1428.

254. El-Zimaity HM, Ramchatesingh J, Saeed MA, Graham DY. Gastric intestinal metaplasia: subtypes and natural history. *J Clin Pathol* 2001;**54**:679.

255. Ricuarte O, Gutierrez O, Cardona H, Kim JG, Graham DY, El-Zimaity HM. Atrophic gastritis in young children and adolescents. *J Clin Pathol* 2005;**58**:1189.

256. Tarpila S, Kekki M, Samloff IM, Sipponen P, Siurala M. Morphology and dynamics of the gastric mucosa in duodenal ulcer patients and their first-degree relatives. *Hepatogastroenterology* 1983;**30**:198.

257. Kelly EJ, Lagopoulos M, Primrose JN. Immunocytochemical localisation of parietal cells and G cells in the developing human stomach. *Gut* 1993;**34**:1057.

258. Cornaggia M, Capella C, Riva C, Finzi G, Solcia E. Electron immunocytochemical localization of pepsinogen I (PgI) in chief cells, mucous-neck cells and transitional mucous-neck/chief cells of the human fundic mucosa. *Histochemistry* 1986; **85**:5.

259. Helpap B, Hattori T, Gedigk P. Repair of gastric ulcer. A cell kinetic study. *Virchows Arch A Pathol Anat Histol* 1981; **392**:159.

260. Hattori T, Helpap B, Gedigk P. The morphology and cell kinetics of pseudopyloric glands. *Virchows Arch B Cell Pathol Incl Mol Pathol* 1982;**39**:31.

261. Filipe MI, Munoz N, Matko I, et al. Intestinal metaplasia types and the risk of gastric cancer: a cohort study in Slovenia. *Int J Cancer* 1994;**57**:324.

262. Rokkas T, Filipe MI, Sladen GE. Detection of an increased incidence of early gastric cancer in patients with intestinal metaplasia type III who are closely followed up. *Gut* 1991;**32**:1110.

263. Huang CB, Xu J, Huang JF, Meng XY. Sulphomucin colonic type intestinal metaplasia and carcinoma in the stomach. A histochemical study of 115 cases obtained by biopsy. *Cancer* 1986;**57**:1370.

264. Filipe MI, Potet F, Bogomoletz WV, et al. Incomplete sulphomucin-secreting intestinal metaplasia for gastric cancer. Preliminary data from a prospective study from three centres. *Gut* 1985;**26**:1319.

265. Silva S, Filipe MI, Pinho A. Variants of intestinal metaplasia in the evolution of chronic atrophic gastritis and gastric ulcer. A follow up study. *Gut* 1990;**31**:1097.

266. Siurala M, Lehtola J, Ihamaki T. Atrophic gastritis and its sequelae. Results of 19–23 years' follow-up examinations. *Scand J Gastroenterol* 1974;**9**:441.

267. Rosch W, Demling L, Elster K. Is chronic gastritis a reversible process? Follow-up study of gastritis by step-wise biopsy. *Acta Hepatogastroenterol (Stuttg)* 1975;**22**:252.

268. Maaroos HI, Salupere V, Uibo R, Kekki M, Sipponen P. Seven-year follow-up study of chronic gastritis in gastric ulcer patients. *Scand J Gastroenterol* 1985;**20**:198.

269. Ihamaki T, Kekki M, Sipponen P, Siurala M. The sequelae and course of chronic gastritis during a 30- to 34-year bioptic follow-up study. *Scand J Gastroenterol* 1985;**20**:485.

270. Villako K, Kekki M, Maaroos HI, et al. Chronic gastritis: progression of inflammation and atrophy in a six-year endoscopic follow-up of a random sample of 142 Estonian urban subjects. *Scand J Gastroenterol Suppl* 1991;**186**:135.

271. Valle J, Kekki M, Sipponen P, Ihamaki T, Siurala M. Long-term course and consequences of *Helicobacter pylori* gastritis. Results of a 32-year follow-up study. *Scand J Gastroenterol* 1996;**31**:546.

272. Kato I, Tominaga S, Ito Y, et al. Atrophic gastritis and stomach cancer risk: cross-sectional analyses. *Jpn J Cancer Res* 1992;**83**:1041.

273. Kato Y, Sugano H, Rubio CA. Classification of intramucosal cysts of the stomach. *Histopathology* 1983;**7**:931.

274. Graham DY, Lew GM, Lechago J. Antral G-cell and D-cell numbers in *Helicobacter pylori* infection: effect of H. pylori eradication. *Gastroenterology* 1993;**104**:1655.

275. Greibe J, Bugge P, Gjorup T, Lauritzen T, Bonnevie O, Wulff HR. Long-term prognosis of duodenal ulcer: follow-up study and survey of doctors' estimates. *BMJ* 1977;**2**:1572.

276. Bardhan KD, Cust G, Hinchliffe RF, Williamson FM, Lyon C, Bose K. Changing pattern of admissions and operations for duodenal ulcer. *Br J Surg* 1989;**76**:230.

277. Kato Y, Kitagawa T, Yanagisawa A, et al. Site-dependent development of complete and incomplete intestinal metaplasia types in the human stomach. *Jpn J Cancer Res* 1992;**83**:178.

278. Ramesar KC, Sanders DS, Hopwood D. Limited value of type III intestinal metaplasia in predicting risk of gastric carcinoma. *J Clin Pathol* 1987;**40**:1287.

279. Doglioni C, Laurino L, Dei Tos AP, et al. Pancreatic (acinar) metaplasia of the gastric mucosa. Histology, ultrastructure, immunocytochemistry, and clinicopathologic correlations of 101 cases. *Am J Surg Pathol* 1993;**17**:1134.

280. el-Zimaity HM, Verghese VJ, Ramchatesingh J, Graham DY. The gastric cardia in gastro-oesophageal disease. *J Clin Pathol* 2000;**53**:619.

281. Boparai V, Rajagopalan J, Triadafilopoulos G. Guide to the use of proton pump inhibitors in adult patients. *Drugs* 2008; **68**:925.

282. Stolte M, Meining A, Schmitz JM, Alexandridis T, Seifert E. Changes in *Helicobacter pylori*-induced gastritis in the antrum and corpus during 12 months of treatment with omeprazole and lansoprazole in patients with gastro-oesophageal reflux disease. *Aliment Pharmacol Ther* 1998;**12**:247.

283. Klinkenberg-Knol EC, Festen HP, Sen JB, et al. Long-term treatment with omeprazole for refractory reflux esophagitis: efficacy and safety. *Ann Intern Med* 1994;**121**:161.

284. Meining A, Bosseckert H, Caspary WF, Nauert C, Stolte M. H₂-receptor antagonists and antacids have an aggravating effect on *Helicobacter pylori* gastritis in duodenal ulcer patients. *Aliment Pharmacol Ther* 1997;**11**:729.

285. Moayyedi P, Wason C, Peacock R, et al. Changing patterns of *Helicobacter pylori* gastritis in long-standing acid suppression. *Helicobacter* 2000;**5**:206.

286. Kuipers EJ, Uyterlinde AM, Pena AS, et al. Increase of *Helicobacter pylori*-associated corpus gastritis during acid suppressive therapy: implications for long-term safety. *Am J Gastroenterol* 1995;**90**:1401.

287. Schenk BE, Kuipers EJ, Nelis GF, et al. Effect of *Helicobacter pylori* eradication on chronic gastritis during omeprazole therapy. *Gut* 2000;**46**:615.

288. Berstad AE, Hatlebakk JG, Maartmann-Moe H, Berstad A, Brandtzaeg P. *Helicobacter pylori* gastritis and epithelial cell proliferation in patients with reflux oesophagitis after treatment with lansoprazole. *Gut* 1997;**41**:740.

289. Eissele R, Brunner G, Simon B, Solcia E, Arnold R. Gastric mucosa during treatment with lansoprazole: *Helicobacter pylori* is a risk factor for argyrophil cell hyperplasia. *Gastroenterology* 1997;**112**:707.

290. Furuta T, Baba S, Takashima M, et al. Effect of *Helicobacter pylori* infection on gastric juice pH. *Scand J Gastroenterol* 1998;**33**:357.

291. Kuipers EJ, Lundell L, Klinkenberg-Knol EC, et al. Atrophic gastritis and *Helicobacter pylori* infection in patients with reflux esophagitis treated with omeprazole or fundoplication. *N Engl J Med* 1996;**334**:1018.

292. Stolte M, Bethke B. Elimination of *Helicobacter pylori* under treatment with omeprazole. *Z Gastroenterol* 1990;**28**:271.

293. Kuipers EJ, Uyterlinde AM, Pena AS, et al. Increase of *Helicobacter pylori*-associated corpus gastritis during acid suppressive therapy: implications for long-term safety. *Am J Gastroenterol* 1995;**90**:1401.

294. Graham DY, Opekun AR, Yamaoka Y, Osato MS, el-Zimaity HM. Early events in proton pump inhibitor-associated exacerbation of corpus gastritis. *Aliment Pharmacol Ther* 2003;**17**:193.

295. Unge P, Gad A, Gnarpe H, Olsson J. Does omeprazole improve antimicrobial therapy directed towards gastric *Campylobacter pylori* in patients with antral gastritis? A pilot study. *Scand J Gastroenterol Suppl* 1989;**167**:49.

296. Klinkenberg-Knol EC, Nelis F, Dent J, et al. Long-term omeprazole treatment in resistant gastroesophageal reflux disease:

efficacy, safety, and influence on gastric mucosa. *Gastroenterology* 2000;**118**:661.

297. Logan RP, Walker MM, Misiewicz JJ, Gummett PA, Karim QN, Baron JH. Changes in the intragastric distribution of *Helicobacter pylori* during treatment with omeprazole. *Gut* 1995; **36**:12.

298. Graham DY, Opekun AR, Hammoud F, et al. Studies regarding the mechanism of false negative urea breath tests with proton pump inhibitors. *Am J Gastroenterol* 2003;**98**:1005.

299. Chourasia D, Misra A, Pandey R, Ghoshal UC. Gastric atrophy and intestinal metaplasia in a patient on long-term proton pump inhibitor therapy. *Trop Gastroenterol* 2008;**29**:172.

300. Cohen H, Weinstein WM, Carmel R. Heterogeneity of gastric histology and function in food cobalamin malabsorption: absence of atrophic gastritis and achlorhydria in some patients with severe malabsorption. *Gut* 2000;**47**:638.

301. Hirschowitz BI, Worthington J, Mohnen J. Vitamin B12 deficiency in hypersecretors during long-term acid suppression with proton pump inhibitors. *Aliment Pharmacol Ther* 2008;**27**: 1110.

302. Cote GA, Howden CW. Potential adverse effects of proton pump inhibitors. *Curr Gastroenterol Rep* 2008;**10**:208.

303. Davidson RJ, Atrah HI, Sewell HF. Longitudinal study of circulating gastric antibodies in pernicious anaemia. *J Clin Pathol* 1989;**42**:1092.

304. Irvine WJ. Immunoassay of gastric intrinsic factor and the titration of antibody to intrinsic factor. *Clin Exp Immunol* 1966; **1**:99.

305. Rose MS, Chanarin I. Dissociation of intrinsic factor from its antibody: application to study of pernicious anaemia gastric juice specimens. *BMJ* 1969;**1**:468.

306. Sourial NA. Rapid protein A assay for intrinsic factor and its binding antibody. *J Clin Pathol* 1988;**41**:568.

307. Desai HG, Dighe PK, Borkar AV. Parietal cell and intrinsic-factor antibodies in Indian subjects. *Scand J Gastroenterol* 1968;**3**:321.

308. Hudak J, Berger Z, Varga L. An assay for serum vitamin-B12 and for intrinsic factor antibody type I by means of hog intrinsic factor. *Acta Med Acad Sci Hung* 1980;**37**:157.

309. Chan JC, Liu HS, Kho BC, et al. Longitudinal study of Chinese patients with pernicious anaemia. *Postgrad Med J* 2008;**84**: 644.

310. Carmel R. Reassessment of the relative prevalences of antibodies to gastric parietal cell and to intrinsic factor in patients with pernicious anaemia: influence of patient age and race. *Clin Exp Immunol* 1992;**89**:74.

311. Carmel R. Ethnic and racial factors in cobalamin metabolism and its disorders. *Semin Hematol* 1999;**36**:88.

312. Carmel R, Green R, Jacobsen DW, Rasmussen K, Florea M, Azen C. Serum cobalamin, homocysteine, and methylmalonic acid concentrations in a multiethnic elderly population: ethnic and sex differences in cobalamin and metabolite abnormalities. *Am J Clin Nutr* 1999;**70**:904.

313. Strickland RG. The Sydney System: auto-immune gastritis. *J Gastroenterol Hepatol* 1991;**6**:238.

314. De Aizpurua HJ, Cosgrove LJ, Ungar B, Toh BH. Autoantibodies cytotoxic to gastric parietal cells in serum of patients with pernicious anaemia. *N Engl J Med* 1983;**309**:625.

315. De Block CE, Van Campenhout CM, De Leeuw IH, et al. Soluble transferrin receptor level: a new marker of iron deficiency anaemia, a common manifestation of gastric auto-immunity in type 1 diabetes. *Diabetes Care* 2000;**23**:1384.

316. Wangel AG, Schiller KF. Diagnostic significance of antibody to intrinsic factor. *BMJ* 1966;**1**:1274.

317. Doniach D, Roitt IM. An Evaluation of gastric and thyroid auto-immunity in relation to hematologic disorders. *Semin Hematol* 1964;**93**:313.

318. Munichoodappa C, Kozak GP. Diabetes mellitus and pernicious anaemia. *Diabetes* 1970;**19**:719.

319. Davis RE, McCann VJ, Stanton KG. Type 1 diabetes and latent pernicious anaemia. *Med J Aust* 1992;**156**:160.

320. Farnam J, Jorizzo JL, Grant JA, Lavastida MT, Ichikawa Y, Daniels JC. Sjogren's syndrome presenting with hypereosinophilia, lymphopenia and circulating immune complexes. *Clin Exp Rheumatol* 1984;**2**:41.

321. De Block CE, De Leeuw IH, Van Gaal LF. Auto-immune gastritis in type 1 diabetes: a clinically oriented review. *J Clin Endocrinol Metab* 2008;**93**:363.

322. Paul I, Reichard RR. Subacute combined degeneration mimicking traumatic spinal cord injury. *Am J Forensic Med Pathol* 2009;**30**:47.

323. Lewin KJ, Dowling F, Wright JP, Taylor KB. Gastric morphology and serum gastrin levels in pernicious anaemia. *Gut* 1976;**17**: 551.

324. Rubio CA. My approach to reporting a gastric biopsy. *J Clin Pathol* 2007;**60**:160.

325. Jhala NC, Montemor M, Jhala D, et al. Pancreatic acinar cell metaplasia in auto-immune gastritis. *Arch Pathol Lab Med* 2003;**127**:854.

326. Odgers RJ, Wangel AG. Abnormalities in IgA-containing mononuclear cells in the gastric lesion of pernicious anaemia. *Lancet* 1968;**ii**:846.

327. Chlumska A, Boudova L, Benes Z, Zamecnik M. Auto-immune gastritis. A clinicopathologic study of 25 cases. *Cesk Patol* 2005;**41**:137.

328. Sjoblom SM, Sipponen P, Karonen SL, Jarvinen HJ. Mucosal argyrophil endocrine cells in pernicious anaemia and upper gastrointestinal carcinoid tumours. *J Clin Pathol* 1989;**42**:371.

329. Kekki M, Samloff IM, Varis K, Ihamaki T. Serum pepsinogen I and serum gastrin in the screening of severe atrophic corpus gastritis. *Scand J Gastroenterol Suppl* 1991;**186**:109.

330. Carmel R. Pepsinogens and other serum markers in pernicious anaemia. *Am J Clin Pathol* 1988;**90**:442.

331. Appelmelk BJ, Faller G, Claeys D, Kirchner T, Vandenbroucke-Grauls CM. Bugs on trial: the case of *Helicobacter pylori* and auto-immunity. *Immunol Today* 1998;**19**:296.

332. Amedei A, Bergman MP, Appelmelk BJ, et al. Molecular mimicry between *Helicobacter pylori* antigens and H+, K+-adenosine triphosphatase in human gastric auto-immunity. *J Exp Med* 2003;**198**:1147.

333. Uibo R, Vorobjova T, Metskula K, Kisand K, Wadstrom T, Kivik T. Association of *Helicobacter pylori* and gastric auto-immunity: a population-based study. *FEMS Immunol Med Microbiol* 1995; **11**:65.

334. Vorobjova T, Faller G, Maaroos HI, et al. Significant increase in antigastric autoantibodies in a long-term follow-up study of H. pylori gastritis. *Virchows Arch* 2000;**437**:37.

335. Vorobjova T, Maaroos HI, Uibo R. Immune response to *Helicobacter pylori* and its association with the dynamics of chronic gastritis in the antrum and corpus. *APMIS* 2008;**116**:465.

336. Faller G, Winter M, Steininger H, et al. Release of antigastric autoantibodies in *Helicobacter pylori* gastritis after cure of infection. *Pathol Res Pract* 1999;**195**:243.

337. Masnou H, Domenech E, Navarro-Llavat M, et al. Pernicious anaemia in triplets. A case report and literature review. *Gastroenterol Hepatol* 2007;**30**:580.

338. Jacobson DL, Gange SJ, Rose NR, Graham NM. Epidemiology and estimated population burden of selected auto-immune dis-

eases in the United States. *Clin Immunol Immunopathol* 1997; **84**:223.

339. De Block CE, De Leeuw IH, Van Gaal LF. High prevalence of manifestations of gastric auto-immunity in parietal cell antibody-positive type 1 (insulin-dependent) diabetic patients. The Belgian Diabetes Registry. *J Clin Endocrinol Metab* 1999; **84**:4062.

340. Segni M, Borrelli O, Pucarelli I, Delle Fave G, Pasquino AM, Annibale B. Early manifestations of gastric auto-immunity in patients with juvenile auto-immune thyroid diseases. *J Clin Endocrinol* Metab 2004;**89**:4944.

341. Korbet SM, Corwin HL. Pernicious anaemia associated with systemic lupus erythematosus. *J Rheumatol* 1986;**13**:193.

342. Veijola LI, Oksanen AM, Sipponen PI, Rautelin HI. Association of auto-immune type atrophic corpus gastritis with *Helicobacter pylori* infection. *World J Gastroenterol* 2010;**16**:83.

343. Imagawa S, Yoshihara M, Ito M, et al. Evaluation of gastric cancer risk using topography of histological gastritis: a large-scaled cross-sectional study. *Dig Dis Sci* 2008;**53**:1818.

344. Meshkinpour H, Orlando RA, Arguello JF, DeMicco MP. Significance of endoscopically visible blood vessels as an index of atrophic gastritis. *Am J Gastroenterol* 1979;**71**:376.

345. Kokkola A, Sjoblom SM, Haapiainen R, Sipponen P, Puolakkainen P, Jarvinen H. The risk of gastric carcinoma and carcinoid tumours in patients with pernicious anaemia. A prospective follow-up study. *Scand J Gastroenterol* 1998;**33**:88.

346. Qvigstad G, Qvigstad T, Westre B, Sandvik AK, Brenna E, Waldum HL. Neuroendocrine differentiation in gastric adeno-carcinomas associated with severe hypergastrinemia and/or pernicious anaemia. *APMIS* 2002;**110**:132.

347. Modlin IM, Lye KD, Kidd M. A 50-year analysis of 562 gastric carcinoids: small tumour or larger problem? *Am J Gastroenterol* 2004;**99**:23.

348. Brinton LA, Gridley G, Hrubec Z, Hoover R, Fraumeni JF Jr. Cancer risk following pernicious anaemia. *Br J Cancer* 1989; **59**:810.

349. Hsing AW, Hansson LE, McLaughlin JK, et al. Pernicious anaemia and subsequent cancer. A population-based cohort study. *Cancer* 1993;**71**:745.

350. Stockbrugger RW, Menon GG, Beilby JO, Mason RR, Cotton PB. Gastroscopic screening in 80 patients with pernicious anaemia. *Gut* 1983;**24**:1141.

351. Borch K. Epidemiologic, clinicopathologic, and economic aspects of gastroscopic screening of patients with pernicious anaemia. *Scand J Gastroenterol* 1986;**21**:21.

352. Lillibridge CB, Brandborg LL, Rubin CE. Childhood pernicious anaemia. Gastrointestinal secretory, histological, and electron microscopic aspects. *Gastroenterology* 1967;**52**:792.

353. Benjamin B. Infantile form of pernicious anaemia: report of a long term study of a case. *Am J Dis Child* 1948;**75**:143.

354. Mollin DL, Baker SJ, Donlach I. Addisonian pernicious anaemia without gastric atrophy in a young man. *Br J Haematol* 1955;**1**: 278.

355. Imerslund O, Bjornstad P. Familial Vitamin B12 malabsorption. *Acta Haematol* 1963;**30**:1.

356. Siurala M. Gastric lesion in some megaloblastic anaemias: with special reference to the mucosal lesion in pernicious tapeworm anaemia. *Acta Med Scand Suppl* 1954;**299**:1.

357. Jevremovic D, Torbenson M, Murray JA, Burgart LJ, Abraham SC. Atrophic auto-immune pangastritis: A distinctive form of antral and fundic gastritis associated with systemic auto-immune disease. *Am J Surg Pathol* 2006;**30**:1412.

358. Mitomi H, Tanabe S, Igarashi M, et al. Auto-immune enteropathy with severe atrophic gastritis and colitis in an adult: pro-posal of a generalized auto-immune disorder of the alimentary tract. *Scand J Gastroenterol* 1998;**33**:716.

359. Strauss RJ, Friedman M, Platt N, Gassner W, Wise L. Gangrene of the stomach: a case of acute necrotizing gastritis. *Am J Surg* 1978;**135**:253.

360. Jung JH, Choi HJ, Yoo J, Kang SJ, Lee KY. Emphysematous gastritis associated with invasive gastric mucormycosis: a case report. *J Korean Med Sci* 2007;**22**:923.

361. Munroe CA, Chen A. Suppurative (phlegmonous) gastritis presenting as a gastric mass. *Dig Dis Sci* 2010;**55**:11.

362. Eliason E, Wright V. Phlegmonous gastritis. *Surg Clin North Am* 1938;**18**:1553.

363. Mittleman RE, Suarez RV. Phlegmonous gastritis associated with the acquired immunodeficiency syndrome/pre-acquired immunodeficiency syndrome. *Arch Pathol Lab Med* 1985;**109**: 765.

364. Zazzo JF, Troche G, Millat B, Aubert A, Bedossa P, Keros L. Phlegmonous gastritis associated with HIV-1 seroconversion. Endoscopic and microscopic evolution. *Dig Dis Sci* 1992;**37**: 1454.

365. Ross DA, Vincenti AC. Acute phlegmonous gastritis: a rare condition with a potentially common cause. *Br J Hosp Med* 1994; **52**:115.

366. LaForce FM. Diffuse phlegmonous gastritis. A rare complication of pneumococcal endocarditis. *Arch Intern Med* 1967; **120**:230.

367. Nevin NC, Eakins D, Clarke SD, Carson DJ. Acute phlegmonous gastritis. *Br J Surg* 1969;**56**:268.

368. Lifton LJ, Schlossberg D. Phlegmonous gastritis after endoscopic polypectomy. *Ann Intern Med* 1982;**97**:373.

369. O'Toole PA, Morris JA. Acute phlegmonous gastritis. *Postgrad Med J* 1988;**64**:315.

370. Miller AI, Smith B, Rogers AI. Phlegmonous gastritis. *Gastroenterology* 1975;**68**:231.

371. Mason EE. Gastrointestinal lesions occurring in uremia. *Ann Intern Med* 1952;**37**:96.

372. Franzin G, Musola R, Mencarelli R. Changes in the mucosa of the stomach and duodenum during immunosuppressive therapy after renal transplantation. *Histopathology* 1982;**6**:439.

373. Boyle JM, Johnston B. Acute upper gastrointestinal hemorrhage in patients with chronic renal disease. *Am J Med* 1983;**75**: 409.

374. Kang JY, Wu AY, Sutherland IH, Vathsala A. Prevalence of peptic ulcer in patients undergoing maintenance hemodialysis. *Dig Dis Sci* 1988;**33**:774.

375. Rank EL, Goldenberg SA, Hasson J, Cartun RW, Grey N. *Treponema pallidum* and *Helicobacter pylori* recovered in a case of chronic active gastritis. *Am J Clin Pathol* 1992;**97**:116.

376. McConnell JB, Stewart WK, Thjodleifsson B, Wormsley KG. Gastric function in chronic renal failure. Effects of maintenance haemodialysis. *Lancet* 1975;**ii**:1121.

377. Doherty CC. Gastric secretion in chronic uraemia and after renal transplantation. *Ir J Med Sci* 1980;**149**:5.

378. Cheli R, Dodero M. [Biopsy and secretion study of the gastric mucosa during chronic uremia]. *Acta Gastroenterol Belg* 1958;**21**: 193.

379. Jaspersen D, Fassbinder W, Heinkele P, et al. Significantly lower prevalence of *Helicobacter pylori* in uremic patients than in patients with normal renal function. *J Gastroenterol* 1995;**30**:585.

380. Wu TT, Hamilton SR. Lymphocytic gastritis: association with etiology and topology. *Am J Surg Pathol* 1999;**23**:153.

381. Dixon MF, Wyatt JI, Burke DA, Rathbone BJ. Lymphocytic gastritis – relationship to *Campylobacter pylori* infection. *J Pathol* 1988;**154**:125.

382. Wolber R, Owen D, DelBuono L, Appelman H, Freeman H. Lymphocytic gastritis in patients with coeliac sprue or sprue-like intestinal disease. *Gastroenterology* 1990;**98**:310.

383. Rutgeerts L, Stuer A, Vandenborre K, Ghillebert G, Tanghe W. Lymphocytic gastritis. Clinical and endoscopic presentation and long-term follow-up. *Acta Gastroenterol Belg* 1995;**58**:238.

384. Weinstein WM. Emerging gastritides. *Curr Gastroenterol Rep* 2001;**3**:523.

385. Haot J, Bogomoletz WV, Jouret A, Mainguet P. Menetrier's disease with lymphocytic gastritis: an unusual association with possible pathogenic implications. *Hum Pathol* 1991;**22**:379.

386. Haot J, Jouret A, Willette M, Gossuin A, Mainguet P. Lymphocytic gastritis – prospective study of its relationship with varioliform gastritis. *Gut* 1990;**31**:282.

387. Lambert R, Andre C, Moulinier B, Bugnon B. Diffuse varioliform gastritis. *Digestion* 1978;**17**:159.

388. Hayat M, Arora DS, Wyatt JI, O'Mahony S, Dixon MF. The pattern of involvement of the gastric mucosa in lymphocytic gastritis is predictive of the presence of duodenal pathology. *J Clin Pathol* 1999;**52**:815.

389. Amenomori M, Umemoto T, Kushima R, Hattori T. Spontaneous remission of hypertrophic lymphocytic gastritis associated with hypoproteinemia. *Intern Med* 1998;**37**:1019.

390. Shimoyama Y, Mukai M, Asato Y, Ochiai A. Clinical and endoscopic improvement of lymphocytic gastritis with eradication of *Helicobacter pylori*. *Gastrointest Endosc* 2001;**54**:251.

391. Hachem CY, El-Zimaity H. A man with rheumatoid arthritis and iron-deficiency anaemia. *MedGenMed* 2007;**9**:64.

392. Weiss AA, Yoshida EM, Poulin M, Gascoyne RD, Owen DA. Massive bleeding from multiple gastric ulcerations in a patient with lymphocytic gastritis and coeliac sprue. *J Clin Gastroenterol* 1997;**25**:354.

393. Haot J, Bogomoletz WV, Jouret A, Mainguet P. Menetrier's disease with lymphocytic gastritis: an unusual association with possible pathogenic implications. *Hum Pathol* 1991;**22**:379.

394. Wu T-T, Hamilton S. Lymphocytic gastritis: association with etiology and topology. *Am J Surg Pathol* 1999;**23**:153.

395. Griffiths AP, Wyatt J, Jack AS, Dixon MF. Lymphocytic gastritis, gastric adenocarcinoma, and primary gastric lymphoma. *J Clin Pathol* 1994;**47**:1123.

396. Wolfsen HC, Carpenter HA, Talley NJ. Menetrier's disease: a form of hypertrophic gastropathy or gastritis? *Gastroenterology* 1993;**104**:1310.

397. Clarke AC, Lee SP, Nicholson GI. Gastritis varioliformis. Chronic erosive gastritis with protein-losing gastropathy. *Am J Gastroenterol* 1977;**68**:599.

398. Hayat M, Arora DS, Dixon MF, Clark B, O'Mahony S. Effects of *Helicobacter pylori* eradication on the natural history of lymphocytic gastritis. *Gut* 1999;**45**:495.

399. Walker NI, Croese J, Clouston AD, Parry M, Loukas A, Prociv P. Eosinophilic enteritis in northeastern Australia. Pathology, association with Ancylostoma caninum, and implications. *Am J Surg Pathol* 1995;**19**:328.

400. Khan S, Orenstein SR. Eosinophilic gastroenteritis: epidemiology, diagnosis and management. *Paediatr Drugs* 2002;**4**:563.

401. Spergel JM, Beausoleil JL, Mascarenhas M, Liacouras CA. The use of skin prick tests and patch tests to identify causative foods in eosinophilic esophagitis. *J Allergy Clin Immunol* 2002;**109**:363.

402. Kelly KJ, Lazenby AJ, Rowe PC, Yardley JH, Perman JA, Sampson HA. Eosinophilic esophagitis attributed to gastroesophageal reflux: improvement with an amino acid-based formula. *Gastroenterology* 1995;**109**:1503.

403. Talley NJ, Shorter RG, Phillips SF, Zinsmeister AR. Eosinophilic gastroenteritis: a clinicopathological study of patients with disease of the mucosa, muscle layer, and subserosal tissues. *Gut* 1990;**31**:54.

404. Johnstone JM, Morson BC. Eosinophilic gastroenteritis. *Histopathology* 1978;**2**:335.

405. Harmon WA, Helman CA. Eosinophilic gastroenteritis and ascites. *J Clin Gastroenterol* 1981;**3**:371.

406. Leinbach GE, Rubin CE. Eosinophilic gastroenteritis: a simple reaction to food allergens? *Gastroenterology* 1970;**59**:874.

407. Klein NC, Hargrove RL, Sleisenger MH, Jeffries GH. Eosinophilic gastroenteritis. *Medicine (Baltimore)* 1970;**49**:299.

408. Blackshaw AJ, Levison DA. Eosinophilic infiltrates of the gastrointestinal tract. *J Clin Pathol* 1986;**39**:1.

409. Griscom NT, Kirkpatrick JA Jr, Girdany BR, Berdon WE, Grand RJ, Mackie GG. Gastric antral narrowing in chronic granulomatous disease of childhood. *Pediatrics* 1974;**54**:456.

410. Kirsch R, Geboes K, Shepherd NA, de Hertogh G, Di Nicola N, Lebel S, Mickys U, Riddell RH. Systemic mastocytosis involving the gastrointestinal tract: clinicopathologic and molecular study of five cases. *Mod Pathol* 2008;**21**:1508.

411. Colletti RB, Trainer TD. Collagenous gastritis. *Gastroenterology* 1989;**97**:1552.

412. Lagorce-Pages C, Fabiani B, Bouvier R, Scoazec JY, Durand L, Flejou JF. Collagenous gastritis: a report of six cases. *Am J Surg Pathol* 2001;**25**:1174.

413. Gopal P, McKenna BJ. The collagenous gastroenteritides: similarities and differences. *Arch Pathol Lab Med* 2010;**134**:1485.

414. Cote JF, Hankard GF, Faure C, et al. Collagenous gastritis revealed by severe anaemia in a child. *Hum Pathol* 1998;**29**:883.

415. Suskind D, Wahbeh G, Murray K, Christie D, Kapur RP. Collagenous gastritis, a new spectrum of disease in pediatric patients: two case reports. *Cases J* 2009;**2**:7511.

416. Leung ST, Chandan VS, Murray JA, Wu TT. Collagenous gastritis: histopathologic features and association with other gastrointestinal diseases. *Am J Surg Pathol* 2009;**33**:788.

417. Temmerman F, Baert F. Collagenous and lymphocytic colitis: systematic review and update of the literature. *Dig Dis* 2009;**27**(suppl 1):137.

418. Haesebrouck F, Pasmans F, Flahou B, et al. Gastric helicobacters in domestic animals and nonhuman primates and their significance for human health. *Clin Microbiol Rev* 2009;**22**:202.

419. McNulty CA, Dent JC, Curry A, et al. New spiral bacterium in gastric mucosa. *J Clin Pathol* 1989;**42**:585.

420. Heilmann KL, Borchard F. Gastritis due to spiral shaped bacteria other than *Helicobacter pylori*: clinical, histological, and ultrastructural findings. *Gut* 1991;**32**:137.

421. Mazzucchelli L, Wilder-Smith CH, Ruchti C, Meyer-Wyss B, Merki HS. Gastrospirillum hominis in asymptomatic, healthy individuals. *Dig Dis Sci* 1993;**38**:2087.

422. Debongnie JC, Donnay M, Mairesse J. Gastrospirillum hominis ('*Helicobacter heilmanii*'): a cause of gastritis, sometimes transient, better diagnosed by touch cytology? *Am J Gastroenterol* 1995;**90**:411.

423. Weber AF, Hasa O, Sautter JH. Some observations concerning the presence of spirilla in the fundic glands of dogs and cats. *Am J Vet Res* 1958;**19**:677.

424. Debongnie JC, Donnay M, Mairesse J, Lamy V, Dekoninck X, Ramdani B. Gastric ulcers and Helicobacter heilmannii. *Eur J Gastroenterol Hepatol* 1998;**10**:251.

425. Yang H, Li X, Xu Z, Zhou D. '*Helicobacter heilmannii*' infection in a patient with gastric cancer. *Dig Dis Sci* 1995;**40**:1013.

426. Lee A, Dent J, Hazell S, McNulty C. Origin of spiral organisms in human gastric antrum. *Lancet* 1988;**i**:300.

427. Dent JC, McNulty CA, Uff JC, Wilkinson SP, Gear MW. Spiral organisms in the gastric antrum. *Lancet* 1987;**ii**:96.

428. Dutz W, Saidi F, Kohout E. Gastric anthrax with massive ascites. *Gut* 1970;**11**:352.

429. El-Zimaity HM, Ramchatesingh J, Clarridge JE, Abudayyeh S, Osato MS, Graham DY. Enterococcus gastritis. *Hum Pathol* 2003;**34**:944.

430. Katzenstein AL, Maksem J. Candidal infection of gastric ulcers. Histology, incidence, and clinical significance. *Am J Clin Pathol* 1979;**71**:137.

431. Fidel PL, Jr., Vazquez JA, Sobel JD. Candida glabrata: review of epidemiology, pathogenesis, and clinical disease with comparison to C. albicans. *Clin Microbiol Rev* 1999;**12**:80.

432. Deal WB, Johnson JE. Gastric phycomycosis. Report of a case and review of the literature. *Gastroenterology* 1969;**57**:579.

433. Fisher JR, Sanowski RA. Disseminated histoplasmosis producing hypertrophic gastric folds. *Am J Dig Dis* 1978;**23**:282.

434. Orchard JL, Luparello F, Brunskill D. Malabsorption syndrome occurring in the course of disseminated histoplasmosis: case report and review of gastrointestinal histoplasmosis. *Am J Med* 1979;**66**:331.

435. Sanguino JC, Rodrigues B, Baptista A, Quina M. Focal lesion of African histoplasmosis presenting as a malignant gastric ulcer. *Hepatogastroenterology* 1996;**43**:771.

436. Bonacini M, Nussbaum J, Ahluwalia C. Gastrointestinal, hepatic, and pancreatic involvement with Cryptococcus neoformans in AIDS. *J Clin Gastroenterol* 1990;**12**:295.

437. Matsuda S, Urata Y, Shiota T, et al. Disseminated infection of Pneumocystis carinii in a patient with the acquired immunodeficiency syndrome. *Virchows Arch A Pathol Anat Histopathol* 1989;**414**:523.

438. Dieterich DT, Lew EA, Bacon DJ, Pearlman KI, Scholes JV. Gastrointestinal pneumocystosis in HIV-infected patients on aerosolized pentamidine: report of five cases and literature review. *Am J Gastroenterol* 1992;**87**:1763.

439. Guarda LA, Stein SA, Cleary KA, Ordonez NG. Human cryptosporidiosis in the acquired immune deficiency syndrome. *Arch Pathol Lab Med* 1983;**107**:562.

440. Rivasi F, Rossi P, Righi E, Pozio E. Gastric cryptosporidiosis: correlation between intensity of infection and histological alterations. *Histopathology* 1999;**34**:405.

441. Misra V, Misra SP, Dwivedi M, Singh PA. Giardia lamblia trophozoites in gastric biopsies. *Indian J Pathol Microbiol* 2006;**49**:519.

442. Oberhuber G, Kastner N, Stolte M. Giardiasis: a histologic analysis of 567 cases. *Scand J Gastroenterol* 1997;**32**:48.

443. Peraire J, Vidal F, ayo E, Razquin S, Richart C. Gastric toxoplasmosis in the acquired immunodeficiency syndrome. *Am J Gastroenterol* 1993;**88**:1464.

444. Grove DI. Human strongyloidiasis. *Adv Parasitol* 1996;**38**:251.

445. Yaldiz M, Hakverdi S, Aslan A, Temiz M, Culha G. Gastric infection with Strongyloides stercoralis: a case report. *Turk J Gastroenterol* 2009;**20**:48.

446. Davison AJ. Herpesvirus systematics. *Vet Microbiol* 2010;**143**:52.

447. Schmidt-Chanasit J, Sauerbrei A. Evolution and world-wide distribution of varicella-zoster virus clades. *Infect Genet Evol* 2011;**11**:1.

448. Ryan JL, Shen YJ, Morgan DR, Thorne LB, Kenney SC, Dominguez RL, Gulley ML. Epstein-Barr virus infection is common in inflamed gastrointestinal mucosa. *Dig Dis Sci* 2012;**57**:1887.

449. Arnar DO, Gudmundsson G, Theodors A, Valtysson G, Sigfusson A, Jonasson JG. Primary cytomegalovirus infection and gastric ulcers in normal host. *Dig Dis Sci* 1991;**36**:108.

450. Yoshinaga M, Nakate S, Motomura S, Sugimura T, Sasaki I, Tsuneyoshi M. Cytomegalovirus-associated gastric ulcerations in a normal host. *Am J Gastroenterol* 1994;**89**:448.

451. Francis ND, Boylston AW, Roberts AH, Parkin JM, Pinching AJ. Cytomegalovirus infection in gastrointestinal tracts of patients infected with HIV-1 or AIDS. *J Clin Pathol* 1989;**42**:1055.

452. Franzin G, Muolo A, Griminelli T. Cytomegalovirus inclusions in the gastroduodenal mucosa of patients after renal transplantation. *Gut* 1981;**22**:698.

453. Henson D. Cytomegalovirus inclusion bodies in the gastrointestinal tract. *Arch Pathol* 1972;**93**:477.

454. Megged O, Schlesinger Y. Cytomegalovirus-associated protein-losing gastropathy in childhood. *Eur J Pediatr* 2008;**167**:1217.

455. Roberts WH, Sneddon JM, Waldman J, Stephens RE. Cytomegalovirus infection of gastrointestinal endothelium demonstrated by simultaneous nucleic acid hybridization and immunohistochemistry. *Arch Pathol Lab Med* 1989;**113**:461.

456. Kakugawa Y, Kami M, Matsuda T, et al. Endoscopic diagnosis of cytomegalovirus gastritis after allogeneic hematopoietic stem cell transplantation. *World J Gastroenterol* 2010;**16**:2907.

457. Lagasse JP, Causse X, Legoux JL, Leyman P, Labarriere D, Brun H. Cytomegalovirus gastritis simulating cancer of the linitis plastica type on endoscopic ultrasonography. *Endoscopy* 1998;**30**:S101.

458. Varsky CG, Correa MC, Sarmiento N, et al. Prevalence and etiology of gastroduodenal ulcer in HIV-positive patients: a comparative study of 497 symptomatic subjects evaluated by endoscopy. *Am J Gastroenterol* 1998;**93**:935.

459. Strayer DS, Phillips GB, Barker KH, Winokur T, DeSchryver-Kecskemeti K. Gastric cytomegalovirus infection in bone marrow transplant patients: an indication of generalized disease. *Cancer* 1981;**48**:1478.

460. Aqel NM, Tanner P, Drury A, Francis ND, Henry K. Cytomegalovirus gastritis with perforation and gastrocolic fistula formation. *Histopathology* 1991;**18**:165.

461. Gazzard BG. HIV disease and the gastroenterologist. *Gut* 1988;**29**:1497.

462. Buss DH, Scharyj M. Herpes virus infection of the esophagus and other visceral organs in adults: incidence and clinical significance. *Am J Med* 1979;**66**:457.

463. Sperling HV, Reed WG. Herpetic gastritis. *Am J Dig Dis* 1977;**22**:1033.

464. Howiler W, Goldberg HI. Gastroesophageal involvement in herpes simplex. *Gastroenterology* 1976;**70**(5 Part 1):775.

465. Nelson AC, Crippin JS. Gastritis secondary to herpes simplex virus. *Am J Gastroenterol* 1997;**92**:2116.

466. Warren KG, Brown SM, Wroblewska Z, Gilden D, Koprowski H, Subak-Sharpe J. Isolation of latent herpes simplex virus from the superior cervical and vagus ganglions of human beings. *N Engl J Med* 1978;**298**:1068.

467. Rand KH, Berns KI, Rayfield MA. Recovery of herpes simplex type 1 from the coeliac ganglion after renal transplantation. *South Med J* 1984;**77**:403.

468. McCluggage WG, Fox JD, Baillie KE, Coyle PV, Jones FG, O'Hara MD. Varicella zoster gastritis in a bone marrow transplant recipient. *J Clin Pathol* 1994;**47**:1054.

469. Toll AD, Malik S, Tuluc M. Ulcerative gastritis secondary to Epstein-Barr viral infection. *Dig Dis Sci* 2010;**55**:218.

470. Gulley ML. Molecular diagnosis of Epstein-Barr virus-related diseases. *J Mol Diagn* 2001;**3**:1.

471. Ectors NL, Dixon MF, Geboes KJ, Rutgeerts PJ, Desmet VJ, Vantrappen GR. Granulomatous gastritis: a morphological and diagnostic approach. *Histopathology* 1993;**23**:55.

472. Shapiro JL, Goldblum JR, Petras RE. A clinicopathologic study of 42 patients with granulomatous gastritis. Is there really an

"idiopathic" granulomatous gastritis? *Am J Surg Pathol* 1996; **20**:462.

473. Maeng L, Lee A, Choi K, Kang CS, Kim KM. Granulomatous gastritis: a clinicopathologic analysis of 18 biopsy cases. *Am J Surg Pathol* 2004;**28**:941.

474. Silverberg MS, Satsangi J, Ahmad T, et al. Toward an integrated clinical, molecular and serological classification of inflammatory bowel disease: Report of a Working Party of the 2005 Montreal World Congress of Gastroenterology. *Can J Gastroenterol* 2005;**19**(suppl A):5.

475. Finder CA, Doman DB, Steinberg WM, Lewicki AM. Crohn's disease of the proximal stomach. *Am J Gastroenterol* 1984;**79**:494.

476. Wright CL, Riddell RH. Histology of the stomach and duodenum in Crohn's disease. *Am J Surg Pathol* 1998;**22**:383.

477. Ruuska T, Vaajalahti P, Arajarvi P, Maki M. Prospective evaluation of upper gastrointestinal mucosal lesions in children with ulcerative colitis and Crohn's disease. *J Pediatr Gastroenterol Nutr* 1994;**19**:181.

478. Lemberg DA, Clarkson CM, Bohane TD, Day AS. Role of esophagogastroduodenoscopy in the initial assessment of children with inflammatory bowel disease. *J Gastroenterol Hepatol* 2005;**20**:1696.

479. Tobin JM, Sinha B, Ramani P, Saleh AR, Murphy MS. Upper gastrointestinal mucosal disease in pediatric Crohn disease and ulcerative colitis: a blinded, controlled study. *J Pediatr Gastroenterol Nutr* 2001;**32**:443.

480. Palmer ED. Note on silent sarcoidosis of the gastric mucosa. *J Lab Clin Med* 1958;**52**:231.

481. Gould SR, Handley AJ, Barnardo DE. Rectal and gastric involvement in a case of sarcoidosis. *Gut* 1973;**14**:971.

482. Croxon S, Chen K, Davidson AR. Sarcoidosis of the stomach. *Digestion* 1987;**38**:193.

483. Afshar K, BoydKing A, Sharma OP, Shigemitsu H. Gastric sarcoidosis and review of the literature. *J Natl Med Assoc* 2010; **102**:419.

484. Marshall JB. Tuberculosis of the gastrointestinal tract and peritoneum. *Am J Gastroenterol* 1993;**88**:989.

485. Braun MM, Byers RH, Heyward WL, et al. Acquired immunodeficiency syndrome and extrapulmonary tuberculosis in the United States. *Arch Intern Med* 1990;**150**:1913.

486. Chazan BI, Aitchison JD. Gastric tuberculosis. *BMJ* 1960;**ii**:1288.

487. Tromba JL, Inglese R, Rieders B, Todaro R. Primary gastric tuberculosis presenting as pyloric outlet obstruction. *Am J Gastroenterol* 1991;**86**:1820.

488. Gupta B, Mathew S, Bhalla S. Pyloric obstruction due to gastric tuberculosis – an endoscopic diagnosis. *Postgrad Med J* 1990; **66**:63.

489. Subei I, Attar B, Schmitt G, Levendoglu H. Primary gastric tuberculosis: a case report and literature review. *Am J Gastroenterol* 1987;**82**:769.

490. Lau CF, Wong AM, Yee KS, Loo CK, Hui PK, Lam KM. A case of colonic tuberculosis mimicking Crohn's disease. *Hong Kong Med J* 1998;**4**:63.

491. Morin ME, Tan A. Diffuse enlargement of gastric folds as a manifestation of secondary syphilis. *Am J Gastroenterol* 1980;**74**:170.

492. Winters HA, Notar-Francesco V, Bromberg K, et al. Gastric syphilis: five recent cases and a review of the literature. *Ann Intern Med* 1992;**116**:314.

493. Mylona EE, Baraboutis IG, Papastamopoulos V, et al. Gastric syphilis: a systematic review of published cases of the last 50 years. *Sex Transm Dis* 2010;**37**:177.

494. Willeford G, Childers JH, Hepner WR Jr. Gumma of the stomach in congenital syphilis. *Pediatrics* 1952;**10**:162.

495. Neafie RC, Marty AM. Unusual infections in humans. *Clin Microbiol Rev* 1993;**6**:34.

496. Fyfe B, Poppiti RJ, Jr., Lubin J, Robinson MJ. Gastric syphilis. Primary diagnosis by gastric biopsy: report of four cases. *Arch Pathol Lab Med* 1993;**117**:820.

497. Inagaki H, Kawai T, Miyata M, Nagaya S, Tateyama H, Eimoto T. Gastric syphilis: polymerase chain reaction detection of treponemal DNA in pseudolymphomatous lesions. *Hum Pathol* 1996;**27**:761.

498. Sherman FE, Moran TJ. Granulomata of stomach. I. Response to injury of muscle and fibrous tissue of wall of human stomach. *Am J Clin Pathol* 1954;**24**:415.

499. Abraham SC, Yardley JH, Wu TT. Erosive injury to the upper gastrointestinal tract in patients receiving iron medication: an underrecognized entity. *Am J Surg Pathol* 1999;**23**:1241.

500. Sandmeier D, Bouzourene H. Does idiopathic granulomatous gastritis exist? *Histopathology* 2005;**46**:352.

501. Yamane T, Uchiyama K, Ishii T, et al. Isolated granulomatous gastritis showing discoloration of lesions after *Helicobacter pylori* eradication. *Dig Endosc* 2010;**22**:140.

502. Kliks MM. Anisakiasis in the western United States: four new case reports from California. *Am J Trop Med Hyg* 1983; **32**:526.

503. Sugimachi K, Inokuchi K, Ooiwa T, Fujino T, Ishii Y. Acute gastric anisakiasis. Analysis of 178 cases. *JAMA* 1985;**253**:1012.

504. Fontaine RE. Anisakiasis from the American perspective. *JAMA* 1985;**253**:1024.

505. Ectors N, Geboes K, Wynants P, Desmet V. Granulomatous gastritis and Whipple's disease. *Am J Gastroenterol* 1992;**87**:509.

506. Wada R, Yagihashi S, Konta R, Ueda T, Izumiyama T. Gastric polyposis caused by multifocal histiocytosis X. *Gut* 1992;**33**:994.

507. Groisman GM, Rosh JR, Harpaz N. Langerhans cell histiocytosis of the stomach. A cause of granulomatous gastritis and gastric polyposis. *Arch Pathol Lab Med* 1994;**118**:1232.

508. Washington K, Stenzel TT, Buckley RH, Gottfried MR. Gastrointestinal pathology in patients with common variable immunodeficiency and X-linked agammaglobulinemia. *Am J Surg Pathol* 1996;**20**:1240.

509. Greenson JK, Trinidad SB, Pfeil SA, et al. Gastric mucosal calcinosis. Calcified aluminium phosphate deposits secondary to containing-containing antacids or sucralfate therapy in organ transplant patients. *Am J Surg Pathol* 1993;**17**:45.

510. Abraham SC, Yardley JH, Wu TT. Erosive injury to the upper gastrointestinal tract in patients receiving iron medication: an under-recognised entity. *Am J Surg Pathol* 1999;**23**:1241.

511. Marginean EC, Bennick M, Cyczk J, et al. Gastric siderosis: patterns and significance. *Am J Surg Pathol* 2006;**30**:514.

512. Iacobuzio-Donahue CA, Lee EL, Abraham SC, et al. Colchicine toxicity: distinct morphologic findings in gastrointestinal biopsies. *Am J Surg Pathol* 2001;**25**:1067.

513. Doria MI Jr, Doria LK, Faintuch J, et al. Gastric mucosal injury after hepatic arterial infusion chemotherapy with floxuridine. A clinical and pathologic study. *Cancer* 1994;**73**:2042.

514. Choi HY, Takeda M. Gastric epithelial atypia following hepatic arterial infusion chemotherapy. *Diagnos Cytopathol* 1985;**1**:241.

515. Petras RE, Hart WR, Bukowski RM. Gastric epithelial atypiaassociated with hepatic arterial infusion chemotherapy. Its distinction from early gastric carcinoma. *Cancer* 1985;**56**:745.

516. Doig RK, Funder JF, Weiden S. Serial gastric biopsy studies in a case of duodenal ulcer treated by deep x-ray therapy. *Med J Aust* 1951;**1**:828.

517. Goldgraber MB, Rubin CE, Palmer WL, Dobson RL, Massey BW. The early gastric response to irradiation; a serial biopsy study. *Gastroenterology* 1954;**27**:1.

518. Wood IJ, Ralston M, Kurrle GR. Irradiation injury to the gastro-intestinal tract: clinical features, management and pathogenesis. *Australas Ann Med* 1963;**12**:143.

519. Sell A, Jensen TS. Acute gastric ulcers induced by radiation. *Acta Radiol Ther Phys Biol* 1966;**4**:289.

520. Novak JM, Collins JT, Donowitz M, et al. Effects of radiation on the human gastrointestinal tract. *J Clin Gastroenterol* 1979;**1**:9.

521. Berthrong M, Fajardo LF. Radiation injury in surgical pathology. Part II. Alimentary tract. *Am J Surg Pathol* 1981;**5**:153.

522. Berthrong M. Pathologic changes secondary to radiation. *World J Surg* 1986;**10**:155.

523. Ogawa F, Mino-Kenudson M, Shimizu M, et al. Gastroduodenitis associated with yttrium 90-microsphere selective internal radiation: an iatrogenic complication in need of recognition. *Arch Pathol Lab Med* 2008;**132**:1734.

524. Bayerdorffer E, Ritter MM, Hatz R, Brooks W, Ruckdeschel G, Stolte M. Healing of protein losing hypertrophic gastropathy by eradication of *Helicobacter pylori* – is *Helicobacter pylori* a pathogenic factor in Menetrier's disease? *Gut* 1994;**35**:701.

525. Murayama Y, Miyagawa J, Shinomura Y, et al. Morphological and functional restoration of parietal cells in *Helicobacter pylori* associated enlarged fold gastritis after eradication. *Gut* 1999; **45**:653.

526. Komorowski RA, Caya JG. Hyperplastic gastropathy. Clinicopathologic correlation. *Am J Surg Pathol* 1991;**15**:577.

CHAPTER 12

Polyps and tumour-like lesions of the stomach

Muriel Genevay[1] and Gregory Y. Lauwers[2]

[1]Service of Clinical Pathology, University Hospitals of Geneva, Geneva, Switzerland
[2]Massachusetts General Hospital; Harvard Medical School, Boston, MA, USA

As most gastric polyps are asymptomatic, they are usually discovered incidentally during an upper endoscopy performed for unrelated reasons. A wide variety of lesions may present as gastric polyps. In many cases, few or no clinical details accompany the specimens. To render a correct diagnosis, the pathologist must first be fully aware of the various entities that may be encountered. Furthermore, the prevalence of gastric polyps has shifted over the years and depends on geographical location. Although some types of polyps may have a somewhat typical appearance at endoscopy, histological assessment remains the only way to determine the type with certainty and confirm, or more likely exclude, the presence of neoplasia.

Epidemiology

The epidemiology of gastric polyps is variable, depending not only on the period of time during which the data were collected but also on the geographical origin of the studies, which in turn is an indication of the prevalence of underlying gastric conditions, such as *Helicobacter pylori* infection. Also, as endoscopy is largely unable to identify a specific diagnosis, only pathology-based series are appropriate to determine the relative frequency of the various types.

Important geographical differences exist in the prevalence of gastric polyps. A retrospective review of 13 000 endoscopies performed in Greece in 1996 yielded 258 gastric polyps (1.2%) [1]. About a third of the patients had more than one polyp and 75.6% had hyperplastic polyps. A large, pathology-based, German study analysed 5515 gastric polyps collected between 1969 and 1989, and found

47% of the lesions to be fundic gland polyps (FGPs) and 28.3% hyperplastic polyps. In the same series, neoplastic polyps, namely gastric adenomas and adenocarcinomas, represented 9% and 7.2% of the polyps, respectively [2]. In 2009, Carmack and colleagues evaluated all gastric polyps obtained over a 12-month period in the USA. In approximately 200 000 patients who underwent an upper endoscopy, 8000 gastric polyps were examined from 7500 patients, with an overall gastric polyp prevalence of 3.75%. In this population, with a 12.3% confirmed prevalence rate of *H. pylori* infection, most gastric polyps were FGPs (77.2%), 14.4% were hyperplastic polyps and only 0.7% were gastric adenomas [3].

Classification of gastric polyps

In the simplest scheme, gastric polyps can be divided into neoplastic and non-neoplastic categories. However, a more practical classification relies on assigning the histogenesis of the polyp first, followed by assessment for neoplastic potential. This classification is summarised in Table 12.1.

Epithelial polyps

Epithelial polyps are the most prevalent type of gastric polyps. These can be further subdivided into non-neoplastic hyperplastic polyps (and variants) and neoplastic polyps, which include adenomas that by definition exhibit dysplasia and carcinoid which are discussed in Chapter 13. Fundic gland (cyst) polyps have traditionally been regarded as

Morson and Dawson's Gastrointestinal Pathology, Fifth Edition. Edited by Neil A. Shepherd, Bryan F. Warren, Geraint T. Williams, Joel K. Greenson, Gregory Y. Lauwers and Marco R. Novelli.

Table 12.1 Classification of gastric polyps

General category	Subtype	Usual location	Malignant potential
Epithelial			
Hyperplastic/inflammatory	Hyperplastic (and variants)	Antrum and lower body	Low[a]
Hamartomatous	Peutz–Jeghers		Low
	Juvenile		Low[a]
	Cowden		Unknown
Neoplastic	Fundic gland polyp	Body fundus	Low[b]
	Polypoid dysplasia (adenoma)	Antrum and body fundus	High
	Neuro-endocrine tumor	Body fundus	Low to moderate
Mesenchymal			
	Inflammatory fibroid polyp	Antrum	None
	Others[c]		
Miscellaneous			
	Cronkhite–Canada		Unknown
	Xanthoma		None
	Gastric heterotopic pancreas		Very low

[a]The risk increases with the size of the polyp.
[b]The risk is higher in syndromic polyps than in sporadic lesions.
[c]These include: gastrointestinal stromal tumour (GIST), smooth muscle tumour, glomus tumour, inflammatory myofibroblastic tumour, lipoma (covered in Chapter 14).

hamartomatous lesions but increasing evidence suggests that they may be neoplastic. Consideration should also be given to early gastric cancers and metastatic tumours, both of which can present as polypoid lesions.

Non-epithelial polyps

The various mesenchymal and stromal elements of the stomach can give rise to nodular proliferations and tumours that manifest endoscopically as 'polyps'. This heterogeneous category comprises spindle cell lesions for which immunohistochemistry is frequently required to establish the final diagnosis. Several entities should be considered in the differential diagnosis of a gastric spindle cell lesion, including inflammatory fibroid polyp (IFP), gastrointestinal stromal tumour (GIST) and inflammatory myofibroblastic tumour (IMT). Less common lesions include nerve sheath tumours such as schwannomas, ganglioneuromas and smooth muscle tumours. Although only IFPs are discussed further here, the interested reader is referred to Chapter 14 for a discussion on GISTs, IMTs and other mesenchymal tumorous lesions.

Fundic gland polyps

Also known as fundic gland cyst polyps, the prevalence of FGPs, which has been reported as ranging from 0.8% to 1.9% of patients, has been seen to increase in the last 10 years, with rates of 3.2% [4,5] to 11% [6] of patients. Today,

they are in fact the most common polyps detected by endoscopists [7] and represent as many as 50% of resected gastric polyps [8].

FGPs fall into two categories based on the clinical circumstances: sporadic cases and syndromic cases that develop in the context of familial adenomatous polyposis (FAP). These subtypes are morphologically similar but differ in demographic distribution, somewhat with regard to associated molecular alterations and definitely in the risk of neoplastic transformation.

Sporadic FGPs are classically reported in middle-aged, predominantly female, patients [4,9]. However, the gender difference has not been uniformly detected, possibly due to the generalised use of proton pump inhibitors (PPIs) [8]. In FAP patients, the prevalence of FGP is much higher than in sporadic cases, up to 88% in some reports [10]. FGPs also occur at a younger age and are equally likely to develop in both genders [10,11]. The demographic features of FGP patients with attenuated forms of FAP are similar.

FGPs are usually completely asymptomatic and discovered in the context of upper endoscopy performed during exploration of gastro-oesophageal reflux disease [4,8,12], which probably explains the high frequency of PPI therapy in these patients [8]. They develop exclusively in the acid-secreting gastric mucosa of the body and corpus. They are small (2–5 mm), rounded, sessile lesions that are covered by benign-looking mucosa. These easily recognisable endoscopic features have led some authors to advise against biopsies when these lesions are observed [7]. FGPs can be single but tend to be multiple. In sporadic cases, there are usually <10 polyps, compared with >50 polyps in syndromic cases, where they may also be confluent and coalesce. The term 'fundic gland polyposis' has been used in that setting. 'Giant' FGPs measuring as much as 80 mm in diameter have been reported [13].

Syndromic and sporadic FGPs, whether or not associated with PPIs, are virtually histologically indistinguishable [9]. They are characterised by cystically dilated oxyntic glands lined by compressed parietal cells, chief cells and mucous neck epithelium. This cystic component is covered by a normal-looking foveolar component (Figures 12.1 and 12.2). Parietal cell hyperplasia, a known consequence of PPI therapy [12,14], characteristically presenting as a protrusion of the parietal cells into the lumen, is commonly noted at the periphery of FGPs associated with PPI therapy. Early in the development of autoimmune atrophic gastritis,

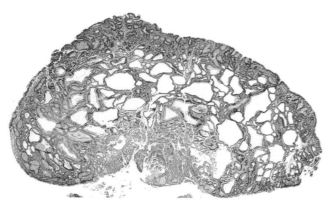

Figure 12.1 Fundic gland polyp: low-power view showing characteristic cystically dilated oxyntic glands.

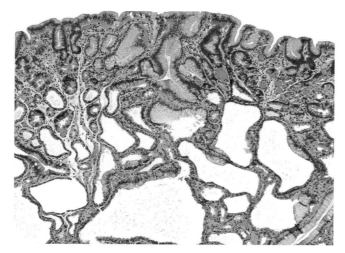

Figure 12.2 Fundic gland polyp: the dilated oxyntic glands are lined by flattened parietal and chief cells. The dilatation reaches the foveolar region, as noted by the lining mucinous foveolar type cells.

patches of preserved oxyntic epithelium, between atrophic mucosa, may result in the development of pseudo-polyps, which can be misinterpreted as FGP by unwary observers. However, cystic glandular elements are absent [15].

Both subtypes of FGPs develop in an otherwise normal gastric mucosa and demonstrate a negative association with *Helicobacter pylori* infection [8–10,16]. This is further supported by reports of the disappearance of FGPs with *H. pylori* infection and their subsequent recurrence after bacterial eradication [17]. This may be due to the action of *H. pylori* on stem cells located in the isthmus of the fundic glands which can differentiate into glandular or foveolar cell lineages [17].

The role of PPIs in the development of FGPs has been debated but evidence supports PPIs being truly implicated in their genesis in a time- and dose-dependent manner [6,9]. Some have even reported that FGPs can regress after the cessation of PPI therapy, confirming its role in FGP development [18]. The fact that the duration of the prescription influences the probability of developing FGP may explain why some have failed to prove a causative role for PPIs [18]. Nevertheless, it may be hypothesised that impairment of acid secretion leads to cystic dilatation of oxyntic glands.

Various immunohistochemical studies have been used to investigate the pathogenesis of FGPs. They are diffusely positive for cytokeratin 7, a marker of de-differentiation [19], typically absent in normal gastric epithelium. They also exhibit a loss of tuberin nuclear expression, which is aberrantly accumulated in cytoplasmic granules with loss of glucocorticoid receptors [20]. The resulting dysregulation in transcriptional activity has been suggested as playing an important role in the development of FGPs [20].

The apparent neoplastic nature of FGPs, for a long time considered to be hamartomatous or hyperplastic in nature, has been revealed by recent molecular analysis [21]. The mechanisms associated with syndromic and sporadic FGPs differ. However, the Wnt signalling pathway is implicated in both, which may explain their morphological similarities. FAP-associated FGPs present with a somatic second-hit mutation of the *APC* gene, which leads to inactivation of both copies of the tumour suppressor gene. This mutation is found in the glandular component as well as in the normal-looking epithelium overlying the cyst [22,23]. This mutation is observed in up to 75% of patients [22,23], independently of the presence of dysplasia [22]. Conversely, sporadic cases are devoid of APC mutations [22,23] and a mutation in the β-catenin gene is noted in 65–91% of cases [21,23]. In this situation, the surrounding gastric mucosa presents a normal molecular profile [21,23]. Notably, when multiple polyps in the same patient are analysed, they reveal different β-catenin mutations, confirming the somatic nature of this mutation [21,23,24]. However, immunohistochemical studies fail to demonstrate a significant accumu-

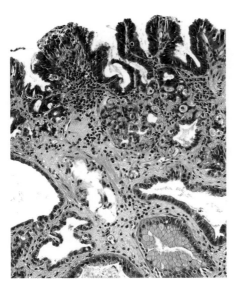

Figure 12.3 Fundic gland polyp with dysplastic transformation involving the surface epithelium.

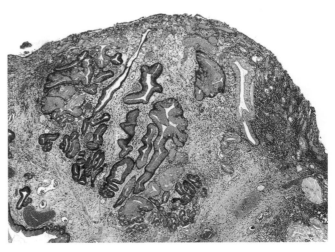

Figure 12.4 Hyperplastic polyp: the polyp is composed of elongated and distorted foveolae within an expanded oedematous and inflamed stroma. As in this case, the surface of hyperplastic polyps frequently is ulcerated.

lation of β-catenin in those cells [21,23]. Methylation of the promoter region of genes p16 and p14, which are classically associated with gastric cancer, has also been observed in a small proportion of FGPs [25]. Interestingly, rare cases of sporadic dysplastic FGP harbour *APC* mutations similar to those observed in syndromic cases, while being negative for β-catenin gene mutations [26,27].

The two pathways may explain the differences in the clinical behaviour of the two subtypes of FGPs. Rare cases of dysplastic sporadic FGPs have been reported [8,27–29], although dysplasia occurs more frequently in FAP patients, with a reported prevalence varying from 25% to 46% [9] (Figure 12.3). In most instances, low grade dysplasia is observed [10], whereas only rare cases of high grade dysplasia are on record [28–30]. Association with gastric cancer is even rarer. The risk of developing dysplasia in syndromic FGP seems to correlate with increased severity of duodenal polyposis, larger polyp size [31] and the presence of antral gastritis [10]. As a result of a report of a higher frequency of colonic adenoma in patients with FGP [11], some authors have recommended that a colonoscopy be performed when FGPs are diagnosed [11,29]. A recent study by Genta et al. confirmed an association between FGPs and colonic adenomas, most commonly for female patients [8].

Hyperplastic polyps

Hyperplastic polyps were once often described as the most common type of gastric polyp, with reported frequencies ranging from 50% to 90% [32–34]. However, a recent study of 8000 gastric polyps found that only 14% of them were hyperplastic [3]. The change reflects increasing rates of PPI

prescription and the simultaneous decrease in the prevalence of *H. pylori* infection [35].

The demographics of hyperplastic polyps are variable. If in most studies a female predominance is reported [21], in others there is a 1:1 sex ratio [36], whereas in others still a male predominance has been noted [35]. Hyperplastic polyps arise in adults (mean age 60 years) and multiple polyps are found in up to 20% of all cases [21].

Most hyperplastic polyps are asymptomatic, but, in some cases, larger, eroded lesions are associated with blood loss and iron deficiency anaemia or abdominal pain [21,37]. Gastric outlet obstruction has also been described for large polyps developing in the antrum and protruding into the duodenal lumen [38,39].

Macroscopically, most hyperplastic polyps are round, sessile lesions which, only after reaching 20 mm, become pedunculated with a lobulated, frequently eroded surface (Figure 12.4). They are typically small, measuring between 5 and 15 mm. Histologically, they consist of hyperplastic and elongated foveolae set in an abundant stroma. Foveolar intraluminal infolding and branching is common (Figure 12.5). Cystic dilatation of the pits is present almost invariably in the deeper parts of the polyp [40]. Sparse, thin bundles of smooth muscle fibres are seen frequently and a variably oedematous lamina propria is infiltrated by both plasma cells and lymphocytes. Lymphoid aggregates with germinal centres may be present.

The lining epithelium consists of a single layer of regularly arranged, usually hypertrophied foveolar epithelium containing abundant neutral mucin. Cuboidal cells with a granular eosinophilic cytoplasm may be observed focally [41,42]. Small groups of pyloric-type glands can be found

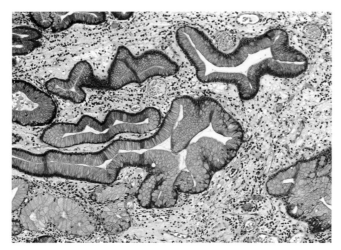

Figure 12.5 Hyperplastic polyp: higher-power view of elongated and branching foveolae lined by a single layer of foveolar mucinous cells and embedded in a vascular and oedematous stroma.

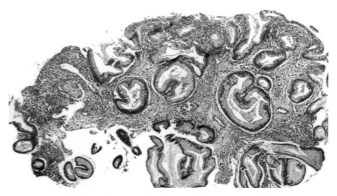

Figure 12.6 Polypoid foveolar hyperplasia: this small lesion measuring about 1 mm in size is regarded as a precursor of hyperplastic polyps. It is composed of inflamed oedematous stroma and exhibits simple elongation of the pit regions without cyst formation.

beneath the proliferating foveolae. Parietal and chief cells are uncommon, even in polyps found in the body mucosa. Focal intestinal metaplasia can occur and, when present, is usually of incomplete type [21,36].

The surface of large hyperplastic polyps frequently is eroded and a cap of fibrinopurulent exudate is commonly produced. Reactive cuboidal atypical epithelium cells with mucin depletion and high nuclear:cytoplasmic ratio may be present, usually associated with acute inflammatory cells and proliferating capillaries. In these areas, mitotically active, bizarre-appearing, reactive stromal cells with hyperchromatic nuclei and prominent nucleoli may be observed, similar to those associated with ulceration at other sites in the gastrointestinal tract [43]. If performed, immunohistochemical studies will reveal increased Ki-67 [36], cyclooxygenase 2 (COX-2) and p21 expression, all consistent with important cellular turnover [36,44,45]. These epithelial and stromal changes should not be construed as evidence of malignancy. The association with acute inflammation and the seamless transition with adjacent surrounding epithelium help in making the appropriate benign diagnosis.

As gastric hyperplastic polyps arise as a hyperproliferative foveolar response to mucosal injury or a chronic inflammatory state, an examination of the surrounding mucosa is necessary [46,47]. Chronic inflammation, observed in 85% of patients, is commonly related to two aetiologies: autoimmune gastritis and *H. pylori*-associated gastritis [48,49]. The risk of developing hyperplastic polyps increases with the severity of gastric mucosal atrophy, especially when it involves the gastric corpus [50]. The role of *H. pylori* infection in the genesis of these polyps is clearly demonstrated by the tendency of gastric hyperplastic polyps to disappear

or regress after *H. pylori* eradication and to reappear on reinfection [51,52]. The development of hyperplastic polyps in the setting of atrophic gastritis could be secondary to the production of gastrin and tumour necrosis factor α (TNF-α), two well-known proliferating factors [50]. A fall in somatostatin levels consequent on a decrease in the number of D-cells resulting from atrophy may also play a role [52]. Solid organ transplantation has been reported as a rare but clear risk factor, with as many as 15% of hyperplastic polyps arising in transplant recipients [53,54]. Finally, post-antrectomy stomachs are also a well-described risk factor.

Variants of hyperplastic polyps

Polypoid foveolar hyperplasia is regarded as a precursor lesion to hyperplastic polyps and is also aetiologically related to chronic mucosal injury. It is commonly noted at the edges of ulcers or erosions. Polypoid foveolar hyperplasia measures 1–2 mm thick and exhibits simple hyperplasia of the gastric foveolae without cystic change and gland distortion (Figure 12.6).

Less common types of hyperplastic polyps have been reported [55]. These include the so-called inverted hyperplastic polyps. This variant is caused by a dense submucosal glandular proliferation with cystic dilatation, covered by a normal-appearing mucosa. Such polyps may be secondary to an injury of the muscularis mucosae, resulting in entrapped gastric glands [56]. They may or may not be associated with gastritis cystica profunda [56] and cancer development [57].

True hyperplastic polyposis of the stomach (the presence of 50 or more hyperplastic polyps) has been described but remains a very rare event. A putative association between hyperplastic polyposis and colorectal cancer has also been

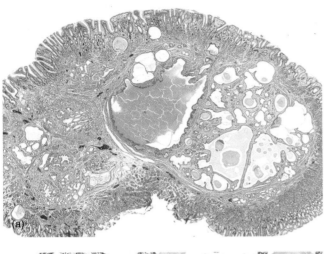

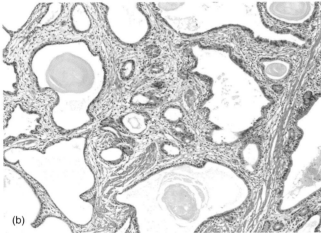

Figure 12.7 Gastritis cystica polyposa: (a) this dome-shaped lesion is formed by epithelial submucosal misplacement with cystic dilatation. (b) The foveolar lining shows a bland morphology devoid of mitotic activity.

suggested [58,59]. Gastritis cystica polyposa/profunda is defined as a hyperplastic polyp showing epithelial misplacement in the muscularis mucosae or more deeply in the submucosa or muscularis propria. It is probably the result of trauma-induced entrapment of glands in the deeper compartments of the gastric wall (frequently seen in post-Billroth I and II gastric stumps). The term 'polyposa' is used when the lesion is mainly intraluminal. 'Gastritis cystica profunda' is the preferred term when most of the lesion is intramural (Figure 12.7a). The main differential diagnosis with these lesions is a well differentiated adenocarcinoma. Bland cytology, absent mitotic activity and a lack of desmoplasia serve as indicators of benign misplaced epithelium (Figure 12.7b).

A recently described variant, termed 'gastric mucosal prolapse polyps', is distinguished by basal glandular ele-

ments, hypertrophic muscle fibres ascending perpendicularly from the muscularis mucosae and thick-walled blood vessels (Figure 12.8). These polyps are more commonly sessile than the typical hyperplastic polyp. The predominantly antral location of gastric mucosal prolapse polyps, in a zone of pronounced peristalsis, suggests that mucosal prolapse plays a role in the development of these polyps [60].

The two main differential diagnoses of gastric hyperplastic polyps are hamartomatous polyps and Ménétrier's disease. The latter diagnosis cannot be made based on histology alone; endoscopic correlation must be made [21]. However, in such cases, the gastric lamina propria is generally devoid of inflammation, which is a frequent feature of gastric hyperplastic polyps. Hamartomatous polyps are generally associated with systemic syndromes such as Cowden's syndrome, Peutz–Jeghers syndrome, juvenile polyposis and Cronkhite–Canada syndrome. Their morphological aspect, characterised by highly dilated glands and ascending smooth muscle fibres, presenting a villous appearance, differs from that of hyperplastic polyps.

Although gastric hyperplastic polyps are benign lesions, dysplastic transformation has been reported in 2–3.3% [36,61] of cases. This may evolve to gastric adenocarcinoma in a small number of cases, with a mean frequency of 2%. Most of the resulting cancers are well differentiated gastric adenocarcinomas but rare cases of signet ring cell carcinoma [62] or papillary carcinoma [63] have been reported. The risk of malignant transformation of these polyps correlates with the size of the polyp [36]. As neoplastic transformation is usually focal within the polyp, it may be missed at endoscopic examination. As a consequence, some authors recommend removing every polyp measuring >20 mm [64]. If dysplasia is observed in a hyperplastic

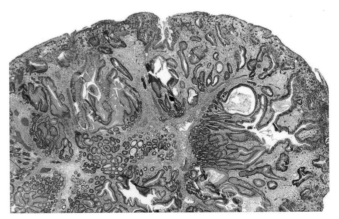

Figure 12.8 Gastric prolapse polyp: this lesion is characterised by thickened and splayed bundles of smooth muscle dissecting toward the mucosa. In other instances, cystic dilatation can be marked. Antral dyskinesia is believed to play a role in the genesis of this polyp.

polyp, it should be considered as a high-risk lesion with a high potential for evolution [65]. Furthermore, as hyperplastic polyps are associated with gastric atrophy and intestinal metaplasia, two well-known risk factors for gastric cancer [49], they should be considered as a surrogate marker for cancer elsewhere in the stomach. Indeed, associated synchronous or metachronous gastric cancer has been reported in 4–6% of cases.

Molecular studies of hyperplastic polyps are limited. Of the two genetic modifications associated with gastric cancer, p53 mutations have been frequently identified in dysplastic or malignant foci of gastric hyperplastic polyps but less commonly *K-ras* mutations [36,65,66]. *H. pylori* eradication may avoid malignant transformation of both gastric mucosa and hyperplastic polyps. In practice, patients with hyperplastic polyps and extensive atrophy and intestinal metaplasia of the surrounding mucosa should be considered at high risk for gastric cancer and should therefore benefit from watchful follow-up.

Adenoma

Gastric adenomas are polypoid lesions composed of tubular and/or villous structures lined by dysplastic epithelium [67,68]. They occur spontaneously or in the context of FAP. We favour using the terms 'polypoid dysplasia' and 'adenoma' interchangeably, regardless of the quality of the surrounding mucosa. The prevalence of gastric adenomas is reported between 0.65% and 3.75% in western countries and 9–27% in Asia, where there is a higher incidence of gastric cancer [2,33,41].

Most adenomas are solitary, exophytic lesions, which can be sessile or pedunculated. They usually measure <20 mm. The risk of malignancy is related to size, grade of dysplasia and villous growth pattern. Larger adenomas are more frequently associated with a component of high grade dysplasia and a significant proportion contain foci of malignant transformation, with an incidence of 40–50% for lesions measuring >20 mm, although even small lesions can contain carcinomatous foci [67,68] (see Chapter 13).

Polyps developing in the setting of polyposis

Polyposis syndromes affect the stomach only rarely and patients usually manifest symptoms unrelated to gastric polyps. However, some cases of juvenile polyposis may affect the stomach alone [69,70]. The hamartomatous polyps detected in juvenile polyposis, Cronkhite–Canada syndrome and Cowden's disease overlap with the histology of hyperplastic polyps, so the diagnosis of a syndromic polyp must rely on a high index of suspicion when polyps are multiple and/or there is an appropriate clinical context [71, 72]. In contrast, gastric polyps detected in patients with Peutz–Jeghers syndrome can be distinguished on the basis of their characteristic morphological features alone.

Juvenile polyps and polyposis

Juvenile polyposis (JP) is a rare (1/100 000) autosomal dominant disease with variable penetrance characterised by the presence of multiple hamartomatous polyps throughout the gut and associated with an increased risk of cancer [73]. One of the following clinical criteria must be met: (1) the presence of at least five juvenile polyps in the colon; (2) the presence of juvenile polyps throughout the gut; or (3) the presence of single or multiple juvenile polyps in a patient with an established family history of JP [74]. The classic belief that the polyps are predominantly located in the colon may be biased by the fact that, until recently, upper gastrointestinal (GI) tract endoscopic screening was performed relatively rarely [75].

Germline mutations of *SMAD4* and *BMPR1A*, two genes that are implicated in the TGFβ-signalling pathway, are the molecular abnormalities most commonly encountered in juvenile polyposis. Each represents about 20% of the genetic alterations detected [73]. Germline mutations of *SMAD4* seem to be associated with a preponderance of gastric polyps [73,76,77] but this genotypic–phenotypic association remains controversial [78]. Some cases of JP have been reported in association with a mutation in the *ENG* gene which is also implicated in the transforming growth factor β (TGF-β)-signalling pathway. In patients with *ENG* mutations, the symptoms of JP develop early in childhood [79].

Juvenile polyps are said to be hamartomatous lesions. They are most often observed in children and young adults. Although usually detected in the colon, they can be seen in the stomach as well. Although gastric juvenile polyps are reported more frequently in the antrum [80], they also have been described in the body and fundus [77,78]. Rare cases of pyloric obstruction due to large antral polyps have been reported [78,81]. When multiple, they can be associated with iron deficiency anaemia [75,78,81] and hypoproteinaemia [75,78,81].

Gastric juvenile polyps are rounded and sessile when small but become pedunculated with a lobular appearance as they enlarge [81,82]. Histologically, they look like their colonic counterparts, composed of a prominent oedematous stroma with an inflammatory cell infiltrate and containing cystically dilated glandular and foveolar elements. The glands are lined with benign-appearing epithelium and filled with mucin. Smooth muscle fibres are not observed in the lamina propria. However, these polyps are often difficult to distinguish from hyperplastic polyps. (Figure 12.9).

Despite the 'hamartomatous' nature of the polyps, patients with JP have a higher risk of developing cancer than the general population, with as many as 38% and

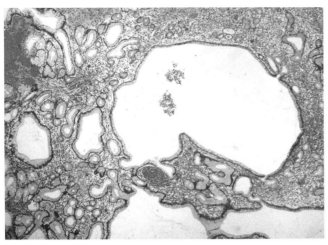

Figure 12.9 Juvenile polyp: the lesion is composed of cystically dilated glandular and foveolar elements lined with benign-appearing epithelium set in a prominent oedematous stroma. Without the benefit of clinical information, this lesion can be easily misdiagnosed as a hyperplastic polyp.

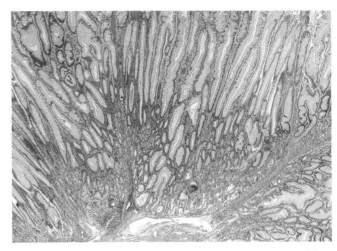

Figure 12.10 Peutz–Jeghers polyp: the lesion is characterised by thin dissecting bands of smooth muscle covered by disorganised foveolae with no cystic changes.

21% of patients developing colorectal and gastric cancer, respectively [75]. Neoplasia seems to develop as part of a dysplasia–carcinoma sequence, with the risk of cancer increasing with the size of the polyps [82]. This propensity to develop cancer justifies follow-up with screening GI endoscopic procedures [75].

Peutz–Jeghers syndrome

Although solitary Peutz–Jeghers polyps are described, they are rare [83,84], and most Peutz–Jeghers polyps are seen in the context of a patient with Peutz–Jeghers syndrome (PJS). This autosomal dominant syndrome is associated with the development of hamartomatous GI polyps, perioral pigmentation and an increased risk of cancer. In 80% of cases, it is caused by a germline mutation of the *STK11/LKB1* gene [85] and its prevalence is estimated at about 1/200 000. The clinical criteria required to establish the diagnosis are: (1) the presence of at least two Peutz–Jeghers polyps; (2) the presence of one polyp and classic pigmentation; or (3) the presence of one polyp along with a family history of Peutz–Jeghers polyps [86].

The hamartomatous polyps of PJS can develop throughout the gut but occur more frequently in the small intestine (90%) than in the colon (78%) or stomach (74%). They have been associated with intestinal intussusceptions, occult bleeding with secondary iron deficiency anaemia and acute abdominal pain [87]. Commonly described as pedunculated elsewhere, Peutz–Jeghers polyps actually tend to be sessile in the stomach [88]. The core of Peutz–Jeghers polyps classically displays branching bundles of smooth muscles emerging from the muscularis mucosae which

are covered by disorganised foveolae with cystic changes (Figure 12.10). However, in the stomach, Peutz–Jeghers polyps usually show thinner and less arborising smooth muscle bundles than their small bowel counterparts and therefore they can easily be mistaken for hyperplastic gastric polyps, particularly on small or superficial biopsies [2,89]. A distinguishing feature is the normal mucosa surrounding Peutz–Jeghers polyps, whereas hyperplastic polyps tend to be surrounded by inflamed mucosa.

The gene *STK11/LKB1*, which is mutated in most patients with PJS, codes for a serine/threonine kinase involved in cell division, differentiation and signal transduction. It also plays a role in the p53-dependent apoptosis pathway. The mutations occur in several loci along the gene. However, truncation mutations, which are observed in about 75% of patients [87], tend to be associated with a higher frequency of gastric involvement and a higher risk of neoplastic transformation than nonsense mutations [87]. COX-2 also has been reported to be upregulated in these polyps, leading some authors to recommend the use of COX-2 inhibitors in patients with severe gastric involvement, with a proven reduction in the number of polyps [90].

The risk of developing GI and extra-intestinal malignancies (genitourinary, pancreatic, mammary and lung) is well established, with as many as 85% of patients with PJS developing cancer by the age of 70 [87]. In these patients, the lifetime risk for gastric cancer has been estimated to be 30% [91]. However, the origin of the gut adenocarcinomas that arise in these patients is still being debated. Some studies have confirmed the hamartomatous nature of the polyps by proving that they are polyclonal [92, 93], whereas other studies have described the development of dysplasia in Peutz–Jeghers polyps [87,88,94]. Regardless, the risk justifies follow-up for these patients, with surveillance starting as early as the age of 8 [87].

Cowden's disease

Cowden's disease, first reported by Lloyd and Denis in 1963 [95], is a rare (1/200 000) autosomal dominant disorder that is a component of *PTEN* hamartoma syndrome. This syndrome includes several disorders, namely Cowden's disease, Bannayan–Riley–Ruvalcaba syndrome, proteus syndrome and all syndromes caused by germline mutations of the tumour suppressor gene *PTEN* (a **p**hosphatase and **t**ensin homologue that is deleted in chromosome TEN, hence the acronym). The mutation is responsible for a combination of mesodermal, endodermal and ectodermal alterations, and results in multiple hamartomas involving various organs.

Gastrointestinal polyps are observed in 35–65% of cases. In the stomach, these polyps resemble hyperplastic polyps [71,96,97] and show foveolar hyperplasia and more basal, cystically dilated glands containing papillary infolding. Smooth muscle fibres may be interspersed among the glands and the cysts sometimes extend into the submucosa [98]. Adenomatous polyps have also occasionally been reported in Cowden's disease [71].

Patients with this condition have an increased risk of breast cancer (most commonly) but urogenital, GI tract and thyroid cancers are reported as well. Cases of gastric cancer are rarely associated [99]. There are no clear guidelines concerning the follow-up of such patients. However, in patients with concurrent *H. pylori* infection, eradication of the bacterium has caused the polyps to regress, thus potentially limiting the risk of malignant transformation [100].

Cronkhite–Canada syndrome

Cronkhite–Canada syndrome is a rare non-inherited GI polyposis with about 400 cases reported in the literature [101]. The pathogenesis is unknown, although some authors have suggested an autoimmune mechanism [102]. The syndrome occurs in the sixth to seventh decades of life and, although examples have been reported worldwide, most cases have been described in Japan. This gut polyposis commonly causes weight loss, malabsorption, diarrhoea, mucus hypersecretion and hypoproteinaemia. Patients also develop ectodermal manifestations, primarily changes in skin pigmentation, alopecia and onychodystrophy.

In the stomach, the polyps are sessile reddish lesions. Histologically, they show marked foveolar hyperplasia with cystic dilated glands, abundant stromal oedema and inflammation [102,103] (Figure 12.11). Cases with dense eosinophilic infiltrate have been reported [104], as well as lesions in which cystically dilated glands invaginate in the

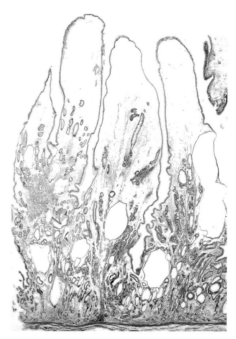

Figure 12.11 Cronkhite–Canada polyp: the finger-like polyps show marked elongation of foveolae and cystic changes with oedematous lamina propria.

submucosa [105]. Cronkhite–Canada syndrome can be difficult to distinguish from other polyposis syndromes, particularly juvenile polyposis, Peutz–Jeghers syndrome and Turcot's disease. Biopsies of the intervening mucosa can be used to distinguish these syndromes, because the gastric mucosa is highly inflamed in Cronkhite–Canada syndrome but not the other diseases [106].

Patients affected by Cronkhite–Canada syndrome have a poor prognosis, with a 5-year mortality rate of 55% due to GI bleeding, sepsis and congestive heart failure. Treatment recommendations are not standardised but oral corticosteroids remain the most common therapy, although surgery is occasionally proposed as well [103]. The risk of cancer remains controversial, even though colorectal and gastric carcinomas seem to be more frequent than in the general population [102,103,107] with an incidence of approximately 5% [108]. In this setting, gastric carcinomas typically have a gastric phenotype [109].

Non-epithelial and malformative polypoid lesions

Inflammatory fibroid polyps

Inflammatory fibroid polyps are rare benign lesions that can be observed throughout the gut in both men and women, primarily as adults. The mean age of patients is 60 years, although cases in children have been reported [110].

These polyps are observed predominantly in the stomach (70%) and ileum (20%) [111,112]. Gastric polyps are typically located in the antrum and occur in approximately 3% of gastric biopsies [2]. Large polyps, which are mostly asymptomatic, may rarely cause anaemia, bleeding and gastric outlet obstruction [113]. Very rare cases of dysphagia have been associated with polyps located unusually at the gastro-oesophageal junction [114,115]. IFPs appear like broad-based submucosal nodules [112] and are either covered by normal-looking mucosa or present apical depressions or ulcerations [116,117] (Figure 12.12a). The submucosal location explains the frequent failure of endoscopic examinations to secure a diagnosis.

Microscopically, inflammatory fibroid polyps show a proliferation of loose spindle cells arranged in short fasci-

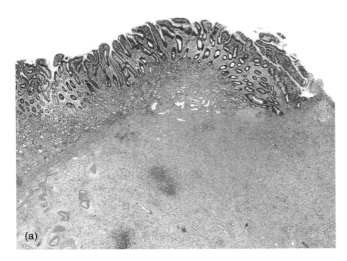

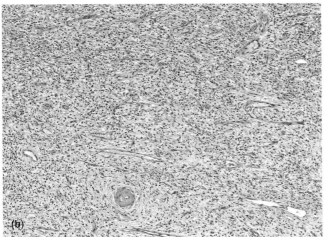

Figure 12.12 Inflammatory fibroid polyp: (a) the lesion appears as a cellular submucosal pathology extending toward the mucosal surface, which is ulcerated. (b) Higher magnification shows the typical bland spindle cell proliferation with numerous eosinophils and mast cells in a vascular background.

cles or whorled structures, commonly in an 'onion-skin' disposition around the abundant capillaries [113,117] (Figure 12.12b). These spindle cells can demonstrate a dense eosinophilic cytoplasm and the mitotic count is usually low. An abundant inflammatory infiltrate dominated by eosinophils is frequently intermixed. The overlying mucosa may have branching foveolae that are elongated and distorted [110]. Despite being centred on the submucosa, involvement of the muscularis mucosae, muscularis propria or even the subserosa has been noted [112], although gastric IFPs tend to be located only in the submucosa and are often much more sharply circumscribed than their ileal equivalents.

Immunohistochemical studies conducted to determine the precise origin of these polyps have demonstrated that the spindle cells are diffusely positive for CD34, CD35, fascin and calponin. Positivity for smooth-muscle actin can be seen, but S100 protein, c-kit, desmin, factor VIII and keratin are consistently negative [118]. With such an immunohistochemical profile, the origin of these cells remains uncertain; possibly they could originate from fibroblastic, myofibroblastic, histiocytic or dendritic cells [118].

The main differential diagnoses for inflammatory fibroid polyps include eosinophilic gastroenteritis, inflammatory pseudo-tumour, haemangio-endothelioma or haemangiopericytoma [113]. They may also be mistaken for malignant tumours on small endoscopic biopsies [111]. Furthermore, the pathogenesis of such lesions remains controversial. For a long time, they were considered to be benign reactive processes that could be in response to an infectious agent, such as *H. pylori* in the stomach, with cases reported to regress after eradication [116,117,119]. However, some recent studies have suggested that, in both gastric and ileal locations, such lesions result from activating mutations of the *PDGFRA* gene, suggesting a neoplastic origin [116,117, 119]. An immunohistochemical positivity for *PDGFRA* has been observed in 95% of intestinal lesions as well. Up to 8% of IFPs have been reported near gastric cancers or adenomas but there is no evidence to believe that these diseases originated from such lesions [120].

Lipoma

Although lipomas are relatively common throughout the GI tract, gastric lipomas are rare, accounting for 2–3% of all benign gastric tumours. They occur equally in both sexes and are more frequently observed in adults, although cases in children have been reported [121,122]. Lipomas typically arise in the antrum and 90% are submucosal. Rare subserosal locations have been reported, although these cases may remain asymptomatic [123]. The two main clinical symptoms of lipomas are abdominal pain and bleeding [124], which can be chronic, leading to anaemia. Other reported symptoms include intussusceptions [125,126],

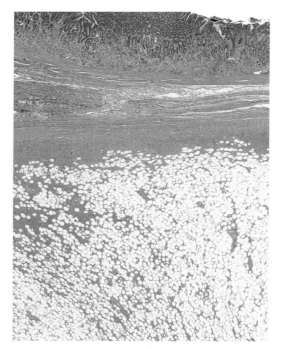

Figure 12.13 Gastric lipoma: benign adipocytes extend through the submucosa and compress the mucosa.

gastric outlet obstruction [127], dyspepsia, vomiting and tachycardia [126].

Gastric lipomas present endoscopically as smooth submucosal lesions protruding into the lumen. Mucosal ulcerations or central depressions are sometimes observed [124]. Reported sizes can be quite variable but some 'giant gastric lipomas', reaching 100 mm in diameter, have been described [125,128]. These encapsulated collections of adipose tissue are composed of mature well differentiated adipocytes that are devoid of atypia (Figure 12.13). Rare cases of 'fibrolipoma', composed of both mature adipose tissue and spindle cell-like fibroblasts, have been described. The overlying mucosa can be inflamed and ulcerated and demonstrate intestinal metaplasia [128]. Lipomas have been reported in association with a variety of other gastric malignancies such as GIST [129] and gastric carcinoma [130].

Xanthoma

Gastric xanthoma, also called 'xanthelasma', is a benign lesion reported in 1–7% of endoscopies [131,132]. They typically develop in the antrum, along the lesser curvature or close to a stoma, on the posterior wall or along the greater curvature, in patients who have had gastric surgery. Rare cases have been reported in the duodenum or in the oesophagus [131]. Xanthomas are small (<10 mm), rounded, yellowish submucosal lesions [132]. They are usually solitary and it is rare to observe multiple lesions, although

there are reports of gastric xanthomatosis [133]. Gastric xanthomas are usually associated with other conditions such as atrophic gastritis [131], chronic gastritis [134], intestinal metaplasia [135], *H. pylori* infection and gastric carcinoma [136].

They correspond to an accumulation of periodic acid–Schiff (PAS)-negative macrophages with vacuolated sudanophilic cytoplasm. The polygonal histiocytes, with a distinct cell membrane and a small centrally located round or oval nucleus, are completely devoid of atypia and lie in a pavement-like arrangement, usually in the upper third of the mucosa [134] (Figure 12.14a). Various lipids (cholesterol, neutral fat, low-density lipoprotein [LDL] and oxidised LDL) have been found within these cells.

The pathogenesis of these lesions is not understood. They are not associated with lipid metabolic disorders [132] but the high percentage of oxidised LDL has lead some authors to conclude that the lesions are secondary to mucosal damage, resulting in macrophage chemotaxis [134]. The main differential diagnoses include gastric signet ring cell carcinoma and the clear-cell variant of gastric carcinoid tumours. There are case reports in which these conditions occur simultaneously. However, the appearance of a xanthoma suggests a benign diagnosis and the immunohistochemical profile (positivity for histiocytic markers such as CD68 with negativity for cytokeratins) should lead the pathologist to the correct diagnosis (Figure 12.14b).

Gastric heterotopic pancreas

Heterotopic pancreas is the second most common pancreatic congenital abnormality after pancreas divisum. Although this entity has been discussed in Chapter 10, it is appropriate that this lesion is also discussed here because it is so commonly polypoid and is an important differential diagnosis of endoscopically detected polyps of the stomach. It is observed in up to 1/500 laparotomies and tends to occur more often in males than in females [137]. This anomaly is defined as the presence of pancreatic tissue devoid of vascular or anatomical communication with the pancreatic gland proper. This tissue usually develops within 50 mm of the pylorus and the submucosa is most commonly involved [137]. The exact pathogenesis has not been determined but it is probably the result of abnormal migration and/or residual rest of pancreatic buds during embryogenesis. The lesions are usually asymptomatic but large lesions (>15 mm) can be associated with abdominal pain, vomiting, gastric outlet obstruction and even dysphagia in the rare cases located near the gastro-oesophageal junction [138,139].

Endoscopically, small (typically approximately 10 mm diameter), rounded submucosal lesions are detected, sometimes with a central nipple-like umbilication. The submucosal location explains the increasing use of echo-endoscopy

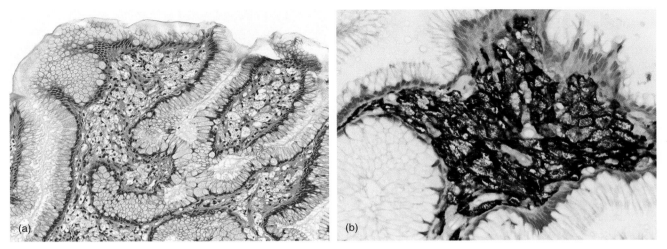

Figure 12.14 Gastric xanthoma: (a) the lesion is composed of loosely packed small foamy histiocytes; (b) the characteristic histology and immunoreactivity to CD68 (a histiocytic marker) distinguish this lesion from signet ring cell carcinoma.

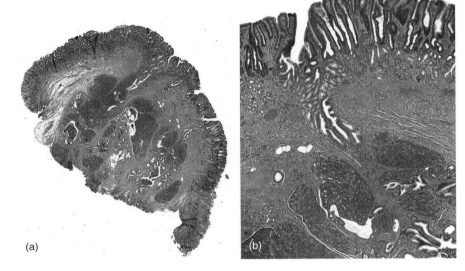

Figure 12.15 Pancreatic heterotopia: (a) the polypoid lesion is formed by acinar and ductular proliferation readily identified under the gastric mucosa. (b) High-power view confirms the benign nature of the acinar and ductular structures extending toward the mucosal surface.

to examine these anomalies, which present as a hypoechoic submucosal mass with small, scattered, heterogeneous signals corresponding to adipose tissue [140] (Figure 12.15a). Anechoic areas that represent duct dilatation can be observed as well. Endoscopic biopsies often fail to provide a diagnosis [141] but endoscopic ultrasonography–fine needle aspiration (EUS-FNA) can be useful in distinguishing ectopic pancreatic tissue from other submucosal lesions, such as GISTs or leiomyoma [138].

Ectopic pancreatic tissue has been classified by the predominant histological composition: type I contains all the components of the pancreatic gland, including ducts, acini and endocrine islets; type II consists of pancreatic ducts only (the canalicular type); type III consists only of acinar tissue (exocrine pancreas); and type IV consists only of

islet cells (the endocrine pancreas) [142] (Figure 12.15b). Several different types can be observed synchronously. In type II, the ducts tend to be dilated and surrounded by an abundant smooth muscle proliferation and have been described as an 'adenomyoma' or 'myoepithelial hamartoma'. In cases of symptomatic lesions or when the diagnosis is uncertain and neoplastic lesions, especially GISTs, require to be excluded, endoscopic resection or limited surgical resection is the treatment of choice.

Ectopic pancreatic tissue can undergo any pathological changes observed in the pancreas, namely acute pancreatitis [143], pseudo-cysts [144], mucinous cysts [145], pancreatic intra-epithelial neoplasia [145], and even ductal adenocarcinoma, acinar cell carcinoma and pancreatic endocrine tumours [146–149].

Ménétrier's disease

Ménétrier's disease is an uncommon acquired clinico-pathological condition, associating diffuse hypertrophic gastropathy, hypochlorhydria and hypoproteinaemia secondary to excessive mucosal protein loss. Given its association with inflammation, it has also been briefly discussed in Chapter 11. It has been described in adults (often men aged 40–60 years) and children. CMV is associated in 70% of children affected [150,151]. In contrast, *H. pylori* is revealed in almost 90% of adult patients with Ménétrier's disease [152]. Interestingly, cases of Ménétrier's disease in children have been reported who had co-infection with CMV and *H. pylori* [153,154]. Finally, a recent case of Ménétrier's disease in an adult with herpes simplex virus (HSV) infection has been reported [155]. One curiosity about the disease is that, in Western countries at least, it appears to be getting much less common with many GI pathologists reporting that they have not seen a case for a considerable time period. This may relate, of course, to improved pathological diagnosis and better identification of conditions that mimic the features of Ménétrier's disease.

Most adult patients show a chronic debilitating course. Conversely, paediatric forms have a self-limited transient course, usually resolving within few months. Vomiting, abdominal pain and oedema are the most common symptoms. Profound hypoproteinaemia with anasarca can also be seen. In addition, patients may develop iron deficiency anaemia from gastric blood loss.

Massively thickened irregular 'cerebriform' gastric folds with large amounts of viscous mucus and superficial erosions are the characteristic macroscopic features (Figure 12.16). These changes are seen in the proximal stomach amid oedematous mucosa, although localised or diffuse

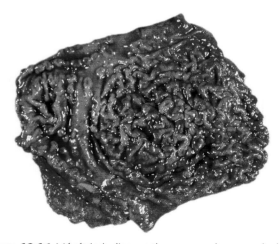

Figure 12.16 Ménétrier's disease: the mucosa shows marked thickening of the gastric rugae of the body and fundus, sparing the antrum.

cases have been reported [156,157]. Localised disease of the gastric antrum, with sparing of the fundus and body, mainly manifested by polyposis and coexisting with glandularis cystica profunda, has also been observed [158]. Based on the macroscopic features of the disease, the differential diagnosis includes diffuse hyperplasia of the oxyntic glandular component (as in Zollinger–Ellison syndrome), hypertrophic gastritis, gastric lymphoma or, rarely, diffuse-type adenocarcinoma. None of these diagnoses is associated with such a severe foveolar hyperplasia, yet the diagnosis may be challenging, because superficial mucosal biopsies may not be representative of the actual pathology.

Microscopically, Ménétrier's disease is characterised by markedly elongated and tortuous foveolae which may be associated with cystic dilatation of the pits and massive over-proliferation of the surface mucus-producing cells (Figure 12.17a,b). The glands may also extend into the submucosa, which may present as gastritis cystica profunda [159,160]. An atrophic or even absent oxyntic glandular component (parietal and chief cells) is frequent. Inflammation is usually scarce but prominent eosinophilia can be observed [157,161]. Histological examination on conventional endoscopic biopsies usually fails to demonstrate the massive foveolar hyperplasia and some authors have recommended obtaining full-thickness biopsies [156,162]. Other changes include a thickened and disorganised muscularis mucosae, with strands of smooth muscles extending into the lamina propria.

The link between Ménétrier's disease and cancer remains controversial and dates from the original paper [163]. Although it is reported that the disease carries an increased risk of subsequent gastric cancer, as high as a 2–15% lifetime risk, the exact risk is unknown and there is no general consensus on endoscopic screening (Figure 12.18). In some cases of gastric adenocarcinoma, the identification of thickened gastric folds at endoscopy, or after radiological examination, has been attributed to Ménétrier's disease but adequate histological confirmation has usually been lacking. In some cases, it is likely that an infiltrating carcinoma gives rise to a hypertrophic mucosal appearance secondarily. In a few cases, however, gastric cancer has been detected several years after the diagnosis of Ménétrier's disease [164].

The pathogenesis of Ménétrier's disease remains uncertain but transforming growth factor α (TGF-α), a ligand for the epidermal growth factor receptor (EGF-R), has been implicated. TGF-α causes dose-dependent in vitro proliferation of gastric epithelial cells and dose-dependent reduction of acid secretion, both of which are hallmarks of the disease. Increased TGF-α levels may be induced by *H. pylori* infection [165,166]. Interestingly, TGF-α immunoreactivity has been shown to be highly upregulated in Ménétrier's disease [167,168]. The best treatment is debated.

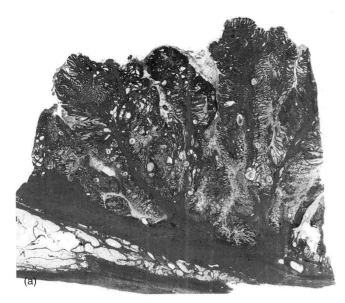

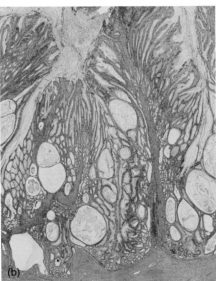

Figure 12.17 Ménétrier's disease: (a) low-power view demonstrating extended gastric folds and rugae. Note, in the middle of the field, an area of dense cellular and glandular proliferation. (b) A higher-power view showing the foveolar and cystic dilatation lined by bland mucin-producing gastric type epithelium.

It seems reasonable to test for, and treat if demonstrated, CMV and *H. pylori* because the disease is known to be associated with these infections. Recently, therapies targeting increased signal of EGF-R have shown to be promising, including octreotide (a somatostatin analogue) and monoclonal antibodies (such as cetuximab) directed against the EGF-R. In refractory or complicated cases, massive bleeding, refractory protein loss or obstructive symptoms, gastrectomy is curative [169–172].

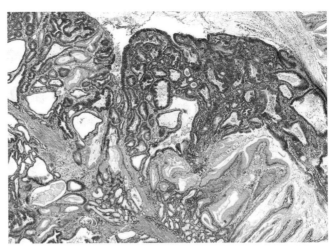

Figure 12.18 Ménétrier's disease: an area of dysplastic transformation (as noted on Figure 12.17a) with back-to-back glandular crowding and obvious nuclear changes.

Polyp-like lesions

Many mucosal gastric nodules may be detected endoscopically. They may represent limited hypertrophy of mucosal, stromal or inflammatory components of the gastric mucosa but rarely constitute well-formed polyps. These conditions are described elsewhere (see Chapters 11, 14, 15 and 16). They include lymphoid proliferations such as polypoid gastritis and lymphoid hyperplasia commonly occurring in the antrum and associated with *H. pylori* infection. Other conditions in this category include secondary neoplasms of the stomach, amyloidosis and Langerhans' cell histiocytosis.

References

1. Archimandritis A, Spiliadis C, Tzivras M, et al. Gastric epithelial polyps: a retrospective endoscopic study of 12974 symptomatic patients. *Ital J Gastroenterol* 1996;**28**:387.
2. Stolte M, Sticht T, Eidt S, Ebert D, Finkenzeller G. Frequency, location, and age and sex distribution of various types of gastric polyp. *Endoscopy* 1994;**26**:659.
3. Carmack SW, Genta RM, Schuler CM, Saboorian MH. The current spectrum of gastric polyps: a 1-year national study of over 120000 patients. *Am J Gastroenterol* 2009;**104**:1524.
4. Samarasam I, Roberts-Thomson J, Brockwell D. Gastric fundic gland polyps: a clinico-pathological study from North West Tasmania. *ANZ J Surg* 2009;**79**:467.
5. Vieth M, Stolte M. Fundic gland polyps are not induced by proton pump inhibitor therapy. *Am J Clin Pathol* 2001;**116**:716.
6. Ally MR, Veerappan GR, Maydonovitch CL, et al. Chronic proton pump inhibitor therapy associated with increased development of fundic gland polyps. *Dig Dis Sci* 2009;**54**:2617.
7. Weston BR, Helper DJ, Rex DK. Positive predictive value of endoscopic features deemed typical of gastric fundic gland polyps. *J Clin Gastroenterol* 2003;**36**:399.
8. Genta RM, Schuler CM, Robiou CI, Lash RH. No association between gastric fundic gland polyps and gastrointestinal

neoplasia in a study of over 100 000 patients. *Clin Gastroenterol Hepatol* 2009;**7**:849.

9. Jalving M, Koornstra JJ, Wesseling J, Boezen HM SDEJ, Kleibeuker JH. Increased risk of fundic gland polyps during long-term proton pump inhibitor therapy. *Aliment Pharmacol Ther* 2006;**24**:1341.

10. Bianchi LK, Burke CA, Bennett AE, Lopez R, Hasson H, Church JM. Fundic gland polyp dysplasia is common in familial adenomatous polyposis. *Clin Gastroenterol Hepatol* 2008;**6**:180.

11. Declich P, Bellone S, Ambrosiani L, et al. Fundic gland polyps: do they arise as a by-product of hypergastrinemia in patients with Zollinger–Ellison syndrome? *Hum Pathol* 2000;**31**:889.

12. Declich P, Bellone S, Porcellati M, et al A. Parietal cell protrusions with fundic gland cysts and fundic gland polyps: are they related or simply similar but distinguishable? *Hum Pathol* 2000; **31**:1536.

13. Winkler A, Hinterleitner TA, Langner C. Giant fundic gland polyp mimicking a gastric malignancy. *Endoscopy* 2007;**39**(suppl 1):E34.

14. Declich P, Ambrosiani L, Bellone S, et al. Parietal cell hyperplasia with deep cystic dilations: a lesion closely mimicking fundic gland polyps. *Am J Gastroenterol* 2000;**95**:566.

15. Krasinskas AM, Abraham SC, Metz DC, Furth EE. Oxyntic mucosa pseudopolyps: a presentation of atrophic autoimmune gastritis. *Am J Surg Pathol* 2003;**27**:236.

16. Shand AG, Taylor AC, Banerjee M, et al. Gastric fundic gland polyps in south-east Scotland: absence of adenomatous polyposis coli gene mutations and a strikingly low prevalence of *Helicobacter pylori* infection. *J Gastroenterol Hepatol* 2002;**17**: 1161.

17. Watanabe N, Seno H, Nakajima T, et al. Regression of fundic gland polyps following acquisition of *Helicobacter pylori*. *Gut* 2002;**51**:742.

18. Kazantsev GB, Schwesinger WH, Heim-Hall J. Spontaneous resolution of multiple fundic gland polyps after cessation of treatment with lansoprazole and Nissen fundoplication: a case report. *Gastrointest Endosc* 2002;**55**:600.

19. Declich P, Tavani E, Bellone S, et al. Sporadic, syndromic, and Zollinger–Ellison syndrome associated fundic gland polyps consistently express cytokeratin 7. *Virchows Arch* 2002;**441**:96.

20. Wei J, Chiriboga L, Yee H, et al. Altered cellular distribution of tuberin and glucocorticoid receptor in sporadic fundic gland polyps. *Mod Pathol* 2002;**15**:862.

21. Abraham SC, Nobukawa B, Giardiello FM, Hamilton SR, Wu TT. Sporadic fundic gland polyps: common gastric polyps arising through activating mutations in the beta-catenin gene. *Am J Pathol* 2001;**158**:1005.

22. Abraham SC, Nobukawa B, Giardiello FM, Hamilton SR, Wu TT. Fundic gland polyps in familial adenomatous polyposis: neoplasms with frequent somatic adenomatous polyposis coli gene alterations. *Am J Pathol* 2000;**157**:747.

23. Sekine S, Shibata T, Yamauchi Y, et al. Beta-catenin mutations in sporadic fundic gland polyps. *Virchows Arch* 2002;**440**:381.

24. Torbenson M, Lee JH, Cruz-Correa M, et al. Sporadic fundic gland polyposis: a clinical, histological, and molecular analysis. *Mod Pathol* 2002;**15**:718.

25. Abraham SC, Park SJ, Cruz-Correa M, et al. Frequent CpG island methylation in sporadic and syndromic gastric fundic gland polyps. *Am J Clin Pathol* 2004;**122**:740.

26. Abraham SC, Park SJ, Mugartegui L, Hamilton SR, Wu TT. Sporadic fundic gland polyps with epithelial dysplasia : evidence for preferential targeting for mutations in the adenomatous polyposis coli gene. *Am J Pathol* 2002;**161**:1735.

27. Jalving M, Koornstra JJ, Boersma-van Ek W, et al. Dysplasia in fundic gland polyps is associated with nuclear beta-catenin expression and relatively high cell turnover rates. *Scand J Gastroenterol* 2003;**38**:916.

28. Jalving M, Koornstra JJ, Gotz JM, et al. High-grade dysplasia in sporadic fundic gland polyps: a case report and review of the literature. *Eur J Gastroenterol Hepatol* 2003;**15**:1229.

29. Stolte M, Vieth M, and Ebert MP. High-grade dysplasia in sporadic fundic gland polyps: clinically relevant or not? *Eur J Gastroenterol Hepatol* 2003;**15**:1153.

30. Sekine S, Shimoda T, Nimura S, et al. High-grade dysplasia associated with fundic gland polyposis in a familial adenomatous polyposis patient, with special reference to APC mutation profiles. *Mod Pathol* 2004;**17**:1421.

31. Garrean S, Hering J, Saied A, Jani J, Espat NJ. Gastric adenocarcinoma arising from fundic gland polyps in a patient with familial adenomatous polyposis syndrome. *Am Surg* 2008;**74**:79.

32. Ming SC, Goldman H. Gastric polyps: a histogenetic classification and its relation to carcinoma. *Cancer* 1965;**18**:721.

33. Nakamura T, Nakano G. Histopathological classification and malignant change in gastric polyps. *J Clin Pathol* 1985;**38**:754.

34. Tomasulo J. Gastric polyps. Histologic types and their relationship to gastric carcinoma. *Cancer* 1971;**27**:1346.

35. Morais DJ, Yamanaka A, Zeitune JM, Andreollo NA. Gastric polyps: a retrospective analysis of 26 000 digestive endoscopies. *Arq Gastroenterol* 2007;**44**:14.

36. Murakami K, Mitomi H, Yamashita K, Tanabe S, Saigenji K, Okayasu I. p53, but not c-Ki-ras, mutation and down-regulation of p21WAF1/CIP1 and cyclin D1 are associated with malignant transformation in gastric hyperplastic polyps. *Am J Clin Pathol* 2001;**115**:224.

37. Al-Haddad M, Ward EM, Bouras EP, Raimondo M. Hyperplastic polyps of the gastric antrum in patients with gastrointestinal blood loss. *Dig Dis Sci* 2007;**52**:105.

38. Alper M, Akcan Y, Belenli O. Large pedunculated antral hyperplastic gastric polyp traversed the bulbus causing outlet obstruction and iron deficiency anemia: endoscopic removal. *World J Gastroenterol* 2003;**9**:633.

39. Gencosmanoglu R, Sen-Oran E, Kurtkaya-Yapicier O, Tozun N. Antral hyperplastic polyp causing intermittent gastric outlet obstruction: case report. *BMC Gastroenterol* 2003;**3**:16.

40. Muller-Lissner SA, Wiebecke B. Investigations of hyperplasiogenous gastric polyps by partial reconstruction. *Pathol Res Pract* 1982;**174**:368.

41. Hattori T. Morphological range of hyperplastic polyps and carcinomas arising in hyperplastic polyps of the stomach. *J Clin Pathol* 1985;**38**:622.

42. Muto T, Ota K. Polypogenesis of gastric mucosa. *Gann* 1970; **61**:435.

43. Dirschmid K, Walser J, Hugel H. Pseudomalignant erosion in hyperplastic gastric polyps. *Cancer* 1984;**54**:2290.

44. Kawada M, Seno H, Wada M, et al. Cyclooxygenase-2 expression and angiogenesis in gastric hyperplastic polyp – association with polyp size. *Digestion* 2003;**67**:20.

45. Nakajima A, Matsuhashi N, Yazaki Y, Oka T, Sugano K. Details of hyperplastic polyps of the stomach shrinking after anti-Helicobacter pylori therapy. *J Gastroenterol* 2000;**35**:372.

46. Abraham SC, Singh VK, Yardley JH, Wu TT. Hyperplastic polyps of the stomach: associations with histologic patterns of gastritis and gastric atrophy. *Am J Surg Pathol* 2001;**25**:500.

47. Dixon MF, O'Connor HJ, Axon AT, King RF, Johnston D. Reflux gastritis: distinct histopathological entity? *J Clin Pathol* 1986;**39**:524.

48. Di Giulio E, Lahner E, Micheletti A, et al. Occurrence and risk factors for benign epithelial gastric polyps in atrophic body gastritis on diagnosis and follow-up. *Aliment Pharmacol Ther* 2005;**21**:567.

49. Dirschmid K, Platz-Baudin C, Stolte M. Why is the hyperplastic polyp a marker for the precancerous condition of the gastric mucosa? *Virchows Arch* 2006;**448**:80.

50. Borch K, Skarsgard J, Franzen L, Mardh S, Rehfeld JF. Benign gastric polyps: morphological and functional origin. *Dig Dis Sci* 2003;**48**:1292.

51. Ji F, Wang ZW, Ning JW, Wang QY, Chen JY, Li YM. Effect of drug treatment on hyperplastic gastric polyps infected with *Helicobacter pylori*: a randomized, controlled trial. *World J Gastroenterol* 2006;**12**:1770.

52. Ohkusa T, Miwa H, Hojo M, et al Endoscopic, histological and serologic findings of gastric hyperplastic polyps after eradication of *Helicobacter pylori*: comparison between responder and non-responder cases. *Digestion* 2003;**68**:57.

53. Amaro R, Neff GW, Karnam US, Tzakis AG, Raskin JB. Acquired hyperplastic gastric polyps in solid organ transplant patients. *Am J Gastroenterol* 2002;**97**:2220.

54. Jewell KD, Toweill DL, Swanson PE, Upton MP, Yeh MM. Gastric hyperplastic polyps in post transplant patients: a clinicopathologic study. *Mod Pathol* 2008;**21**:1108.

55. Kamata Y, Kurotaki H, Onodera T, Nishida N. An unusual heterotopia of pyloric glands of the stomach with inverted downgrowth. *Acta Pathol Jpn* 1993;**43**:192.

56. Yamashita M, Hirokawa M, Nakasono M, et al. Gastric inverted hyperplastic polyp. Report of four cases and relation to gastritis cystica profunda. *APMIS* 2002;**110**:717.

57. Kono T, Imai Y, Ichihara T, et al. Adenocarcinoma arising in gastric inverted hyperplastic polyp: a case report and review of the literature. *Pathol Res Pract* 2007;**203**:53.

58. Hu TL, Hsu JT, Chen HM, Chen MF. Diffuse gastric polyposis: report of a case. *J Formos Med Assoc* 2002;**101**:712.

59. Niv Y, Delpre G, Sperber AD, Sandbank J, Zirkin H. Hyperplastic gastric polyposis, hypergastrinaemia and colorectal neoplasia: a description of four cases. *Eur J Gastroenterol Hepatol* 2003;**15**:1361.

60. Gonzalez-Obeso E, Fujita H, Deshpande V, et al. Gastric 'hyperplastic polyps', a heterogeneous clinicopathological group including a distinct subset best categorized as mucosal prolapse polyp. *Am J Surg Pathol* 2011;**35**:1248.

61. Hizawa K, Fuchigami T, Iida M, et al. Possible neoplastic transformation within gastric hyperplastic polyp. Application of endoscopic polypectomy. *Surg Endosc* 1995;**9**:714.

62. Hirasaki S, Suzuki S, Kanzaki H, Fujita K, Matsumura S, Matsumoto E. Minute signet ring cell carcinoma occurring in gastric hyperplastic polyp. *World J Gastroenterol* 2007;**13**:5779.

63. Hirasaki S, Kanzaki H, Fujita K, et al. Papillary adenocarcinoma occurring in a gastric hyperplastic polyp observed by magnifying endoscopy and treated with endoscopic mucosal resection. *Intern Med* 2008;**47**:949.

64. Carmack SW, Genta RM, Graham DY, Lauwers GY. Management of gastric polyps: a pathology-based guide for gastroenterologists. *Nat Rev Gastroenterol Hepatol* 2009;**6**:331.

65. Yao T, Kajiwara M, Kuroiwa S, et al. Malignant transformation of gastric hyperplastic polyps: alteration of phenotypes, proliferative activity, and p53 expression. *Hum Pathol* 2002;**33**:1016.

66. Lauwers GY, Wahl SJ, Melamed J, Rojas-Corona RR. p53 expression in precancerous gastric lesions: an immunohistochemical study of PAb 1801 monoclonal antibody on adenomatous and hyperplastic gastric polyps. *Am J Gastroenterol* 1993;**88**:1916.

67. Park do Y, Lauwers GY. Gastric polyps: classification and management. *Arch Pathol Lab Med* 2008;**132**:633.

68. Watanabe H, Jass JR, Sobin LH, eds. Histological typing of oesophageal and gastric tumors. In: *Histological Typing of Oesophageal and Gastric Tumours*. Berlin: Springer-Verlag, 1990: 34.

69. Dunlop MG. Guidance on gastrointestinal surveillance for hereditary non-polyposis colorectal cancer, familial adenomatous polyposis, juvenile polyposis, and Peutz–Jeghers syndrome. *Gut* 2002;**51**(suppl 5):V21.

70. Hizawa K, Iida M, Yao T, Aoyagi K, Fujishima M. Juvenile polyposis of the stomach: clinicopathological features and its malignant potential. *J Clin Pathol* 1997;**50**:771.

71. Hizawa K, Iida M, Matsumoto T, et al. Gastrointestinal manifestations of Cowden's disease. Report of four cases. *J Clin Gastroenterol* 1994;**18**:13.

72. Johnson GK, Soergel KH, Hensley GT, Dodds WJ, Hogan WJ. Cronkite–Canada syndrome: gastrointestinal pathophysiology and morphology. *Gastroenterology* 1972;**63**:140.

73. Friedl W, Uhlhaas S, Schulmann K, et al. Juvenile polyposis: massive gastric polyposis is more common in *MADH4* mutation carriers than in *BMPR1A* mutation carriers. *Hum Genet* 2002;**111**:108.

74. Jass JR, Williams CB, Bussey HJ, Morson BC. Juvenile polyposis – a precancerous condition. *Histopathology* 1988;**13**:619.

75. Howe JR, Mitros FA, Summers RW. The risk of gastrointestinal carcinoma in familial juvenile polyposis. *Ann Surg Oncol* 1998;**5**:751.

76. Pintiliciuc OG, Heresbach D, de-Lajarte-Thirouard AS, et al. Gastric involvement in juvenile polyposis associated with germline SMAD4 mutations: an entity characterized by a mixed hypertrophic and polypoid gastropathy. *Gastroenterol Clin Biol* 2008;**32**:445.

77. Shikata K, Kukita Y, Matsumoto T, et al. Gastric juvenile polyposis associated with germline SMAD4 mutation. *Am J Med Genet A* 2005;**134**:326.

78. Yamashita K, Saito M, Itoh M, et al. Juvenile polyposis complicated with protein losing gastropathy. *Intern Med* 2009;**48**:335.

79. Sweet K, Willis J, Zhou XP, et al. Molecular classification of patients with unexplained hamartomatous and hyperplastic polyposis. *JAMA* 2005;**294**:2465.

80. Jarvinen HJ, Sipponen P. Gastroduodenal polyps in familial adenomatous and juvenile polyposis. *Endoscopy* 1986;**18**:230.

81. Covarrubias DJ, Huprich JE. Best cases from the AFIP. Juvenile polyposis of the stomach. Armed Forces Institute of Pathology. *Radiographics* 2002;**22**:415.

82. Coffin CM, Dehner LP. What is a juvenile polyp? An analysis based on 21 patients with solitary and multiple polyps. *Arch Pathol Lab Med* 1996;**120**:1032.

83. Kantarcioglu M, Kilciler G, Turan I, et al. Solitary Peutz–Jeghers-type hamartomatous polyp as a cause of recurrent acute pancreatitis. *Endoscopy* 2009;**41** Suppl 2:E117.

84. Oncel M, Remzi FH, Church JM, Goldblum JR, Zutshi M, Fazio VW. Course and follow-up of solitary Peutz-Jeghers polyps: a case series. *Int J Colorectal Dis* 2003;**18**:33.

85. Volikos E, Robinson J, Aittomaki K, et al. LKB1 exonic and whole gene deletions are a common cause of Peutz–Jeghers syndrome. *J Med Genet* 2006;**43**:e18.

86. Tomlinson IP, Houlston RS. Peutz–Jeghers syndrome. *J Med Genet* 1997;**34**:1007.

87. Salloch H, Reinacher-Schick A, Schulmann K, et al. Truncating mutations in Peutz–Jeghers syndrome are associated with more polyps, surgical interventions and cancers. *Int J Colorectal Dis*, **25**:97.

88. Lin J, Chen M, Lei W, Law W, Hu C. Eradication of diffuse gastric Peutz–Jeghers polyps by unsedated transnasal snare polypectomy and argon plasma coagulation. *Endoscopy* 2009;**41** Suppl 2:E207.

89. Burkart AL, Sheridan T, Lewin M, Fenton H, Ali NJ, Montgomery E. Do sporadic Peutz–Jeghers polyps exist? Experience of a large teaching hospital. *Am J Surg Pathol* 2007;**31**:1209.

90. Udd L, Katajisto P, Rossi DJ, et al. Suppression of Peutz–Jeghers polyposis by inhibition of cyclooxygenase-2. *Gastroenterology* 2004;**127**:1030.

91. Giardiello FM, Brensinger JD, Tersmette AC, et al. Very high risk of cancer in familial Peutz–Jeghers syndrome. *Gastroenterology* 2000;**119**:1447.

92. de Leng WW, Jansen M, Keller JJ, et al. Peutz–Jeghers syndrome polyps are polyclonal with expanded progenitor cell compartment. *Gut* 2007;**56**:1475.

93. Jansen M, de Leng WW, Baas AF, et al. Mucosal prolapse in the pathogenesis of Peutz–Jeghers polyposis. *Gut* 2006;**55**:1.

94. Ben Brahim E, Jouini R, Khayat O, et al. Adenomatous transformation in hamartomatous polyps cases of two patients with Peutz-Jeghers syndrome. *Int J Colorectal Dis* 2009;**24**:1361.

95. Lloyd KM, 2nd, Dennis M. Cowden's disease. A possible new symptom complex with multiple system involvement. *Ann Intern Med* 1963;**58**:136.

96. Campos FG, Habr-Gama A, Kiss DR, et al. Cowden syndrome: report of two cases and review of clinical presentation and management of a rare colorectal polyposis. *Curr Surg* 2006;**63**:15.

97. Vasovcak P, Krepelova A, Puchmajerova, et al. A novel mutation of *PTEN* gene in a patient with Cowden syndrome with excessive papillomatosis of the lips, discrete cutaneous lesions, and gastrointestinal polyposis. *Eur J Gastroenterol Hepatol* 2007;**19**:513.

98. Carlson GJ, Nivatvongs S, Snover DC. Colorectal polyps in Cowden's disease (multiple hamartoma syndrome). *Am J Surg Pathol* 1984;**8**:763.

99. Hamby LS, Lee EY, Schwartz RW. Parathyroid adenoma and gastric carcinoma as manifestations of Cowden's disease. *Surgery* 1995;**118**:115.

100. Isomoto H, Furusu H, Ohnita K, Takehara Y, Wen CY, Kohno S. Effect of *Helicobacter pylori* eradication on gastric hyperplastic polyposis in Cowden's disease. *World J Gastroenterol* 2005;**11**:1567.

101. Cronkhite LW, Jr, Canada WJ. Generalized gastrointestinal polyposis: an unusual syndrome of polyposis, pigmentation, alopecia and onychotrophia. *N Engl J Med* 1955;**252**:1011.

102. Takeuchi Y, Yoshikawa M, Tsukamoto N, et al. Cronkhite–Canada syndrome with colon cancer, portal thrombosis, high titer of antinuclear antibodies, and membranous glomerulonephritis. *J Gastroenterol* 2003;**38**:791.

103. Yamaguchi K, Ogata Y, Akagi Y, et al. Cronkhite–Canada syndrome associated with advanced rectal cancer treated by a subtotal colectomy: report of a case. *Surg Today* 2001;**31**:521.

104. Anderson RD, Patel R, Hamilton JK, Boland CR. Cronkhite–Canada syndrome presenting as eosinophilic gastroenteritis. *Proc Bayl Univ Med Cent* 2006;**19**:209.

105. Ward EM, Wolfsen HC, Raimondo M. Novel endosonographic findings in Cronkhite–Canada syndrome. *Endoscopy* 2003;**35**:464.

106. Samet JD, Horton KM, Fishman EK, Iacobuzio-Donahue CA. Cronkhite–Canada syndrome: Gastric involvement diagnosed by MDCT. *Case Report Med* 2009;**2009**:148795.

107. Watanabe T, Kudo M, Shirane H, et al. Cronkhite–Canada syndrome associated with triple gastric cancers: a case report. *Gastrointest Endosc* 1999;**50**:688.

108. Egawa T, Kubota T, Otani Y, et al. Surgically treated Cronkhite-Canada syndrome associated with gastric cancer. *Gastric Cancer* 2000;**3**:156.

109. Karasawa H, Miura K, Ishida K, et al. Cronkhite–Canada syndrome complicated with huge intramucosal gastric cancer. *Gastric Cancer* 2009;**12**:113.

110. Chongsrisawat V, Yimyeam P, Wisedopas N, Viravaidya D, Poovorawan Y. Unusual manifestations of gastric inflammatory fibroid polyp in a child. *World J Gastroenterol* 2004;**10**:460.

111. Ozolek JA, Sasatomi E, Swalsky PA, Rao U, Krasinskas A, Finkelstein SD. Inflammatory fibroid polyps of the gastrointestinal tract: clinical, pathologic, and molecular characteristics. *Appl Immunohistochem Mol Morphol* 2004;**12**:59.

112. Santos Gda C, Alves VA, Wakamatsu A, Zucoloto S. Inflammatory fibroid polyp: an immunohistochemical study. *Arq Gastroenterol* 2004;**41**:104.

113. Paikos D, Moschos J, Tzilves D, et al. Inflammatory fibroid polyp or Vanek's tumour. *Dig Surg* 2007;**24**:231.

114. Yamane T, Uchiyama K, Ishii T, et al. Case of inflammatory fibroid polyp of the esophagogastric junction. *Dig Endosc* 2009;**21**:97.

115. Zinkiewicz K, Zgodzinski W, Dabrowski A, Szumilo J, Cwik G, Wallner G. Recurrent inflammatory fibroid polyp of cardia: a case report. *World J Gastroenterol* 2004;**10**:767.

116. Matsuhashi N, Nakajima A, Nomura S, Kaminishi M. Inflammatory fibroid polyps of the stomach and Helicobacter pylori. *J Gastroenterol Hepatol* 2004;**19**:346.

117. Nishiyama Y, Koyama S, Andoh A, et al. Gastric inflammatory fibroid polyp treated with Helicobacter pylori eradication therapy. *Intern Med* 2003;**42**:263.

118. Pantanowitz L, Antonioli DA, Pinkus GS, Shahsafaei A, Odze RD. Inflammatory fibroid polyps of the gastrointestinal tract: evidence for a dendritic cell origin. *Am J Surg Pathol* 2004;**28**:107.

119. Hirasaki S, Matsubara M, Ikeda F, Taniguchi H, Suzuki S. Gastric inflammatory fibroid polyp treated with Helicobacter pylori eradication therapy. *Intern Med* 2007;**46**:855.

120. Mori M, Tamura S, Enjoji M, Sugimachi K. Concomitant presence of inflammatory fibroid polyp and carcinoma or adenoma in the stomach. *Arch Pathol Lab Med* 1988;**112**:829.

121. Alberti D, Grazioli L, Orizio P, et al. Asymptomatic giant gastric lipoma: What to do? *Am J Gastroenterol* 1999;**94**:3634.

122. Antoniou D, Soutis M, Stefanaki K, Christopoulos-Geroulanos G. Gastric fibrolipoma causing bleeding in a child. *Eur J Pediatr Surg* 2007;**17**:282.

123. Krasniqi AS, Hoxha FT, Bicaj BX, et al. Symptomatic subserosal gastric lipoma successfully treated with enucleation. *World J Gastroenterol* 2008;**14**:5930.

124. Thompson WM, Kende AI, Levy AD. Imaging characteristics of gastric lipomas in 16 adult and pediatric patients. *Am J Roentgenol* 2003;**181**:981.

125. Moues CM, Steenvoorde P, Viersma JH, van Groningen K, de Bruine JF. Jejunal intussusception of a gastric lipoma: a review of literature. *Dig Surg* 2002;**19**:418.

126. Vinces FY, Ciacci J, Sperling DC, Epstein S. Gastroduodenal intussusception secondary to a gastric lipoma. *Can J Gastroenterol* 2005;**19**:107.

127. Ha JP, Tang CN, Cheung HY, Yang GP, Li MK. An unusual cause of gastric outlet obstruction. *Gut* 2007;**56**:967.

128. Zak Y, Biagini B, Moore H, Desantis M, Ghosh BC. Submucosal resection of giant gastric lipoma. *J Surg Oncol* 2006;**94**:63.

129. Al-Brahim N, Radhi J, Gately J. Synchronous epithelioid stromal tumour and lipoma in the stomach. *Can J Gastroenterol* 2003;**17**:374.

130. Yamamoto T, Imakiire K, Hashiguchi S, et al. A rare case of gastric lipoma with early gastric cancer. *Intern Med* 2004;**43**:1039.

131. Gursoy S, Yurci A, Torun E, et al. An uncommon lesion: gastric xanthelasma. *Turk J Gastroenterol* 2005;**16**:167.

132. Yi SY. Dyslipidemia and H pylori in gastric xanthomatosis. *World J Gastroenterol* 2007;**13**:4598.

133. Jeong YS, Park H, Lee DY, Lee SI, Park C. Gastric xanthomatosis. *Gastrointest Endosc* 2004;**59**:399.

134. Kaiserling E, Heinle H, Itabe H, Takano T, Remmele W. Lipid islands in human gastric mucosa: morphological and immunohistochemical findings. *Gastroenterology* 1996;**110**:369.

135. Gravina AG, Iacono A, Alagia I, D'Armiento FP, Sansone S, Romano M. Gastric xanthomatosis associated with gastric intestinal metaplasia in a dyspeptic patient. *Dig Liver Dis* 2009; **41**:765.

136. Muraoka A, Suehiro I, Fujii M, et al. Type IIa early gastric cancer with proliferation of xanthoma cells. *J Gastroenterol* 1998; **33**:326.

137. Lai EC, Tompkins RK. Heterotopic pancreas. Review of a 26 year experience. *Am J Surg* 1986;**151**:697.

138. Rodriguez FJ, Abraham SC, Allen MS, Sebo TJ. Fine-needle aspiration cytology findings from a case of pancreatic heterotopia at the gastroesophageal junction. *Diagn Cytopathol* 2004; **31**:175.

139. Shalaby M, Kochman ML, Lichtenstein GR. Heterotopic pancreas presenting as dysphagia. *Am J Gastroenterol* 2002;**97**:1046.

140. Kim JH, Lim JS, Lee YC, et al. Endosonographic features of gastric ectopic pancreases distinguishable from mesenchymal tumors. *J Gastroenterol Hepatol* 2008;**23**:e301.

141. Ormarsson OT, Gudmundsdottir I, Marvik R. Diagnosis and treatment of gastric heterotopic pancreas. *World J Surg* 2006; **30**:1682.

142. Hammock L, Jorda M. Gastric endocrine pancreatic heterotopia. *Arch Pathol Lab Med* 2002;**126**:464.

143. Hirasaki S, Tanimizu M, Moriwaki T, Nasu J. Acute pancreatitis occurring in gastric aberrant pancreas treated with surgery and proved by histological examination. *Intern Med* 2005;**44**:1169.

144. Mulholland KC, Wallace WD, Epanomeritakis E, Hall SR. Pseudocyst formation in gastric ectopic pancreas. *JOP* 2004;**5**:498.

145. Kaufman A, Storey D, Lee CS, Murali R. Mucinous cyst exhibiting severe dysplasia in gastric heterotopic pancreas associated with gastrointestinal stromal tumour. *World J Gastroenterol* 2007; **13**:5781.

146. Osanai M, Miyokawa N, Tamaki T, Yonekawa M, Kawamura A, Sawada N. Adenocarcinoma arising in gastric heterotopic pancreas: clinicopathological and immunohistochemical study with genetic analysis of a case. *Pathol Int* 2001;**51**:549.

147. Song DE, Kwon Y, Kim KR, Oh ST, Kim JS. Adenocarcinoma arising in gastric heterotopic pancreas: a case report. *J Korean Med Sci* 2004;**19**:145.

148. Chetty R, Weinreb I. Gastric neuroendocrine carcinoma arising from heterotopic pancreatic tissue. *J Clin Pathol* 2004;**57**:314.

149. Mizuno Y, Sumi Y, Nachi S, et al. Acinar cell carcinoma arising from an ectopic pancreas. *Surg Today* 2007;**37**:704.

150. Cieslak TJ, Mullett CT, Puntel RA, Latimer JS. Ménétrier's disease associated with cytomegalovirus infection in children: report of two cases and review of the literature. *Pediatr Infect Dis J* 1993;**12**:340.

151. Occena RO, Taylor SF, Robinson CC, Sokol RJ. Association of cytomegalovirus with Ménétrier's disease in childhood: report of two new cases with a review of literature. *J Pediatr Gastroenterol Nutr* 1993;**17**:217.

152. Bayerdorffer E, Ritter MM, Hatz R, Brooks W, Ruckdeschel G, Stolte M. Healing of protein losing hypertrophic gastropathy by eradication of *Helicobacter pylori* – is *Helicobacter pylori* a pathogenic factor in Ménétrier's disease? *Gut* 1994;**35**:701.

153. Iwama I, Kagimoto S, Takano T, Sekijima T, Kishimoto H, Oba A. Case of pediatric Ménétrier disease with cytomegalovirus and *Helicobacter pylori* co-infection. *Pediatr Int*, **52**:e200.

154. Tokuhara D, Okano Y, Asou K, Tamamori A, Yamano T. Cytomegalovirus and *Helicobacter pylori* co-infection in a child with Ménétrier disease. *Eur J Pediatr* 2007;**166**:63.

155. Jun DW, Kim DH, Kim SH, Song MH, Lee HH, Jo YJ, Park YS. Ménétrier's disease associated with herpes infection: response to treatment with acyclovir. *Gastrointest Endosc* 2007;**65**:1092.

156. Sanchez C, Brody F, Pucci E, Bashir S. Laparoscopic total gastrectomy for Ménétrier's disease. *J Laparoendosc Adv Surg Tech A* 2007;**17**:32.

157. Hemmings CT. Ménétrier's disease in a patient with ulcerative colitis: a case report and review of the literature. *Pathology* 2007; **39**:282.

158. Lim JK, Jang YJ, Jung MK, Ryeom HK, Kim GC, Bae J. Ménétrier disease manifested by polyposis in the gastric antrum and coexisting with gastritis cystica profunda. *Gastrointest Endosc*.

159. Fenoglio-Preiser C, Noffsinger AE, Stemmermann GN, Lantz PE, Isaacson PG, eds. The non-neoplastic stomach. In: *Gastrointestinal Pathology: An atlas and text*, 3rd edn. Philadelphia: Lippincott Williams & Wilkins, 2008: 206.

160. Kurland J, DuBois S, Behling C, Savides T. Severe upper-GI bleed caused by gastritis cystica profunda. *Gastrointest Endosc* 2006;**63**:716.

161. Wolfsen HC, Carpenter HA, Talley NJ. Ménétrier's disease: a form of hypertrophic gastropathy or gastritis? *Gastroenterology* 1993;**104**:1310.

162. Brautbar A, Paz J, Hadas-Halpern I, et al. Ménétrier's disease presenting as an acute protein-losing gastroenteropathy in a 27-year-old man with Gaucher disease. *Eur J Gastroenterol Hepatol* 2005;**17**:679.

163. Chusid EL, Hirsch RL, Colcher H. Spectrum of hypertrophic gastropathy: giant rugal folds, polyposis, and carcinoma of the stomach – case report and review of the literature. *Arch Intern Med* 1964;**114**:621.

164. Wood MG, Bates C, Brown RC, Losowsky MS. Intramucosal carcinoma of the gastric antrum complicating Ménétrier's disease. *J Clin Pathol* 1983;**36**:1071.

165. Madsen LG, Taskiran M, Madsen JL, Bytzer P. Ménétrier's disease and *Helicobacter pylori*: normalization of gastrointestinal protein loss after eradication therapy. *Dig Dis Sci* 1999;**44**:2307.

166. Simon L, Feher I, Salamon A, Vadasz E. Reversible protein-losing hypertrophic gastropathy: causal relationship with *Helicobacter pylori* infection, or simple coincidence? *Am J Gastroenterol* 2000;**95**:1091.

167. Bluth RF, Carpenter HA, Pittelkow MR, Page DL, Coffey RJ. Immunolocalization of transforming growth factor-alpha in normal and diseased human gastric mucosa. *Hum Pathol* 1995; **26**:1333.

168. Dempsey PJ, Goldenring JR, Soroka CJ, et al. Possible role of transforming growth factor alpha in the pathogenesis of Ménétrier's disease: supportive evidence form humans and transgenic mice. *Gastroenterology* 1992;**103**:1950.

169. Burdick JS, Chung E, Tanner G, et al. Treatment of Ménétrier's disease with a monoclonal antibody against the epidermal growth factor receptor. *N Engl J Med* 2000;**343**:1697.

170. Rothenberg M, Pai R, Stuart K. Successful use of octreotide to treat Ménétrier's disease: a rare cause of abdominal pain, weight loss, edema, and hypoalbuminemia. *Dig Dis Sci* 2009; **54**:1403.

171. Toubia N, Schubert ML. Ménétrier's disease. *Curr Treat Options Gastroenterol* 2008;**11**:103.

172. Coffey RJ, Washington MK, Corless CL, Heinrich MC. Ménétrier disease and gastrointestinal stromal tumors: hyperproliferative disorders of the stomach. *J Clin Invest* 2007;**117**:70.

CHAPTER 13

Epithelial tumours of the stomach

Fátima Carneiro[1] and Gregory Y. Lauwers[2]

[1]Faculty of Medicine of the University of Porto, Centro Hospitalar de São João and IPATIMUP, Porto, Portugal
[2]Massachusetts General Hospital and Harvard Medical School, Boston, MA, USA

Benign epithelial tumours

Dysplasia/intra-epithelial neoplasia

Gastric dysplasia represents the penultimate stage of the gastric carcinogenesis sequence [1]. It is characterised by cellular atypia reflective of abnormal differentiation and disorganised glandular architecture. Determination of the correct diagnosis and grade of dysplasia is critical because it predicts the risk of both malignant transformation and metachronous gastric cancer [1].

In the early 1980s, dysplasia was defined as unequivocally neoplastic epithelium [2] and graded in a two-tier system: low grade and high grade dysplasia. The term 'indefinite for dysplasia' (IFD) was coined for epithelia that were neither unequivocally dysplastic nor unequivocally non-dysplastic. However, diagnostic criteria and grading schemes have evolved differently worldwide and there are disagreements between western and Japanese pathologists [3,4], e.g. in Japan, non-invasive intramucosal neoplastic lesions with high grade cellular and architectural atypia are termed 'non-invasive intramucosal carcinoma', whereas the same lesions are diagnosed as high grade dysplasia by most pathologists in the west.

In an attempt to resolve these differences, a consensus nomenclature (the 'Vienna classification') was proposed in 1999 [5] and subsequently updated in 2003 [6]. This original Vienna classification comprises five categories:

1. Negative for neoplasia
2. Indefinite for neoplasia
3. Non-invasive low grade neoplasia

4. Non-invasive high grade neoplasia, including three different types of lesions: high grade adenoma/dysplasia, non-invasive carcinoma (carcinoma *in situ*) and suspicion of invasion
5. Invasive neoplasia, including intramucosal carcinoma as well as carcinoma invasive into the submucosa or beyond.

The updated version, presented in 2003, takes into account improvement in endoscopic techniques and their management implications. Consequently, non-invasive, high grade, pre-malignant lesions, without invasion of the lamina propria, and invasive adenocarcinomas confined to the lamina propria, were placed in the single diagnostic category 4 (Table 13.1).

Recently, the World Health Organization (WHO) reiterated the classification of dysplasia/intra-epithelial neoplasia. Acknowledging widespread use of both 'dysplasia' and 'intra-epithelial neoplasia' (IEN), it uses these terms as synonymous. The following categories should thus be considered.

Indefinite for intra-epithelial neoplasia/dysplasia

This term represents a pragmatic solution to an ambiguous morphological pattern but it is not a final diagnosis. It should not be seen as a diagnostic failure but, rather, as the response to a real practical issue. The use of this category is favoured where there is doubt as to whether a lesion is neoplastic or non-neoplastic (i.e. reactive or regenerative), particularly in small biopsies exhibiting inflammation. Regenerative changes can be mistaken for intra-epithelial neoplasia/dysplasia, especially in reactive gastritis and at

Morson and Dawson's Gastrointestinal Pathology, Fifth Edition. Edited by Neil A. Shepherd, Bryan F. Warren, Geraint T. Williams, Joel K. Greenson, Gregory Y. Lauwers and Marco R. Novelli.

Table 13.1 The Vienna classification of gastrointestinal epithelial neoplasia

Vienna classification, 1999 [5]	Updated Vienna classification, 2003 [6]
Negative for neoplasia/dysplasia (category 1)	No neoplasia (category 1)
Indefinite for neoplasia/dysplasia (category 2)	Indefinite for neoplasia (category 2)
Non-invasive low grade neoplasia (low grade adenoma/dysplasia) (category 3)	Low grade adenoma/dysplasia (category 3)
High grade adenoma/dysplasia (category 4.1)	High grade adenoma/dysplasia (category 4.1)
Non-invasive carcinoma (carcinoma *in situ*) (category 4.2)	Non-invasive carcinoma (carcinoma *in situ*) (category 4.2)
Suspicion of invasive carcinoma (category 4.3)	Suspicion for invasive carcinoma (category 4.3)
Intramucosal carcinoma (category 5.1)	Intramucosal carcinoma (category 4.4)
Submucosal carcinoma or beyond (category 5.2)	Submucosal invasive carcinoma or beyond (category 5)

the edge of a benign ulcer or in the postoperative stomach. The distinction between regenerative atypia and low grade intra-epithelial neoplasia/dysplasia can be difficult and is reflected in the significant inter-observer variation reported in the diagnosis of dysplasia. In such cases, the dilemma may be solved by cutting to deeper levels, obtaining additional biopsies or considering all possible aetiologies. Foveolar hyperplasia may show irregular and tortuous tubular structures with epithelial mucus depletion, a high nucleus:cytoplasm ratio and loss of cellular polarity. Enlarged, hyperchromatic nuclei associated with prominent mitoses, if present, are usually located near the proliferative zone in the mucus–neck region. The glands may appear closely packed and lined by cells with large, hyperchromatic, basally located nuclei. Importantly, the cytoarchitectural alterations tend to decrease from the base of the glands towards the superficial portion (Figure 13.1).

Intra-epithelial neoplasia/dysplasia

This category comprises unequivocally neoplastic epithelial proliferations characterised by variable cellular and architectural atypia but without convincing evidence of invasion. Intra-epithelial neoplasia (gastric epithelial dysplasia) can have polypoid, flat, or slightly depressed growth patterns; the flat or slightly depressed patterns may show an irregular appearance on chromoendoscopy or microvasculature anomalies on narrow-band imaging, which are not apparent with conventional white-light endoscopy (Figure 13.2).

In Europe and North America, the term 'adenoma' has been applied when the neoplastic proliferation produces a discrete, protruding lesion. Histologically, gastric adeno-

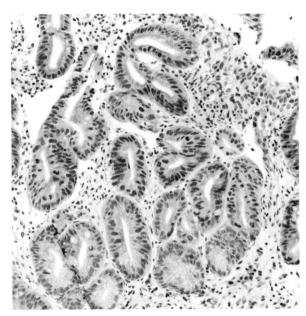

Figure 13.1 Indefinite for dysplasia: the disorganised pits and glands show limited branching. The nuclei are hyperchromatic with limited stratification and overlapping. However, the stromal inflammation raises the suspicion of an atypical regenerative process.

mas may have a tubular, villous or tubulovillous architecture. The larger they are, the more likely they are to be villous. However, in Japan, 'adenomas' include all gross types (i.e. flat, elevated and depressed).

Most cases have an intestinal phenotype (adenomatous, type I) resembling colonic adenomas with crowded, tubular glands, lined by atypical columnar cells with overlapping, pencillate, hyperchromatic and/or pleomorphic nuclei with pseudostratification and inconspicuous nucleoli, mucin depletion and lack of surface maturation [7] (Figure 13.3). Other variants include a gastric phenotype (foveolar or pyloric phenotype, type II) in which the cells are cuboidal or low columnar, with clear or eosinophilic cytoplasm and show round-to-oval nuclei [7] (Figure 13.4). Differentiation towards goblet, Paneth and enterochromaffin cells can be seen. It is frequently focal and can occur with no architectural disorganisation in the mucosa. The two types may be distinguished by mucin, CD10 and cdx-2 expres-sion (intestinal/adenomatous: MUC2, CD10 and cdx-2; gastric/foveolar: MUC5AC, absence of CD10 and low expression of cdx-2) [8–10], as well as by background changes in the gastric mucosa [11]. Cases with hybrid differentiation may also occur [9]. Finally, a pyloric adenomatous variant has been noted. These lesions are frequently observed in the body/fundus of elderly patients and are commonly associated with autoimmune gastritis. The lesions are characterised by eosinophilic cuboidal cells with finely granular cytoplasm with round nuclei and limited mitotic activity (Figure 13.5).

Further, the exceedingly rare tubule neck (or globoid) dysplasia is believed to be a precursor of sporadic diffuse-type gastric carcinoma [12]. The features of this subtype are ill-defined but it is generally believed to be composed of disorganised cells with rounded nuclei and other cells assuming signet-ring cell features, but limited by the basement membrane and noted in the glandular neck region.

Low and high grade intra-epithelial neoplasia/dysplasia

Low grade intra-epithelial neoplasia/dysplasia shows minimal architectural disarray and only mild to moderate cytological atypia. The nuclei are elongated, polarised and basally located and mitotic activity is mild to moderate. For polypoid lesions, the term 'low grade adenoma' can be used (Figure 13.3).

High grade intra-epithelial neoplasia/dysplasia shows neoplastic cells that are usually cuboidal rather than columnar, with a high nucleus:cytoplasm ratio, prominent amphophilic nucleoli, more pronounced architectural disarray and numerous mitoses, which can be atypical. (Figure 13.6). Increased mitotic activity in itself is not pathognomonic of intra-epithelial neoplasia/dysplasia, because it is seen in regenerating epithelium as well. Importantly, the

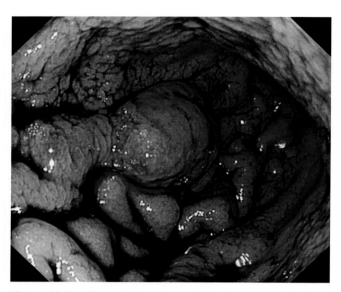

Figure 13.2 Endoscopic appearance of gastric dysplasia: the contour of the raised lesion with a congested mucosa is easily recognised when chromoendoscopy is performed (courtesy of Dr Shinichi Ban).

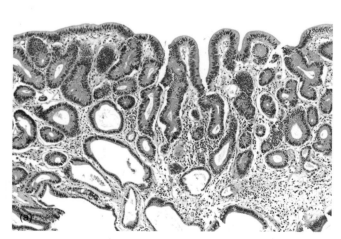

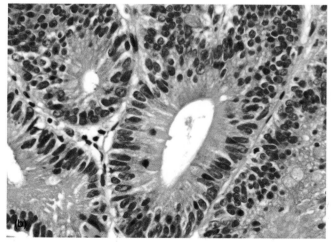

Figure 13.3 Low grade dysplasia (adenomatous type): (a) there is limited architectural disarray. (b) Mucin depletion is notable along with pencillate hyperchromatic nuclei with no stratification.

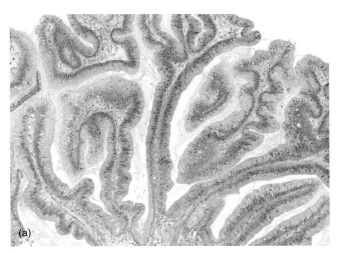
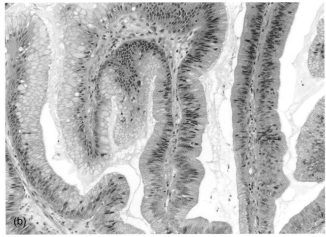

Figure 13.4 Low grade dysplasia (foveolar type): (a) the lesion is characterised by epithelial fronds with serrated contours. (b) The lining epithelium, composed of columnar cells with varying amounts of apical mucin, retains a distinctly foveolar phenotype.

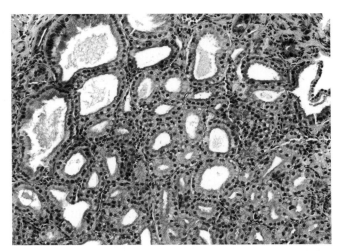

Figure 13.5 Pyloric type dysplasia: the lesion displays back-to-back glands lined by small cuboidal faintly eosinophilic cells. In this example of low dysplasia, the cells have small hyperchromatic nuclei.

nuclei frequently extend towards the luminal half of the cell and nuclear polarity is usually lost. For polypoid lesions, the term 'high grade adenoma' can be used. In general, the diagnosis of high grade intra-epithelial neoplasia/dysplasia is more reproducible than the diagnosis of low grade lesions.

Intramucosal invasive neoplasia/intramucosal carcinoma

Intramucosal invasive neoplasia defines carcinomas that infiltrate the lamina propria. It is distinguished from intra-epithelial neoplasia/dysplasia not only by desmoplastic changes which can be minimal or absent but also by distinct structural anomalies, such as marked glandular crowding, excessive branching and budding. Intraluminal necrotic

debris is common. Single infiltrating cells can also be seen within the lamina propria in the absence of desmoplasia. The neoplastic cells in intramucosal invasive neoplasia are usually cuboidal with a high nucleus:cytoplasm ratio. Round nuclei with prominent nucleoli and marked loss of polarity are common. Mitoses are usually numerous and atypical mitoses can be identified (Figure 13.7).

The management of intra-epithelial neoplasia/dysplasia and intramucosal adenocarcinoma

The diagnosis of gastric intra-epithelial neoplasia/dysplasia alerts the gastroenterologist that the patient has an increased, albeit variable, risk of progression to gastric cancer. Progression to adenocarcinoma has been reported as 0–23% for low grade intra-epithelial neoplasia/dysplasia, within a mean interval of 10 months to 4 years. In contrast, the rate of malignant transformation for high grade lesions is in the range 60–85% over a median interval of 4–48 months [13–19]. However, a diagnosis of carcinoma within a year or less of a diagnosis of intra-epithelial neoplasia/dysplasia is more likely to represent failure to recognise a pre-existing cancer rather than true neoplastic progression [14–16].

Given the low rate of malignant transformation of low grade intra-epithelial neoplasia/dysplasia, endoscopic resection with annual endoscopic surveillance with re-biopsy is typically performed [20,21]. Patients who have high grade intra-epithelial neoplasia/dysplasia, large adenomatous polyps or well differentiated intramucosal adenocarcinomas no more than 20 mm in size should undergo definitive therapy, which can be achieved by endoscopic mucosal resection, obviating the need for surgical resection in many cases [22,23]. Mucosal lesions that are not amenable to endoscopic resection are best managed with surgical resection.

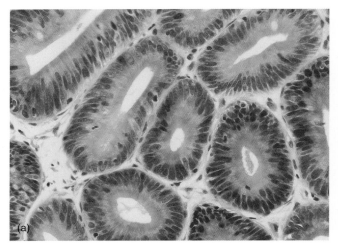 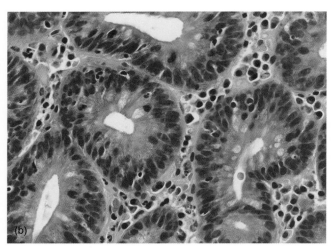

Figure 13.6 Low and high grade dysplasia (adenomatous type): (a) the basally located pencillate hyperchromatic nuclei with limited stratification are characteristic of low grade dysplasia. (b) High grade lesions display larger, rounder nuclei and increased mitotic activity.

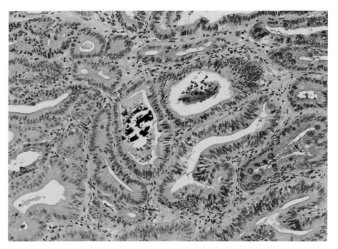

Figure 13.7 Intramucosal adenocarcinoma: the diagnosis is based not only on the high grade nuclear features but also on the marked architectural disarray with back-to-back and merging glands. Note also the intra-glandular necrosis.

The diagnosis of intramucosal carcinoma indicates that there is an increased risk of lymphatic invasion and lymph node metastasis. However, novel endoscopic techniques allow treatment without open surgery, particularly for lesions ≤20 mm in size and for those that are well differentiated with no lymphatic invasion [22].

Malignant epithelial tumours

Adenocarcinoma

Adenocarcinomas of the stomach are a biologically and genetically heterogeneous group of malignant epithelial neoplasms resulting from multifactorial environmental and genetic aetiologies. They are characterised by broad morphological heterogeneity in architectural and growth patterns, cell differentiation and histogenesis.

Epidemiology

Gastric cancer accounts for 10% of cancers worldwide [24]. However, the distribution is uneven, from areas of high incidence (>60 per 100 000 males) as in eastern Asia, eastern Europe and Latin America, to zones of low incidence (<15 per 100 000 population) as in North America, northern Europe, and most countries in Africa and south-east Asia [25]. In regions of high incidence, cancers of the antrum and pylorus are most common, whereas cancers of the proximal stomach and the oesophago-gastric junction (OGJ) are more common in countries with a low incidence [26].

Notably, OGJ adenocarcinoma shares many epidemiological characteristics with cancers of the distal oesophagus and of the proximal stomach. Incidence rates are higher among Caucasians, in men compared to women and in older patients [27]. The incidence of this type of tumour increased markedly in the second half of the twentieth century [28] in both the USA [29,30] and Europe [31], in parallel with rising incidence of adenocarcinomas of the lower oesophagus [32,33].

Gastric carcinoma in young patients

Less than 10% of gastric cancer patients present with the disease before age 45 years (early onset gastric cancer) [34,35]. In this group of patients, the male:female ratio is approximately equal or shows female predominance. Furthermore, most tumours are usually of diffuse type [34,36–38]. Once considered to be associated with poor prognosis [39], recent studies show that young gastric cancer patients no longer present with more advanced disease than elderly patients and overall survival is better in young patients with resectable tumour [37,38]. Several studies point to a pathogenesis of early onset gastric cancer different from that of sporadic cancers occurring at a later age [35,40–46]. In some populations an association has been found between virulent strains of *Helicobacter pylori* (*H. pylori*) and the development of early onset cancers [47,48]. Furthermore, 10–25% of young patients with gastric cancer have a positive family history, suggesting the aetiological importance of genetic factors. Among these are hereditary cancers in individuals with germline mutations of the E-cadherin gene [49].

Aetiology and pathogenesis

Gastric carcinogenesis is a multistep and multifactorial process which, in many cases, appears to involve a progression from normal mucosa through chronic gastritis, atrophic gastritis and intestinal metaplasia to dysplasia and carcinoma, a sequence of events that has been designated as the Correa cascade of multi-step gastric carcinogenesis [50,51]. A number of precancerous conditions have been recognised, such as atrophic gastritis and intestinal metaplasia due to *H. pylori* infection or autoimmunity, gastric ulcers, gastric polyps, previous gastric surgery and Ménétrier's disease. There also are putative associations with environmental agents such as dietary constituents and the formation of carcinogenic *N*-nitroso compounds within the stomach. In a minority of cases, there is good evidence for an inherited disposition.

Chronic gastritis and intestinal metaplasia

An association has been demonstrated between chronic gastritis, particularly atrophic gastritis with intestinal metaplasia, and gastric cancer, particularly in areas of high incidence [50–52]. Epidemiologically, the prevalence of chronic atrophic gastritis within populations correlates closely with the incidence and death rate from gastric cancer [51–53] and, in follow-up studies, atrophic gastritis has been shown to precede the development of malignancy [54,55]. Conditions that predispose to gastric cancer, such as pernicious anaemia and the postoperative stomach, are frequently characterised by extensive atrophic gastritis and intestinal metaplasia.

As a result of the heterogeneity of intestinal metaplasia, interest has focused on the significance of its different subtypes. Although all three types are associated with gastric cancer, type III intestinal metaplasia, which is the least common and characterised by the presence of columnar mucous cells containing sulphomucins, is the most closely associated, especially with intestinal-type adenocarcinoma [56,57]. However, type III metaplasia is considered to be a marker neither sensitive nor specific enough to be used in routine practice for selecting individuals for gastric cancer surveillance [58,59].

Several classification schemes of chronic gastritis have been developed in an attempt to combine topographic, morphological and aetiological information into a reporting system including both grading and staging of gastritis [60,61]. In the Sydney classification system, several features of inflammation, atrophy and intestinal metaplasia, are assessed individually. A visual analogue scale was added to facilitate grading but agreement is limited [62–65]. To date, three histopathology indices have been proposed to evaluate the cancer risk associated with atrophic gastritis: the Gastric Risk Index [66], the OLGA (Operative Link for Gastritis Assessment) system [67] and the Baylor system [68]. Recently, a long-term follow-up study provides the first evidence that OLGA staging conveys relevant information on the clinico-pathological outcome of gastritis [69]. It also has been suggested that, based on OLGA staging and *H. pylori* status, patients could be stratified and managed confidently according to their cancer risk [69].

The two main types of intestinal metaplasia that have been described are 'complete' (i.e. 'small intestinal type' or type I) and 'incomplete' (types IIA/II and IIB/III) [70,71]. Complete-type intestinal metaplasia shows decreased expression of gastric mucins (MUC1, MUC5AC and MUC6) and expression of MUC2, an intestinal mucin. In contrast, in incomplete intestinal metaplasia, gastric mucins are co-expressed with MUC2. These expression patterns show that incomplete intestinal metaplasia has a mixed gastric and intestinal phenotype, reflecting an aberrant differentiation programme [72]. Some studies indicate a positive correlation of the degree of incomplete intestinal metaplasia, the extent of intestinal metaplasia and the risk of progression to carcinoma [57,73–75]. However, these associations have not been confirmed [76–78]. Furthermore, some authors also claim that intestinal metaplasia is a 'para-cancerous' lesion and not pre-cancerous [79].

Another pattern of metaplasia, spasmolytic polypeptide-expressing metaplasia (SPEM), expresses trefoil factor family 2 spasmolytic polypeptide and is associated with oxyntic atrophy. SPEM characteristically develops in the gastric body and fundus, shares biochemical features with pseudo-pyloric metaplasia and is strongly associated with chronic *H. pylori* infection and gastric adenocarcinoma. It is believed to represent another pathway to gastric neoplasia [80].

Helicobacter pylori infection and gastric cancer

H. pylori has an important role in gastric carcinogenesis, because almost all non-cardiac gastric cancers develop from a background of *H. pylori*-infected mucosa [81,82]. In 1994, the WHO categorised the bacterium as a group 1 carcinogen for gastric cancer [83] based on results of epidemiological studies that were available at that time [84–87], and later confirmed [88–90]. In a meta-analysis evaluating prospective studies in individuals tested at least

10 years before diagnosis, the odds ratio for cancer risk was 5.9 (95% confidence interval [CI] 3.4–10.3) [91].

The causal link between *H. pylori* and gastric cancer is supported by animal models [92–95], as well as experimental studies showing that *H. pylori* eradication has a prophylactic effect on gastric cancer risk [96–98]. However, the prophylactic effect of such eradication in humans remains controversial [99,100] and a meta-analysis of four randomised intervention studies with gastric cancer incidence as a secondary outcome showed a non-statistically significant overall odds ratio of 0.67 (95%CI 0.42–1.07) [101]. However, it was shown that, in patients with early gastric cancer, the eradication of *H. pylori* after endoscopic resection reduced the development of metachronous gastric cancer [102,103].

Factors associated with colonisation and pathogenicity of *H. pylori* comprise outer membrane proteins, including BabA, SabA, OipA, AlpA/B and homB [104–106], as well as the virulence factors cagA, in the cag pathogenicity island (cagPAI), and the vacuolating cytotoxin vacA [107–109]. Polymorphic determinants influencing the expression of vacA cytotoxin include the signal region (s1 and s2), mid-region (m1 and m2), intermediary region (i1 and i2), and d region (d1 and d2) [110–112]. Strains producing the cagA protein that induces a greater degree of inflammation are associated with gastric pre-cancerous lesions and a greater risk of developing 'non-cardia' cancer [113,114]. Although the risk of gastric cancer in some countries of Europe and North America has been related to vacA genotype [115,116], such relationships have not been observed in east Asian countries, suggesting that the consequences of vacuolating activity are locale dependent [112].

Cytokines modulate the severity and extent of gastritis caused by *H. pylori*. Polymorphisms of the interleukin 1β gene (*IL-1β*) (initiation and amplification of inflammatory response) and the IL-1-receptor antagonist gene (*IL-1RN*) (modulation of inflammation) are associated with susceptibility to carcinogenesis associated with *H. pylori* [117]. It has been suggested that in individuals with alleles that predispose to inflammation, infection with *H. pylori* may cause increased production of gastric IL-1β, leading to severe and sustained inflammation and thus an increased risk of developing cancer [118–120].

H. pylori infection also has been associated with modified expression of specific oncogenes or tumour-suppressor genes, such as *CTNNB1* (β-catenin), *CCND1* (cyclin D1), *TP73* (p73) and *CDKN1B* (p27) [121–123]. Finally, the role of bone marrow-derived cells (BMDCs), in the re-population of damaged gastric mucosa, has shown to be associated with the development of intestinal metaplasia and gastric cancer [124,125].

Diet

Diet plays an important role in gastric carcinogenesis, especially for intestinal-type adenocarcinoma. Low intake of fresh fruit and vegetables, low levels of vitamin C, vitamin E and carotenoids, has been shown to increase cancer risk, especially in *H. pylori*-infected individuals [126–128]. Mechanistically, vitamins C and E inhibit the formation of *N*-nitroso compounds [129] and scavenge oxygen-derived free radicals but it is uncertain whether these represent the primary mechanisms of their protective effect. A recent meta-analysis of randomised trials comparing the effect of anti-oxidant supplements (β-carotene, vitamin A, vitamin C, vitamin E and selenium, alone or in combination) with placebo or no intervention did not show a significant protective effect on the incidence of gastric cancer [130]. Notably, the results seem to be influenced by whether the trials are performed in well-nourished populations or in those likely to have nutritional deficiencies [131]. However, high plasma concentrations of carotenoids, retinol and α-tocopherol were found to be associated with reduced risk of gastric cancer [132].

High intake of salt-preserved foods (a probable mucosal irritant) and/or smoked foods [133,134] is a risk factor for gastric cancer, particularly in combination with *H. pylori* infection [127,134,135]. Intake of all meat, red meat and processed meat, is also associated with an increased risk of 'non-cardia' cancer [136]. The so-called 'Mediterranean diet' was shown to be associated with a significant reduction in the risk of incident gastric cancer; it is defined as the high consumption of fruit, vegetables, cereals, legumes, nuts and seeds, and seafood, with olive oil as the main fat source, moderate alcohol consumption (particularly red wine), a low-to-moderate consumption of dairy products (mainly cheese and yogurt) and a relatively low consumption of red and processed meat [137]. Furthermore, citrus fruit was observed to have a probable protective effect, mainly on 'cardia' cancer [138]. Finally, it was shown that cereal fibre consumption could reduce the risk of diffuse-type gastric cancer [139].

Smoking

An association has been shown between smoking and stomach cancer that could not be explained by bias or confounding factors [140,141]. Smoking also potentiates the carcinogenic effect of infection with cagA-positive *H. pylori* [142–144].

Autoimmune gastritis and pernicious anaemia

Pernicious anaemia is associated with an increased risk of gastric dysplasia and gastric carcinoma [145–147]. However, the magnitude of the risk is debated; it is reported by some to be around three times that of the general population [148–152], although a large US population-based cohort study found an incidence of gastric cancer of only 1.2%, similar to that of the general population [153].

There also is an increased incidence of mucosal polyps in autoimmune gastritis, and some of these show adenomatous dysplasia of the glandular epithelium [154]. Furthermore, there is a well-established increased risk of developing neuro-endocrine tumours/carcinoids [155,156] which arise as a result of the proliferative effect of longstanding hypergastrinaemia on gastric fundic enterochromaffin-like (ECL) cells [157] (see below).

Gastric polyps and cancer

Gastric epithelial polyps may be classified as neoplastic and non-neoplastic, the former encompassing adenomatous polyps (intestinal type), gastric-type adenomas (pyloric gland adenomas and foveolar-type adenomas) and fundic gland polyps. Non-neoplastic polyps of the stomach include hyperplastic polyps, hamartomatous polyps (Peutz–Jeghers, juvenile and Cronkhite–Canada syndrome-associated polyps) and miscellaneous lesions with a polypoid growth pattern [158,159]. They are more comprehensively covered in Chapter 12 (see 'Polyps developing in the setting of polyposis') and this section addresses mainly their cancer risk and association.

Hyperplastic polyps Hyperplastic polyps are discussed in Chapter 12 (see 'Hyperplastic polyps'). Malignant transformation, although rare, is well documented [160–164]. Intramucosal carcinoma may be found in up to 2%, especially in lesions >20 mm in diameter [161,165]. Diffuse gastric cancer in a setting of hyperplastic polyposis has been described in a Portuguese family [160].

Fundic gland (cyst) polyps Fundic gland (cyst) polyps may occur sporadically, in patients with familial adenomatous polyposis (FAP) [159] or as a familial condition confined to the stomach with no colorectal polyposis [166]. They also affect patients receiving long-term treatment with proton pump inhibitors [167,168]. Although sporadic fundic gland polyps have very weak malignant potential and the frequency of dysplasia is very low [169,170], fundic gland polyps developing in patients with FAP develop intra-epithelial neoplasia/dysplasia in up to 48% of cases, but carcinomas remain extremely rare [171,172].

The operated stomach and cancer

Patients with a gastric stump after previous gastric surgery have an increased risk of developing gastric cancer compared with the general population [173,174]. This risk increases, usually after 15–25 years [175–178]. It is higher after Billroth II gastrectomy and in those who have undergone surgery for gastric ulcer, whereas those operated on for duodenal ulcer are at a lower risk [179]. Bile reflux and secondary reactive gastritis, observed in post-gastrectomy gastric stumps [180], are likely to play a role in promoting gastric carcinogenesis in this situation: it is often associated with intestinal metaplasia, the prevalence of which increases with higher concentrations of bile in the gastric juice [181,182]. A high frequency of dysplasia was reported in gastric stump biopsies [183,184] but some of this may represent the florid regenerative atypia now recognised to occur in reactive gastritis. The development of hyperplastic polyps, either single or multiple, may play a role in the genesis of stump cancer close to the stoma [185].

Hypertrophic gastropathy and gastritis, including Ménétrier's disease

The incidence of carcinoma complicating Ménétrier's disease has been reported as 8–10% [186]. However, establishing the diagnosis can be difficult. In some cases, a finding of thickened gastric folds at endoscopy, or on radiological examination at the time of diagnosis of gastric cancer, has been attributed to Ménétrier's disease but histological confirmation can be lacking. Furthermore, it is equally possible that an infiltrating carcinoma has given rise to the appearances secondarily. Nevertheless, there are reports of early gastric cancer occurring synchronously with histologically proven Ménétrier's disease [187–189].

Peptic ulcer disease

It is well established that chronic duodenal ulcer is associated with a reduced risk of gastric cancer [190]. The association between chronic gastric ulcer and cancer is less clear. However, in a study of Swedish patients with gastric ulcer who did not undergo surgery, it was observed that the incidence of gastric cancer was almost twice the expected rate during an average follow-up of 9 years [191]. This was particularly true for women and patients with ulcers in the body of the stomach compared with those with pre-pyloric ulcers. Interestingly, eradication of *H. pylori* is associated with decreased risk of gastric cancer in patients with peptic ulcer disease [192].

Genetic predisposition and hereditary syndromes

First-degree relatives of patients with gastric cancer are almost three times as likely as the general population to develop gastric cancer themselves [193]. This may be partly attributable to *H. pylori* infection being common in families and to the potential role of *IL-1* gene polymorphisms [117,118]. Susceptibility to carcinogens may play a role as well, e.g. polymorphisms of genes encoding for glutathione *S*-transferase enzymes, known to metabolise tobacco-related carcinogens and *N*-acetyltransferase 1, increase the risk of gastric cancer development [194,195]. There is also evidence of familial clustering: about 10% of stomach cancers show evidence of a familial component and approximately 1–3% of gastric cancers are a result of an inherited predisposition [196–198].

Macroscopic features and topography of gastric adenocarcinoma

The OGJ corresponds to the level at which the oesophagus ends and the stomach begins. The OGJ can be described in many ways: the end of the tubular oesophagus, the squamo-columnar junction, the peritoneal reflection, the angle of His, the proximal limit of gastric rugal folds, the distal limit of squamous epithelium, the proximal limit of gastric oxyntic mucosa, the distal limit of the lower oesophageal sphincter and the distal limit of palisading vessels [199–202]. The proximal stomach is often referred to as the 'cardia' but the histology of this region is controversial. Some suggest that the 'cardia' is composed of pure oxyntic glands and others propose that it may be composed of pure mucous glands or a mixture of mucous glands and oxyntic glands [203–206].

The various classification systems that have been proposed for OGJ tumours [207,208] have generally been based on the location of the tumour epicentre in relation to the OGJ, such as the Siewert classification [208]. According to the WHO classification [209]:

1. Adenocarcinomas that cross the OGJ are considered to be adenocarcinomas of the OGJ, regardless of where the bulk of the tumour lies.

2. Adenocarcinomas located entirely above the OGJ are considered to represent oesophageal carcinomas.

3. Adenocarcinomas located entirely below the OGJ are considered to be gastric in origin.

For the third group, the use of the ambiguous and often misleading term 'carcinoma of the gastric cardia' is discouraged in favour of 'carcinoma of the proximal stomach.' The seventh edition of the TNM classification of the American Joint Committee on Cancer proposes that cancers with an epicentre in the lower oesophagus or OGJ or within the proximal 50 mm of the stomach but extending into the OGJ be staged as primary oesophageal adenocarcinoma, whereas other tumours of the proximal stomach be staged as gastric cancer.

Interestingly, a recent study evaluating Chinese patients indicated that, in this specific population, proximal gastric cancers extending into the OGJ are better staged as gastric cancer [210]. This is not completely surprising, because epidemiological studies indicate that OGJ tumours can be divided into two groups. In the west, most lesions are associated with gastro-oesophageal reflux disease (GORD) and other characteristics similar to adenocarcinoma arising in Barrett's oesophagus (see Chapters 5 and 7). However, in parts of Asia, e.g. in China, but also for a subset of tumours diagnosed in the west, neoplasms of the proximal stomach arise in a setting of chronic atrophic gastritis with *H. pylori* infection and are similar to distal gastric cancer.

Advanced gastric carcinomas can display various gross appearances. Borrmann's classification remains the most widely used and divides gastric carcinomas into four distinct types: polypoid carcinoma (type I), fungating carcinoma (type II), ulcerating carcinoma (type III), diffusely infiltrating carcinoma (type IV) and unclassifiable (type V) [211] (Figure 13.8).

Polypoid and fungating tumours typically consist of friable, ulcerated masses that bleed easily and project from

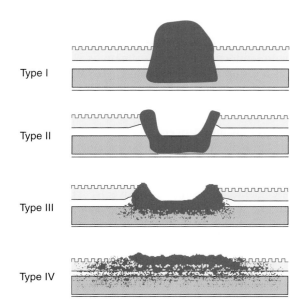

Figure 13.8 The five categories of the Borrmann classification for advanced carcinoma is as follows: type I: polypoid; type II: fungating, ulcerated with sharp raised margins; type III: ulcerated with poorly defined infiltrative margins; type IV: infiltrative, predominantly intramural lesion, poorly demarcated; and type V: unclassifiable (not shown).

a broad base in the gastric lumen. They tend to develop in the body of the stomach, in the region of the greater curvature, posterior wall or fundus (Figure 13.9b).

Ulcerated tumours occur frequently in the OGJ, antrum or lesser curvature. They can differ from benign ulcers by an irregular margin with raised borders and thickened, uneven and indurated surrounding mucosa (Figure 13.9a). The ulcer base is necrotic, shaggy and often nodular. Mucosal folds radiating from the crater are irregular and frequently show club-like thickening and fusion. Malignant ulcers tend to be larger than their benign counterparts. However, many malignant ulcers lack these typical features and, therefore, endoscopic appearance is not a sufficiently reliable guide to diagnosis [212] and should be complemented by biopsies.

Invasive adenocarcinoma may spread superficially in the mucosa and submucosa, giving rise to plaque-like lesions with flattening of the rugal folds. In some cases, superficial ulceration supervenes. Frequently, however, the infiltration involves the entire thickness of the wall, usually over a limited area but sometimes extensively, to produce the so-called linitis plastica or 'leather-bottle' stomach. In these cases, the wall assumes a stiff consistency due to an extensive desmoplastic response to tumour cells. In such cases, there is usually no visible localised growth. A characteristic feature, at endoscopy, of this tumour type is that, because of the diffuse involvement of the stomach, it fails to inflate, in marked contrast to the normal stomach.

Other gastric carcinomas, irrespective of histological type, may secrete considerable amounts of mucin, which

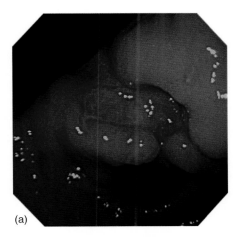

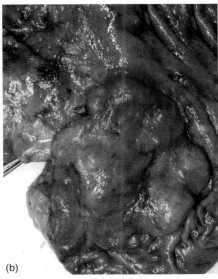

Figure 13.9 Gross appearance of gastric adenocarcinoma:
(a) Borrmann type III: the ulcerated neoplasm is surrounded by
thickened gastric folds indicating infiltration in the surrounding wall.
(b) Borrmann type I: the polypoid tumour is sharply demarcated
from the surrounding mucosa. (Courtesy of Dr Hiroshi Fujita.)

gives the tumour a gelatinous appearance to the naked eye.
These are sometimes referred to as mucinous or colloid
carcinomas.

Microscopic features

Despite epidemiological differences, adenocarcinomas of
the proximal and distal stomach show similar microscopic
features. The histological classification of gastric adenocarcinoma is challenging because of intratumoral variations in
architecture and/or differentiation and several histological
classifications have been proposed over the years.

The WHO classification

The WHO classification, which does not take into account
histogenesis and differentiation, recognises five main types of
adenocarcinomas, as well as rare variants [213] (Table 13.2).

Table 13.2 The World Health Organization classification of
epithelial tumours of the stomach [213]

Malignancy-associated and premalignant lesions
Glandular intraepithelial neoplasia (dysplasia), low grade
Glandular intraepithelial neoplasia (dysplasia), high grade
Adenoma

Adenocarcinoma
Papillary adenocarcinoma
Tubular adenocarcinoma
Mucinous adenocarcinoma
Poorly cohesive carcinoma (including signet ring cell carcinoma
and other variants)
Mixed carcinoma
Adenosquamous carcinoma
Squamous cell carcinoma
Hepatoid adenocarcinoma
Carcinoma with lymphoid stroma (medullary carcinoma)
Undifferentiated carcinoma
Hereditary diffuse gastric cancer

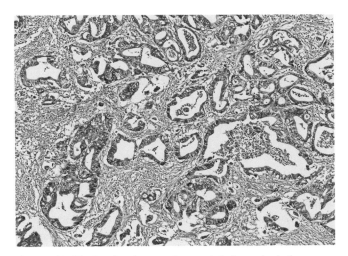

Figure 13.10 Gastric adenocarcinoma, tubular variant: the
neoplasm is composed of irregularly shaped tubules lined by
columnar neoplastic cells.

Tubular adenocarcinoma This type consists of tubular structures, branching glands or acinar structures surrounded by
various degrees of desmoplasia. Individual neoplastic cells
can be columnar, cuboidal or flattened by prominent intraluminal mucin. A clear cell variant has also been recognised. Nuclear atypia ranging from low to high grade
can be seen [214,215]. A poorly differentiated variant, composed of compact infiltrative sheets of tumour cells, has
been called solid carcinoma. At the other end of the spectrum, very well differentiated gastric adenocarcinoma has
been described. These tumours develop mainly in the body
of the stomach; they show mild cytological atypia and
limited architectural distortion (Figure 13.10).

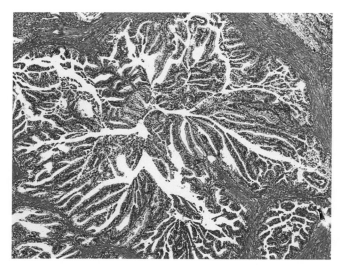

Figure 13.11 Gastric adenocarcinoma, papillary variant: the anastomosing fibrovascular cores lined by neoplastic cells are characteristic of this type.

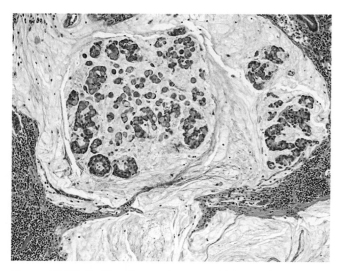

Figure 13.12 Gastric adenocarcinoma, mucinous variant: scattered signet-ring cells are noted in the abundant mucinous lake.

Papillary adenocarcinoma Typically, this tumour grows as an exophytic polypoid mass with sharply demarcated invading edge; these adenocarcinomas are composed of pointed or blunted papillary epithelial processes with fibrovascular cores. Tubulocystic formation may be observed but the papillary pattern predominates. The neoplastic cells tend to maintain their polarity and the degree of cellular atypia and mitotic index can vary significantly. A dense acute and chronic inflammatory infiltrate can be noted (Figure 13.11).

Mucinous adenocarcinoma Mucinous adenocarcinomas (also described as mucoid or colloid carcinomas) are composed of malignant epithelium mixed with extracellular mucinous pools. Marked heterogeneity can be seen in some tumours, with the epithelial component forming glands whereas, in others, disaggregated ribbons or clusters of signet-ring cells float in lakes of mucin (Figure 13.12).

Poorly cohesive carcinomas, including signet-ring cell carcinoma Discohesive tumours were previously inaccurately included in a general category of signet-ring cell carcinoma even in cases in which signet-ring cells were not identified. The new WHO classification recognises that a general category of poorly cohesive tumours better reflects the wide diversity of tumours composed of neoplastic cells which are isolated or arranged in small aggregates and may display various morphologies. These encompass:
• Signet-ring cell type, a tumour composed predominantly or exclusively of signet-ring cells characterised by a central, optically clear, globoid droplet of cytoplasmic mucin with an eccentrically placed nucleus (Figure 13.13a). The cells may form a lace-like or delicate microtrabecular pattern (usually when intramucosal) or are accompanied by marked

desmoplasia in deeper levels of the gastric wall. In some cases, signet-ring cells may be restricted to the superficial aspect of the mucosa with a transition towards other variants of discohesive cells within the deeper levels of the gastric wall. Tumours composed predominantly of signet-ring cells are more common in younger patients and in the distal stomach [216].
• Other cellular variants, including tumours composed of neoplastic cells resembling histiocytes or lymphocytes; others have deeply eosinophilic cytoplasm sometimes mimicking plasma cells [217] (Figure 13.13b). Some poorly cohesive cells may show significant nuclear irregularity, including particularly bizarre nuclei. Finally, a mixture of the different cell types can be seen, including signet-ring cells.

Mixed carcinoma These adenocarcinomas show a mixture of morphologically identifiable glandular (tubular/papillary) and poorly cohesive cellular histological components (Figure 13.14a). Mixed carcinomas have been shown to be clonal [218,219]] and the phenotypic divergence has been attributed to somatic mutation in the E-cadherin gene (*CDH1*), restricted to the poorly cohesive component [220] (Figure 13.14b). Enhanced promoter CpG island hypermethylation also has been implicated in the histogenesis of mixed carcinoma [221].

Grading of gastric adenocarcinoma

Grading applies primarily to tubular and papillary carcinomas, whereas other types of gastric carcinoma are not graded [213]. Well differentiated adenocarcinomas are composed of preserved glands, sometimes resembling metaplastic intestinal epithelium. Poorly differentiated

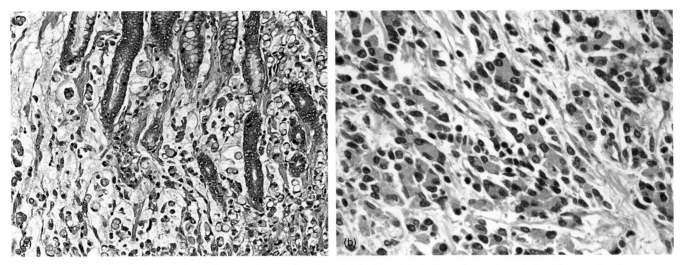

Figure 13.13 Poorly cohesive gastric carcinoma: signet-cell variant: (a) in this subtype the cells are characterised by prominent intracytoplasmic mucin. (b) In this second example the cells have a plasmacytoid appearance.

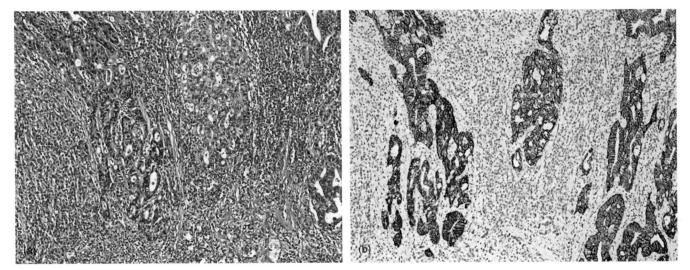

Figure 13.14 Mixed gastric adenocarcinoma: (a) the neoplasm is composed of tubular and poorly cohesive components. (b) E-cadherin immunostain underscores the loss of expression in the poorly cohesive component.

adenocarcinomas are composed of irregular glandular structures that are recognised with difficulty. Moderately differentiated adenocarcinomas display features intermediate between well and poorly differentiated. Given the notorious inter-observer variability in grading lesions, we favour gastric cancers being reported as low grade (well and moderately differentiated) or high grade (poorly differentiated).

The Lauren classification

The Lauren classification [222] maintains historical value, because it has proved useful in evaluating the natural history of gastric carcinoma, especially with regard to its association with environmental factors, incidence trends and precursors. The tumours are classified into one of

two major types: intestinal or diffuse. Tumours that contain approximately equal quantities of intestinal and diffuse components are called mixed carcinomas. Carcinomas that are too undifferentiated to fit neatly into either category are placed in the indeterminate category.

Intestinal carcinomas

These neoplasms form glands of various degrees of differentiation, sometimes with poorly differentiated tumour areas. The glandular epithelium consists of large pleomorphic cells with hyperchromatic nuclei, often with numerous mitoses. Mucin secretion is variable and occurs either focally in the cytoplasm of scattered cells or extracellularly in the lumina of neoplastic glands. Intestinal carcinomas typically arise on a background of intestinal metaplasia. At the cellular level, despite being classified as intestinal, the neoplastic cells may show morphological or immunological evidence, not only of intestinal differentiation, but also of gastric, gastrointestinal, unclassifiable or null differentiation, underscoring the inadequacies of this classification.

Diffuse carcinomas

These tumours are classified as 'poorly cohesive carcinomas, including signet-ring cell carcinoma' in the new WHO classification. In this type, poorly cohesive cells diffusely infiltrate the gastric wall with little or no gland formation. Mucin secretion is common, and can be widespread throughout the tumour. Desmoplastic connective tissue proliferation is usually more marked than in intestinal cancers and inflammatory cell infiltration less prominent.

Of the 1344 tumours originally described by Lauren, 53% were intestinal and 33% diffuse, and the remainder included tumours that contained equal proportions of intestinal and diffuse types (mixed) or that were undifferentiated with a solid growth pattern. The decreasing incidence of gastric cancer appears to result from a reduction in intestinal-type tumours, whereas diffuse tumours remain constant.

The related classification of Mulligan is based on cell differentiation and recognises a third subtype, pylorocardiac gland type, characterised by glands of various sizes lined by stratified or singly oriented cylindrical cells that often show striking vacuolisation or clear cell changes [223]. Notably, it occurs predominantly in the 'cardia' or pylorus.

Other classifications

A classification proposed by Ming [224] is based on the pattern of growth and invasion at the advancing edge, dividing tumours into an expanding type (about 67%), for those composed of discrete tumour nodules with pushing edge, and an infiltrative type (about 33%), for those formed of widely infiltrative tumour cells with poor inflammatory cell response and desmoplasia.

The Goseki classification The Goseki classification [225] is a four-grade scheme based on tubular differentiation and intracellular mucin production: group I consists of well differentiated tubules with poor intracellular mucin production; group II consists of well differentiated tubules and plentiful intracellular mucin; group III has poorly differentiated tubules and poor intracellular mucin; and group IV tumours are made up of poorly differentiated tubules and plentiful intracellular mucin. Notably, prognostic value has been attributed to this classification system [225,226].

The dawn of phenotypic classification

In 1997, Carneiro and colleagues proposed a classification [227] based on four histotypes:

- Glandular and isolated cell carcinomas (roughly equivalent to the intestinal and diffuse carcinomas of the Lauren classification)
- A solid variety (composed of sheets, trabeculae or islands of undifferentiated cells with no glandular formation)
- A mixed type that consists of a mixture of glandular and isolated cell types.

This classification first underscored that the designation of intestinal carcinoma is a misnomer, because a large proportion of those tumours displays a gastric phenotype, as demonstrated by mucins and trefoil factors peptides expression (discussed below). This classification was shown to have a prognostic significance [228], whereas other studies have also shown that mixed carcinomas have distinct patterns of invasion and are more aggressive than pure types [219,229].

An increasing interest in cell differentiation has allowed for a better understanding of tumour histogenesis. Contributions emerged from ultrastructural [230] and immunohistochemical studies using markers of cell differentiation, such as the following:

- Markers of surface gastric epithelium (foveolar cells): mucin MUC5AC and trefoil peptide TFF1
- Markers of mucous neck cell, pyloric gland and Brunner's gland cells: mucin MUC6 and trefoil peptide TFF2
- Markers of intestinal cells: mucin MUC2, cdx-2 and CD10.

Consequently, gastric carcinomas can be divided into four phenotypes:

1. Gastric
2. Mixed gastric and intestinal
3. Intestinal
4. Unclassifiable or null phenotype devoid of the expression of these markers [231–233] (Figure 13.15).

The mixed phenotype may be further subdivided into gastric predominant type and intestinal predominant type. In addition, pepsinogen-1 staining has been used to distinguish mucous neck/pseudo-pyloric type from true pyloric type [233]. Importantly, all these phenotypes can be noted in the so-called intestinal carcinomas of the Lauren classification. These findings challenge the classic proposed histogenetic pathway from chronic atrophic gastritis through intestinal metaplasia to intestinal-type carcinoma [227,234–236] and also show the phenotype impacts on prognosis, although the proportion of each variant differs in various studies [237–239].

Relative merits of the different classifications

The number of classifications indirectly demonstrates that none of the current schemes is fully satisfactory. None offers ease of use and reproducibility, along with prognostic relevance and a relationship to the histogenesis and perhaps the aetiology of the tumours, e.g. the WHO and Lauren classifications are widely used but are of little prog-

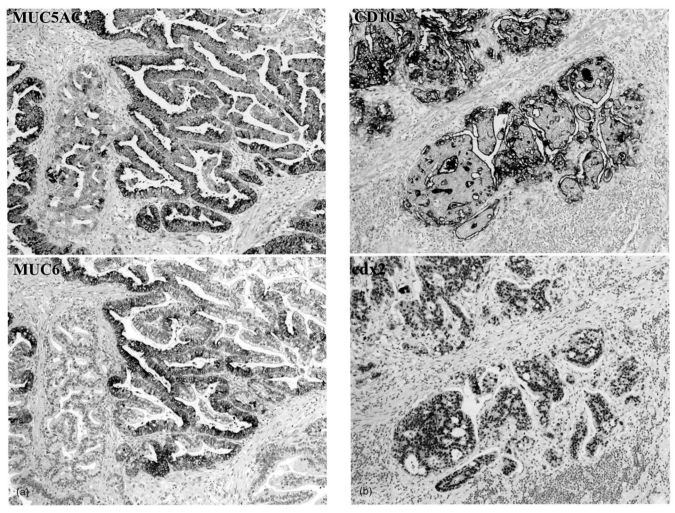

Figure 13.15 (a) Tubular gastric adenocarcinoma with a gastric immunophenotype demonstrated by MUC5-AC (above) and MUC6 positivity. (b) Tubular gastric adenocarcinoma with an intestinal immunophenotype demonstrated by CD10 (above) and cdx-2 positivity.

nostic value. One drawback of both classifications is that many carcinomas are heterogeneous and contain a variety of tumour patterns, and assessment of the predominant component is difficult.

In contrast, some have indicated that the Ming classification is of prognostic value, in that expanding tumours have considerably better prognosis than similarly advanced carcinomas of the infiltrative type [240,241]. Others have claimed prognostic value and high reproducibility for the Goseki classification, with types II and IV (both mucin rich) having a worse prognosis than type I and III tumours (mucin poor) [226,242]. The proponents of the Carneiro classification found that mixed-type tumours have a much worse prognosis than the other subtypes and multivariate analysis showed the classification to have independent prognostic significance that was second only to TNM

staging [227,228]. Also, there has been a suggestion that the phenotypic classification of gastric cancer, related to the histogenesis and the aetiology, impacts on prognosis.

Unusual variants of gastric carcinoma
Uncommon histological variants represent about 5% of gastric cancers.

Adenosquamous and squamous cell carcinoma
The diagnosis of primary adenosquamous carcinoma requires the presence of a neoplastic squamous component characterised by keratin pearl formation and intercellular bridges, in addition to the glandular element [243] (Figure 13.16). The transition between the elements may be abrupt or there may be intermingling of squamous foci within neoplastic glands [243,244]. Ultrastructural evaluation of

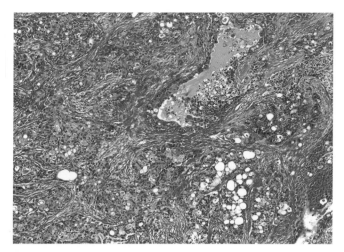

Figure 13.16 Adenosquamous gastric adenocarcinoma: the squamous differentiation is predominant with admixed residual glandular structures.

tumour cells shows evidence of both squamous and adenosquamous differentiation, supporting the view that this neoplastic type arises from a multipotential common stem cell [245]. These tumours occur most often in the antrum, and most examples present as advanced carcinomas, although rare cases of early gastric cancer (EGC) have been reported [246]. Lymphovascular permeation is common and the prognosis poor [243,246–248], although some exhibit a favourable response to chemotherapy [249]. Metastases usually contain both glandular and squamous components but, in some instances, only one component may be present. Of note, tumours with a distinct boundary between components may represent a rare collision tumour. Exceptionally, rare tumours containing discrete foci of benign-appearing squamous metaplasia have been observed and termed 'adenocarcinomas with squamous differentiation' or adenoacanthoma.

Pure squamous cell carcinomas develop rarely in the stomach [247,250], affect men four times as often as women [251,252], are usually diagnosed at a late stage and have a poor prognosis [251]. Of note, a glandular component is often present when such tumours are extensively sampled [243]. At the OGJ and in the proximal stomach, caudal extension of an oesophageal squamous cell carcinoma should be excluded. Pure squamous cell carcinomas of the stomach possibly arise from squamous metaplasia of an adenocarcinoma, from heterotopic squamous epithelium or from multipotential stem cells showing bidirectional differentiation [246,251]. Gastric squamous cell carcinomas have also been described as a complication of gastric involvement in tertiary syphilis [253], after ingestion of corrosive acids [254] and after long-term cyclophosphamide therapy [255].

Hepatoid adenocarcinoma

A small number of gastric adenocarcinomas contain variable amounts of tumour cells resembling hepatocellular carcinoma, usually interspersed with areas of more typical adenocarcinoma. These tumours may produce large amounts of α-fetoprotein (AFP) which is detectable in the serum and can be demonstrated by immunohistochemistry [256]. Molecular evidence supports the clonal origin of hepatoid adenocarcinoma and coexistent adenocarcinoma [257]. Hepatoid adenocarcinoma usually occurs in patients aged >50 and, although occasional early cases have been detected [258,259], most are advanced bulky polypoid tumours with ulceration and areas of necrosis and haemorrhage. The antrum appears to be the most common site of hepatoid adenocarcinoma, followed by the fundus and, occasionally, the cardia [258].

These tumours are commonly heterogeneous, with hepatoid foci intermingled with adenocarcinoma, often showing a papillary pattern, and less differentiated areas containing bizarre giant cells and spindle cells [256,260]. The characteristic hepatoid features are of large, polygonal cells with prominent eosinophilic cytoplasm, resembling hepatocellular carcinoma [256,261], arranged in trabeculae, wide sheets or glandular structures (Figure 13.17a). These also may contain periodic acid–Schiff (PAS)–diastase-resistant hyaline globules [258,260] (Figure 13.17b). Of note, based on the immunohistochemical expression of CD10, MUC2, MUC5AC, MUC6 and cdx-2, Kumashiro et al. suggested that these tumours arise from carcinomas with an intestinal phenotype [262]. Clinically, a characteristic of these neoplasms is the extensive vascular infiltration, reflected in the high incidence of liver metastases, lymph node metastases and a poorer prognosis compared with conventional gastric adenocarcinoma [256,259,263,264].

Immunohistochemical and *in situ* hybridisation studies have documented albumin, AFP, α1-antichymotrypsin and bile production within the tumour cells [261,265,266]. Positivity for AFP on immunohistochemistry can be demonstrated usually, but not invariably, and over-expression of *p53* has been described [260]. Of interest, gene expression profiling recently identified PLUNC (**p**alate, **lu**ng and **n**asal epithelium **c**arcinoma-associated protein) as a marker for gastric hepatoid adenocarcinoma [267]. Other types of gastric tumour may also produce AFP, including well differentiated papillary/tubular adenocarcinoma with clear cytoplasm, yolk sac tumour-like carcinoma and fetal-type adenocarcinoma [261,265].

It may be difficult to distinguish a liver metastasis from gastric hepatoid adenocarcinoma and a primary hepatocellular carcinoma (HCC) in a liver biopsy. Yet it has been reported that immunostaining for Hep-Par-1, CK19 or CK20 is useful, with most HCCs showing extensive staining of Hep-Par-1, whereas only focal staining of Hep-Par-1 is observed in gastric hepatoid adenocarcinoma [268].

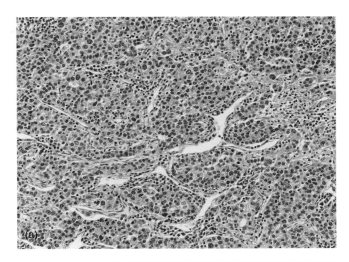

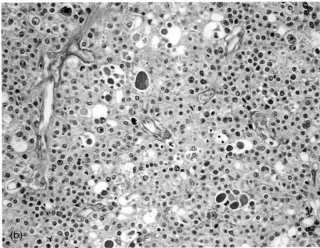

Figure 13.17 Hepatoid gastric adenocarcinoma: (a) characteristically, this tumour shows a trabecular growth pattern and rare gland like spaces. (b) Periodic acid–Schiff-positive and diastase-resistant intracytoplasmic eosinophilic globules can be seen in some cases.

Choriocarcinoma

A small number of gastric tumours, affecting both sexes, have been reported in which areas of choriocarcinoma containing syncytioblast and cytotrophoblast occur in association with poorly differentiated adenocarcinoma with no evidence of primary choriocarcinoma elsewhere [269,270]. The tumour often contains widespread areas of haemorrhagic necrosis that can be seen with the naked eye [271,272]. The commonly accepted pathogenic explanation is that these tumours represent choriocarcinomatous differentiation or transformation of conventional adenocarcinoma [273]. Immunohistochemical evidence of human chorionic gonadotrophin (hCG) expression within trophoblastic areas has been shown [272–275] and markedly elevated levels of circulating hCG are often present [273,274,276]. In occasional cases, other germ-cell tumour-like elements may coexist, such as embryonal carcinoma and yolk sac tumour [276,277]. Metastases to the liver and lung are common and the prognosis is typically poor, with survival a matter of months after diagnosis [270,272,278].

Among these rarities, only two cases of pure gastric yolk sac tumour have been reported [279]. Recent publications have described a case of choriocarcinoma admixed with an AFP-producing adenocarcinoma and 'separated' adenocarcinoma [280], as well as a case of combined choriocarcinoma, neuro-endocrine cell carcinoma and tubular adenocarcinoma [281].

Gastric carcinoma with lymphoid stroma

Epstein–Barr virus (EBV) is detected in up to 18% of gastric carcinomas [282]. Among these, a subset of tumours has been described under several synonyms, such as medullary carcinoma with lymphocytic infiltration [283], gastric carcinoma with lymphoid stroma [284], undifferentiated gastric carcinoma with intense lymphocytic infiltrate [285] and lymphoepithelioma-like carcinoma [286]. Such tumours are more frequent in eastern Asia than in the West and they display certain distinctive macroscopic and histological characteristics [283,284]. Over 80% of these tumours are related to EBV infection [287]. On gross examination, the tumours commonly involve the proximal stomach and are usually ulcerated with a well-circumscribed edge. Necrosis or haemorrhages are notably absent. Histologically, the tumours usually have a well-demarcated pushing rather than infiltrating margin. They are typically composed of irregular sheets, trabeculae, ill-defined tubules or syncytia of polygonal cells embedded within a prominent lymphocytic infiltrate, with occasional lymphoid follicles.

Other histological variants of EBV-positive gastric carcinomas are observed. These include tumours frequently composed of tubulo-glandular formation, with limited desmoplasia, a smaller number of lymphocytes than tumour cells and prominent, patchy lymphoid follicles with active germinal centres, as well conventional adenocarcinomas with scant lymphocytic infiltrate. Immunophenotypic analysis reveals that CD8-positive cytotoxic T lymphocytes form the predominant component of the infiltrate, which also contains B lymphocytes, plasma cells, neutrophils and eosinophils (Figure 13.18). Rarely, giant cells are observed [288]. The lymphocytic infiltrate may be so intense that a diagnosis of gastric lymphoma may be considered until the tumour cells proper are confirmed by immunostaining for epithelial markers.

Gastric carcinoma with lymphoid stroma occurs predominantly in the proximal stomach [289], including in the stump of patients with previous subtotal gastrectomy [290]. The age at presentation is slightly younger than in conventional carcinoma and men are affected more often

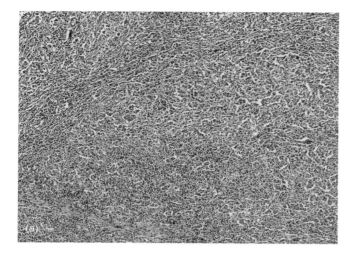

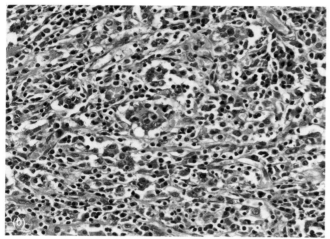

Figure 13.18 Gastric carcinoma with lymphoid stroma: (a) this neoplasm is composed of solid sheets of polygonal epithelial cells, (b) intermixed with a prominent lymphocytic infiltrate.

than women [283,284,289]. The prognosis is reportedly better than that for typical gastric cancers [283,286,290,291], possibly as a result of the immunological factors at play in the associated lymphocytic infiltrate.

It is not clear whether EBV plays a direct role in carcinogenesis or is simply a secondary infection [292] but infection probably occurs early in the process because EBV can be found in adjacent dysplasia [293], although it has not been observed in normal gastric mucosa or intestinal metaplasia [294]. In a recent meta-analysis, it was observed that these tumours are associated with CpG island methylator (CIMP) high status, but not with *H. pylori* infection, *p53* expression or *TP53* mutation [289]. A sequence of events within the mucosa has been proposed [295]: EBV infection of certain gastric stem cells; expression of viral latent genes; abnormality of signal pathways caused by viral gene products; DNA methylation-mediated repression of tumour

suppressor genes; and monoclonal growth of EBV-infected cells through interaction with other aetiological factors [295]. EBV infection can be demonstrated in tumour cells by *in situ* hybridisation or polymerase chain reaction (PCR) [296]. EBV genomic sequences have also been identified, much less rarely, in conventional gastric carcinomas, raising the possibility that EBV infection may contribute to gastric carcinogenesis [297].

Recently Song et al. reported that the pattern of host inflammatory response was important in predicting survival. In their series, in addition to the typical lympho-epithelial-like variant of EBV-associated gastric carcinoma, cancers with a Crohn's disease-like inflammatory response had a similarly improved prognosis compared with EBV-positive cancers without lymphoid follicles [298].

Small cell carcinoma This tumour is considered in the section on endocrine cell tumours (see below).

Gastric carcinosarcoma and gastroblastoma

Gastric carcinosarcomas are composed of admixed adeno-carcinomatous and sarcomatous elements. The latter may include elements of chondrosarcomatous, osteosarcomatous, rhabdomyosarcomatous or leiomyosarcomatous differentiation [299–302]. Cases have been reported in the OGJ and gastric stump [303,304]. Neoplasms combining adenosquamous and neuro-endocrine components have also been reported [305–308]. Most cases present as large polypoid tumours and are associated with a poor outcome [309]. Of note, a case has been reported of gastric adenosarcoma composed of benign tubular and cystic glands embedded in a leiomyosarcomatous stroma [310].

Recently, a distinctive epithelial and mesenchymal biphasic tumour ('gastroblastoma') has been described in young adults [311,312]. These tumours are characterised by mixed spindle and epithelial cellular elements. Neither the epithelial nor the mesenchymal component display sufficient atypia to be diagnosed as a carcinosarcoma or other malignancy [312]. They are considered more fully in Chapter 14 (see Gastroblastoma).

Micropapillary carcinoma

Micropapillary carcinoma (MPC) is a rare, distinctive tumour characterised by irregular small clusters of tumour cells lying within clear lacunar spaces and simulating lymphatic or vascular channels (Figure 13.19). Most gastric MPCs arise from tubular or papillary adenocarcinomas with an incidence of about 6%. The proportion of micropapillary carcinoma component is reported to range from 5% to 80%. MPC carcinoma is an aggressive neoplasm, with a high incidence of lymphovascular invasion and nodal metastasis and a higher TNM stage. The overall 5-year survival rates for patients with MPC are significantly worse than those with non-MPC carcinomas [313,314].

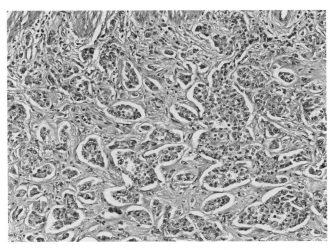

Figure 13.19 Micropapillary variant of gastric adenocarcinoma: the tumour consists of small clusters of neoplastic cells surrounded by clear spaces resembling lymphatic tumour emboli.

Parietal cell carcinoma

These exceedingly rare tumours have been reported to present as bulky lesions involving both the gastric body and the antrum [315]. Histologically, they have an expanding rather than an infiltrating growth pattern and are composed of sheets of cells that may contain small gland-like clefts. The tumour cells resemble acid-secreting parietal cells in that they have eosinophilic granular cytoplasm and stain positively with PTAH (phosphotungstic acid haematoxylin) and Luxol fast blue. They also are positive for parietal cell-specific antibodies, to H^+/K^+ ATPase and human milk fat globule-2, and ultrastructural evaluation reveals numerous mitochondria and intracellular canaliculi [315–317]. Focal parietal cell differentiation has been reported in a well differentiated (gland-forming) EGC [318]. Lymph node metastases occur but are not extensive. It has been suggested that the prognosis of parietal cell carcinoma is better than that for usual gastric carcinomas [316]. Some cases of oncocytic gastric carcinomas negative for anti-parietal cell antibodies have been reported [319].

Gastric mucoepidermoid carcinoma

These neoplasms are exceedingly rare and morphologically present the characteristic admixture of mucus-producing and squamous epithelia [320].

Paneth cell carcinomas

These neoplasms are characterised by a predominance of Paneth cells, characteristically showing eosinophilic cytoplasmic granules that are positive for lysozyme by immunohistochemistry [321,322]. Of note, neoplastic Paneth cells can be identified dispersed among typical gastric adenocarcinomas [323,324].

Gastric malignant rhabdoid tumour

Gastric malignant rhabdoid tumours are composed of poorly cohesive, round-to-polygonal cells characterised by eosinophilic or clear cytoplasm and large nuclei with predominant nucleoli. The neoplastic cells show strong cellular immunoreactivity for vimentin and can also show cytokeratin, epithelial membrane antigen and focal neuron-specific enolase (NSE) positivity but are negative for carcinoembryonic antigen (CEA) [325–327]. The prognosis of these tumours is dismal.

Undifferentiated carcinoma

This terminology is used to categorise carcinomas lacking any differentiated features but showing an epithelial phenotype at least in part (e.g. by cytokeratin expression). They fall into the indeterminate category of the Lauren classification.

Staging gastric cancer

Early gastric cancer

Early gastric cancer is an invasive carcinoma limited to the mucosa or submucosa, regardless of nodal status. The term 'early' does not imply a stage in the genesis of the cancer but means that these are gastric cancers that can often be cured [328]. However, if untreated, 63% of EGCs progress to advanced tumours within 5 years [329].

Countries with a high incidence of gastric cancer and in which asymptomatic patients are screened have a high incidence of EGCs, ranging from 30% to 50% in east Asia [330,331], with lower figures for the West (16–24%) [332–334]. Most EGCs measure from 20 mm to 50 mm and are localised on the lesser curvature and around the angulus [23,335]. Some EGCs can remain confined to the superficial layers for several years, although potentially expanding laterally to a considerable degree, whereas others penetrate the gastric wall rapidly and can then invade into the submucosa, when they are only about 3–5 mm in size [336,337]. Minute EGCs that measure <5 mm in diameter and superficial spreading EGCs with neoplastic cells spreading over large areas can be observed [338] .

Endoscopists divide EGCs into three types based on the endoscopic appearance. These are protruded (type I), superficial (type II) and excavated (type III) (Japanese classification) (Figure 13.20). Type II accounts for 80% of EGCs and is further subdivided into IIa (elevated type), IIb (flat type), and IIc (depressed type), the last being the most common [339].

Most EGCs are well differentiated glandular carcinomas. This is particularly true for small (<20 mm) lesions. However, when the size of the tumour increases and submucosal invasion develops, histological diversity with mixed

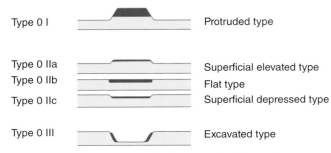

Type 0 I		Protruded type
Type 0 IIa		Superficial elevated type
Type 0 IIb		Flat type
Type 0 IIc		Superficial depressed type
Type 0 III		Excavated type

Figure 13.20 Macroscopic classification of early gastric carcinoma. The categories of early gastric carcinoma, defined as limited to mucosa and/or submucosa, are as noted in the diagram: I, protuberant; IIa, flat, superficially elevated; IIb, flat, not elevated; IIc, flat, slightly depressed; and III, excavated (full thickness of submucosa).

or poorly differentiated components is common. There is also a correlation with the endoscopic appearances. Tubular and papillary variants represent over 50% and 30% of EGCs and are usually types I and II. Signet-ring cell carcinoma and poorly differentiated carcinoma represent 25% and 15% of the cases and are usually depressed or ulcerated (types IIc and III) [23,339,340].

The biopsy diagnosis of EGC may be challenging. A small number of signet-ring cells infiltrating the lamina propria can be overlooked easily but their detection can be facilitated by special stains [341]. Conversely, muciphages and the finely vacuolated cells of a gastric xanthoma/xanthelasma (see Chapter 12) may be mistaken for signet-ring cell carcinoma. In such cases, careful attention to the nuclear morphology and the use of immunohistochemical epithelial and macrophage markers are helpful.

For gland-forming neoplasms, the distinction between high grade intra-epithelial neoplasia/dysplasia and well differentiated tubular carcinoma, especially of type I and IIa EGCs, can be virtually impossible to make on biopsy material. Furthermore, there is good evidence that a proportion of type I and IIa EGCs result from malignant change in an adenoma [341,342]. Fortunately, the distinction between high grade intra-epithelial neoplasia/dysplasia and well differentiated tubular carcinoma has become of limited clinical interest because these two conditions should be managed endoscopically. The location, size and configuration of the lesion and the patient's physical condition are now the important features guiding the therapeutic decision.

Careful histological assessment of submucosal invasion, particularly the depth of invasion, is important in evaluating resected EGCs because it correlates with the likelihood of lymph node metastasis [343]. Submucosal invasion

occurs in about 50% of all cases, a figure that varies remarkably little between series [340], and is least common in flat (type IIb) lesions [344]. Lymph node metastasis occurs in 10–20% of all EGCs [330,340,343] and correlates with the depth of submucosal invasion and increasing tumour diameter [340,343,345,346]. Accordingly, endoscopic mucosal resection alone is recommended for well or moderately differentiated tumours that are not ulcerated, are <30 mm in diameter and in which subsequent histological examination confirms no submucosal invasion, no lymphovascular invasion and complete local excision [347]. Endoscopic submucosal dissection allows a more extensive excision of the submucosa and is currently promoted as a valid therapeutic approach for differentiated (intestinal) EGCs if they are not ulcerated (whatever the size), they are ulcerated and ≤30 mm in size, they are invasive and ≤30 mm in size and the depth of invasion is superficially submucosal (<500 μm) with no lymphovascular invasion [348]. However, recent data contest the safety of these extended criteria, reporting a high level of nodal metastasis [349].

Patterns of spread

Gastric carcinomas can spread by direct extension to adjacent organs, lymphatic and/or haematogenous spread or peritoneal dissemination.

Direct extension of tumour

According to the primary site, penetration of the serosa may result in direct spread to the pancreas, liver, spleen, transverse colon and greater omentum, and often leads to early transperitoneal dissemination. Tumours at the OGJ infiltrate within the wall into the lower end of the oesophagus whereas distal tumours, particularly discohesive neoplasms, not uncommonly show microscopic extension into the duodenum [350]. Widespread direct spread is particularly common in poorly cohesive carcinomas, which frequently show extensive spread on the serosal surface, well beyond the macroscopically visible tumour. Intramural permeation of small lymphovascular vessels is widespread in these neoplasms with a high propensity to invade the duodenum via either submucosal or subserosal routes or the submucosal lymphatics [351]. Consequently, frozen section examination of margins is desirable, particularly when the clearance is <40 mm, to ensure completeness of resection.

Lymphatic spread

The incidence of lymph node metastatic disease increases with the depth of tumour invasion [352] and occurs with equal frequency regardless of histological type. The distribution varies according to the location of the tumour.

Involvement of nodes along the lesser and greater curves is common and extension to the next zone is often seen (e.g. along the left gastric, common hepatic and coeliac arteries). Distant spread may involve para-aortic and mesenteric nodes. Tumours of the mid-portion of the stomach may give rise to metastases in pancreatic and splenic nodes and lesions of the proximal stomach can metastasise to mediastinal lymph nodes. It is important for the surgeon to perform an exhaustive lymphadenectomy and for the pathologist to examine all lymph nodes, however small, because even the smallest node may be involved by metastatic disease and there is good evidence that prognosis depends on the number of nodes involved [353]. Further, the ratio of metastatic to examined nodes (node ratio) has been suggested as an independent prognostic factor [354].

Haematogenous spread

Spread via the bloodstream occurs from invasion of tributaries of the portal venous system and may occur even in the absence of lymph node involvement. Metastases can occur in almost any organ but are most commonly seen in the liver, followed by the lung, peritoneum, adrenal glands, skin and ovaries; the last can also be involved because of transperitoneal spread. The distribution of metastases is also dictated, to some extent, by the histological tumour type. Gland-forming carcinomas are more likely to give rise to liver metastases by haematogenous spread than poorly cohesive carcinomas. Poorly cohesive carcinomas are more likely to involve the peritoneum than gland-forming carcinomas. They also tend to disseminate more widely, infiltrating lungs more extensively than the nodal metastases associated with gland-forming tumours and more often involving unusual sites such as the kidney, spleen, uterus and meninges [355,356]. Peritoneal involvement is more common in younger patients. In carcinomas showing unusual metastatic distribution, e.g. gland-forming carcinomas involving the peritoneum or poorly cohesive carcinomas involving the liver, the primary often shows a mixed histological pattern [357].

Transperitoneal spread

Secondary tumour deposits are common in the omentum, peritoneum and mesentery but are rare over the spleen. Secondary ovarian deposits are well known as one form of Krukenberg's tumour for which bloodstream spread is at least as likely a cause as transperitoneal spread. Krukenberg's tumours are more frequently associated with diffuse primary carcinomas than gland-forming tumours. However, the presence of signet-ring cells within an ovarian mucinous tumour should not automatically exclude the extremely rare primary ovarian tumour [358].

Staging and prognosis of advanced gastric cancer

The TNM staging for carcinoma of the stomach was substantially modified in 2009, as seen in Table 13.3 [359,360]. Major changes include the subdivision of T1 to delineate mucosal and submucosal depth of invasion, the alteration of stages T2a and T2b into T2 (muscularis propria) and T3 (subserosa) and the re-definition of T3 and T4 to T4a (penetrates serosa) and T4b (invades adjacent structures). Consequently, the TNM categories are now almost identical to those for the oesophagus and OGJ, except that N3 (metastasis in seven or more regional lymph nodes) is divided into N3a (7–15 nodes) and N3b (≥16 nodes) for gastric carcinomas but not for oesophageal carcinomas [359,360].

For adenocarcinomas of the OGJ, staging is based on the location of the epicentre. A tumour that extends into the oesophagus and whose centre is located within 50 mm of the OGJ is staged according to the scheme for oesophageal carcinoma. Tumours with an epicentre in the stomach >50 mm from the OGJ or those within 50 mm of the OGJ without extension into the oesophagus are staged according to the scheme for gastric carcinoma [359,360]. However, this proposal has already been contested [210].

Prognosis

In Japan, the 5-year survival rate for T2 adenocarcinoma is 60–80% and decreases to 50% for T3 tumours [361,362]. Lower survival rates have been observed in the West [363]. Female sex and Japanese ethnicity have been associated with a survival advantage [364]. Higher frequency of early stage carcinomas, accurate staging and surgical expertise has also been associated with improved survival in Japan compared with western nations [365, 366].

At the time of diagnosis, most patients with advanced carcinoma have lymph node metastatic disease for which only palliative surgery can be considered [367]. Lymphatic and vascular invasion, often seen in advanced cases, specifically carry a poor prognosis. In patients with involvement of 1–6 lymph nodes, the 5-year survival rate is 46%, compared with 30% in patients with 7–15 lymph nodes involved [368]. The extent of the regional lymphadenectomy performed and the quality of lymph node evaluation are salient. Patients undergoing a 'curative' gastrectomy but limited lymph-node dissection (D1/D0) have an overall 5-year survival rate of only 23%, versus more than 50% for those undergoing a more aggressive lymphadenectomy (D2) [369]. Furthermore, adequate N staging requires that at least 15 lymph nodes to be examined and, thus, careful examination of surgical resection specimens by pathologists.

Table 13.3 TNM classification of tumours of the stomach [359,360]

Carcinoma of the stomach

T	**Primary tumour**	
TX	Primary tumour cannot be assessed	
T0	No evidence of primary tumour	
Tis	Carcinoma *in situ*: intraepithelial tumour without invasion of the lamina propria, high grade dysplasia	
T1	Tumour invades lamina propria, muscularis mucosae or submucosa	
	T1a	Tumour invades lamina propria or muscularis mucosae
	T1b	Tumour invades submucosa
T2	Tumour invades muscularis propria	
T3	Tumour invades subserosa	
T4	Tumour perforates serosa or invades adjacent structures	
	T4a	Tumour perforates serosa (visceral peritoneum)
	T4b	Tumour invades adjacent structures
N	**Regional lymph nodes**	
NX	Regional lymph nodes cannot be assessed	
N0	No regional lymph-node metastasis	
N1	Metastasis in 1–2 regional lymph nodes	
N2	Metastasis in 3–6 regional lymph nodes	
N3	Metastasis in ≥7 regional lymph nodes	
	N3a	Metastasis in 7–15 regional lymph nodes
	N3b	Metastasis in 16 or more regional lymph nodes
M	**Distant metastasis**	
M0	No distant metastasis	
M1	Distant metastasis	

Stage grouping

Stage	T	N	M
Stage 0	Tis	N0	M0
Stage IA	T1	N0	M0
Stage IB	T2	N0	M0
	T1	N1	M0
Stage IIA	T3	N0	M0
	T2	N1	M0
	T1	N2	M0
Stage IIB	T4a	N0	M0
	T3	N1	M0
	T2	N2	M0
	T1	N3	M0
Stage IIIA	T4a	N1	M0
	T3	N2	M0
	T2	N3	M0
Stage IIIB	T4b	N0, N1	M0
	T4a	N2	M0
	T3	N3	M0
Stage IIIC	T4a	N3	M0
	T4b	N2,N3	M0
Stage IV	Any T	Any N	M1

In resectable cases, complete tumour removal with negative margins is important [370]. In addition, the depth of invasion, the number of positive lymph nodes and postoperative complications are important independent prognostic factors [371]. After curative resection, recurrence is locoregional (resection margins, surgical bed and/or regional lymph nodes) in 40% of cases and systemic (liver and peritoneum) in 60% [372–374]. Whether distal adenocarcinomas have a better prognosis compared with proximal carcinomas is debated [366,375]. Saito and colleagues have reported a 5-year survival rate of 62% in patients with carcinoma of the 'cardia' versus 83% for those with carcinoma of the lower third of the stomach [376]. In another series, however, the prognoses were equally grim, with 28% and 29% survival rates, respectively [375].

Histological features and prognosis

The value of histological typing in predicting prognosis is controversial. Whether the prognosis for diffuse carcinoma (Lauren classification) is or is not worse than that for intestinal carcinoma is debated [226,242]. Recently, it has been suggested that diffuse carcinomas encompass lesions with different prognoses, such as a low grade desmoplastic subtype (with no or scarce angio-lympho-neuroinvasion) and a high grade subtype (with anaplastic cells) [377]. The prognosis is particularly bad for children and young adults with poorly cohesive carcinoma, for whom diagnosis is often delayed [378,379]. Some investigations have shown that only the Goseki classification [226] adds additional prognostic information to the TNM stage [226,242] with 5-year survival of patients with mucus-rich (Goseki II and IV) T3 tumours being significantly worse than that for patients with mucus-poor (Goseki I and III) T3 tumours (18% versus 53%; p <0.003) [226]. Some patients with medullary carcinoma have a better prognosis than those with other histological types; some of them are Lynch syndrome patients with microsatellite instability, a feature associated with better survival.

Hereditary gastric cancer syndromes

About 10% of gastric cancer can be qualified as familial and several inherited cancer predisposition syndromes have been associated with increased risk of gastric cancers. These include FAP, Lynch syndrome [380–382], Li–Fraumeni syndrome and Peutz–Jeghers syndrome.

In the setting of FAP, there is an increased risk of gastric cancer [383]. A Korean study claimed that patients with FAP have a sevenfold increased risk of gastric cancer [384]. Adenocarcinoma develops extremely rarely in fundic gland polyps but may be more common in the rarer gastric adenoma. In Lynch syndrome, resulting from germline mutation of one of the DNA-mismatch repair genes, there

is also an increased frequency of gastric cancers, namely in carriers of the *hMLH1* and *hMSH2* mutations [380,381]. The tumours arise at an earlier age than sporadic neoplasms and most are of intestinal type, even though coincidental *H. pylori* infection is relatively uncommon [385].

Gastric cancer is also observed in the Li–Fraumeni syndrome with germline mutation of *TP53* [386]. Gastrointestinal cancers are rare, representing less than 10% of malignancies associated with the syndrome, but gastric cancer represents 50% of the cases. It was also reported recently that, among patients with Peutz–Jeghers syndrome, those with frameshift mutations in the *STK11* gene develop aggressive gastric cancers [387]. Furthermore, a novel germline mutation of the *LKB1* gene was reported in a patient with sporadic Peutz–Jeghers syndrome with early onset gastric cancer [388].

Gastric cancer has also been described in gastric hyperplastic polyposis, an inherited autosomal dominant syndrome characterised by the presence of hyperplastic gastric polyposis, severe psoriasis and a high incidence of gastric cancer of the diffuse type [160,389].

Criteria for familial gastric cancer

Among individuals with familial aggregation, there are cases in which the histopathology of the tumours is unknown that are simply designated as familial gastric cancer (FGC) whereas there are cases in which the histopathology of one or more gastric cancers can be characterised, including hereditary diffuse gastric cancer (HDGC), familial diffuse gastric cancer (FDGC) and familial intestinal gastric cancer (FIGC).

Hereditary diffuse gastric cancer

Hereditary diffuse gastric cancer (HDGC) is an autosomal dominant cancer susceptibility syndrome characterised by signet-ring cell (diffuse) gastric cancer and lobular breast cancer. The genetic basis of this syndrome was discovered in 1998 by Guilford et al. [390], who studied three Maori kindreds in New Zealand with multi-generational, diffuse gastric cancer, in which germline mutations of the E-cadherin (*CDH1*) gene (OMIM no. 192090) were identified by linkage analysis and mutation screening.

On the basis of clinical criteria, the International Gastric Cancer Linkage Consortium (IGCLC) defined families with HDGC syndrome as meeting one of two criteria:
1. Two or more documented cases of diffuse gastric cancer in first- or second-degree relatives with at least one being diagnosed before the age of 50 years
2. Three or more cases of documented diffuse gastric cancer in first- or second-degree relatives, independent of age of diagnosis [391].
Women in these families have an elevated risk of lobular breast cancer [392–396]. The IGCLC criteria for genetic

testing were updated in 2010 [397]. An alternative genetically based nomenclature has been proposed, in which the term 'HDGC' is restricted to families with germline mutations in the *CDH1* gene [390,398].

In clinically defined HDGC, *CDH1* mutations are detected in 30–40% of cases [198,395,399]. Most (75–80%) are truncating mutations and the remainder are missense mutations [400,401]. In addition to point mutations, large germline deletions have been found in 6.5% of HDGC families who tested negatively for point mutations [399]. Unlike the somatic mutations in *CDH1*, which occur in sporadic gastric cancers and cluster around exons 7 and 8, the germline mutations in *CDH1* in HDGC families span the whole length of the gene and no hot spots have been identified.

In HDGC, the *CDH1* gene can be inactivated by a number of mechanisms. Most frequently, this occurs via promoter hypermethylation (epigenetic modification) and less frequently by loss of heterozygosity (LOH) and *CDH1* mutations [402–404]. An intragenic deletion in the wild-type allele is also reported [405]. Humar et al. [406] have suggested that the initiation of diffuse gastric cancer seems to occur at the proliferative zone of the gastric epithelium and correlates with absent or reduced expression of junctional proteins, activation of the c-Src system and epithelial–mesenchymal transition. In about two-thirds of HDGC patients, *CDH1* germline mutations are not identified. Germline mutations in *TP53* were detected in two studies of families with gastric cancer and no mutation in *CDH1* [407,408].

Clinical features of HDGC

The age of onset of clinically significant diffuse gastric cancer may be extremely variable (with a range of 14–85 years), even within families. The age at which to offer genetic testing to at-risk relatives should take into consideration the earliest age of cancer onset in that family. Testing from the late teens or early 20s is favoured in families with early onset gastric cancer [395]. Current guidelines recommend that asymptomatic carriers of *CDH1* mutations be offered prophylactic gastrectomy or, for selected groups, annual endoscopic surveillance, as risk-reduction strategies. Surveillance is recommended for individuals aged <20 years, for those aged >20 years who elect to delay surgery, for those for whom prophylactic gastrectomy (biopsy negative) is unacceptable but gastrectomy with curative intent (biopsy positive) is acceptable, and for those with mutations of undetermined significance (e.g. missense) [395,409]. Total gastrectomy is recommended in at-risk family members aged >20 years who have a *CDH1* mutation [400]. In biopsy-positive individuals, a curative total gastrectomy is advised, regardless of age.

Histopathology of HDGC

Early stage HDGC in *CDH1* mutation carriers is characterised by multiple *foci* of invasive (T1a) signet-ring cell carcinoma in the superficial gastric mucosa (Figure 13.21a), with no nodal metastases [400,410–412]. Mapping of the entire gastric mucosa, performed in many stomachs from kindred with different *CDH1* mutations [400,410, 412–417], showed that there is wide variation in the number of T1a foci observed in these stomachs, both within and between kindreds, ranging from one focus [413] to hundreds of tiny foci [400,412]. Histological examination of the entire gastric mucosa is required before the absence of neoplasia can be claimed. The cause of this variation in number of foci is currently unknown. Early invasive carcinoma is not restricted to any topographical region in the stomach [410,413–415]. The signet-ring cell (diffuse) carcinomas observed in asymptomatic *CDH1* mutation carriers show absent or reduced staining for E-cadherin [410,411,413], in keeping with a clonal origin of the cancer foci, indicating that the second *CDH1* allele has been down-regulated or lost.

Two precursors (Tis) to T1a signet-ring cell carcinoma are recognised in HDGC:

1. Pagetoid spread of signet-ring cells below the preserved epithelium of glands and foveolae but within the basal membrane (Figure 13.21b)

2. *In situ* signet ring cell carcinoma, corresponding to the presence of signet-ring cells within the basal membrane, substituting for normal epithelial cells, generally with hyperchromatic and depolarised nuclei (Figure 13.21c) [413].

In these lesions, E-cadherin immuno-expression is reduced or absent [198,413]. Confirmation of *in situ* carcinoma by an independent histopathologist with experience in this area is strongly recommended.

GAPPS syndrome

Recently, a new hereditary syndrome has been identified: '**g**astric **a**denocarcinoma and **p**roximal **p**olyposis of the **s**tomach' (GAPPS), characterised by the autosomal dominant transmission of fundic gland polyposis, including areas of dysplasia or intestinal-type gastric adenocarcinoma, restricted to the proximal stomach, and with no evidence of colorectal or duodenal polyposis or other heritable gastrointestinal cancer syndromes [418].

Molecular aspects of gastric carcinoma

Gastric carcinoma is the result of accumulated genomic damage affecting cellular functions essential for cancer development, the so-called hallmarks of cancer: self-sufficiency in growth signals, escape from anti-growth signals, apoptosis resistance, sustained replicative potential, angiogenesis induction and invasive or metastatic potential [419]. These genomic changes arise through three genomic instability pathways: microsatellite instability (MSI), chromosomal instability (CIN) [420] and a CpG

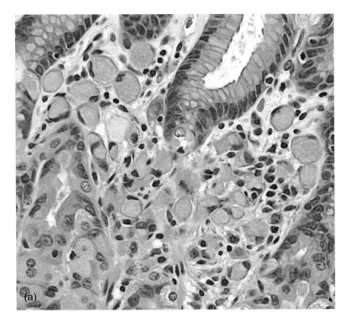

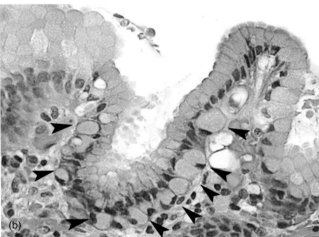

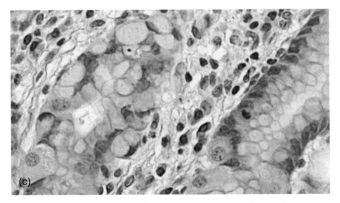

Figure 13.21 Microscopic lesions characteristic of hereditary diffuse gastric cancer: (a) typical invasive focus of T1a intramucosal signet-ring cell (diffuse) carcinoma; (b) Pagetoid spread of signet-ring cells (arrow heads) representing Tis; and (c) signet-ring cell carcinoma *in situ* (Tis).

islands methylation phenotype (CIMP) [421]. Furthermore, genetic and epigenetic changes affect oncogenes and tumour suppressor genes (Table 13.4).

Microsatellite instability

The MSI or mutator phenotype is caused by defects in the MMR system responsible for the correction of mismatches that occur during DNA replication. In gastric cancer, MSI is mainly caused by epigenetic silencing (promoter methylation) of the *MLH1* gene [422]. Somatic mutations of MMR genes are very rare in sporadic gastric cancer [423]. MSI is observed in 5–10% of diffuse carcinomas and in 15–40% of intestinal carcinomas. Gastric carcinomas with a high level of MSI (MSI high) are characterised by antral location, intestinal phenotype and an expanding growth pattern. MSI-high tumours show a better prognosis than MSI-low ones [424–426]. Several reports have shown a relation between MSI and tumour multiplicity [425].

Chromosomal instability

About 80% of sporadic adenomas show chromosomal instability, resulting in numerical (gains, losses and amplifications) or structural (e.g. translocations) changes of parts or whole chromosomes, with aneuploidy. In contrast with MSI, the mechanism underlying chromosomal instability is not well known. Errors in mitotic chromosomal segregation and the mitotic spindle checkpoint have been implicated. Mechanisms and genes involved in these processes have been reviewed by Aguilera and Gomez-Gonzalez [427]. In gastric cancer, the most frequently reported numerical aberrations, by comparative genomic hybridisation are gains of chromosomes 3q, 7q, 8q, 13q, 17q and 20q, and losses on chromosomes 4q, 5q, 6p, 9p, 17p and 18q. Consistent high-level amplifications are located on chromosomes 7q, 8p, 8q, 17q, 19q and 20q [428].

CpG islands methylator phenotype

CIMP is a third pattern of genomic instability, characterised by hypermethylation of gene promoters, leading to gene silencing. Much overlap between MSI and CIMP has been observed in gastric cancer, suggesting that MSI is a confounding factor [429]. Irrespective of CIMP being a separate pathway in gastric carcinogenesis, the presence of hypermethylation of important genes could be clinically relevant, because methylation can be reverted by DNA methyltransferase.

Hypermethylation has been observed in the following genes, among others: *CDKN2A*, *RARB* and *RUNX3*. *CDKN2A* (p16) gene hypermethylation is seen in 12–30% of gastric carcinomas and reduced expression of the gene correlates with depth of invasion and metastasis in some studies [430]. Hypermethylation with reduced expression of the retinoic acid receptor β (*RARB*) gene is restricted to intestinal carcinomas and observed in 60–65% of the cases [431]. Hypermethylation of *RUNX3* (a member of

Table 13.4 Frequency of the most common genetic alterations found in gastric carcinomas

Gene	Alteration	Frequency[a] Intestinal carcinoma (%)	Diffuse carcinoma (%)
APC	LOH, mutations	30–40	<2
BCL2	Over-expression	–	10–30
CDH1	Mutations, hypermethylation, LOH	–	>50
CDKN1B (p27Kip1)	Reduced expression	40–50[b]	
CTNNB1 (β-catenin)	Mutations	17–27	
Cyclin E	Over-expression	15–20[b]	
DCC	LOH	60	<1
ERBB2	Amplification	9–15	<1
FGFR2 (K-SAM)	Amplification	–	35[c]
KRAS	Mutations	1–28[d]	<1
MET (c-MET)	Amplification	20–40[b]	
MYC (cMYC)	Over-expression	40–45[b]	
PTEN	LOH, mutations	20–30[e]	
RB1	Reduced expression	–	30[b]
TP53	Mutations, LOH	25–40[f]	0–21[f]

LOH, loss of heterozygosity.

[a]The frequencies are presented according to the two major histotypes of the Lauren classification, i.e. 'intestinal' and 'diffuse' (roughly corresponding to the 'well differentiated' and 'poorly differentiated' carcinomas of the Japanese classification), as reported in the relevant cited literature.

[b]Correlates with prognosis and/or more advanced disease.

[c]Present only in advanced cases.

[d]Mostly occurring in carcinomas with microsatellite instability.

[e]Associated with invasion and metastasis.

[f]Frequent in aneuploid (60–70%) but rare in diploid carcinoma.

the RUNX family that plays a role in transforming growth factor β [TGF-β] signalling) is observed in 45–65% of gastric cancers, sometimes accompanied by reduced expression of *RUNX3* in adjoining non-neoplastic gastric mucosa [432]. Biallelic inactivation of *RUNX3* can also be caused by homozygous deletion and, rarely, by mutation [433].

Acetylation and demethylation

Aberrant acetylation is frequently detected in H3 and H4 histone genes, in both the promoter and coding regions, and is associated with reduced expression of *CDKN1A* in gastric carcinoma [434]. Demethylation of genes such as melanoma antigen family (MAGE) and synuclein-γ (*SNCG*) has been described in gastric cancer, the former associated with advanced adenocarcinoma and a bad prognosis, the latter with lymph node metastasis [435,436].

Tumour-suppressor genes

Many tumour-suppressor genes have been implicated in gastric carcinoma development, including *APC* [437–440] and *DCC* [441,442] in intestinal-type carcinomas, as well as *CDH1* [443–448] and *RB1* [449] in diffuse carcinomas. Other tumour-suppressor genes are altered in both types

of gastric carcinoma, such as *PTEN* [450] and *TP53* [439, 451–453], although the latter is more common in intestinal-type carcinoma.

Oncogenes

Some oncogenes are preferentially altered in a specific type of gastric cancer, such as *HER2* [454–456] and *KRAS* [457–460] in intestinal type. *HER2* over-expression and/or amplification is present in about 20% of gastric cancers [461]. There is current interest in the immunohistochemical (IHC) and *in situ* hybridisation (ISH) detection of HER2 expression in gastric cancer because there is some evidence that these tumours may respond well to therapy with the humanised monoclonal antibody trastuzumab (Herceptin), as shown in the ToGA trial [462]. Compared with breast carcinoma, HER2 positivity in gastric cancer is frequently heterogeneous and there is a less stringent correlation between *HER2* amplification and protein over-expression [461]. The European Medicines Agency (EMEA) recommends HER2 testing by immunohistochemistry as a first evaluation assay, followed by fluorescence ISH (FISH) in IHC2-positive cases [463]. The presence of five intensely positive neoplastic cells in a biopsy or, at least 10% in a surgical specimen, is necessary for an IHC3-positive score. Notably, U shaped or lateral staining is more common than completeness of membrane staining in gastric cancer [461,464]. EMEA recommends that Herceptin should be used only in patients with metastatic gastric cancer whose tumours have HER2 over-expression as defined by an IHC2-positive and a confirmatory FISH-positive result, or IHC3 positive, as determined by an accurate and validated assay [463] (Figure 13.22).

Some oncogenes are altered preferentially in diffuse carcinoma, such as *BCL2* [465,466] and *FGFR2* (formerly *K-sam*) [467,468]. Other oncogenes are altered both in intestinal and diffuse carcinomas, including *CTNNB1* (encoding β-catenin) [469], *MET* [470] and *MYC* [471,472]. The expression of genes involved in the regulation of the cell cycle is also deregulated in gastric cancer, e.g. *CDKN1B* [473–475] and cyclin E [476].

Endocrine cell tumours

Gastric endocrine cell tumours are relatively uncommon neoplasms. The normal stomach contains five types of endocrine cells, including somatostatin-producing D cells, gastrin-producing G cells, histamine-producing enterochromaffin-like (ECL) cells, serotonin-producing enterochromaffin cells and ghrelin-producing cells. Endocrine neoplasms are generally recognised by their histological pattern, immunopositivity for cytosolic (e.g. NSE, protein gene product [PGP] 9.5 or CD56), vesicle (synaptophysin) or secretory granule (chromogranin) markers, immunohistochemistry, or ISH for specific peptide hormones or their characteristic ultrastructural features.

Some increase in incidence of gastric endocrine cell tumours has been reported in recent years, probably as a result of more widespread use of endoscopy. Gastric endocrine cell tumours increased from 0.5% to about 2% of gastric malignancies in one study [477]. Studies based on endoscopic techniques and increased awareness of neuro-endocrine tumours suggest that the gastric tumours account for 11–41% of all gastrointestinal endocrine tumours [478] and its incidence has shown an incremental increasing trend in the last three decades [479].

The older term of gastric 'carcinoid' is, in most circles, not now recommended. Further there is considerable controversy over whether these tumours should be termed 'endocrine (cell) tumours' or 'neuro-endocrine tumours'. The terms are used interchangeably here because of the different classifications. Gastric endocrine cell tumours are currently classified as (neuro-)endocrine tumours (NETs), (neuro-) endocrine carcinomas (NECs) and mixed adeno-neuro-endocrine carcinomas (MANECs), the last displaying exocrine and endocrine components, with one component exceeding 30%. NETs are also described in the literature as carcinoids and well differentiated endocrine tumour/carcinoma [480]; synonyms for NECs include poorly differentiated endocrine carcinomas, high grade neuro-endocrine carcinoma, and small and large cell endocrine carcinomas.

Most (neuro-)endocrine neoplasms of the stomach are NETs: well differentiated, non-functioning ECL cell tumours (ECL-cell NETs) that arise predominantly in the corpus–fundus region [480]. They encompass three distinct types: type I, tumours associated with autoimmune chronic atrophic gastritis (A-CAG); type II, tumours associated with multiple endocrine neoplasia type 1 (MEN-1) and Zollinger–Ellison syndrome (ZES); and type III, sporadic tumours. Serotonin-producing EC cell, gastrin cell, ghrelin cell or adrenocorticotrophic hormone (ACTH) cell NETs are very rare and may arise in both the corpus–fundus and the antrum. NECs and MANECs are also rare and may arise in any part of the stomach.

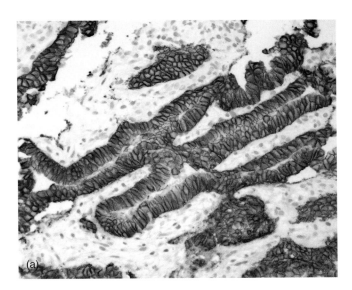

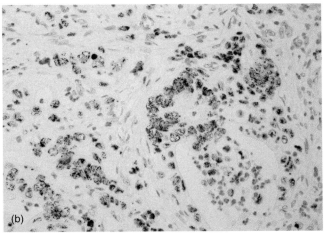

Figure 13.22 Adenocarcinoma of the stomach showing strong HER2 staining in most cells: (a) note that in this example, the staining in many cells is not limited to basolateral membranous reactivity but to the entire membrane. (b) Example of uniform *HER2* gene amplification by bright field *in situ* hybridisation. (Courtesy of Dr P. Kumarasinghe, University of Western Australia, Perth, WA, Australia.)

Recently, a three-tier grading system has been proposed. The following criteria are used: G1 (grade 1), with a mitotic count of <2 per 10 high power field (hpf) and/or ≤2% Ki67 index; G2, with a mitotic count of 2–20/10 hpf and/or 3–20% Ki67 index; and G3, with a mitotic count >20/10 hpf and/or >20% Ki67 index [481,482]. The mitotic count is calculated in at least 50 hpf (hpf = 2 mm^2) and the Ki67 index is based on the percentage positivity in 500–2000 cells in areas of highest nuclear labelling (hot spots). In cases of discrepancy in the criteria, use of the higher grade is suggested. This scheme has been shown to be of prognostic value [483,484].

Type I gastric ECL cell NETs

These are found in the body–fundus mucosa or at the antral–corpus junction [485] on a background of autoimmune chronic atrophic gastritis (A-CAG). They are frequently multiple (in 60% of cases) [486]. They represent 74% of all gastric NETs and occur more often in females. Clinical signs include achlorhydria and, less frequently, pernicious anaemia. Hypergastrinaemia or antral gastrin cell hyperplasia is observed in all cases of A-CAG associated with ECL cell tumours [487]. ECL cell hyperplasia and/or dysplasia is invariably present in the surrounding mucosa [486]. The tumours usually present as small nodular polypoid lesions, commonly <10 mm and virtually never >20 mm in size. They are usually confined to the mucosa and/or the submucosa [488,489] (Figure 13.23) and the muscularis propria is involved in only a minority of cases.

Microscopically, type I NETs are composed of small uniform cuboidal cells arranged in trabecular aggregates. The nuclei are monomorphic with inconspicuous nucleoli and abundant, eosinophilic cytoplasm (Figure 13.24).

Mitoses are almost absent and angio-invasion is infrequent [490]. Larger lesions (measuring >20 mm but sometimes 1–20 mm tumours) occasionally metastasise to local lymph nodes or, very rarely, spread to the liver [486,491]. Only exceptional tumour-related deaths are observed with type I NETs. Spontaneous regression is well recorded [492]. However, antrectomy to remove the main source of gastrin production or more extensive resection to remove as many tumours as possible (especially if >10 mm in size or G2) proved to cure about 80% of patients [493]. Nevertheless current recommendations for the management of these tumours suggest conservatism, with endoscopic removal of larger lesions (by endoscopic mucosal resection [EMR] or endoscopic submucosal dissection [ESD]) and surveillance of multiple smaller lesions, unless there is clinical or histological evidence to suggest a more aggressive phenotype.

Type II ECL cell NETs

These are associated with MEN-1 and Zollinger–Ellison syndrome. These tumours are located in the body–fundus mucosa or the body–antrum junction. They represent about 6% of all gastric NETs and show no gender predilection. These lesions are similar to those associated with chronic atrophic gastritis, in that they are frequently multiple, usually <15 mm in diameter and confined to the mucosa or submucosa. They also are accompanied by ECL cell hyperplasia in the surrounding mucosa [486,494]. In general, they also have a good prognosis. However, in some instances, larger tumours (>20 mm) may show atypical histological features such as nuclear pleomorphism and prominent mitoses: these lesions may be aggressive and associated with a poor prognosis [495]. In addition to the

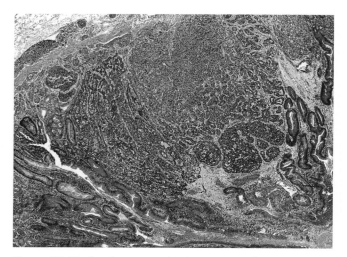

Figure 13.23 Gastric neuro-endocrine tumours: the expansile lesion displays a predominantly intramucosal growth pattern with only focal submucosal invasion.

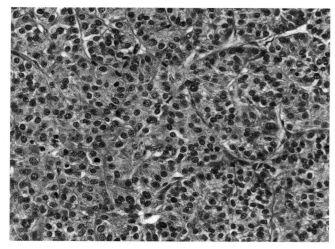

Figure 13.24 Cytology of gastric neuro-endocrine tumours: the solid nests are composed of uniform small cuboidal cells devoid of significant atypia.

multiple NETs, hypertrophic–hypersecretory gastropathy and high levels of circulating gastrin are critical diagnostic findings [490]. In most cases, a gastrin-producing tumour will be found in the duodenum or in the pancreas [496].

Type III ECL cell NETs

These are sporadic and usually a single neoplasm. They are also located in the body–fundus or body–antrum junctional mucosa. In over a third of cases, the tumour is >20 mm in size. Infiltration of the muscularis propria and the serosa is found in more than 50% of cases [486]. Type III NETs account for about 13% of all gastric neuro-endocrine neoplasms and are observed mainly in men [486]. These tumours develop in mucosa devoid of ECL cell hyperplasia/dysplasia and may present with symptoms similar to those of an adenocarcinoma. Although most are non-functioning and show evidence of ECL cell differentiation, rare functional metastasising tumours give rise to a carcinoid syndrome due to the release of histamine and serotonin (5-hydroxytryptamine) [497,498].

Type IV ECL cell NETs

Only three cases have been reported [499–501]. These neoplasms are small and multiple, and located in a hypertrophic body–fundus mucosa with prominent rugae reflecting florid parietal cell hyperplasia. As type I and II ECL cell NETs, these tumours develop in a background of ECL cell hyperplasia and hypergastrinaemia. However, this subtype is believed to result from a primary defect of acid secretion by parietal cells [499,500]. Microscopically, the parietal cells are vacuolated, with cytoplasmic protrusions into cystically distended oxyntic glands, some containing inspissated eosinophilic material.

NETs composed of other cell types

Enterochromaffin- and ACTH-, gastrin- or ghrelin-producing tumours represent less than 1% of all gastric neuro-endocrine neoplasms. EC cell NET are rare tumours, occasionally associated with carcinoid syndrome [502]. Rare cases of NETs have been observed associated with Cushing's syndrome as a result of ectopic secretion of ACTH [503]. Gastrin cell NET is also an uncommon tumour that may present associated with Zollinger–Ellison syndrome due to overproduction of gastrin, and may thus be defined as a gastrinoma. The sole functioning ghrelin cell tumour so far described was located in the corpus [504].

Neuro-endocrine carcinomas

These account for 6–16% of gastric neuro-endocrine neoplasms [486,490]. They may form a large fungating mass deeply infiltrating the gastric wall, and are often metastatic to the lymph nodes and liver [505]. NECs are high grade malignant tumours that show cellular pleomorphism and a variable spectrum of histology, ranging from obvious

NETs to tumours resembling small cell (oat cell) carcinoma which may be found in different areas of the same lesion. These highly malignant tumours are composed of poorly formed trabeculae, nests or sheets of anaplastic round, polyhedral to spindle cells, small to fairly large in size, and reactive for general neuro-endocrine markers, including chromogranin A, synaptophysin, neural cell adhesion molecule (N-CAM), PGP9.5 and/or NSE [487, 490, 506, 507]. Multifocal necrosis and a high mitotic rate (>20 mitoses/10 hpf) are observed, thus fulfilling a G3 grade.

Depending mainly on the amount of cytoplasm, two subtypes have been identified – small cell and large cell – similar to the corresponding lung cancers. Small cell variant shows solid organoid or trabecular patterns and small tumour cells with round or fusiform nuclei, little cytoplasm and finely granular nuclear chromatin, but few nucleoli. Occasional rosettes are present and there may be peripheral palisading. The tumour cells are usually pleomorphic and larger than the classic oat cell type [508]. The main differential diagnosis is poorly differentiated adenocarcinoma and malignant lymphoma. Paraneoplastic syndromes are seldom detected in small cell gastric NECs (Figure 13.25).

A large cell variant presents with organoid, trabecular or pseudo-glandular patterns. The cells have a prominent eosinophilic cytoplasm, coarse nuclear chromatin and numerous nucleoli. Mixed neuro-endocrine (especially of large cell type) and non-neuro-endocrine cancer may also be found [507]. Conversely, ordinary cancer foci are frequently observed in the intramucosal component of NECs [487]. Evidence for progression from NET (G1 and G2) to high grade (G3) NEC has been noted only rarely. All observations indicate that gastric NEC is a distinct, highly malignant cancer that has to be clearly distinguished from NET.

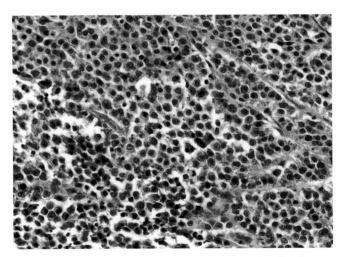

Figure 13.25 Gastric neuro-endocrine carcinoma (small cell type): prominent apoptosis and necrosis are characteristic of the neoplasm.

Guidelines have been established for standards of care of neuro-endocrine tumours [509]. Minimum requirements for reporting are the exact site and size, and the distance from the resection margins (for resection specimens). Microscopically, the number of mitoses counted per 10 hpf, the number of high power fields assessed and the Ki67 index percentage are essential. Endocrine function assessment should be provided upon specific clinical request. Finally, the diagnosis should classify the lesion (NET or NEC), and provide the grade (G1, G2 or G3) and the relevant TNM stage.

Precursor lesions of gastric neuro-endocrine neoplasms

ECL cell NET types I and II develop through a sequence of hyperplasia (simple, linear, micronodular and adenomatoid), dysplasia and neoplasia. These changes are directly related to the trophic effect of hypergastrinaemia caused by the hypochlorhydria/achlorhydria which results from severe chronic atrophic gastritis. The hypergastrinaemia initially induces hyperplasia of intraglandular ECL cells that is first linear (contiguous endocrine cells confined within the gland basement membrane) and then 'nodular' (small micronodular cellular aggregates escaping into the lamina propria). These changes can be difficult to detect on routine haematoxylin and eosin stain and immunohistochemistry is useful. Dysplasia is characterised by enlarging or fusing micronodules with microinvasion or newly formed stroma. When the nodules increase in size to >0.5 mm or invade the submucosa, the lesion is classified as a microcarcinoid (<5 mm) or plain 'carcinoid' (≥5 mm). Linear hyperplasia or more advanced changes have been shown to represent a risk factor for the development of gastric ECL cell tumours in patients with MEN-1–Zollinger–Ellison syndrome [510], and dysplastic lesions markedly increased the risk of developing ECL cell tumours [511] (Figure 13.26).

ECL cell hyperplasia secondary to hypergastrinaemia may also occur in patients receiving long-term treatment with proton pump inhibitors, especially if there is concomitant *H. pylori* infection [512,513]. However, NETs have not been observed to develop in this clinical setting.

Allelic loss at the *MEN1* gene locus has been demonstrated in neuro-endocrine neoplasms occurring in MEN, suggesting that the gene behaves as a classic tumour suppressor gene in this scenario [514].

Mixed adeno-neuro-endocrine carcinomas

Small numbers of scattered endocrine cells are not uncommonly detected in conventional gastric adenocarcinomas [515]. Alternatively, gastric MANECs are mixed carcinomas with a NET cell component composing at least 30% of

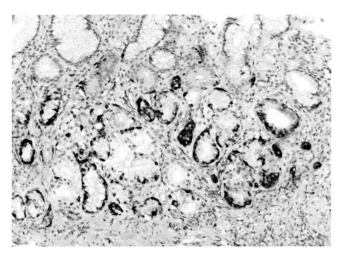

Figure 13.26 Precursor lesion of neuro-endocrine tumours: the chromogranin stain highlights the diffuse linear (chain-forming) and micronodular enterochromaffin-like cell hyperplasia.

the whole neoplasm. The neuro-endocrine component of the tumours usually consists of an NEC, often of large cell type [506], and rarely by a NET [516,517]. Conversely, the exocrine component may vary from well differentiated to a diffuse signet-ring cell carcinoma [506,516–519]. Gastric MANEC displays a distinct immunophenotype with expression of neuro-endocrine markers restricted to the neuro-endocrine component only, possibly also with expression of CEA in a fraction of cases [506,516,517,519]. In most cases, the clinical behaviour is aggressive.

Secondary carcinoma in the stomach

Various types of neoplasms can metastasise to the stomach by lymphatic and haematogenous spread, direct extension or intraperitoneal dissemination. The reported prevalence of haematogenous spread is between 1.7 and 5.4% [520–523]. Metastatic deposits often appear as raised, volcano-like lesions, covered by normal mucosa with central ulceration. In other instances, the metastasis forms a polypoid mass or a necrotic ulcer. Other metastatic tumours such as lobular carcinoma of the breast may diffusely infiltrate the wall of the stomach, simulating linitis plastica [524].

The most common primary neoplasms to show secondary spread to the stomach are malignant melanomas. Other common primary tumour sites are the breast, oesophagus, lung and pancreas [523,525,526]. Gastric metastases are reported in up to 30% of disseminated malignant melanoma (Figure 13.27) and 12% of breast cancers (Figure 13.28). About two-thirds of breast cancer metastases to the stomach are lobular carcinomas [527,528], and the interval between a primary breast tumour and presentation of gastric metas-

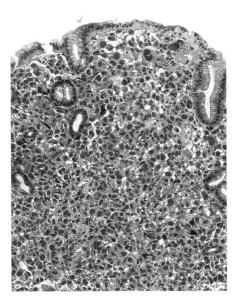

Figure 13.27 Metastatic malignant melanoma to stomach: the normal epithelium is in stark contrast with the subjacent atypical neoplastic cells. The diagnosis was confirmed by *HMB-45* positivity.

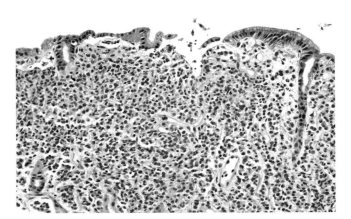

Figure 13.28 Metastatic breast carcinoma to the stomach: the proven *GCDFP15*-positive metastatic carcinoma shows Indian filing and epithelial clustering similar to the original lobular breast carcinoma. This lesion could easily be mistaken for a poorly cohesive gastric carcinoma.

tases is often considerable, averaging around 6 years [529]. Metastases from primary neoplasms of the kidney, testis, uterus, ovary and colon have also been described [522,530].

In most cases, the metastasis is located within the submucosa or muscularis propria, with little or no involvement of the mucosa. The lack of an *in situ* component within the mucosa may also serve as a clue that the neo-

plasm is a metastasis. Lewin and Appelman have described an unusual pattern of mucosal infiltration by secondary carcinoma where tumour cells form nests and appear to grow within the contours of mucosal glands [338]. Immunohistochemistry may help to differentiate a primary gastric carcinoma from secondary carcinoma from a variety of primary sites, e.g. metastases from breast may be positive for gross cystic disease fluid protein and oestrogen/ progesterone receptors but negative for cdx-2, villin and Hep-Par-1. Lung-derived tumour may be positive for thyroid transcription factor-1 (TTF-1) and carcinomas from the liver, kidney and prostate may be negative for keratins 7 and 20 but positive for, respectively, HepPar-1 antibody and glypican 3, paired box gene 8 (PAX8) and prostate-specific antigen [531–535].

References

1. Lauwers GY, Srivastava A. Gastric preneoplastic lesions and epithelial dysplasia. *Gastroenterol Clin North Am* 2007;**36**:813.
2. Riddell RH, Goldman H, Ransohoff DF, et al. Dysplasia in inflammatory bowel disease: standardized classification with provisional clinical applications. *Hum Pathol* 1983;**14**:931.
3. Lauwers GY, Shimizu M, Correa P, et al. Evaluation of gastric biopsies for neoplasia: differences between Japanese and Western pathologists. *Am J Surg Pathol* 1999;**23**:511.
4. Schlemper RJ, Kato Y, Stolte M. Review of histological classifications of gastrointestinal epithelial neoplasia: differences in diagnosis of early carcinomas between Japanese and Western pathologists. *J Gastroenterol* 2001;**36**:445.
5. Schlemper RJ, Riddell RH, Kato Y, et al. The Vienna classification of gastrointestinal epithelial neoplasia. *Gut* 2000;**47**:251.
6. Stolte M. The new Vienna classification of epithelial neoplasia of the gastrointestinal tract: advantages and disadvantages. *Virchows Arch* 2003;**442**:99.
7. Jass JR. A classification of gastric dysplasia. *Histopathology* 1983;**7**:181.
8. Nogueira AM, Machado JC, Carneiro F, Reis CA, Gott P, Sobrinho-Simoes M. Patterns of expression of trefoil peptides and mucins in gastric polyps with and without malignant transformation. *J Pathol* 1999;**187**:541.
9. Park do Y, Srivastava A, Kim GH, et al. Adenomatous and foveolar gastric dysplasia: distinct patterns of mucin expression and background intestinal metaplasia. *Am J Surg Pathol* 2008;**32**:524.
10. Park do Y, Srivastava A, Kim GH, et al. CDX2 expression in the intestinal-type gastric epithelial neoplasia: frequency and significance. *Mod Pathol* 2010;**23**:54.
11. Abraham SC, Montgomery EA, Singh VK, Yardley JH, Wu TT. Gastric adenomas: intestinal-type and gastric-type adenomas differ in the risk of adenocarcinoma and presence of background mucosal pathology. *Am J Surg Pathol* 2002;**26**:1276.
12. Ghandur-Mnaymneh L, Paz J, Roldan E, Cassady J. Dysplasia of nonmetaplastic gastric mucosa. A proposal for its classification and its possible relationship to diffuse-type gastric carcinoma. *Am J Surg Pathol* 1988;**12**:96.
13. Lansdown M, Quirke P, Dixon MF, Axon AT, Johnston D. High grade dysplasia of the gastric mucosa: a marker for gastric carcinoma. *Gut* 1990;**31**:977.
14. Di Gregorio C, Morandi P, Fante R, De Gaetani C. Gastric dysplasia. A follow-up study. *Am J Gastroenterol* 1993;**88**:1714.

15. Rugge M, Farinati F, Di Mario F, Baffa R, Valiante F, Cardin F. Gastric epithelial dysplasia: a prospective multicenter follow-up study from the Interdisciplinary Group on Gastric Epithelial Dysplasia. *Hum Pathol* 1991;**22**:1002.

16. Saraga EP, Gardiol D, Costa J. Gastric dysplasia. A histological follow-up study. *Am J Surg Pathol* 1987;**11**:788.

17. Fertitta AM, Comin U, Terruzzi V, et al., Gastrointestinal Endoscopic Pathology Study Group. Clinical significance of gastric dysplasia: a multicenter follow-up study. *Endoscopy* 1993;**25**:265.

18. Kokkola A, Haapiainen R, Laxen F, et al. Risk of gastric carcinoma in patients with mucosal dysplasia associated with atrophic gastritis: a follow up study. *J Clin Pathol* 1996;**49**:979.

19. Yamada H, Ikegami M, Shimoda T, Takagi N, Maruyama M. Long-term follow-up study of gastric adenoma/dysplasia. *Endoscopy* 2004;**36**:390.

20. Weinstein WM, Goldstein NS. Gastric dysplasia and its management. *Gastroenterology* 1994;**107**:1543.

21. Rugge M, Nitti D, Farinati F, di Mario F, Genta RM. Non-invasive neoplasia of the stomach. *Eur J Gastroenterol Hepatol* 2005;**17**:1191.

22. Nakajima T. Gastric cancer treatment guidelines in Japan. *Gastric Cancer* 2002;**5**:1.

23. Gotoda T. Endoscopic resection of early gastric cancer. *Gastric Cancer* 2007;**10**:1.

24. Ferlay J, Bray F, Pisani P, Parkin M. *Cancer Incidence, mortality and prevalence worldwide.* Globocan 2002. IARC CancerBase, No. 5. Lyon: IARC, 2004.

25. Curado MP, Edwards B, Shin HR, Storm H, Ferlay J, Heanue M, eds. *Cancer Incidence in Five Continents.* IARC: Lyon, 2007.

26. Parkin DM. The global health burden of infection-associated cancers in the year 2002. *Int J Cancer* 2006;**118**:3030.

27. Keeney S, Bauer TL. Epidemiology of adenocarcinoma of the esophagogastric junction. *Surg Oncol Clin N Am* 2006;**15**:687.

28. Zheng T, Mayne ST, Holford TR, et al. The time trend and age-period-cohort effects on incidence of adenocarcinoma of the stomach in Connecticut from 1955 to 1989. *Cancer* 1993;**72**:330.

29. Blot WJ, Devesa SS, Kneller RW, Fraumeni JF, Jr. Rising incidence of adenocarcinoma of the esophagus and gastric cardia. *JAMA* 1991;**265**:1287.

30. Pohl H, Welch HG. The role of overdiagnosis and reclassification in the marked increase of esophageal adenocarcinoma incidence. *J Natl Cancer Inst* 2005;**97**:142.

31. Botterweck AA, Schouten LJ, Volovics A, Dorant E, van Den Brandt PA. Trends in incidence of adenocarcinoma of the oesophagus and gastric cardia in ten European countries. *Int J Epidemiol* 2000;**29**:645.

32. Pera M, Manterola C, Vidal O, Grande L. Epidemiology of esophageal adenocarcinoma. *J Surg Oncol* 2005;**92**:151.

33. Brown LM, Devesa SS, Chow WH. Incidence of adenocarcinoma of the esophagus among white Americans by sex, stage, and age. *J Natl Cancer Inst* 2008;**100**:1184.

34. Kokkola A, Sipponen P. Gastric carcinoma in young adults. *Hepatogastroenterology* 2001;**48**:1552.

35. Milne AN, Sitarz R, Carvalho R, Carneiro F, Offerhaus GJ. Early onset gastric cancer: on the road to unraveling gastric carcinogenesis. *Curr Mol Med* 2007;**7**:15.

36. Koea JB, Karpeh MS, Brennan MF. Gastric cancer in young patients: demographic, clinicopathological, and prognostic factors in 92 patients. *Ann Surg Oncol* 2000;**7**:346.

37. Moreira H, Pinto-de-Sousa J, Carneiro F, Cardoso de Oliveira M, Pimenta A. Early onset gastric cancer no longer presents as an advanced disease with ominous prognosis. *Dig Surg* 2009;**26**:215.

38. Park JC, Lee YC, Kim JH, et al. Clinicopathological aspects and prognostic value with respect to age: an analysis of 3,362 consecutive gastric cancer patients. *J Surg Oncol* 2009;**99**:395.

39. Theuer CP, de Virgilio C, Keese G, et al. Gastric adenocarcinoma in patients 40 years of age or younger. *Am J Surg* 1996;**172**:473.

40. Seruca R, Sobrinho-Simoes M. Assessment of microsatellite alterations in young patients with gastric adenocarcinoma. *Cancer* 1997;**80**:1358.

41. Hayden JD, Cawkwell L, Dixon MF, et al. A comparison of microsatellite instability in early onset gastric carcinomas from relatively low and high incidence European populations. *Int J Cancer* 2000;**85**:189.

42. Lim S, Lee HS, Kim HS, Kim YI, Kim WH. Alteration of E-cadherin-mediated adhesion protein is common, but microsatellite instability is uncommon in young age gastric cancers. *Histopathology* 2003;**42**:128.

43. Milne AN, Carvalho R, Morsink FM, et al. Early-onset gastric cancers have a different molecular expression profile than conventional gastric cancers. *Mod Pathol* 2006;**19**:564.

44. Carvalho R, Milne AN, Polak M, Offerhaus GJ, Weterman MA. A novel region of amplification at 11p12–13 in gastric cancer, revealed by representational difference analysis, is associated with overexpression of CD44v6, especially in early-onset gastric carcinomas. *Genes Chromosomes Cancer* 2006;**45**:967.

45. Buffart TE, Carvalho B, Hopmans E, et al. Gastric cancers in young and elderly patients show different genomic profiles. *J Pathol* 2007;**211**:45.

46. Silva EM, Begnami MD, Fregnani JH, et al. Cadherin-catenin adhesion system and mucin expression: a comparison between young and older patients with gastric carcinoma. *Gastric Cancer* 2008;**11**:149.

47. Rugge M, Busatto G, Cassaro M, et al. Patients younger than 40 years with gastric carcinoma: *Helicobacter pylori* genotype and associated gastritis phenotype. *Cancer* 1999;**85**:2506.

48. Koshida Y, Koizumi W, Sasabe M, Katoh Y, Okayasu I. Association of *Helicobacter pylori*-dependent gastritis with gastric carcinomas in young Japanese patients: histopathological comparison of diffuse and intestinal type cancer cases. *Histopathology* 2000;**37**:124.

49. Huntsman DG, Carneiro F, Lewis FR, et al. Early gastric cancer in young, asymptomatic carriers of germ-line E-cadherin mutations. *N Engl J Med* 2001;**344**:1904.

50. Correa P. A human model of gastric carcinogenesis. *Cancer Res* 1988;**48**:3554.

51. Correa P. Human gastric carcinogenesis: a multistep and multifactorial process – First American Cancer Society Award Lecture on Cancer Epidemiology and Prevention. *Cancer Res* 1992;**52**:6735.

52. Imai T, Kubo T, Watanabe H. Chronic gastritis in Japanese with reference to high incidence of gastric carcinoma. *J Natl Cancer Inst* 1971;**47**:179.

53. Correa P, Cuello C, Duque E. Carcinoma and intestinal metaplasia of the stomach in Colombian migrants. *J Natl Cancer Inst* 1970;**44**:297.

54. Siurala M, Varis K, Wiljasalo M. Studies of patients with atrophic gastritis: a 10–15-year follow-up. *Scand J Gastroenterol* 1966;**1**:40.

55. Walker IR, Strickland RG, Ungar B, Mackay IR. Simple atrophic gastritis and gastric carcinoma. *Gut* 1971;**12**:906.

56. Jass JR. Role of intestinal metaplasia in the histogenesis of gastric carcinoma. *J Clin Pathol* 1980;**33**:801.

57. Filipe MI, Munoz N, Matko I, et al. Intestinal metaplasia types and the risk of gastric cancer: a cohort study in Slovenia. *Int J Cancer* 1994;**57**:324.

58. Ectors N, Dixon MF. The prognostic value of sulphomucin positive intestinal metaplasia in the development of gastric cancer. *Histopathology* 1986;**10**:1271.

59. Antonioli DA. Precursors of gastric carcinoma: a critical review with a brief description of early (curable) gastric cancer. *Hum Pathol* 1994;**25**:994.

60. Price AB. The Sydney System: histological division. *J Gastroenterol Hepatol* 1991;**6**:209.

61. Dixon MF, Genta RM, Yardley JH, Correa P. Classification and grading of gastritis. The updated Sydney System. International Workshop on the Histopathology of Gastritis, Houston, 1994. *Am J Surg Pathol* 1996;**20**:1161.

62. El-Zimaity HM, Graham DY, al-Assi MT, et al. Interobserver variation in the histopathological assessment of *Helicobacter pylori* gastritis. *Hum Pathol* 1996;**27**:35.

63. Offerhaus GJ, Price AB, Haot J, et al. Observer agreement on the grading of gastric atrophy. *Histopathology* 1999;**34**:320.

64. Chen XY, van der Hulst RW, Bruno MJ, et al. Interobserver variation in the histopathological scoring of *Helicobacter pylori* related gastritis. *J Clin Pathol* 1999;**52**:612.

65. Rugge M, Correa P, Dixon MF, et al. Gastric mucosal atrophy: interobserver consistency using new criteria for classification and grading. *Aliment Pharmacol Ther* 2002;**16**:1249.

66. Meining A, Bayerdorffer E, Muller P, et al. Gastric carcinoma risk index in patients infected with *Helicobacter pylori*. *Virchows Arch* 1998;**432**:311.

67. Rugge M, Meggio A, Pennelli G, et al. Gastritis staging in clinical practice: the OLGA staging system. *Gut* 2007;**56**:631.

68. Graham DY, Nurgalieva ZZ, El-Zimaity HM, et al. Noninvasive versus histologic detection of gastric atrophy in a Hispanic population in North America. *Clin Gastroenterol Hepatol* 2006;**4**:306.

69. Rugge M, de Boni M, Pennelli G, et al. Gastritis OLGA-staging and gastric cancer risk: a twelve-year clinico-pathological follow-up study. *Aliment Pharmacol Ther* 2010;**31**:1104.

70. Filipe MI, Potet F, Bogomoletz WV, et al. Incomplete sulphomucin-secreting intestinal metaplasia for gastric cancer. Preliminary data from a prospective study from three centres. *Gut* 1985;**26**:1319.

71. Filipe MI, Jass JR, eds. Intestinal metaplasia subtypes and cancer risk. In: *Gastric Carcinoma*. London: Churchill Livingstone, 1986: 87.

72. Reis CA, David L, Correa P, et al. Intestinal metaplasia of human stomach displays distinct patterns of mucin (MUC1, MUC2, MUC5AC, and MUC6) expression. *Cancer Res* 1999;**59**:1003.

73. Rokkas T, Filipe MI, Sladen GE. Detection of an increased incidence of early gastric cancer in patients with intestinal metaplasia type III who are closely followed up. *Gut* 1991;**32**:1110.

74. Rubio CA, Jonasson J, Nesi G, et al. Extensive intestinal metaplasia in gastric carcinoma and in other lesions requiring surgery: a study of 3,421 gastrectomy specimens from dwellers of the Atlantic and Pacific basins. *J Clin Pathol* 2005;**58**:1271.

75. de Vries AC, Haringsma J, de Vries RA, et al. The use of clinical, histologic, and serologic parameters to predict the intragastric extent of intestinal metaplasia: a recommendation for routine practice. *Gastrointest Endosc* 2009;**70**:18.

76. El-Zimaity HM, Ramchatesingh J, Saeed MA, Graham DY. Gastric intestinal metaplasia: subtypes and natural history. *J Clin Pathol* 2001;**54**:679.

77. Smith JL, Dixon MF. Is subtyping of intestinal metaplasia in the upper gastrointestinal tract a worthwhile exercise? An evaluation of current mucin histochemical stains. *Br J Biomed Sci* 2003;**60**:180.

78. Kang KP, Lee HS, Kim N, et al. Role of intestinal metaplasia subtyping in the risk of gastric cancer in Korea. *J Gastroenterol Hepatol* 2009;**24**:140.

79. Kakinoki R, Kushima R, Matsubara A, et al. Re-evaluation of histogenesis of gastric carcinomas: a comparative histopathological study between *Helicobacter pylori*-negative and *H. pylori*-positive cases. *Dig Dis Sci* 2009;**54**:614.

80. Gutierrez-Gonzalez L, Wright NA. Biology of intestinal metaplasia in 2008: more than a simple phenotypic alteration. *Dig Liver Dis* 2008;**40**:510.

81. Uemura N, Okamoto S, Yamamoto S, et al. *Helicobacter pylori* infection and the development of gastric cancer. *N Engl J Med* 2001;**345**:784.

82. Malfertheiner P, Bornschein J, Selgrad M. Role of *Helicobacter pylori* infection in gastric cancer pathogenesis: a chance for prevention. *J Dig Dis* 2010;**11**:2.

83. International Agency for Research on Cancer. Schistosomes, liver flukes and *Helicobacter pylori*. Lyon: IARC 1994.

84. Forman D, Newell DG, Fullerton F, et al. Association between infection with *Helicobacter pylori* and risk of gastric cancer: evidence from a prospective investigation. *BMJ* 1991;**302**:1302.

85. Nomura A, Stemmermann GN, Chyou PH, Kato I, Perez-Perez GI, Blaser MJ. *Helicobacter pylori* infection and gastric carcinoma among Japanese Americans in Hawaii. *N Engl J Med* 1991;**325**:1132.

86. Parsonnet J, Friedman GD, Vandersteen DP, et al. *Helicobacter pylori* infection and the risk of gastric carcinoma. *N Engl J Med* 1991;**325**:1127.

87. Asaka M, Kimura T, Kato M, et al. Possible role of *Helicobacter pylori* infection in early gastric cancer development. *Cancer* 1994;**73**:2691.

88. Huang JQ, Sridhar S, Chen Y, Hunt RH. Meta-analysis of the relationship between *Helicobacter pylori* seropositivity and gastric cancer. *Gastroenterology* 1998;**114**:1169.

89. Danesh J. *Helicobacter pylori* infection and gastric cancer: systematic review of the epidemiological studies. *Aliment Pharmacol Ther* 1999;**13**:851.

90. Eslick GD, Lim LL, Byles JE, Xia HH, Talley NJ. Association of *Helicobacter pylori* infection with gastric carcinoma: a metaanalysis. *Am J Gastroenterol* 1999;**94**:2373.

91. Helicobacter and Cancer Collaborative Group. Gastric cancer and *Helicobacter pylori*: a combined analysis of 12 case control studies nested within prospective cohorts. *Gut* 2001;**49**:347.

92. Watanabe T, Tada M, Nagai H, Sasaki S, Nakao M. *Helicobacter pylori* infection induces gastric cancer in mongolian gerbils. *Gastroenterology* 1998;**115**:642.

93. Honda S, Fujioka T, Tokieda M, Satoh R, Nishizono A, Nasu M. Development of *Helicobacter pylori*-induced gastric carcinoma in Mongolian gerbils. *Cancer Res* 1998;**58**:4255.

94. Sugiyama A, Maruta F, Ikeno T, et al. *Helicobacter pylori* infection enhances N-methyl-N-nitrosourea-induced stomach carcinogenesis in the Mongolian gerbil. *Cancer Res* 1998;**58**:2067.

95. Shimizu N, Inada K, Nakanishi H, et al. *Helicobacter pylori* infection enhances glandular stomach carcinogenesis in Mongolian gerbils treated with chemical carcinogens. *Carcinogenesis* 1999;**20**:669.

96. Shimizu N, Ikehara Y, Inada K, et al. Eradication diminishes enhancing effects of *Helicobacter pylori* infection on glandular stomach carcinogenesis in Mongolian gerbils. *Cancer Res* 2000;**60**:1512.

97. Nozaki K, Shimizu N, Ikehara Y, et al. Effect of early eradication on *Helicobacter pylori*-related gastric carcinogenesis in Mongolian gerbils. *Cancer Sci* 2003;**94**:235.

98. Maruta F, Sugiyama A, Ishizone S, Miyagawa S, Ota H, Katsuyama T. Eradication of *Helicobacter pylori* decreases mucosal

alterations linked to gastric carcinogenesis in Mongolian gerbils. *J Gastroenterol* 2005;**40**:104.

99. Wong BC, Lam SK, Wong WM, et al. *Helicobacter pylori* eradication to prevent gastric cancer in a high-risk region of China: a randomized controlled trial. *JAMA* 2004;**291**:187.

100. Take S, Mizuno M, Ishiki K, et al. The effect of eradicating *Helicobacter pylori* on the development of gastric cancer in patients with peptic ulcer disease. *Am J Gastroenterol* 2005;**100**:1037.

101. Fuccio L, Zagari RM, Minardi ME, Bazzoli F. Systematic review: *Helicobacter pylori* eradication for the prevention of gastric cancer. *Aliment Pharmacol Ther* 2007;**25**:133.

102. Uemura N, Mukai T, Okamoto S, et al. Effect of *Helicobacter pylori* eradication on subsequent development of cancer after endoscopic resection of early gastric cancer. *Cancer Epidemiol Biomarkers Prev* 1997;**6**:639.

103. Fukase K, Kato M, Kikuchi S, et al. Effect of eradication of *Helicobacter pylori* on incidence of metachronous gastric carcinoma after endoscopic resection of early gastric cancer: an open-label, randomised controlled trial. *Lancet* 2008;**372**:392.

104. Mahdavi J, Sonden B, Hurtig M, et al. *Helicobacter pylori* SabA adhesin in persistent infection and chronic inflammation. *Science* 2002;**297**:573.

105. Jung SW, Sugimoto M, Graham DY, Yamaoka Y. homB status of *Helicobacter pylori* as a novel marker to distinguish gastric cancer from duodenal ulcer. *J Clin Microbiol* 2009;**47**:3241.

106. Odenbreit S, Swoboda K, Barwig I, et al. Outer membrane protein expression profile in *Helicobacter pylori* clinical isolates. *Infect Immun* 2009;**77**:3782.

107. Atherton JC, Cao P, Peek RM, Jr., Tummuru MK, Blaser MJ, Cover TL. Mosaicism in vacuolating cytotoxin alleles of *Helicobacter pylori*. Association of specific vacA types with cytotoxin production and peptic ulceration. *J Biol Chem* 1995;**270**:17771.

108. Censini S, Lange C, Xiang Z, et al. cag, a pathogenicity island of *Helicobacter pylori*, encodes type I-specific and disease-associated virulence factors. *Proc Natl Acad Sci U S A* 1996;**93**:14648.

109. Basso D, Zambon CF, Letley DP, et al. Clinical relevance of *Helicobacter pylori* cagA and vacA gene polymorphisms. *Gastroenterology* 2008;**135**:91.

110. Nogueira C, Figueiredo C, Carneiro F, et al. *Helicobacter pylori* genotypes may determine gastric histopathology. *Am J Pathol* 2001;**158**:647.

111. Rhead JL, Letley DP, Mohammadi M, et al. A new *Helicobacter pylori* vacuolating cytotoxin determinant, the intermediate region, is associated with gastric cancer. *Gastroenterology* 2007;**133**:926.

112. Ogiwara H, Sugimoto M, Ohno T, et al. Role of deletion located between the intermediate and middle regions of the *Helicobacter pylori* vacA gene in cases of gastroduodenal diseases. *J Clin Microbiol* 2009;**47**:3493.

113. Palli D, Masala G, Del Giudice G, et al. CagA+ *Helicobacter pylori* infection and gastric cancer risk in the EPIC-EURGAST study. *Int J Cancer* 2007;**120**:859.

114. Plummer M, van Doorn LJ, Franceschi S, et al. *Helicobacter pylori* cytotoxin-associated genotype and gastric precancerous lesions. *J Natl Cancer Inst* 2007;**99**:1328.

115. Figueiredo C, Van Doorn LJ, Nogueira C, et al. *Helicobacter pylori* genotypes are associated with clinical outcome in Portuguese patients and show a high prevalence of infections with multiple strains. *Scand J Gastroenterol* 2001;**36**:128.

116. Hussein NR, Mohammadi M, Talebkhan Y, et al. Differences in virulence markers between *Helicobacter pylori* strains from Iraq and those from Iran: potential importance of regional differences in *H. pylori*-associated disease. *J Clin Microbiol* 2008;**46**:1774.

117. El-Omar EM, Carrington M, Chow WH, et al. Interleukin-1 polymorphisms associated with increased risk of gastric cancer. *Nature* 2000;**404**:398.

118. El-Omar EM. The importance of interleukin 1beta in *Helicobacter pylori* associated disease. *Gut* 2001;**48**:743.

119. El-Omar EM, Carrington M, Chow WH, et al. The role of interleukin-1 polymorphisms in the pathogenesis of gastric cancer. *Nature* 2001;**412**:99.

120. Figueiredo C, Machado JC, Pharoah P, et al. *Helicobacter pylori* and interleukin 1 genotyping: an opportunity to identify high-risk individuals for gastric carcinoma. *J Natl Cancer Inst* 2002;**94**:1680.

121. Eguchi H, Herschenhous N, Kuzushita N, Moss SF. *Helicobacter pylori* increases proteasome-mediated degradation of p27(kip1) in gastric epithelial cells. *Cancer Res* 2003;**63**:4739.

122. Franco AT, Israel DA, Washington MK, et al. Activation of beta-catenin by carcinogenic *Helicobacter pylori*. *Proc Natl Acad Sci U S A* 2005;**102**:10646.

123. Wei J, O'Brien D, Vilgelm A, et al. Interaction of *Helicobacter pylori* with gastric epithelial cells is mediated by the p53 protein family. *Gastroenterology* 2008;**134**:1412.

124. Houghton J, Stoicov C, Nomura S, et al. Gastric cancer originating from bone marrow-derived cells. *Science* 2004;**306**:1568.

125. Correa P, Houghton J. Carcinogenesis of *Helicobacter pylori*. *Gastroenterology* 2007;**133**:659.

126. Ekstrom AM, Serafini M, Nyren O, Hansson LE, Ye W, Wolk A. Dietary antioxidant intake and the risk of cardia cancer and noncardia cancer of the intestinal and diffuse types: a population-based case-control study in Sweden. *Int J Cancer* 2000;**87**:133.

127. Epplein M, Nomura AM, Hankin JH, et al. Association of *Helicobacter pylori* infection and diet on the risk of gastric cancer: a case-control study in Hawaii. *Cancer Causes Control* 2008;**19**:869.

128. Kono S, Hirohata T. Nutrition and stomach cancer. *Cancer Causes Control* 1996;**7**:41.

129. Mirvish SS. Effects of vitamins C and E on N-nitroso compound formation, carcinogenesis, and cancer. *Cancer* 1986;**58**:1842.

130. Bjelakovic G, Nikolova D, Simonetti RG, Gluud C. Systematic review: primary and secondary prevention of gastrointestinal cancers with antioxidant supplements. *Aliment Pharmacol Ther* 2008;**28**:689.

131. Qiao YL, Dawsey SM, Kamangar F, et al. Total and cancer mortality after supplementation with vitamins and minerals: follow-up of the Linxian General Population Nutrition Intervention Trial. *J Natl Cancer Inst* 2009;**101**:507.

132. Jenab M, Riboli E, Ferrari P, et al. Plasma and dietary carotenoid, retinol and tocopherol levels and the risk of gastric adenocarcinomas in the European prospective investigation into cancer and nutrition. *Br J Cancer* 2006;**95**:406.

133. Lee SA, Kang D, Shim KN, Choe JW, Hong WS, Choi H. Effect of diet and *Helicobacter pylori* infection to the risk of early gastric cancer. *J Epidemiol* 2003;**13**:162.

134. Shikata K, Kiyohara Y, Kubo M, et al. A prospective study of dietary salt intake and gastric cancer incidence in a defined Japanese population: the Hisayama study. *Int J Cancer* 2006;**119**:196.

135. Phukan RK, Narain K, Zomawia E, Hazarika NC, Mahanta J. Dietary habits and stomach cancer in Mizoram, India. *J Gastroenterol* 2006;**41**:418.

136. Gonzalez CA, Jakszyn P, Pera G, et al. Meat intake and risk of stomach and esophageal adenocarcinoma within the European Prospective Investigation Into Cancer and Nutrition (EPIC). *J Natl Cancer Inst* 2006;**98**:345.

137. Buckland G, Agudo A, Lujan L, et al. Adherence to a Mediterranean diet and risk of gastric adenocarcinoma within the

European Prospective Investigation into Cancer and Nutrition (EPIC) cohort study. *Am J Clin Nutr* 2010;**91**:381.

138. Gonzalez CA, Pera G, Agudo A, et al. Fruit and vegetable intake and the risk of stomach and oesophagus adenocarcinoma in the European Prospective Investigation into Cancer and Nutrition (EPIC-EURGAST). *Int J Cancer* 2006;**118**:2559.

139. M AM, Pera G, Agudo A, et al. Cereal fiber intake may reduce risk of gastric adenocarcinomas: the EPIC-EURGAST study. *Int J Cancer* 2007;**121**:1618.

140. Gonzalez CA, Pera G, Agudo A, et al. Smoking and the risk of gastric cancer in the European Prospective Investigation Into Cancer and Nutrition (EPIC). *Int J Cancer* 2003;**107**:629.

141. International Agency for research on Cancer. *Tobacco Smoke and Involuntary Smoking*. IARC Monographs on the Evaluation of the Carcinogenic Risks to Humans, Vol 83. Lyon: IARC, 2004.

142. Brenner H, Arndt V, Bode G, Stegmaier C, Ziegler H, Stumer T. Risk of gastric cancer among smokers infected with *Helicobacter pylori*. *Int J Cancer* 2002;**98**:446.

143. Siman JH, Forsgren A, Berglund G, Floren CH. Tobacco smoking increases the risk for gastric adenocarcinoma among *Helicobacter pylori*-infected individuals. *Scand J Gastroenterol* 2001;**36**:208.

144. Zaridze D, Borisova E, Maximovitch D, Chkhikvadze V. Alcohol consumption, smoking and risk of gastric cancer: case-control study from Moscow, Russia. *Cancer Causes Control* 2000;**11**:363.

145. Armbrecht U, Stockbrugger RW, Rode J, Menon GG, Cotton PB. Development of gastric dysplasia in pernicious anaemia: a clinical and endoscopic follow up study of 80 patients. *Gut* 1990;**31**:1105.

146. Mosbech J, Videbaek A. Mortality from and risk of gastric carcinoma among patients with pernicious anaemia. *Br Med J* 1950;**2**:390.

147. Magnus HA. A re-assessment of the gastric lesion in pernicious anaemia. *J Clin Pathol* 1958;**11**:289.

148. Brinton LA, Gridley G, Hrubec Z, Hoover R, Fraumeni JF, Jr. Cancer risk following pernicious anaemia. *Br J Cancer* 1989;**59**:810.

149. Hsing AW, Hansson LE, McLaughlin JK, et al. Pernicious anemia and subsequent cancer. A population-based cohort study. *Cancer* 1993;**71**:745.

150. Mellemkjaer L, Gridley G, Moller H, et al. Pernicious anaemia and cancer risk in Denmark. *Br J Cancer* 1996;**73**:998.

151. Karlson BM, Ekbom A, Wacholder S, McLaughlin JK, Hsing AW. Cancer of the upper gastrointestinal tract among patients with pernicious anemia: a case-cohort study. *Scand J Gastroenterol* 2000;**35**:847.

152. Ye W, Nyren O. Risk of cancers of the oesophagus and stomach by histology or subsite in patients hospitalised for pernicious anaemia. *Gut* 2003;**52**:938.

153. Schafer LW, Larson DE, Melton LJ 3rd, Higgins JA, Zinsmeister AR. Risk of development of gastric carcinoma in patients with pernicious anemia: a population-based study in Rochester, Minnesota. *Mayo Clin Proc* 1985;**60**:444.

154. Stockbrugger RW, Menon GG, Beilby JO, Mason RR, Cotton PB. Gastroscopic screening in 80 patients with pernicious anaemia. *Gut* 1983;**24**:1141.

155. Solcia E, Rindi G, Fiocca R, et al. Distinct patterns of chronic gastritis associated with carcinoid and cancer and their role in tumorigenesis. *Yale J Biol Med* 1992;**65**:793.

156. Kokkola A, Sjoblom SM, Haapiainen R, Sipponen P, Puolakkainen P, Jarvinen H. The risk of gastric carcinoma and carcinoid tumours in patients with pernicious anaemia. A prospective follow-up study. *Scand J Gastroenterol* 1998;**33**:88.

157. Bordi C, D'Adda T, Azzoni C, Pilato FP, Caruana P. Hypergastrinemia and gastric enterochromaffin-like cells. *Am J Surg Pathol* 1995;**19**(suppl 1):S8.

158. Carmack SW, Genta RM, Graham DY, Lauwers GY. Management of gastric polyps: a pathology-based guide for gastroenterologists. *Nat Rev Gastroenterol Hepatol* 2009;**6**:331.

159. Park do Y, Lauwers GY. Gastric polyps: classification and management. *Arch Pathol Lab Med* 2008;**132**:633.

160. Carneiro F, David L, Seruca R, Castedo S, Nesland JM, Sobrinho-Simoes M. Hyperplastic polyposis and diffuse carcinoma of the stomach. A study of a family. *Cancer* 1993;**72**:323.

161. Orlowska J, Jarosz D, Pachlewski J, Butruk E. Malignant transformation of benign epithelial gastric polyps. *Am J Gastroenterol* 1995;**90**:2152.

162. Carneiro F, Sobrinho-Simoes M. Signet ring cell carcinoma in hyperplastic polyp. *Scand J Gastroenterol* 1996;**31**:95.

163. Zea-Iriarte WL, Sekine I, Itsuno M, et al. Carcinoma in gastric hyperplastic polyps. A phenotypic study. *Dig Dis Sci* 1996;**41**:377.

164. Stolte M. Hyperplastic polyps of the stomach: associations with histologic patterns of gastritis and gastric atrophy. *Am J Surg Pathol* 2001;**25**:1342.

165. Daibo M, Itabashi M, Hirota T. Malignant transformation of gastric hyperplastic polyps. *Am J Gastroenterol* 1987;**82**:1016.

166. Tsuchikame N, Ishimaru Y, Ohshima S, Takahashi M. Three familial cases of fundic gland polyposis without polyposis coli. *Virchows Arch A Pathol Anat Histopathol* 1993;**422**:337.

167. Fossmark R, Jianu CS, Martinsen TC, Qvigstad G, Syversen U, Waldum HL. Serum gastrin and chromogranin A levels in patients with fundic gland polyps caused by long-term proton-pump inhibition. *Scand J Gastroenterol* 2008;**43**:20.

168. Ally MR, Veerappan GR, Maydonovitch CL, et al. Chronic proton pump inhibitor therapy associated with increased development of fundic gland polyps. *Dig Dis Sci* 2009;**54**:2617.

169. Jalving M, Koornstra JJ, Gotz JM, et al. High-grade dysplasia in sporadic fundic gland polyps: a case report and review of the literature. *Eur J Gastroenterol Hepatol* 2003;**15**:1229.

170. Stolte M, Vieth M, Ebert MP. High-grade dysplasia in sporadic fundic gland polyps: clinically relevant or not? *Eur J Gastroenterol Hepatol* 2003;**15**:1153.

171. Attard TM, Giardiello FM, Argani P, Cuffari C. Fundic gland polyposis with high-grade dysplasia in a child with attenuated familial adenomatous polyposis and familial gastric cancer. *J Pediatr Gastroenterol Nutr* 2001;**32**:215.

172. Abraham SC, Park SJ, Mugartegui L, Hamilton SR, Wu TT. Sporadic fundic gland polyps with epithelial dysplasia : evidence for preferential targeting for mutations in the adenomatous polyposis coli gene. *Am J Pathol* 2002;**161**:1735.

173. Viste A, Bjornestad E, Opheim P, et al. Risk of carcinoma following gastric operations for benign disease. A historical cohort study of 3470 patients. *Lancet* 1986;**2**:502.

174. Offerhaus GJ, Tersmette AC, Huibregtse K, et al. Mortality caused by stomach cancer after remote partial gastrectomy for benign conditions: 40 years of follow up of an Amsterdam cohort of 2633 postgastrectomy patients. *Gut* 1988;**29**:1588.

175. Caygill CP, Hill MJ, Hall CN, Kirkham JS, Northfield TC. Increased risk of cancer at multiple sites after gastric surgery for peptic ulcer. *Gut* 1987;**28**:924.

176. Toftgaard C. Gastric cancer after peptic ulcer surgery. A historic prospective cohort investigation. *Ann Surg* 1989;**210**:159.

177. Safatle-Ribeiro AV, Ribeiro U Jr, Reynolds JC. Gastric stump cancer: what is the risk? *Dig Dis* 1998;**16**:159.

178. La Vecchia C, Negri E, D'Avanzo B, Moller H, Franceschi S. Partial gastrectomy and subsequent gastric cancer risk. *J Epidemiol Community Health* 1992;**46**:12.

214 | Stomach

179. Tersmette AC, Offerhaus GJ, Tersmette KW, et al. Meta-analysis of the risk of gastric stump cancer: detection of high risk patient subsets for stomach cancer after remote partial gastrectomy for benign conditions. *Cancer Res* 1990;**50**:6486.

180. Dixon MF, O'Connor HJ, Axon AT, King RF, Johnston D. Reflux gastritis: distinct histopathological entity? *J Clin Pathol* 1986;**39**:524.

181. Sobala GM, O'Connor HJ, Dewar EP, King RF, Axon AT, Dixon MF. Bile reflux and intestinal metaplasia in gastric mucosa. *J Clin Pathol* 1993;**46**:235.

182. Kaminishi M, Shimizu N, Yamaguchi H, Hashimoto M, Sakai S, Oohara T. Different carcinogenesis in the gastric remnant after gastrectomy for gastric cancer. *Cancer* 1996;**77**:1646.

183. Offerhaus GJ, van de Stadt J, Huibregtse K, Tersmette AC, Tytgat GN. The mucosa of the gastric remnant harboring malignancy. Histologic findings in the biopsy specimens of 504 asymptomatic patients 15 to 46 years after partial gastrectomy with emphasis on nonmalignant lesions. *Cancer* 1989;**64**:698.

184. Stael von Holstein C, Hammar E, Eriksson S, Huldt B. Clinical significance of dysplasia in gastric remnant biopsy specimens. *Cancer* 1993;**72**:1532.

185. Stemmermann GN, Hayashi T. Hyperplastic polyps of the gastric mucosa adjacent to gastroenterostomy stomas. *Am J Clin Pathol* 1979;**71**:341.

186. Scharschmidt BF. The natural history of hypertrophic gastrophy (Menetrier's disease). Report of a case with 16 year follow-up and review of 120 cases from the literature. *Am J Med* 1977;**63**:644.

187. Wood MG, Bates C, Brown RC, Losowsky MS. Intramucosal carcinoma of the gastric antrum complicating Menetrier's disease. *J Clin Pathol* 1983;**36**:1071.

188. Meuwissen SG, Ridwan BU, Hasper HJ, Innemee G. Hypertrophic protein-losing gastropathy. A retrospective analysis of 40 cases in The Netherlands. The Dutch Menetrier Study Group. *Scand J Gastroenterol Suppl* 1992;**194**:1.

189. Johnson MI, Spark JI, Ambrose NS, Wyatt JI. Early gastric cancer in a patient with Menetrier's disease, lymphocytic gastritis and *Helicobacter pylori*. *Eur J Gastroenterol Hepatol* 1995;**7**:187.

190. Hole DJ, Quigley EM, Gillis CR, Watkinson G. Peptic ulcer and cancer: an examination of the relationship between chronic peptic ulcer and gastric carcinoma. *Scand J Gastroenterol* 1987;**22**:17.

191. Hansson LE, Nyren O, Hsing AW, et al. The risk of stomach cancer in patients with gastric or duodenal ulcer disease. *N Engl J Med* 1996;**335**:242.

192. Wu CY, Kuo KN, Wu MS, Chen YJ, Wang CB, Lin JT. Early *Helicobacter pylori* eradication decreases risk of gastric cancer in patients with peptic ulcer disease. *Gastroenterology* 2009;**137**:1641.

193. La Vecchia C, Negri E, Franceschi S, Gentile A. Family history and the risk of stomach and colorectal cancer. *Cancer* 1992;**70**:50.

194. Saadat M. Genetic polymorphisms of glutathione S-transferase T1 (GSTT1) and susceptibility to gastric cancer: a meta-analysis. *Cancer Sci* 2006;**97**:505.

195. Wideroff L, Vaughan TL, Farin FM, et al. GST, NAT1, CYP1A1 polymorphisms and risk of esophageal and gastric adenocarcinomas. *Cancer Detect Prev* 2007;**31**:233.

196. Palli D, Galli M, Caporaso NE, et al. Family history and risk of stomach cancer in Italy. *Cancer Epidemiol Biomarkers Prev* 1994;**3**:15.

197. Fitzgerald RC, Caldas C. Familial gastric cancer – clinical management. *Best Pract Res Clin Gastroenterol* 2006;**20**:735.

198. Oliveira C, Seruca R, Carneiro F. Hereditary gastric cancer. *Best Pract Res Clin Gastroenterol* 2009;**23**:147.

199. McClave SA, Boyce HW, Jr., Gottfried MR. Early diagnosis of columnar-lined esophagus: a new endoscopic diagnostic criterion. *Gastrointest Endosc* 1987;**33**:413.

200. Choi DW, Oh SN, Baek SJ, et al. Endoscopically observed lower esophageal capillary patterns. *Korean J Intern Med* 2002;**17**:245.

201. Nakanishi Y, Saka M, Eguchi T, Sekine S, Taniguchi H, Shimoda T. Distribution and significance of the oesophageal and gastric cardiac mucosae: a study of 131 operation specimens. *Histopathology* 2007;**51**:515.

202. Vianna A, Hayes PC, Moscoso G, et al. Normal venous circulation of the gastroesophageal junction. A route to understanding varices. *Gastroenterology* 1987;**93**:876.

203. Chandrasoma PT, Der R, Ma Y, Dalton P, Taira M. Histology of the gastroesophageal junction: an autopsy study. *Am J Surg Pathol* 2000;**24**:402.

204. Chandrasoma PT, Der R, Ma Y, Peters J, Demeester T. Histologic classification of patients based on mapping biopsies of the gastroesophageal junction. *Am J Surg Pathol* 2003;**27**:929.

205. Chandrasoma P. Controversies of the cardiac mucosa and Barrett's oesophagus. *Histopathology* 2005;**46**:361.

206. Odze RD. Pathology of the gastroesophageal junction. *Semin Diagn Pathol* 2005;**22**:256.

207. Kalish RJ, Clancy PE, Orringer MB, Appelman HD. Clinical, epidemiologic, and morphologic comparison between adenocarcinomas arising in Barrett's esophageal mucosa and in the gastric cardia. *Gastroenterology* 1984;**86**:461.

208. Siewert JR, Stein HJ. Classification of adenocarcinoma of the oesophagogastric junction. *Br J Surg* 1998;**85**:1457.

209. Odze RD, Fléjou J-F, Boffetta P, Höfler H, Montgomery E, Spechler SJ. Tumours of the oesophagogastric junction. In: Bosman FT, Carneiro F, Hruban RH, Theise ND (eds), *WHO Classification of Tumours of the Digestive System*. Lyon: IARC Press, 2010: 40.

210. Huang Q, Shi J, Feng A, et al. Gastric cardiac carcinomas involving the esophagus are more adequately staged as gastric cancers by the 7th edition of the American Joint Commission on Cancer Staging System. *Mod Pathol* 2011;**24**:138.

211. Borrmann R. Geshwuelste des Magens und Duodenum. In: Henke F, Lubarsch O (eds), *Handbuch des speziellen Pathologischen Anatomie und Histologie*, vol 4. Berlin: Springer-Verlag, 1926: 865.

212. Dekker W, Tytgat GN. Diagnostic accuracy of fiberendoscopy in the detection of upper intestinal malignancy. A follow-up analysis. *Gastroenterology* 1977;**73**:710.

213. Lauwers GY, Carneiro F, Graham DY, et al. Gastric carcinoma. In: Bosman FT, Carneiro F, Hruban RH, Theise ND (eds), *Classification of Tumours of the Digestive System*. Lyon: IARC Press, 2010: 48.

214. Endoh Y, Tamura G, Motoyama T, Ajioka Y, Watanabe H. Well-differentiated adenocarcinoma mimicking complete-type intestinal metaplasia in the stomach. *Hum Pathol* 1999;**30**:826.

215. Yao T, Utsunomiya T, Oya M, Nishiyama K, Tsuneyoshi M. Extremely well-differentiated adenocarcinoma of the stomach: clinicopathological and immunohistochemical features. *World J Gastroenterol* 2006;**12**:2510.

216. Wang HH, Antonioli DA, Goldman H. Comparative features of esophageal and gastric adenocarcinomas: recent changes in type and frequency. *Hum Pathol* 1986;**17**:482.

217. Gupta R, Arora R, Das P, Singh MK. Deeply eosinophilic cell variant of signet-ring type of gastric carcinoma: a diagnostic dilemma. *Int J Clin Oncol* 2008;**13**:181.

218. Carvalho B, Buffart TE, Reis RM, et al. Mixed gastric carcinomas show similar chromosomal aberrations in both their diffuse and glandular components. *Cell Oncol* 2006;**28**:283.

219. Zheng HC, Li XH, Hara T, et al. Mixed-type gastric carcinomas exhibit more aggressive features and indicate the histogenesis of carcinomas. *Virchows Arch* 2008;**452**:525.

220. Machado JC, Soares P, Carneiro F, et al. E-cadherin gene mutations provide a genetic basis for the phenotypic divergence of mixed gastric carcinomas. *Lab Invest* 1999;**79**:459.

221. Park SY, Kook MC, Kim YW, Cho NY, Kim TY, Kang GH. Mixed-type gastric cancer and its association with high-frequency CpG island hypermethylation. *Virchows Arch* 2010;**456**:625.

222. Lauren P. The two histological main types of gastric carcinoma: diffuse and so-called intestinal-type carcinoma. an attempt at a histo-clinical classification. *Acta Pathol Microbiol Scand* 1965;**64**:31.

223. Mulligan RM. Histogenesis and biologic behavior of gastric carcinoma. *Pathol Annu* 1972;**7**:349.

224. Ming SC. Gastric carcinoma. A pathobiological classification. *Cancer* 1977;**39**:2475.

225. Goseki N, Takizawa T, Koike M. Differences in the mode of the extension of gastric cancer classified by histological type: new histological classification of gastric carcinoma. *Gut* 1992;**33**:606.

226. Martin IG, Dixon MF, Sue-Ling H, Axon AT, Johnston D. Goseki histological grading of gastric cancer is an important predictor of outcome. *Gut* 1994;**35**:758.

227. Carneiro F. Classification of gastric carcinoma. *Curr Diag Pathol* 1997;**4**:5.

228. Carneiro F, Seixas M, Sobrinho-Simoes M. New elements for an updated classification of the carcinomas of the stomach. *Pathol Res Pract* 1995;**191**:571.

229. Stelzner S, Emmrich P. The mixed type in Lauren's classification of gastric carcinoma. Histologic description and biologic behavior. *Gen Diagn Pathol* 1997;**143**:39.

230. Fiocca R, Villani L, Tenti P, et al. Characterization of four main cell types in gastric cancer: foveolar, mucopeptic, intestinal columnar and goblet cells. An histopathologic, histochemical and ultrastructural study of 'early' and 'advanced' tumours. *Pathol Res Pract* 1987;**182**:308.

231. Machado JC, Carneiro F, Ribeiro P, Blin N, Sobrinho-Simoes M. pS2 protein expression in gastric carcinoma. An immunohistochemical and immunoradiometric study. *Eur J Cancer* 1996;**32A**:1585.

232. Machado JC, Nogueira AM, Carneiro F, Reis CA, Sobrinho-Simoes M. Gastric carcinoma exhibits distinct types of cell differentiation: an immunohistochemical study of trefoil peptides (TFF1 and TFF2) and mucins (MUC1, MUC2, MUC5AC, and MUC6). *J Pathol* 2000;**190**:437.

233. Kushima R, Vieth M, Borchard F, Stolte M, Mukaisho K, Hattori T. Gastric-type well-differentiated adenocarcinoma and pyloric gland adenoma of the stomach. *Gastric Cancer* 2006;**9**:177.

234. Kushima R, Hattori T. Histogenesis and characteristics of gastric-type adenocarcinomas in the stomach. *J Cancer Res Clin Oncol* 1993;**120**:103.

235. Tsukashita S, Kushima R, Bamba M, Sugihara H, Hattori T. MUC gene expression and histogenesis of adenocarcinoma of the stomach. *Int J Cancer* 2001;**94**:166.

236. Shiroshita H, Watanabe H, Ajioka Y, Watanabe G, Nishikura K, Kitano S. Re-evaluation of mucin phenotypes of gastric minute well-differentiated-type adenocarcinomas using a series of HGM, MUC5AC, MUC6, M-GGMC, MUC2 and CD10 stains. *Pathol Int* 2004;**54**:311.

237. Wakatsuki K, Yamada Y, Narikiyo M, et al. Clinicopathological and prognostic significance of mucin phenotype in gastric cancer. *J Surg Oncol* 2008;**98**:124.

238. Lee OJ, Kim HJ, Kim JR, Watanabe H. The prognostic significance of the mucin phenotype of gastric adenocarcinoma and its relationship with histologic classifications. *Oncol Rep* 2009;**21**:387.

239. Han HS, Lee SY, Lee KY, et al. Unclassified mucin phenotype of gastric adenocarcinoma exhibits the highest invasiveness. *J Gastroenterol Hepatol* 2009;**24**:658.

240. Shennib H, Lough J, Klein HW, Hampson LG. Gastric carcinoma: intestinal metaplasia and tumor growth patterns as indicators of prognosis. *Surgery* 1986;**100**:774.

241. Roy P, Piard F, Dusserre-Guion L, Martin L, Michiels-Marzais D, Faivre J. Prognostic comparison of the pathological classifications of gastric cancer: a population-based study. *Histopathology* 1998;**33**:304.

242. Songun I, van de Velde CJ, Arends JW, et al. Classification of gastric carcinoma using the Goseki system provides prognostic information additional to TNM staging. *Cancer* 1999;**85**:2114.

243. Mori M, Iwashita A, Enjoji M. Adenosquamous carcinoma of the stomach. A clinicopathologic analysis of 28 cases. *Cancer* 1986;**57**:333.

244. Donald KJ. Adenocarcinoma of the pyloric antrum with extensive squamous differentiation. *J Clin Pathol* 1967;**20**:136.

245. Mori M, Fukuda T, Enjoji M. Adenosquamous carcinoma of the stomach. Histogenetic and ultrastructural studies. *Gastroenterology* 1987;**92**:1078.

246. Yoshida K, Manabe T, Tsunoda T, Kimoto M, Tadaoka Y, Shimizu M. Early gastric cancer of adenosquamous carcinoma type: report of a case and review of literature. *Jpn J Clin Oncol* 1996;**26**:252.

247. Boswell JT, Helwig EB. Squamous cell carcinoma and adenoacanthoma of the stomach. A clinicopathologic study. *Cancer* 1965;**18**:181.

248. Namatame K, Ookubo M, Suzuki K, et al. [A clinicopathological study of five cases of adenosquamous carcinoma of the stomach.] *Gan No Rinsho* 1986;**32**:170.

249. Ikeda E, Shigematsu T, Hidaka K, et al. [A case of adenosquamous gastric carcinoma successfully treated with TS-1, low-dose CDDP and docetaxel as neoadjuvant chemotherapy.] *Gan To Kagaku Ryoho* 2007;**34**:423.

250. Bonnheim DC, Sarac OK, Fett W. Primary squamous cell carcinoma of the stomach. *Am J Gastroenterol* 1985;**80**:91.

251. Marubashi S, Yano H, Monden T, et al. Primary squamous cell carcinoma of the stomach. *Gastric Cancer* 1999;**2**:136.

252. Won OH, Farman J, Krishnan MN, Iyer SK, Vuletin JC. Squamous cell carcinoma of the stomach. *Am J Gastroenterol* 1978;**69**:594.

253. Vaughan WP, Straus FH, 2nd, Paloyan D. Squamous carcinoma of the stomach after luetic linitis plastica. *Gastroenterology* 1977;**72**:945.

254. Eaton H, Tennekoon GE. Squamous carcinoma of the stomach following corrosive acid burns. *Br J Surg* 1972;**59**:382.

255. McLoughlin GA, Cave-Bigley DJ, Tagore V, Kirkham N. Cyclophosphamide and pure squamous-cell carcinoma of the stomach. *Br Med J* 1980;**280**:524.

256. Ishikura H, Kirimoto K, Shamoto M, et al. Hepatoid adenocarcinomas of the stomach. An analysis of seven cases. *Cancer* 1986;**58**:119.

257. Akiyama S, Tamura G, Endoh Y, et al. Histogenesis of hepatoid adenocarcinoma of the stomach: molecular evidence of identical origin with coexistent tubular adenocarcinoma. *Int J Cancer* 2003;**106**:510.

258. Nagai E, Ueyama T, Yao T, Tsuneyoshi M. Hepatoid adenocarcinoma of the stomach. A clinicopathologic and immunohistochemical analysis. *Cancer* 1993;**72**:1827.

259. Chang YC, Nagasue N, Kohno H, et al. Clinicopathologic features and long-term results of alpha-fetoprotein-producing gastric cancer. *Am J Gastroenterol* 1990;**85**:1480.

260. Petrella T, Montagnon J, Roignot P, et al. Alphafetoprotein-producing gastric adenocarcinoma. *Histopathology* 1995;**26**:171.

261. Motoyama T, Aizawa K, Watanabe H, Fukase M, Saito K. alpha-Fetoprotein producing gastric carcinomas: a comparative study of three different subtypes. *Acta Pathol Jpn* 1993;**43**:654.

262. Kumashiro Y, Yao T, Aishima S, et al. Hepatoid adenocarcinoma of the stomach: histogenesis and progression in association with intestinal phenotype. *Hum Pathol* 2007;**38**:857.

263. Ishikura H, Kishimoto T, Andachi H, Kakuta Y, Yoshiki T. Gastrointestinal hepatoid adenocarcinoma: venous permeation and mimicry of hepatocellular carcinoma, a report of four cases. *Histopathology* 1997;**31**:47.

264. Liu X, Cheng Y, Sheng W, et al. Analysis of clinicopathologic features and prognostic factors in hepatoid adenocarcinoma of the stomach. *Am J Surg Pathol* 2010;**34**:1465.

265. Inagawa S, Shimazaki J, Hori M, et al. Hepatoid adenocarcinoma of the stomach. *Gastric Cancer* 2001;**4**:43.

266. Supriatna Y, Kishimoto T, Uno T, Nagai Y, Ishikura H. Evidence for hepatocellular differentiation in alpha-fetoprotein-negative gastric adenocarcinoma with hepatoid morphology: a study with in situ hybridisation for albumin mRNA. *Pathology* 2005;**37**:211.

267. Sentani K, Oue N, Sakamoto N, et al. Gene expression profiling with microarray and SAGE identifies PLUNC as a marker for hepatoid adenocarcinoma of the stomach. *Mod Pathol* 2008; **21**:464.

268. Terracciano LM, Glatz K, Mhawech P, et al. Hepatoid adenocarcinoma with liver metastasis mimicking hepatocellular carcinoma: an immunohistochemical and molecular study of eight cases. *Am J Surg Pathol* 2003;**27**:1302.

269. Wurzel J, Brooks JJ. Primary gastric choriocarcinoma: immunohistochemistry, postmortem documentation, and hormonal effects in a postmenopausal female. *Cancer* 1981;**48**:2756.

270. Kobayashi A, Hasebe T, Endo Y, et al. Primary gastric choriocarcinoma: two case reports and a pooled analysis of 53 cases. *Gastric Cancer* 2005;**8**:178.

271. Imai Y, Kawabe T, Takahashi M, et al. A case of primary gastric choriocarcinoma and a review of the Japanese literature. *J Gastroenterol* 1994;**29**:642.

272. Saigo PE, Brigati DJ, Sternberg SS, Rosen PP, Turnbull AD. Primary gastric choriocarcinoma. An immunohistological study. *Am J Surg Pathol* 1981;**5**:333.

273. Liu AY, Chan WY, Ng EK, et al. Gastric choriocarcinoma shows characteristics of adenocarcinoma and gestational choriocarcinoma: a comparative genomic hybridization and fluorescence in situ hybridization study. *Diagn Mol Pathol* 2001;**10**:161.

274. Smith FR, Barkin JS, Hensley G. Choriocarcinoma of the stomach. *Am J Gastroenterol* 1980;**73**:45.

275. Yonezawa S, Maruyama I, Tanaka S, Nakamura T, Sato E. Immunohistochemical localization of thrombomodulin in chorionic diseases of the uterus and choriocarcinoma of the stomach. A comparative study with the distribution of human chorionic gonadotropin. *Cancer* 1988;**62**:569.

276. Krulewski T, Cohen LB. Choriocarcinoma of the stomach: pathogenesis and clinical characteristics. *Am J Gastroenterol* 1988;**83**:1172.

277. Garcia RL, Ghali VS. Gastric choriocarcinoma and yolk sac tumor in a man: observations about its possible origin. *Hum Pathol* 1985;**16**:955.

278. Jindrak K, Bochetto JF, Alpert LI. Primary gastric choriocarcinoma: case report with review of world literature. *Hum Pathol* 1976;**7**:595.

279. Kanai M, Torii A, Hamada A, et al. Pure gastric yolk sac tumor that was diagnosed after curative resection: case report and review of literature. *Int J Gastrointest Cancer* 2005;**35**:77.

280. Eom BW, Jung SY, Yoon H, et al. Gastric choriocarcinoma admixed with an alpha-fetoprotein-producing adenocarcinoma and separated adenocarcinoma. *World J Gastroenterol* 2009; **15**:5106.

281. Hirano Y, Hara T, Nozawa H, et al. Combined choriocarcinoma, neuroendocrine cell carcinoma and tubular adenocarcinoma in the stomach. *World J Gastroenterol* 2008;**14**:3269.

282. Young LS, Rickinson AB. Epstein-Barr virus: 40 years on. *Nat Rev Cancer* 2004;**4**:757.

283. Minamoto T, Mai M, Watanabe K, et al. Medullary carcinoma with lymphocytic infiltration of the stomach. Clinicopathologic study of 27 cases and immunohistochemical analysis of the subpopulations of infiltrating lymphocytes in the tumor. *Cancer* 1990;**66**:945.

284. Watanabe H, Enjoji M, Imai T. Gastric carcinoma with lymphoid stroma. Its morphologic characteristics and prognostic correlations. *Cancer* 1976;**38**:232.

285. Shibata D, Tokunaga M, Uemura Y, Sato E, Tanaka S, Weiss LM. Association of Epstein–Barr virus with undifferentiated gastric carcinomas with intense lymphoid infiltration. Lymphoepithelioma-like carcinoma. *Am J Pathol* 1991;**139**:469.

286. Wang HH, Wu MS, Shun CT, Wang HP, Lin CC, Lin JT. Lymphoepithelioma-like carcinoma of the stomach: a subset of gastric carcinoma with distinct clinicopathological features and high prevalence of Epstein–Barr virus infection. *Hepatogastroenterology* 1999;**46**:1214.

287. Murphy G, Pfeiffer R, Camargo MC, Rabkin CS. Meta-analysis shows that prevalence of Epstein–Barr virus-positive gastric cancer differs based on sex and anatomic location. *Gastroenterology* 2009;**137**:824.

288. Willems S, Carneiro F, Geboes K. Gastric carcinoma with osteoclast-like giant cells and lymphoepithelioma-like carcinoma of the stomach: two of a kind? *Histopathology* 2005;**47**:331.

289. Lee JH, Kim SH, Han SH, An JS, Lee ES, Kim YS. Clinicopathological and molecular characteristics of Epstein–Barr virus-associated gastric carcinoma: a meta-analysis. *J Gastroenterol Hepatol* 2009;**24**:354.

290. Yamamoto N, Tokunaga M, Uemura Y, et al. Epstein–Barr virus and gastric remnant cancer. *Cancer* 1994;**74**:805.

291. Matsunou H, Konishi F, Hori H, et al. Characteristics of Epstein–Barr virus-associated gastric carcinoma with lymphoid stroma in Japan. *Cancer* 1996;**77**:1998.

292. Fukayama M, Chong JM, Kaizaki Y. Epstein–Barr virus and gastric carcinoma. *Gastric Cancer* 1998;**1**:104.

293. Gulley ML, Pulitzer DR, Eagan PA, Schneider BG. Epstein–Barr virus infection is an early event in gastric carcinogenesis and is independent of bcl-2 expression and p53 accumulation. *Hum Pathol* 1996;**27**:20.

294. Truong CD, Feng W, Li W, et al. Characteristics of Epstein–Barr virus-associated gastric cancer: a study of 235 cases at a comprehensive cancer center in U.S.A. *J Exp Clin Cancer Res* 2009; **28**:14.

295. Fukayama M, Hino R, Uozaki H. Epstein–Barr virus and gastric carcinoma: virus-host interactions leading to carcinoma. *Cancer Sci* 2008;**99**:1726.

296. Chang MS, Kim WH, Kim CW, Kim YI. Epstein–Barr virus in gastric carcinomas with lymphoid stroma. *Histopathology* 2000;**37**:309.

297. Shibata D, Weiss LM. Epstein–Barr virus-associated gastric adenocarcinoma. *Am J Pathol* 1992;**140**:769.

298. Song HJ, Srivastava A, Lee J, et al. Host inflammatory response predicts survival of patients with Epstein–Barr virus-associated gastric carcinoma. *Gastroenterology* 2010;**139**:84.

299. Cho KJ, Myong NH, Choi DW, Jang JJ. Carcinosarcoma of the stomach. A case report with light microscopic, immuno-

histochemical, and electron microscopic study. *APMIS* 1990; **98**:991.

300. Nakayama Y, Murayama H, Iwasaki H, et al. Gastric carcinosarcoma (sarcomatoid carcinoma) with rhabdomyoblastic and osteoblastic differentiation. *Pathol Int* 1997;**47**:557.

301. Sato Y, Shimozono T, Kawano S, et al. Gastric carcinosarcoma, coexistence of adenosquamous carcinoma and rhabdomyosarcoma: a case report. *Histopathology* 2001;**39**:543.

302. Randjelovic T, Filipovic B, Babic D, Cemerikic V. Carcinosarcoma of the stomach: a case report and review of the literature. *World J Gastroenterol* 2007;**13**:5533.

303. Solerio D, Ruffini E, Camandona M, Raggio E, Castellano I, Dei Poli M. Carcinosarcoma of the esophagogastric junction. *Tumori* 2008;**94**:416.

304. Matsukuma S, Wada R, Hase K, Sakai Y, Ogata S, Kuwabara N. Gastric stump carcinosarcoma with rhabdomyosarcomatous differentiation. *Pathol Int* 1997;**47**:73.

305. Tsuneyama K, Sasaki M, Sabit A, et al. A case report of gastric carcinosarcoma with rhabdomyosarcomatous and neuroendocrinal differentiation. *Pathol Res Pract* 1999;**195**:93.

306. Yamazaki K. A gastric carcinosarcoma with neuroendocrine cell differentiation and undifferentiated spindle-shaped sarcoma component possibly progressing from the conventional tubular adenocarcinoma;an immunohistochemical and ultrastructural study. *Virchows Arch* 2003;**442**:77.

307. Teramachi K, Kanomata N, Hasebe T, Ishii G, Sugito M, Ochiai A. Carcinosarcoma (pure endocrine cell carcinoma with sarcoma components) of the stomach. *Pathol Int* 2003;**53**:552.

308. Kuroda N, Oonishi K, Iwamura S, et al. Gastric carcinosarcoma with neuroendocrine differentiation as the carcinoma component and leiomyosarcomatous and myofibroblastic differentiation as the sarcomatous component. *APMIS* 2006;**114**:234.

309. Ikeda Y, Kosugi S, Nishikura K, et al. Gastric carcinosarcoma presenting as a huge epigastric mass. *Gastric Cancer* 2007; **10**:63.

310. Kallakury BV, Bui HX, delRosario A, Wallace J, Solis OG, Ross JS. Primary gastric adenosarcoma. *Arch Pathol Lab Med* 1993; **117**:299.

311. Miettinen M, Dow N, Lasota J, Sobin LH. A distinctive novel epitheliomesenchymal biphasic tumor of the stomach in young adults ('gastroblastoma'): a series of 3 cases. *Am J Surg Pathol* 2009;**33**:1370.

312. Shin DH, Lee JH, Kang HJ, et al. Novel epitheliomesenchymal biphasic stomach tumour (gastroblastoma) in a 9-year-old: morphological, usltrastructural and immunohistochemical findings. *J Clin Pathol* 2010;**63**:270.

313. Eom DW, Kang GH, Han SH, et al. Gastric micropapillary carcinoma: A distinct subtype with a significantly worse prognosis in TNM stages I and II. *Am J Surg Pathol* 2011;**35**:84.

314. Roh JH, Srivastava A, Lauwers GY, et al. Micropapillary carcinoma of stomach: a clinicopathologic and immunohistochemical study of 11 cases. *Am J Surg Pathol* 2010;**34**:1139.

315. Capella C, Frigerio B, Cornaggia M, Solcia E, Pinzon-Trujillo Y, Chejfec G. Gastric parietal cell carcinoma – a newly recognized entity: light microscopic and ultrastructural features. *Histopathology* 1984;**8**:813.

316. Byrne D, Holley MP, Cuschieri A. Parietal cell carcinoma of the stomach: association with long-term survival after curative resection. *Br J Cancer* 1988;**58**:85.

317. Yang GY, Liao J, Cassai ND, Smolka AJ, Sidhu GS. Parietal cell carcinoma of gastric cardia: immunophenotype and ultrastructure. *Ultrastruct Pathol* 2003;**27**:87.

318. Caruso RA, Fabiano V, Rigoli L, Inferrera A. Focal parietal cell differentiation in a well-differentiated (intestinal-type) early gastric cancer. *Ultrastruct Pathol* 2000;**24**:417.

319. Takubo K, Honma N, Sawabe M, et al. Oncocytic adenocarcinoma of the stomach: parietal cell carcinoma. *Am J Surg Pathol* 2002;**26**:458.

320. Hayashi I, Muto Y, Fujii Y, Morimatsu M. Mucoepidermoid carcinoma of the stomach. *J Surg Oncol* 1987;**34**:94.

321. Kazzaz BA, Eulderink F. Paneth cell-rich carcinoma of the stomach. *Histopathology* 1989;**15**:303.

322. Ooi A, Nakanishi I, Itoh T, Ueda H, Mai M. Predominant Paneth cell differentiation in an intestinal type gastric cancer. *Pathol Res Pract* 1991;**187**:220.

323. Lev R, DeNucci TD. Neoplastic Paneth cells in the stomach. Report of two cases and review of the literature. *Arch Pathol Lab Med* 1989;**113**:129.

324. Caruso RA, Famulari C. Neoplastic Paneth cells in adenocarcinoma of the stomach: a case report. *Hepatogastroenterology* 1992;**39**:264.

325. Ueyama T, Nagai E, Yao T, Tsuneyoshi M. Vimentin-positive gastric carcinomas with rhabdoid features. A clinicopathologic and immunohistochemical study. *Am J Surg Pathol* 1993;**17**:813.

326. Pinto JA, Gonzalez Alfonso JE, Gonzalez L, Stevenson N. Well differentiated gastric adenocarcinoma with rhabdoid areas: a case report with immunohistochemical analysis. *Pathol Res Pract* 1997;**193**:801.

327. Rivera-Hueto F, Rios-Martin JJ, Dominguez-Triano R, Herrerias-Gutierrez JM. Early gastric stump carcinoma with rhabdoid features. Case report. *Pathol Res Pract* 1999;**195**:841.

328. Murakami T, ed. Pathomorphological diagnosis: definition and growth classification of early gastric cancer. In: *Gann Monograph on Cancer Research II*. Tokyo: University of Tokyo Press, 1971: 53.

329. Tsukuma H, Mishima T, Oshima A. Prospective study of 'early' gastric cancer. *Int J Cancer* 1983;**31**:421.

330. Ohta H, Noguchi Y, Takagi K, Nishi M, Kajitani T, Kato Y. Early gastric carcinoma with special reference to macroscopic classification. *Cancer* 1987;**60**:1099.

331. Hisamichi S, Sugawara N. Mass screening for gastric cancer by X-ray examination. *Jpn J Clin Oncol* 1984;**14**:211.

332. Green PH, O'Toole KM, Weinberg LM, Goldfarb JP. Early gastric cancer. *Gastroenterology* 1981;**81**:247.

333. Carter KJ, Schaffer HA, Ritchie WP Jr. Early gastric cancer. *Ann Surg* 1984;**199**:604.

334. Grigioni WF, D'Errico A, Milani M, et al. Early gastric cancer. Clinico-pathological analysis of 125 cases of early gastric cancer (EGC). *Acta Pathol Jpn* 1984;**34**:979.

335. Ming SC. Malignant epithelial tumors of the stomach In: Ming SC, Goldman H (eds), *Pathology of the Gastrointestinal Tract*, 2nd edn. Baltimore, MA: Williams & Wilkins, 1998.

336. Oohara T, Tohma H, Takezoe K, et al. Minute gastric cancers less than 5 mm in diameter. *Cancer* 1982;**50**:801.

337. Kodama Y, Inokuchi K, Soejima K, Matsusaka T, Okamura T. Growth patterns and prognosis in early gastric carcinoma. Superficially spreading and penetrating growth types. *Cancer* 1983;**51**:320.

338. Lewin KJ, Appelman HD. Tumors of the esophagus and stomach. In: *Atlas of Tumour Pathology*, Fascicle 18. Washington: AFIP, 1996: 282.

339. Xuan ZX, Ueyama T, Yao T, Tsuneyoshi M. Time trends of early gastric carcinoma. A clinicopathologic analysis of 2846 cases. *Cancer* 1993;**72**:2889.

340. Everett SM, Axon AT. Early gastric cancer in Europe. *Gut* 1997; **41**:142.

341. Yamashina M. A variant of early gastric carcinoma. Histologic and histochemical studies of early signet ring cell carcinomas discovered beneath preserved surface epithelium. *Cancer* 1986; **58**:1333.

342. Johansen A. Elevated early gastric carcinoma. Differential diagnosis as regards adenomatous polyps. *Pathol Res Pract* 1979; **164**:316.

343. Yasuda K, Shiraishi N, Suematsu T, Yamaguchi K, Adachi Y, Kitano S. Rate of detection of lymph node metastasis is correlated with the depth of submucosal invasion in early stage gastric carcinoma. *Cancer* 1999;**85**:2119.

344. Fukutomi H, Sakita T. Analysis of early gastric cancer cases collected from major hospitals and institutes in Japan. *Jpn J Clin Oncol* 1984;**14**:169.

345. Kurihara N, Kubota T, Otani Y, et al. Lymph node metastasis of early gastric cancer with submucosal invasion. *Br J Surg* 1998;**85**:835.

346. Ishigami S, Hokita S, Natsugoe S, et al. Carcinomatous infiltration into the submucosa as a predictor of lymph node involvement in early gastric cancer. *World J Surg* 1998;**22**:1056.

347. Ono H, Kondo H, Gotoda T, et al. Endoscopic mucosal resection for treatment of early gastric cancer. *Gut* 2001;**48**:225.

348. Gotoda T, Yanagisawa A, Sasako M, et al. Incidence of lymph node metastasis from early gastric cancer: estimation with a large number of cases at two large centers. *Gastric Cancer* 2000;**3**:219.

349. Kang HJ, Kim DH, Jeon TY, et al. Lymph node metastasis from intestinal-type early gastric cancer: experience in a single institution and reassessment of the extended criteria for endoscopic submucosal dissection. *Gastrointest Endosc* 2010;**72**:508.

350. Zinninger MM, Collins WT. Extension of carcinoma of the stomach into the duodenum and esophagus. *Ann Surg* 1949; **130**:557.

351. Fernet P, Azar HA, Stout AP. Intramural (tubal) spread of linitis plastica along the alimentary tract. *Gastroenterology* 1965; **48**:419.

352. Maruyama K, Gunven P, Okabayashi K, Sasako M, Kinoshita T. Lymph node metastases of gastric cancer. General pattern in 1931 patients. *Ann Surg* 1989;**210**:596.

353. Ahn HS, Lee HJ, Hahn S, et al. Evaluation of the Seventh American Joint Committee on Cancer/International Union Against Cancer Classification of gastric adenocarcinoma in comparison with the sixth classification. *Cancer* 2010;**116**: 5592.

354. Maduekwe UN, Lauwers GY, Fernandez-Del-Castillo C, et al. New metastatic lymph node ratio system reduces stage migration in patients undergoing D1 lymphadenectomy for gastric adenocarcinoma. *Ann Surg Oncol* 2010;**17**:1267.

355. Duarte I, Llanos O. Patterns of metastases in intestinal and diffuse types of carcinoma of the stomach. *Hum Pathol* 1981; **12**:237.

356. Esaki Y, Hirayama R, Hirokawa K. A comparison of patterns of metastasis in gastric cancer by histologic type and age. *Cancer* 1990;**65**:2086.

357. Mori M, Sakaguchi H, Akazawa K, Tsuneyoshi M, Sueishi K, Sugimachi K. Correlation between metastatic site, histological type, and serum tumor markers of gastric carcinoma. *Hum Pathol* 1995;**26**:504.

358. McCluggage WG, Young RH. Primary ovarian mucinous tumors with signet ring cells: report of 3 cases with discussion of so-called primary Krukenberg tumor. *Am J Surg Pathol* 2008; **32**:1373.

359. Edge SB, Byrd DR, Compton CC, Fritz AG, Greene FL, Trotti A. *AJCC Cancer Staging Manual*. New York: Springer, 2009.

360. Sobin LH, Gospodarowicz MK, Wittekind C. *TNM Classification of Malignant Tumours*. Oxford: Wiley-Blackwell, 2009.

361. Ishigami S, Natsugoe S, Miyazono F, et al. Clinical merit of subdividing gastric cancer according to invasion of the muscularis propria. *Hepatogastroenterology* 2004;**51**:869.

362. Yoshikawa K, Maruyama K. Characteristics of gastric cancer invading to the proper muscle layer – with special reference to mortality and cause of death. *Jpn J Clin Oncol* 1985;**15**:499.

363. Harrison JC, Dean PJ, Vander Zwaag R, el-Zeky F, Wruble LD. Adenocarcinoma of the stomach with invasion limited to the muscularis propria. *Hum Pathol* 1991;**22**:111.

364. Hundahl SA, Phillips JL, Menck HR. The National Cancer Data Base Report on poor survival of U.S. gastric carcinoma patients treated with gastrectomy: Fifth Edition American Joint Committee on Cancer staging, proximal disease, and the 'different disease' hypothesis. *Cancer* 2000;**88**:921.

365. Reid-Lombardo KM, Gay G, Patel-Parekh L, Ajani JA, Donohue JH. Treatment of gastric adenocarcinoma may differ among hospital types in the United States, a report from theNational Cancer Data Base. *J Gastrointest Surg* 2007;**11**:410.

366. Noguchi Y, Yoshikawa T, Tsuburaya A, Motohashi H, Karpeh MS, Brennan MF. Is gastric carcinoma different between Japan and the United States? *Cancer* 2000;**89**:2237.

367. Fielding JW, Roginski C, Ellis DJ, et al. Clinicopathological staging of gastric cancer. *Br J Surg* 1984;**71**:677.

368. Roder JD, Bottcher K, Busch R, Wittekind C, Hermanek P, Siewert JR, German Gastric Cancer Study Group. Classification of regional lymph node metastasis from gastric carcinoma. *Cancer* 1998;**82**:621.

369. Kappas AM, Fatouros M, Roukos DH. Is it time to change surgical strategy for gastric cancer in the United States? *Ann Surg Oncol* 2004;**11**:727.

370. Bizer LS. Adenocarcinoma of the stomach: current results of treatment. *Cancer* 1983;**51**:743.

371. Siewert JR, Bottcher K, Stein HJ, Roder JD. Relevant prognostic factors in gastric cancer: ten-year results of the German Gastric Cancer Study. *Ann Surg* 1998;**228**:449.

372. Wanebo HJ, Kennedy BJ, Chmiel J, Steele G Jr, Winchester D, Osteen R. Cancer of the stomach. A patient care study by the American College of Surgeons. *Ann Surg* 1993;**218**:583.

373. Karpeh MS, Leon L, Klimstra D, Brennan MF. Lymph node staging in gastric cancer: is location more important than Number? An analysis of 1,038 patients. *Ann Surg* 2000;**232**:362.

374. Landry J, Tepper JE, Wood WC, Moulton EO, Koerner F, Sullinger J. Patterns of failure following curative resection of gastric carcinoma. *Int J Radiat Oncol Biol Phys* 1990;**19**:1357.

375. Cunningham SC, Kamangar F, Kim MP, et al. Survival after gastric adenocarcinoma resection: eighteen-year experience at a single institution. *J Gastrointest Surg* 2005;**9**:718.

376. Saito H, Fukumoto Y, Osaki T, et al. Distinct recurrence pattern and outcome of adenocarcinoma of the gastric cardia in comparison with carcinoma of other regions of the stomach. *World J Surg* 2006;**30**:1864.

377. Chiaravalli AM, Klersy C, Tava F, et al. Lower- and higher-grade subtypes of diffuse gastric cancer. *Hum Pathol* 2009; **40**:1591.

378. Radi MJ, Fenoglio-Preiser CM, Bartow SA, Key CR, Pathak DR. Gastric carcinoma in the young: a clinicopathological and immunohistochemical study. *Am J Gastroenterol* 1986;**81**:747.

379. Umeyama K, Sowa M, Kamino K, Kato Y, Satake K. Gastric carcinoma in young adults in Japan. *Anticancer Res* 1982;**2**:283.

380. Vasen HF, Stormorken A, Menko FH, et al. MSH2 mutation carriers are at higher risk of cancer than MLH1 mutation carriers: a study of hereditary nonpolyposis colorectal cancer families. *J Clin Oncol* 2001;**19**:4074.

381. Capelle LG, Van Grieken NC, Lingsma HF, et al. Risk and epidemiological time trends of gastric cancer in Lynch syndrome carriers in the Netherlands. *Gastroenterology* 2010;**138**:487.

382. Lynch HT, Lynch PM, Lanspa SJ, Snyder CL, Lynch JF, Boland CR. Review of the Lynch syndrome: history, molecular genet-

ics, screening, differential diagnosis, and medicolegal ramifications. *Clin Genet* 2009;**76**:1.

383. Jagelman DG, DeCosse JJ, Bussey HJ. Upper gastrointestinal cancer in familial adenomatous polyposis. *Lancet* 1988;**1**:1149.

384. Park JG, Park KJ, Ahn YO, et al. Risk of gastric cancer among Korean familial adenomatous polyposis patients. Report of three cases. *Dis Colon Rectum* 1992;**35**:996.

385. Aarnio M, Salovaara R, Aaltonen LA, Mecklin JP, Jarvinen HJ. Features of gastric cancer in hereditary non-polyposis colorectal cancer syndrome. *Int J Cancer* 1997;**74**:551.

386. Varley JM, McGown G, Thorncroft M, et al. An extended Li–Fraumeni kindred with gastric carcinoma and a codon 175 mutation in TP53. *J Med Genet* 1995;**32**:942.

387. Shinmura K, Goto M, Tao H, et al. A novel STK11 germline mutation in two siblings with Peutz–Jeghers syndrome complicated by primary gastric cancer. *Clin Genet* 2005;**67**:81.

388. Takahashi M, Sakayori M, Takahashi S, et al. A novel germline mutation of the LKB1 gene in a patient with Peutz-Jeghers syndrome with early-onset gastric cancer. *J Gastroenterol* 2004;**39**:1210.

389. Seruca R, Carneiro F, Castedo S, David L, Lopes C, Sobrinho-Simoes M. Familial gastric polyposis revisited. Autosomal dominant inheritance confirmed. *Cancer Genet Cytogenet* 1991;**53**:97.

390. Guilford P, Hopkins J, Harraway J, et al. E-cadherin germline mutations in familial gastric cancer. *Nature* 1998;**392**:402.

391. Caldas C, Carneiro F, Lynch HT, et al. Familial gastric cancer: overview and guidelines for management. *J Med Genet* 1999;**36**:873.

392. Keller G, Vogelsang H, Becker I, et al. Diffuse type gastric and lobular breast carcinoma in a familial gastric cancer patient with an E-cadherin germline mutation. *Am J Pathol* 1999;**155**:337.

393. Brooks-Wilson AR, Kaurah P, Suriano G, et al. Germline E-cadherin mutations in hereditary diffuse gastric cancer: assessment of 42 new families and review of genetic screening criteria. *J Med Genet* 2004;**41**:508.

394. Suriano G, Yew S, Ferreira P, et al. Characterization of a recurrent germ line mutation of the E-cadherin gene: implications for genetic testing and clinical management. *Clin Cancer Res* 2005;**11**:5401.

395. Kaurah P, MacMillan A, Boyd N, et al. Founder and recurrent CDH1 mutations in families with hereditary diffuse gastric cancer. *JAMA* 2007;**297**:2360.

396. Schrader KA, Masciari S, Boyd N, et al. Hereditary diffuse gastric cancer: association with lobular breast cancer. *Fam Cancer* 2008;**7**:73.

397. Fitzgerald RC, Hardwick R, Huntsman D, et al. Hereditary diffuse gastric cancer: updated consensus guidelines for clinical management and directions for future research. *J Med Genet* 2010;**47**:436.

398. Guilford PJ, Hopkins JB, Grady WM, et al. E-cadherin germline mutations define an inherited cancer syndrome dominated by diffuse gastric cancer. *Hum Mutat* 1999;**14**:249.

399. Oliveira C, Senz J, Kaurah P, et al. Germline CDH1 deletions in hereditary diffuse gastric cancer families. *Hum Mol Genet* 2009;**18**:1545.

400. Blair V, Martin I, Shaw D, et al. Hereditary diffuse gastric cancer: diagnosis and management. *Clin Gastroenterol Hepatol* 2006;**4**:262.

401. Carneiro F, Oliveira C, Suriano G, Seruca R. Molecular pathology of familial gastric cancer, with an emphasis on hereditary diffuse gastric cancer. *J Clin Pathol* 2008;**61**:25.

402. Grady WM, Willis J, Guilford PJ, et al. Methylation of the CDH1 promoter as the second genetic hit in hereditary diffuse gastric cancer. *Nat Genet* 2000;**26**:16.

403. Oliveira C, Sousa S, Pinheiro H, et al. Quantification of epigenetic and genetic 2nd hits in CDH1 during hereditary diffuse gastric cancer syndrome progression. *Gastroenterology* 2009;**136**:2137.

404. Barber M, Murrell A, Ito Y, et al. Mechanisms and sequelae of E-cadherin silencing in hereditary diffuse gastric cancer. *J Pathol* 2008;**216**:295.

405. Oliveira C, de Bruin J, Nabais S, et al. Intragenic deletion of CDH1 as the inactivating mechanism of the wild-type allele in an HDGC tumour. *Oncogene* 2004;**23**:2236.

406. Humar B, Fukuzawa R, Blair V, et al. Destabilized adhesion in the gastric proliferative zone and c-Src kinase activation mark the development of early diffuse gastric cancer. *Cancer Res* 2007;**67**:2480.

407. Oliveira C, Ferreira P, Nabais S, et al. E-Cadherin (CDH1) and p53 rather than SMAD4 and Caspase-10 germline mutations contribute to genetic predisposition in Portuguese gastric cancer patients. *Eur J Cancer* 2004;**40**:1897.

408. Keller G, Vogelsang H, Becker I, et al. Germline mutations of the E-cadherin(CDH1) and TP53 genes, rather than of RUNX3 and HPP1, contribute to genetic predisposition in German gastric cancer patients. *J Med Genet* 2004;**41**:e89.

409. Shaw D, Blair V, Framp A, et al. Chromoendoscopic surveillance in hereditary diffuse gastric cancer: an alternative to prophylactic gastrectomy? *Gut* 2005;**54**:461.

410. Richards FM, McKee SA, Rajpar MH, et al. Germline E-cadherin gene (CDH1) mutations predispose to familial gastric cancer and colorectal cancer. *Hum Mol Genet* 1999;**8**:607.

411. Chun YS, Lindor NM, Smyrk TC, et al. Germline E-cadherin gene mutations: is prophylactic total gastrectomy indicated? *Cancer* 2001;**92**:181.

412. Charlton A, Blair V, Shaw D, Parry S, Guilford P, Martin IG. Hereditary diffuse gastric cancer: predominance of multiple foci of signet ring cell carcinoma in distal stomach and transitional zone. *Gut* 2004;**53**:814.

413. Carneiro F, Huntsman DG, Smyrk TC, et al. Model of the early development of diffuse gastric cancer in E-cadherin mutation carriers and its implications for patient screening. *J Pathol* 2004;**203**:681.

414. Barber ME, Save V, Carneiro F, et al. Histopathological and molecular analysis of gastrectomy specimens from hereditary diffuse gastric cancer patients has implications for endoscopic surveillance of individuals at risk. *J Pathol* 2008;**216**:286.

415. Rogers WM, Dobo E, Norton JA, et al. Risk-reducing total gastrectomy for germline mutations in E-cadherin (CDH1): pathologic findings with clinical implications. *Am J Surg Pathol* 2008;**32**:799.

416. Norton JA, Ham CM, Van Dam J, et al. CDH1 truncating mutations in the E-cadherin gene: an indication for total gastrectomy to treat hereditary diffuse gastric cancer. *Ann Surg* 2007;**245**:873.

417. Hebbard PC, Macmillan A, Huntsman D, et al. Prophylactic total gastrectomy (PTG) for hereditary diffuse gastric cancer (HDGC): the Newfoundland experience with 23 patients. *Ann Surg Oncol* 2009;**16**:1890.

418. Worthley DL, Phillips KD, Wayte N, et al. Gastric adenocarcinoma and proximal polyposis of the stomach (GAPPS): a new autosomal dominant syndrome. *Gut* 2012;**61**:774.

419. Hanahan D, Weinberg RA. The hallmarks of cancer. *Cell* 2000;**100**:57.

420. Lengauer C, Kinzler KW, Vogelstein B. Genetic instabilities in human cancers. *Nature* 1998;**396**:643.

421. Ottini L, Falchetti M, Lupi R, et al. Patterns of genomic instability in gastric cancer: clinical implications and perspectives. *Ann Oncol* 2006;**17**(suppl 7):vii97.

422. Carneiro F, Oliveira C, Leite M, Seruca R. Molecular targets and biological modifiers in gastric cancer. *Semin Diagn Pathol* 2008;**25**:274.

423. Pinto M, Wu Y, Mensink RG, Cirnes L, Seruca R, Hofstra RM. Somatic mutations in mismatch repair genes in sporadic gastric carcinomas are not a cause but a consequence of the mutator phenotype. *Cancer Genet Cytogenet* 2008;**180**:110.

424. dos Santos NR, Seruca R, Constancia M, Seixas M, Sobrinho-Simoes M. Microsatellite instability at multiple loci in gastric carcinoma: clinicopathologic implications and prognosis. *Gastroenterology* 1996;**110**:38.

425. Lee HS, Choi SI, Lee HK, et al. Distinct clinical features and outcomes of gastric cancers with microsatellite instability. *Mod Pathol* 2002;**15**:632.

426. Beghelli S, de Manzoni G, Barbi S, et al. Microsatellite instability in gastric cancer is associated with better prognosis in only stage II cancers. *Surgery* 2006;**139**:347.

427. Aguilera A, Gomez-Gonzalez B. Genome instability: a mechanistic view of its causes and consequences. *Nat Rev Genet* 2008;**9**:204.

428. Hartgrink HH, Jansen EP, van Grieken NC, van de Velde CJ. Gastric cancer. *Lancet* 2009;**374**:477.

429. Carvalho B, Pinto M, Cirnes L, et al. Concurrent hypermethylation of gene promoters is associated with a MSI-H phenotype and diploidy in gastric carcinomas. *Eur J Cancer* 2003;**39**:1222.

430. Becker KF, Keller G, Hoefler H. The use of molecular biology in diagnosis and prognosis of gastric cancer. *Surg Oncol* 2000;**9**:5.

431. Hayashi K, Yokozaki H, Goodison S, et al. Inactivation of retinoic acid receptor beta by promoter CpG hypermethylation in gastric cancer. *Differentiation* 2001;**68**:13.

432. Nakase Y, Sakakura C, Miyagawa K, et al. Frequent loss of RUNX3 gene expression in remnant stomach cancer and adjacent mucosa with special reference to topography. *Br J Cancer* 2005;**92**:562.

433. Li QL, Ito K, Sakakura C, et al. Causal relationship between the loss of RUNX3 expression and gastric cancer. *Cell* 2002;**109**:113.

434. Mitani Y, Oue N, Hamai Y, et al. Histone H3 acetylation is associated with reduced p21(WAF1/CIP1) expression by gastric carcinoma. *J Pathol* 2005;**205**:65.

435. Honda T, Tamura G, Waki T, et al. Demethylation of MAGE promoters during gastric cancer progression. *Br J Cancer* 2004;**90**:838.

436. Yanagawa N, Tamura G, Honda T, Endoh M, Nishizuka S, Motoyama T. Demethylation of the synuclein gamma gene CpG island in primary gastric cancers and gastric cancer cell lines. *Clin Cancer Res* 2004;**10**:2447.

437. Nakatsuru S, Yanagisawa A, Ichii S, et al. Somatic mutation of the APC gene in gastric cancer: frequent mutations in very well differentiated adenocarcinoma and signet-ring cell carcinoma. *Hum Mol Genet* 1992;**1**:559.

438. Tamura G, Maesawa C, Suzuki Y, et al. Mutations of the APC gene occur during early stages of gastric adenoma development. *Cancer Res* 1994;**54**:1149.

439. Seruca R, David L, Castedo S, Veiga I, Borresen AL, Sobrinho-Simoes M. p53 alterations in gastric carcinoma: a study of 56 primary tumors and 204 nodal metastases. *Cancer Genet Cytogenet* 1994;**75**:45.

440. Lee JH, Abraham SC, Kim HS, et al. Inverse relationship between APC gene mutation in gastric adenomas and development of adenocarcinoma. *Am J Pathol* 2002;**161**:611.

441. Nishizuka S, Tamura G, Terashima M, Satodate R. Loss of heterozygosity during the development and progression of differentiated adenocarcinoma of the stomach. *J Pathol* 1998;**185**:38.

442. Uchino S, Tsuda H, Noguchi M, et al. Frequent loss of heterozygosity at the DCC locus in gastric cancer. *Cancer Res* 1992;**52**:3099.

443. Becker KF, Atkinson MJ, Reich U, et al. E-cadherin gene mutations provide clues to diffuse type gastric carcinomas. *Cancer Res* 1994;**54**:3845.

444. Jawhari A, Jordan S, Poole S, Browne P, Pignatelli M, Farthing MJ. Abnormal immunoreactivity of the E-cadherin-catenin complex in gastric carcinoma: relationship with patient survival. *Gastroenterology* 1997;**112**:46.

445. Machado JC, Carneiro F, Beck S, et al. E-cadherin expression is correlated with the isolated cell diffuse histotype and with features of biological aggressiveness of gastric carcinoma. *Int J Surg Pathol* 1998;**6**:135.

446. Ascano JJ, Frierson H, Jr., Moskaluk CA, et al. Inactivation of the E-cadherin gene in sporadic diffuse-type gastric cancer. *Mod Pathol* 2001;**14**:942.

447. Machado JC, Oliveira C, Carvalho R, et al. E-cadherin gene (CDH1) promoter methylation as the second hit in sporadic diffuse gastric carcinoma. *Oncogene* 2001;**20**:1525.

448. Chan AO. E-cadherin in gastric cancer. *World J Gastroenterol* 2006;**12**:199.

449. Feakins RM, Nickols CD, Bidd H, Walton SJ. Abnormal expression of pRb, p16, and cyclin D1 in gastric adenocarcinoma and its lymph node metastases: relationship with pathological features and survival. *Hum Pathol* 2003;**34**:1276.

450. Li YL, Tian Z, Wu DY, Fu BY, Xin Y. Loss of heterozygosity on 10q23.3 and mutation of tumor suppressor gene PTEN in gastric cancer and precancerous lesions. *World J Gastroenterol* 2005;**11**:285.

451. Kakeji Y, Korenaga D, Tsujitani S, et al. Gastric cancer with p53 overexpression has high potential for metastasising to lymph nodes. *Br J Cancer* 1993;**67**:589.

452. Yonemura Y, Fushida S, Tsugawa K, et al. Correlation of p53 expression and proliferative activity in gastric cancer. *Anal Cell Pathol* 1993;**5**:277.

453. Ikeguchi M, Saito H, Kondo A, Tsujitani S, Maeta M, Kaibara N. Mutated p53 protein expression and proliferative activity in advanced gastric cancer. *Hepatogastroenterology* 1999;**46**:2648.

454. Oda N, Tsujino T, Tsuda T, et al. DNA ploidy pattern and amplification of ERBB and ERBB2 genes in human gastric carcinomas. *Virchows Arch B Cell Pathol Incl Mol Pathol* 1990;**58**:273.

455. Varis A, Zaika A, Puolakkainen P, et al. Coamplified and overexpressed genes at ERBB2 locus in gastric cancer. *Int J Cancer* 2004;**109**:548.

456. Barros-Silva JD, Leitao D, Afonso L, et al. Association of ERBB2 gene status with histopathological parameters and disease-specific survival in gastric carcinoma patients. *Br J Cancer* 2009;**100**:487.

457. Brennetot C, Duval A, Hamelin R, et al. Frequent Ki-ras mutations in gastric tumors of the MSI phenotype. *Gastroenterology* 2003;**125**:1282.

458. Kim IJ, Park JH, Kang HC, et al. Mutational analysis of BRAF and K-ras in gastric cancers: absence of BRAF mutations in gastric cancers. *Hum Genet* 2003;**114**:118.

459. Oliveira C, Pinto M, Duval A, et al. BRAF mutations characterize colon but not gastric cancer with mismatch repair deficiency. *Oncogene* 2003;**22**:9192.

460. Wu M, Semba S, Oue N, Ikehara N, Yasui W, Yokozaki H. BRAF/K-ras mutation, microsatellite instability, and promoter hypermethylation of hMLH1/MGMT in human gastric carcinomas. *Gastric Cancer* 2004;**7**:246.

461. Ruschoff J, Dietel M, Baretton G, et al. HER2 diagnostics in gastric cancer-guideline validation and development of stand-

ardized immunohistochemical testing. *Virchows Arch* 2010; **457**:299.

462. Bang YJ, Van Cutsem E, Feyereislova A, et al. Trastuzumab in combination with chemotherapy versus chemotherapy alone for treatment of HER2-positive advanced gastric or gastro-oesophageal junction cancer (ToGA): a phase 3, open-label, randomised controlled trial. *Lancet* 2010;**376**:687.

463. European Medicines Agency. Opinion. 2009. Available at: www.emea.europa.eu/pdfs/human/opinion/Herceptin_82246709en.pdf. (accessed May 9, 2012).

464. Albarello L, Pecciarini L, Doglioni C. HER2 testing in gastric cancer. *Adv Anat Pathol* 2011;**18**:53.

465. Ayhan A, Yasui W, Yokozaki H, Seto M, Ueda R, Tahara E. Loss of heterozygosity at the bcl-2 gene locus and expression of bcl-2 in human gastric and colorectal carcinomas. *Jpn J Cancer Res* 1994;**85**:584.

466. Lee HK, Lee HS, Yang HK, et al. Prognostic significance of Bcl-2 and p53 expression in gastric cancer. *Int J Colorectal Dis* 2003; **18**:518.

467. Hattori Y, Odagiri H, Nakatani H, et al. K-sam, an amplified gene in stomach cancer, is a member of the heparin-binding growth factor receptor genes. *Proc Natl Acad Sci U S A* 1990; **87**:5983.

468. Smith MG, Hold GL, Tahara E, El-Omar EM. Cellular and molecular aspects of gastric cancer. *World J Gastroenterol* 2006; **12**:2979.

469. Wang L, Zhang F, Wu PP, Jiang XC, Zheng L, Yu YY. Disordered beta-catenin expression and E-cadherin/CDH1 promoter methylation in gastric carcinoma. *World J Gastroenterol* 2006; **12**:4228.

470. Kuniyasu H, Yasui W, Kitadai Y, Yokozaki H, Ito H, Tahara E. Frequent amplification of the c-met gene in scirrhous type stomach cancer. *Biochem Biophys Res Commun* 1992;**189**:227.

471. Kozma L, Kiss I, Hajdu J, Szentkereszty Z, Szakall S, Ember I. C-myc amplification and cluster analysis in human gastric carcinoma. *Anticancer Res* 2001;**21**:707.

472. Calcagno DQ, Leal MF, Seabra AD, et al. Interrelationship between chromosome 8 aneuploidy, C-MYC amplification and increased expression in individuals from northern Brazil with gastric adenocarcinoma. *World J Gastroenterol* 2006;**12**:6207.

473. Yasui W, Kudo Y, Semba S, Yokozaki H, Tahara E. Reduced expression of cyclin-dependent kinase inhibitor p27Kip1 is associated with advanced stage and invasiveness of gastric carcinomas. *Jpn J Cancer Res* 1997;**88**:625.

474. Xiangming C, Natsugoe S, Takao S, et al. The cooperative role of p27 with cyclin E in the prognosis of advanced gastric carcinoma. *Cancer* 2000;**89**:1214.

475. Kim DH, Lee HI, Nam ES, et al. Reduced expression of the cell-cycle inhibitor p27Kip1 is associated with progression and lymph node metastasis of gastric carcinoma. *Histopathology* 2000;**36**:245.

476. Akama Y, Yasui W, Yokozaki H, et al. Frequent amplification of the cyclin E gene in human gastric carcinomas. *Jpn J Cancer Res* 1995;**86**:617.

477. Modlin IM, Lye KD, Kidd M. A 50-year analysis of 562 gastric carcinoids: small tumor or larger problem? *Am J Gastroenterol* 2004;**99**:23.

478. Sjoblom SM. Clinical presentation and prognosis of gastrointestinal carcinoid tumours. *Scand J Gastroenterol* 1988;**23**:779.

479. Yao JC, Hassan M, Phan A, et al. One hundred years after 'carcinoid': epidemiology of and prognostic factors for neuroendocrine tumors in 35,825 cases in the United States. *J Clin Oncol* 2008;**26**:3063.

480. Solcia E, Kloppel G, Sobin LH. *Histological Typing of Endocrine Tumours*. Berlin: Springer-Verlag, 2000.

481. Rindi G, Kloppel G, Alhman H, et al. TNM staging of foregut (neuro)endocrine tumors: a consensus proposal including a grading system. *Virchows Arch* 2006;**449**:395.

482. Rindi G, Kloppel G, Couvelard A, et al. TNM staging of midgut and hindgut (neuro)endocrine tumors: a consensus proposal including a grading system. *Virchows Arch* 2007;**451**:757.

483. Ekeblad S, Skogseid B, Dunder K, Oberg K, Eriksson B. Prognostic factors and survival in 324 patients with pancreatic endocrine tumor treated at a single institution. *Clin Cancer Res* 2008; **14**:7798.

484. Fischer L, Kleeff J, Esposito I, et al. Clinical outcome and long-term survival in 118 consecutive patients with neuroendocrine tumours of the pancreas. *Br J Surg* 2008;**95**:627.

485. Bordi C, Yu JY, Baggi MT, et al. Gastric carcinoids and their precursor lesions. A histologic and immunohistochemical study of 23 cases. *Cancer* 1991;**67**:663.

486. Rindi G, Bordi C, Rappel S, La Rosa S, Stolte M, Solcia E. Gastric carcinoids and neuroendocrine carcinomas: pathogenesis, pathology, and behavior. *World J Surg* 1996;**20**:168.

487. Rindi G, Luinetti O, Cornaggia M, Capella C, Solcia E. Three subtypes of gastric argyrophil carcinoid and the gastric neuroendocrine carcinoma: a clinicopathologic study. *Gastroenterology* 1993;**104**:994.

488. Rindi G. Clinicopathologic aspects of gastric neuroendocrine tumors. *Am J Surg Pathol* 1995;**19** Suppl 1:S20.

489. Gough DB, Thompson GB, Crotty TB, et al. Diverse clinical and pathologic features of gastric carcinoid and the relevance of hypergastrinemia. *World J Surg* 1994;**18**:473.

490. Rindi G, Azzoni C, La Rosa S, et al. ECL cell tumor and poorly differentiated endocrine carcinoma of the stomach: prognostic evaluation by pathological analysis. *Gastroenterology* 1999;**116**: 532.

491. Davies MG, O'Dowd G, McEntee GP, Hennessy TP. Primary gastric carcinoids: a view on management. *Br J Surg* 1990;**77**:1013.

492. Harvey RF. Spontaneous resolution of multifocal gastric enterochromaffin-like cell carcinoid tumours. *Lancet* 1988;**i**:821.

493. Ruszniewski P, Delle Fave G, Cadiot G, et al. Well-differentiated gastric tumors/carcinomas. *Neuroendocrinology* 2006;**84**:158.

494. Solcia E, Capella C, Fiocca R, Rindi G, Rosai J. Gastric argyrophil carcinoidosis in patients with Zollinger-Ellison syndrome due to type 1 multiple endocrine neoplasia. A newly recognized association. *Am J Surg Pathol* 1990;**14**:503.

495. Bordi C, Falchetti A, Azzoni C, et al. Aggressive forms of gastric neuroendocrine tumors in multiple endocrine neoplasia type I. *Am J Surg Pathol* 1997;**21**:1075.

496. Watson RG, Johnston CF, O'Hare MM, et al. The frequency of gastrointestinal endocrine tumours in a well-defined population – Northern Ireland 1970–1985. *Q J Med* 1989;**72**:647.

497. Oates JA, Sjoerdsma A. A unique syndrome associated with secretion of 5-hydroxytryptophan by metastatic gastric carcinoids. *Am J Med* 1962;**32**:333.

498. Roberts LJ, 2nd, Bloomgarden ZT, Marney SR, Jr., Rabin D, Oates JA. Histamine release from a gastric carcinoid: provocation by pentagastrin and inhibition by somatostatin. *Gastroenterology* 1983;**84**:272.

499. Ooi A, Ota M, Katsuda S, Nakanishi I, Sugawara H, Takahashi I. An unusual case of multiple gastric carcinoids associated with diffuse endocrine cell hyperplasia and parietal cell hypertrophy. *Endocr Pathol* 1995;**6**:229.

500. Abraham SC, Carney JA, Ooi A, Choti MA, Argani P. Achlorhydria, parietal cell hyperplasia, and multiple gastric carcinoids: a new disorder. *Am J Surg Pathol* 2005;**29**:969.

501. Nakata K, Aishima S, Ichimiya H, et al. Unusual multiple gastric carcinoids with hypergastrinemia: report of a case. *Surg Today* 2010;**40**:267.

502. Christodoulopoulos JB, Klotz AP. Carcinoid syndrome with primary carcinoid tumor of the stomach. *Gastroenterology* 1961;**40**:429.

503. Hirata Y, Sakamoto N, Yamamoto H, Matsukura S, Imura H, Okada S. Gastric carcinoid with ectopic production of ACTH and beta-MSH. *Cancer* 1976;**37**:377.

504. Tsolakis AV, Portela-Gomes GM, Stridsberg M, et al. Malignant gastric ghrelinoma with hyperghrelinemia. *J Clin Endocrinol Metab* 2004;**89**:3739.

505. Chejfec G, Gould VE. Malignant gastric neuroendogrinomas. Ultrastructural and biochemical characterization of their secretory activity. *Hum Pathol* 1977;**8**:433.

506. Jiang SX, Mikami T, Umezawa A, Saegusa M, Kameya T, Okayasu I. Gastric large cell neuroendocrine carcinomas: a distinct clinicopathologic entity. *Am J Surg Pathol* 2006;**30**:945.

507. Shia J, Tang LH, Weiser MR, et al. Is nonsmall cell type high-grade neuroendocrine carcinoma of the tubular gastrointestinal tract a distinct disease entity? *Am J Surg Pathol* 2008;**32**:719.

508. Matsui K, Kitagawa M, Miwa A, Kuroda Y, Tsuji M. Small cell carcinoma of the stomach: a clinicopathologic study of 17 cases. *Am J Gastroenterol* 1991;**86**:1167.

509. Kloppel G, Couvelard A, Perren A, et al. ENETS Consensus Guidelines for the Standards of Care in Neuroendocrine Tumors: towards a standardized approach to the diagnosis of gastroenteropancreatic neuroendocrine tumors and their prognostic stratification. *Neuroendocrinology* 2009;**90**:162.

510. Berna MJ, Annibale B, Marignani M, et al. A prospective study of gastric carcinoids and enterochromaffin-like cell changes in multiple endocrine neoplasia type 1 and Zollinger–Ellison syndrome: identification of risk factors. *J Clin Endocrinol Metab* 2008;**93**:1582.

511. Annibale B, Azzoni C, Corleto VD, et al. Atrophic body gastritis patients with enterochromaffin-like cell dysplasia are at increased risk for the development of type I gastric carcinoid. *Eur J Gastroenterol Hepatol* 2001;**13**:1449.

512. Lamberts R, Creutzfeldt W, Struber HG, Brunner G, Solcia E. Long-term omeprazole therapy in peptic ulcer disease: gastrin, endocrine cell growth, and gastritis. *Gastroenterology* 1993;**104**:1356.

513. Eissele R, Brunner G, Simon B, Solcia E, Arnold R. Gastric mucosa during treatment with lansoprazole: *Helicobacter pylori* is a risk factor for argyrophil cell hyperplasia. *Gastroenterology* 1997;**112**:707.

514. Cadiot G, Laurent-Puig P, Thuille B, Lehy T, Mignon M, Olschwang S. Is the multiple endocrine neoplasia type 1 gene a suppressor for fundic argyrophil tumors in the Zollinger–Ellison syndrome? *Gastroenterology* 1993;**105**:579.

515. Bonar SF, Sweeney EC. The prevalence, prognostic significance and hormonal content of endocrine cells in gastric cancer. *Histopathology* 1986;**10**:53.

516. Caruso ML, Pilato FP, D'Adda T, et al. Composite carcinoid–adenocarcinoma of the stomach associated with multiple gastric carcinoids and nonantral gastric atrophy. *Cancer* 1989;**64**:1534.

517. Kim KM, Kim MJ, Cho BK, Choi SW, Rhyu MG. Genetic evidence for the multi-step progression of mixed glandular-neuroendocrine gastric carcinomas. *Virchows Arch* 2002;**440**:85.

518. Yang GC, Rotterdam H. Mixed (composite) glandular–endocrine cell carcinoma of the stomach. Report of a case and review of literature. *Am J Surg Pathol* 1991;**15**:592.

519. Rayhan N, Sano T, Qian ZR, Obari AK, Hirokawa M. Histological and immunohistochemical study of composite neuroendocrine–exocrine carcinomas of the stomach. *J Med Invest* 2005;**52**:191.

520. Menuck LS, Amberg JR. Metastatic disease involving the stomach. *Am J Dig Dis* 1975;**20**:903.

521. Telerman A, Gerard B, Van den Heule B, Bleiberg H. Gastrointestinal metastases from extra-abdominal tumors. *Endoscopy* 1985;**17**:99.

522. Green LK. Hematogenous metastases to the stomach. A review of 67 cases. *Cancer* 1990;**65**:1596.

523. Oda, Kondo H, Yamao T, et al. Metastatic tumors to the stomach: analysis of 54 patients diagnosed at endoscopy and 347 autopsy cases. *Endoscopy* 2001;**33**:507.

524. Cormier WJ, Gaffey TA, Welch JM, Welch JS, Edmonson JH. Linitis plastica caused by metastatic lobular carcinoma of the breast. *Mayo Clin Proc* 1980;**55**:747.

525. Washington K, McDonagh D. Secondary tumors of the gastrointestinal tract: surgical pathologic findings and comparison with autopsy survey. *Mod Pathol* 1995;**8**:427.

526. De Palma GD, Masone S, Rega M, et al. Metastatic tumors to the stomach: clinical and endoscopic features. *World J Gastroenterol* 2006;**12**:7326.

527. McLemore EC, Pockaj BA, Reynolds C, et al. Breast cancer: presentation and intervention in women with gastrointestinal metastasis and carcinomatosis. *Ann Surg Oncol* 2005;**12**:886.

528. Taal BG, Peterse H, Boot H. Clinical presentation, endoscopic features, and treatment of gastric metastases from breast carcinoma. *Cancer* 2000;**89**:2214.

529. Schwarz RE, Klimstra DS, Turnbull AD. Metastatic breast cancer masquerading as gastrointestinal primary. *Am J Gastroenterol* 1998;**93**:111.

530. Campoli PM, Ejima FH, Cardoso DM, et al. Metastatic cancer to the stomach. *Gastric Cancer* 2006;**9**:19.

531. Chu P, Wu E, Weiss LM. Cytokeratin 7 and cytokeratin 20 expression in epithelial neoplasms: a survey of 435 cases. *Mod Pathol* 2000;**13**:962.

532. O'Connell FP, Wang HH, Odze RD. Utility of immunohistochemistry in distinguishing primary adenocarcinomas from metastatic breast carcinomas in the gastrointestinal tract. *Arch Pathol Lab Med* 2005;**129**:338.

533. Oien KA. Pathologic evaluation of unknown primary cancer. *Semin Oncol* 2009;**36**:8.

534. Tong GX, Yu WM, Beaubier NT, et al. Expression of PAX8 in normal and neoplastic renal tissues: an immunohistochemical study. *Mod Pathol* 2009;**22**:1218.

535. Park SY, Kim BH, Kim JH, Lee S, Kang GH. Panels of immunohistochemical markers help determine primary sites of metastatic adenocarcinoma. *Arch Pathol Lab Med* 2007;**131**:1561.

Stromal tumours of the stomach

Erinn Downs-Kelly, Brian P. Rubin and John R. Goldblum

Cleveland Clinic, Cleveland, OH, USA

Gastric mesenchymal neoplasms can be broadly conceptualised into two groups. One group is composed of tumours that are histologically identical to their counterparts in soft tissue (e.g. leiomyomas and schwannomas), accounting for about 5% of gastric mesenchymal neoplasms. The other group is composed of gastrointestinal stromal tumours (GISTs), a histologically heterogeneous group of tumours that suggest a broad differential diagnosis. GISTs may occur anywhere in the gastrointestinal tract but are most common in the stomach (approximately 60%) and small bowel (roughly 30%). Approximately 10% arise in other parts of the gastrointestinal tract (oesophagus, colon and rectum) and a small percentage are extra-gastrointestinal, arising in the mesentery, omentum, retroperitoneum or pelvis [1,2]. GISTs account for about 95% of gastric mesenchymal neoplasms. The recognition and diagnosis of these lesions is important because they may follow an aggressive clinical course and their common molecular alterations allow for targeted therapy with small molecule tyrosine kinase inhibitors. Given that GISTs compose the vast majority of gastric mesenchymal neoplasms, much of this chapter is devoted to this topic.

Gastrointestinal stromal tumours

Pathogenesis and common molecular findings

The concept of GISTs has changed significantly over the past 20 years with the accumulation of ultrastructural and immunohistochemical findings and the elucidation of the molecular events that drive the proliferation of these tumours. Once thought to represent smooth muscle neoplasms [3–5], GISTs are now known to share features with interstitial cells of Cajal, based on ultrastructural findings and immunophenotyping [6–11]. Interstitial cells of Cajal are present within the interstitium of the muscularis propria throughout the gastrointestinal tract and serve a pacemaker function by generating and propagating electrical slow waves of depolarisation, effectively coordinating peristalsis [8–10,12,13]. The current hypothesis is that GISTs arise from either the interstitial cells of Cajal or a common progenitor stem cell [14].

CD117 or c-KIT (KIT) is a receptor tyrosine kinase that plays a role in the development and maintenance of interstitial cells of Cajal [7,15]. The binding of the KIT ligand leads ultimately to the phosphorylation of signal transduction proteins that modulate cell proliferation and inhibit apoptosis [16,17]. Studies have established that activating mutations of the KIT gene are present in about 75–80% of GISTs and play a fundamental role in their development [18–20]. The activating mutations most commonly involve the juxta-membrane domain in exon 11, resulting in ligand-independent activation of tyrosine kinase activity and ultimately promoting proliferation and cell survival [21–24]. Less commonly, mutations in exon 9 (extracellular domain) and exons 13 and 17 (kinase domains) have been identified [25,26] (Figure 14.1). Approximately 7% of GISTs harbour a mutation in platelet-derived growth factor receptor α (PDGFRA), a homologous receptor tyrosine kinase [27,28]. KIT and PDGFRA mutations are mutually exclusive and, taken together, are found in about 85–90% of all GISTs. These mutations have been detected in small, incidentally

Morson and Dawson's Gastrointestinal Pathology, Fifth Edition. Edited by Neil A. Shepherd, Bryan F. Warren, Geraint T. Williams, Joel K. Greenson, Gregory Y. Lauwers and Marco R. Novelli.

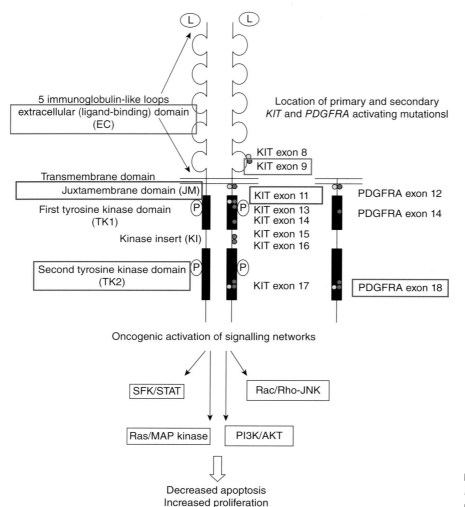

Figure 14.1 Molecular biology: *KIT* and *PDGFRA* (platelet-derived growth factor receptor α).

identified, gastrointestinal stromal tumours, suggesting that they occur as an early event in tumorigenesis [29,30]. Mutations in *KIT* have not been identified in tumours that are within the histological differential diagnosis of GISTs, including leiomyomas, leiomyosarcomas, intra-abdominal desmoids/fibromatoses and schwannomas.

Clinical features

Although once thought to be rare, approximately 4500–6000 GISTs are now diagnosed annually within the USA alone [31,32]. Data from Europe report that the annual incidence is roughly 7–19 cases per million [33–35]. GISTs occur in relatively equal proportions between the sexes and arise in a wide age range, although approximately 75% are diagnosed in patients aged >50 years [36]. Presentation is typically dependent on size and location within the stomach. GISTs may be discovered incidentally on routine endoscopy or found within resection specimens removed

for unrelated reasons such as gastric carcinoma [29,37]. If a tumour is large enough, the presenting symptoms may include early satiety, bloating and gastrointestinal bleeding, with subsequent anaemia and fatigue [38]. Most GISTs are uninodular and centred on the bowel wall. However, multi-focal nodules are well described (Figure 14.2). The tumour may develop as a polypoid mass and ulcerate the overlying mucosa or grow exophytically and protrude towards the serosal aspect. Some GISTs are predominantly extramural and may be attached to the stomach by only a thin stalk of tissue.

GISTs that behave in an aggressive fashion have an expected pattern of metastatic spread to the liver and serosal seeding within the abdominal cavity [36]. Metastatic disease to the lungs occurs in particularly advanced cases [36,39]. Historically, nodal metastases in GISTs are extremely uncommon (noted in less than 1% of cases). A recent study evaluating GISTs arising in the setting of the Carney triad reported gastric lymph node metastases in 29% of patients with metastatic disease. This and many other aspects of Carney triad GISTs led the authors to conclude that they are clinically and behaviourally different than sporadic GISTs [40] (see 'GIST syndromes' below).

Pathological features

GISTs are typically well circumscribed and, although they may be surrounded by a thin rim of fibrous tissue, they are not encapsulated. On cut section, the lesions are usually solid, firm, white masses that may show areas of haemorrhage, necrosis or cystic change, features that are not indicative of malignancy in GISTs (see Figure 14.2a).

The morphology varies greatly with spindle cell, epithelioid or mixed spindle and epithelioid cell types [31]. Epithelioid and mixed cell type GISTs are most commonly encountered in the stomach compared with other gastrointestinal sites [41,42]. However, epithelioid GISTs still make up the minority of gastric GISTs.

Spindle cell GISTs are composed of hypercellular, uniform spindle cells with generous pale to eosinophilic fibrillary cytoplasm. The cells are consistent in size and shape. The nuclei contain evenly distributed chromatin and inconspicuous nucleoli. Perinuclear vacuoles are often present and indent the nucleus at one pole (Figure 14.3). Such vacuoles were originally considered to be highly characteristic of smooth muscle tumours of the gut but it is now realised that they are a particular feature of GISTs. The cells are typically arranged in short fascicles but other architectural patterns such as broad sweeping sheets and a herring-bone pattern can also be seen. Occasional cases also show palisading similar to that seen in schwannomas. The spindle cells are frequently separated by hyalinised, myxoid or focally calcified stroma [43].

Epithelioid GISTs are composed predominately of cells with distinct borders arranged in nests and sheets. The nuclei are round with small nucleoli, although scattered multinucleated giant cells or cells with bizarre nuclei may be present [44]. Cells with abundant eosinophilic cytoplasm and an eccentrically placed nucleus are common (Figure 14.4). These may have a superficial resemblance to large plasma cells. Stromal alterations including liquefaction, hyalinisation and calcification may be seen.

Immunohistochemical features

CD117 (KIT), the product of the *KIT* gene, has been identified as a sensitive marker of GISTs from all sites and is

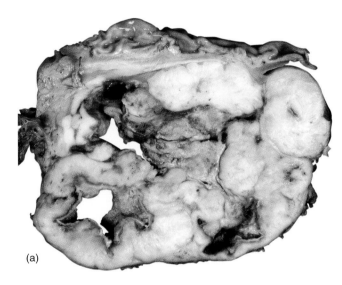

(a)

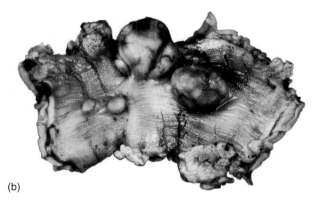

(b)

Figure 14.2 (a) Single large gastric gastrointestinal stromal tumour (GIST): the cross-section demonstrates the distinct firm poly-lobulated white mass which shows areas of haemorrhage, necrosis and cystic change. (b) Multiple GISTs distributed along the subserosa of the stomach.

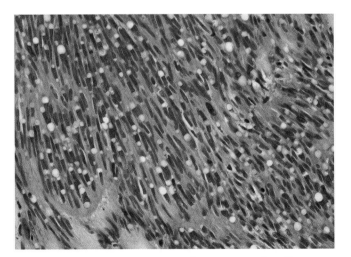

Figure 14.3 Gastrointestinal stromal tumour, spindle cell type, composed of uniform spindle cells with pale-to-eosinophilic fibrillary cytoplasm. The cells are uniform in size and shape, with prominent perinuclear vacuoles that indent the nucleus at one pole. The nuclei are also uniform with evenly distributed chromatin and inconspicuous nucleoli.

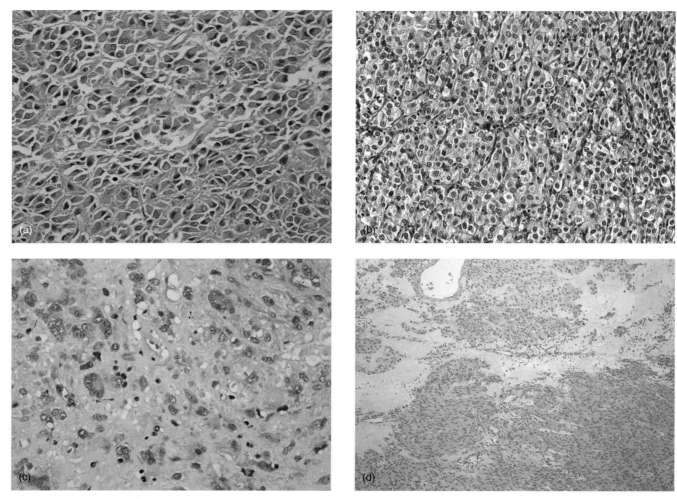

Figure 14.4 Gastrointestinal stromal tumour (GIST), epithelioid cell type, has a cellular arrangement that may vary between different areas of the same tumour with cells arranged in sheets or nests. (a) In this case, a sheet-like architecture is composed of cells with ample eosinophilic cytoplasm and an eccentrically located nucleus. Typically the nuclei are round with small nucleoli. (b) In a case like this one the cells are deceptively epithelial looking. (c) Multinucleated giant cells are not uncommon in epithelioid GISTs and in this example are deposited in a myxoid stroma. (d) Mixed spindle cell and epithelioid GIST with the upper half of the image composed of an epithelioid cell population and the lower half of a typical spindle cell population.

expressed in up to 95% of GISTs [45]. The pattern of immunoreactivity is typically diffuse and pancytoplasmic. However, membranous staining and a perinuclear dot-like immunoreactivity have been described in epithelioid GISTs (Figure 14.5). Approximately 5% of GISTs do not express KIT [46,47]; often the subset of KIT-negative GISTs that contain a *PDGFRA* mutation do not react with antibodies to KIT [20]. These tumours frequently have epithelioid morphology and are located within the stomach. CD34, a haematopoietic stem cell marker, is expressed in roughly 70% of GISTs [48,49]. *KIT* and *PDGFRA* mutation analysis, which can be performed on paraffin-embedded and formalin-fixed tissue, may be helpful in the diagnosis of KIT-immunonegative GISTs.

Approximately 20–30% of GISTs are positive for smooth muscle actin, 5% may show some positivity for S100 protein and 1–2% are positive for desmin or cytokeratin [6,31,45]. Desmin staining is typically limited to scattered tumour cells with more prominent staining noted within epithelioid GISTs. The pathologist should not mistake native muscularis propria, positive for desmin and apparently within the tumour, for focal positive staining in the tumour itself, because such entrapped muscularis is a common feature of GISTs.

Gene expression profiling studies of GISTs identified *Discovered on GIST-1 (DOG1)* transcripts [50] and the corresponding protein has been shown to be a calcium-regulated chloride channel protein [51,52]. In initial studies, antibod-

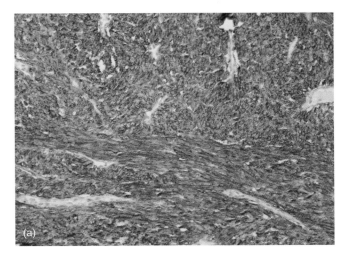

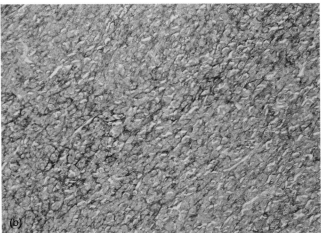

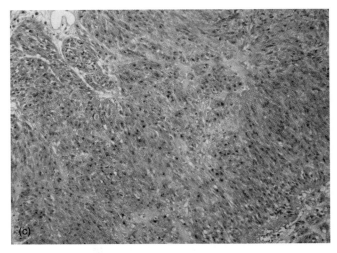

Figure 14.5 Different patterns of KIT staining in gastrointestinal stromal tumours (GISTs): (a) diffuse and strong immunoreactivity in a spindle cell GIST; (b) membranous pattern of staining; and (c) perinuclear dot-like staining.

ies to the corresponding protein appeared to be immunoreactive with GISTs regardless of the *KIT/PDGFRA* mutational status [53,54]. A study evaluating expression of DOG1 in a large series of GISTs and non-GISTs found that the sensitivity of *DOG1* was similar to KIT in GISTs (both roughly 94%). However, *DOG1* positivity was also identified in a small subset of mesenchymal tumours including leiomyomas and synovial sarcomas [55]. Gene expression studies have also identified protein kinase C theta as consistently overexpressed in GISTs [56,57]. Initial immunohistochemical studies have reported that this protein is sensitive and specific for the diagnosis of GIST [58].

Differential diagnosis of GISTs

Spindle cell GISTs have to be distinguished from other spindle cell proliferations of the gastrointestinal tract, including smooth muscle neoplasms, nerve sheath tumours, inflammatory fibroid polyps and intra-abdominal fibromatoses (desmoid tumours).

True smooth muscle tumours of the gastrointestinal tract are much less common than GISTs. Similar to soft tissue leiomyomas and leiomyosarcomas, gastrointestinal smooth muscle neoplasms are composed of elongated cells with 'cigar-shaped' nuclei, eosinophilic fibrillary cytoplasm and a fascicular architecture. The cells are strongly and diffusely immunoreactive for actin (smooth muscle actin and muscle-specific actin) and are often immunoreactive for desmin although there is no expression of KIT [39,59].

Benign and malignant nerve sheath tumours are also rare in the gastrointestinal tract. Schwannomas occur much more commonly in the stomach than neurofibromas and may be histologically similar to spindle cell GISTs. Schwannomas are composed of a proliferation of diffuse, S100 protein-immunoreactive, wavy, spindled cells with an associated peripheral lymphoid cuff. Very rarely, a malignant peripheral nerve sheath tumour may arise in the gastrointestinal tract and will resemble its counterparts in the peripheral soft tissues. Unlike GISTs, these lesions do not express KIT and are variably immunoreactive for S100 protein.

Inflammatory fibroid polyps (IFPs) are benign lesions seen in adults that occur as solitary or multiple polyps arising in the submucosa. Although IFPs have been noted throughout the gastrointestinal tract [60], they have a propensity for the stomach, especially the antrum, and the ileum. These mesenchymal lesions are composed of bland spindle cells, granulation tissue-like vessels and prominent eosinophils, and admixed mast cells, plasma cells and lymphocytes. Typically, a concentric whorling of the spindle cells in an 'onion-skin pattern' around blood vessels is noted. Although the spindle cells are negative for KIT, the scattered mast cells will be immunoreactive. A potential confusion with GIST arises from the fact that the spindle cells and vessels are immunoreactive for CD34 [61]. Additional confusion with GISTs may arise as well due to the fact that IFPs have been found to harbour gain-of-function mutations in *PDGFRA* within the same genomic hot spots as those identified within GISTs that lack an activating *KIT* mutation [62]. Despite having similar activating mutations, IFPs are benign whereas GISTs have the capacity to metastasise; this has led some to conclude that additional genetic alterations are required for the malignant progression of GISTs [62].

Intra-abdominal fibromatosis (desmoid tumour) is the most common primary tumour of the mesentery. Mesenteric fibromatosis may originate from the gastrocolic ligament and omentum and have a similar growth pattern to that of some GISTs. Histologically, mesenteric fibromatosis are composed of cytologically bland and monotonous spindled or stellate-shaped cells that are evenly deposited in a collagenous or sometimes myxoid stroma. The cells are arranged in long sweeping fascicles that have projections extending into the surrounding soft tissue. Scattered keloid-type collagen fibres may be present, as are dilated thin-walled vessels. Immunohistochemically, the spindle cells of fibromatosis are immunoreactive for vimentin, smooth muscle actin and muscle-specific actin. The lesional cells frequently have β-catenin nuclear immunoreactivity [63] and are usually negative for KIT, although one group has reported KIT immunoreactivity in these tumours [64]. Based on personal experience, when KIT is positive in desmoid fibromatosis, it is usually very weak in comparison to the strong staining seen in GIST.

GISTs with epithelioid features may be confused with lymphoma, melanoma, neuro-endocrine tumours and carcinoma, especially in small biopsies, necessitating immunohistochemical analysis. It is worth noting that the expression of KIT has been identified in a small subset of melanomas [65–67] and exclusion of the possibility of melanoma by performing a panel of immunohistochemical stains that include S100 protein, HMB-45 and/or Melan-A is warranted. Rare examples of epithelioid GISTs may show focal cytokeratin immunoreactivity, so the co-expression of either CD34 or KIT becomes essential to avoid misdiagnosing such cases as carcinoma. Epithelioid GISTs containing *PDGFRA* mutations may express CD34 in the absence of KIT.

Prognostic indicators

The most important prognostic biomarkers for GIST are mitotic rate, size and anatomical location and these features define the Miettinen criteria for risk stratification (Table 14.1). These criteria establish a risk of progressive disease, defined as either metastatic disease or tumour-related death, and have been endorsed by the College of American

Table 14.1 Miettinen criteria for risk assessment of primary gastric gastrointestinal stromal tumours[a]

Mitotic index	Size (cm)	Risk of progressive disease (%)
≤5/50 hpf	≤2	None (0)
	>2 but ≤5	Very low (1.9)
	>5 but ≤10	Low (3.6)
	>10	Moderate (10)
>5/50 hpf	≤2	None (small number of cases)
	>2 but ≤5	Moderate (16)
	>5 but ≤10	High (55)
	>10	High (86)

hpf, high power fields.
[a]Data based on the long-term follow-up of 1074 gastric gastrointestinal stromal tumours in the pre-imatinib era [41].

Pathologists and the National Comprehensive Cancer Network. The Miettinen criteria are an expansion of the National Institutes of Health (NIH) consensus document which defined relative risk of aggressive behaviour in GISTs utilising tumour size and mitotic counts [31]. Although reproducible, the NIH approach is an oversimplification because GISTs from different sites within the gastrointestinal tract have differing behaviour [41,68,69]. The criteria are based on large Armed Forces Institute of Pathology (AFIP) studies evaluating how the clinicopathological features of GISTs within different sites (gastric, small intestinal, duodenal and rectal locations) affected prognosis in the pre-imatinib era [39,41,59,70]. For gastric GISTs, the Miettinen criteria for risk stratification were developed from a series of 1074 patients with about 14 years of follow-up data [41].

To assign an accurate risk of progressive disease a thorough mitotic count should be performed, evaluating a total area of 5 mm^2. It should be noted that, for modern wide-field microscopes with wide-field eye-pieces, the mitotic count correlating with the total area of 5 mm^2 is obtained from 20 high power fields (hpf) [6]. Careful gross examination of GISTs with regard to measuring greatest tumour dimension is important for risk stratification, especially when a tumour is almost 50 mm in size, e.g. a gastric GIST with more than five mitotic figures per high power field, measuring >20 but ≤50 mm has a moderate (16%) risk of progressive disease, whereas one measuring >50 but ≤100 mm has a high (55%) risk of progressive disease.

Other factors that have been reported in the literature to be associated with poor outcome have included tumour necrosis, mucosal invasion and ulceration [41,71,72]. Tumour rupture, either spontaneous or at the time of surgery, increases the risk of recurrence with intra-abdominal seeding

[73,74]. Patients whose complete resection is complicated by tumour rupture have been shown to have a significantly shortened survival compared with patients with complete resection without tumour rupture [74–76].

Treatment

The main treatment goal for a localised GIST is complete surgical resection with negative margins and preservation of an intact pseudo-capsule. As mentioned previously, tumour rupture places the patient at a high risk for recurrence.

Tyrosine kinase inhibitors play a pivotal role in the management of metastatic or unresectable disease. Imatinib is a small molecule tyrosine kinase inhibitor with a structure that mimics ATP and binds competitively to the intracellular portion of KIT, inhibiting signalling. This molecule also targets PDGFRA. Tumour genotype has been shown to correlate with response to imatinib, e.g. tumours with exon 11 *KIT* mutations have shown the best imatinib response rates whereas tumours with no *KIT* mutation or those with a *PDGFRA D842V* mutation were less likely to have a favourable or a sustained response to imatinib [20,77]. Other studies have suggested that patients with exon 9 *KIT* mutations may benefit from the use of higher-dose imatinib [78,79]. Some patients with GISTs may develop amplification of *KIT* or secondary mutations in *KIT* or *PDGFRA* that infer tumour resistance to imatinib [80–83]. In these resistant tumours, alternative kinase inhibitors, such as sunitinib, are being used.

GIST syndromes

Familial GISTs and those associated with neurofibromatosis type I (NF-1) and the Carney triad have been well described. Familial GISTs arise from heritable mutations in exon 8, 11 or 13 of *KIT* and in exon 12 of *PDGFRA* [84–91]. Tumours are often multiple, typically involve the stomach and small bowel and may develop as early as an age of 18 years. A background of diffuse hyperplasia of the interstitial cells of Cajal has been noted in the adjacent gut wall and some patients also have pigmented macules on the skin of the perineum, axilla, hands and face, as well as evidence of mastocytosis (urticaria pigmentosa), which is associated with activating *KIT* mutations [90,92].

A small subset of patients with NF-1 will develop GISTs [93–95]: the incidence from a Swedish study [93] was found to be 7% of NF1 patients. The lesions are typically present within the small bowel and are multifocal with a background of interstitial cell of Cajal hyperplasia. Most of these GISTs have been shown to lack either *KIT* or *PDGFRA* mutations [95,96].

The Carney triad, the rare tumour syndrome occurring chiefly in girls and young women, consists of gastric GISTs (typically an epithelioid cell type), paraganglioma and pulmonary chondroma [97]. Thus far, mutations in *KIT* and *PDGFRA* have not been identified in this subset of GISTs [98]. As mentioned above, recent literature suggests that GISTs in the setting of the Carney triad are quite different from sporadic GISTs [40]. Zhang et al. evaluated 104 GISTs arising in the Carney triad and found that the lesions were most commonly antrum-based, multifocal and composed of epithelioid cells. Of the 61 cases evaluated with KIT immunohistochemistry, 100% were positive. Interestingly, lymph node metastases were identified in 29% of patients with metastatic disease [40].

Tumours of neural origin

Schwannomas

Schwannomas (neurilemmomas) are uncommon in the gastrointestinal tract but are most commonly encountered in the stomach [99], followed by the colon and rectum [100]. They occur primarily during middle to late adulthood with a peak in the sixth decade. An association with neurofibromatosis is not common, with only one report of an NF-1 patient identified with a gastric schwannoma [96,101,102]. These benign neoplasms typically involve the submucosa and the muscularis propria, although some have an intraluminal polypoid component. The overlying mucosa may be intact or ulcerated.

Although schwannomas are grossly well circumscribed, gastrointestinal schwannomas are devoid of a true capsule. The cellularity of these lesions varies in different portions of the tumour. Some areas may be highly cellular and contain aborted fascicles or whorls, whereas other less cellular areas may have a prominent hyalinised or myxoid stroma. The nuclear palisading, Verocay bodies and thick-walled vessels typically seen in peripheral schwannomas may be present but are often inconspicuous. Unlike their soft tissue counterparts, gastric schwannomas have a discontinuous cuff of lymphoid cells with or without germinal centre formation at the periphery of the lesion which is often the initial clue to the diagnosis (Figure 14.6). Scattered lymphocytes and plasma cells are often found within the tumour. The spindle cells composing the lesions have wavy or 'buckled' nuclei and occasional intranuclear inclusions. Scattered cells with nuclear atypia may be present but mitotic activity is usually low (<5 mitoses/50 hpf). Although predominantly spindled, rare cases are composed of epithelioid cells [100]. Similar to their soft tissue counterparts, schwannomas of the stomach are strongly and diffusely immunoreactive for S100 protein and glial fibrillary acidic protein (GFAP); some may show focal CD34 staining. KIT and muscle markers are negative.

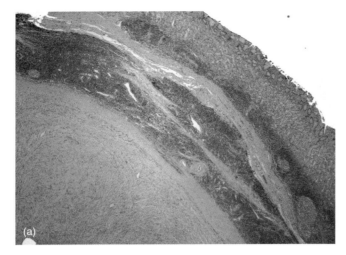

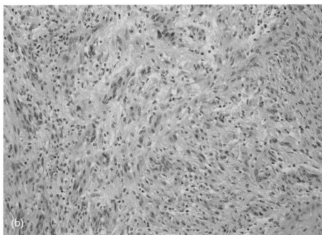

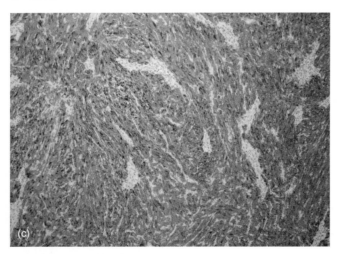

Figure 14.6 (a) Example of a gastric schwannoma demonstrating the circumscription and prominent lymphoid cuff at the periphery of the lesion. (b) The lesion is composed of spindle cells with wavy or 'buckled' nuclei and scattered lymphocytes and plasma cells. (c) Diffuse S100 protein immunoreactivity.

Granular cell tumours

Most granular cell tumours of the gut occur in the oesophagus. However, there are rare descriptions of them occurring in the stomach [103]. Granular cell tumours are predominantly located in the submucosa but may involve the muscularis propria, muscularis mucosae and mucosa. The lesional cells are plump and epithelioid or spindled with abundant eosinophilic granular cytoplasm that contains numerous periodic acid–Schiff (PAS)-positive, diastase-resistant phagolysosomes. The nuclei may be small and hyperchromatic or large with open chromatin. The cells may be arranged in nests with intervening fibrous tissue or broad sheets (Figure 14.7). These lesions are immunoreactive for S100 protein and neuron-specific enolase. Often the pan-macrophage marker CD68 is also immunoreactive, given the numerous lysosomes [104,105].

Virtually all of these lesions behave in a clinically benign fashion. However, rare examples of malignant granular cell tumours have been described in the soft tissues and one could extrapolate these findings to granular cell tumours within other sites. Fanburg-Smith et al. evaluated six histological variables within granular cells tumours that they considered potentially indicative of malignancy, including necrosis, vesicular nuclei with large nucleoli, increased mitotic rate (>2 mitoses/10 hpf at 200 × magnification), spindling of tumour cells, a high nuclear:cytoplasmic (N:C) ratio and pleomorphism. Of these histological factors, necrosis, spindling, increased N:C ratio and vesicular nuclei with large nucleoli were statistically significant whereas multivariate analysis of these histological features showed that spindling, increased N:C ratio and vesicular nuclei with large nucleoli were the features most likely to lead to a malignant classification [106].

Tumours of smooth muscle origin

Smooth muscle tumours of the gastrointestinal tract arise from the muscularis mucosae or muscularis propria and are much less common than GISTs. These tumours are characterised by positive staining for a variety of muscle markers, including actin and desmin. Smooth muscle tumours are consistently negative for KIT.

Leiomyomas

Leiomyomas of the gastrointestinal tract that come to clinical attention occur predominantly in the oesophagus, colon and rectum and are rare in the stomach and small intestine [39,59]. However, Abraham et al. identified small incidental leiomyomas (mean diameter 1.7 mm) in 47% of patients undergoing oesophago-gastrectomy for oesophageal or oesophago-gastric junction carcinomas, with most of these lesions identified on the gastric side of the junction [37].

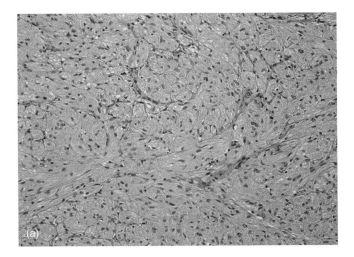

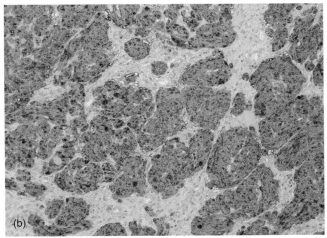

Figure 14.7 Granular cell tumour: (a) composed of epithelioid cells with small uniform nuclei and abundant eosinophilic granular cytoplasm arranged in sheets and nests. (b) Example of S100 protein immunoreactivity in a granular cell tumour.

Most leiomyomas have been discovered incidentally during evaluations for other processes [107]. Grossly or endoscopically leiomyomas may have a pedunculated appearance. Histologically, gastrointestinal leiomyomas, regardless of their site of origin, are characterised by a proliferation of bland spindle-shaped cells with elongate 'cigar-shaped' nuclei and eosinophilic fibrillary cytoplasm. The lesions are of low or moderate cellularity and have a fascicular architecture. They are uniformly positive for both smooth muscle actin and desmin and negative for KIT. Mitotic activity is either absent or minimal (0–1/50 hpf). These lesions uniformly behave in a benign fashion.

Leiomyosarcomas

True leiomyosarcomas of the gastrointestinal tract are rare and have not been well studied. Most previously published studies of 'leiomyosarcomas of the gastrointestinal tract' were in fact GISTs. Similar to GISTs, these tumours typically occur in older patients and most arise as luminal polypoid growths [108].

Histologically, leiomyosarcomas of the gastrointestinal tract resemble their soft tissue counterparts. These moderate-to-hypercellular tumours may have a fascicular architecture and are composed of cells with eosinophilic fibrillary cytoplasm and cytologically atypical elongate nuclei which are enlarged and hyperchromatic (Figure 14.8). Atypia is paramount in separating benign from malignant smooth muscle tumours with mitotic activity frequently paralleling the atypia. Generalised malignant features extrapolated from retroperitoneal and abdominal lesions considered to be leiomyosarcomas include a minimum mitotic rate of 1–4/10 hpf, some degree of nuclear atypia and coagulative necrosis [109,110]. Immunohistochemistry usually ensures their recognition as true smooth muscle tumours because most of these lesions are immunoreactive for actin, h-caldesmon and desmin. Focal immunoreactivity for CD34 and epithelial membrane antigen (EMA) has been described, although KIT is consistently negative.

Given the rarity of these tumours and the fact that many reported series have included GISTs, the clinical behaviour of this group of tumours is poorly defined. Therefore histological grading based on the FNCLCC (French Fédération Nationale des Centres de Lutte Contre le Cancer) system may offer some utility, because this grading schema has shown good correlation with overall and metastasis-free survival in the setting of primary untreated soft tissue tumours. The FNCLCC system incorporates the degree of tumour differentiation, mitotic rate and amount of tumour necrosis to assign a histological grade of 1–3 [111].

Smooth muscle tumours of uncertain malignant potential

Some smooth muscle tumours do not fit neatly into either the leiomyoma or the leiomyosarcoma category histologically. As stated above, identifying atypia within a smooth muscle tumour should raise concern for malignancy. However, cases that have been well sampled and contain only focal atypia without the presence of mitotic activity may be most appropriately designated as a smooth muscle tumour of uncertain malignant potential.

Vascular tumours

Glomus tumours

Glomus tumours are composed of modified smooth muscle cells, representing a counterpart of the perivascular glomus body. These tumours occur most commonly in the

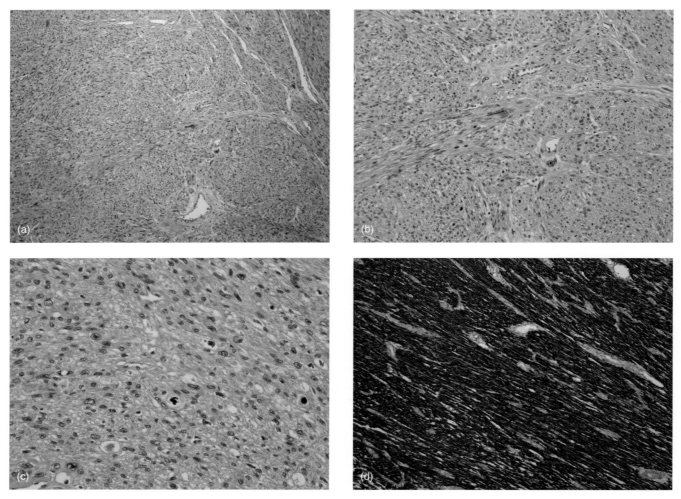

Figure 14.8 Leiomyosarcoma, intermediate grade: (a) with a fascicular architecture composed of cells with eosinophilic fibrillary cytoplasm and scattered nuclear atypia. (b) Most of the neoplasm is composed of elongate cigar-shaped nuclei whereas rare cells with marked nuclear atypia and prominent nucleoli are present within the centre of the image as are (c) mitotic figures. (d) There is strong and diffuse positivity for desmin immunohistochemically.

peripheral soft tissues but those arising within the gastrointestinal tract are found most commonly within the stomach [112]. Miettinen and colleagues have reviewed the largest series of gastrointestinal glomus tumours and, of the 32 tumours studied, only one was not located within the stomach [113]. These tumours have a strong predilection for women and the median age is 55 years. Patients typically present with gastrointestinal bleeding or ulcer-like symptoms.

Gastric glomus tumours are histologically similar to their peripheral soft tissue counterparts and are characterised by the distinctive glomus cell, which has a round uniform shape and a discrete round nucleus surrounded by pale-to-eosinophilic cytoplasm. The cells are often arranged around prominent dilated haemangio-pericytoma-like vascular spaces in a myxoid or hyalinised stroma (Figure 14.9). Mitotic activity is typically low (<5/50 hpf). The neoplastic cells are immunoreactive for muscle markers such as smooth muscle actin and calponin, whereas there is variable expression of desmin and no expression of S100 protein or KIT.

Most glomus tumours in the stomach behave in a clinically benign fashion. In the study by Miettinen et al., follow-up of 32 gastrointestinal glomus tumours revealed only one patient who developed metastatic disease [113]. In this case, the primary tumour had cytological atypia with focal areas of spindle cell morphology and vascular invasion. Long-term follow-up of the remaining patients has shown that all have remained disease-free.

Angiosarcoma and Kaposi's sarcoma

Angiosarcoma of the gastrointestinal tract is an exceedingly rare tumour and most have been described in case

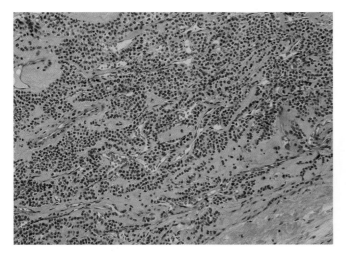

Figure 14.9 Glomus tumour composed of uniform cells with round, centrally located nuclei and pale-to-clear cytoplasm arranged around prominent dilated haemangiopericytoma-like vascular spaces.

reports and small series [114]. Involvement of the stomach has been reported mainly secondary to metastatic spread [115]. Angiosarcoma is composed of spindled or epithelioid cells which form primitive vascular channels that dissect through the involved tissue. Immunohistochemically, the vascular endothelial markers, CD31, CD34 and von Willebrand's factor, are typically expressed and the epithelioid variants may show significant cytokeratin immunoreactivity [114].

Kaposi's sarcoma (KS) is seen in the setting of immunosuppression and is the most common gastrointestinal malignancy in AIDS [116]. Since the advent of highly active anti-retroviral therapy (HAART), the incidence of Kaposi's sarcoma has been dramatically reduced but not eliminated. Patients may be asymptomatic or experience weight loss, nausea, vomiting, gastrointestinal bleeding and/or diarrhoea [117]. The endoscopic appearance ranges from multiple purple maculopapular lesions to larger nodular and polypoid tumours [118,119]. Histologically, Kaposi's sarcoma is composed of monomorphic spindle cells, which are separated by slit-like vessels and arranged in vague fascicles. Frequently, PAS-positive, diastase-resistant hyaline globules may be present, both within and without the lesional cells. Human herpesvirus 8 (HHV8) has been identified as the causative agent of Kaposi's sarcoma. Commercially available antibodies to latency-associated nuclear antigen (LAN-1), a protein encoded by HHV8, have shown excellent sensitivity and specificity in identifying Kaposi's sarcoma [120,121]. The vascular marker CD31 is also typically expressed. Some examples of Kaposi's sarcoma in the gut may show immunoreactivity for CD117/c-KIT, providing some potential diagnostic confusion with GISTs.

Tumours of adipose tissue

Lipomas

Primary lipomatous tumours of the stomach are exceptionally rare and resemble lipomas at peripheral sites. Many are identified incidentally. However, occasional lipomas arising within the stomach have come to clinical attention due to haemorrhage from ulceration [122,123]. They are usually centred in the submucosa and often compress the overlying muscularis mucosae. If large enough, the lesions may cause reactive changes within the adjacent mucosa. Histologically, these tumours are composed of mature adipocytes of uniform size and lack fibrous septa, nuclear hyperchromasia or cytological atypia (Figure 14.10).

Liposarcomas

Liposarcomas involving the gastrointestinal tract are exceptionally rare and most represent secondary involvement from retroperitoneal liposarcomas. Well differentiated liposarcomas/atypical lipomatous tumours (WDLS/ALT) are characterised by enlarged hyperchromatic nuclei that may be identified either between adipocytes or within fibrous septa. WDLS/ALT may undergo progression to a de-differentiated liposarcoma that most commonly resembles a pleomorphic undifferentiated sarcoma. From a cytogenetic standpoint, WDLS/ALT is typified by giant marker and ring chromosomes [124,125] which contain amplified sequences of 12q13-15 resulting in amplification of the *MDM2* gene (12q14). In cases of potential WDLS/ALT that lack diagnostic cytological atypia, fluorescence *in situ* hybridisation to identify the presence of *MDM2* gene amplification can be an extremely useful ancillary study [126].

Other mesenchymal tumours

It is important to remember that the overwhelming majority (>95%) of gastric mesenchymal neoplasms will be accounted for by GISTs, schwannomas and leiomyomas. However some interesting and noteworthy lesions have been described in the stomach more recently.

Plexiform angiomyxoid myofibroblastic tumour of the stomach

Case reports and small series have described a distinct entity termed 'plexiform angiomyxoid myofibroblastic tumour of the stomach' which appears to behave in a benign fashion [127–131]. Most of these tumours have involved the antrum and pyloric region, with presenting features including anaemia, gastric ulcer and pyloric obstruction. The lesions have been described as having

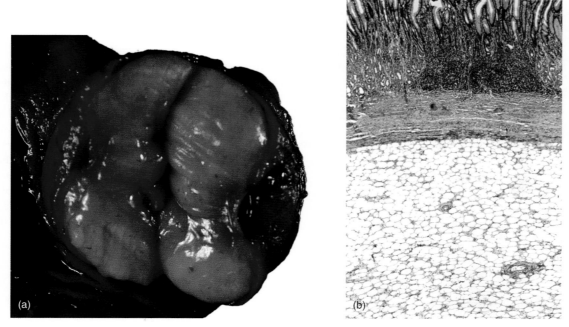

Figure 14.10 (a) This large primary lipoma of the stomach was clinically mistaken for a gastrointestinal stromal tumour (GIST). (b) The lesion is centred in the submucosa and composed of mature adipocytes,

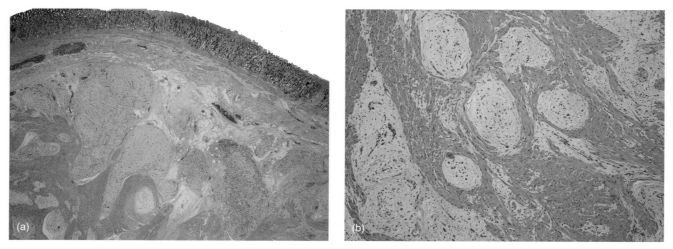

Figure 14.11 Plexiform angiomyxoid myofibroblastic tumour of the stomach showing (a) the typical involvement of the muscularis propria by multiple discontinuous nodules which are (b) pauci-cellular, predominantly myxoid and composed of bland spindle cells. (Case courtesy of Dr Yan Zhao.)

intraluminal, intramural and serosal extragastric components, forming multiple submesothelial nodules with a characteristic gelatinous or mucoid appearance grossly [131]. Histologically, these lesions have a distinct plexiform and multi-nodular appearance at low power with discontinuous myxoid nodules interspersed within the muscularis propria (Figure 14.11). The myxoid nodules are relatively hypocellular and composed of uniform bland spindle cells, frequently with an arborising capillary network (Figure 14.12). By immunohistochemistry, these lesions have consistently shown immunoreactivity within the spindled cells for smooth muscle actin and HHF-35 and variable expression of desmin, although none of the lesions has shown expression of KIT, CD34, S100 protein, EMA or cytokeratin AE1/AE3 [127–131]. Miettinen et al. have reviewed the largest series with long-term follow-up after excision and found that ulceration, mucosal invasion and vascular invasion were not indicative of an adverse outcome [131].

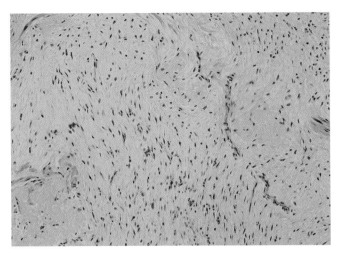

Figure 14.12 Plexiform angiomyxoid myofibroblastic tumour of the stomach with bland spindle cells within a myxoid background and linear capillaries that have a tendency to arborise.

Clear cell sarcoma of the stomach

Clear cell sarcoma (CCS), first described by Enzinger in 1965, is most commonly identified as a neoplasm arising in and adjacent to tendons and aponeuroses of the distal extremities [132]. However, CCS arising within the gastrointestinal tract has been noted in children and adults, primarily within the small bowel and stomach [133–136]. Similar to soft tissue CCSs, gastrointestinal CCSs have a nested architecture due to prominent fibrous tissue septa that divide the tumour. The oval-to-spindled cells composing the lesion are fairly uniform and have clear-to-eosinophilic cytoplasm, nuclei with vesicular chromatin and prominent nucleoli (Figure 14.13). Gastrointestinal CCSs often have osteoclast-like giant cells whereas soft tissue CCSs have multi-nucleated tumour giant cells with peripherally placed nuclei.

Virtually all soft tissue and gastrointestinal CCSs express S100 protein, with most soft tissue CCSs showing additional evidence of melanin production with the expression of HMB-45, Melan-A and MiTF [137–139], and ultrastructural evidence of melanocytic differentiation [137,140]. Most gastrointestinal CCSs lack evidence of melanin production by immunohistochemistry [135]. Soft tissue and gastrointestinal CCSs are cytogenetically similar, with both lesions having an alteration of EWS (22q12). Most soft tissue CCSs have a t(12,22)(q13;q12), resulting in an EWS–ATF1 fusion protein [141–143], whereas several gastrointestinal CCSs have been shown to harbour a EWS–CREB1 fusion protein [144].

The number of cases with follow-up is limited. However, gastrointestinal CCSs appear to have aggressive behaviour with frequent regional lymph node and liver metastases [135].

Synovial sarcoma of the stomach

Synovial sarcoma typically occurs in the extremities and histologically may be monophasic, biphasic or poorly differentiated. These lesions are typified by a characteristic t(X;18)(p11;q11) that results in a SYT–SSX fusion transcript. Rare cases of synovial sarcoma have been documented within the gastrointestinal tract [145,146]. Makhlouf et al. compiled 10 gastric synovial sarcomas, the largest series to date. They reported a roughly equal gender distribution, a mean age of 52 and a mean tumour size of 30 mm [146]. Histologically, nine of the lesions were monophasic, with one having a poorly differentiated component, and the tenth lesion was biphasic. The SYT–SSX fusion transcript was identified in all cases tested. Similar to their peripheral counterparts, focal cytokeratin or EMA expression was noted; there was no expression of CD34 or KIT. The prognosis was variable and appeared to depend on tumour size and differentiation, with large tumours and those containing a poorly differentiated component having aggressive behaviour [146].

Gastroblastoma

Two groups have recently published reports of a novel epithelio-mesenchymal biphasic tumour of the stomach or so called 'gastroblastoma' [147,148]. In both accounts, the lesions occurred in a young population (age range 9–30 years) and measured from 50 mm to 150 mm. The biphasic components include uniform spindled cells in diffuse sheets and epithelial cells in clusters or cords, with rare glandular structures with small lumina. The epithelial components express cytokeratin AE1/AE3 and low-molecular-weight cytokeratin, whereas high-molecular-weight cytokeratin was negative. EMA expression was variable in the two studies. The spindle cell component was immunoreactivity for CD10, although there was no expression of CD34 or KIT. Importantly, none of these lesions had evidence of a SYT gene rearrangement, distinguishing them from synovial sarcoma. In the series by Miettinen et al., no recurrent or metastatic disease has been noted in follow-up at 3.5, 5 and 14 years. However, given the limited number of cases, the prognosis of gastroblastoma is uncertain and the authors of this series suggest that these lesions should be considered low grade malignant [147].

Calcifying fibrous tumour of the stomach

Calcifying fibrous tumour (CFT) is a rare benign tumour characterised histologically by hyalinised fibrous tissue with a variable lymphoplasmacytic inflammatory cell infiltrate, bland fibroblasts and psammomatous and/or dystrophic calcifications. CFT most commonly develops in the

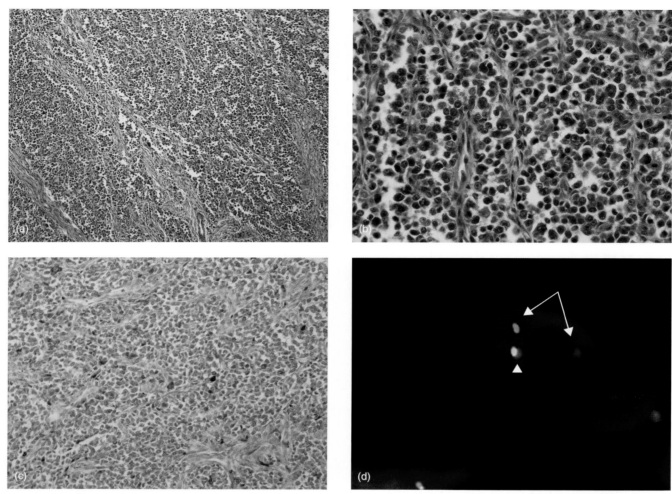

Figure 14.13 Clear cell sarcoma (CCS): (a) the typical nested architecture secondary to prominent fibrous septa that divide the tumour. (b) The cells composing the lesion are fairly uniform with clear-to-eosinophilic cytoplasm, nuclei with vesicular chromatin and prominent nucleoli. (c) S100 immunoreactivity within a gastrointestinal CCS. (d) A fluorescence *in situ* hybridisation assay using a break-apart probe for rearrangements in *EWS* (22q12) shows evidence of an *EWS* rearrangement, with the arrows highlighting a split signal (translocated) and the arrowhead denoting a fused (normal) signal within the same cell. (Case courtesy of Dr David Schuetze.)

abdominal cavity and peritoneum [149]. Their occurrence within the gastrointestinal tract is rare and Agaimy et al. [150] have published the largest case series of gastric CFTs to date. In their series, most gastric CFTs were identified incidentally post mortem or during the investigation or treatment of a different disease process. The lesions predominantly arose within the body of the stomach and involved the muscularis propria with a mean size of around 20 mm. In contrast to peritoneal CFTs, which are commonly multifocal, gastric CFTs are unifocal. Some authors have proposed that CFTs may represent a sclerosing phase of inflammatory myofibroblastic tumour (IMT). However, the characteristic expression of ALK-1 present in IMTs has not been identified in two series specifically addressing this in CFTs [151,152]. Immunohistochemically, gastric CFTs are negative for S100 protein, smooth muscle actin, KIT, desmin, ALK-1 and h-caldesmon, whereas molecular analysis has not identified mutations within *KIT* or *PDGFRA* [150]. Although follow-up is limited, recurrences and metastatic disease have not been documented.

References

1. Miettinen M, Monihan JM, Sarlomo-Rikala M, et al. Gastrointestinal stromal tumors/smooth muscle tumors (GISTs) primary in the omentum and mesentery: clinicopathologic and immunohistochemical study of 26 cases. *Am J Surg Pathol* 1999;**23**:1109.
2. Reith JD, Goldblum JR, Lyles RH, Weiss SW. Extragastrointestinal (soft tissue) stromal tumors: an analysis of 48 cases with emphasis on histologic predictors of outcome. *Mod Pathol* 2000;**13**:577.

3. Golden T, Stout AP. Smooth muscle tumors of the gastrointestinal tract and retroperitoneal tissues. *Surg Gynecol Obstet* 1941;**73**:784.

4. Evans HL. Smooth muscle tumors of the gastrointestinal tract. A study of 56 cases followed for a minimum of 10 years. *Cancer* 1985;**56**:2242.

5. Appelman HD. Smooth muscle tumors of the gastrointestinal tract. What we know now that Stout didn't know. *Am J Surg Pathol* 1986;**10**(suppl 1):83.

6. Kindblom LG, Remotti HE, Aldenborg F, Meis-Kindblom JM. Gastrointestinal pacemaker cell tumor (GIPACT): gastrointestinal stromal tumors show phenotypic characteristics of the interstitial cells of Cajal. *Am J Pathol* 1998;**152**:1259.

7. Huizinga JD, Thuneberg L, Kluppel M, et al. W/kit gene required for interstitial cells of Cajal and for intestinal pacemaker activity. *Nature* 1995;**373**:347.

8. Kluppel M, Huizinga JD, Malysz J, Bernstein A. Developmental origin and Kit-dependent development of the interstitial cells of Cajal in the mammalian small intestine. *Dev Dyn* 1998;**211**:60.

9. Sanders KM. A case for interstitial cells of Cajal as pacemakers and mediators of neurotransmission in the gastrointestinal tract. *Gastroenterology* 1996;**11**:492.

10. Thuneberg L. Interstitial cells of Cajal: intestinal pacemaker cells? *Adv Anat Embryol Cell Biol* 1982;**71**:1.

11. Chan JK. Mesenchymal tumors of the gastrointestinal tract: a paradise for acronyms (STUMP, GIST, GANT and now GIPACT), implication of c-kit in genesis and yet another of the many emerging roles of the interstitial cell of Cajal in the pathogenesis of gastrointestinal diseases? *Adv Anat Pathol* 1999;**6**:19.

12. Lee JC, Thuneberg L, Berezin I, Huizinga JD. Generation of slow waves in membrane potential is an intrinsic property of interstitial cells of Cajal. *Am J Physiol* 1999;**277**(2 Part 1):G409.

13. Rumessen JJ, Thuneberg L. Interstitial cells of Cajal in human small intestine. Ultrastructural identification and organization between the main smooth muscle layers. *Gastroenterology* 1991;**100**(5 Part 1):1417.

14. Miettinen M, Sarlomo-Rikala M, Lasota J. Gastrointestinal stromal tumors: recent advances in understanding of their biology. *Hum Pathol* 1999;**30**:1213.

15. Maeda H, Yamagata A, Nishikawa S, et al. Requirement of c-kit for development of intestinal pacemaker system. *Development* 1992;**116**:369.

16. Ronnstrand L. Signal transduction via the stem cell factor receptor/c-Kit. *Cell Mol Life Sci* 2004;**61**:2535.

17. Blume-Jensen P, Claesson-Welsh L, Siegbahn A, et al. Activation of the human c-kit product by ligand-induced dimerization mediates circular actin reorganization and chemotaxis. *EMBO J* 1991;**10**:4121.

18. Hirota S, Isozaki K, Moriyama Y, et al. Gain-of-function mutations of c-kit in human gastrointestinal stromal tumors. *Science* 1998;**279**:577.

19. Rubin BP, Singer S, Tsao C, et al. KIT activation is a ubiquitous feature of gastrointestinal stromal tumors. *Cancer Res* 2001;**61**:8118.

20. Heinrich MC, Corless CL, Demetri GD, et al. Kinase mutations and imatinib response in patients with metastatic gastrointestinal stromal tumor. *J Clin Oncol* 2003;**21**:4342.

21. Mol CD, Dougan DR, Schneider TR, et al. Structural basis for the autoinhibition and STI-571 inhibition of c-Kit tyrosine kinase. *J Biol Chem* 2004;**279**:31655.

22. Chan PM, Ilangumaran S, La Rose J, Chakrabartty A, Rottapel R. Autoinhibition of the kit receptor tyrosine kinase by the cytosolic juxtamembrane region. *Mol Cell Biol* 2003;**23**:3067.

23. Kitayama H, Kanakura Y, Furitsu T, et al. Constitutively activating mutations of c-kit receptor tyrosine kinase confer factor-independent growth and tumorigenicity of factor-dependent hematopoietic cell lines. *Blood* 1995;**85**:790.

24. Ma Y, Cunningham ME, Wang X, et al. Inhibition of spontaneous receptor phosphorylation by residues in a putative alpha-helix in the KIT intracellular juxtamembrane region. *J Biol Chem* 1999;**274**:13399.

25. Lasota J, Wozniak A, Sarlomo-Rikala M, et al. Mutations in exons 9 and 13 of KIT gene are rare events in gastrointestinal stromal tumors. A study of 200 cases. *Am J Pathol* 2000;**157**:1091.

26. Lux ML, Rubin BP, Biase TL, et al. KIT extracellular and kinase domain mutations in gastrointestinal stromal tumors. *Am J Pathol* 2000;**156**:791.

27. Heinrich MC, Corless CL, Duensing A, et al. PDGFRA activating mutations in gastrointestinal stromal tumors. *Science* 2003;**299**:708.

28. Hirota S, Ohashi A, Nishida T, et al. Gain-of-function mutations of platelet-derived growth factor receptor alpha gene in gastrointestinal stromal tumors. *Gastroenterology* 2003;**125**:6607.

29. Corless CL, McGreevey L, Haley A, Town A, Heinrich MC. KIT mutations are common in incidental gastrointestinal stromal tumors one centimeter or less in size. *Am J Pathol* 2002;**160**:1567.

30. Agaimy A, Wunsch PH, Hofstaedter F, et al. Minute gastric sclerosing stromal tumors (GIST tumorlets) are common in adults and frequently show c-KIT mutations. *Am J Surg Pathol* 2007;**31**:113.

31. Fletcher CD, Berman JJ, Corless C, et al. Diagnosis of gastrointestinal stromal tumors: A consensus approach. *Hum Pathol* 2002;**33**:459.

32. Kindblom LG, Meis-Kindblom JM, Bumming P. Incidence, prevalence, phenotype and biologic spectrum of gastrointestinal stromal cell tumors (GIST) – a population-based study of 600 cases *Ann Oncol* 2002;**13**(suppl 5):157.

33. Mucciarini C, Rossi G, Bertolini F, et al. Incidence and clinicopathologic features of gastrointestinal stromal tumors. A population-based study. *BMC Cancer* 2007;**7**:230.

34. Nilsson B, Bumming P, Meis-Kindblom JM, et al. Gastrointestinal stromal tumors: the incidence, prevalence, clinical course and prognostication in the preimatinib mesylate era – a population-based study in western Sweden. *Cancer* 2005;**103**:821.

35. Steigen SE, Eide TJ. Trends in incidence and survival of mesenchymal neoplasm of the digestive tract within a defined population of northern Norway. *APMIS* 2006;**114**:192.

36. DeMatteo RP, Lewis JJ, Leung D, et al. Two hundred gastrointestinal stromal tumors: recurrence patterns and prognostic factors for survival. *Ann Surg* 2000;**231**:51.

37. Abraham SC, Krasinskas AM, Hofstetter WL, Swisher SG, Wu TT. 'Seedling' mesenchymal tumors (gastrointestinal stromal tumors and leiomyomas) are common incidental tumors of the esophagogastric junction. *Am J Surg Pathol* 2007;**31**:1629.

38. Demetri GD, Benjamin RS, Blanke CD, et al. NCCN Task Force report: management of patients with gastrointestinal stromal tumor (GIST) – update of the NCCN clinical practice guidelines. *J Natl Compr Canc Netw* 2007;**5**(suppl 2):S1;quiz S30.

39. Miettinen M, Furlong M, Sarlomo-Rikala M, et al. Gastrointestinal stromal tumors, intramural leiomyomas and leiomyosarcomas in the rectum and anus: a clinicopathologic, immunohistochemical and molecular genetic study of 144 cases. *Am J Surg Pathol* 2001;**25**:1121.

40. Zhang L, Smyrk TC, Young WF Jr, Stratakis CA, Carney JA. Gastric stromal tumors in Carney triad are different clinically, pathologically and behaviorally from sporadic gastric gastrointestinal stromal tumors: findings in 104 cases. *Am J Surg Pathol* 2010;**34**:53.

41. Miettinen M, Sobin LH, Lasota J. Gastrointestinal stromal tumors of the stomach: a clinicopathologic, immunohistochemical and

molecular genetic study of 1765 cases with long-term follow-up. *Am J Surg Pathol* 2005;**29**:52.

42. Wasag B, Debiec-Rychter M, Pauwels P, et al. Differential expression of KIT/PDGFRA mutant isoforms in epithelioid and mixed variants of gastrointestinal stromal tumors depends predominantly on the tumor site. *Mod Pathol* 2004;**17**:889.

43. Trupiano JK, Stewart RE, Misick C, Appelman HD, Goldblum JR. Gastric stromal tumors: a clinicopathologic study of 77 cases with correlation of features with nonaggressive and aggressive clinical behaviors. *Am J Surg Pathol* 2002;**26**:705.

44. Cornog JL Jr. Gastric leiomyoblastoma. A clinical and ultrastructural study. *Cancer* 1974;**34**:711.

45. Sarlomo-Rikala M, Kovatich AJ, Barusevicius A, Miettinen M. CD117: a sensitive marker for gastrointestinal stromal tumors that is more specific than CD34. *Mod Pathol* 1998;**11**:728.

46. Medeiros F, Corless CL, Duensing A, et al. KIT-negative gastrointestinal stromal tumors: proof of concept and therapeutic implications. *Am J Surg Pathol* 2004;**28**:889.

47. Debiec-Rychter M, Wasag B, Stul M, et al. Gastrointestinal stromal tumours (GISTs) negative for KIT (CD117 antigen) immunoreactivity. *J Pathol* 2004;**202**:430.

48. van de Rijn M, Hendrickson MR, Rouse RV. CD34 expression by gastrointestinal tract stromal tumors. *Hum Pathol* 1994;**25**:766.

49. Miettinen M, Virolainen M, Maarit Sarlomo R. Gastrointestinal stromal tumors – value of CD34 antigen in their identification and separation from true leiomyomas and schwannomas. *Am J Surg Pathol* 1995;**19**:207.

50. West RB, Corless CL, Chen X, et al. The novel marker, DOG1, is expressed ubiquitously in gastrointestinal stromal tumors irrespective of KIT or PDGFRA mutation status. *Am J Pathol* 2004;**165**:107.

51. Caputo A, Caci E, Ferrera L, et al. TMEM16A, a membrane protein associated with calcium-dependent chloride channel activity. *Science* 2008;**322**:590.

52. Yang YD, Cho H, Koo JY, et al. TMEM16A confers receptor-activated calcium-dependent chloride conductance. *Nature* 2008;**455**:1210.

53. Espinosa I, Lee CH, Kim MK, et al. A novel monoclonal antibody against DOG1 is a sensitive and specific marker for gastrointestinal stromal tumors. *Am J Surg Pathol* 2008;**32**:210.

54. Liegl B, Hornick JL, Corless CL, Fletcher CD. Monoclonal antibody DOG1.1 shows higher sensitivity than KIT in the diagnosis of gastrointestinal stromal tumors, including unusual subtypes. *Am J Surg Pathol* 2009;**33**:437.

55. Miettinen M, Wang ZF, Lasota J. DOG1 antibody in the differential diagnosis of gastrointestinal stromal tumors: a study of 1840 cases. *Am J Surg Pathol* 2009;**33**:1401.

56. Nielsen TO, West RB, Linn SC, et al. Molecular characterisation of soft tissue tumours: a gene expression study. *Lancet* 2002;**359**:1301.

57. Allander SV, Nupponen NN, Ringner M, et al. Gastrointestinal stromal tumors with KIT mutations exhibit a remarkably homogeneous gene expression profile. *Cancer Res* 2001;**61**:8624.

58. Blay P, Astudillo A, Buesa JM, et al. Protein kinase C theta is highly expressed in gastrointestinal stromal tumors but not in other mesenchymal neoplasias. *Clin Cancer Res* 2004;**10**:4089.

59. Miettinen M, Kopczynski J, Makhlouf HR, et al. Gastrointestinal stromal tumors, intramural leiomyomas and leiomyosarcomas in the duodenum: a clinicopathologic, immunohistochemical and molecular genetic study of 167 cases. *Am J Surg Pathol* 2003;**27**:625.

60. Johnstone JM, Morson BC. Inflammatory fibroid polyp of the gastrointestinal tract. *Histopathology* 1978;**2**:349.

61. Hasegawa T, Yang P, Kagawa N, Hirose T, Sano T. CD34 expression by inflammatory fibroid polyps of the stomach. *Mod Pathol* 1997;**10**:451.

62. Schildhaus HU, Cavlar T, Binot E, et al. Inflammatory fibroid polyps harbour mutations in the platelet-derived growth factor receptor alpha (*PDGFRA*) gene. *J Pathol* 2008;**216**:176.

63. Bhattacharya B, Dilworth HP, Iacobuzio-Donahue C, et al. Nuclear beta-catenin expression distinguishes deep fibromatosis from other benign and malignant fibroblastic and myofibroblastic lesions. *Am J Surg Pathol* 2005;**29**:653.

64. Yantiss RK, Spiro IJ, Compton CC, Rosenberg AE. Gastrointestinal stromal tumor versus intra-abdominal fibromatosis of the bowel wall: a clinically important differential diagnosis. *Am J Surg Pathol* 2000;**24**:947.

65. Went PT, Dirnhofer S, Bundi M, et al. Prevalence of KIT expression in human tumors. *J Clin Oncol* 2004;**22**:4514.

66. Willmore-Payne C, Holden JA, Tripp S, Layfield LJ. Human malignant melanoma: detection of BRAF- and c-kit-activating mutations by high-resolution amplicon melting analysis. *Hum Pathol* 2005;**36**:486.

67. Antonescu CR, Busam KJ, Francone TD, et al. L576P KIT mutation in anal melanomas correlates with KIT protein expression and is sensitive to specific kinase inhibition. *Int J Cancer* 2007;**121**:257.

68. Miettinen M, Lasota J. Gastrointestinal stromal tumors – definition, clinical, histological, immunohistochemical and molecular genetic features and differential diagnosis. *Virchows Arch* 2001;**438**:1.

69. Rubin BP, Heinrich MC, Corless CL. Gastrointestinal stromal tumour. *Lancet* 2007;**369**:1731.

70. Miettinen M, Makhlouf H, Sobin LH, Lasota J. Gastrointestinal stromal tumors of the jejunum and ileum: a clinicopathologic, immunohistochemical and molecular genetic study of 906 cases before imatinib with long-term follow-up. *Am J Surg Pathol* 2006;**30**:477.

71. Koay MH, Goh YW, Iacopetta B, et al. Gastrointestinal stromal tumours (GISTs): a clinicopathological and molecular study of 66 cases. *Pathology* 2005;**37**:22.

72. Tryggvason G, Gislason HG, Magnusson MK, Jonasson JG. Gastrointestinal stromal tumors in Iceland, 1990–2003: the Icelandic GIST study, a population-based incidence and pathologic risk stratification study. *Int J Cancer* 2005;**117**:289.

73. Takahashi T, Nakajima K, Nishitani A, et al. An enhanced risk-group stratification system for more practical prognostication of clinically malignant gastrointestinal stromal tumors. *Int J Clin Oncol* 2007;**12**:369.

74. Ng EH, Pollock RE, Romsdahl MM. Prognostic implications of patterns of failure for gastrointestinal leiomyosarcomas. *Cancer* 1992;**69**:1334.

75. Ng EH, Pollock RE, Munsell MF, Atkinson EN, Romsdahl MM. Prognostic factors influencing survival in gastrointestinal leiomyosarcomas. Implications for surgical management and staging. *Ann Surg* 1992;**215**:68.

76. Rutkowski P, Nowecki ZI, Michej W, et al. Risk criteria and prognostic factors for predicting recurrences after resection of primary gastrointestinal stromal tumor. *Ann Surg Oncol* 2007;**14**:2018.

77. Debiec-Rychter M, Dumez H, Judson I, et al. Use of c-KIT/PDGFRA mutational analysis to predict the clinical response to imatinib in patients with advanced gastrointestinal stromal tumours entered on phase I and II studies of the EORTC Soft Tissue and Bone Sarcoma Group. *Eur J Cancer* 2004;**40**:689.

78. Debiec-Rychter M, Sciot R, Le Cesne A, et al. KIT mutations and dose selection for imatinib in patients with advanced gastrointestinal stromal tumours. *Eur J Cancer* 2006;**42**:1093.

79. Heinrich MC, Owzar K, Corless CL, et al. Correlation of kinase genotype and clinical outcome in the North American Intergroup Phase III Trial of imatinib mesylate for treatment of advanced gastrointestinal stromal tumor: CALGB 150105 Study by Cancer and Leukemia Group B and Southwest Oncology Group. *J Clin Oncol* 2008;**26**:5360.

80. Heinrich MC, Corless CL, Blanke CD, et al. Molecular correlates of imatinib resistance in gastrointestinal stromal tumors. *J Clin Oncol* 2006;**24**:4764.

81. Antonescu CR, Besmer P, Guo T, et al. Acquired resistance to imatinib in gastrointestinal stromal tumor occurs through secondary gene mutation. *Clin Cancer Res* 2005;**11**:4182.

82. Chen LL, Trent JC, Wu EF, et al. A missense mutation in KIT kinase domain 1 correlates with imatinib resistance in gastrointestinal stromal tumors. *Cancer Res* 2004;**64**:5913.

83. Debiec-Rychter M, Cools J, Dumez H, et al. Mechanisms of resistance to imatinib mesylate in gastrointestinal stromal tumors and activity of the PKC412 inhibitor against imatinib-resistant mutants. *Gastroenterology* 2005;**128**:270.

84. Maeyama H, Hidaka E, Ota H, Minami S, et al. Familial gastrointestinal stromal tumor with hyperpigmentation: association with a germline mutation of the c-kit gene. *Gastroenterology* 2001;**120**:210.

85. Isozaki K, Terris B, Belghiti J, et al. Germline-activating mutation in the kinase domain of KIT gene in familial gastrointestinal stromal tumors. *Am J Pathol* 2000;**157**:1581.

86. Beghini A, Tibiletti MG, Roversi G, et al. Germline mutation in the juxtamembrane domain of the kit gene in a family with gastrointestinal stromal tumors and urticaria pigmentosa. *Cancer* 2001;**92**:657.

87. Chompret A, Kannengiesser C, Barrois M, et al. PDGFRA germline mutation in a family with multiple cases of gastrointestinal stromal tumor. *Gastroenterology* 2004;**126**:318.

88. Hirota S, Okazaki T, Kitamura Y, et al. Cause of familial and multiple gastrointestinal autonomic nerve tumors with hyperplasia of interstitial cells of Cajal is germline mutation of the c-kit gene. *Am J Surg Pathol* 2000;**24**:326.

89. Li FP, Fletcher JA, Heinrich MC, et al. Familial gastrointestinal stromal tumor syndrome: phenotypic and molecular features in a kindred. *J Clin Oncol* 2005;**23**:2735.

90. Carballo M, Roig I, Aguilar F, et al. Novel c-KIT germline mutation in a family with gastrointestinal stromal tumors and cutaneous hyperpigmentation. *Am J Med Genet A* 2005;**132**:361.

91. Lasota J, Miettinen M. A new familial GIST identified. *Am J Surg Pathol* 2006;**30**:1342.

92. Hartmann K, Wardelmann E, Ma Y, et al. Novel germline mutation of KIT associated with familial gastrointestinal stromal tumors and mastocytosis. *Gastroenterology* 2005;**129**:1042.

93. Zoller ME, Rembeck B, Oden A, Samuelsson M, Angervall L. Malignant and benign tumors in patients with neurofibromatosis type 1 in a defined Swedish population. *Cancer* 1997;**79**:2125.

94. Min KW, Balaton AJ. Small intestinal stromal tumors with skeinoid fibers in neurofibromatosis: report of four cases with ultrastructural study of skeinoid fibers from paraffin blocks. *Ultrastruct Pathol* 1993;**17**:307.

95. Yantiss RK, Rosenberg AE, Sarran L, Besmer P, Antonescu CR. Multiple gastrointestinal stromal tumors in type I neurofibromatosis: a pathologic and molecular study. *Mod Pathol* 2005;**18**:475.

96. Takazawa Y, Sakurai S, Sakuma Y, et al. Gastrointestinal stromal tumors of neurofibromatosis type I (von Recklinghausen's disease). *Am J Surg Pathol* 2005;**29**:755.

97. Carney JA. Gastric stromal sarcoma, pulmonary chondroma and extra-adrenal paraganglioma (Carney Triad): natural history, adrenocortical component and possible familial occurrence. *Mayo Clin Proc* 1999;**74**:543.

98. Diment J, Tamborini E, Casali P, Gronchi A, Carney JA, Colecchia M. Carney triad: case report and molecular analysis of gastric tumor. *Hum Pathol* 2005;**36**:112.

99. Sarlomo-Rikala M, Miettinen M. Gastric schwannoma – a clinicopathological analysis of six cases. *Histopathology* 1995;**27**:355.

100. Miettinen M, Shekitka KM, Sobin LH. Schwannomas in the colon and rectum: a clinicopathologic and immunohistochemical study of 20 cases. *Am J Surg Pathol* 2001;**25**:846.

101. Daimaru Y, Kido H, Hashimoto H, Enjoji M. Benign schwannoma of the gastrointestinal tract: a clinicopathologic and immunohistochemical study. *Hum Pathol* 1988;**19**:257.

102. Agaimy A, Markl B, Kitz J, et al. Peripheral nerve sheath tumors of the gastrointestinal tract: a multicenter study of 58 patients including NF1-associated gastric schwannoma and unusual morphologic variants. *Virchows Arch* 2010;**456**:411.

103. Johnston J, Helwig EB. Granular cell tumors of the gastrointestinal tract and perianal region: a study of 74 cases. *Dig Dis Sci* 1981;**26**:807.

104. Filie AC, Lage JM, Azumi N. Immunoreactivity of S100 protein, alpha-1-antitrypsin and CD68 in adult and congenital granular cell tumors. *Mod Pathol* 1996;**9**:888.

105. Kurtin PJ, Bonin DM. Immunohistochemical demonstration of the lysosome-associated glycoprotein CD68 (KP-1) in granular cell tumors and schwannomas. *Hum Pathol* 1994;**25**:1172.

106. Fanburg-Smith JC, Meis-Kindblom JM, Fante R, Kindblom LG. Malignant granular cell tumor of soft tissue: diagnostic criteria and clinicopathologic correlation. *Am J Surg Pathol* 1998;**22**:779.

107. Agaimy A, Wunsch PH. True smooth muscle neoplasms of the gastrointestinal tract: morphological spectrum and classification in a series of 85 cases from a single institute. *Langenbecks Arch Surg* 2007;**392**:75.

108. Miettinen M, Sarlomo-Rikala M, Sobin LH, Lasota J. Gastrointestinal stromal tumors and leiomyosarcomas in the colon: a clinicopathologic, immunohistochemical and molecular genetic study of 44 cases. *Am J Surg Pathol* 2000;**24**:1339.

109. Hashimoto H, Tsuneyoshi M, Enjoji M. Malignant smooth muscle tumors of the retroperitoneum and mesentery: a clinicopathologic analysis of 44 cases. *J Surg Oncol* 1985;**28**:177.

110. Rajani B, Smith TA, Reith JD, Goldblum JR. Retroperitoneal leiomyosarcomas unassociated with the gastrointestinal tract: a clinicopathologic analysis of 17 cases. *Mod Pathol* 1999;**12**:21.

111. Trojani M, Contesso G, Coindre JM, et al. Soft tissue sarcomas of adults: study of pathological prognostic variables and definition of a histopathological grading system. *Int J Cancer* 1984;**33**:37.

112. Lee HW, Lee JJ, Yang DH, Lee BH. A clinicopathologic study of glomus tumor of the stomach. *J Clin Gastroenterol* 2006;**40**:717.

113. Miettinen M, Paal E, Lasota J, Sobin LH. Gastrointestinal glomus tumors: a clinicopathologic, immunohistochemical and molecular genetic study of 32 cases. *Am J Surg Pathol* 2002;**26**:301.

114. Allison KH, Yoder BJ, Bronner MP, Goldblum JR, Rubin BP. Angiosarcoma involving the gastrointestinal tract: a series of primary and metastatic cases. *Am J Surg Pathol* 2004;**28**:298.

115. Kim TO, Kim GH, Heo J, Kang DH, Song GA, Cho M. Metastasis of hepatic angiosarcoma to the stomach. *J Gastroenterol* 2005;**40**:1003.

116. Danzig JB, Brandt LJ, Reinus JF, Klein RS. Gastrointestinal malignancy in patients with AIDS. *Am J Gastroenterol* 1991;**86**:715.

117. Friedman SL, Wright TL, Altman DF. Gastrointestinal Kaposi's sarcoma in patients with acquired immunodeficiency syndrome. Endoscopic and autopsy findings. *Gastroenterology* 1985;**89**:102.

118. Parente F, Cernuschi M, Orlando G, et al. Kaposi's sarcoma and AIDS: frequency of gastrointestinal involvement and its effect on survival. A prospective study in a heterogeneous population. *Scand J Gastroenterol* 1991;**26**:1007.

119. Weprin L, Zollinger R, Clausen K, Thomas FB. Kaposi's sarcoma: endoscopic observations of gastric and colon involvement. *J Clin Gastroenterol* 1982;**4**:357.

120. Cheuk W, Wong KO, Wong CS, et al. Immunostaining for human herpesvirus 8 latent nuclear antigen-1 helps distinguish Kaposi sarcoma from its mimickers. *Am J Clin Pathol* 2004;**121**:335.

121. Patel RM, Goldblum JR, Hsi ED. Immunohistochemical detection of human herpes virus-8 latent nuclear antigen-1 is useful in the diagnosis of Kaposi sarcoma. *Mod Pathol* 2004;**17**:456.

122. Bijlani RS, Kulkarni VM, Shahani RB, et al. Gastric lipoma presenting as obstruction and hematemesis. *J Postgrad Med* 1993;**39**:42.

123. Alberti D, Grazioli L Orizio P, et al. Asymptomatic giant gastric lipoma: What to do? *Am J Gastroenterol* 1999;**94**:3634.

124. Fletcher CD, Akerman M, Dal Cin P, et al. Correlation between clinicopathological features and karyotype in lipomatous tumors. A report of 178 cases from the Chromosomes and Morphology (CHAMP) Collaborative Study Group. *Am J Pathol* 1996;**148**:623.

125. Rosai J, Akerman M, Dal Cin P, et al. Combined morphologic and karyotypic study of 59 atypical lipomatous tumors. Evaluation of their relationship and differential diagnosis with other adipose tissue tumors (a report of the CHAMP Study Group). *Am J Surg Pathol* 1996;**20**:1182.

126. Weaver J, Downs-Kelly E, Goldblum JR, et al. Fluorescence in situ hybridization for MDM2 gene amplification as a diagnostic tool in lipomatous neoplasms. *Mod Pathol* 2008;**21**:9439.

127. Galant C, Rousseau E, Ho Minh Duc DK, Pauwels P. Re: Plexiform angiomyxoid myofibroblastic tumor of the stomach. *Am J Surg Pathol* 2008;**32**:1910;author reply 1912.

128. Rau TT, Hartmann A, Dietmaier W, et al. Plexiform angiomyxoid myofibroblastic tumour: differential diagnosis of gastrointestinal stromal tumour in the stomach. *J Clin Pathol* 2008;**61**:1136.

129. Takahashi Y, Shimizu S, Ishida T, et al. Plexiform angiomyxoid myofibroblastic tumor of the stomach. *Am J Surg Pathol* 2007;**31**:724.

130. Yoshida A, Klimstra DS, Antonescu CR. Plexiform angiomyxoid tumor of the stomach. *Am J Surg Pathol* 2008;**32**:1910;author reply 1912.

131. Miettinen M, Makhlouf HR, Sobin LH, Lasota J. Plexiform fibromyxoma: a distinctive benign gastric antral neoplasm not to be confused with a myxoid GIST. *Am J Surg Pathol* 2009;**33**:1624.

132. Enzinger FM. Clear cell sarcoma of tendons and aponeuroses. An analysis of 21 cases. *Cancer* 1965;**18**:1163.

133. Pauwels P, Debiec-Rychter M, Sciot R, et al. Clear cell sarcoma of the stomach. *Histopathology* 2002;**41**:526.

134. Huang W, Zhang X, Li D, et al. Osteoclast-rich tumor of the gastrointestinal tract with features resembling those of clear cell sarcoma of soft parts. *Virchows Arch* 2006;**448**:200.

135. Zambrano E, Reyes-Mugica M, Franchi A, Rosai J. An osteoclast-rich tumor of the gastrointestinal tract with features resembling clear cell sarcoma of soft parts: reports of 6 cases of a GIST simulator. *Int J Surg Pathol* 2003;**11**:75.

136. Lagmay JP, Ranalli M, Arcila M, Baker P. Clear cell sarcoma of the stomach. *Pediatr Blood Cancer* 2009;**53**:214.

137. Kindblom LG, Lodding P, Angervall L. Clear-cell sarcoma of tendons and aponeuroses. An immunohistochemical and electron microscopic analysis indicating neural crest origin. *Virchows Arch A Pathol Anat Histopathol* 1983;**401**:109.

138. Mechtersheimer G, Tilgen W, Klar E, Moller P. Clear cell sarcoma of tendons and aponeuroses: case presentation with special reference to immunohistochemical findings. *Hum Pathol* 1989;**20**:914.

139. Swanson PE, Wick MR. Clear cell sarcoma. An immunohistochemical analysis of six cases and comparison with other epithelioid neoplasms of soft tissue. *Arch Pathol Lab Med* 1989;**113**:55.

140. Sara AS, Evans HL, Benjamin RS. Malignant melanoma of soft parts (clear cell sarcoma). A study of 17 cases, with emphasis on prognostic factors. *Cancer* 1990;**65**:367.

141. Lyle PL, Amato CM, Fitzpatrick JE, Robinson WA. Gastrointestinal melanoma or clear cell sarcoma? Molecular evaluation of 7 cases previously diagnosed as malignant melanoma. *Am J Surg Pathol* 2008;**32**:858.

142. Covinsky M, Gong S, Rajaram V, Perry A, Pfeifer J. EWS-ATF1 fusion transcripts in gastrointestinal tumors previously diagnosed as malignant melanoma. *Hum Pathol* 2005;**36**:74.

143. Sandberg AA, Bridge JA. Updates on the cytogenetics and molecular genetics of bone and soft tissue tumors: clear cell sarcoma (malignant melanoma of soft parts). *Cancer Genet Cytogenet* 2001;**130**:1.

144. Antonescu CR, Nafa K, Segal NH, Dal Cin P, Ladanyi M. EWS-CREB1: a recurrent variant fusion in clear cell sarcoma – association with gastrointestinal location and absence of melanocytic differentiation. *Clin Cancer Res* 2006;**12**:5356.

145. Billings SD, Meisner LF, Cummings OW, Tejada E. Synovial sarcoma of the upper digestive tract: a report of two cases with demonstration of the X;18 translocation by fluorescence *in situ* hybridization. *Mod Pathol* 2000;**13**:68.

146. Makhlouf HR, Ahrens W, Agarwal B, et al. Synovial sarcoma of the stomach: a clinicopathologic, immunohistochemical and molecular genetic study of 10 cases. *Am J Surg Pathol* 2008;**32**:275.

147. Miettinen M, Dow N, Lasota J, Sobin LH. A distinctive novel epitheliomesenchymal biphasic tumor of the stomach in young adults ('gastroblastoma'): a series of 3 cases. *Am J Surg Pathol* 2009;**33**:1370.

148. Shin DH, Lee JH, Kang HJ, et al. Novel epitheliomesenchymal biphasic stomach tumour (gastroblastoma) in a 9-year-old: morphological, ultrastructural and immunohistochemical findings. *J Clin Pathol* 2010;**63**:270.

149. Zamecnik M, Michal M, Boudova L, et al. CD34 expression in calcifying fibrous pseudotumours. *Histopathology* 2000;**46**:346.

150. Agaimy A, Bihl MP, Tornillo L, et al. Calcifying fibrous tumor of the stomach: clinicopathologic and molecular study of seven cases with literature review and reappraisal of histiogenesis. *Am J Surg Pathol* 2010;**34**:271.

151. Hill KA, Gonzalez-Crussi F, Chou PM. Calcifying fibrous pseudotumor versus inflammatory myofibroblastic tumor: a histological and immunohistochemical comparison. *Mod Pathol* 2001;**14**:784.

152. Sigel JE, Smith TA, Reight JD, Goldblum JR. Immunohistochemical analysis of anaplastic lymphoma kinase expression in deep soft tissue calcifying fibrous pseudotumor: evidence of a late sclerosing stage of inflammatory myofibroblastic tumor? *Ann Diagn Pathol* 2001;**5**:10.

CHAPTER 15

Lymphoid tumours of the stomach

Laurence de Leval

Centre Hospitalier Universitaire Vaudois, Lausanne, Switzerland

Introduction

The gastric mucosa is normally devoid of organised lymphoid tissue and any lymphoid proliferations represent pathological conditions broadly categorised as either benign lymphoid proliferations or malignant lymphomas. In this chapter, neoplastic lymphoproliferations are emphasised and benign lymphoid proliferations considered only in the context of the differential diagnosis. Lymphomas in the stomach may occur as either a primary gastric disease or secondary involvement from systemic disease. This distinction is relevant from a clinical and therapeutic prospective but is marked with controversy over the definition of primary extra-nodal lymphoma. Dawson's original criteria for primary gastric lymphoma [1] required the main disease to present in the stomach, with or without involvement of regional lymph nodes. Later, these criteria were relaxed to allow for contiguous involvement of other organs (i.e. liver, spleen) and for distant nodal disease, provided that the gastric lesion was the presenting site and constituted the bulk of the disease to which primary treatment needed to be directed [2,3].

Primary gastric lymphomas

Incidence and distribution

The gastrointestinal tract accounts for 30–50% of primary extra-nodal lymphomas and the stomach is the site most commonly involved (50–60% of cases) [2]. Although the overall incidence of non-epithelial tumours of the stomach is low compared with epithelial tumours, non-Hodgkin's lymphoma is the second most common neoplasm of the stomach, following adenocarcinoma [4]. In contrast, gastric involvement by Hodgkin's lymphoma is exceedingly rare [5]. However, in childhood, when the overall incidence of gastric tumours is low, lymphomas are the most common tumour type [6].

The incidence of non-Hodgkin's lymphomas has been reported to be increasing in recent decades, especially in extra-nodal forms [7]. Accordingly, there is evidence that primary gastric lymphoma is increasing in prevalence in western nations. However, the real increase is uncertain because of improvements in diagnostic procedures over the same period of time [8,9]. In fact, epidemiological studies also reveal considerable geographical variation in the prevalence of gastric lymphomas, perhaps related to variations in *Helicobacter pylori* colonisation, e.g. the incidence of gastric lymphoma in north-eastern Italy is more than 10 times higher than in England and Wales [10].

The classification of primary gastric lymphomas

Except for some organ-specific lymphomas and rare entities, most non-Hodgkin's lymphoma types listed in the WHO classification arise in the stomach with a marked preponderance of B-cell lymphomas. However, the relative prevalence of the various subtypes is considerably different from that of systemic lymphomas. The two most common primary gastric lymphomas, diffuse large B-cell lymphoma (DLBCL) and marginal zone lymphoma of the mucosa-associated lymphoid tissue (MALT) type (MALT lymphoma), together account for the vast majority of cases, whereas other lymphomas commonly associated

Morson and Dawson's Gastrointestinal Pathology, Fifth Edition. Edited by Neil A. Shepherd, Bryan F. Warren, Geraint T. Williams, Joel K. Greenson, Gregory Y. Lauwers and Marco R. Novelli.
© 2013 Blackwell Publishing Ltd. Published 2013 by Blackwell Publishing Ltd.

with nodal disease occur only rarely as primary gastric neoplasms [11,12]. Primary Hodgkin's lymphoma of the stomach is vanishingly rare and any suggested cases should be treated with extreme scepticism. The main histological types of primary gastric lymphoma are listed in Table 15.1.

General considerations on diagnostic procedures

The diagnosis of gastric lymphoma can be established on biopsy in the vast majority of cases but ascertaining the specific type requires an adequate number of biopsies from both macroscopically abnormal and normal mucosa. This

is of cardinal importance, because subtyping and grading of gastric lymphomas have been shown to be inaccurate in about 25% of cases in a multicentric study performed in the early 1990s [13].

Staging of gastric lymphoma

Establishing the anatomical extent of primary gastric lymphoma is important for therapeutic and prognostic purposes. However, there is little agreement on the most appropriate staging system and various different systems are currently used. The Ann Arbor system, originally developed for nodal lymphoma, is not optimal for primary extra-nodal lymphomas and several modifications have been proposed [14,15]. The Musshoff system, proposed in 1977, combines information on involvement of the wall of the gut (stage I_E) with involvement of local lymph nodes (stage II_{1E}), regional lymph nodes (stage II_{2E}), thoracic lymph nodes (stage III) and the spleen (stage III_S), whereas stage IV indicates dissemination to bone marrow and non-lymphoid viscera [14]. In 1993, an international workshop in Lugano proposed stage II_E for serosal penetration without lymph node involvement, in addition to the original definition of stage II as lymph node involvement [15].

In 2004, the European Gastro-Intestinal Lymphoma Study Group proposed the Paris staging system for primary gastrointestinal lymphomas, based on the TNM staging system for epithelial tumours [16]. A comparison of the staging systems currently in use is presented in Table 15.2.

General recommendations for staging procedures after the biopsy-proven diagnosis of gastric lymphoma are summarised in Table 15.3 [17]. Specific investigations may be required for specific subtypes. The general physical examination is often normal. However, special attention should be paid to the upper aerodigestive tract in order to exclude

---

Table 15.1 The main histological types of primary gastric lymphoma

B-cell lymphomas
Diffuse large B-cell lymphoma
  With MALT component
  Without MALT component
Marginal zone B-cell lymphoma of MALT type
Mantle cell lymphoma (malignant lymphomatous polyposis)
Burkitt's lymphoma

Miscellaneous rare types
T/NK-cell lymphomas
HTLV-1-associated adult T-cell lymphoma/leukaemia
Peripheral T-cell lymphoma, not otherwise specified
Anaplastic large cell lymphoma
Immunodeficiency-related lymphoproliferative diseases
HIV-associated lymphoproliferations
Post-transplant lymphoproliferative disorders
Congenital immunodeficiency lymphoproliferative diseases

HTLV-1, human T-lymphotropic virus; MALT, mucosa-associated lymphoid tissue; NK, natural killer.

Table 15.2 Staging systems for gastric lymphoma

Lymphoma extension	Musshoff system [14]	Lugano classification [15]	Paris staging system [16]
Gastric mucosa	I_{E1}	I[a]	T1m N0 M0
Gastric submucosa	I_{E2}	I	T1sm N0 M0
Gastric muscularis propria or subserosa	I_{E2}	I	T2 N0 M0
Penetration of gastric serosa without involvement of adjacent organs	I_{E2}	II_E	T3 N0 M0
Involvement of adjacent organs or structures	I_E	II_E	T4 N0 M0
Involvement of regional lymph nodes (peri-gastric and along the celiac artery)	II_{E1}	II_1	T1–3 N1 M0
Involvement of abdominal lymph nodes beyond the regional area	II_{E2}	II_2	T1–3 N2 M0
Involvement of extra-abdominal lymph nodes	III_E	IV	T1–4 N3 M0
Non-contiguous involvement of separate sites in the gastrointestinal tract	III_E	I	T1–4 N0–3 M1
Non-contiguous involvement of other tissues	IV_E	IV	T1–4 N0–3 M2
Bone marrow involvement	IV_E	IV	T1–4 N0–3 B1

[a]Stage I in the Lugano system is defined as disease confined to the gastrointestinal tract, including single primary or multiple non-contiguous foci.

Table 15.3 Investigative procedures at diagnosis for gastric lymphoma

Physical examination
   Upper aerodigestive tract
   Other MALT sites
Upper and lower gastrointestinal endoscopy with biopsies
CT scan (abdomen and chest)
Endoscopic ultrasonography
Positron emission tomography
Bone marrow examination
Laboratory studies: blood cell counts, lactate dehydrogenase and β_2-microglobulin serum levels

MALT, mucosa-associated lymphoid tissue.

synchronous involvement of Waldeyer's ring, which has been reported occasionally [18–20]. In the case of gastric MALT lymphoma, other sites sometimes involved by MALT should be examined (thyroid, salivary glands, conjunctiva), because simultaneous extra-digestive involvement occurs in about 10% of cases [21]. An endoscopic evaluation including, at least, meticulous oesophago-gastro-duodenoscopy is recommended. Lower intestinal endoscopy may also reveal additional foci of disease, especially in MALT lymphoma, whereas the procedure is optional for high grade tumours. Computed tomography (CT) scans of the abdomen and chest should also be performed to seek potential lymph node involvement and/or focal visceral lesions.

Endoscopic ultrasonography (EUS) is integrated into current standard staging procedures because it has proven highly useful for discerning the depth of invasion into the gastric wall and the presence of peri-gastric lymph nodes [22]. In some cases, the imaging pattern can evoke a specific histological type (e.g. diffuse superficial infiltration being more indicative of MALT lymphoma, whereas the presence of masses tends to correlate with high grade histology) [23]. Moreover, EUS has prognostic value in MALT lymphomas, as a greater depth of infiltration is associated with a greater risk of nodal involvement and a lesser chance of response to antibiotic therapy. The relevance of EUS in follow-up of gastric lymphoma is more controversial: some authors have found a correlation between normalisation of the EUS findings and the evolution of the histological lesions, whereas others could not confirm these observations [22].

The usefulness of [18F]fluoro-deoxyglucose positron emission tomography (18FDG-PET) has been documented for gastric DLBCLs because its sensitivity and specificity exceed that of CT [17,23]. One study reported that a higher intensity of uptake at diagnosis correlated with adverse prognosis [24]. It remains to be clarified whether residual 18FDG uptake on PET during follow-up is predictive of prognosis [24,25]. In contrast, 18FDG-PET for staging of MALT lymphomas is more controversial, because the degree of uptake is usually less evident and the signals more difficult to interpret [23].

Staging bone marrow aspiration and biopsy must be performed irrespective of histological type but lymphomatous involvement of bone marrow is infrequent (10–20% of gastric MALT lymphomas) [26,27].

Extra-nodal marginal zone lymphoma of MALT type (MALT lymphoma)

The concept that some extra-nodal, low grade, B-cell lymphomas are related to MALT was developed in the early 1980s by Isaacson and Wright, who observed that many primary gastrointestinal lymphomas recapitulate the histo-morphological features of lymphoid aggregates in the gut, as with Peyer's patches, rather than those of nodal lymphoid tissue, and are characterised by a distinctive indolent clinical course, possibly related to the homing properties of MALT B cells [28–30]. Investigation of other low grade B-cell lymphomas arising in diverse mucosal sites reinforced this concept and resulted in the establishment of the term 'MALT lymphoma' [29,31–33]. This category of B-cell lymphoma, which is formally termed 'extra-nodal marginal zone lymphoma of mucosa-associated lymphoid tissue' in the current WHO classification of tumours of lymphoid tissues, comprises 7–8% of all B-cell lymphomas and arises in a wide range of extra-nodal sites, most commonly involving the stomach (70% of cases) [34,35].

MALT lymphomas only rarely arise from native MALT: generally, they arise from MALT resulting from a chronic inflammatory disorder driven by an autoimmune process and/or infection. There is now compelling evidence that acquired MALT in the stomach, caused primarily by *H. pylori*-induced chronic active gastritis, provides the seed bed for MALT lymphoma [34,36].

Clinical features

Gastric MALT lymphoma occurs predominantly in male individuals over 50 years, with a peak incidence in the seventh decade, but cases have been reported in patients in their 30s or even younger [11,12,36,37]. Symptoms are non-specific but include abdominal pain, dyspepsia, bloating and heartburn, and resemble those of chronic gastritis or peptic ulcer disease. Bleeding, vomiting and weight loss are reported in fewer than a third of patients [37]. Systemic symptoms are uncommon.

Endoscopic and macroscopic features

The antrum is the most common site for gastric MALT lymphoma but any part of the stomach can be involved and multifocal involvement is common at the microscopic level [38]. Various endoscopic appearances can be observed such

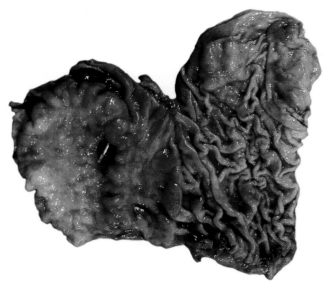

Figure 15.1 Macroscopic appearance of gastric mucosa-associated lymphoid tissue lymphoma surgically resected because of uncontrollable bleeding. The lymphoma formed one large elevated and ulcerated tumour mass and additional lesions manifested as mucosal fold thickening and nodularity. An endoscopic clip, to try to control bleeding, is seen in the base of a lymphoma-induced ulcer.

as ulcerative lesions, subtle features such as mucosal granularity and rugal fold thickening, and/or diffusely infiltrative, ill-defined lesions [3]. Occasionally, MALT lymphomas may form localised polypoid tumours [39]. However, in some cases, the mucosa may appear macroscopically normal or with slight petechiae only [37]. Deep infiltration, mass formation and ulceration occur (Figure 15.1) but less frequently than in high grade lymphomas.

Microscopic features

The histopathology of low grade MALT lymphoma closely recapitulates the characteristic features of normal intestinal Peyer's patches [40], which comprise lymphoid follicles composed of a reactive germinal centre surrounded by a mantle zone of small lymphocytes and a broad outer marginal zone in which most of the cells are small- to medium-sized B cells resembling germinal centre centrocytes (centrocyte-like cells) or monocytes (monocytoid B cells). The marginal zone extends towards the mucosal surface to form lympho-epithelial lesions that are a defining feature of MALT.

The diagnosis of MALT relies on three features reminiscent of Peyer's patches:
1. A diffuse and/or nodular infiltrate of neoplastic lymphoid B cells cytologically resembling marginal zone B cells and showing a marginal zone distribution

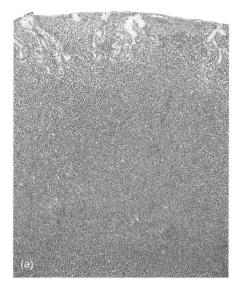

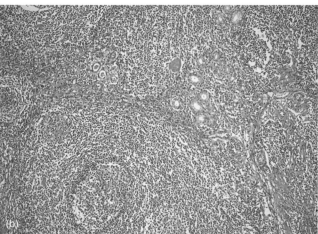

Figure 15.2 Patterns of infiltration of the neoplastic cells in gastric mucosa-associated lymphoid tissue lymphoma: (a) diffuse obliterative infiltrate throughout the mucosa and submucosa; (b) diffuse spread into the lamina propria from the marginal zone around reactive follicles.

2. Lympho-epithelial lesions
3. Reactive lymphoid follicles with germinal centres [3,35].

The neoplastic cells surround follicles corresponding to the marginal zone and spread diffusely into the surrounding mucosa (Figure 15.2). There is marked cytological variation, both within a given case and between cases. Most neoplastic cells are small lymphoid cells with irregular nuclei and scant cytoplasm (centrocyte-like cells). Some show features of medium-sized monocytoid cells, with abundant pale cytoplasm, well-defined cell membranes and round-to-oval, smoothly contoured nuclei. The proportion of cells with these features varies. In some tumours, there is a relatively monotonous population, whereas, in others, there is a mixture of cell types (Figure 15.3).

The neoplastic infiltrate also usually contains scattered, large, transformed blastic cells resembling centroblasts or immunoblasts. Plasma cell differentiation is seen in about 30% of cases and tends to be more prominent in the more superficial part of the lymphoma beneath the surface epithelium (Figure 15.4). The neoplastic plasma cells may appear as normal mature plasma cells, have crystalline inclusions in the cytoplasm and possess nuclei with Dutcher bodies. In some cases, intracytoplasmic immunoglobulin may be so abundant that the nucleus is pushed to one side and the cell resembles the signet-ring cells of diffuse-type adenocarcinoma [41].

Lympho-epithelial lesions (LELs) are an important and characteristic feature of gastric MALT lymphoma (Figure 15.5). LELs, which are reminiscent of the physiological involvement of dome epithelium seen in Peyer's patches, are defined as the invasion of individual crypts by aggregates (three or more) of neoplastic cells, eventually leading to degenerative changes or destruction and disintegration of the crypt epithelium. The degenerative changes manifest as eosinophilic and/or oncocytic changes. The number of LELs is variable: they are usually easily found but, occasionally, they are scarce and require a careful search that may be aided by immunohistochemical tools, especially cytokeratin immunohistochemistry, which highlights the associated epithelial destruction. Notably, although LELs in a lymphoproliferative lesion of the stomach are highly suggestive of MALT lymphoma, they are not specific for a diagnosis of malignancy and may be seen in non-MALT lymphomas as well.

An important component of MALT lymphomas are reactive lymphoid follicles, around which the neoplastic cells tend to be distributed. Moreover, neoplastic MALT lymphoid cells may invade the reactive germinal centres, producing so-called follicular colonisation (Figure 15.6) [42]. Eventually, the lymphoma may completely overrun and destroy the lymphoid follicles, leading to a nodular pattern and, sometimes, a resemblance to follicular lymphoma. Within the germinal centres, the neoplastic cells may undergo marked plasma cell differentiation or show blast cell transformation.

Gastric MALT lymphoma is usually multifocal and microscopic tumour foci may be seen throughout the gastric mucosa at a distance from the main tumour mass (Figure 15.7) [38]. Regional lymph node involvement may be subtle, because the lymphoma cells initially localise to the marginal zones without architectural distortion. Further involvement is characterised by marginal zone cells spreading to the interfollicular areas and producing confluent sheets of lymphoma cells. Follicular colonisation may also be seen in lymph nodes and mimic follicular lymphoma [35]. Gastric MALT lymphoma has also been shown to

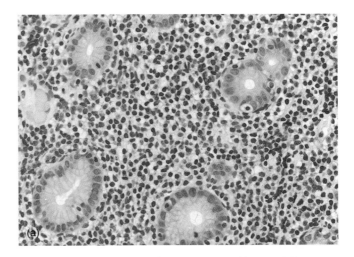

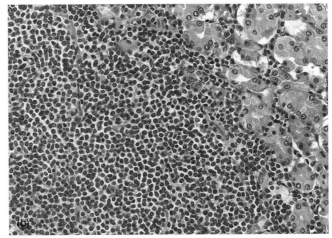

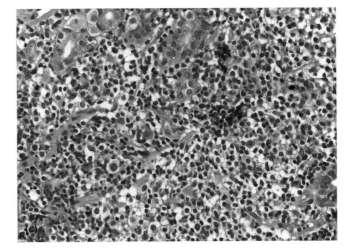

Figure 15.3 Cytological aspects of gastric mucosa-associated lymphoid tissue lymphoma: (a) small lymphoid cells with irregular nuclei and scant cytoplasm (centrocyte-like cells); (b) small lymphoid cells with more regular nuclei; and (c) small- to medium-sized lymphoid cells with abundant clear cytoplasm and scattered large blastic cells.

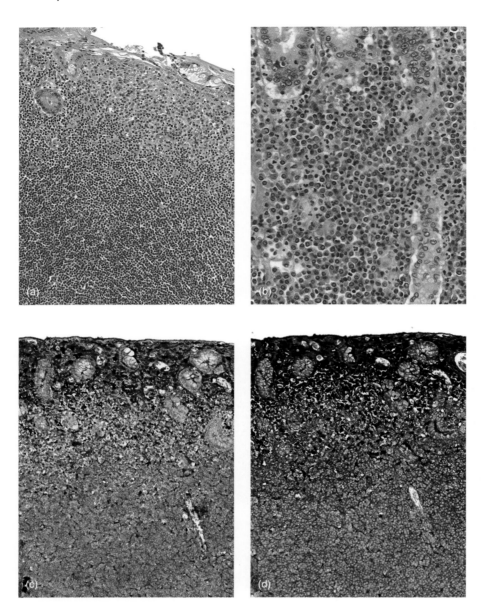

Figure 15.4 Gastric mucosa-associated lymphoid tissue lymphoma with plasma cell differentiation. The cells with plasma cell differentiation preferentially distribute in the upper mucosa (a) and frequently contain nuclear inclusions (Dutcher bodies) (b). There is monotypic λ light chain expression in both the lymphoid and plasma cell components (c, d); κ and λ, immunoperoxidase.

disseminate preferentially to the marginal zone of the spleen [43]. Bone marrow involvement is infrequent (10–20% of cases) and occurs as inter-trabecular aggregates of neoplastic B cells [27].

Immunophenotype and the normal cell counterpart

The neoplastic cells of MALT lymphoma show immunophenotypic similarities to normal marginal zone B cells. They express CD20 and other B-cell antigens and are negative for CD5, with few exceptions [44,45]. They usually express IgM and are generally negative for IgD [46]. Occasional cases are positive for IgG or IgA. Monotypic immunoglobulin with light chain restriction is expressed at the membrane and, to a lesser extent, in the cytoplasm, according to the degree of plasmacytic differentiation. About half the cases show aberrant co-expression of CD43. No specific immunohistochemical marker has yet been identified for MALT lymphoma, and so a panel of immunostains is necessary to exclude other lymphomas. MALT lymphoma cells are BCL2+ BCL6– CD10– cyclinD1– [35].

CD21, CD23 and CD35 are useful for highlighting follicular dendritic cells. Whereas reactive germinal centres are typically associated with tight, dense, follicular, dendritic cell meshworks, neoplastic follicular colonisation may be associated with large expanded irregular aggregates of follicular dendritic cells. An IgD stain may be useful for demonstrating IgD+ mantle zones and delineating IgD– marginal zones. Cytokeratin immunohistochemistry is also

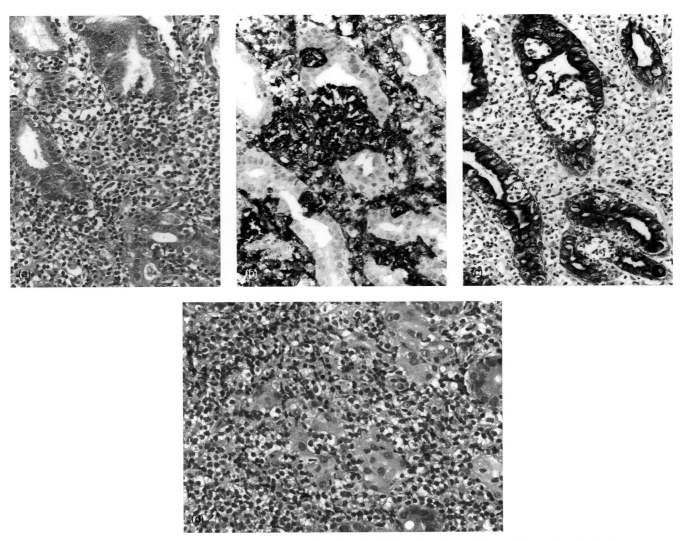

Figure 15.5 Lympho-epithelial lesions in gastric mucosa-associated lymphoid tissue lymphoma. The gastric crypts and glands are infiltrated and disrupted by lymphoid neoplastic cells which form small aggregates within the epithelium (a). Immunostains for (b) CD20 and (c) cytokeratins show the disruption of the epithelial structures by CD20+ cells. (d) The degenerative changes of the epithelium manifest as oncocytic changes.

useful for demonstrating the epithelial destruction associated with LELs. Non-neoplastic reactive T cells, highlighted by CD3 and CD5, are usually found in substantial numbers. Ig heavy and light chains are rearranged and show somatic hypermutation of their variable regions, consistent with derivation from a post-germinal centre memory B cell [47,48].

Pathogenesis of gastric MALT lymphoma

Association with chronic *H. pylori* infection

Epidemiological, cell biological and therapeutic studies provide evidence of a strong link between *H. pylori* infection and gastric MALT lymphoma [10,49]. In most cases of gastric MALT lymphoma, *H. pylori* can be demonstrated

[50,51]. Some studies have shown a lower incidence of this association but the density and detectability of *H. pylori* may decrease as the lymphoma progresses from chronic gastritis [10,51,52]. More direct evidence of the role of *H. pylori*, in the pathogenesis of gastric lymphoma, is provided by in vitro studies showing that the growth of lymphoma can be sustained in culture by *H. pylori* strain-specific T cells when crude lymphoma cultures are exposed to the organism [53]. Finally, following an initial study by Wotherspoon et al., several groups have confirmed that eradication of *H. pylori* with antibiotics induces regression of gastric MALT lymphoma in about 75% of cases [54–56].

From an immunological perspective, specificity for *H. pylori* relies on intra-tumoral T-cells and the T-cell stimulation of lymphoma B cells is dependent on intercellular contacts

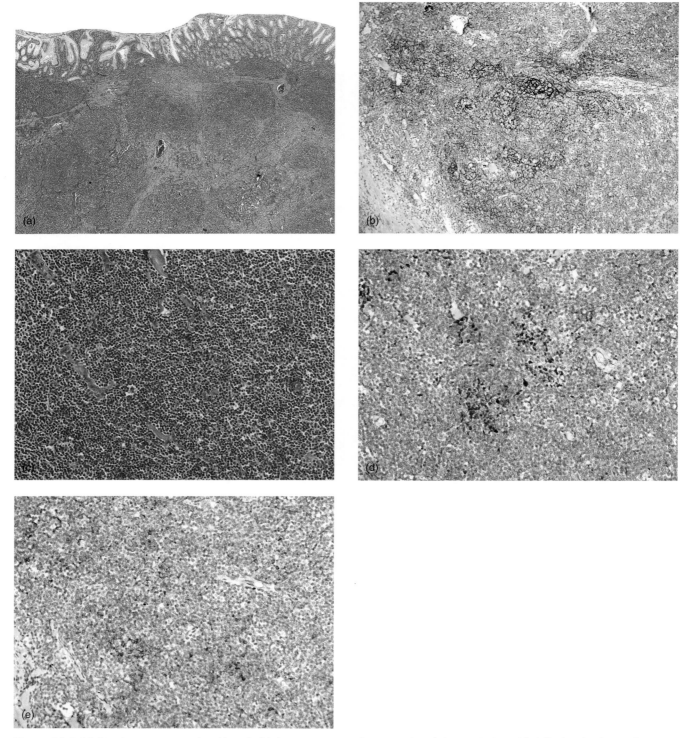

Figure 15.6 (a) Gastric mucosa-associated lymphoid tissue (MALT) lymphoma with a nodular pattern and extensive follicular colonisation. (b) The low-power view shows a lymphomatous infiltrate consisting of large lymphoid nodules. These correspond to large follicular structures, as evidenced by CD21 staining, demonstrating their association with follicular dendritic cell meshworks. (c) The nodules are composed of a monotonous population of small lymphoid cells corresponding mostly to MALT lymphoma cells. (d, e) Small foci of residual germinal centre cells are demonstrated with BCL6 (d) and CD10 (e) immunostains.

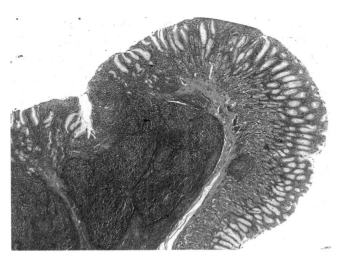

Figure 15.7 Low-power view of a gastric mucosa-associated lymphoid tissue lymphoma showing a small mucosal focus of lymphoma distant from the main lesion.

involving CD40 and additional co-stimulatory molecules [57,58]. Despite proliferation of gastric MALT lymphoma cells after *H. pylori* stimulation, tumour-derived immunoglobulin does not recognise *H. pylori* but does recognise various autoantigens [59], suggesting that gastric MALT lymphoma cells are transformed from autoreactive B cells which are induced after *H. pylori* infection. The rearranged immunoglobulin gene of gastric MALT lymphoma carries somatic hypermutations, with a pattern indicative of antigen selection and evidence of ongoing mutations, suggesting that tumour cell growth is partially driven by direct antigen stimulation [48]. Thus, *H. pylori* infection stimulates lymphomatous B cells through both indirect (via T cells) and direct (autoantigen) mechanisms. The rate of ongoing mutations appears to decline over the progression of the disease, implying that the role of direct antigen stimulation may decrease during tumour evolution [34].

Genetic and molecular alterations
A number of genetic and epigenetic alterations have been identified in gastric MALT lymphomas, including chromosomal translocations, trisomies and chromosomal imbalances, *p53* locus of heterozygosity (LOH)/mutations, and p15 and p16 promoter hypermethylation.

Chromosomal translocations Two translocations [t(11;18) (q21;q21) and t(1;14)(p22;q32)] have been reported in association with gastric MALT lymphomas. Remarkably, these translocations seem to promote lymphomatous development through a shared mechanism resulting in the activation of the nuclear factor κB (NF-κB), a transcription factor that regulates genes involved in lymphocytic proliferation and survival. Physiologically, both the caspase-like protein MALT1 and the adaptor molecule BCL10 are involved in

a cascade triggered by antigen receptor stimulation that ultimately leads to NF-κB activation. In gastric MALT lymphoma, the t(11;18) translocation causes reciprocal fusion of the *API2* gene (encoding an inhibitor of apoptosis family member) and the *MALT1* gene, resulting in the expression of an API2–MALT1 fusion protein that is believed to self-oligomerise [60], whereas the t(1;14) translocation results in over-expression of *BCL10* as a result of juxtaposition to the *IGH* enhancer. In both cases, the over-expressed oncoproteins seem to act at least partly through aberrant activation of NF-κB [61]. Another translocation, specifically associated with MALT lymphomas, which results in MALT1 over-expression, t(14;18)(q32;q21), is found mostly in lymphomas at non-gastric sites [62–64].

The t(11;18)(q21;q21) translocation, specifically associated with extra-nodal marginal zone lymphomas of MALT types, is identified in about 25–30% of primary gastric lymphomas. When present, this translocation is almost always the only cytogenetic abnormality, in contrast to t(11;18)-negative tumours, which often show other alterations such as trisomies or allelic imbalances [65,66]. The t(11;18) translocation is significantly associated with cytotoxin-associated antigen A (cagA)-positive strains of *H. pylori* and may be related to direct DNA damage by oxidative reactive species released by neutrophils that characterise the host response to this bacterial strain [67].

Importantly, t(11;18)-positive gastric MALT lymphomas do not respond to *H. pylori* eradication [68,69], are frequently at an advanced stage and rarely undergo high grade transformation [70], suggesting that t(11;18)-positive MALT lymphomas are a distinct subgroup of MALT lymphomas [66]. This translocation occurs with high frequency among the minority of gastric MALT lymphomas with no evidence of *H. pylori* infection [71]. The t(11;18)(q21;q21) translocation can be detected in routinely processed endoscopic biopsies by fluorescence *in situ* hybridisation (FISH) or reverse-transcriptase polymerase chain reaction (rtPCR) assays [69,72]. Cases harbouring the t(11;18) translocation show moderate aberrant nuclear staining for BCL10. However, this pattern is also seen in translocation-negative cases and thus cannot be used as a surrogate to identify translocation-positive cases [73].

The t(1;14)(p22;q32) translocation, which is also specific for MALT lymphomas, is detected in only 4% of gastric MALT lymphomas [67,74]. Cases harbouring this translocation show strong aberrant nuclear BCL10 staining that is more intense than in cases with t(11;18)(q21;q21) (Figure 15.8) [73,75].

Other genetic and molecular alterations Chromosomal numerical aberrations such as trisomies 3 and 18 are frequently seen in t(11;18)-negative tumours and those carrying t(1;14) [65,76]. A comparative genomic hybridisation study also revealed recurrent gains of entire or major parts of a chromosome (in chromosomes 12 and 22, and at 9q34) and

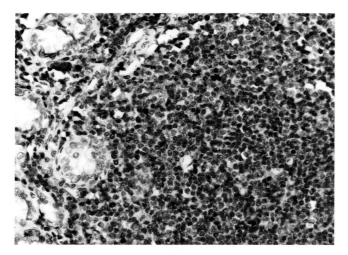

Figure 15.8 Strong expression of BCL10 in a gastric mucosa-associated lymphoid tissue lymphoma harbouring a t(1;11) translocation.

identified a few target genes mapping to loci involved in the modulation of NF-κB activation (*TRAF2* and *CARD9* at 9q34 and *MALT1* at 18q21) [77]. Whereas t(14;18)(q32;q21) (*MALT1/IGH*) is notably rare in gastric MALT lymphomas, extra copies of the *MALT1* gene are a frequent aberration in t(11;18)-negative cases and appear to predict an adverse outcome [64].

Several studies have shown aberrant hypermethylation of CpG islands in the promoter region of multiple genes, including some with tumour suppressor activities (*p16*, *p57*, *MGMT*, *ATM*), in *H. pylori* infection and MALT lymphomas, with a higher load of alterations in cases with high grade transformation. Thus, epigenetic inactivation of these genes may play a role in the progression of MALT lymphomas [78–80].

Dissemination and multifocality of gastric MALT lymphoma

Gastric MALT lymphoma is considered a localised disease with an indolent course. At presentation, most cases are restricted to the gastric wall, predominantly involving the mucosa and submucosa, but may spread into the muscularis propria and, less commonly, into the subserosa. Most cases are therefore stage I$_E$, whereas local lymph node involvement (stage II$_E$) occurs in a minority of cases (15–30%) [26,81]. However, recent studies using detailed and comprehensive staging protocols have revealed both local progression and systemic dissemination more frequently than originally believed.

MALT lymphoma of the stomach is multifocal. Although there may be a predominant lesion, numerous clonally identical, remote, microscopic foci often can be demonstrated even in macroscopically normal regions [38,82]. Moreover, clonally identical cells can even be detected by

PCR in reactive lymphoid tissue showing no evidence of lymphoma [82].

Gastric MALT lymphomas have a propensity to disseminate to other parts of the gastrointestinal mucosa and the splenic marginal zone, which may reflect the homing receptor profile of the tumour cells [43,83,84]. Dissemination to the bone marrow, demonstrated by classic staging methods, is present in about 10% of cases [27] but, in a recent study, PCR methods for clonality detection detected a circulating clone in almost half the patients with early stage disease as assessed by conventional techniques [85].

Differential diagnosis

MALT lymphoma versus reactive lymphoid hyperplasia (gastritis)

The most common challenge in the diagnosis of gastric MALT lymphoma is differentiating it from *H. pylori*-associated gastritis. Longstanding severe infection results in chronic active gastritis and the production of lymphoid follicles with germinal centres. These may have prominent marginal zones and, occasionally, some marginal zone cells infiltrate the juxtaposed glands, creating small IELs adjacent to the lymphoid follicle (Figure 15.9). However 'chronic follicular gastritis' lacks the sheet-like morphology of MALT-type lymphoma.

In favour of lymphoma is the presence, on routinely stained sections, of an expansile, destructive infiltrate with loss of normal architecture, with the cytological features of the infiltrating cells (with the appearance of marginal zone cells rather than small lymphocytes), Dutcher bodies, infiltration of the muscularis mucosae (Figure 15.10) and well-formed LELs adding further diagnostic evidence. However, many biopsies lack some of these features. In 1993, Wotherspoon et al. developed a useful scoring system (Table 15.4) [54]. Additional immunohistochemical studies are helpful by revealing monotypic immunoglobulin expression and/or co-expression of CD43 by B cells. Furthermore, determining B-cell clonality by a PCR-based method helps resolve difficult cases [86]. Nevertheless, some cases remain ambiguous, even with stains for B- and T-cell markers (see Immunophenotype above).

MALT lymphoma versus other small B-cell lymphomas

As a result of differences in clinical behaviour and management, it is important to differentiate MALT lymphoma from other small B-cell lymphomas that may present in the stomach, including mantle cell lymphoma, small lymphocytic lymphoma/chronic lymphocytic leukaemia and follicular lymphoma. The main differential diagnosis of MALT lymphoma is mantle cell lymphoma (MCL), which has a tropism for mucosal involvement of the gastrointestinal tract and may present with gastric involvement. MCL may display histopathological features similar to those of MALT lymphoma (Figure 15.11), including the presence of occasional LELs. MCL is characterised by a diffuse and/

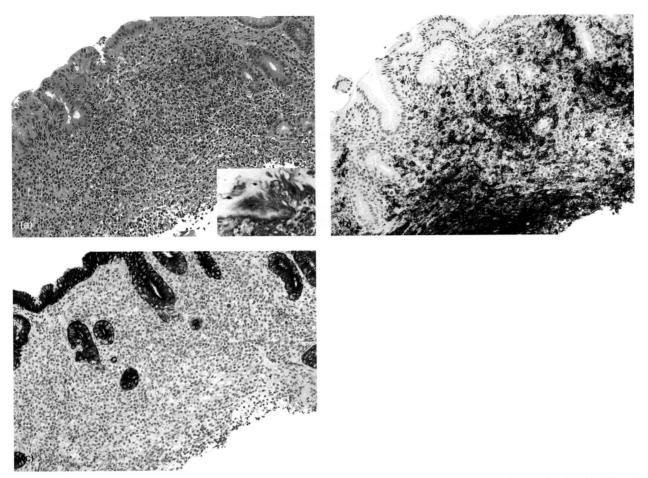

Figure 15.9 (a) *Helicobacter pylori*-associated gastritis with an atypical lymphoid infiltrate; inset: Giemsa stain showing *H. pylori*; (b, c) a few lympho-epithelial lesions as demonstrated by CD20 (b) and cytokeratin (c) immunostains.

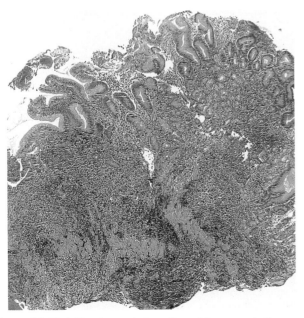

Figure 15.10 Infiltration and disruption of the muscularis mucosae in gastric mucosa-associated lymphoid tissue lymphoma.

or vaguely nodular monotonous infiltrate of small lymphoid cells with irregular nuclei and scant cytoplasm. The infiltrate may surround small, residual, reactive germinal centres. In classic MCL, plasmacytic differentiation and large blastic cells are not found. Distinctive immunophenotypic features include positivity for CD5 and IgD, and nuclear expression of cyclin D1 as a consequence of the t(11;14) (q13;q32) translocation (Figure 15.12) [87].

Lymphocytic lymphoma/chronic lymphocytic leukaemia (CLL) involving the gastric mucosa may be confused with MALT lymphoma but the cytological features are different, because CLL cells comprise small lymphocytes with round nuclei and occasional pro-lymphocytes. Additional distinguishing features include the absence of reactive follicles, the usual absence of LELs and immunophenotypic features of CLL (CD5+ CD23+ IgD+).

Follicular lymphoma is rarely encountered in the stomach and most cases represent secondary involvement of the stomach from systemic disease. MALT lymphoma shares the presence of follicular structures in association with follicular dendritic cells and a mixed cytological composition comprising small lymphoid cells with scattered larger cells. However,

Table 15.4 Wotherspoon scoring system for gastric lymphoid infiltrates

Score	Diagnosis	Histological features
0	Normal	Scattered plasma cells in lamina propria, no lymphoid follicles
1	Chronic active gastritis	Small clusters of lymphocytes in lamina propria, no lymphoid follicles, no lympho-epithelial lesions
2	Chronic active gastritis with florid lymphoid follicle formation	Prominent lymphoid follicles with a surrounding mantle zone and plasma cells, no lympho-epithelial lesions
3	Suspicious lymphoid infiltrate, probably reactive	Lymphoid follicles surrounded by small lymphocytes that infiltrate diffusely in lamina propria and occasionally into the epithelium
4	Suspicious lymphoid infiltrate, probably lymphoma	Lymphoid follicles surrounded by marginal zone cells that infiltrate diffusely in lamina propria and into the epithelium in small groups
5	MALT lymphoma	Presence of dense diffuse infiltrate of marginal zone cells in lamina propria with prominent lympho-epithelial lesions

MALT, mucosa-associated lymphoid tissue.

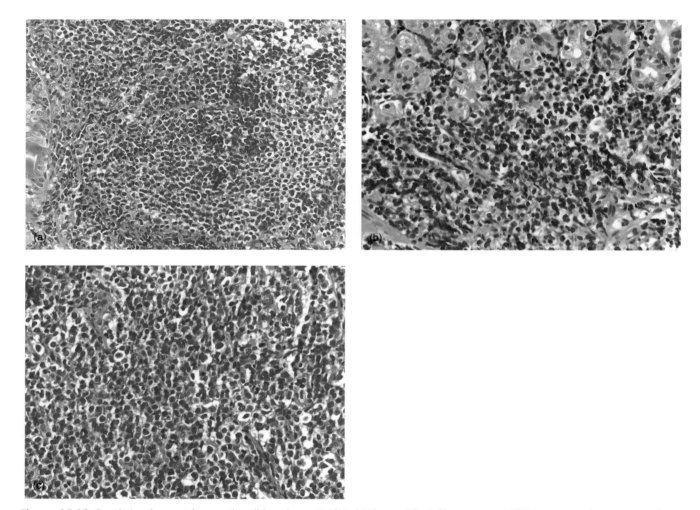

Figure 15.11 Gastric involvement by mantle cell lymphoma (MCL): (a) the nodular infiltrate seen in MCL, corresponding to a mantle zone pattern around an atrophic germinal centre, may resemble a marginal zone pattern. (b) The small irregular neoplastic cells of MCL resemble centrocyte-like cells of gastric mucosa-associated lymphoid tissue (MALT) lymphoma. (c) In this case, clear cell morphology and the presence of blastic cells are overlapping features with MALT lymphoma.

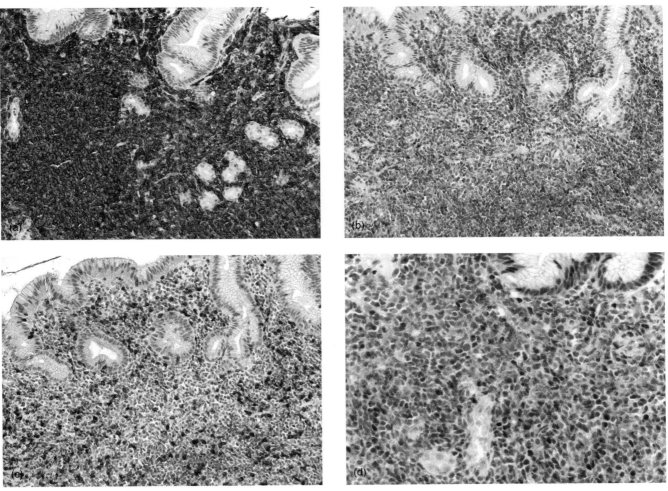

Figure 15.12 Immunophenotyping of mantle cell lymphoma (MCL): (a) the neoplastic cells of MCL are positive for CD20, with co-expression of (b) CD5 (compare with (c) CD3) and show nuclear expression of (d) cyclin D1.

its phenotype differs from that of the neoplastic cells of follicular lymphoma, which are CD10+ BCL2+ BCL6+.

MALT lymphoma with increased large cells versus transformation to diffuse large B-cell lymphoma

Transformation of MALT lymphoma to a DLBCL is diagnosed when sheets or confluent clusters of large, transformed cells are found outside follicles in a background of MALT lymphoma. Clusters of at least 20 cells are needed to consider large cell transformation. Conversely, diffusely scattered large cells, representing 5–10% or even up to 20% of the total population, are not associated with a worse prognosis, as long as they do not form clusters [81,88,89]. Before considering large cell transformation, the possibility that the large cells represent residual reactive germinal centre cells or large neoplastic cells confined to colonised follicles must be excluded. Immunohistochemical stains for follicular dendritic cell meshworks (CD21, CD23) may be helpful to delineate the underlying architecture.

MALT lymphoma versus plasma cell neoplasia

The stomach is an uncommon site for extra-medullary plasmacytomas or dissemination of multiple myeloma [90]. However, MALT lymphoma with extensive plasma cell differentiation may suggest the alternative diagnosis of a plasma cell neoplasm. In favour of lymphoma are the presence of a component of B lymphocytes, Dutcher's bodies, LELs and reactive lymphoid follicles, and the expression of IgM by the neoplastic cells (although a minority of MALT lymphomas express other heavy chains, and plasma cell neoplasms may infrequently be IgM+).

MALT lymphoma versus poorly preserved high grade lymphoma

In small biopsies with crush artefact harbouring DLBCL or Burkitt's lymphoma, there may be distortion leading to the impression of a small cell tumour. The presence of apoptotic debris, necrosis and/or numerous mitotic figures should raise the suspicion of a high grade malignancy.

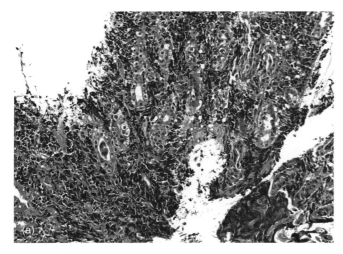

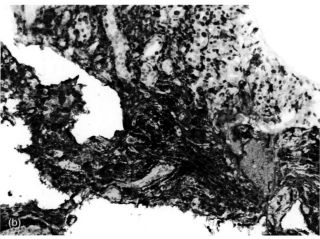

Figure 15.13 (a) Crushed gastric biopsy showing a dense lymphoid infiltrate that is difficult to characterise by morphology. (b) A high proliferation fraction shown by Ki67 immunostaining indicates a high grade neoplasm.

Staining with Ki67 is helpful for identifying highly proliferative tumours (Figure 15.13). Clinical information, such as the endoscopic appearance of the tumour and/or its apparent growth rate, can also provide evidence for the correct diagnosis.

Treatment and prognosis

Although surgery was once widely recommended as first-line treatment for gastric MALT lymphoma, more conservative approaches are currently preferred, because retrospective analyses have shown equal efficacy with lower morbidity [23,55,91]. The indications for surgery are now restricted to acute presentations such as bleeding or perforation.

At present, the standard treatment for early stage, *H. pylori*-positive, MALT gastric lymphoma is eradication of *H. pylori* through a combination of antibiotics and proton pump inhibitors. *H. pylori* eradication induces lymphoma regression and long-term remission in about 75% of cases, with the time to complete response varying from 3 months to more than 1 year. Translocation t(11;18)-positive cases and peri-gastric lymphadenopathy are the main negative predictors of response. For patients who respond to antibiotic therapy, there is no evidence to justify additional treatment. Most patients with histological residual disease after successful *H. pylori* eradication will have a favourable course without additional treatment, but lifelong surveillance is mandatory to detect late relapses (6–22%) and metachronous gastric cancer.

Controversy persists over the treatment of early stage disease with *H. pylori*-negative MALT lymphoma or *H. pylori*-positive tumours unresponsive to antibiotics. A few reports suggest that antibiotic therapy may be efficient in some cases of *H. pylori*-negative MALT lymphomas. Cases unresponsive to antibiotics may benefit from local radiotherapy, providing good disease control and 77% disease-free survival at 5 years. Treatment with oral alkylating agents leads to remission rates of 60–75%, with poorer response rates in t(11;18)-positive cases [92]. Nucleoside analogues represent another therapeutic option. Rituximab, a chimaeric antibody directed against CD20, has shown efficacy in MALT lymphoma, and its combination with chlorambucil was successfully tested for the treatment of patients with t(11;18)-positive gastric MALT lymphomas [93]. In all patients with disease that is locally advanced or has spread systemically, systemic therapy is recommended with cytotoxic agents, alone or in combination. The combination of rituximab and chemotherapy is currently under evaluation by the International Extranodal Lymphoma Study Group. Overall, the survival rate for patients with gastric MALT lymphoma is approximately 90% at 5 years [94].

Post-treatment evaluation of gastric MALT lymphoma

Follow-up for gastric MALT lymphoma includes serial gastroscopy (and/or EUS, if abnormal at diagnosis) with histological assessment of multiple biopsies from all parts of the stomach [95]. Biopsies are usually taken every 3–6 months for the first 2 years and yearly thereafter.

Morphological assessment

A good histological response to treatment is characterised by regression of the diffuse lymphoid infiltrate, LELs with frequent persistence of small basal aggregates of lymphocytes and an 'empty' lamina propria composed of loose

Table 15.5 GELA histological grading system for post-treatment assessment of gastric MALT lymphoma

Score		Lymphoid infiltrate	LEL	Stromal changes
CR	Complete histological remission	Absent or scattered plasma cells and small lymphoid cells in the lamina propria	Absent	Normal or 'empty' lamina propria and/or fibrosis
pMRD	Probable minimal residual disease	Aggregates of lymphoid cells or lymphoid nodules in the lamina propria/muscularis mucosae and/or submucosa	Absent	'Empty' lamina propria and/or fibrosis
rRD	Responding residual disease	Dense, diffuse or nodular extension around glands in the lamina propria	Focal or absent	Focal 'empty' lamina propria and/or fibrosis
NC	No change	Dense, diffuse or nodular	Usually present	No changes

LEL, lympho-epithelial lesion. MALT, mucosa-associated lymphoid tissue.
(Reproduced from Copie-Bergman C, Gaulard P, Lavergne-Slove A, Brousse N, Flejou JF, Dordonne K, et al. Proposal for a new histological grading system for post-treatment evaluation of gastric MALT lymphoma. Gut. 2003 Nov;52(11):1656, with permission from BMJ Publishing Group Ltd).

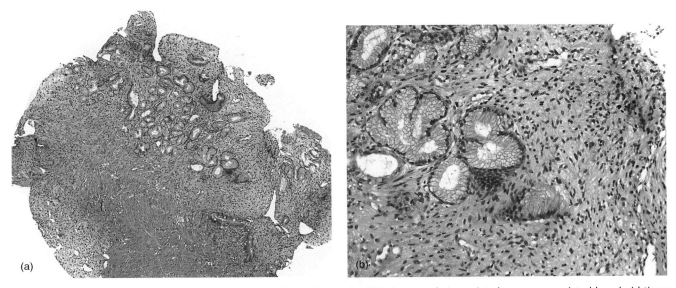

Figure 15.14 Complete histological remission after antibiotic therapy for *Helicobacter pylori*-associated mucosa-associated lymphoid tissue lymphoma: (a) 'empty' lamina propria characterised by loss of epithelial structures and a pauci-cellular lamina propria devoid of lymphoid aggregates; (b) fibrotic lamina propria.

connective tissue with scattered plasma cells and glandular loss [96,97]. In order to standardise the pathological evaluation of follow-up gastric biopsies, the Groupe d'Etude des Lymphomes de l'Adulte (GELA) has proposed a grading system based on histological features, independent of immunohistochemical or molecular studies (Table 15.5) [97]. The morphological features are classified into four categories: complete histological remission (Figure 15.14), probable minimal residual disease (Figure 15.15), respond-

ing residual disease and no change. The category of 'probable minimal residual disease' is of uncertain significance, as half of these cases are associated with a clonal *IGH* gene rearrangement by PCR, but it is not an indication for further treatment and, as it is not associated with active disease, it can be considered as a state of remission.

Most patients who achieve complete remission and 'probable minimal residual disease' remain in remission, although relapse occurs in about 20% of patients, whether

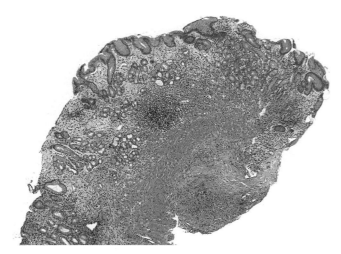

Figure 15.15 Probable minimal residual disease after antibiotic therapy for *Helicobacter pylori*-associated mucosa-associated lymphoid tissue lymphoma: small limited lymphoid infiltrate in the deep mucosa in association with stromal changes.

or not in association with *H. pylori* reinfection [98]. Relapses may occur several years after initial remission and can be focal. In *H. pylori*-positive relapses, antibiotic therapy usually results in a further remission. In some cases, the disease may wax and wane with apparent relapses that are self-limiting and transient, and may not require additional therapy. For these reasons, and because of variations due to sampling, at least two sets of gastric biopsies with the same findings are recommended to establish true remission.

Long-term endoscopic follow-up of gastric MALT lymphoma patients is also recommended to detect pre-neoplastic or neoplastic changes of the gastric epithelium, because the association of gastric adenocarcinoma and MALT lymphoma occurs more often than would be expected by chance [99,100]. The most common scenario is the synchronous development of both neoplasms (Figure 15.16) but there are also reports of gastric adenocarcinomas developing several years after remission of MALT lymphoma [101,102].

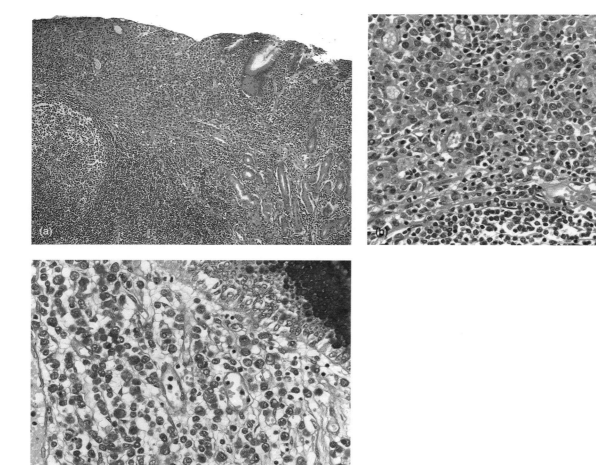

Figure 15.16 (a) Synchronous gastric mucosa-associated lymphoid tissue (MALT) lymphoma and gastric adenocarcinoma of the diffuse type. The MALT lymphoma is seen abutting the more superficial carcinoma. (b) Carcinoma cells, some with signet ring cell features, are seen adjacent to the rim of a lymphoid follicle. (c) Intracytoplasmic mucus, demonstrated by a periodic acid–Schiff stain, is seen in the carcinoma cells.

Molecular studies

Several studies have investigated the utility of PCR-based tests for assessing B-cell clonality in follow-up gastric biopsies after antibiotic therapy. In up to half of cases, B-cell monoclonality persists despite apparent histological complete response or probable minimal residual disease, whereas, in others, clonality disappears with time [103–105]. In some studies, patients in histological remission and persistent monoclonality were more prone to relapse than those with polyclonal results [105], but other investigators have found no such correlation [106]. More recently, some authors have suggested that molecular monitoring of MALT lymphomas with *API2–MALT1* rearrangement, using assays specifically designed for the detection of t(11;18), may be more sensitive than PCR for *IGH* rearrangement [107,108]. The difficulty in interpreting molecular data is compounded by the occurrence of sampling artefacts, false negatives and conflicting reports on the detection of monoclonality of histologically reactive infiltrates [96,109]. Therefore, although molecular monitoring is under further evaluation in clinical trials, there is currently no evidence to recommend it in the routine post-treatment follow-up of gastric MALT lymphoma.

Primary gastric diffuse large B-cell lymphoma

DLBCL is the most common form of primary gastric lymphoma, closely followed in frequency by MALT lymphoma [11,12]. It has been argued that this may not reflect its true incidence, because many cases of low grade MALT-type lymphomas may have been misidentified in the past as 'pseudo-lymphoma'. Moreover, further challenges are posed by the spectrum of cytological composition found in low grade MALT lymphomas, the lack of precise criteria for defining high grade transformation and the inappropriate use of the term 'high grade MALT-type malignant lymphoma', a designation that is not recognised in the current WHO classification of haematopoietic neoplasms.

Clinical features

Primary gastric DLBCL shows a male predominance and occurs at a median age of 55 years. The clinical presentation is non-specific and overlaps with that of other benign or malignant conditions. Most patients report epigastric pain or dyspepsia. Weight loss is common, usually as a consequence of the dyspepsia. Bleeding and perforation are rare presenting features [110]. The duration of symptoms before diagnosis varies.

Endoscopic and macroscopic features

DLBCL is usually, but not exclusively, associated with a mass lesion (Figure 15.17). The antrum is the most common

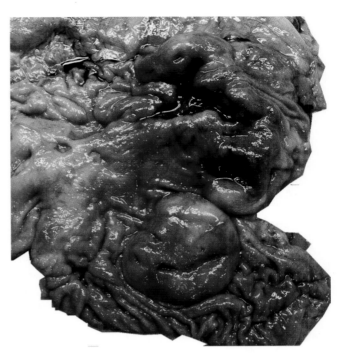

Figure 15.17 Primary gastric diffuse large B-cell lymphoma massively involving the stomach as an ulcero-infiltrative lesion and forming a voluminous polypoid mass.

site but any part of the stomach may be involved. Mass lesions are likely to show ulceration, but, occasionally, more diffuse infiltration with an intact mucosa is seen. A polypoid pattern may also be encountered. Marked thickening of the gastric wall, as seen on CT or EUS, is more common in DLBCL than in MALT lymphomas, and there is usually preservation of the peri-gastric fat. Local lymph node involvement is common and at least 50% of tumours will be at least stage II$_E$ [6,94].

Microscopic features

DLBCL is defined by the presence of compact aggregates or sheet-like proliferation of large atypical lymphoid cells; these have nuclei at least twice the size of a small lymphocyte, usually larger than tissue macrophages (Figure 15.18a). The nuclei are round, lobated or irregular, with nucleoli. The cytoplasm is variably abundant. In most cases, the predominant cells resemble either centroblasts or immunoblasts, and there is often a mixture of both. Occasional cases show large, bizarre and often multinucleated cells. The large cells infiltrate in sheets between the glands, which ultimately atrophy and disappear, but invasion of individual glands and formation of LELs are uncommon (Figure 15.19) [111].

DLBCL of the stomach may be seen as the sole tumour component or in association with MALT lymphoma. When DLBCL is seen in association with MALT lymphoma,

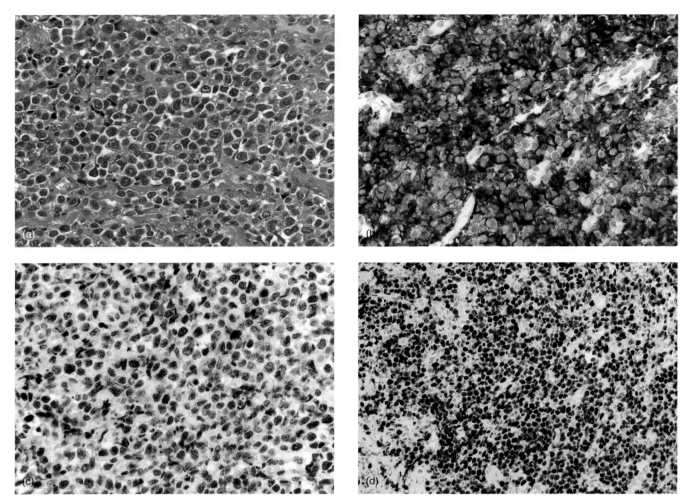

Figure 15.18 Gastric diffuse large B-cell lymphoma: this tumour, composed of large lymphoid cells with (a) centroblastic features and expression of (b) CD20, had a non-germinal centre-like immunophenotype with absent CD10 expression (not shown), weak expression of (c) BCL6 and (d) strong MUM1 positivity.

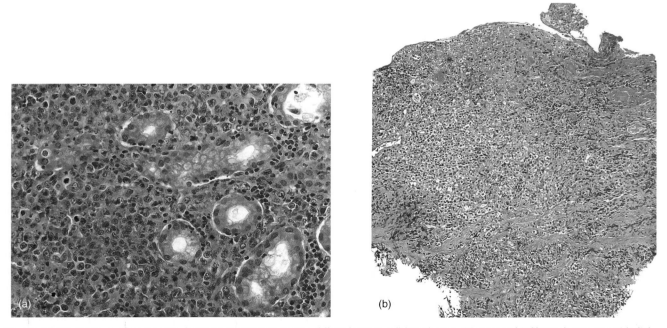

Figure 15.19 Patterns of gastric involvement in primary gastric diffuse large B-cell lymphoma: (a) mucosal infiltrate between epithelial structures with no evidence of lympho-epithelial lesions; (b) diffuse replacement of the glandular structures.

the extent of the secondary high grade component varies. Some cases comprise small foci of cohesive sheets of large transformed cells, whereas others are characterised by a predominance of large cell lymphoma with only minor residual foci of small cell lymphoma which may be difficult to identify [112]. In some cases in which only a large cell component is seen, the MALT component may have been completely overgrown by the DLBCL, but others represent true primary DLBCL [36].

Immunohistochemistry

Similar to DLBCL occurring elsewhere, the tumour cells express CD20 and other pan-B-cell antigens (CD19, CD22, CD79a, Pax-5) (Figure 15.18b). The transformed cells express surface and/or cytoplasmic immunoglobulin, usually IgM. When DLBCL coexists with a low grade component, both components show the same light chain restriction and identical Ig gene rearrangements, supporting the view that the DLBCL represents a transformation of the small B-cell component [113,114]. A variable number of CD3+ reactive T cells are scattered throughout the tumour. Residual follicular dendritic cell meshworks, highlighted by CD21 or CD23, are probably remnants of reactive follicles overrun by the lymphoma and suggest transformation from MALT lymphoma.

DLBCLs arising from low grade MALT lymphoma are characteristically negative for BCL2 and negative for CD10 but, in contrast to MALT lymphoma, usually express BCL6 [36,115]. Conversely, new gastric DLBCL may express CD10 and/or BCL2. However, there are no reliable immunophenotypic features distinguishing gastric lymphomas arising anew from those that have transformed from MALT lymphomas.

Different published series show a highly variable proportion of gastric DLBCL cases when they are classified into germinal centre B-cell (GCB)-like and non-GCB-like categories based on the expression of CD10, BCL6 and MUM1, according to Hans's algorithm [116]. Some authors have found a predominance of non-GCB-like tumours (Figure 15.18c,d), interpreted as reflective of the frequent derivation of gastric DLBCL from MALT lymphomas [117,118], whereas others have found the opposite [119] and, in the largest study by Nakamura et al., the proportion of GCB-like and non-GCB-like DLBCLs was similar, irrespective of the presence of a MALT component [120]. The prognostic value of immunophenotyping DLBCL into GCB-like and non-GCB-like subgroups remains controversial. Three studies have shown a positive prognostic value in primary gastric DLBCL for CD10 positivity [111,121], bcl6 expression [117] and GCB immunophenotype [117], whereas others found no correlation between prognosis and either single differentiation markers or combined immunophenotype [119,120].

Pathogenesis

As mentioned above, it is believed that many cases arise by transformation of pre-existing low grade MALT lymphomas, a concept supported by the finding of the same clonal *IGH* rearrangement in both large cell and small cell components in cases with mixed histology. Interestingly, MALT-specific translocations such as t(11;18)/*API2–MALT1* have been demonstrated rarely in cases of gastric DLBCL [120], and it has been suggested that t(11;18)-positive MALT lymphomas are less prone to transformation than translocation-negative MALT lymphomas. However, Toracchio et al. have found a similar frequency of t(11;18)-positive cases in gastric low grade MALT lymphomas and DLBCLs [122]. Conversely, in some cases of t(11;18)-positive transformed MALT lymphomas, the translocation may be found in the small cell component only, suggesting that, in a subset of these cases, the large cell lymphoma developed independently [120,123].

Compared with nodal DLBCL, *BCL2* gene rearrangements are extremely rare in primary gastric DLBCL [120]. In contrast, rearrangements of *BCL6* have been reported in up to 48% of gastric DLBCLs and were found to predict increased likelihood of complete remission and better survival [124]. Unlike *BCL6* rearrangements, hypermutations of *BCL6* do not appear to affect prognosis [125]. In another large FISH-based study of 141 DLBCLs of the stomach (including 58 with associated MALT lymphoma and 83 without MALT lymphoma), translocations involving *IGH* were detected in 32% of the cases. Their partner genes included *BCL6* in a third of the cases with *c-MYC* and *FOXP1* in a minority of cases. Partner genes were undetected/unknown in 50% of the cases. Translocations involving *IGH* were an independent prognostic factor for better overall and event-free survival [120]. One study has documented frequent LOH at 6q in sites of putative tumour suppressor genes and less frequent LOH of other tumour suppressor genes, including *TP53* and *APC* [126].

Differential diagnosis

The criteria for distinguishing DLBCL from MALT lymphoma were discussed earlier. Another potential issue is differentiating DLBCL from Burkitt's lymphoma, which is discussed in the next section. DLBCLs may be difficult to distinguish from poorly differentiated carcinomas, especially in poorly preserved biopsy specimens and in rare cases where the malignant lymphoid cells have the appearance of signet-ring cells, but this differential diagnosis is easily clarified by histochemical and immunohistochemical studies.

Treatment and prognosis

DLBCLs usually present at a more advanced stage than MALT lymphomas and their prognosis is worse [94]. There are conflicting reports as to whether the presence of an associated low grade component influences the outcome of primary gastric DLBCLs [89] but, in a large international study of follow-up data for 138 patients, the overall survival and event-free survival rates at 5 years were 76% and 58%, respectively, and no difference was observed according to the presence of an associated low grade component [120].

Currently, the treatment of choice for gastric DLBCLs, as for DLBCLs in general, consists of anthracycline-based combination chemotherapy plus rituximab [110]. Although the impact of rituximab has not been examined for primary gastric DLBCLs specifically, the therapeutic benefit of immunotherapy in DLBCLs has been proved [127]. Surgery, which until recently was considered the primary treatment of choice, is now generally used only for patients with major complications such as bleeding and/or perforation at diagnosis. [29] The role of consolidation radiation therapy is debated but it has been associated with a lower recurrence rate in some series. The role of *H. pylori* infection and eradication in primary gastric DLBCLs is controversial but the bacterium is detected in 35% of the cases and more commonly in cases arising in association with MALT lymphoma (65% vs 15% in pure DLBCLs) [89]. In addition to chemotherapy, *H. pylori* should always be eradicated, and there are even reports of series of patients with early stage DLBCL arising in MALT lymphoma in which a significant proportion achieved complete and durable remission after antibiotic therapy [128–130].

Other primary gastric lymphomas

DLBCLs and MALT lymphomas together account for more than 85% of primary gastric lymphomas. Although virtually any type of lymphoma may primarily involve the stomach, only the most commonly encountered are discussed.

Mantle cell lymphoma

Mantle cell lymphoma affects middle-aged to older adults with a male predominance [87]. As a primary gastrointestinal disease, it may present as innumerable mucosal polyps, so-called multiple lymphomatous polyposis [131, 132]. Any portion of the gastrointestinal tract may be involved but the ileo-caecal region is usually the main site. Gastric involvement manifests as large cerebroid folds. Staging frequently reveals widespread extra-intestinal disease (stage IV). Conversely, microscopic gastrointestinal tract involvement is extremely frequent (84%) in patients with systemic mantle cell lymphoma. Thus, it is not clear whether multiple lymphomatous polyposis is a different entity from gastrointestinal tract involvement in peripheral mantle cell lymphoma. It has been suggested that expression of the mucosal homing receptor alpha4-beta7 by the neoplastic cells is associated with digestive tract involvement [133].

Microscopically, mantle cell lymphoma is composed of a diffuse or vaguely nodular infiltrate of small- to medium-sized lymphocytes with irregular nuclei and scant cytoplasm. Scattered epithelioid histiocytes may be dispersed among the neoplastic cells. Atrophic germinal centre remnants may be seen within some nodules. The lymphoma cells tend to displace and obliterate glandular structures, but LELs are not a typical feature, even if the gland destruction can mimic them. The neoplastic cells are CD20+, CD79a+, CD5+, CD43+, cyclinD1+ and BCL2+, usually lack CD10, CD23 and BCL6, and show monotypic immunoglobulin expression (usually IgM+ IgD+, with λ more frequent than κ). Cyclin D1 is over-expressed as a consequence of *CCND1* gene rearrangement, usually to the *IGH* locus, but variant translocations may occur. Rare cases of mantle cell lymphoma, about 5%, do not harbour such a rearrangement and are negative for cyclin D1, but such cases should be diagnosed with extreme caution.

Burkitt's lymphoma

Burkitt's lymphoma is a highly aggressive neoplasm composed of mature B cells with very high proliferative activity, preferentially affecting children and young adults [134]. Three clinical variants are recognised: endemic, sporadic and immune deficiency associated. Burkitt's lymphoma has a predilection for extra-nodal sites, especially the ileo-caecal region, which is the most common site of involvement for the sporadic disease. Primary gastric Burkitt's lymphoma is rare compared with other lymphoma types and its true incidence is not defined [135]. One study found a better outcome for patients with gastric Burkitt's lymphoma compared with non-gastric Burkitt's lymphoma, especially when the disease was localised to the stomach [135].

The tumours are often bulky, sometimes with ulceration, and usually sited in the gastric body or antrum. Microscopically, there is a diffuse infiltrate of uniform, medium-sized lymphoid cells containing round nuclei with granular chromatin and several nucleoli, and a rim of basophilic cytoplasm. Mitotic figures are usually numerous, with abundant apoptotic activity and scattered, tingible, body macrophages imparting a 'starry-sky' pattern (Figure 15.20a). A subset of cases shows plasmacytoid differentiation. The neoplastic cells are CD20+, IgM+, CD10+, BCL2– and BCL6+, with a proliferation fraction approaching 100% (Figure 15.20b–f). The tumour cells are positive for the Epstein–Barr virus (EBV) in most endemic cases and in a subset of the other clinical variants.

The characteristic cytogenetic abnormality is rearrangement of the *c-MYC* gene to either the Ig heavy chain gene or the κ or λ light chain gene. The differential diagnosis with diffuse large B-cell lymphoma may be difficult, especially in adult patients (Figure 15.21) [136,137]. Several

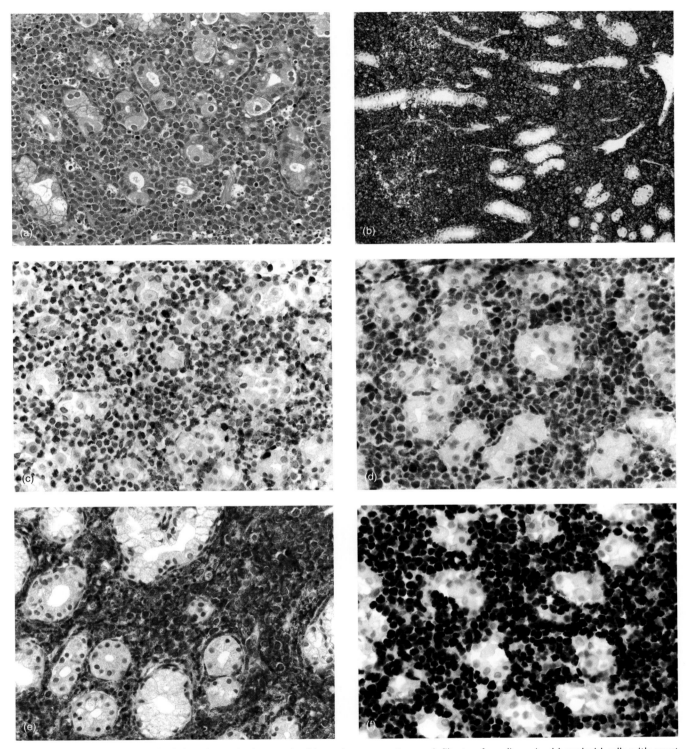

Figure 15.20 (a) Gastric Burkitt's lymphoma is characterised by a dense monotonous infiltrate of medium-sized lymphoid cells with scant cytoplasm, numerous mitoses and apoptotic bodies and a starry-sky appearance. The lymphoid cells are (b) CD20+, (c) negative for BCL2 (compare with few reactive T cells which are BCL2 positive), strongly positive for (d) BCL6 and (e) CD10, and almost 100% of nuclei are (f) Ki67-positive.

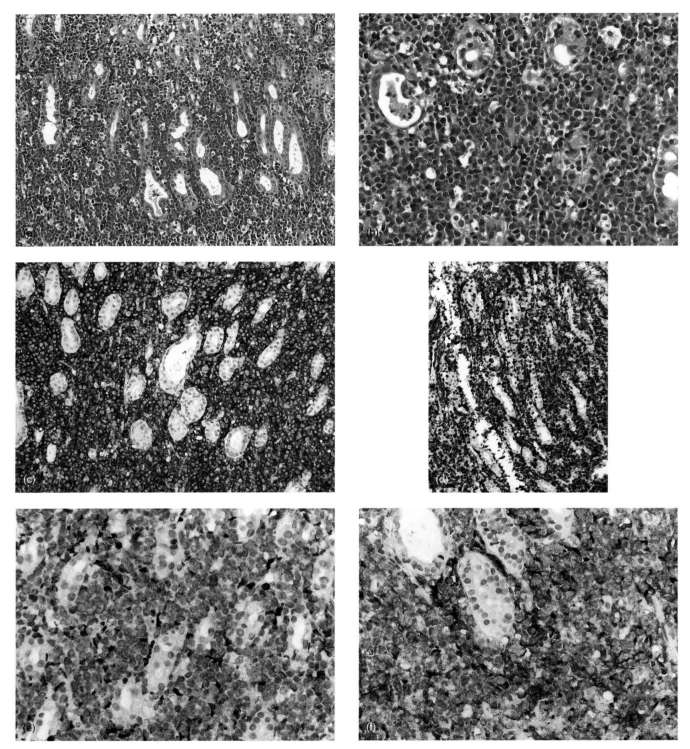

Figure 15.21 B-cell lymphoma with features intermediate between diffuse large B-cell lymphoma and Burkitt's lymphoma. (a) The tumour cells densely infiltrate the mucosa with a focally prominent starry sky pattern. (b) The tumour is composed of medium-sized and occasional larger lymphoid cells, suggestive of Burkitt's lymphoma, but with slightly more pleomorphism including blastic cells with moderately prominent nucleoli. The neoplastic cells are (c) CD20+ with (d) a Ki67 labelling index of almost 100%, are faintly positive for (e) BCL2 and show weak expression of (f) CD10. By genetic analyses, this case, in an elderly patient, was shown to have a *cMYC* gene rearrangement in a complex karyotype.

reports have documented the presence of *H. pylori* in gastric mucosa involved by Burkitt's lymphoma [138,139]. More recently, complete remission after eradication of *H. pylori* has been reported, suggesting a role for the bacterium in the pathogenesis of gastric Burkitt's lymphoma, and the importance of seeking and eradicating the bacterium in combination with conventional chemotherapy [140].

Peripheral T-cell lymphomas

Primary gastric T-cell lymphoma is rare. Although its precise incidence is unknown, it appears to show geographical variations, especially with respect to specific histotypes. Many case series and case reports are from Japan, where human T-lymphotrophic virus-1 (HTLV-1) infection is endemic. Gastric lymphoma associated with HTLV-1 may represent the primary manifestation of adult T-cell leukaemia/lymphoma (ATLL) and is generally associated with an extremely poor prognosis [141,142]. There is also a high frequency of gastric involvement by systemic ATLL at an advanced stage [143].

Gastric lymphomas associated with HTLV-1 often present as ulcerated masses in the middle or upper corpus, or are more widely distributed. Microscopically, the cytology ranges from monomorphic to polymorphic, and may comprise medium-sized cells with round or irregular nuclei and medium- to large-sized cells or cells with anaplastic morphology. The lymphoma cells express T-cell antigens, are usually CD4+, CD7− and CD8−, strongly express CD25 and are positive for *FoxP3*, a feature of regulatory T cells [144].

Primary gastric T-cell lymphomas without HTLV-1 infection mostly fall into the category of peripheral T-cell lymphoma, not otherwise specified. The majority display large cell morphology or, less commonly, comprise a population of small- to medium-sized lymphoid cells [145,146]. Tumours composed of smaller cells may show clear cell features and epithelio-tropism, potentially mimicking the LELs of MALT B-cell lymphoma [147]. The neoplastic infiltrates may show a pronounced eosinophilia that may partially obscure the neoplastic cells [148]. Most T-cell lymphomas show a helper-inducer phenotype (CD4+, CD8−), although occasional examples of suppressor-cytotoxic phenotype (CD4−, CD8±, TIA-1+, granzyme B+) do occur [146,149]. A subset of the latter with the immunophenotype of IELs may express CD103 and/or show enteropathy-like features, and represent gastric localisations of enteropathy-associated T-cell lymphoma (Figure 15.22). Expression of CD30 by the tumour cells is frequently detected and almost universal in cases with large cell morphology [145,146]. However, few cases present the constellation of features typical of anaplastic large cell lymphoma and cases positive for ALK are exceedingly rare [145].

A few cases of gastric T-cell lymphomas are positive for EBV and a larger proportion occur in association with *H. pylori* infection. It is unknown whether these associations bear any causal relationship to the development of T-cell lymphoma. In general, the outcome of patients with primary gastric T-cell lymphoma is better than that of patients with intestinal enteropathy-associated lymphomas, e.g. a 57% 5-year survival rate was reported in a retrospective analysis from Japan [145].

Gastric lymphoma in abnormal immune states

Lymphomas in HIV-positive individuals comprise a high proportion of cases with extra-nodal presentation and often involve the gastrointestinal tract. However, the stomach is involved relatively infrequently compared with the colon, rectum and small intestine [150]. Most cases are high grade B-cell lymphomas, classified as diffuse large B-cell lymphomas or Burkitt's lymphomas, and show an association with EBV infection more commonly than those occurring in the HIV-negative population. Rare cases of *H. pylori*-associated gastric marginal zone lymphomas have also been reported [151].

Post-transplant lympho-proliferative disorders (PTLDs) may also occur in the stomach They are classified as early lesions, polymorphic PTLDs, monomorphic PTLDs and classic Hodgkin's lymphoma type [152]. The polymorphic and monomorphic PTLDs of B-cell lineage are most frequently encountered in the gastrointestinal tract. A few cases of EBV-negative gastric MALT lymphomas have also been reported in allograft recipients [153].

Secondary lymphomatous involvement

Secondary involvement of the stomach by non-Hodgkin's lymphoma is common in clinical practice and postmortem examinations, estimated to be about 25–30% in prospective analyses [154]. Any type of non-Hodgkin's lymphoma arising elsewhere may disseminate to the stomach. Histologically, secondary involvement by high grade B-cell neoplasms may be impossible to distinguish from primary gastric lymphoma (Figure 15.23). The presence of a low grade component and LELs may be helpful in identifying primary gastric neoplasms but, in general, clinical features and history are crucial to definitive categorisation as primary versus secondary involvement.

Miscellaneous haematological malignancies

Acute myeloblastic leukaemia may present as a myeloid sarcoma in the stomach [155] and, as the cells have plasmacytoid features, it may mimic primary lymphoma or even myeloma. Chloroacetate esterase demonstration and lysozyme immunohistochemistry are useful diagnostic tests.

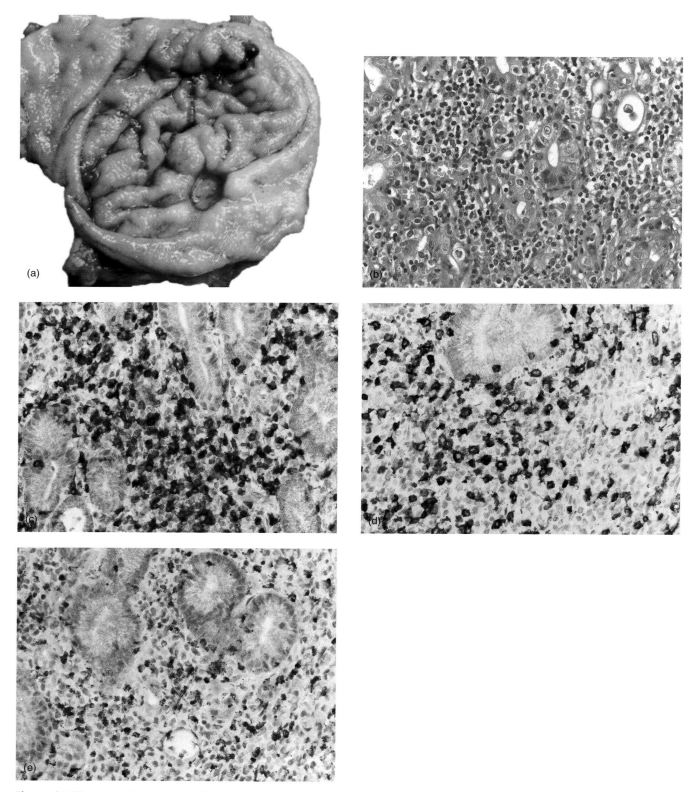

Figure 15.22 Enteropathy-associated T-cell lymphoma involving the stomach. (a) The lesion manifested as an indurated ulcer in a patient with history of coeliac disease. (b) A polymorphic atypical lymphoid infiltrate is seen in the gastric mucosa, admixed with eosinophils. The atypical lymphoid cells are (c) CD3+, with co-expression of (d) CD8 and contain (e) cytotoxic granules (granzyme-B).

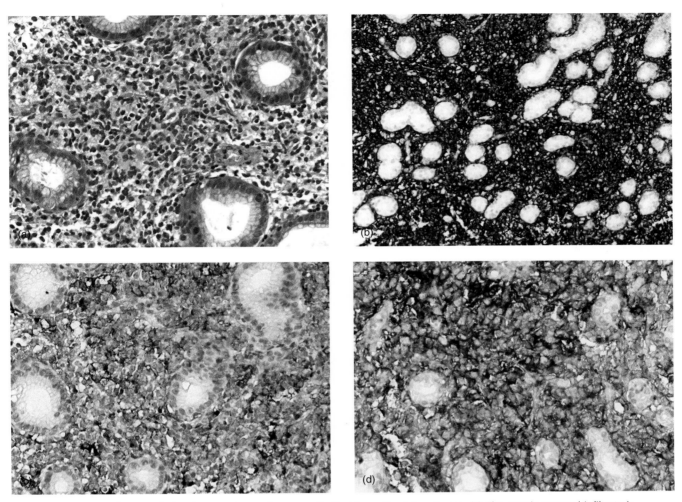

Figure 15.23 Secondary gastric involvement by a primary mediastinal large B-cell lymphoma. (a) The gastric mucosal infiltrate is morphologically indistinguishable from primary gastric lymphoma, although the cells are somewhat smaller than in primary gastric diffuse large B-cell lymphoma. (b) The lymphoid cells are strongly CD20+. Co-expression of (c) CD23 and (d) CD30 are features typically seen in a subset of primary mediastinal large B-cell lymphomas.

References

1. Dawson IM, Cornes JS, Morson BC. Primary malignant lymphoid tumours of the intestinal tract. Report of 37 cases with a study of factors influencing prognosis. *Br J Surg* 1961;**49**:80.
2. d'Amore F, Christensen BE, Brincker H, et al. Clinicopathological features and prognostic factors in extranodal non-Hodgkin lymphomas. Danish LYFO Study Group. *Eur J Cancer* 1991;**27**:1201.
3. Isaacson PG. Gastrointestinal lymphoma. *Hum Pathol* 1994;**25**:1020.
4. Hockey MS, Powell J, Crocker J, Fielding JW. Primary gastric lymphoma. *Br J Surg* 1987;**74**:483.
5. Venizelos I, Tamiolakis D, Bolioti S, et al. Primary gastric Hodgkin's lymphoma: a case report and review of the literature. *Leuk Lymphoma* 2005;**46**:147.
6. Ghai S, Pattison J, Ghai S, O'Malley ME, Khalili K, Stephens M. Primary gastrointestinal lymphoma: spectrum of imaging findings with pathologic correlation. *Radiographics* 2007;**27**:1371.
7. Chiu BC, Weisenburger DD. An update of the epidemiology of non-Hodgkin's lymphoma. *Clin Lymphoma* 2003;**4**:161.
8. Severson RK, Davis S. Increasing incidence of primary gastric lymphoma. *Cancer* 1990;**66**:1283.
9. Gurney KA, Cartwright RA, Gilman EA. Descriptive epidemiology of gastrointestinal non-Hodgkin's lymphoma in a population-based registry. *Br J Cancer* 1999;**79**:1929.
10. Doglioni C, Wotherspoon AC, Moschini A, de Boni M, Isaacson PG. High incidence of primary gastric lymphoma in northeastern Italy. *Lancet* 1992;**339**:834.
11. Koch P, del Valle F, Berdel WE, et al. Primary gastrointestinal non-Hodgkin's lymphoma: I. Anatomic and histologic distribution, clinical features and survival data of 371 patients registered in the German Multicenter Study GIT NHL 01/92. *J Clin Oncol* 2001;**19**:3861.
12. Papaxoinis G, Papageorgiou S, Rontogianni D, et al. A Hellenic Cooperative Oncology Group study (HeCOG). Primary gastrointestinal non-Hodgkin's lymphoma: a clinicopathologic study of 128 cases in Greece. *Leuk Lymphoma* 2006;**47**:2140.

13. Fischbach W, Dragosics B, Kolve-Goebeler ME, et al. The German-Austrian Gastrointestinal Lymphoma Study Group. Primary gastric B-cell lymphoma: results of a prospective multicenter study. *Gastroenterology* 2000;**119**:1191.

14. Musshoff K. [Clinical staging classification of non-Hodgkin's lymphomas (author's transl).] *Strahlentherapie* 1977;**153**:218.

15. Rohatiner A, d'Amore F, Coiffier B, et al. Report on a workshop convened to discuss the pathological and staging classifications of gastrointestinal tract lymphoma. *Ann Oncol* 1994;**5**:397.

16. Ruskone-Fourmestraux A, Dragosics B, Morgner A, Wotherspoon A, De Jong D. Paris staging system for primary gastrointestinal lymphomas. *Gut* 2003;**52**:912.

17. Boot H. Diagnosis and staging in gastrointestinal lymphoma. *Best Practice Res Clin Gastroenterol* 2010;**24**:3.

18. Gospodarowicz MK, Sutcliffe SB, Brown TC, Chua T, Bush RS. Patterns of disease in localized extranodal lymphomas. *J Clin Oncol* 1987;**5**:875.

19. Zucca E, Roggero E, Bertoni F, Conconi A, Cavalli F. Primary extranodal non-Hodgkin's lymphomas. Part 2: Head and neck, central nervous system and other less common sites. *Ann Oncol* 1999;**10**:1023.

20. Krol AD, Le Cessie S, Snijder S, Kluin-Nelemans JC, Kluin PM, Noorduk EM. Waldeyer's ring lymphomas: a clinical study from the Comprehensive Cancer Center West population based NHL registry. *Leuk Lymphoma* 2001;**42**:1005.

21. Raderer M, Wohrer S, Streubel B, et al. Assessment of disease dissemination in gastric compared with extragastric mucosa-associated lymphoid tissue lymphoma using extensive staging: a single-center experience. *J Clin Oncol* 2006 1;**24**:3136.

22. Fischbach W, Al-Taie O. Staging role of EUS. *Best Practice Res Clin Gastroenterol* 2010;**24**:13.

23. Ferrucci PF, Zucca E. Primary gastric lymphoma pathogenesis and treatment: what has changed over the past 10 years? *Br J Haematol* 2007;**136**:521.

24. Yi JH, Kim SJ, Choi JY, Ko YH, Kim BT, Kim WS. (18)F-FDG uptake and its clinical relevance in primary gastric lymphoma. *Hematol Oncol* 2010;**28**:57.

25. Kumar R, Xiu Y, Potenta S, et al. ^{18}F-FDG PET for evaluation of the treatment response in patients with gastrointestinal tract lymphomas. *J Nucl Med* 2004;**45**:1796.

26. Zucca E, Bertoni F, Roggero E, Cavalli F. The gastric marginal zone B-cell lymphoma of MALT type. *Blood* 2000 15;**96**:410.

27. Thieblemont C, Berger F, Dumontet C, et al. Mucosa-associated lymphoid tissue lymphoma is a disseminated disease in one third of 158 patients analyzed. *Blood* 2000;**95**:802.

28. Isaacson P, Wright D. Malignant lymphoma of mucosa associated lymphoid tissue. A distinctive B cell lymphoma. *Cancer* 1983;**52**:1410.

29. Isaacson P, Wright DH. Extranodal malignant lymphoma arising from mucosa-associated lymphoid tissue. *Cancer* 1984;**53**:2515.

30. Spencer J, Finn T, Pulford K, Mason D, Isaacson P. The human gut contains a novel population of B lymphocytes which resemble marginal zone cells. *Clin Exp Immunol* 1985;**62**:607.

31. Hyjek E, Isaacson PG. Primary B cell lymphoma of the thyroid and its relationship to Hashimoto's thyroiditis. *Hum Pathol* 1988;**19**:1315.

32. Hyjek E, Smith WJ, Isaacson PG. Primary B-cell lymphoma of salivary glands and its relationship to myoepithelial sialadenitis. *Hum Pathol* 1988;**19**:766.

33. Addis BJ, Hyjek E, Isaacson PG. Primary pulmonary lymphoma: a re-appraisal of its histogenesis and its relationship to pseudolymphoma and lymphoid interstitial pneumonia. *Histopathology* 1988;**13**:1.

34. Isaacson PG, Du MQ. MALT lymphoma: from morphology to molecules. *Nat Rev Cancer* 2004;**4**:644.

35. Isaacson P, Chott A, Nakamura S, Müller-Hermelink H, Harris N, Swerdlow S. Extranodal marginal zone lymphoma of mucosa-associated lymphoid tissue (MALT lymphoma). In: Swerdlow S, Campo E, Harris N, et al. (eds), *WHO Classification of Tumours of Haematopoietic and Lymphoid Tissues*. Lyon: International Agency for Research on Cancer, 2008: 214.

36. Isaacson PG, Du MQ. Gastrointestinal lymphoma: where morphology meets molecular biology. *J Pathol* 2005;**205**:255.

37. Andriani A, Zullo A, Di Raimondo F, et al. Clinical and endoscopic presentation of primary gastric lymphoma: a multicentre study. *Aliment Pharmacol Therap* 2006;**23**:721.

38. Wotherspoon A, Doglioni C, Isaacson P. Gastric B cell lymphoma of mucosa-associated lymphoid tissue is a multifocal disease. *Histopathology* 1992;**20**:29.

39. Yokoi T, Nakamura T, Kasugai K, et al. Primary low grade gastric mucosa-associated lymphoid tissue (MALT) lymphoma with polypoid appearance. Polypoid gastric MALT lymphoma: A clinicopathologic study of eight cases. *Pathol Int* 1999;**49**:702.

40. Isaacson PG, Spencer J. Malignant lymphoma of mucosa-associated lymphoid tissue. *Histopathology* 1987;**11**:445.

41. Zamboni G, Franzin G, Scarpa A, et al. Carcinoma-like signet-ring cells in gastric mucosa-associated lymphoid tissue (MALT) lymphoma. *Am J Surg Pathol* 1996;**20**:588.

42. Isaacson P, Wotherspoon A, Diss T, Pan L. Follicular colonization in B-cell lymphoma of mucosa-associated lymphoid tissue. *Am J Surg Pathol* 1991;**15**:819.

43. Du MQ, Peng HZ, Dogan A, et al. Preferential dissemination of B-cell gastric mucosa-associated lymphoid tissue (MALT) lymphoma to the splenic marginal zone. *Blood* 1997 15;**90**:4071.

44. Ferry JA, Yang WI, Zukerberg LR, Wotherspoon AC, Arnold A, Harris NL. CD5+ extranodal marginal zone B-cell (MALT) lymphoma. A low grade neoplasm with a propensity for bone marrow involvement and relapse. *Am J Clin Pathol* 1996;**105**:31.

45. Ballesteros E, Osborne BM, Matsushima AY. CD5+ low grade marginal zone B-cell lymphomas with localized presentation. *Am J Surg Pathol* 1998;**22**:201.

46. Isaacson P, Spencer J. Malignant lymphoma of mucosa-associated lymphoid tissue. *Histopathology* 1987;**11**:445.

47. Qin Y, Greiner A, Trunk MJ, Schmausser B, Ott MM, Muller-Hermelink HK. Somatic hypermutation in low grade mucosa-associated lymphoid tissue-type B-cell lymphoma. *Blood* 1995;**86**:3528.

48. Du M, Diss TC, Xu C, Peng H, Isaacson PG, Pan L. Ongoing mutation in MALT lymphoma immunoglobulin gene suggests that antigen stimulation plays a role in the clonal expansion. *Leukemia* 1996;**10**:1190.

49. Parsonnet J, Hansen S, Rodriguez L, et al. Helicobacter pylori infection and gastric lymphoma. *N Engl J Med* 1994;**330**:1267.

50. Wotherspoon A, Ortiz-Hidalgo C, Falzon M, Isaacson P. *Helicobacter pylori*-associated gastritis and primary B-cell gastric lymphoma. *Lancet* 1991;**338**:1175.

51. Nakamura S, Yao T, Aoyagi K, Iida M, Fujishima M, Tsuneyoshi M. *Helicobacter pylori* and primary gastric lymphoma. A histopathologic and immunohistochemical analysis of 237 patients. *Cancer* 1997;**79**:3.

52. Nakamura S, Aoyagi K, Furuse M, et al. B-cell monoclonality precedes the development of gastric MALT lymphoma in *Helicobacter pylori*-associated chronic gastritis. *Am J Pathol* 1998; **152**:1271.

53. Hussell T, Isaacson P, Crabtree J, Spencer J. The response of cells from low grade B-cell gastric lymphomas of mucosa-associated lymphoid tissue to *Helicobacter pylori*. *Lancet* 1993; **342**:571.

54. Wotherspoon A, Doglioni C, Diss T, et al. Regression of primary low grade B-cell gastric lymphoma of mucosa-associated lymphoid tissue type after eradication of *Helicobacter pylori*. *Lancet* 1993;**342**:575.

55. Raderer M, Isaacson PG. Extranodal lymphoma of MALT-type: perspective at the beginning of the 21st century. *Expert Rev Anticancer Ther* 2001;**1**:53.

56. Bertoni F, Zucca E. State-of-the-art therapeutics: marginal-zone lymphoma. *J Clin Oncol* 2005;**23**:6415.

57. Hussell T, Isaacson PG, Crabtree JE, Spencer J. *Helicobacter pylori*-specific tumour-infiltrating T cells provide contact dependent help for the growth of malignant B cells in low grade gastric lymphoma of mucosa-associated lymphoid tissue. *J Pathol* 1996;**178**:122.

58. Greiner A, Knorr C, Qin Y, et al. Low grade B cell lymphomas of mucosa-associated lymphoid tissue (MALT-type) require CD40-mediated signaling and Th2-type cytokines for in vitro growth and differentiation. *Am J Pathol* 1997;**150**: 1583.

59. Hussell T, Isaacson PG, Crabtree JE, Dogan A, Spencer J. Immunoglobulin specificity of low grade B cell gastrointestinal lymphoma of mucosa-associated lymphoid tissue (MALT) type. *Am J Pathol* 1993;**142**:285.

60. Dierlamm J, Baens M, Wlodarska I, et al. The apoptosis inhibitor gene API2 and a novel 18q gene, MLT, are recurrently rearranged in the t(11;18)(q21;q21)p6ssociated with mucosa-associated lymphoid tissue lymphomas. *Blood* 1999 1;**93**:3601.

61. Lucas PC, Yonezumi M, Inohara N, et al. Bcl10 and MALT1, independent targets of chromosomal translocation in malt lymphoma, cooperate in a novel NF-kappa B signaling pathway. *J Biol Chem* 2001;**276**:19012.

62. Streubel B, Lamprecht A, Dierlamm J, et al. T(14;18)(q32;q21) involving IGH and MALT1 is a frequent chromosomal aberration in MALT lymphoma. *Blood* 2003;**101**:2335.

63. Streubel B, Simonitsch-Klupp I, Mullauer L, et al. Variable frequencies of MALT lymphoma-associated genetic aberrations in MALT lymphomas of different sites. *Leukemia* 2004;**18**: 1722.

64. Nakamura S, Ye H, Bacon CM, et al. Clinical impact of genetic aberrations in gastric MALT lymphoma: a comprehensive analysis using interphase fluorescence in situ hybridisation. *Gut* 2007;**56**:1358.

65. Remstein ED, Kurtin PJ, James CD, Wang XY, Meyer RG, Dewald GW. Mucosa-associated lymphoid tissue lymphomas with t(11;18)(q21;q21) and mucosa-associated lymphoid tissue lymphomas with aneuploidy develop along different pathogenetic pathways. *Am J Pathol* 2002;**161**:63.

66. Starostik P, Patzner J, Greiner A, et al. Gastric marginal zone B-cell lymphomas of MALT type develop along 2 distinct pathogenetic pathways. *Blood* 2002;**99**:3.

67. Ye H, Liu H, Attygalle A, et al. Variable frequencies of t(11;18)(q21;q21) in MALT lymphomas of different sites: significant association with CagA strains of *H. pylori* in gastric MALT lymphoma. *Blood* 2003;**102**:1012.

68. Liu H, Ruskon-Fourmestraux A, Lavergne-Slove A, et al. Resistance of t(11;18) positive gastric mucosa-associated lymphoid tissue lymphoma to *Helicobacter pylori* eradication therapy. *Lancet* 2001;**357**:39.

69. Liu H, Ye H, Ruskone-Fourmestraux A, et al. t(11;18) is a marker for all stage gastric MALT lymphomas that will not respond to H. pylori eradication. *Gastroenterology* 2002;**122**:1286.

70. Ott G, Katzenberger T, Greiner A, et al. The t(11;18)(q21;q21) chromosome translocation is a frequent and specific aberration in low grade but not high grade malignant non-Hodgkin's lymphomas of the mucosa-associated lymphoid tissue (MALT-) type. *Cancer Res* 1997;**57**:3944.

71. Ye H, Liu H, Raderer M, et al. High incidence of t(11;18)(q21;q21) in *Helicobacter pylori*-negative gastric MALT lymphoma. *Blood* 2003;**101**:2547.

72. Dierlamm J, Baens M, Stefanova-Ouzounova M, et al. Detection of t(11;18)(q21;q21) by interphase fluorescence in situ hybridization using API2 and MLT specific probes. *Blood* 2000;**96**: 2215.

73. Ye H, Dogan A, Karran L, et al. *BCL10* expression in normal and neoplastic lymphoid tissue. Nuclear localization in MALT lymphoma. *Am J Pathol* 2000;**157**:1147.

74. Wotherspoon AC, Pan LX, Diss TC, Isaacson PG. Cytogenetic study of B-cell lymphoma of mucosa-associated lymphoid tissue. *Cancer Genet Cytogenet* 1992;**58**:35.

75. Ye H, Gong L, Liu H, et al. MALT lymphoma with t(14;18)(q32;q21)/IGH-MALT1 is characterized by strong cytoplasmic MALT1 and BCL10 expression. *J Pathol* 2005;**205**:293.

76. Auer IA, Gascoyne RD, Connors JM, et al. t(11;18)(q21;q21) is the most common translocation in Malt lymphomas. *Ann Oncol* 1997;**8**:979.

77. Zhou Y, Ye H, tin-Subero JI, et al. Distinct comparative genomic hybridisation profiles in gastric mucosa-associated lymphoid tissue lymphomas with and without t(11;18)(q21;q21). *Br J Haematol* 2006;**133**:35.

78. Min KO, Seo EJ, Kwon HJ, et al. Methylation of p16(INK4A) and p57(KIP2) are involved in the development and progression of gastric MALT lymphomas. *Mod Pathol* 2006;**19**:141.

79. Huang Q, Su X, Ai L, Li M, Fan CY, Weiss LM. Promoter hypermethylation of multiple genes in gastric lymphoma. *Leuk Lymphoma* 2007;**48**:1988.

80. Kondo T, Oka T, Sato H, et al. Accumulation of aberrant CpG hypermethylation by Helicobacter pylori infection promotes development and progression of gastric MALT lymphoma. *Int J Oncol* 2009;**35**:547.

81. Hsi ED, Eisbruch A, Greenson JK, Singleton TP, Ross CW, Schnitzer B. Classification of primary gastric lymphomas according to histologic features. *Am J Surg Pathol* 1998;**22**:17.

82. Du MQ, Diss TC, Dogan A, et al. Clone-specific PCR reveals wide dissemination of gastric MALT lymphoma to the gastric mucosa. *J Pathol* 2000;**192**:488.

83. Du MQ, Xu CF, Diss TC, et al. Intestinal dissemination of gastric MALT lymphoma occurs following antigen mediated tumour clonal expansion. *Blood* 1996;**88**(suppl 1):671a.

84. Dogan A, Du M, Koulis A, Briskin MJ, Isaacson PG. Expression of lymphocyte homing receptors and vascular addressins in low grade gastric B-cell lymphomas of mucosa-associated lymphoid tissue. *Am J Pathol* 1997;**151**:1361.

85. Siakantaris MP, Pangalis GA, Dimitriadou E, et al. Early-stage gastric MALT lymphoma: is it a truly localized disease? *The Oncologist* 2009;**14**:148.

86. Hummel M, Oeschger S, Barth TF, et al. Wotherspoon criteria combined with B cell clonality analysis by advanced polymerase chain reaction technology discriminates covert gastric marginal zone lymphoma from chronic gastritis. *Gut* 2006;**55**: 782.

87. Swerdlow S, Campo E, Seto M, Müller-Hermelink H. Mantle cell lymphoma. In: Swerdlow S, Campo E, Harris N, et al. (eds), *WHO Classification of Tumours of Haematopoietic and Lymphoid Tissues.* Lyon: International Agency for Research on Cancer, 2008: 229.

88. de Jong D, Boot H, Taal B. Histological grading with clinical relevance in gastric mucosa-associated lymphoid tissue (MALT) lymphoma. *Recent Results Cancer Res* 2000;**156**:27.

89. Ferreri AJ, Freschi M, Dell'Oro S, Viale E, Villa E, Ponzoni M. Prognostic significance of the histopathologic recognition of low- and high grade components in stage I-II B-cell gastric lymphomas. *Am J Surg Pathol* 2001;**25**:95.

90. Stasi R, Evangelista ML, Brunetti M, et al. Primary gastric plasmacytoma and *Helicobacter pylori* infection. *J Clin Oncol* 2009;**27**:150.

91. Ferreri AJ, Ernberg I, Copie-Bergman C. Infectious agents and lymphoma development: molecular and clinical aspects. *J Intern Med* 2009;**265**:421.

92. Levy M, Copie-Bergman C, Gameiro C, et al. Prognostic value of translocation t(11;18) in tumoral response of low grade gastric lymphoma of mucosa-associated lymphoid tissue type to oral chemotherapy. *J Clin Oncol* 2005;**23**:5061.

93. Levy M, Copie-Bergman C, Molinier-Frenkel V, et al. Treatment of t(11;18)-positive gastric mucosa-associated lymphoid tissue lymphoma with rituximab and chlorambucil: clinical, histological and molecular follow-up. *Leuk Lymphoma* 2010;**51**:284.

94. Cogliatti S, Schmid U, Schumacher U, et al. Primary B-cell gastric lymphoma: a clinicopathological study of 145 patients. *Gastroenterology* 1991;**101**:1159.

95. Boot H, de Jong D. Diagnosis, treatment decisions and follow up in primary gastric lymphoma. *Gut* 2002;**51**:621.

96. Savio A, Franzin G, Wotherspoon AC, et al. Diagnosis and post-treatment follow-up of Helicobacter pylori-positive gastric lymphoma of mucosa-associated lymphoid tissue: histology, polymerase chain reaction, or both? *Blood* 1996 15;**87**:1255.

97. Copie-Bergman C, Gaulard P, Lavergne-Slove A, et al. Proposal for a new histological grading system for post-treatment evaluation of gastric MALT lymphoma. *Gut* 2003;**52**:1656.

98. Raderer M, Streubel B, Woehrer S, et al. High relapse rate in patients with MALT lymphoma warrants lifelong follow-up. *Clin Cancer Res* 2005;**11**:3349.

99. Wotherspoon AC, Isaacson PG. Synchronous adenocarcinoma and low grade B-cell lymphoma of mucosa associated lymphoid tissue (MALT) of the stomach. *Histopathology* 1995;**27**:325.

100. Goteri G, Ranaldi R, Rezai B, Baccarini MG, Bearzi I. Synchronous mucosa-associated lymphoid tissue lymphoma and adenocarcinoma of the stomach. *Am J Surg Pathol* 1997;**21**:505.

101. Morgner A, Miehlke S, Stolte M, et al. Development of early gastric cancer 4 and 5 years after complete remission of *Helicobacter pylori* associated gastric low grade marginal zone B cell lymphoma of MALT type. *World J Gastroenterol* 2001;**7**:248.

102. Copie-Bergman C, Locher C, Levy M, et al. Metachronous gastric MALT lymphoma and early gastric cancer: is residual lymphoma a risk factor for the development of gastric carcinoma? *Ann Oncol* 2005;**16**:1232.

103. Thiede C, Wundisch T, Alpen B, et al. Long-term persistence of monoclonal B cells after cure of *Helicobacter pylori* infection and complete histologic remission in gastric mucosa-associated lymphoid tissue B-cell lymphoma. *J Clin Oncol* 2001;**19**:1600.

104. Bertoni F, Conconi A, Capella C, et al. Molecular follow-up in gastric mucosa-associated lymphoid tissue lymphomas: early analysis of the LY03 cooperative trial. *Blood* 2002;**99**:2541.

105. Wundisch T, Thiede C, Morgner A, et al. Long-term follow-up of gastric MALT lymphoma after *Helicobacter pylori* eradication. *J Clin Oncol* 2005;**23**:8018.

106. Montalban C, Santon A, Redondo C, et al. Long-term persistence of molecular disease after histological remission in low grade gastric MALT lymphoma treated with *H. pylori* eradication. Lack of association with translocation t(11;18): a 10-year updated follow-up of a prospective study. *Ann Oncol* 2005;**16**:1539.

107. Salar A, Bellosillo B, Serrano S, Besses C. Persistent residual disease in t(11;18)(q21;q21) positive gastric mucosa-associated lymphoid tissue lymphoma treated with chemotherapy or rituximab. *J Clin Oncol* 2005;**23**:7361; author reply 2–3.

108. Streubel B, Huber D, Wohrer S, Chott A, Raderer M. Reverse transcription-PCR for t(11;18)(q21;q21) staging and monitoring in mucosa-associated lymphoid tissue lymphoma. *Clin Cancer Res* 2006;**12**(20 Part 1):6023.

109. Wundisch T, Neubauer A, Stolte M, Ritter M, Thiede C. B-cell monoclonality is associated with lymphoid follicles in gastritis. *Am J Surg Pathol* 2003;**27**:882.

110. Ferreri AJ, Montalban C. Primary diffuse large B-cell lymphoma of the stomach. *Crit Rev Oncol/Hematol* 2007;**63**:65.

111. Takeshita M, Iwashita A, Kurihara K, et al. Histologic and immunohistologic findings and prognosis of 40 cases of gastric large B-cell lymphoma. *Am J Surg Pathol* 2000;**24**:1641.

112. de Jong D, J B, van Heerde P, Hart A. Histological grading in gastric lymphoma: pretreatment criteria and clinical relevance. *Gastroenterology* 1997;**112**:1466.

113. Chan J, Ng C, Isaacson P. Relationship between high grade lymphoma and low grade B-cell mucosa-associated lymphoid tissue lymphoma (MALToma) of the stomach. *Am J Pathol* 1990;**136**:1153.

114. Peng H, Du M, Diss TC, Isaacson PG, Pan L. Genetic evidence for a clonal link between low and high grade components in gastric MALT B-cell lymphoma. *Histopathology* 1997;**30**:425.

115. Omonishi K, Yoshino T, Sakuma I, Kobayashi K, Moriyama M, Akagi T. bcl-6 protein is identified in high grade but not low grade mucosa- associated lymphoid tissue lymphomas of the stomach. *Mod Pathol* 1998;**11**:181.

116. Hans CP, Weisenburger DD, Greiner TC, et al. Confirmation of the molecular classification of diffuse large B-cell lymphoma by immunohistochemistry using a tissue microarray. *Blood* 2004;**103**:275.

117. Chen YW, Hu XT, Liang AC, et al. High BCL6 expression predicts better prognosis, independent of BCL6 translocation status, translocation partner, or BCL6-deregulating mutations, in gastric lymphoma. *Blood* 2006;**108**:2373.

118. Connor J, Ashton-Key M. Gastric and intestinal diffuse large B-cell lymphomas are clinically and immunophenotypically different. An immunohistochemical and clinical study. *Histopathology* 2007;**51**:697.

119. Mitchell KA, Finn WG, Owens SR. Differences in germinal centre and non-germinal centre phenotype in gastric and intestinal diffuse large B-cell lymphomas. *Leuk Lymphoma* 2008;**49**:1717.

120. Nakamura S, Ye H, Bacon CM, et al. Translocations involving the immunoglobulin heavy chain gene locus predict better survival in gastric diffuse large B-cell lymphoma. *Clin Cancer Res* 2008;**14**:3002.

121. Ponzoni M, Ferreri AJ, Pruneri G, et al. Prognostic value of bcl-6, CD10 and CD38 immunoreactivity in stage I–II gastric lymphomas: identification of a subset of CD10+ large B-cell lymphomas with a favorable outcome. *Int J Cancer* 2003;**106**:288.

122. Toracchio S, Ota H, de Jong D, Wotherspoon A, Rugge M, Graham DY, et al. Translocation t(11;18)(q21;q21) in gastric B-cell lymphomas. *Cancer Sci* 2009;**100**:881.

123. Chuang SS, Lee C, Hamoudi RA, et al. High frequency of t(11;18) in gastric mucosa-associated lymphoid tissue lymphomas in Taiwan, including one patient with high grade transformation. *Br J Haematol* 2003;**120**:97.

124. Liang R, Chan WP, Kwong YL, Xu WS, Srivastava G, Ho FC. High incidence of BCL-6 gene rearrangement in diffuse large B-cell lymphoma of primary gastric origin. *Cancer Genet Cytogenet* 1997;**97**:114.

125. Liang R, Chan WP, Kwong YL, et al. *Bcl-6* gene hypermutations in diffuse large B-cell lymphoma of primary gastric origin. *Br J Haematol* 1997;**99**:668.

126. Starostik P, Greiner A, Schultz A, et al. Genetic aberrations common in gastric high grade large B-cell lymphoma. *Blood* 2000;**95**:1180.

127. Coiffier B. State-of-the-art therapeutics: diffuse large B-cell lymphoma. *J Clin Oncol* 2005;**23**:6387.

128. Morgner A, Miehlke S, Fischbach W, et al. Complete remission of primary high grade B-cell gastric lymphoma after cure of *Helicobacter pylori* infection. *J Clin Oncol* 2001 1;**19**:2041.

129. Chen LT, Lin JT, Shyu RY, et al. Prospective study of *Helicobacter pylori* eradication therapy in stage I(E) high grade mucosa-associated lymphoid tissue lymphoma of the stomach. *J Clin Oncol* 2001;**19**:4245.

130. Charton-Bain MC, Brousset P, Bouabdallah R, et al. Variation in the histological pattern of nodal involvement by gamma/delta T-cell lymphoma. *Histopathology* 2000;**36**:233.

131. Ruskone-Fourmestraux A, Delmer A, Lavergne A, et al. Groupe D'etude des Lymphomes Digestifs. Multiple lymphomatous polyposis of the gastrointestinal tract: prospective clinicopathologic study of 31 cases. *Gastroenterology* 1997;**112**:7.

132. Ruskone-Fourmestraux A, Audouin J. Primary gastrointestinal tract mantle cell lymphoma as multiple lymphomatous polyposis. *Best Practice Res Clin Gastroenterol* 2010;**24**:35.

133. Geissmann F, Ruskone-Fourmestraux A, Hermine O, et al. Homing receptor alpha4beta7 integrin expression predicts digestive tract involvement in mantle cell lymphoma. *Am J Pathol* 1998;**153**:1701.

134. Leoncini L, Raphael M, Stein H, Harris N, Jaffe E, Kluin P. Burkitt lymphoma. In: Swerdlow S, Campo E, Harris N, et al. (eds), *WHO Classification of Tumours of Haematopoietic and Lymphoid Tissues*. Lyon: International Agency for Research on Cancer, 2008.

135. Park YH, Kim WS, Kang HJ, et al. Gastric Burkitt lymphoma is a distinct subtype that has superior outcomes to other types of Burkitt lymphoma/leukemia. *Ann Hematol* 2006;**85**:285.

136. de Leval L, Hasserjian RP. Diffuse large B-cell lymphomas and Burkitt lymphoma. *Hematol Oncol Clin North Am* 2009;**23**:791.

137. Hasserjian RP, Ott G, Elenitoba-Johnson KS, Balague-Ponz O, de Jong D, de Leval L. Commentary on the WHO classification of tumours of lymphoid tissues (2008): 'Gray zone' lymphomas overlapping with Burkitt lymphoma or classical Hodgkin lymphoma. *J Hematopathol* 2009;**2**:89.

138. Moschovi M, Menegas D, Stefanaki K, Constantinidou CV, Tzortzatou-Stathopoulou F. Primary gastric Burkitt lymphoma in childhood: associated with *Helicobacter pylori*? *Med Pediatr Oncol* 2003;**41**:444.

139. Grewal SS, Hunt JP, O'Connor SC, Gianturco LE, Richardson MW, Lehmann LE. *Helicobacter pylori* associated gastric Burkitt lymphoma. *Pediatr Blood Cancer* 2008;**50**:888.

140. Baumgaertner I, Copie-Bergman C, Levy M, et al. Complete remission of gastric Burkitt's lymphoma after eradication of *Helicobacter pylori*. *World J Gastroenterol* 2009;**15**:5746.

141. Tanaka K, Nakamura S, Matsumoto T, et al. Long-term remission of primary gastric T cell lymphoma associated with human T lymphotropic virus type 1: a report of two cases and review of the literature. *Intern Med* 2007;**46**:1783.

142. Ohshima K. Pathological features of diseases associated with human T-cell leukemia virus type I. *Cancer Sci* 2007;**98**:772.

143. Sakata H, Iwakiri R, Koyama T, et al. Human T-cell lymphotropic virus-associated primary gastric lymphoma. *Dig Dis Sci* 2001;**46**:1381.

144. Ohshima k, Jaffe E, Kikuchi M. Adult T-cell leukaemia/lymphoma. In: Swerdlow S, Campo E, Harris N, et al. (eds), *WHO Classification of Tumours of Haematopoietic and Lymphoid Tissues*. Lyon: International Agency for Research on Cancer, 2008: 281.

145. Kawamoto K, Nakamura S, Iwashita A, et al. Clinicopathological characteristics of primary gastric T-cell lymphoma. *Histopathology* 2009;**55**:641.

146. Iwamizu-Watanabe S, Yamashita Y, Yatabe Y, Nakamura S, Mori N. Frequent expression of CD30 antigen in the primary gastric non-B, non-Hodgkin lymphomas. *Pathol Int* 2004;**54**:503.

147. Holanda D, Zhao MY, Rapoport AP, Garofalo M, Chen Q, Zhao XF. Primary gastric T cell lymphoma mimicking marginal zone B cell lymphoma of mucosa-associated lymphoid tissue. *J Hematopathol* 2008;**1**:29.

148. Shimada-Hiratsuka M, Fukayama M, Hayashi Y, et al. Primary gastric T-cell lymphoma with and without human T-lymphotropic virus type 1. *Cancer* 1997;**80**:292.

149. Banerjee D, Walton JC, Jory TA, Crukley C, Meek M. Primary gastric T-cell lymphoma of suppressor-cytotoxic (CD8+) phenotype: discordant expression of T-cell receptor subunit beta F1, CD7and CD3 antigens. *Hum Pathol* 1990;**21**:872.

150. Beck PL, Gill MJ, Sutherland LR. HIV-associated non-Hodgkin's lymphoma of the gastrointestinal tract. *Am J Gastroenterol* 1996;**91**:2377.

151. Wotherspoon AC, Diss TC, Pan L, Singh N, Whelan J, Isaacson PG. Low grade gastric B-cell lymphoma of mucosa associated lymphoid tissue in immunocompromised patients. *Histopathology* 1996;**28**:129.

152. Swerdlow S, Webber S, Chadburn A, Ferry J. Post-transplant lymphoproliferative disorders. In: Swerdlow S, Campo E, Harris N, et al. (eds), *WHO Classification of Tumours of Haematopoietic and Lymphoid Tissues*. Lyon: International Agency for Research on Cancer, 2008: 343.

153. Hsi ED, Singleton TP, Swinnen L, Dunphy CH, Alkan S. Mucosa-associated lymphoid tissue-type lymphomas occurring in post-transplantation patients. *Am J Surg Pathol* 2000;**24**:100.

154. Fischbach W, Kestel W, Kirchner T, Mossner J, Wilms K. Malignant lymphomas of the upper gastrointestinal tract. Results of a prospective study in 103 patients. *Cancer* 1992 1;**70**:1075.

155. Brugo EA, Marshall RB, Riberi AM, Pautasso OE. Preleukemic granulocytic sarcomas of the gastrointestinal tract. Report of two cases. *Am J Clin Pathol* 1977;**68**:616.

CHAPTER 16

Miscellaneous conditions

Do-Youn Park¹ and Michio Shimizu²
¹Pusan National University College of Medicine, Pusan National University Hospital, Busan, Republic of Korea
²Saitama Medical University, Saitama International Medical Center, Saitama, Japan

Acute gastric dilatation

Acute spontaneous gastric dilatation is rare and occurs mainly in patients with post-operative complications and eating disorders [1,2]. Other associated conditions and causes include severe trauma [3], acute pancreatitis [4], diabetes mellitus [5], especially in diabetic ketoacidosis [6], drugs [7], Duchenne muscular dystrophy [8] and Prader–Willi syndrome. It has also been reported after endoscopic procedures, including insertion of a percutaneous endoscopic gastrostomy (PEG) feeding tube [9] or after injection sclerotherapy of oesophageal and gastric varices [10]. The dilatation is due to gas and gastric hypersecretion. The onset is usually rapid, leading to regurgitation of small amounts of fluid, shock and collapse [11]. Gastric rupture is unusual but, when it occurs, it may be fatal [12] (Figure 16.1).

Motility disorders

Adult pyloric obstruction

In its most common form, adult pyloric obstruction is related to hypertrophic stenosis of the pylorus due to previous pre-pyloric, pyloric or duodenal ulceration, tumour or extrinsic adhesions [13–16]. Occasionally, it may be related to eosinophilic gastroenteritis. In the latter scenario, it is secondary to fibrosis of the circular muscle and not muscular hypertrophy.

Rare adult cases of congenital diaphragms at the pyloric ring, comprising mucosa, muscularis mucosae and submucosa and responsible for obstruction, have been described [17]. A similar pathology has been described in a patient taking non-steroidal anti-inflammatory drugs [18], resembling diaphragm disease seen elsewhere in the gastrointes-

tinal tract, especially in the small intestine (see 'Diaphragm disease', Chapter 20) [19].

The literature reports only about 200 cases of primary adult hypertrophic pyloric stenosis. It is characterised by total or segmental hypertrophy of the circular muscle coat of pylorus without obvious disease [20,21]. Most cases seem to represent infantile pyloric stenosis persisting into adulthood and show findings macroscopically and microscopically similar to the infantile form. Clinically, it is especially important to differentiate such primary disease from secondary pyloric stenosis, such as that caused by peptic ulceration and tumours.

Gastric motility disorders associated with neuromuscular disorders

Gastroparesis is a chronic disorder of peristalsis featuring delayed gastric emptying without evidence of a mechanical cause of obstruction. Drugs including opioids, anticholinergics and tricyclic antidepressants have been implicated. Other causes include surgery, especially vagotomy, severe diabetic mellitus and generalised neuromuscular disorders [22]. Patients with muscular dystrophy, such as Duchenne muscular dystrophy, mitochondrial myopathies, the polyneuropathy, ophthalmoplegia and leukoencephalopathy syndrome (so-called POLYP syndrome) [23] and patients with oculo-gastrointestinal muscular dystrophy are included in this group, along with progressive muscular dystrophy. The appearance of the stomach in progressive muscular dystrophy is similar to that seen in the oesophagus and small bowel with smooth muscle fibrosis [24].

Patients with Friedreich's ataxia may have repetitive uncoordinated gastric contractions and these may be seen

Morson and Dawson's Gastrointestinal Pathology, Fifth Edition. Edited by Neil A. Shepherd, Bryan F. Warren,
Geraint T. Williams, Joel K. Greenson, Gregory Y. Lauwers and Marco R. Novelli.
© 2013 Blackwell Publishing Ltd. Published 2013 by Blackwell Publishing Ltd.

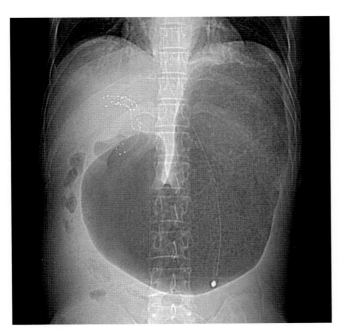

Figure 16.1 Gastric dilatation: this plain abdominal radiograph demonstrates a stomach markedly distended by air.

throughout the gastrointestinal tract. The myenteric plexus usually shows a reduction in neuron numbers and the presence of eosinophilic nuclear inclusions, similar to those seen elsewhere in the nervous system in these patients. Myotonic dystrophy patients may suffer delayed gastric emptying and, in this autosomal dominant inherited condition, the gastrointestinal effects may precede the classic systemic features [25]. The nerves appear normal but there is smooth muscle atrophy with fatty replacement and fibrosis. Surviving smooth muscle fibres may appear pleomorphic, oedematous and hypereosinophilic, with nuclear pyknosis and perinuclear vacuolation.

Post-viral gastroparesis

Gastric outlet obstruction has been reported to follow viral illnesses in previously healthy young to middle-aged adults. These cases are not well characterised, because the histology has not been studied. The nature of the precipitating viral infection, suspected because of the presence of antibodies against neurotrophic viruses such as cytomegalovirus (CMV) and Epstein–Barr virus (EBV), is not always confirmed [26,27]. Post-viral gastroparesis usually has an acute onset and resolves rapidly, a feature not seen in idiopathic gastroparesis [27,28].

Familial visceral myopathies

There are several different types of familial visceral myopathy, all of which are uncommon. They are inherited

and characterised by histological findings of degeneration, thinning and fibrous replacement of the smooth muscle of the gastrointestinal tract. Some of these also involve the smooth muscle of the bladder. Although the histological features are similar in these different disorders, the pattern of inheritance and involvement of the organs vary. Schuffler has subdivided them into types I–IV. Type I shows an autosomal dominant inheritance and the others are autosomal recessive [29]. Type I does not involve the stomach. Its effects are seen in the oesophagus, duodenum, colon and bladder. Type II is associated with gastric and jejunoileal dilatation and the presence of multiple diverticula in the small bowel. The duodenum is usually spared. Ptosis and ophthalmoplegia also occur in this variety. Type III results in marked dilatation of the whole gastrointestinal tract [30]. In Type IV, there is gastroparesis and a narrow small intestine without diverticula. The histological features, in all of these forms of visceral myopathy, include marked vacuolar degeneration with a characteristic honeycomb appearance of the longitudinal muscle and hypertrophy of the circular muscle coat. The smooth muscle cells are reported to include spheroidal inclusions that are grey on haematoxylin and eosin (H&E) staining and periodic acid–Schiff (PAS) positive.

Non-familial visceral myopathies

These conditions may occur sporadically without obvious inheritance. Patients may present at all ages with pseudo-obstruction involving the whole gastrointestinal tract. Unlike inherited conditions, the sporadic varieties may show an inflammatory infiltrate in the smooth muscle layers [31].

Systemic sclerosis

Involvement of the gastrointestinal tract is common in systemic sclerosis. Involvement of the oesophagus, with gastro-oesophageal reflux and dysphagia, is the most common gastrointestinal manifestation (see Chapter 3, 'Progressive systemic sclerosis') [32,33]. Gastric emptying is significantly delayed in about half the scleroderma patients.

Motility disorders in patients with malignancy

Tumour-associated gastric paresis may be due to the local effects of neoplasia, the systemic effects of tumour or the effect of therapy, both radiotherapy and chemotherapy [34–36]. Local effects of vagal infiltration by tumour cells may be contributory, as may the stiffness of the gastric wall due to tumour infiltration. Gastroparesis may be seen in patients with brain-stem or posterior fossa tumours, and in association with small cell carcinoma of the lung, breast and ovarian carcinoma or thymoma, among others [37–39]. The para-neoplastic neuropathy is related to the development of pro-neuronal nuclear and cytoplasmic autoantibodies, such as anti-Hu antibodies. Ganglionitis and subsequent aganglionosis are the hallmark of the histopathological changes.

A related condition, *autoimmune gastrointestinal dysmotility*, has been reported outside the context of para-neoplastic manifestations. It is associated with the idiopathic development of antibodies to ganglionic neuronal acetylcholine receptor and N-type voltage-gated calcium channel. A favourable response to acetyl cholinesterase inhibitors has been demonstrated [40].

Amyloidosis

Gastric amyloidosis (Figure 16.2) may occur in isolation or as part of generalised amyloidosis [41]. About 10% of patients with systemic amyloidosis show gastric involvement [42]. Amyloid deposition is usually seen in submucosal small- to medium-sized blood vessels in the gastric wall. It may manifest clinically as gastric outlet obstruction, in the form of submucosal tumour or by infiltration of the whole gastric wall to give a rigid, non-distensible and non-collapsible stomach which resembles the 'leather-bottle' stomach of diffuse gastric carcinoma. The causes, associations and diagnostic issues are the same as elsewhere in the gastrointestinal tract and are more fully discussed in Chapter 40 (see 'Amyloidosis').

Gastric bezoars

A bezoar is a mass of foreign material in the stomach or intestine [43]. In the stomach, they are mainly one of two types, a trichobezoar (comprising hair) or a phytobezoar (comprising vegetable matter). Very occasionally, bezoars comprise enteric-coated and sustained-release medications, so-called pharmacobezoars [44]. Factors associated with the development of gastric bezoars are psychiatric disorders, dental problems, vagotomy and gastric outlet obstruction [44,45]. In young people and psychiatric patients, trichobezoars consisting of balls or mats of swallowed hair are most common (Figure 16.3) [46]. Rapunzel's syndrome refers to the extension of the hair mass through the pylorus into the duodenum, similar to the mane of hair associated

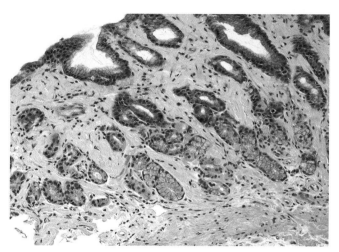

Figure 16.2 Gastric amyloidosis: in this example, the lamina propria is largely replaced by amorphous amyloid material, which compresses the gastric glands. There is no inflammation.

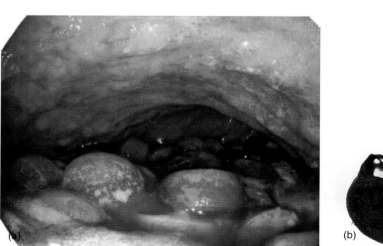

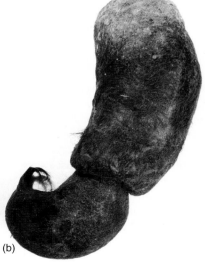

Figure 16.3 (a) An endoscopic image demonstrating a pharmacobezoar composed of nifedipine sustained-release tablets. (Courtesy of Drs W. Brugge and B. Abu Dayyeh, Massachusetts General Hospital.) (b) A huge gastric trichobezoar that fills and expands the lumen of the stomach.

with the Grimm's fairytale character [47]. Occasionally, other unusual substances eaten by psychiatric patients may form bezoars. In adults, phytobezoars composed of indigestible vegetable matter (often persimmon) are the rule. Combined bezoars (trichophytobezoars) rarely occur. Identification of the cause of the bezoar has been helped by the use of analytical techniques, including X-ray energy spectroscopy [48]. Complications such as acute intestinal obstruction, ulceration and bleeding have been reported.

Gastric hyalinisation

This is a rare condition characterised by marked thickening of the submucosa and the muscle coats of the stomach with increased submucosal collagen, whereas the blood vessels are normal. In some cases the thickened stomach resembles linitis plastica. Gastric hyalinisation has been observed after patients received therapeutic irradiation and/or cytotoxic chemotherapy [49–50]. Other cases have followed corrosive injury [50]. One case was associated with chronic peptic ulcer disease but, in others, the cause remains obscure [51]. The condition may be distinguished from systemic sclerosis by the absence of appropriate clinical or serological features or the lack of involvement of other parts of the gut and the fact that changes in the muscle coat are relatively minor.

Pseudo-lipomatosis

Pseudo-lipomatosis is characterised by the presence of small multiple gas-filled cysts in the gastric mucosa [52]. In an analysis of 909 endoscopic biopsies from the corpus of the stomach, 3% of specimens revealed the changes of pseudo-lipomatosis [53]. The pathogenesis of this lesion is unknown. Although as yet unproven, it seems likely that pseudo-lipomatosis, in the stomach, has the same aetiology as its intestinal equivalent, namely the result of endoscopic air insufflation.

Pseudo-xanthoma elasticum

Pseudo-xanthoma elasticum is a rare inherited elastic tissue disorder with degeneration of elastic fibres. The main clinical features are characteristic skin lesions, retinal angioid streaks and occlusive cardiovascular disease [54]. Gastric haemorrhage is a rare manifestation that may occasionally require gastrectomy [55]. Endoscopically, there are usually yellow submucosal nodules resembling xanthomas in the skin [56,57] and histology shows degenerative changes in gastric submucosal arterioles with elastic lamina degeneration and dystrophic calcification. Angiography, which may demonstrate angiomatous malformation, aneurysmal dilatation and narrowing or occlusion of visceral arteries, can aid the diagnosis. The stomach is not usually affected in isolation in pseudo-xanthoma elasticum [58].

Graft-versus-host disease

Graft-versus-host disease (GVHD) is a complication of allogeneic haematopoietic cell transplantation or blood transfusion, particularly in immunocompromised patients, and frequently affects the gastrointestinal tract, the second most commonly involved organ system [59,60]. The diagnosis of GVHD requires a synthesis of clinical, laboratory and histological findings. It may occur in acute or chronic forms, the acute phase commonly occurring within 100 days of transplantation, although it can be diagnosed beyond that time point. It usually manifests with a skin rash and gastrointestinal symptoms of nausea, vomiting, abdominal pain and diarrhoea. In practice, it should be noted that the morphological features of GVHD may be subtle, are characteristically focal and often require a diligent search over many sections from the biopsy. Patients with GVHD have involvement of stomach, small intestine and colorectum in 66% of cases. In practice, gastric biopsies are less sensitive (72%) than duodenal (79%) and rectal biopsies (95%) for the diagnosis of gastrointestinal involvement by GVHD, whereas their negative predictive value is 45% [59].

Endoscopically, the stomach is normal in most cases but may be erythematous with erosions [59,61] and show prominent vascular ectasia [62]. The cardinal histological finding is enhanced apoptosis, especially in the mucous neck cells of the gastric foveolae of body mucosa and antral glands, associated with granular debris within the glands and varying degrees of glandular attenuation and loss [63] (Figure 16.4). Lymphocytic infiltration can be seen and an acute inflammatory reaction may be present, but it is now seen less often than in the past because of the earlier diagnosis and treatment of GVHD. Graft-versus-host changes may also coexist with other forms of pre-existing gastritis, such as that induced by *Helicobacter pylori*.

A careful search for CMV inclusions (supplemented by immunohistochemistry) is mandatory because CMV infection, which can occur concomitantly, may mimic GVHD [64,65]. Other infections such as with *Aspergillus* species and secondary pseudo-membranous gastritis may complicate gastric GVHD [66].

Various drugs, including proton pump inhibitors and mycophenolate mofetil, can cause GVHD-like mucosal injury, including enhanced apoptosis [66–68]. Practically, the histological diagnosis of acute GVHD needs to be made with caution in the immediate post-transplantation period (before 20 days post-transplantation), because cytoreductive-conditioning regimens may produce similar histological changes.

Several immune deficiency disorders can also mimic GVHD including HIV infection, common variable immunodeficiency (CVID) syndrome and IPEX (immunodysregulation, polyendocrinopathy, enteropathy and X-linked inheritance) syndrome [69,70].

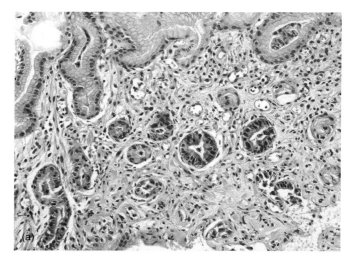

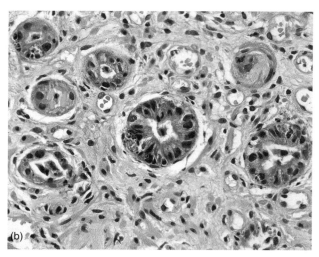

Figure 16.4 Graft-versus-host disease: (a) the lamina propria is sparsely infiltrated by lymphocytes and the gastric pits and glands show varying degrees of epithelial attenuation and loss. (b) Higher magnification emphasises the damaged withering glands, epithelial injury and numerous apoptotic bodies.

Chronic GVHD is seen between 3 and 13 months after transplantation in approximately a third of patients [61]. Some of the clinical features may resemble systemic sclerosis [71]. The histological changes are not specific or diagnostic, but there is glandular atrophy and lamina propria fibrosis.

Vascular disorders

Angiodysplasia

Angiodysplasia may be isolated in the stomach but is more commonly part of a generalised gastrointestinal angiodysplasia. The lesions occur more commonly in the colon and are discussed in Chapter 36 (see 'Angioectasia/ angiodysplasia').

Dieulafoy's disease

First reported in the nineteenth century, the lesions of Dieulafoy are vascular abnormalities characterised by persistent large calibre arteries in the mucosa or, more frequently, in the submucosa of the stomach [72,73]. Their true incidence is unclear because quiescent Dieulafoy's lesions are easily overlooked on endoscopy and bleeding lesions are occasionally misidentified. However, these lesions can be the source of considerable gastric haemorrhage [74,75].

The usual presentation is with profound, occasionally recurrent, sometimes fatal, gastric haemorrhage. Most patients are in the fifth decade and men are affected twice as often as women [74]. The lesions are frequently noted in the proximal stomach [73]. Microscopically, there is an unusually large, tortuous and aneurysmal artery in the base of a small, well-circumscribed ulcer between 2mm and 5mm in diameter. The surrounding gastric mucosa is usually

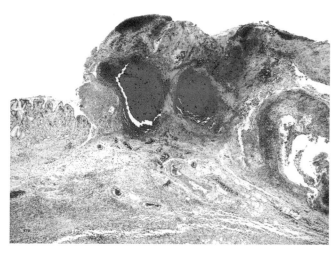

Figure 16.5 Dieulafoy's disease: a ruptured dilated artery is seen close to the epithelial surface. Erosion, as well as haemorrhage, is also observed.

normal [75] (Figure 16.5). The abnormal vessel is thought to represent a congenital calibre-persistent submucosal artery [76]. Similar lesions have been diagnosed in the small and large bowel. Dieulafoy's lesions are now routinely successfully managed endoscopically [73].

Gastric antral vascular ectasia ('watermelon stomach')

Gastric antral vascular ectasia (GAVE) is a not uncommon disorder characterised by dilated intramucosal blood vessels. It shows distinctive endoscopic features, with parallel, longitudinal red stripes situated on hyperplastic mucosal folds and radiating outward from the pylorus

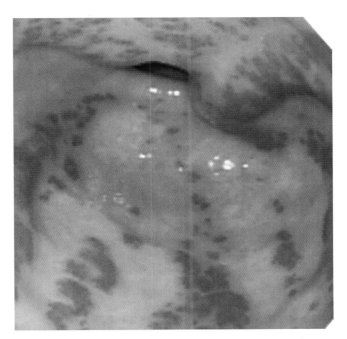

Figure 16.6 Endoscopic appearance of gastric antral vascular ectasia (GAVE): the characteristic endoscopic features with parallel, red, longitudinal stripes situated along the hyperplastic antral mucosal folds.

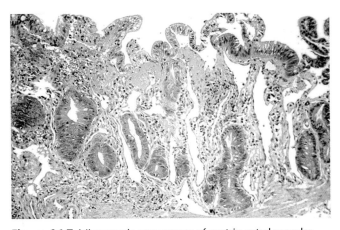

Figure 16.7 Microscopic appearance of gastric antral vascular ectasia (GAVE) with dilated, tortuous mucosal capillaries and numerous fibrin thrombi.

in a spoke-wheel pattern which resembles the surface of a watermelon [77] (Figure 16.6). GAVE is estimated to cause up to 4% of all non-variceal upper gastrointestinal bleeding [78]. The pathological changes associated with GAVE are covered more fully in Chapter 11.

GAVE is associated with a variety of medical conditions, such as autoimmune connective tissue disorders, cirrhosis, bone marrow transplantation and chronic renal failure [78,79]. Its pathogenesis is not fully explained. Some have proposed that abnormal gastric peristalsis draws the mucosa into the characteristic longitudinal folds, with mechanical prolapse leading to mucosal regenerative changes, including

vessel ectasia and increased smooth muscle, whereas vessel injury and local blood flow stasis are responsible for local thrombogenesis [80]. GAVE may present with persistent iron deficiency anaemia and gastrointestinal haemorrhage, predominantly affecting women [77,78,81].

Histologically, the longitudinal stripes in the mucosa demonstrate ectatic, tortuous intramucosal capillaries with fibrin thrombi and fibromuscular hyperplasia of the lamina propria (Figure 16.7). Regenerative/hyperplastic epithelial changes are also common, similar to those seen in reactive/chemical gastritis [82].

The diagnosis of GAVE can be easily missed on small biopsy specimens. Fibromuscular hyperplasia of the lamina propria and epithelial regeneration are not specific and the thrombi can be subtle. Consequently, a diagnosis of chemical gastropathy/reactive gastritis can be readily rendered instead, underscoring the need for correlation with the endoscopic appearances. It is also important to differentiate GAVE from portal hypertensive gastropathy (PHG) because it does not respond to measures that reduce portal pressures. The distinction from PHG is not always easy because the latter does not always display the characteristic mosaic or snake-skin appearance. Furthermore both entities can present with non-specific diffuse gastric erythema. The use of CD61 (platelet marker) immunohistochemistry has been promoted to reveal the thrombi, including in cases initially diagnosed as PHG on biopsies and in which active gastritis was obscuring the recognition of ectatic vessels [80].

Endoscopic ablation (by Nd:YAG laser or argon plasma coagulation) is the treatment of choice. Pharmacological therapy with oestrogen (and/or progesterone) or tranexamic acid can be used if endoscopic measures have failed. Surgical antrectomy is reserved for unresponsive cases [78].

References

1. Adson DE, Mitchell JE, Trenkner SW. The superior mesenteric artery syndrome and acute gastric dilatation in eating disorders: a report of two cases and a review of the literature. *Int J Eat Disord* 1997;**21**:103.
2. Mahajna A, Mitkal S, Krausz MM. Postoperative gastric dilatation causing abdominal compartment syndrome. *World J Emerg Surg* 2008;**3**:7.
3. Cogbill TH, Bintz M, Johnson JA, Strutt PJ. Acute gastric dilatation after trauma. *J Trauma* 1987;**27**:1113.
4. Murray WJ. Massive gastric distension in acute pancreatitis – a report of two cases. *Postgrad Med J* 1984;**60**:631.
5. Nagai T, Yokoo M, Tomizawa T, Mori M. Acute gastric dilatation accompanied by diabetes mellitus. *Intern Med* 2001;**40**:320.
6. Magee MF, Bhatt BA. Management of decompensated diabetes. Diabetic ketoacidosis and hyperglycaemic hyperosmolar syndrome. *Crit Care Clin* 2001;**17**:75.
7. Sarici SU, Yurdatok M, Unal S. Acute gastric dilatation complicating the use of mydriatics in a preterm newborn. *Pediatr Radiol* 2001;**31**:581.
8. Bensen ES, Jaffe KM, Tarr PI. Acute gastric dilatation in Duchenne muscular dystrophy: a case report and review of the literature. *Arch Phys Med Rehabil* 1996;**77**:512.

9. Vautier G, Scott BB. Early acute gastric dilatation following percutaneous endoscopic gastrostomy. *Gastrointest Endosc* 1995; **42**:189.

10. Sabanathan K, Dean J, Carr-Locke D, Pohl JE. Acute gastric dilatation after injection sclerotherapy. *Lancet* 1984;**i**:1240.

11. Watanabe S, Terazawa K, Asari M, Matsubara K, Shiono H, Shimizu K. An autopsy case of sudden death due to acute gastric dilatation without rupture. *Forensic Sci Int* 2008;**18**:e6.

12. Sinicina I, Pankratz H, Büttner A, Mall G. Death due to neurogenic shock following gastric rupture in an anorexia nervosa patient. *Forensic Sci Int* 2005;**155**:7.

13. Ger R. Postoperative extrinsic pyloric stenosis. *BMJ* 1964; **ii**:294.

14. Balint JA, Spence MP. Pyloric stenosis. *BMJ* 1959;**i**:890.

15. Howe CT, Spence MP. Pyloric stenosis in adults. *Postgrad Med J* 1960;**36**:743.

16. Knoght CD. Hypertrophic pyloric stenosis in the adult. *Ann Surg* 1961;**153**:899.

17. Chamberlain D, Addison NV. Adult pyloric obstruction due to a mucosal diaphragm. Report on 2 cases. *BMJ* 1959;**ii**:1381.

18. Warren BF, Shepherd NA. Iatrogenic pathology of the gastrointestinal tract. In: Kirkham N, Hall P (eds), *Progress in Pathology*. Edinburgh: Churchill Livingstone, 1995: 31.

19. Lang J, Price AB, Levi AJ, Burke M, Gumpel JM, Bjarnason I. Diaphragm like disease of the small intestine induced by non steroidal anti-inflammatory drugs. *J Clin Pathol* 1988;**41**;516.

20. McLaughlin RT, Madding GF. Primary pyloric hypertrophy in the adult. *Ann Surg* 1962;**104**:874.

21. Hellan M, Lee T, Lerner T. Diagnosis and therapy of primary hypertrophic pyloric stenosis in adults: case report and review of literature. *J Gastrointest Surg* 2006;**10**:265.

22. Horowitz M, Su YC, Rayner CK, Jones KL. Gastroparesis: prevalence, clinical significance and treatment. *Can J Gastroenterol* 2001;**15**:805.

23. Simon LT, Dikram S, Horoupian DS, et al. Polyneuropathy, ophthalmoplegia, leukoencephalopathy and intestinal pseudoobstruction: POLYP syndrome. *Ann Neurol* 1990;**28**:349.

24. Bevans M. Changes in the musculature of the gastrointestinal tract and the myocardium in progressive muscular dystrophy. *Arch Pathol* 1945;**40**:225.

25. Bellini M, Alduini P, Costa F, et al. Gastric emptying in myotonic dystrophic patients. *Dig Liver Dis* 2002;**34**:484.

26. Oh JJ, Kim OH. Gastroparesis after a presumed viral illness: clinical and laboratory features and natural history. *Mayo Clin Proc* 1990;**65**:636.

27. Naftali T, Yishai R, Zangen T, Levine A. Post-infectious gastroparesis: clinical and electrogastrographic aspects. *J Gastroenterol Hepatol* 2007;**22**:1423.

28. Bityutskiy LP, Soykan I, McCallum RW. Viral gastroparesis: a subgroup of idiopathic gastroparesis – clinical characteristics and long-term outcomes. *Am J Gastroenterol* 1997;**92**:1501.

29. Schuffler MD, Pope CE. Studies of idiopathic intestinal pseudoobstruction 2. Hereditary hollow visceral myopathy: family studies. *Gastroenterology* 1977;**73**:339.

30. Fenoglio-Preisser CM, Noffsinger AE, Stemmermann GN, Lantz PE, Listrom MB, Rilke FO. *Gastrointestinal Pathology: An atlas and text*. New York: Lippincott-Raven, 1999: 622.

31. Moore SW, Schneider JW, Kaschula RD. Non-familial visceral myopathy: clinical and pathologic features of degenerative leiomyopathy. *Pediatr Surg Int* 2002;**18**:6.

32. Sjogren R. Gastrointestinal motility disorders in scleroderma. *Arthritis Rheum* 1994;**37**:1265.

33. Domsic R, Fasanella K, Bielefeldt K. Gastrointestinal manifestations of systemic sclerosis. *Dig Dis Sci* 2008;**53**:1163.

34. Shivshanker K, Bennett RW, Haynie TP. Tumour associated gastroparesis: correction with metoclopramide. *Am J Surg* 1983; **145**:221.

35. Layer P, Demol P, Hotz J, Goebell H. Gastroparesis after radiation. *Dig Dis Sci* 1986;**31**:1377.

36. Choe AI, Ziessman HA, Fleischer DE. Tumour associated gastroparesis with esophageal carcinoma. Use of intravenous metoclopramide during radionuclide gastric emptying studies to predict clinical response. *Dig Dis Sci* 1989;**34**:1132.

37. Schobinger-Clément S, Gerber HA, Stallmach T. Autoaggressive inflammation of the myenteric plexus resulting in intestinal pseudoobstruction. *Am J Surg Pathol* 1999;**23**:602.

38. Hejazi RA, Zhang D, McCallum RW. Gastroparesis, pseudoachalasia and impaired intestinal motility as paraneoplastic manifestations of small cell lung cancer. *Am J Med Sci* 2009;**338**:69.

39. Drukker CA, Heij HA, Wijnaendts LC, Verbeke JI, Kaspers GJ. Paraneoplastic gastro-intestinal anti-Hu syndrome in neuroblastoma. *Pediatr Blood Cancer* 2009;**52**:396.

40. Pasha SF, Lunsford TN, Lennon VA. Autoimmune gastrointestinal dysmotility treated successfully with pyridostigmine. *Gastroenterology* 2006;**131**:1592.

41. Usui M, Matsuda S, Suzuki H, Hirata K, Ogura Y, Shiraishi T. Gastric amyloidosis with massive bleeding requiring emergency surgery. *J Gastroenterol* 2000;**35**:924.

42. Ebert EC, Nagar M. Gastrointestinal manifestations of amyloidosis. *Am J Gastroenterol* 2008;**103**:776.

43. De Bakey M. Bezoars and concretions. *Surgery* 1938;**4**:934.

44. Stack PE, Thomas E. Pharmacobezoar: an evolving new entity. *Dig Dis* 1995;**13**:356.

45. Fenoglio-Preisser CM, Noffsinger AE, Stemmermann GN, Lantz PE, Listrom MB, Rilke FO. *Gastrointestinal Pathology: An atlas and text*. New York: Lippincott-Raven, 1999: 233.

46. Singh A, Khanna RC, Jolly SS. Three unusual cases of trichobezoar. *Gastroenterology* 1961;**40**:441.

47. Gonuguntla V, Joshi DD. Rapunzel syndrome: a comprehensive review of an unusual case of trichobezoar. *Clin Med Res* 2009;**7**:99.

48. Levison DA, Crocker PR, Boxall TA, Randall KJ. Coconut matting bezoar identified by a combined analytical approach. *J Clin Pathol* 1986;**39**:172.

49. Smith JC, Bolande RP. Radiation and drug induced hyalinisation of the stomach. *Arch Pathol* 1965;**79**:310.

50. Kazsuba A, Vitéz A, Gáll J, Máthé L, Ludmány E, Krasznai G. Gastric hyalinization as a possible consequence of corrosive injury. *Endoscopy* 2000;**32**:356.

51. McGregor DH, Haque AU. Gastric hyalinization associated with peptic ulceration. *Arch Pathol Lab Med* 1982;**106**:472.

52. Stebbing J, Wyatt JI. Gastric pseudolipomatosis. *Histopathology* 1998;**33**:394.

53. Alper M, Akcan Y, Belenli OK, Cukur S, Aksoy KA, Suna M. Gastric pseudolipomatosis, usual or unusual? Re-evaluation of 909 endoscopic gastric biopsies. *World J Gastroenterol* 2003;**9**:2846.

54. Bonotto G, Tonetto F, Baraglia E, et al. [Pseudoxanthoma elasticum. A rare cause of upper digestive hemorrhage.] *Minerva Chir* 1992;**47**:1641.

55. Morgan AA. Recurrent gastrointestinal haemorrhage: an unusual cause. *Am J Gastroenterol* 1982;**77**:925.

56. Costopanagiotou E, Spyrou S, Farantos C, Kostopanagiotou G, Smymiotis V. An unusual cause of massive gastric bleeding in a young patient. *Am J Gastroenterol* 2000;**95**:2400.

57. Spinzi G, Strocchi E, Imperiali G, Sangiovanni A, Terruzzi V, Minoli G. Pseudoxanthoma elasticum: a rare cause of gastrointestinal bleeding. *Am J Gastroenterol* 1996;**91**:1631.

58. Belli A, Cawthorne S. Visceral angiographic findings in pseudoxanthoma elasticum. *Br J Radiol* 1988;**61**:368.

59. Ross WA, Ghosh S, Dekovich AA, et al. Endoscopic biopsy diagnosis of acute gastrointestinal graft-versus-host disease: rectosigmoid biopsies are more sensitive than upper gastrointestinal biopsies. *Am J Gastroenterol* 2008;**103**:982.

60. Snover DC, Weisdorf SA, Vercellotti GM, et al. A histopathologic study of gastric and small intestinal graft-versus host disease following allogenic bone marrow transplantation. *Hum Pathol* 1985;**16**:387.

61. McDonald GB, Shulman HM, Sullivan KM, Spencer GD. Intestinal and hepatic complications of human bone marrow transplantation. *Gastroenterology* 1986;**90**:460.

62. Marmaduke DP, Greenson JK, Cunningham I, Herderick EE, Cornhill JF. Gastric vascular ectasia in patients undergoing bone marrow transplantation. *Am J Clin Pathol* 1994;**102**:708.

63. Snover DC. Graft versus host disease of the gastrointestinal tract. *Am J Surg Pathol* 1991;**14**:101.

64. Washington K, Bentley RC, Green A, Olson J, Treem WR, Krigman HR. Graft versus host disease: a blinded histologic study. *Am J Surg Pathol* 1997;**21**:1037.

65. Washington K, Jagasia M. Pathology of graft-versus-host disease in the gastrointestinal tract. *Hum Pathol* 2009;**40**:909.

66. Yong S, Attal H, Chedjfec G. Pseudomembranous gastritis: a novel complication of Aspergillus infection in a patient with a bone marrow transplant and graft versus host disease. *Arch Pathol Lab Med* 2000;**124**:619.

67. Parfitt JR, Jayakumar S, Driman DK. Mycophenolate mofetil-related gastrointestinal mucosal injury: variable injury patterns, including graft-versus-host disease-like changes. *Am J Surg Pathol* 2008;**32**:1367.

68. Welch DC, Wirth PS, Goldenring JR, Ness E, Jagasia M, Washington K. Gastric graft-versus-host disease revisited: does proton pump inhibitor therapy affect endoscopic gastric biopsy interpretation? *Am J Surg Pathol* 2006;**30**:444.

69. Patey-Mariaud de Serre N, Canioni D, Ganousse S, et al. Digestive histopathological presentation of IPEX syndrome. *Mod Pathol* 2009;**22**:92.

70. Daniels JA, Lederman HM, Maitra A, Montgomery EA. Gastrointestinal tract pathology in patients with common variable immunodeficiency (CVID): a clinicopathologic study and review. *Am J Surg Pathol* 2007;**31**:1800.

71. Shulman HM, Sullivan KM, Weiden Pl, et al. Chronic graft versus host syndrome in man. A long term clinicopathologic study of 20 Seattle patients. *Am J Med* 1980;**69**:204.

72. Dieulafoy G. Exulceratio simplex: l'intervention surgicale dans les hematemeses foudroyantes consecutives a l'exulceration simple de l'estomac. *Bull Acad Med* 1898;**49**:49.

73. Schmulewitz N, Baillie J. Dieulafoy lesions: a review of 6 years of experience at a tertiary referral center. *Am J Gastroenterol* 2001;**96**:1688.

74. Veldhuyzen van Zanten SJO, Bartelsman JFWM, Schipper MEI, Tytgat GNJ. Recurrent massive haematemesis from Dieulafoy malformations: a review of 101 cases. *Gut* 1986;**27**:213.

75. Mortensen NJMcC, Mountford RA, Davies JD, Jeans WD. Dieulafoy's disease: a distinctive arteriovenous malformation causing massive gastric haemorrhage. *Br J Surg* 1983;**70**:76.

76. Miko TL, Thomazy VA. The calibre persistent artery of the stomach: a unifying approach to gastric aneurysm, Dieulafoy's lesion and submucosal arterial malformation. *Hum Pathol* 1988;**19**:914.

77. Jabbari M, Cherry R, Lough JI, et al. Gastric antral vascular ectasia: the watermelon stomach. *Gastroenterology* 1984;**87**:165.

78. Selinger CP, Ang YS. Gastric antral vascular ectasia (GAVE): an update on clinical presentation, pathophysiology and treatment. *Digestion* 2008;**77**:131.

79. Ward EM, Raimondo M, Rosser BG, Wallace MB, Dickson RD. Prevalence and natural history of gastric antral vascular ectasia in patients undergoing orthotopic liver transplantation. *J Clin Gastroenterol* 2004;**38**:898.

80. Westerhoff M, Tretiakova M, Hovan L, Miller J, Noffsinger A, Hart J. CD61, CD31, and CD34 improve diagnostic accuracy in gastric antral vascular ectasia and portal hypertensive gastropathy: an immunohistochemical and digital morphometric study. *Am J Surg Pathol*. 2010;**34**:494.

81. Suit PF, Petras RE, Bauer TW, et al. Gastric antral vascular ectasia. A histologic and morphometric study of 'watermelon stomach'. *Am J Surg Pathol* 1987;**11**:750.

82. Fenoglio-Preisser CM, Noffsinger AE, Stemmermann GN, Lantz PE, Listrom MB, Rilke FO. *Gastrointestinal Pathology: An atlas and text*. New York: Lippincott-Raven, 1999: 225.

PART 3

Small Intestine

Normal small intestine: anatomy, specimen dissection and histology relevant to pathological practice

Robert E. Petras

AmeriPath, Inc., Oakwood Village; Northeast Ohio Medical University, Rootstown, OH, USA

Gross anatomy

The small intestine is a multiply coiled tubular organ, located predominantly within the abdominal cavity. It extends from the gastric pylorus to its insertion into the large intestine at the junction of the caecum and ascending colon. The adult small bowel varies in length. Measurements taken post mortem have ranged from 3000 mm to 9000 mm [1]. The presence of muscle tone in the longitudinal layer of the muscularis propria/externa in the small intestine has resulted in shorter lengths in vivo, usually averaging 6000–7000 mm [2]. In infants, the small bowel generally measures three to seven times the crown-to-heel length [3]. The overall length of fetal/infant small bowel at 19–27 weeks' gestation is 1420 ± 220 mm, increasing to 3040 ± 440 mm by 35 weeks [4]. Three subdivisions of the small intestine – the duodenum, jejunum and ileum – are recognised and defined by various anatomical features and relationships.

The duodenum, the most proximal portion of the small bowel, was so named because it is approximately 12 fingers in breadth. It measures approximately 200–250 mm in length and extends from the gastric pylorus to the duodeno-jejunal flexure. Except for the most proximal few centimetres, the duodenum is a retroperitoneal fixed structure forming a C-shape around the head of the pancreas [5]. It consists of four parts:

1. The first portion, often referred to as the duodenal cap or bulb
2. The descending or second portion into which the biliary and pancreatic ducts empty their contents, usually through a common orifice at the major duodenal papilla

3. The horizontal or third portion
4. The ascending or fourth portion, which veers forwards and upwards to the level of the second lumbar vertebra, terminating at the duodeno-jejunal junction.

This junction is fixed by a strip of fibromuscular tissue referred to as the ligament of Treitz [6,7]. At this point, the small intestine acquires a mesentery and continues distally as the jejunum.

The small bowel distal to the ligament of Treitz is arbitrarily divided into the jejunum (the proximal 40%) and the ileum (the distal 60%) which terminates at the ileo-caecal valve [8]. There is no discrete demarcation point dividing jejunum from ileum. However, several features become gradually more apparent from proximal to distal. The proximal jejunum has a thicker wall and is about double the diameter of the terminal ileum. The jejunum has more prominent permanent circular folds, the plicae circulares (also known as valvulae conniventes or folds of Kerckring) that can be palpated at surgery [9]. The amount of mesenteric fat is greater in the ileum. Most of the jejunum lies within the upper abdominal cavity, whereas the ileum is generally located within the lower abdominal cavity and pelvis [9].

The arterial blood supply to the small intestine originates from the coeliac axis and the superior mesenteric artery [9, 10]. The duodenum is supplied by the superior pancreatico-duodenal branch of the gastro-duodenal artery, deriving from the coeliac axis, whereas the fourth portion of the duodenum and the remainder of the small bowel are supplied by the superior mesenteric artery, which forms numerous arcades within the mesentery, allowing for rich collateral circulation. The veins drain into the portal system. The

Morson and Dawson's Gastrointestinal Pathology, Fifth Edition. Edited by Neil A. Shepherd, Bryan F. Warren, Geraint T. Williams, Joel K. Greenson, Gregory Y. Lauwers and Marco R. Novelli.
© 2013 Blackwell Publishing Ltd. Published 2013 by Blackwell Publishing Ltd.

lymphatics follow the arterial supply and flow into regional lymphatics and lymph nodes [10]. The mucosal microcirculation has been described in detail in relationship to countercurrent effects [11]. Capillaries and lymphatic lacteals traverse the villi and are difficult, if not impossible, to distinguish from each other except after a fatty meal when the latter dilate. If required, immunohistochemistry with D2-40 antibody will selectively stain lymphatic endothelium. The lacteals of adjacent villi interconnect. In the lower portion of the villus, lacteals fuse to form a wider sinus. From there, one to three lymphatic vessels drain into the lymphatic network of the submucosa [12].

Sympathetic nervous innervation of the small bowel tends to be adrenergic, inhibitory, and derived from the coeliac and superior mesenteric plexuses. The parasympathetic input is cholinergic and excitatory, and comes from distal branches of the vagus nerve [9].

Physiology

A detailed discussion of small bowel physiology is beyond the scope of this book. Briefly, however, the small bowel has digestive, absorptive, secretory and immunological functions, the most important of which is processing and absorption of nutrients [13,14]. Pancreatic enzymes act on ingested carbohydrates and proteins to produce smaller-sized molecules for ingestion. The brush border created by apical microvilli on absorptive enterocytes contains an array of peptidases and carbohydrases. Protein oligopeptides are hydrolysed to amino acids by these peptidases. A small amount of unhydrolysed protein can be absorbed unchanged [15,16]. Aminopeptidases can be demonstrated histochemically and by immunohistochemistry although this is rarely needed clinically [17,18]. Carbohydrates are ingested as polysaccharides, oligosaccharides or disaccharides. All are broken down to monosaccharides for absorption by brush border saccharidases [19].

Almost all dietary fat is ingested as water-insoluble triglycerides [20]. These are emulsified and hydrolysed in the small bowel lumen by combination with bile salt and pancreatic lipase, to create free fatty acids and monoglycerides that can diffuse across the lipid-soluble plasma membrane. Most lipids undergo intracytoplasmic resynthesis to triglycerides, with direct packaging within chylomicrons and release into regional lymphatics [9,20].

Water, electrolytes, vitamins, minerals and various drugs are also absorbed at particular points along the mucosa of the small intestine [9], so the integrity of the small bowel is essential to health and nutrition as well as appropriate drug handling. There are some regional differences in absorption, e.g. calcium and iron are absorbed proximally within the small intestine whereas magnesium and vitamin B12 (cobalamin) are preferentially absorbed in the ileum [21].

Microscopic anatomy

Regional histological differences exist within the small bowel (see below) but the general structure is consistent throughout. The small bowel wall is divided into four layers; the mucosa, submucosa, muscularis propria/externa and serosa.

Mucosa

Architectural adaptation within the small bowel is specifically designed to augment absorption [22,23]. One of these is the formation of permanent circular folds, the plicae circulares, coursing perpendicular to the long axis of the bowel. These folds are composed of mucosa-covered submucosal cores, which traverse almost the entire circumference of the bowel and overlap with adjacent permanent folds (Figure 17.1). These enhance the surface area and attenuate the forward flow of intestinal contents, thereby extending contact time with the absorptive surfaces.

The mucosa is made up of epithelium, a supporting lamina propria and the muscularis mucosae. The epithelium and lamina propria form finger- or leaf-like intraluminal projections called villi. Villi line the entire small bowel and are the most important adaptational change to enhance surface area [22,24,25] (Figure 17.2). Each villus is covered by epithelium and contains a lamina propria core of connective tissue, which itself contains a centrally located lacteal, an arteriovenous capillary network and migrating inflammatory cell populations [12,26–29]. Normal villi may

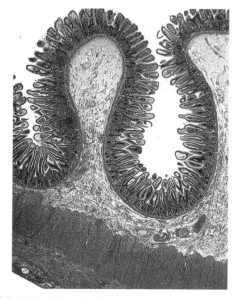

Figure 17.1 The plicae circulares or permanent folds of the small bowel are made up of a submucosal core and the mucosal surface.

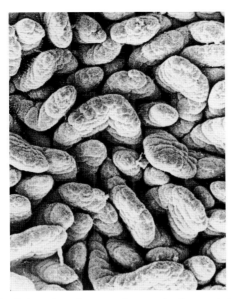

Figure 17.2 Scanning electron micrograph of normal duodenum. Finger- and leaf-like (spade-shaped) villi are present. Finger-like projections are more common in the distal small bowel whereas spade-shaped villi predominate within the duodenum.

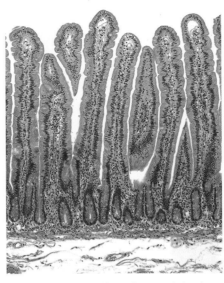

Figure 17.3 Normal jejunal villi are long and slender mucosal projections composed of a lamina propria core covered by epithelial cells. The intestinal glands (crypts) are located at the base of the mucosa. The crypts lie between adjacent villi and are also surrounded by lamina propria.

branch and branches can connect to form bridges, especially in the duodenum and proximal jejunum. The tubular invaginations that surround the villi and extend to the muscularis mucosae are referred to as the crypts of Lieberkühn. The lamina propria of the villous core is continuous with the lamina propria surrounding the crypts. The ratio of villus length to crypt length varies from about 3:1 to 5:1 [9,22] (Figure 17.3).

Mucosal components

Epithelium

The villi are principally lined by an absorptive epithelial cell which is tall and columnar with a basally located round to oval nucleus and an eosinophilic cytoplasm (Figure 17.4). The apical surface is covered by a brush border that is also eosinophilic, somewhat refractile and stains positively with periodic acid–Schiff (PAS) stain or an Alcian blue/PAS combination stain (Figure 17.5). The brush border is ultrastructurally composed of microvilli and a glycocalyx or fuzzy coat [9,29–32] (Figure 17.6). The microvillus–glycocalyx complex houses the peptidases and disaccharidases and also probably provides a barrier to micro-organisms and luminal foreign material [33]. Goblet cells are found scattered along the lining of the villi. They have a characteristic apical mucin droplet and an attenuated basally oriented nucleus (Figure 17.4). Using an Alcian blue/PAS combination stain, the mucin appears blue–purple and is composed predominantly of sialomucins (Figure 17.5). The number of goblet cells increases

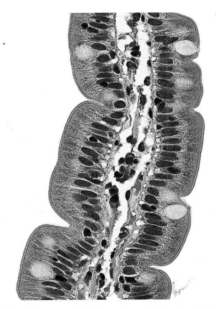

Figure 17.4 High magnification view of jejunal villi: columnar absorptive cells and goblet cells (with apical clear vacuoles) cover the villous surface. Each cell type has a basally located nucleus that is round to oval. The brush border extends from the absorptive cell and appears refractile. Note the scattered intra-epithelial lymphocytes among and between the epithelium.

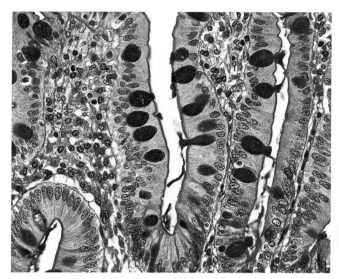

Figure 17.5 The combined Alcian blue and periodic acid–Schiff stain highlights the red-staining microvillous membrane–glycocalyx complex along the luminal surface of the absorptive cells. The thin subepithelial basement membrane is also weakly PAS positive. The goblet cells which contain both neutral and acid mucins also stain blue-purple.

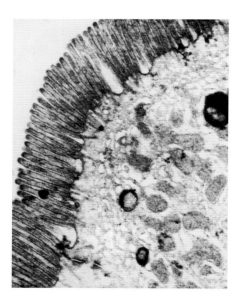

Figure 17.6 Transmission electron micrograph of the microvilli on the luminal surface of the absorptive enterocyte. The glycocalyx, the filamentous layer overlying the microvilli, has been artefactually removed during processing.

with distal progression through the small intestine. Scattered endocrine cells may also be seen lining the villi but are much more abundant within the crypt epithelium.

Intra-epithelial lymphocytes lie between surface epithelial cells just above the basement membrane and usually number approximately 20 per 100 enterocytes [9,34,35] (see

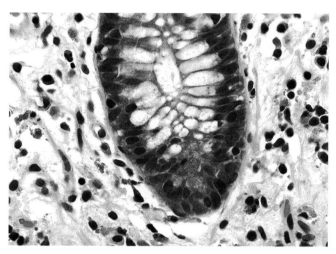

Figure 17.7 A single crypt surrounded by lamina propria that contains migratory inflammatory cells. Typically, absorptive, goblet, endocrine (with infranuclear darker eosinophilic granules) and Paneth cells (with larger lighter-coloured eosinophilic supranuclear granules) can be found.

Figure 17.4). Intra-epithelial lymphocytes mark as T cells and most are of the CD8-positive T-suppressor/cytotoxic subset [36–38]. Approximately 5–30% bear a γδ T-cell receptor (TCR) and lack CD4 and CD8 or are only CD8 positive [38]. CD4-negative, CD8-negative intra-epithelial lymphocytes are more common in the ileum [38]. Increased numbers of intra-epithelial lymphocytes may be seen in a number of disorders, including coeliac disease/sprue, tropical sprue and giardiasis [39,40].

The epithelium found in the crypts primarily functions in cell renewal (Figure 17.7). As a result, mitotic figures are frequently encountered (normal range: 1–12 mitoses per crypt) [41]. The crypt contains goblet cells as well as undifferentiated columnar cells, some of which are stem cells [42]. These stem cells give rise to the four epithelial cell types that can be identified within the mucosa; absorptive, goblet, endocrine and Paneth. Differentiation and maturation of absorptive epithelia occurs in approximately 4 days as the cells migrate from the crypt to the villous tip where they are eventually shed, presumably through apoptosis [42–45]. The exception, Paneth cells, migrate downward and stay in the crypt base longer [42,46]. Complex molecular pathways, especially involving Wnt signalling, play key roles in proliferation and differentiation [47].

Endocrine cells are relatively abundant in the crypts and often demonstrate infranuclear eosinophilic granules that can be seen on haematoxylin and eosin (H&E) staining (Figure 17.7). Identification is more readily accomplished using immunohistochemistry for non-specific markers of endocrine cells, such as chromogranin and synaptophysin (Figure 17.8) or by precise identification of specific

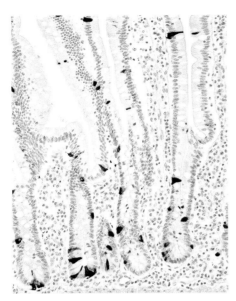

Figure 17.8 Immunohistochemistry for chromogranin highlights numerous endocrine cells within the crypt and scattered along the villus.

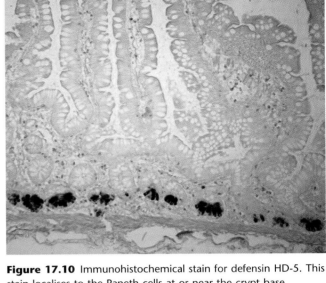

Figure 17.10 Immunohistochemical stain for defensin HD-5. This stain localises to the Paneth cells at or near the crypt base.

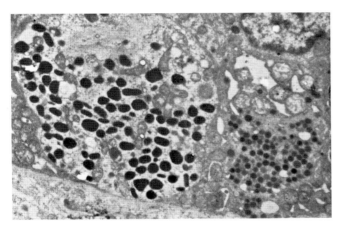

Figure 17.9 Transmission electron micrograph of the duodenum showing a serotonin (5HT)-secreting cell with characteristic dense pleomorphic granules (left) and a second endocrine cell (right), probably a secretin-containing cell with small round granules of varying density.

endocrine chemical content [48–50]. Endocrine cells are of two morphological types: the 'open' type has a pyramidal shape that tapers towards and communicates with the lumen; a 'closed' type is spindled in shape and has no luminal connection [51]. Electron microscopy can be used to identify neuro-endocrine-type granules, and even types of neuro-endocrine granules, but this is rarely used clinically (Figure 17.9).

At least 16 types of endocrine cells have been detected in the gastrointestinal tract [49,52] and some have a pre-

dominant regional distribution, e.g. serotonin, vasoactive intestinal peptide (VIP), encephalin and somatostatin-containing cells are diffusely distributed throughout the gut. Cells containing cholecystokinin, secretin, gastric inhibitory polypeptide and motilin are usually found proximally in the small intestine, whereas enteroglucagon-, substance P- and neurotensin-containing cells are seen in greater frequency in the distal small intestine [49,52].

Paneth cells are normally found only in the crypts [53] (see Figure 17.7). These cells demonstrate a pyramidal shape with the apex pointing towards the lumen. The cytoplasm contains supranuclear, intensely eosinophilic, relatively large granules that are easily identified on H&E-stained sections. The rounded nucleus is often nucleolated. These cells contain lysozyme, defensins and immunoglobulins, and can be capable of phagocytic activity. Paneth cell α-defensin HD-5 is active against bacteria. This fact and the location of Paneth cells suggest that they may function as a protector of the stem cells and regulate intestinal microbials [54,55] (Figure 17.10). Intra-epithelial lymphocytes are occasionally seen in the crypts. Other inflammatory cells, such as neutrophils and eosinophils, within crypt or villous epithelium, often indicate a pathological state [9,56].

Carcinoembryonic antigen (CEA) and CD10 can be demonstrated by immunohistochemistry on the apical surface of the cells, covering the villi and within the crypts. These antigens localise to the glycocalyx and are sometimes used to demonstrate pathological conditions, such as microvillous inclusion disease [57–59].

Lamina propria

Each villus has a central connective tissue core that is continuous with connective tissue surrounding the crypts. This lamina propria functions structurally and immunologically. It contains the arterioles, venules, capillaries, lymphatics, smooth muscle and inflammatory cells (see Figures 17.4, 17.5 and 17.7]. The crypt and villus epithelium rest on the lamina propria and are separated from it by a basement membrane, a slender eosinophilic band that can be highlighted with a PAS stain (see Figure 17.5). A mesenchymal cell layer immediately beneath the epithelial cells (the pericryptal fibroblastic sheath) has been described [60].

A conspicuous feature within the lamina propria is abundant inflammatory cells including plasma cells, lymphocytes, eosinophils, histiocytes and mast cells. Plasma cells are the most abundant inflammatory cell. Most contain immunoglobulin A (IgA) with some containing IgM. IgG-containing plasma cells are usually scant [61–63]. T and B lymphocytes are also present. The predominant T cell (60–70%) expresses the CD4 helper/inducer immunophenotype [64–66], with almost all expressing the αβ TCR [36]. CD8-positive T cells account for 30–40% of T cells within the lamina propria [38]. Lymphocytes can aggregate into nodules and many with germinal centres are scattered throughout the small bowel with the highest concentration in the ileum. These may function similarly to Peyer's patches as a site for induction of a mucosal immune response [67].

Histiocytes or macrophages are fewer in number in the lamina propria and usually cluster near the luminal aspect of the villus, where they may function as antigen-presenting cells. Scattered eosinophils and mast cells are normally found within the lamina propria but the role played by these cells types in normal small bowel is uncertain [9]. Occasionally, in normal individuals and certain disease processes, such as Crohn's disease, ganglion cells may be found within the lamina propria. Care must be taken not to confuse these ganglion cells with a cytomegalovirus cytopathic effect.

Muscularis mucosae

The muscularis mucosae represents the outermost layer of the mucosa and is composed of elastic fibres and smooth muscle. The latter is arranged into an inner circular and outer longitudinal layer (Figure 17.11). The muscularis mucosae may not be distinct in all places, especially in the duodenum where Brunner's glands are concentrated and immediately adjacent to mucosal lymphoid aggregates [9].

Submucosa

The submucosa, located between the muscularis mucosae and muscularis propria/externa is composed of loose paucicellular connective tissue, including collagen and elastic

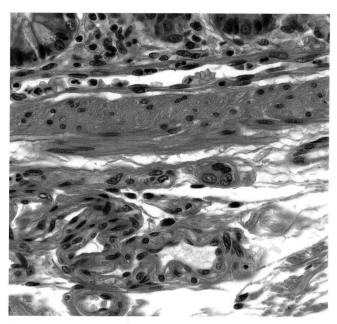

Figure 17.11 This high magnification view highlights the inner circular and outer longitudinal layers of smooth muscle that make up the muscularis mucosae. Neural structures of Meissner's plexus in the superficial submucosa are also illustrated.

fibres and related fibroblasts [9] (see Figure 17.1). The submucosa contains scattered inflammatory cells and adipose tissue. It also contains blood vessels, lymphatics and neural structures, including Meissner's plexuses [68] (Figure 17.11). These plexuses contain neurons, seen on H&E as large oval cells with abundant eosinophilic cytoplasm and a large vesicular nucleus containing a single, often prominent, nucleolus. Abundant Schwann cells, axons, dendrites and glial-like cells, immunoreactive for S100 protein, are also found within the plexuses.

Muscularis propria/externa

The muscularis propria/externa is the outer smooth muscle layer that surrounds the submucosa. It is covered externally by the subserosal or adventitial connective tissue and then, in most places, by a serosal layer. The two smooth muscle layers are arranged as inner circular and outer longitudinal bands separated by the myenteric plexus of Auerbach (Figure 17.12). Blood vessels, nerves and lymphatics course through the muscularis propria.

Auerbach's plexus is similar in composition to Meissner's plexus. Interstitial cells of Cajal form a meshwork around Auerbach's plexus and within the smooth muscle layer of the muscularis propria. These pacemaker cells require special staining (e.g. CD117 and CD34 immunostains) for visualisation [69,70] (Figure 17.13). At least three

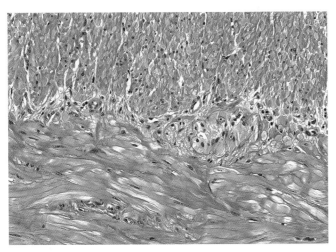

Figure 17.12 Muscularis propria: the ganglia of the mesenteric plexus of Auerbach separate the inner circular (above) and outer longitudinal (below) bands of smooth muscle that make up the bulk of the muscularis propria.

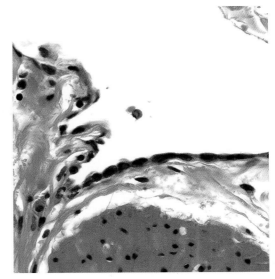

Figure 17.14 The serosa consists of a thin fibrous layer covered by a single layer of mesothelial cells. The mesothelium is often partially or totally denuded in surgical resection specimens.

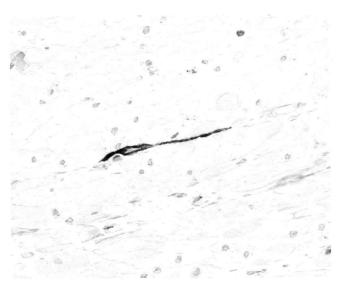

Figure 17.13 An interstitial cell of Cajal as demonstrated by CD117 (c-kit) immunostain.

distinct subsets of interstitial cells of Cajal are identified by electron microscopy [71] but this is not important in clinical practice. These cells are necessary for propagation of the slow waves that are an essential element of peristalsis [72].

Serosa and subserosa

The serosa envelops almost all the small bowel. Its outermost layer consists of a single row of cuboidal mesothelial cells resting upon a well-developed elastic membrane (Figure 17.14). The subserosal connective tissue lies between the serosa and muscularis propria, and contains collagen, elastin, adipose tissue, blood vessels and lymphatics. This layer is typically devoid of lymphoid tissue [9].

Distinctive regional characteristics

Duodenum

The gastro-duodenal junction is poorly demarcated histologically [73]. Irregular strips of antral mucosa can extend 1–2 mm into the anatomical duodenum followed by a 2- or 3-mm segment of 'transitional' epithelium which appears as a combination of antral and typical small bowel mucosa. This can sometimes be appreciated on H&E staining but is better demonstrated with an Alcian blue/PAS combination stain [9] (Figure 17.15). The villi are typically broader and shorter than those in the jejunum or ileum (Figure 17.16).

Brunner's glands begin just distal to the gastro-duodenal junction and gradually decrease in size and distribution distally, and are often used as a histological marker of the duodenum [74]. These are lobular collections of tubulo-alveolar glands predominantly located within the submucosa. However, on average, a third of Brunner's glands occur above the muscularis mucosae [75]. Brunner's glands are lined by cuboidal cells, with pale uniform cytoplasm and an oval, basally oriented nucleus. The cytoplasm typically contains neutral mucus. Scattered endocrine and Paneth cells can be seen within Brunner's glands. These glands drain by way of ducts lined by similar epithelium to the glands into the crypts of Lieberkühn at various levels (Figure 17.17).

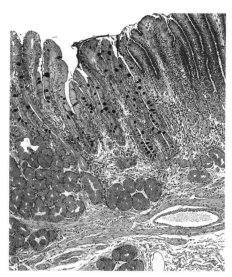

Figure 17.15 The gastro-duodenal junction. Note the transition from periodic acid–Schiff (PAS)-positive (red) gastric epithelium (right) to the villous mucosal architecture of the duodenum (left) lined by Alcian blue/PAS-positive goblet cells and luminal PAS-positive absorptive enterocytes. Brunner's glands and pyloric glands are composed of cells containing neutral PAS-positive mucin. A villus near the junction discloses both usual small intestinal type epithelium and PAS-positive foveolar epithelium. This finding is considered normal near the gastro-duodenal junction. At more distal sites in the duodenum, this transitional type epithelium is called gastric foveolar metaplasia.

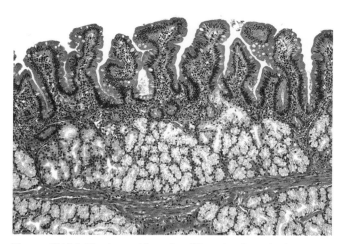

Figure 17.16 Shorter and broader villi predominate in the duodenum. Underlying Brunner's glands are a distinctive feature of the duodenum.

Jejunum

The jejunum is the least distinctive segment of the small bowel. Characteristic features include prominent plicae circulares, a larger villus:crypt ratio approaching 5:1 and prominent serration to the villous profile [9] (Figure 17.18).

Ileum

Unique features of the ileum include the junction with the large bowel, a high concentration of lymphoid aggregates and the deposition of pigment [9].

The ileum protrudes for about 20 mm into the large bowel at the ileo-caecal valve. This nipple-like extension of ileum is encircled by the colon [76]. The mucosa in this transition zone demonstrates a gradual loss of villi and eventually blends into the columnar-type mucosa of

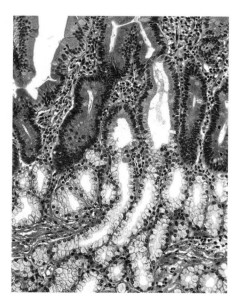

Figure 17.17 Submucosal Brunner's gland lobules drain via a duct that traverses the muscularis mucosae and opens into nearby crypts. Paneth cells can occasionally be seen lining Brunner's glands.

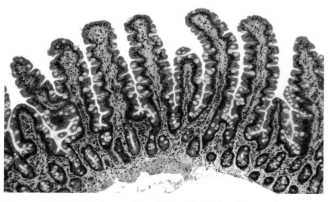

Figure 17.18 Histology of small bowel obtained by endoscopic biopsy from the distal duodenum/proximal jejunum. Note the saw-tooth serrations along the sides of the villi.

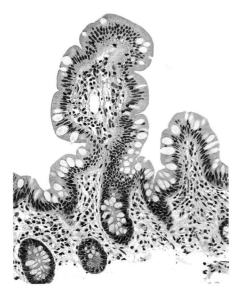

Figure 17.19 The ileal mucosal villi appear shorter and more slender compared with the jejunal villi (see Figure 17.18). Ileal villi are lined by more numerous goblet cells and fewer absorptive cells. The villi show less serration when compared with those in the jejunum.

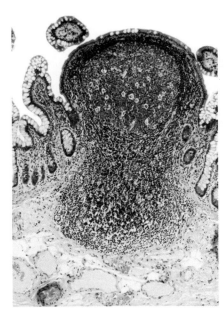

Figure 17.20 An organised lymphoid aggregate demonstrates the four zones, which include the germinal centre, dense monotonous small lymphocytic mantle zone, less dense dome area and T-cell-rich interfollicular zone. The epithelium overlying the lymphoid aggregate is flat without villi and lined by the follicle-associated epithelium.

the colon. The ileo-caecal valve typically shows increased amounts of smooth muscle extending from the circular layer of muscularis propria into the submucosa, and contains abundant submucosal fat which is roughly proportional to the adipose tissue content seen in the rest of the abdomen [77]. The ileo-caecal valve functions not as a true valve but as a sphincter [8].

The ileal mucosa demonstrates fewer plicae circulares and has an increased concentration of goblet cells compared with the duodenum and jejunum. The villi are shorter and typically show less serration than in the more proximal small bowel mucosa. The villi are also less straight, so tangential cuts can be seen in normal samples [78] (Figure 17.19).

The ileum contains increased lymphoid tissue. Specialised aggregates of lymphoid tissue called Peyer's patches are located in an anti-mesenteric location; these increase in size as an individual approaches puberty and then gradually reduce in number [79]. Peyer's patches occupy the mucosa and a variable portion of the submucosa (Figure 17.20). Four distinct cellular compartments have been described: the follicle, dome, follicular-associated epithelium and interfollicular region [80]. Lymphoid follicles within Peyer's patch typically contain germinal centres populated by numerous IgA-positive B cells and scattered CD4-positive T cells, macrophages and follicular dendritic cells [78,81]. The surrounding mantle zone contains small B lymphocytes. The dome area between the follicle and the surface epithelium contains B cells, macrophages, dendritic cells and plasma cells [38].

The villi over lymphoid aggregates are often poorly formed or absent (Figure 17.20). A specialised lympho-epithelium, the follicle-associated epithelium [78], overlies Peyer's patches and probably solitary lymphoid follicles as well. The follicle-associated epithelium has fewer goblet cells and contains M cells [82], which histologically resemble flattened enterocytes and ultrastructurally have modified microvilli or microfolds (from which the cell name is derived) and lack a terminal web [83,84]. The M cells transport luminal antigen into the adjacent extracellular space, giving access to immunocompetent cells. Therefore, these M cells play a key role in mucosa-based immunity, antigen tolerance and pathological states [85]. There are typically increased intra-epithelial lymphocytes within the M cell zone. Finally, the interfollicular zone resembles that seen in a lymph node and is composed predominantly of CD4-positive T cells and post-capillary venules [12,38,78].

Irregular deposits of granular black pigment are commonly found in the deeper portions of Peyer's patches, especially in the terminal ileum (Figure 17.21). This pigment is within histiocytes sited in the basal aspect of Peyer's patch and is environmentally derived. It has been shown to contain compounds such as silicates, aluminium and titanium. The pigments are inert and have no known clinical significance [86,87]. Nevertheless the demonstration

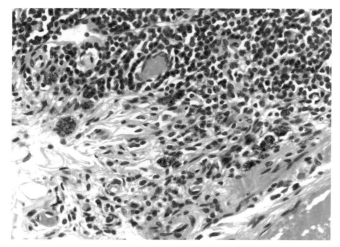

Figure 17.21 Dense brown–black pigment is usually found in macrophages at the basal aspect of Peyer's patches. In biopsies of ileal reservoirs and in other post-surgical situations, its presence can be useful to signify that the mucosa is of ileal type (rather than colonic/rectal) when there are villous atrophic changes.

of this black pigment can be used, in biopsy practice, to show that the biopsy derives from the true ileum. This is especially useful in the histological assessment of ileal reservoir/pouch biopsies, particularly when adaptive and inflammatory changes have concealed other discriminative features.

References

1. Underhill BML. Intestinal length in man. *BMJ* 1955;**ii**:1243.
2. Hirsch J, Ahrens EH, Blankenhorn DH. Measurement of human intestinal length in vivo. *Gastroenterology* 1956;**31**:274.
3. Reiquam CW, Allen RP, Akers DR. Normal and abnormal small bowel lengths. An analysis of 389 autopsy cases in infants and children. *Am J Dis Child* 1965;**109**:447.
4. Touloukian RJ, Walker-Smith GJ. Normal intestinal length in pre-term infants. *J Pediatr Surg* 1983;**18**:720.
5. Thorek P. *Anatomy in Surgery*, 3rd edn. New York: Springer-Verlag, 1985.
6. Riddell RH, Petras RE, Williams GT, Sobin LH. Tumors of the intestines. In: *Atlas of Tumor Pathology*, Third Series Fascicle no. 32. Washington DC: Armed Forces Institute of Pathology, 2003: 1.
7. Costacurta L. Anatomical and functional aspects of the human suspensory muscle of the duodenum. *Acta Anat (Basel)* 1972; **82**:34.
8. Gazet JC, Jarrett RJ. The ileocaeco-colic sphincter. Studies in vitro in man, monkey, cat and dog. *Br J Surg* 1964;**51**:368.
9. Gramlich TL, Petras RE. Small Intestine. In: Mills SE (ed.), *Histology for Pathologists*, 3rd edn. Philadelphia, PA: Lippincott Williams & Wilkins, 2006: 603.
10. Parks DA, Jacobson ED. Physiology of the splanchnic circulation. *Arch Intern Med* 1985;**145**:1278.
11. Granger DN, Barrowman JA. Microcirculation of the alimentary tract, II. Pathophysiology of edema. *Gastroenterology* 1983;**84**:1035.
12. Ohtani O, Ohtani Y. Organization and developmental aspects of lymphatic vessels. *Arch Histol Cytol* 2008;**71**:1.
13. Lucas M. Physiology of the small intestine. *Curr Opinion Gastroenterol* 1985;**1**:203.
14. Clark ML. Small intestinal pathophysiology. *Curr Opinion Gastroenterol* 1985;**1**:212.
15. Freeman HJ, Sleisenger MH, Kim YS. Human protein digestion and absorption; normal mechanisms and protein-energy malnutrition. *Clin Gastroenterol* 1983;**12**:357.
16. Nicholson JA, Peters TJ. Subcellular distribution of di- and tripeptidase activity in human jejunum. *Clin Sci Mol Med* 1977; **52**:168.
17. Feracci H, Bernadac A, Gorvel JP, Maroux S. Localization by immunofluorescence and histochemical labelling of a aminopeptidase N in relation to its biosynthesis in rabbit and pig enterocytes. *Gastroenterology* 1982;**82**:317.
18. Lojda Z. The histochemical demonstration of brush border endopeptidase. *Histochemistry* 1979;**64**:205.
19. Ravich WJ, Bayless TM. Carbohydrate absorption and malabsorption. *Clin Gastroenterol* 1983;**12**:335.
20. Glickman RM. Fat absorption and malabsorption. *Clin Gastroenterol* 1983;**12**:323.
21. Farrell JJ. Digestion and absorption of nutrients and vitamins. In: Feldman M, Friedman LS, Brandt LJ (eds), *Sleisenger and Fordtran's Gastrointestinal and Liver Disease*, 8th edn. Philadelphia, PA: Saunders, Elsevier, 2006: 2147.
22. Rubin W. The epithelial 'membrane' of the small intestine. *Am J Clin Nutr* 1971;**24**:45.
23. Wilson JP. Surface area of the small intestine in man. *Gut* 1967;**8**:618.
24. Toner PG, Carr KE. The use of scanning electron microscopy in the study of the intestinal villi. *J Pathol* 1969;**97**:611.
25. Holmes R, Hourihane DO, Booth CC. The mucosa of the small intestine. *Postgrad Med J* 1961;**37**:717.
26. Trier JS, Madara JL. Functional morphology of the mucosa of the small intestine. In: Johnson LR (ed.), *Physiology of the Gastrointestinal Tract*, 2nd edn. New York: Raven Press, 1987: 1209.
27. Dobbins WO. The intestinal mucosal lymphatic in man. A light and electron microscopic study. *Gastroenterology* 1966;**51**: 994.
28. Golab B, Szkudlarek R. Lymphatic vessels of the duodenum-deep network. *Folia Morphol (Warsz)* 1981;**39**:263.
29. Sinclair TS, Jones DA, Kumar PJ, Phillips AD. The microvillus in adult jejunal mucosa – an electron microscopic study. *Histopathology* 1984;**8**:739.
30. Trier JS, Rubin CE. Electron microscopy of the small intestine: a review. *Gastroenterology* 1965;**49**:574.
31. Trier JS. The surface coat of gastrointestinal epithelial cells. *Gastroenterology* 1969;**56**:618.
32. Dobbins WO III. Morphologic and functional correlates of intestinal brush borders. *Am J Med Sci* 1969;**258**:150.
33. Poley JR. Loss of the glycocalyx of enterocytes in small intestine: a feature detected by scanning electron microscopy in children with gastrointestinal intolerance to dietary protein. *J Pediatr Gastroenterol Nutr* 1988;**7**:386.
34. Dobbins WO III. Human intestinal intra-epithelial lymphocytes. *Gut* 1986;**27**:972.
35. Ferguson A, Murray D. Quantitation of intra-epithelial lymphocytes in human jejunum. *Gut* 1971;**12**:988.
36. Cerf-Bensussan N, Schneeberger EE, Bhan AK. Immunohistologic and immunoelectron microscopic characterization of the mucosal lymphocytes of human small intestine by the use of monoclonal antibodies. *J Immunol* 1983;**130**:2615.

37. Greenwood JH, Austin LL, Dobbins WO III. In vitro characterization of human intestinal intra-epithelial lymphocytes. *Gastroenterology* 1983;**85**:1023.

38. Wittig BM, Zeitz M. The gut as an organ of immunology. *Int J Colorectal Dis* 2003;**18**:181.

39. Petras R, Gramlich T. Non-neoplastic intestinal diseases. In: Mills SE (ed.), *Sternberg's Diagnostic Surgical Pathology*, 5th edn. New York: Lippincott, Williams & Wilkins, 2010: 1313.

40. Kakar S, Nehra V, Murray JA, Dayharsh GA, Burgart LJ. Significance of intra-epithelial lymphocytosis in small bowel biopsy samples with normal mucosal architecture. *Am J Gastroenterol* 2003;**98**:2027.

41. Ferguson A, Sutherland A, MacDonald TT, Allan F. Technique for microdissection and measurement in biopsies of human small intestine. *J Clin Pathol* 1977;**30**:1068.

42. Garrison AP, Helmrath MA, Dekaney CM. Intestinal stem cells. *J Pediatr Gastroenterol Nutr* 2009;**49**:2.

43. Watson AJM. Necrosis and apoptosis in the gastrointestinal tract. *Gut* 1995;**37**:165.

44. de Santa Barbara P, van den Brink GR, Roberts DJ. Development and differentiation of the intestinal epithelium. *CMLS, Cell Mol Life Sci* 2003;**60**:1322.

45. Reed JC. Mechanisms of apoptosis. *Am J Pathol* 2000;**157**: 1415.

46. Williamson RC. Intestinal adaptation [first of two parts]. Structural, functional, and cytokinetic changes. *N Engl J Med* 1978; **298**:1393.

47. Ahuja V, Dieckgraefe BK, Anant S. Molecular biology of the small intestine. *Curr Opin Gastroenterol* 2006;**22**:90.

48. Facer P, Bishop AE, Lloyd RV, Wilson BS, Hennessy RJ, Polak JM. Chromogranin: a newly recognised marker for endocrine cells of the human gastrointestinal tract. *Gastroenterology* 1985; **89**:1366.

49. Sjolund K, Sanden G, Hakanson R, Sundler F. Endocrine cells in human intestine: an immunocytochemical study. *Gastroenterology* 1983;**85**:1120.

50. Buffa R, Rindi G, Sessa F, et al. Synaptophysin immunoreactivity and small clear vesicles in neuroendocrine cells and related tumours. *Mol Cell Probes* 1987;**1**:367.

51. Lewin KJ. The endocrine cells of the gastrointestinal tract: the normal endocrine cells and their hyperplasias. In: Sommers SC, Rosen PP, Fechner RE (eds), *Pathology Annual*. Part 1. Norwalk, CT: Appleton-Century-Crofts, 1986: 1.

52. Liddle RA. Peptide hormones of the gastrointestinal tract. In: Feldman M, Friedman LS, Brandt LJ (eds), *Sleisenger and Fordtran's Gastrointestinal and Liver Disease*, 8th edn. Philadelphia, PA: Saunders, Elsevier, 2006: 6.

53. Lewin K. The Paneth cell in disease. *Gut* 1969;**10**:804.

54. Wehkamp J, Fellermann K, Herrlinger KR, Bevins CL, Stange EF. Mechanisms of disease: defensins in gastrointestinal diseases. *Nat Clin Pract Gastroenterol Hepatol* 2005;**2**:406.

55. Wehkamp J, Salzman NH, Porter E, et al. Reduced Paneth cell alpha-defensins in ileal Crohn's disease. *Proc Natl Acad Sci U S A* 2005;**102**:18129.

56. Jenkins D, Goodall A, Scott BB. T-lymphocyte populations in normal and coeliac small intestinal mucosa defined by monoclonal antibodies. *Gut* 1986;**27**:1330.

57. Isaacson P, Judd MA. Carcinoembryonic antigen (CEA) in the normal human small intestine: a light and electron microscopic study. *Gut* 1977;**18**:786.

58. Groisman GM, Ben-Izhak O, Schwersenz A, et al. The value of polyclonal carcinoembryonic antigen immunostaining in the diagnosis of microvillous inclusion disease. *Hum Pathol* 1993; **24**:1232.

59. Groisman GM, Amar M, Livne E. CD10: a valuable tool for the light microscopic diagnosis of microvillous inclusion disease (familial microvillous atrophy). *Am J Surg Pathol* 2002;**26**:902.

60. Parker FG, Barnes EN, Kaye GI. The pericryptal fibroblast sheath. IV. Replication, migration and differentiation of the subepithelial fibroblasts of the crypt and villus of the rabbit jejunum. *Gastroenterology* 1974;**67**:607.

61. Chiba M, Ohta H, Nagasaki A, Arakawa H, Masamune O. Lymphoid cell subsets in normal human small intestine. *Gastroenterol Jpn* 1986;**21**:336.

62. Kingston D, Pearson JR, Penna FJ. Plasma cell counts of human jejunal biopsy specimens examined by immunofluorescence and immunoperoxidase techniques; a comparative study. *J Clin Pathol* 1981;**34**:381.

63. Husband AJ, Gowans JLN. The origin and antigen dependent distribution of IgA-containing cells in the intestine. *J Exp Med* 1978;**148**:1146.

64. MacDonald TT, Pender SL. Lamina propria T cells. *Chem Immunol* 1998;**71**:103.

65. Clancy R, Cripps A, Chipchase H. Regulation of human gut lymphocytes by T lymphocytes. *Gut* 1984;**25**:47.

66. Brandtzaeg P, Halstensen TS, Kett K, et al. Immunobiology and immunopathology of human gut mucosa: humoral immunity and intra-epithelial lymphocytes. *Gastroenterology* 1989;**97**: 1562.

67. Lorenz RG, Newberry RD. Isolated lymphoid follicles can function as sites for induction of mucosal immune responses. *Ann N Y Acad Sci* 2004;**1029**:44.

68. Gershon MD, Erde SM. The nervous system of the gut. *Gastroenterology* 1981;**80**:1571.

69. Krishnamurthy S, Schuffler MD. Pathology of neuromuscular disorders of the small intestine and colon. *Gastroenterology* 1987;**93**:610.

70. Streutker CJ, Huizinga JD, Driman DK, Riddell RH. Interstitial cells of Cajal in health and disease. Part I: normal ICC structure and function with associated motility disorders. *Histopathology* 2007;**50**:176.

71. Farrugia G. Interstitial cells of Cajal in health and disease. *Neurogastroenterol Motil* 2008;**20**(suppl 1):54.

72. Hagger R, Finlayson C, Jeffrey I, Kumar D. Role of the interstitial cells of Cajal in the control of gut motility. *Br J Surg* 1997;**84**:445.

73. Lawson HH. The duodenal mucosa in health and disease. A clinical and experimental study. *Surg Ann* 1989;**21**:157.

74. Dandalides SM, Carey WD, Petras RE, Achkar E. Endoscopic small bowel mucosal biopsy: a controlled trial evaluating forceps size and biopsy location in the diagnosis of normal and abnormal mucosal architecture. *Gastrointest Endosc* 1989;**35**:197.

75. Robertson HE. The pathology of Brunner's glands. *Arch Pathol* 1941;**31**:112.

76. Rosenberg JC, DiDio LJ. Anatomic and clinical aspects of the junction of the ileum with the large intestine. *Dis Colon Rectum* 1970;**13**:220.

77. Axelsson C, Andersen JA. Lipohyperplasia of the ileocaecal region. *Acta Chir Scand* 1974;**140**:649.

78. Cuvelier C, Demetter P, Mielants H, Veys EM, DeVos M. Interpretation of ileal biopsies: morphological features in normal and diseased mucosa. *Histopathology* 2001;**38**:1.

79. Cornes JS. Number, size, and distribution of Peyer's patches in the human small intestine. Part I. The development of Peyer's patches. Part II. The effect of age on Peyer's patches. *Gut* 1965; **6**:225.

80. Bjerke K, Brandtzaeg P, Fausa O. T cell distribution is different in follicle-associated epithelium of human Peyer's patches and villous epithelium. *Clin Exp Immunol* 1988;**74**:270.

81. Spencer J, Finn T, Isaacson PG. Human Peyer's patches: an immunohistochemical study. *Gut* 1986;**27**:405.

82. Owen RI, Jones AL. Epithelial cell specialization within human Peyer's patches: an ultrastructural study of intestinal lymphoid follicles. *Gastroenterology* 1974;**66**:189.

83. Bhalla DK, Owen RL. Cell renewal and migration in lymphoid follicles of Peyer's patches and cecum: an autoradiographic study in mice. *Gastroenterology* 1982;**82**:232.

84. Bye WH, Allan CH, Trier JS. Structure, distribution and origin of M cells in Peyer's patches of mouse ileum. *Gastroenterology* 1984;**86**:789.

85. Wolf JL, Bye WA. The membranous epithelial (M) cell and the mucosal immune system. *Annu Rev Med* 1984;**35**:95.

86. Shepherd NA, Crocker PR, Smith AP, Levison DA. Exogenous pigment in Peyer's patches. *Hum Pathol* 1987;**18**:50.

87. Urbanski SJ, Arsenault AL, Green FH, Habert G. Pigment resembling atmospheric dust in Peyer's patches. *Mod Pathol* 1989;**2**:222.

CHAPTER 18

Congenital abnormalities of the small intestine

Claude Cuvelier

Ghent University, Ghent, Belgium

Congenital anomalies of the small intestine include a variety of different malformations such as Meckel's diverticulum, atresia, malrotation, duplication and Hirschsprung's disease. They are commonly associated with other anomalies elsewhere [1]. Most serious developmental abnormalities reveal themselves at birth or during early childhood [2,3]. They present as obstructions, with perforation and peritonitis as likely complications. Those that are less severe, and most hamartomas, present later with less dramatic symptoms, although intussusception is relatively more common. To understand many of the developmental anomalies in the small bowel, its development and rotation are briefly reviewed [4–6].

Normal development

As there are individual differences in development between fetuses, and it is not always possible to know the exact date of fertilisation, especially when this has to be deduced from the date of the last menstrual period, Table 18.1 gives a rough approximation of the relationship between gestational age and embryo length. In the 1.5- to 3.0-mm stage (week 4), the head and somites appear. The notochord develops and the mesoderm grows into the embryonic disc and separates ectoderm from endoderm except at the *buccopharyngeal membrane* anteriorly and the *cloacal membrane* posteriorly. The head and tail now curve ventrally and the *cloacal membrane* comes to lie on the ventral surface. Failure of the mesodermal ingrowth may result in non-separation of neural and gut elements and so to those duplications associated with defects of spinal cord and vertebrae.

By this stage the former yolk sac, seen in longitudinal section, is shaped somewhat like a mushroom; its anterior limb lies between the developing central nervous system and the heart, where it forms the primitive foregut, whereas the posterior limb lies in the tail fold and forms the primitive hindgut. The central portion, which will form the midgut, is in free communication through a wide opening, the vitello-intestinal duct, with the remains of the yolk sac, which is now outside the embryo. As the embryo grows the body becomes bounded by definitive folds that form the ventral body wall and narrow the broad body stalk, which will later form the umbilical cord and, between the 23- and 60-mm stages, will contain the midgut in a physiological hernia.

The foregut is at first short and lies in close apposition to the developing vertebrae, from which it becomes suspended by a short dorsal mesentery. It has its own arterial blood supply from the coeliac axis and from this develops the oesophagus, stomach, first part of the duodenum, trachea and respiratory system. The dorsal wall of the stomach grows relatively more rapidly than the ventral, producing the greater curve. The stomach rotates to the left, causing a slight deviation of the lower oesophagus to the left and of the duodenum to the right. The oesophageal and duodenal mesenteries are later absorbed and these organs become anchored to the posterior thoracic and abdominal walls. The hindgut is suspended by a similar mesentery and is supplied by the inferior mesenteric artery; from it develop the descending colon, sigmoid colon and rectum.

The midgut develops into the third and fourth parts of the duodenum, jejunum, ileum, caecum, appendix, ascending

Table 18.1 Approximate relationship between fetal age and embryo length

Age after fertilisation (days)	Embryo length (mm)
22	1.5–2.0
25	2.5–3.5
30	6.0–7.5
35	12–15
40	20–23
45	24–28
50	29–34
55	35–41
60	42–50
70	53–67
84	80–95
98	110–130
112	130–150
126	155–180
140 (20 weeks)	175–205

colon and transverse colon, supplied by the superior mesenteric artery. At the 5- to 12-mm stage the midgut begins to lengthen and become tubular, at first growing away from the vertebral axis in the sagittal plane and later becoming coiled, which induces development of the dorsal mesentery, in which the superior mesenteric artery runs. By the 14- to 23-mm stage, due to lack of intra-abdominal space resulting partly from the rapid growth of the liver and also by the marked elongation of the gut itself, the midgut is extruded into the umbilical cord as a physiological hernia. The caecum develops on its caudal limb and the vitello-intestinal duct lies at its apex. Further growth in a purely sagittal plane now becomes impossible and rotation begins. It is completed as the bowel returns to the abdominal cavity at the 50- to 60-mm stage. This process may be divided into phases that are most easily followed by taking a piece of flexible rubber tubing, marking it into cranial and caudal loops, and using it as a model, as follows:

• Phase 1: the cranial (ventral) loop of bowel rotates to the fetal right and caudally. The caudal (dorsal) loop, on which lies the caecum, is correspondingly displaced upwards and to the fetal left through 90° (this is an anti-clockwise rotation around the superior mesenteric artery when the embryo is viewed from the front). It takes place between weeks 6 and 10.

• Phase 2: this takes place at the end of phase 1, at about week 10, when there is room for the bowel to return to the abdominal cavity. The cranial (ventral) loop of small bowel re-enters first and passes to the fetal right of the superior mesenteric artery; it then rotates through a further 180°, making a total rotation of 270°. The caecum, which returns

last, has a similar rotation and comes to lie to the fetal right of the umbilicus, in front of the small bowel. The future transverse colon lies across the abdomen in front of the superior mesenteric artery and the mesenteric attachment, although it is no longer thought that its further growth is responsible for pushing the caecum down into the right iliac fossa [7]. The descending colon is displaced to the left and comes to lie in the left loin. When rotation is complete the small intestine is approximately six times as long as the large.

• Phase 3: this is a phase of fixation. The mesenteries of the caecum, and ascending and descending colons shorten and become absorbed, leaving those parts of the large bowel attached to the posterior abdominal wall. The transverse and sigmoid colons retain a full mesentery.

Small intestinal development

A number of studies are available on the mucosal development of human fetuses [6,8–15]. At the 10- to 20-mm stage the small bowel is lined by a layer of cubical cells, two to four cells thick around a central lumen. These cells proliferate and some become vacuolated. The duodenum can appear occluded for a time but there is probably never occlusion below this level. The structural development of the small intestinal mucosa is determined by the expression of products of the so-called homoeobox, or *HOX*, genes [16], particularly *CDX-1* and *CDX-2*. Contact of the epithelial cells with their environment causes up-regulation of growth factors, transforming growth factor (TGF)-α, TGF-β, epidermal growth factor (EGF) and hepatocyte growth factor (HGF), which stimulate cell proliferation. Rudimentary microvilli appear on the luminal cells at the 35- to 40-mm stage [11,12]. This is followed by villus formation which becomes complete by the 80- to 90-mm stage [13,15]. Some workers have considered that villi are produced by the vacuolation and breakdown of intervening cells [16], but recent findings demonstrate the crucial involvement of Wnt signalling in the development and homoeostasis of the intestine [17,18].

Surface enterocytes differentiate on the developing villi, and alkaline phosphatase, aminopeptidases, adenosine triphosphatase and succinate dehydrogenase become demonstrable histochemically as early as the 25-mm stage [10] and are followed by lactase and other disaccharidases [14,15], at first in equal concentrations throughout the bowel but later showing regional differences with higher concentrations of sucrase and lactase in the jejunum. Mucin granules and goblet cells appear at the same time. Crypts are formed by bud-like down-growths into the surrounding mesenchyme at the 50- to 60-mm stage [13,15]. Endocrine cells containing gastrin, secretin, motilin, gastric inhibitory peptide (GIP), vasoactive intestinal polypeptide (VIP), enteroglucagon and somatostatin have been recognised as early as the 40- to 45-mm stage [19], and are said to have an adult distribution by 175–205 mm. Paneth cells have been present in our own material by 110–130 mm.

Lymphoid follicles first appear in the mucosa at 110–150 mm and recognisable Peyer's patches by 175–205 mm [20]. Cells that may be membranous (M) cells have been described at 130–150 mm [13]. The circular muscle coat appears first in the duodenum at the 30-mm stage and extends distally throughout the small bowel; the longitudinal coat follows at the 60- to 75-mm stage and the muscularis mucosae much later at about week 20. An intramuscular ganglionic plexus is present at 35–40 mm and a submucosal plexus at 60 mm [21]. Neurotensin and VIP can be demonstrated at the 80- to 90-mm stage. The myenteric plexus appears to be fully formed in the 60-mm fetus but there is doubt about the functionality of the innervation before birth, at least in dogs [22].

Malformations

Knowledge of the development of the human small intestine has advanced greatly, due to the availability of suitable material for study following the legalisation of abortions. There has not as yet been corresponding advance in the understanding of many human bowel malformations.

Comparatively few congenital anomalies in the bowel are genetically inherited; examples are mucoviscidosis and anomalies associated with certain chromosomal trisomies [5]. A good, although now somewhat dated, review is available [2]. Very few anomalies are linked to known environmental factors, such as maternal rubella. There is, however, considerable evidence that many are associated with interference with the blood supply at critical periods in development, between weeks 3 and 8, although we do not know the primary causative factor for the interruption. A small study that compared children with congenital anomalies of the mesentery with normal children, using postmortem arteriography, showed a significant number of vascular aberrations in the affected children [23].

Malrotation and malfixation

Minor degrees of malrotation and, more commonly, malfixation are not uncommon [2,3,24]. The more severe forms are rare [24–28]. Their importance lies in their secondary effects, particularly volvulus and obstruction. The recognised types are described below.

Reversed rotation

In phase 1 the ventral and dorsal loops rotate to the fetal left through 90° instead of to the fetal right. The caecum still comes to lie in the right iliac fossa but the small bowel is now ventral (superficial) to the transverse colon, which often passes through an aperture in the small bowel mesen-

tery. The caecum and ascending colon may retain a mesentery and fail to become fixed [28,29].

Failure of the small bowel to rotate fully

This is a failure in phase 2, following a normal phase 1. As the small bowel returns to the abdomen it remains on the right side without rotation. The caecum also fails to rotate, retains its mesentery and lies in either the left iliac fossa or the midline. The ascending colon also retains its mesentery and lies just to the left of the midline behind the greater curve of the stomach. A shortened loop of transverse colon connects it to a normally situated descending colon. The whole bowel from duodenum to splenic flexure is unanchored and supported by a single mesentery with a very narrow base, prone to volvulus. Symptoms of appendicitis can be central or left sided [28,30,31].

Other rotational anomalies

After a normal phase 1, the caecum may undergo normal rotation but retain a mesentery, while the small bowel does not rotate further [30] or undergoes reverse rotation, in which case the caecum will come to lie in the pyloric region [32,33].

Anomalies of fixation

After normal rotation, the caecum initially lies over the right kidney. It may become fixed here or, conversely, delay in absorption of the mesentery may result in a pelvic caecum or a mobile ascending colon. Abnormal peritoneal bands may be found between caecum or ascending colon and the posterior abdominal wall; they are clinically important because they often cross and compress the duodenum [26,34].

Consequences of failures of rotation or fixation

There may be an unusually long mesentery extending from the duodenum to the splenic flexure and arising from an abnormally narrow base. Volvulus leading to duodenal obstruction and the formation of varices, with haemorrhage due to involvement of superior mesenteric vessels, can occur [35]. Duodenal obstruction can result from direct pressure of a malrotated caecum or from abnormal peritoneal bands. These result from imperfect mesenteric absorption and can also act as potential sacs for internal hernias. Such bands often coexist with volvulus and must always be looked for. It should be remembered that the above abnormalities may not be present in isolation. Even after apparently adequate surgical correction of a malrotation, persistent pseudo-obstruction frequently occurs [36]. This may be due to other congenital mechanical anomalies or defective intrinsic innervation.

Situs inversus and Kartagener's syndrome

Some form of situs inversus occurs once in every 1400 births [37]. It may be complete, when thoracic and abdominal organs are both involved but more commonly involves the abdominal viscera only. When complete it can be associated with bronchiectasis and abnormal nasal ciliary dyskinesia, so-called Kartagener's syndrome. Reversals of position can cause difficulties in diagnosis but do not directly predispose to pathological complications.

Omphalocoele (exomphalos) and related defects

Omphalocoele and exomphalos are commonly used as synonyms and are not separated here. A physiological hernial sac composed of amnion is normally present from the 10- to 60-mm stage and becomes obliterated after the intestine returns to the body cavity. The most common form of omphalocoele results from a persistence of this sac, which usually contains a variable length of ileum, the caecum and part of the ascending colon, usually unrotated [38–40]. Liver, spleen and stomach can also be present within it. The sac may persist because its neck becomes abnormally narrowed or the bowel adheres to it before the end of week 10, or as a result of undue enlargement of the liver, all of which hinder the normal return of the bowel.

Other defects include herniation of the bowel into the umbilical cord through an umbilical ring that has failed to close and non-formation of the fetal part of the umbilical cord because of defective condensation of mesenchyme around the attachment of the cord to the embryo. This condition is allied to complete eventration, in which a large sac forms that occupies much of the abdominal wall above and below the umbilicus, and contains gut and other abdominal viscera. These defects, which resemble omphalocoele clinically and in their appearance, are not due to the persistence of a physiological hernia. They must also be distinguished from upper and lower abdominal and para-umbilical hernias, which are associated with malformations of the abdominal wall, covered by skin and lined by peritoneum, and not of primary umbilical origin. Cases are also described in which, in the absence of hernia or exomphalos, the bowel is surrounded by an adherent sac or encapsulation of peritoneum thought to be derived from the primitive peritoneum lining the physiological hernial sac, which has become adherent some time in the 20- to 60-mm stage [41,42]. This condition is distinct from that of abdominal cocooning. The association of abdominal muscle defects with malformations of the gut is well recognised [43].

Maldevelopment

Aplasia and agenesis

Complete absence of the small bowel is not, to our knowledge, recorded but would clearly be incompatible with life.

The term 'aplasia' is used in the literature in two ways: to describe a short but otherwise normal small bowel in adults [44] or children [45] or to indicate a solid cord of tissue of variable length, without a lumen [46–48]. The latter is probably more correctly considered as an acquired atresia due to interference with the blood supply (see below).

Atresias and stenoses

We use the term 'atresia', which means 'non-perforated', to describe a congenital anomaly that can involve any part of the gut and in which there is complete discontinuity of the lumen over a variable length of bowel. We use the term 'stenosis' to indicate a narrowing of the lumen without complete obliteration. About 60% of all cases presenting as stenoses, and a higher proportion with duodenal obstruction, result from extrinsic causes, such as peritoneal bands or an annular pancreas [49].

The incidence of intrinsic atresias and stenoses together varies in different series from 1 in 2000 to 1 in 6000 live births [50]. Sex incidence is equal and there is rarely any evidence of a familial predisposition [51]. Atresias are more common than stenoses and may be single or multiple. They are often associated with mesenteric defects; 60% occur in the ileum and 40% in the duodenum (Figure 18.1) or upper jejunum, where they often give rise to maternal hydramnios [52]. There is an association with a single umbilical artery and with Down's syndrome [53]. Stenoses are more common in the duodenum than elsewhere and are usually single [54]. Occasional multiple stenoses are accompanied by malrotation. They are important because the malrotation may be diagnosed and corrected, and the stenosis missed [55].

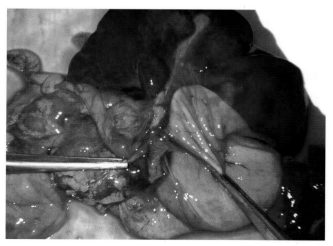

Figure 18.1 Duodenal atresia without formation of a lumen. The duodenal bulb on the right is dilated because of the atresia.

There are three main types of atresia [56,57]:

1. Type 1: an imperforate septum, covered on both sides by mucosa and often with smooth muscle in the septal wall, stretches across an otherwise continuous bowel.

2. Type 2: a variable length of bowel is replaced by a thin cord of fibromuscular tissue; there may or may not be an associated defect in the mesentery.

3. Type 3: two blind ends of bowel are separated by a gap with a corresponding mesenteric defect.

These types may coexist and any may be single or multiple. A variety has been described with a segmental absence of muscle coats but with normal ganglion cells [58].

There are two main types of stenosis.

1. Type 1: a septum identical to that seen in type 1 atresia is present but with a central perforation of variable size.

2. Type 2: the lumen of the bowel is uniformly narrowed over a variable length but all the coats are more or less normally formed.

Studies on the histology of atresias and stenoses are few. Mucosal ulceration with replacement of the lamina propria by granulation tissue containing haemosiderin-filled macrophages has been described – a finding that supports the suggestion that an interruption of blood supply is causative [59,60]. The mucosa may regenerate simple crypts, but not villi, and the muscularis mucosae and submucosa often show distortion with fibrosis. In complete atresia the bowel proximally is dilated and can become gangrenous, whereas distally it is collapsed and small. When stenoses are multiple, the intervening normal segments are usually dilated (Figure 18.2).

There have been numerous theories as to the cause of atresias and stenoses [5,61]. Suggestions that developing epithelial cells normally occlude the lumen at one stage of development and fail to break down [62] or that, at some stage, epithelial proliferation fails to keep pace with longitudinal growth [63] appear to be excluded by the finding of bile, squames and lanugo hairs distal to atretic segments. This indicates that a lumen was originally present and subsequently became occluded and that atresia developed after the 20-mm stage [64]. The currently accepted explanation, supported by experimental evidence from the ligature of mesenteric vessels in dogs [56,65] and sheep [66], is that local interruption of the blood supply occurs, due to either intrauterine intussusception [67] or splanchnic shunting of blood in intrapartum asphyxia [60]. In stenoses involving long segments of intestine, Hirschsprung's disease must always be excluded.

Idiopathic dilatation of small bowel

Idiopathic segmental dilatation of the small bowel is described [68] but its aetiology remains undetermined. Ganglion cells appear to be normal. Occasional cases of unexplained megaduodenum are also recorded [69].

Duplications, diverticula and cysts

In few fields in pathology has so much speculative literature been written based on so little concrete evidence as on the nature and genesis of these lesions. We refer the interested reader to the few valuable general surveys in the field [70–76].

Duplications

Duplication is defined as the complete or partial doubling of a variable length of intestine. The anomaly is always congenital. The duplicated segment may possess its own independent mesentery but is more commonly included in the mesentery of the normal bowel. It may communicate with the normal bowel at either or both ends or not at all, when it may be regarded as a cyst (see below). It is normally lined by intestinal epithelium and usually possesses a submucosa and an inner circular muscle coat. The longitudinal muscle coat is frequently incomplete [77] but a myenteric plexus is usually present. Gastric epithelial heterotopia is common [78]. Examples of triplication have been recorded [79].

Diverticula

We define a diverticulum as an out-pouching of mucosa into or through the muscle coats. It can be congenital or acquired. Congenital diverticula are often out-pouchings of the full-thickness intestinal wall including muscle coats. Those of foregut origin arise in the duodenum. They may be small and localised; when large they may either pass upward behind the stomach, through a separate opening

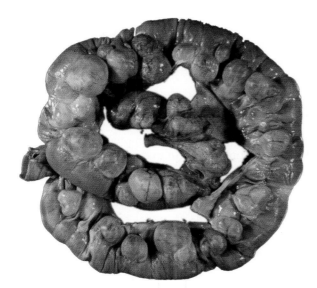

Figure 18.2 Multiple jejunal diverticula.

in the diaphragm to enter the right thoracic cavity where they are often attached to a defective thoracic vertebra [80], or penetrate the pancreas along the line of fusion between its ventral and dorsal components [81]. The majority, which are of midgut origin, and vary in size from small to the so-called giant diverticula, are not associated with vertebral anomalies. In all varieties, heterotopic gastric mucosa is extremely common.

Multiple jejunal diverticula are not uncommon, especially in postmortem examination practice. They are mainly asymptomatic and often discovered only incidentally during investigation for other conditions. However, they may be a cause of bacterial overgrowth syndrome and should always be considered in such cases because they are difficult to diagnose without the aid of either specialist radiology or enteroscopy (see 'Bacterial overgrowth syndrome', Chapter 22). They are typically wide-necked and, unlike Meckel's diverticula, tend to lie close to the mesentery of the small bowel (see Figure 18.2).

Cysts

Enterogenous cysts are common. They are found incorporated into the bowel wall, lying on its serosal aspect or in the mesentery, posterior mediastinum or pelvis, detached and separate from the tract. Those cysts that lie within the bowel wall can be submucosal, intramuscular or subserosal in position and may secondarily invaginate into the lumen, producing symptoms and signs of obstruction, especially in the duodenum or at the ileo-caecal valve. Those that are detached are usually surrounded by smooth muscle and, if they are of foregut origin, may be associated with anomalies of spinal cord and vertebrae. All types of cyst have a mucosal lining of alimentary-type epithelium that may be more primitive than the normal. The presence of ciliated cells in the epithelial lining is not uncommon.

Rarely cysts, fistulae, sinus tracks or diverticula, lined by alimentary-type epithelium and often surrounded by smooth muscle, are found either beneath the skin that covers the dorsal vertebral spines or opening on to it. There is always an associated vertebral defect, sometimes with local duplication of the spinal cord. It is clear that endoderm giving rise to bowel has failed to separate from ectoderm giving rise to skin and spinal cord, and that mesoderm has failed to grow inward to form normal vertebrae. Cysts containing alimentary epithelium described in the spinal cord are of similar origin [82].

Complications of diverticula and cysts

Diverticula can be associated with stagnant loop syndromes, disturbed bowel ecology bacterial overgrowth syndrome and signs of malabsorption (see 'Bacterial overgrowth syndrome', Chapter 22). Intussusception, intraluminal obstruction, infarction [83], perforation and haemorrhage have all been described.

Causative factors of diverticula and cysts

Earlier theories must be discarded, including imperfect luminal recanalisation and the outgrowth of epithelium through the bowel wall [84]. Many diverticula and cysts of foregut and hindgut origin are associated with vertebral anomalies or the Klippel–Feil syndrome [70,72,74]; midgut anomalies do not have this association but are otherwise similar.

It seems logical to consider one embryological concept to explain them all. In the 2- to 4-mm embryo, the endoderm, which forms the roof of the yolk sac and is destined to give rise to the future foregut and hindgut, is in contact with the ectoderm, which forms the floor of the amniotic sac and will give rise to the neural crest and tube. The two communicate through the neurenteric canal. This canal normally closes and the notochord grows forward to become intercalated with the endoderm and separate it from the ectoderm. Mesoderm grows inward to surround the notochord and form the future vertebrae and surrounding muscle; this separates the ectoderm and endoderm still further. At the same time the midgut develops from the yolk sac and thus has no relationship to the ectoderm. Failure of separation of ectoderm from endoderm at this early stage would explain the formation of diverticula and cysts of the foregut and hindgut, and their association with spinal cord abnormalities. Failure of mesoderm to grow inwards would explain the vertebral anomalies [85,86] and development of the midgut from the yolk sac, which is unrelated to the ectoderm, provides the reason for the non-association of neural and vertebral anomalies with midgut anomalies.

That the development of diverticula may also be linked to genetic defects is suggested by their infrequent but significant association with Marfan's syndrome [87].

Duodenocolic fistulae

Examples of fistulae between the third part of the duodenum and the transverse colon are described which are thought to have developed at the time of physiological herniation [88].

Anomalies of the vitello-intestinal duct

This duct, also known as the omphalo-mesenteric duct, links the developing midgut to the yolk sac. It is normally obliterated and disappears at about the 7-mm stage although its distal end can be recognised as a fibrous strand in most umbilical cords at birth. Remnants of it persist in a number of individuals.

Meckel's diverticulum

Meckel's diverticulum is the persisting proximal part of the vitello-intestinal duct. It is present equally in males and females in 1–4% of the population but causes symptoms much more commonly in men [89,90]. It lies on the anti-mesenteric border of the ileum, some 300 mm from the ileo-caecal valve in infants and some 900 mm from it in adults. It varies from 20 mm to 80 mm in length and usually possesses a narrow lumen, which is patent throughout, although the opening into the bowel is occasionally valvular or occluded. The tip is usually free but may be attached to the umbilicus by the remains of the vitello-intestinal duct, which can be fibrous or have a wholly or partially patent lumen. The lining mucosa is small intestinal, although patches of heterotopic gastric epithelium, containing pepsinogen- or acid-secreting cells, are common. Large intestinal-type epithelium is rare. Pancreatic tissue is frequently present in the wall [89] (Figure 18.3).

Symptoms occur in about 20% of individuals and are numerous and diverse [91]. Acid secretion may lead to peptic ulceration with haemorrhage and perforation, either in the diverticulum itself or in the adjacent ileum. A cord that anchors the diverticulum to the umbilicus can give rise to volvulus or obstruction. The diverticulum may invaginate and act as the starting point for an intussusception [92]. We have seen very occasional examples of inverted Meckel's diverticula actually presenting as colonic polyps due to intussusception through the ileo-caecal valve. In one exceptional case, colonoscopic biopsies of the 'polyp' revealed (heterotopic) gastric-type mucosa and caused considerable consternation.

Meckel's diverticulum may herniate into an internal sac or be perforated by a foreign body [93]. Enteroliths may form in it, pass out and obstruct the ileum [94]. It may become inflamed and adhesions may form. Tumours, usually leiomyomas, gastrointestinal stromal tumours

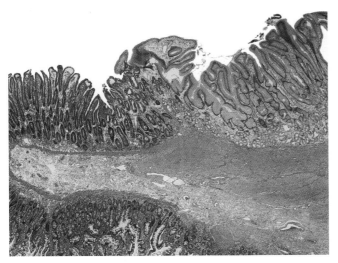

Figure 18.3 Meckel's diverticulum lined partly by gastric body-type mucosa.

or endocrine cell tumours, are rare [95–98]. Endometriosis and regional enteritis involving the diverticulum have both been described [99].

Complete or partial patency of the vitello-intestinal duct

Closure of the duct is complete by week 10 of embryonic life. The duct may remain patent throughout, giving rise to an umbilical fistula. Segments may remain patent, producing cysts, or the umbilical end may remain patent, producing a sinus that may contain pancreatic tissue in its wall and be lined by gastric, duodenal or ileal mucosa [100]. The mucosal lining sometimes undergoes hyperplasia, producing one form of umbilical polyp. An open duct at the umbilicus can cause an umbilical fistula with loss of faecal material from the umbilicus.

The intestinal lesions of cystic fibrosis (mucoviscidosis)

In about 15% of babies with neonatal intestinal obstruction there is a thick putty-like mass of meconium in the terminal ileum, adhering to the mucosa and resisting onward propulsion by peristalsis [101], a condition usually described as meconium ileus. Most patients have or will develop other stigmata of cystic fibrosis [102]. Conversely, although only some 10% of babies with cystic fibrosis present with meconium ileus at birth, many show suggestive mucosal changes on small intestinal or rectal biopsy [67,103–107]. In a small number, the ileum perforates in the antenatal period and meconium peritonitis develops. A good general review of all the gastrointestinal manifestations of cystic fibrosis is available [108].

The disease is a generalised disorder of exocrine glands, including sweat glands, inherited as an autosomal recessive genetic condition. Either patients synthesise an abnormal glycoprotein that is more viscid than normal mucin or there is a variation of polymerisation in normal mucin which increases its viscosity. More recently it has also become apparent that the transport of HCO_3^- is defective. As HCO_3^- secretion is impaired in cystic fibrosis, mucins in affected organs tend to remain aggregated, poorly soluble and less transportable [102,109–112]. Carcinoembryonic antigen and an α-glycoprotein (Mec-6) may also be reduced in concentration and measurement of these may be a useful screening procedure [113]. As the exocrine pancreas is also affected, there is a theoretical possibility that a lack of pancreatic enzymes may prevent breakdown of the thick meconium, but the abnormality of the mucin itself is the most significant factor. Some patients have associated intestinal atresia, probably as a result of inspissated meconium producing ischaemic ulceration by pressure, followed by scarring, rather than as a separate anomaly [114].

In babies with meconium ileus, the terminal ileum is enlarged and often congested; the small intestine proximally is dilated but the large intestine often appears empty and shrunken. The lower ileum is filled with greenish-grey meconium with the consistency of putty, which adheres to the mucosal surface and is difficult to remove manually (Figure 18.4). The bowel content above this meconium is usually fluid. Microscopic appearances are the same whether or not ileus is present, although they vary in degree from patient to patient. There are streaks and pools of mucin between villi and within crypts which are often distended (Figure 18.5). This mucin is predominantly acid non-sulphated (sialomucin) and does not differ histochemically from normal ileal mucin. Goblet cells are distended but not increased in number. Villus flattening is common but this probably results from a secondary pressure effect. There may be evidence of previous meconium peritonitis.

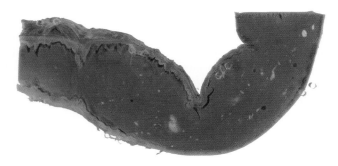

Figure 18.4 Terminal ileum from a 4-day-old child who had cystic fibrosis with meconium ileus. The tenacious putty-like material is clearly shown.

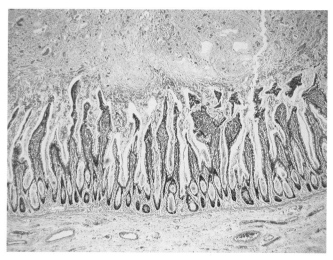

Figure 18.5 Section from the terminal ileum of an infant with cystic fibrosis, showing inspissated mucin and debris in the crypts, between the villi and in the lumen.

Similar appearances are found in Brunner's glands and in rectal biopsies, although in the latter there is usually less mucin present on the mucosal surface. Muciphages have not, surprisingly, been a feature in either the lamina propria or the submucosa.

Histochemical studies on rectal biopsies have shown no quantitative differences from normal [115] and there are apparently no differences from normal individuals in stereological studies [116]. As both parents must carry the recessive gene concerned, one of the authors of this text has created (with informed consent) an unpublished study of rectal biopsies from a number of parents in an attempt to identify the carrier state; no diagnostic histological or histochemical changes were found.

Some patients with cystic fibrosis develop intestinal obstruction later in childhood [102,107,117,118] or even in adult life [119,120], a condition termed 'meconium ileus equivalent' or 'meconium plugging'. They present with small intestinal obstruction, a palpable mass in the right iliac fossa and the presence of 'bubbly' intestinal contents on straight radiograph. Intussusception occurs with increased frequency [121].

Meconium plug syndrome

In a small number of babies who present with small intestinal obstruction, plugs of meconium are present but the mucosa is histologically normal and there are no other stigmata of cystic fibrosis [122]. If the viscid meconium is washed out, no sequelae usually follow. The cause of the plugging is uncertain. A similar syndrome may occur in the large intestine, sometimes in association with Hirschsprung's disease [123].

Fetal and neonatal peritonitis

Peritonitis in neonates and evidence of peritonitis *in utero* in stillbirths are rare but well recognised [124,125]. Both are related to perforation, usually in zones of distension proximal to an obstruction, but sometimes without obvious cause. The peritonitis can be infective or sterile, due to irritation by meconium. In infections there is an acute inflammatory reaction with numerous pus cells and the site of perforation is usually obvious. In meconium peritonitis, which is often associated with cystic fibrosis, there is granulation tissue formation leading to fibrosis with formation of adhesions and the site of perforation may not be detectable. Swallowed fetal squames from the vernix caseosa can sometimes be seen in the reparative tissue.

Heterotopias and heteroplasias

Heterotopia is the presence of a particular type of tissue in a place where it is not normally found. Under the term 'heterotopia', we include the term 'heteroplasia', which some authors reserve for the anomalous differentiation of a developing tissue, e.g. the development of gastric epithelium in Meckel's diverticulum [126]. We separate both of these from metaplasia, which we regard as a change of one type of fully developed tissue to another, usually as a result of inflammation or 'irritation'. The pyloric gland metaplasia (or ulcer-associated cell lineage) described in a number of inflammatory disorders, including Crohn's disease, falls into this group. This is a novel EGF-secreting cell lineage induced by the human EGF homologue, urogastrone, to stimulate ulcer healing throughout the gut [127].

There are a number of useful reviews of what are probably true heterotopias in the small intestine [126,128–133]. The heterotopic epithelium is nearly always gastric, of either body or antrum type, or pancreatic. In rats it has been shown that under-expression of cdx-2 protein, as a result of haplodeletion of the gene, inhibits small intestinal differentiation and causes a shift of phenotype to a more proximal type of mucosa [134]. Heterotopic gastric mucosa has rarely been described in the normal small bowel [135,136]. Cases of polypoid gastric heterotopia of the jejunum can occur (Figure 18.6). Heterotopic gastric mucosa is not uncommon in Meckel's diverticula (see Figure 18.3) or in other persisting parts of the vitello-intestinal duct and in duplications, diverticula and cysts.

Most pathologists now consider that full-thickness body-type mucosa, seen as small nodules in the first part of the duodenum, represents a true heterotopia rather than metaplasia [129–131]. The immunohistochemical demonstration of cells synthesising gastrin may be helpful in deciding whether pyloric-type mucosa is heterotopic or metaplastic [137]. Examples of gastric-type epithelium seen in the duodenum in association with gastric peptic ulcer, Zollinger–Ellison syndrome and hyperacidity are almost certainly metaplastic [138].

Heterotopic pancreatic tissue is most common in the duodenum, where it lies in the submucosa or muscle coat and projects into the lumen as elevations that occasionally become pedunculated. It has been alternatively named periampullary myoepithelial hamartoma. These are most common around the ampulla of Vater and microscopically consist of normal pancreatic tissue in which islets are often present [139,140]. They may be the origin of at least some duodenal islet cell neoplasms. Heterotopic pancreas is also found in Meckel's diverticulum (see Figure 18.3).

Hamartomas

Hamartomas are not primarily neoplastic lesions, although some have neoplastic potential. They are primarily malformations of epithelial and/or of connective tissue. They tend, however, to be polypoid and/or resemble neoplasms both clinically and in their gross appearance, and have to be distinguished from them, usually on microscopic grounds. For this reason they are discussed in Chapter 23 (see 'Hamartomas').

Aganglionosis of the small bowel

Hirschsprung's disease is primarily a colorectal disease and is mainly considered in Chapter 33 (see 'Hirschsprung's disease'). It involves embryogenesis and developmental abnormalities of the large intestine (including the anal region). However, in about 5% of patients with Hirschsprung's disease, the aganglionic segment extends proximally to involve the small intestine [141]. These patients present with intestinal obstruction without evidence of megacolon, and the diagnosis must be considered in all babies with neonatal obstruction for which no mechanical cause can be found. In this form of the disease a full-thickness small intestinal biopsy is essential. Ganglion cells are absent in both plexuses but nerve trunks do not always show hypertrophy and palisading. Acetylcholinesterase techniques, for thickened nerves in mucosa, are therefore not reliable.

Patients have been described in whom both ganglion cells and nerve trunks are absent [142]. This is probably a developmental anomaly related to Hirschsprung's disease, but may have resulted from temporary ischaemia during the normal phases of bowel rotation with selective damage to ganglion cells [143]. In some patients with the very rare condition of total aganglionosis of small bowel [144–145], the disorder may be inherited as an autosomal recessive characteristic.

Under the name 'adynamic ileus with dilatation' occasional patients are described with persistent non-motility of small and large bowel, clinically resembling Hirschsprung's disease, in whom ganglion cells were normal [146].

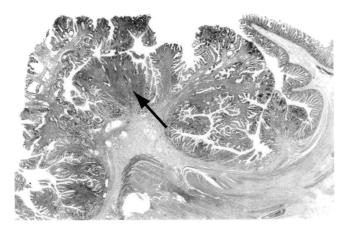

Figure 18.6 Polypoid gastric heterotopia: section of a polyp that was obstructing the jejunum. Much of the epithelium in the polyp is of gastric type and there is a focus of gastric body glands (arrowed).

The defect here may be in the central nervous stem and the condition may be related to that of idiopathic dilatation described above (see 'Idiopathic dilatation of the small intestine').

References

1. Evans PR, Polani N. Congenital malformations in a postmortem series. *Teratology* 1980;**22**:207.
2. Santulli TV, Amoury RA. Congenital anomalies of the gastrointestinal tract. *Pediatr Clinics North Am* 1967;**14**:21.
3. Silverberg M, Davidson M. Paediatric gastroenterology. A review. *Gastroenterology* 1970;**58**:229.
4. Rubin DC. Intestinal morphogenesis. *Curr Opin Gastroenterol* 2007;**23**:111.
5. Louw JH. The pathogenesis of congenital abnormalities of the digestive tract. *S Afr Med J* 1967;**2**:1057.
6. Montgomery RK, Mulberg AE, Grand RJ. Development of the human gastrointestinal tract: twenty years of progress. *Gastroenterology* 1999;**116**:702.
7. Fitzgerald MJT, Nolan JP, O'Neill MN. The formation of the ascending colon. *Irish J Med Sci* 1971;**140**:258.
8. McLin VA, Henning SJ, Jamrich M. The role of the visceral mesoderm in the development of the gastrointestinal tract. *Gastroenterology* 2009;**136**:2074.
9. Ménard D. Functional development of the human gastrointestinal tract: Hormone and growth factor-mediated regulatory mechanisms. *Can J Gastroenterol* 2004;**18**:39.
10. Desdicioglu K, Malas MA, Evcil EH. Development of the fetal duodenum: a postmortem study. *Fetal Diagn Ther* 2009;**26**:16.
11. Kelley R. An ultrastructural and cytochemical study of developing small intestine in man. *J Embryol Exp Morph* 1973;**29**:411.
12. Varkonyi T, Gergely G, Varro V. The ultrastructure of the small intestinal mucosa in the developing human fetus. *Scand J Gastroenterol* 1974;**9**:495.
13. Moxey PC, Trier JS. Specialised cell types in the human fetal small intestine. *Anat Rec* 1978;**191**:269.
14. Sato T, Mushiake S, Kato Y, et al. The Rab8 GTPase regulates apical protein localization in intestinal cells. *Nature* 2007;**448**:366.
15. Lacroix B, Kedinger M, Simon-Assmann P, Haffen K. Early organogenesis of human small intestine: scanning electron microscopy and brush border enzymology. *Gut* 1984;**25**:925.
16. Walters JR, Howard A, Rumble HE, Prathalingam SR, Shaw-Smith CJ, Lagon S. Differences in expression of homeobox transcription factors in proximal and distal human small intestine. *Gastroenterology* 1997;**113**:472.
17. Ahuja V, Dieckgraefe BK, Anant S. Molecular biology of the small intestine. *Curr Opin Gastroenterology* 2006;**22**:90.
18. Gregorieff A, Pinto D, Begthel H, Destrée O, Kielman M, Clevers H. Expression pattern of Wnt signaling components in the adult intestine. *Gastroenterology* 2005;**129**:626.
19. Koldovsky O. Longitudinal specialization of the small intestine: developmental aspects. *Gastroenterology* 1983;**85**:1436.
20. Newberry RD, Lorenz RG. Organizing a mucosal defense. *Immunol Rev* 2005;**206**:6.
21. Read JB, Burnstock G. The development of adrenergic innervation and chromaffin cells in human fetal gut. *Dev Biol* 1970;**22**:513.
22. Daniel EE, Wang YF. Control systems of gastrointestinal motility are immature at birth in dogs. *Neurogastroenterol Motil* 1999;**11**:375.
23. Jimenez FA, Reiner L. Arteriographic findings in congenital abnormalities of the mesentery and intestines. *Surg Gynecol Obstet* 1961;**113**:346.
24. McIntosh R, Donovan EJ. Disturbances of rotation of the intestinal tract. *Am J Dis Child* 1939;**57**:116.
25. Kluth D, Jaeschke-Melli S, Fiegel H. The embryology of gut rotation. *Semin Pediatr Surg* 2003;**12**:275.
26. Strouse PJ. Disorders of intestinal rotation and fixation ('malrotation'). *Pediatr Radiol* 2004;**34**:837.
27. Moran Penco JM, Cardenal Murillo J, Hernandez A, et al. Anomalies of intestinal rotation and fixation: consequences of late diagnosis beyond two years of age. *Pediatr Surg Int* 2007;**23**:723.
28. Söderlund S. Anomalies of midgut rotation and fixation. *Acta Paediatr (Stockh) Suppl* 1962;**135**:225.
29. Glasgow EF. Unsuspected malrotation of gut in an adult male. *Lancet* 1962;**i**:621.
30. Rixford E. Failure of primary rotation of the intestine (left-sided colon) in relation to intestinal obstruction. *Ann Surg* 1920;**72**:114.
31. Thorlakson PHT, Monie IW, Thorlakson TK. Anomalous peritoneal encapsulation of the small intestine. A report of 3 cases. *Br J Surg* 1953;**40**:490.
32. Denzer BS. Congenital duodenal obstruction, malrotation of the intestine: report of case. *Am J Dis Child* 1922;**24**:534.
33. Eggers C. Non rotation of the large intestine. *Ann Surg* 1922;**75**:757.
34. Waugh GE. The morbid consequences of a mobile ascending colon with a record of 180 operations. *Br J Surg* 1920;**7**:343.
35. Park RW, Watkins JB. Mesenteric vascular occlusion and varices complicating midgut malrotation. *Gastroenterology* 1979;**77**:565.
36. Devane SP, Coombes R, Smith VV, et al. Persistent gastrointestinal symptoms after correction of malrotation. *Arch Dis Child* 1992;**67**:218.
37. Leigh MW, Pittman JE, Carson JL, et al. Clinical and genetic aspects of primary ciliary dyskinesia/Kartagener syndrome. *Genet Med* 2009;**11**:473.
38. Soper RT, Green EW. Omphalocoele. *Surg Gynecol Obstet* 1961;**113**:501.
39. Eckstein HB. Exomphalos. A review of 100 cases. *Br J Surg* 1963;**50**:405.
40. Langer JC. Abdominal wall defects. *World J Surg* 2003;**27**:117.
41. Lewin K, McCarthy LJ. Peritoneal encapsulation of the small intestine. *Gastroenterology* 1970;**59**:270.
42. Sieck JO, Cowgill R, Larkworthy W. Peritoneal encapsulation and abdominal cocoon. Case reports and a review of the literature. *Gastroenterology* 1983;**84**:1597.
43. Wilson RD, Johnson MP. Congenital abdominal wall defects: an update. *Fetal Diagn Ther* 2004;**19**:385.
44. Raeburn C, Brafield AJ. A short small intestine associated with fibrosis of the liver. *Lancet* 1956;**i**:884.
45. Hamilton JR, Reilly BJ, Morecki R. Short small intestine associated with malrotation: a newly described congenital cause of intestinal malabsorption. *Gastroenterology* 1969;**56**:124.
46. Bennington JL, Haber SL. The embryologic significance of an undifferentiated intestinal tract. *J Pediatr* 1964;**64**:735.
47. Besner GE, Bates GD, Boesel CP, Singh V, Welty SE, Corpron CA. Total absence of the small bowel in a premature neonate. *Pediatr Surg Int* 2005;**21**:396.
48. Hasosah M, Lemberg DA, Skarsgard E, Schreiber R. Congenital short bowel syndrome: a case report and review of the literature. *Can J Gastroenterol* 2008;**22**:71.
49. Muracka I, Ohno Y, Kobayashi K, Honda R, Kubo T, Kanematsu T. Preduodenal position of the common bile duct associated with annular pancreas: case report and literature review. *Pancreas* 2005;**31**:283.
50. Moore TC, Stokes GE. Congenital stenosis and atresia of the small intestine. *Surg Gynecol Obstet* 1953;**97**:719.

51. Mishalany HG, Najjar FB. Familial jejunal atresia: three cases in one family. *J Pediatr* 1968;**73**:753.

52. Grosfeld JL, Rescoria FJ. Duodenal atresia and stenosis: reassessment of treatment and outcome based on antenatal diagnosis, pathologic variance, and long-term follow-up. *World J Surg* 1993;**17**:301.

53. Stringer MD, Brereton RJ, Drake DP, Wright VM. Double duodenal atresia/stenosis: a report of four cases. *J Pediatr Surg* 1992;**27**:576.

54. Ehrenpreis T, Sandblom P. Duodenal atresia and stenosis. *Acta Paediatr (Stockh)* 1949;**38**:109.

55. Knutrud O, Eek S. Combined intrinsic duodenal obstruction and malrotation. *Acta Chir Scand* 1960;**119**:506.

56. Louw JH. Congenital intestinal atresia and stenosis in the newborn. *Ann R Coll Surg* 1959;**25**:209.

57. Willis RA. *The Borderland of Embryology and Pathology*, 2nd edn. London: Butterworths, 1962: 187.

58. Alvarez SP, Greco MA, Geneiser NB. Small intestinal atresia and segmental absence of muscle coats. *Hum Pathol* 1982;**13**:948.

59. Louw JH. Congenital intestinal atresia and severe stenosis in the new born. *S Afr J Clin Sci* 1952;**3**:109.

60. DeSa DJ. Congenital stenosis and atresia of the jejunum and ileum. *J Clin Pathol* 1972;**25**:1063.

61. Walker K, Badawi N, Hamid CH, et al. A population-based study of the outcome after small bowel atresia/stenosis in New South Wales and the Australian Capital Territory, Australia 1992–2003. *J Pediatr Surg* 2008;**43**:484.

62. Feggetter S. Congenital intestinal atresia. *Br J Surg* 1955;**42**:378.

63. Morison JE. *Fetal and Neonatal Pathology*, 2nd edn. London: Butterworths, 1963.

64. Santulli TV, Blanc WA. Congenital atresia of the intestine. Pathogenesis and treatment. *Ann Surg* 1961;**154**:939.

65. Louw JH, Barnard CN. Congenital intestinal atresia: observations on its origin. *Lancet* 1955;**ii**:1065.

66. Abrams JS. Experimental intestinal atresia. *Surgery* 1968;**64**:185.

67. Gaillard D, Bouvier R, Scheiner C, Meconium ileus and intestinal atresia in fetuses and neonates. *Pediatr Pathol Lab Med* 1996;**16**:25.

68. Sjölin S, Thoren L. Segmental dilatation of the small intestine. *Arch Dis Child* 1962;**37**:422.

69. Basilisco G. Hereditary megaduodenum. *Am J Gastroenterol* 1997;**92**:150.

70. McLetchie NGB, Purves JK, Saunders RL. The genesis of gastric and certain intestinal diverticula and enterogenous cysts. *Surg Gynecol Obstet* 1954;**99**:135.

71. Rhaney K, Barclay GP. Enterogenous cysts and congenital diverticula of the alimentary canal with abnormalities of the vertebral column and spinal cord. *J Pathol Bacteriol* 1959;**77**:457.

72. Smith JR. Accessory enteric formations. A classification and nomenclature. *Arch Dis Child* 1960;**35**:87.

73. Bentley JRF, Smith JR. Developmental posterior enteric remnants and spinal malformations. *Arch Dis Child* 1960;**35**:76.

74. Anderson MC, Silverman WW, Shields TW. Duplications of the alimentary tract in the adult. *Arch Surg* 1962;**85**:94.

75. Bower RJ, Sieber WK, Kieseweter WB. Alimentary tract duplications in children. *Ann Surg* 1978;**188**:669.

76. Avni F, Kalifa G, Sauvegrain J. Gastric and duodenal duplications in infants and children. *Ann Radiol* 1980;**23**:195.

77. Gross RE, Holcomb GW Jr, Farber S. Duplications of the alimentary tract. *Pediatrics* 1952;**9**:449.

78. Tribi B, Aschi G, Mitterbaure G, Novacek G, Vogelsang H, Chott A. Severe malabsorption due to refractory celiac disease complicated by extensive gastric heterotopia of the jejunum. *Am J Surg Pathol* 2004;**28**:262.

79. Basu R, Forshall I, Rickham PP. Duplications of the alimentary tract. *Br J Surg* 1966;**47**:477.

80. Goldberg HM, Johnson TP. Posterior abdominothoracic enteric duplication. *Br J Surg* 1963;**50**:445.

81. Suda K, Mizuguchi K, Matsumoto M. A histopathological study on the etiology of duodenal diverticulum related to the fusion of the pancreatic anlage. *Am J Gastroenterol* 1983;**78**:335.

82. Yoshino MT, Meakem TJ, Hamilton A, Carter LP. Intraspinal enterogenous cyst. *Am J Roentgenol* 1992;**159**:904.

83. Fan ST, Lau WY, Pang SW. Infarction of a duodenal duplication cyst. *Am J Gastroenterol* 1985;**80**:337.

84. Lewis FT, Thyng FW. The regular occurrence of intestinal diverticula in embryos of the pig, rabbit and man. *Am J Anat* 1908;**7**:505.

85. Chang SH, Morrison L, Shaffner L, Crowe JE. Intrathoracic gastrogenic cysts and hemoptysis. *J Pediatr* 1976;**88**:594.

86. Abell MR. Mediastinal cysts. *Arch Pathol* 1956;**61**:360.

87. de Silva DG, Gunawardena TP, Law FM. Unusual complications in siblings with marfanoid phenotype. *Arch Dis Child* 1996;**75**:247.

88. McQuaide JR, Naidoo G. Benign duodenocolic fistula. A report of 3 cases. *S Afr Med J* 1979;**55**:600.

89. Söderland S. Meckel's diverticulum. A clinical and histologic study. *Acta Chir Scand Suppl* 1959;**248**.

90. Jackson RH, Bird AR. Meckel's diverticulum in childhood. *BMJ* 1961;**ii**:1399.

91. Ker H. A muckle of Meckels. *Lancet* 1962;**i**:617.

92. McKenzie G, Gault EW, Wood IJ. Meckel's diverticulum: invagination causing recurrent ileal obstruction. *Aust N Z J Surg* 1966;**35**:272.

93. Sagar J, Kumar V, Shah Dk. Meckel's diverticulum: a systematic review. *J R Soc Med* 2006;**99**:501.

94. Bergland RL, Gump F, Price JB Jr. An unusual complication of Meckel's diverticulum seen in older patients. *Ann Surg* 1963;**158**:6.

95. Doyle JL, Severance AO. Carcinoid tumours of Meckel's diverticulum. *Cancer* 1966;**19**:1591.

96. Freeman GC. Adenocarcinoma in a Meckel's diverticulum with perforation. *Arch Surg* 1957;**75**:158.

97. Jones EL, Thompson H, Williams JA. Argentaffin-cell tumour of Meckel's diverticulum. A report of 2 cases and review of the literature. *Br J Surg* 1972;**59**:213.

98. Chandramohan K, Agarwal M, Gurjar G, et al. Gastrointestinal tumour in Meckel's diverticulum. *World J Surg Oncol* 2007;**5**:50.

99. Won KH. Endometriosis, mucocele and regional enteritis of Meckel's diverticulum. *Arch Surg* 1969;**98**:209.

100. Vane DW, West KW, Grosfeld JL. Vitelline duct anomalies. Experience with 217 childhood cases. *Arch Surg* 1987;**122**:542.

101. Burge D, Drewett M, Meconium plug obstruction. *Pediatr Surg Int* 2004;**20**:108.

102. Robertson MB, Choe KA, Joseph PM. Review of the abdominal manifestations of cystic fibrosis in the adult patient. *Radiographics* 2006;**26**:679.

103. Riedel BD. Gastrointestinal manifestations of cystic fibrosis. *Pediatr Ann* 1997;**26**:235.

104. Modolell I, Alvarez A, Guarner L, De Gracia J, Malagelada JR. Gastrointestinal, liver, and pancreatic involvement in adult patients with cystic fibrosis. *Pancreas* 2001;**22**:395.

105. Modolell I, Guarner L, Malagelada JR. Digestive system involvement in cystic fibrosis. *Pancreatology* 2002;**2**:12.

106. Nick JA, Rodman DM. Manifestations of cystic fibrosis diagnosed in adulthood. *Curr Opin Pulmonol Med* 2005;**11**:513.

107. Chaudry G, Navarro OM, Levine DS, Oudjihane K. Abdominal manifestations of cystic fibrosis in children. *Pediatr Radiol* 2006;**36**:233.

108. Fields TM, Michel SJ, Butler CL, Kriss VM, Albers SL. Abdominal manifestations of cystic fibrosis in older children and adults. *Am J Roentgenol* 2008;**187**:1199.

109. Blanck C, Okmian L, Robbe H. Mucoviscidosis and intestinal atresia. A study of 4 cases in the same family. *Acta Paediatr (Stockh)* 1965;**54**:557.

110. Lewis MJ, Lewis EH 3rd, Amos JA, Tsongalis GJ. Cystic fibrosis. *Am J Clin Pathol* 2003;**120**:S3.

111. Quinton PM. Cystic fibrosis: impaired bicarbonate secretion and mucoviscidosis. *Lancet* 2008;**372**:415.

112. Rubin BK. Mucus, phlegm, and sputum in cystic fibrosis. *Respir Care* 2009;**54**:726.

113. Ryley HC. Distribution of non-plasma protein components in meconium from healthy and cystic fibrosis neonates. *J Clin Pathol* 1981;**34**:179.

114. Bernstein J, Vawter G, Harris GBC, Young V, Hillman LS. The occurrence of intestinal atresia in new born with meconium ileus. *Am J Dis Child* 1960;**99**:804.

115. Johansen PG, Kay R. Histochemistry of the rectal mucosa in cystic fibrosis of the pancreas. *J Pathol* 1969;**99**:299.

116. Hage E, Anderson U. Light and electron microscopical studies of rectal biopsies in cystic fibrosis. *Acta Pathol Microbiol Scand* 1972;**80**:345.

117. Fanconi A. Postneonataler Kotileus bei cystischer Pancreasfibrose. *Helvt Paediat Acta* 1960;**15**:566.

118. Cordonnier JK, Izant RJ Jr. Meconium ileus equivalent. *Surgery* 1963;**54**:667.

119. Speck K, Charles A. Distal intestinal obstruction syndrome in adults with cystic fibrosis: a surgical perspective. *Arch Surg* 2008;**143**:601.

120. Morton JR, Ansari N, Glanville AR, Meagher AP, Lord RV. Distal intestinal obstruction syndrome (DIOS) in patients with cystic fibrosis after lung transplantation. *J Gastrointest Surg* 2009;**13**:1448.

121. Eggermont E, de Boeck K. Small intestinal abnormalities in cystic fibrosis patients. *Eur J Pediatr* 1991;**150**:824.

122. Loening-Baucke V, Kimura K. Failure to pass meconium: diagnosing neonatal intestinal obstruction. *Am Fam Physician* 1999;**60**:2043.

123. Swischuk LE. Meconium plug syndrome: a cause of neonatal intestinal obstruction. *Am J Roentgenol* 1968;**103**:339.

124. Davis JR, Miller HS, Feng JD. Vernix caseosa peritonitis: report of two cases with antenatal onset. *Am J Clin Pathol* 1998;**109**:696.

125. Drut R. Squamous cell peritonitis associated with hydrometrocolpos in a multimalformed newborn. *Fetal Pediatr Pathol* 2005;**24**:161.

126. Cserni G. Gastric pathology in Meckel's diverticulum. Review of cases resected between 1965 and 1995. *Am J Clin Pathol* 1996;**106**:782.

127. Wright NA, Pike C, Elia G. Induction of a novel epidermal growth factor-secreting cell lineage by mucosal ulceration in human gastrointestinal stem cells. *Nature* 1990;**343**:82.

128. Rubin W, Ross LL, Jeffries GH. Sleisenger. Intestinal heterotopia. A fine structural study. *Lab Invest* 1966;**15**:1024.

129. Lessels AM, Martin DF. Heterotopic gastric mucosa in the duodenum. *J Clin Pathol* 1982;**35**:591.

130. Spiller RC, Shousha S, Barrison IG. Heterotopic gastric tissue in the duodenum: a report of 8 cases. *Dig Dis Sci* 1982;**27**:880.

131. Kundrotas LW, Camara DS, Meenaghan MA, Montes M, Wosick WF, Weiser MM. Heterotopic gastric mucosa: a case report. *Am J Gastroenterol* 1985;**80**:253.

132. Cserni G. Proliferative epithelial changes in ectopic gastric mucosa of Meckel's diverticula. *Pathol Oncol Res* 1998;**4**:130.

133. Tribl B, Aschi G, Mitterbauer G, Novacek G, Vogelsang H, Chott A. Severe malabsorption due to refractory celiac disease complicated by extensive gastric heterotopia of the jejunum. *Am J Surg Pathol* 2004;**28**:262.

134. Beck F, Chawengsaksophak K, Waring Playford RJ, Furness JB. Reprogramming of intestinal differentiation and intercalary regeneration in Cdx2 mutant mice. *Proc Natl Acad Sci USA* 1999;**96**:7381.

135. Gore I, Williams WJ. Adenomatous polyp of the jejunum composed of gastric mucosa. *Cancer* 1953;**6**:164.

136. Nawaz K, Graham DY, Fechner RE, Eiband JM. Gastric heterotopia in the ileum with ulceration and bleeding. *Gastroenterology* 1974;**66**:113.

137. Dayal Y, Wolfe HJ. Gastrin-producing cells in ectopic gastric mucosa of developmental and metaplastic origin. *Gastroenterology* 1978;**75**:655.

138. James AH. Gastric epithelium in the duodenum. *Gut* 1964;**5**:285.

139. Contini S, Zinicola R, Bonati L, Caruana P. Heterotopic pancreas in the ampulla of Vater. *Minerva Chir* 2003;**58**:405.

140. Levy AD, Hobbs CM. From the archives of the AFIP. Meckel diverticulum: radiologic features with pathologic correlation. *Radiographics* 2004;**24**:565.

141. Walkor AW, Kempson RL, Ternberg JL. Aganglionosis of the small intestine. *Surgery* 1966;**60**:449.

142. Gariepy CE. Developmental disorders of the enteric nervous system genetic and molecular basis. *J Pediatr Gastroenterol Nutr* 2004;**39**:5.

143. Earlam RJ. A vascular cause for aganglionic bowel. A new hypothesis. *Am J Dig Dis* 1972;**17**:255.

144. Saperstein L, Pollack J, Beck AR. Total intestinal aganglionosis. *Mt Sinai Med J* 1980;**47**:72.

145. Ruttenstock E, Puri. A meta-analysis of clinical outcome in patients with total intestinal aganglionosis. *Pediatr Surg Int* 2009;**25**:833.

146. Ehrenpreis T, Bentley JFR, Nixon HH. Seminar on pseudo Hirschsprung's disease and related disorders. *Arch Dis Child* 1966;**41**:143.

CHAPTER 19

Muscular and mechanical disorders of the small intestine

Paola Domizio and Joanne E. Martin

Barts and the London School of Medicine and Dentistry, Queen Mary University of London; The Royal London Hospital, London, UK

Many of the mechanical disorders of the small bowel are associated with anomalies of rotation and mesenteric resorption or are abnormalities in development. The small bowel, apart from the first three parts of the duodenum, is entirely suspended from a mesentery that arises from a relatively narrow base, through which the superior mesenteric artery enters and the superior mesenteric vein drains. The bowel and mesentery are, within limits, freely mobile. Apart from congenital atresias and stenoses (see Chapter 18), most purely mechanical effects in this group arise as the result of herniation of the bowel or torsion of the mesentery, for which there may or may not be a recognisable antecedent cause. They usually result in acute intestinal obstruction, with the risk of haemorrhagic infarction due to vascular obstruction. The principal conditions in each group are described below.

Intussusception

Intussusception is the telescopic invagination of a variable length of the intestine into the intestine immediately distal to it. Once initiated, the invaginated segment, called the intussusceptum, is propelled distally by the peristaltic activity of the ensheathing outer bowel or intussuscipiens (Figure 19.1). The process is usually triggered by the presence of a 'mass' of poorly propagated material within the intestinal lumen. Most often this is a bolus of firmly adherent ingested material or a polypoid lesion of the intestinal wall itself. The presence of this intraluminal mass gives rise to increased peristaltic activity which propels the obstruction distally, taking with it the attached bowel wall. This

initiates the intussusception, which is then perpetuated by further peristaltic activity, until it is terminated by stretching of the mesentery of the intussusceptum and the consequent complete intestinal obstruction. Although it is customary to regard intussusception as a distal propulsion of invaginated intestine, retrograde intussusceptions have been recorded [1].

Intussusception occurs most commonly in childhood, with an incidence of between 1 and 4 cases per 1000 live births [2,3]. It is likely that the incidence is greater than this because many intussusceptions may be self-correcting and never diagnosed. Boys outnumber girls by about 2:1, and this proportion rises with the age of onset. The condition is rare in the neonatal period, becomes increasingly common from 3 months to 6 months and is infrequent after the age of 3 years [3,4]. Multiple or single intussusceptions are occasionally seen in the small bowel at necropsy on babies and children; they are rarely associated with antemortem obstructive symptoms or visible change in the bowel, and are considered to be agonal and of no clinical significance.

In many children intussusception occurs for no obvious reason [3,5,6,7] and, although up to 50% may be linked to viral infection [8], occasional examples appear to be triggered by foreign bodies such as bezoars, Meckel's diverticula, intestinal tumours or polyps, such as Peutz–Jeghers polyps. Well-nourished children are affected more commonly than poorly nourished ones and the condition is said to occur more commonly in siblings than would be expected by chance [2]. Many children with 'idiopathic' intussusception often have mesenteric adenitis, sometimes

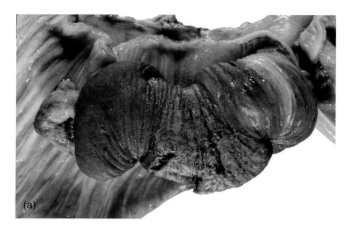

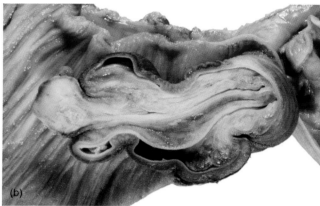

Figure 19.1 (a) Intussusception in the terminal ileum: (a) a necrotic nodular mass at the tip of a haemorrhagic intussusceptum. (b) This is seen on slicing to be a discrete nodule and appears to be an inverted Meckel's diverticulum.

associated with adenovirus infection, although an association with rotavirus and immunisation has been postulated [3,7,8]. Intussusception is a frequent cause of abdominal pain and melaena in Henoch–Schönlein purpura. Other cases have been associated with an excess intake of fluids [9]. Intussusception due to heterotopic pancreas in the small bowel has also been described [10]. There is an increased incidence of intussusception in cystic fibrosis [11], possibly related to the tenacious, adherent intestinal contents typical of this condition.

The usual site of intussusception in childhood is the ileum close to the ileo-caecal valve, most likely related to the abundant lymphoid tissue at this site. Hyperplasia of lymphoid tissue, possibly due to viral infection or antigenic stimulation from intestinal contents, results in its protrusion into the lumen of the terminal ileum, triggering the process of intussusception which then becomes self-perpetuating [12]. The leading point of the intussusceptum frequently reaches the transverse colon. Additional factors

are probably involved, however, because the high frequency of childhood ileal lymphoid hyperplasia continues well beyond the age of 5 years, when the incidence of intussusception falls markedly. Childhood ileo-ileal intussusception is less common and, in our experience, jejunal intussusceptions are rare unless there is a particular anatomical abnormality.

Intussusception in adults is rare and, although some cases are idiopathic [4,13,14], an organic cause is found in the vast majority. In contrast to childhood cases, adult intussusception is frequently chronic and recurrent. Among the more common causes are swallowed foreign bodies, polypoid epithelial tumours (especially Peutz–Jeghers polyps and endocrine tumours/carcinoids), tumours of connective tissue in the bowel wall (especially submucosal lipomas and inflammatory fibroid polyps), metastatic tumours (especially metastatic malignant melanoma, which characteristically causes multiple submucosal polypoid masses), Meckel's diverticula (see Figure 19.1) and gastroenterostomy sites [14,15]. Viral infection has also been associated with adult intussusception [14,16]. Intussusception in adults is less commonly ileo-caecal than in children and other varieties, including gastroduodenal intussusception, occur [17].

Early symptoms of intussusception are those of obstruction: if an appreciable length of mesentery is drawn into the ensheathing bowel the venous return may be occluded, and ischaemic necrosis with perforation and peritonitis supervenes. On macroscopic examination of a longitudinally sectioned specimen, three definite layers can be distinguished, namely the outermost investing *intussuscipiens* and the entering (inner) and returning (outer) layers of the invaginated *intussusceptum*. The intussusceptum itself is oedematous and engorged; if its vasculature has been severely compromised, it may appear black from infarction. Microscopically the picture is one of developing haemorrhagic necrosis of both inner coats, often with acute inflammatory changes on the peritoneal surface. It is important to examine the apex of the intussusceptum histologically to determine whether a polyp or tumour is the cause of the intussusception and to identify its nature. Ischaemic necrosis may make this difficult.

Internal (intra-abdominal) hernia

Obstruction of bowel associated with an internal hernia accounts for between 1 and 5% of all cases of intestinal obstruction [18,19]. The most common type is entrapment of a loop of intestine within a so-called paraduodenal hernia, where there is a protrusion of peritoneum beneath the inferior mesenteric vein and left colic artery [20]. Various other types occur, including those through the foramen of Winslow [21], and are well classified [22]. A small but important group is those in which bowel herniates through a mesenteric or omental defect [23,24]. The most common sites for these are in the terminal ileal region or the transverse mesocolon. Most internal hernias are developmental in origin, although some have been associated with trauma or previous abdominal surgery [18].

The complications of internal hernias occur in adults more commonly than in children. They include strangulation of bowel with ischaemic necrosis, perforation with peritonitis and/or incomplete small intestinal obstruction when part of the circumference of the bowel is involved in a so-called Richter's hernia.

Volvulus

Volvulus is defined as a twist of a loop of bowel to such a degree that obstruction occurs to either the lumen or the blood supply or to both. In the western world it accounts for only a small proportion of all cases of small intestinal obstruction, without predilection for sex or age. Aetiological factors include a congenitally long mesentery with a narrow base, congenital omental and mesenteric bands, and acquired inflammatory or post-operative adhesions [25,26]. Nevertheless, in some parts of the world, e.g. Iran [27], small intestinal volvulus is much more common, possibly related to a high-residue diet. A study from Afghanistan has found that hospital admissions for small intestinal volvulus were much more common during the religious period of Ramadan, a time of daylight fasting and the consumption of a single, large, high-residue meal in the evening [26]. A related condition is intestinal knotting, such as ileo-sigmoid knotting or compound volvulus, in which two loops of bowel twist around each other, with the ileum wrapping around the sigmoid colon [28].

Symptoms of small intestinal volvulus are those of obstruction, often with disproportionate shock requiring early operation. The mortality rate in adults is over 10% and, even when surgery is successful, in both adults and children, long-term complications may follow, including short bowel syndrome, which can be severe enough to require transplantation [29–31]. Findings in the resected intestine depend largely on whether there is partial or complete venous obstruction with or without arterial obstruction. The bowel involved is distended and gas-producing organisms frequently proliferate. Haemorrhagic infarction and necrosis are common.

Chronic volvulus can lead to repeated episodes of relatively mild ischaemia with the formation of granulation tissue in the submucosa. There is patchy mucosal ulceration and dense fibrosis, often extending into the mesenteric tissues, although the muscularis of the small intestine is relatively spared. A stricture may then form, the histology of which can be difficult to distinguish from ischaemic stricture due to other causes and from Crohn's disease.

Perforation and rupture

Small intestinal perforations in adults may follow ingestion of foreign bodies, peptic or other ulceration, chronic inflammatory bowel disease, thinning and weakening of the bowel wall due to systemic sclerosis [32] or diverticula, or follow obstruction of the bowel lumen from a large number of causes. Meconium ileus is an additional cause in infancy whereas trauma, often of a blunt nature, may produce a single laceration on the anti-mesenteric surface of the ileum in both adults and children [33]. The usual consequence is peritonitis or local abscess formation, and shock is often a concomitant feature. Blast injury can produce multiple perforations of the intestine as the shock wave travels across the air–fluid interfaces present [34].

Small intestinal obstruction

The mechanical causes of small intestinal obstruction are often divided into those situated within the lumen, those within the bowel wall and extramural causes. The last are almost always diseases of the peritoneum and include congenital mesenteric or omental bands, peritonitis and associated peritoneal adhesions [35] and primary or secondary tumours of the peritoneal cavity. Intramural causes include congenital atresias, inflammatory conditions such as Crohn's disease, tuberculosis or drug-induced stenoses, ischaemic strictures, irradiation damage and polypoid or infiltrative neoplasms. They are described in other chapters.

The most common luminal cause of mechanical small intestinal obstruction is a bolus of food, almost always of fruit or vegetable origin [36,37]. Persimmons are the most common offender in America but oranges, peaches, grapefruit, apples, raw figs, mushrooms and coconuts have all been incriminated. Macaroni, sauerkraut, onion and tomato skins, potato skin and peanuts are among the vegetable foods reported to cause obstruction. Predisposing factors include false teeth, previous gastrectomy [38] and intestinal adhesions but inadequate mastication and bolting of large amounts of food are key factors. Bolus obstruction due to food can lead to mucosal ulceration and perforation, with release of food into the submucosa, muscle coats and even the abdominal cavity, to give rise to so-called food granulomas. Abscesses follow perforation of sharp objects, such as undigested peanuts, into the mesenteric attachment of the gut. A variety of food bolus obstruction in neonates is called the milk curd syndrome. In this condition, which usually occurs during week 2 of life in babies fed with artificial milk products, impaction of thick milk curds in the terminal ileum produces acute intestinal obstruction [39].

Ingested therapeutic agents may also give rise to obstruction. Barium sulphate used for radiological imaging is probably the most common luminal blocker but obstruction may result from warfarin-induced haemorrhage into the bowel wall or hormone-related thrombosis of vasculature [40]. Bezoars, concretions formed within the stomach from ingested hairs, vegetables or other materials (see Chapter 16), may also give rise to small intestinal obstruction after fragmentation and, in parts of the world where roundworm (*Ascaris lumbricoides*) infestation is endemic, a mass of worms may form an obstructing bolus [41].

Swallowed foreign bodies are not infrequently the cause of mechanical small intestinal obstruction, especially in children, people with mental health problems and people in prison. The variety of articles involved is vast but among the most common are dentures, bones, pins, coins, screws and nails. The vast majority of swallowed objects that can negotiate the gastro-oesophageal junction will traverse the remainder of the alimentary tract with little difficulty, although potential sites of obstruction are the second part of the duodenum and the terminal ileum. Experimental studies suggest that soft, malleable objects are more dangerous than hard ones [42]. Drug traffickers may use ingested balloons or condoms filled with illicit drugs to avoid detection at customs points. Offenders place themselves in great personal danger, not only from intestinal obstruction, but also from lethal drug overdose following rupture of the balloons [43].

Luminal obstruction of the small intestine may also be of 'endogenous' origin. Two varieties are well described: meconium ileus and gallstone ileus. Meconium ileus almost always occurs in infants with cystic fibrosis (mucoviscidosis), in whom the abnormally viscid mucus secreted into the gut lumen makes meconium tenacious and liable to cause obstruction, notably in the mid- or terminal ileum [44]. The mucin hyperviscosity is due to decreased fluid and increased chloride ion secretion as a result of defective cystic fibrosis transmembrane conductance regulator (CFTR), with modifiers influencing the phenotype. Occasionally, intestinal obstruction develops during fetal life, leading to intrauterine perforation and meconium peritonitis. Intestinal obstruction may also occur in older children or adults with cystic fibrosis. It has been called 'meconium ileus equivalent', and 'distal intestinal obstruction syndrome' (DIOS) predominantly occurs in the ileo-caecal region [45] and appears to be more prevalent with increased longevity following advances in treatment, including lung transplantation [46].

Gallstone ileus, on the other hand, is a disease of adults, in most instances in elderly women [47]. It is said to account for about 1–2% of all cases of adult small intestinal obstruction [48]. Patients have underlying gallbladder disease and the obstructing gallstone, which is almost always >25 mm in diameter, lodges in the terminal ileum. It usually reaches the small intestinal lumen through a cholecystoduodenal fistula, although in rare instances a small stone passing

down the biliary tree may grow within the intestinal lumen (a so-called enterolith) until it reaches obstructing proportions [49]. As multiple gallstones are common in cholelithiasis, it is not infrequent for patients with gallstone ileus to have recurrent attacks of intestinal obstruction unless any additional stones are removed during surgery for the first attack [50].

Intestinal pseudo-obstruction

Although many cases of small intestinal obstruction are caused by some recognisable mechanical obstructing lesion, this is not always so. When no localised lesion is apparent, the name intestinal pseudo-obstruction is given. The functional obstruction is due to a failure of intestinal propulsion, caused by either disorders of intestinal smooth muscle or innervation of the bowel, or by both. Intestinal pseudo-obstruction may be divided into acute and chronic forms.

Acute intestinal pseudo-obstruction (paralytic ileus)

By far the most common variety of small intestinal pseudo-obstruction is so-called paralytic (or adynamic) ileus. This acute, usually self-limiting, condition is typically a complication of peritoneal irritation, from acute peritonitis, trauma or abdominal surgery. Rarer causes are metabolic disturbances (especially hypokalaemia, uraemia, diabetic ketoacidosis and myxoedema), spinal injuries and the use of ganglion-blocking drugs. The clinical picture is one of acute small intestinal obstruction with abdominal distension, vomiting and absent bowel sounds. In most cases the whole of the small intestine is affected and on gross examination it is distended by gas and a watery brown faeculent fluid [51]. The wall is thin and often dusky in appearance.

The aetiology of the smooth muscle paralysis in ileus is poorly understood but is probably multifactorial. There is evidence that post-operative ileus is at least partly related to changes in autonomic nervous function, from either over-stimulation of the splanchnic sympathetic system or damage to cholinergic fibres [52] due to surgical manipulation of the mesentery. More recent research has indicated that mast cell degranulation may contribute to this condition through neuro-immune mechanisms [53,54]. Contributing factors may include electrolyte imbalance and the use of anaesthetic agents. Abnormalities of autonomic function are also important when ileus is associated with acute peritonitis, when toxins absorbed through the inflamed peritoneal membrane and anoxia due to vascular stasis contribute to the smooth muscle dysfunction.

Chronic intestinal pseudo-obstruction

Chronic intestinal pseudo-obstruction manifests clinically by recurrent attacks of nausea, vomiting, abdominal pain and distension, which vary greatly in their frequency, severity and duration [55]. These attacks are the result of acute or subacute functional obstruction of the small intestine but motility studies in the intervening 'asymptomatic' periods usually show an impaired propulsive capacity of the intestinal smooth muscle. In many cases, they also show a more widespread abnormality of motor function of the whole alimentary tract than would be suspected from the clinical features, such that subclinical involvement of the oesophagus, colon and, less frequently, the stomach are quite common. Nevertheless localised functional obstruction in some patients leads to segmental dilatation of one part of the small intestine, resulting in so-called mega-duodenum or mega-jejunum whereas in others it leads to the formation of intestinal diverticula [56].

The abnormality of propulsive action frequently predisposes to overgrowth of colonic-type micro-organisms within the affected small bowel, leading to malabsorption. Sometimes this complication may even produce more clinical effects than the underlying motor disorder. Involvement of the whole gastrointestinal tract is common and sometimes there are similar disorders of motility in other organs, notably the urinary bladder [57]. Malabsorption may also lead to the accumulation of lipofuscin (ceroid) pigment within the smooth muscle coats of the intestine, giving the appearance of the so-called 'brown bowel syndrome' (Figure 19.2), although, with the advent of total parenteral nutrition, this is now rare.

Chronic intestinal pseudo-obstruction may result from a wide variety of disease processes, many of which are neuromuscular in origin (Tables 19.1 and 19.2). The classification of this heterogeneous group of disorders has in the past lacked standardisation, leading to confusion in terminology, in both research literature and diagnostic practice. To resolve these difficulties an international working group has reported a consensus classification of gastrointestinal neuromuscular disorders, based on histopathological phenotypes, termed 'The London Classification'. A version of this classification is listed in Table 19.2. The same working group has also reported comprehensive guidelines for the

Table 19.1 Examples of secondary and systemic causes of chronic small intestinal pseudo-obstruction

Collagen diseases
  Scleroderma
  Dermatomyositis
  Mixed connective tissue disease

Systemic muscle disease
  Myotonic dystrophy
  Muscular dystrophy

Mitochondrial disease

Vasculitis

Amyloidosis

Infective
  Chagas' disease
  Cytomegalovirus
  Dog hookworm
  JC virus

Immunological
  Paraneoplastic
  Crohn's disease
  Increase in mast cells

Metabolic disorders
  Diabetes mellitus
  Hypothyroidism

Drug-induced
  Psychotropic drugs (phenothiazines, tricyclic antidepressants, anti-cholinergic drugs)
  Anti-neoplastic drugs (vinca alkaloids, daunorubicin)
  Warfarin
  Hormones [40]

handling and histopathological examination of all specimen types, from mucosal biopsies to resection specimens, from patients with gastrointestinal motility disorders [58]. In addition to routine stains, a range of special stains should be carried out, including stains to look for amyloid,

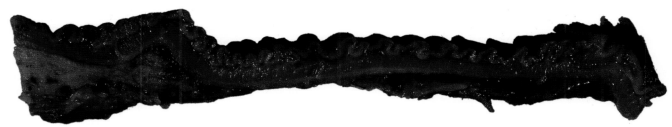

Figure 19.2 Brown bowel syndrome: a segment of involved small intestine cut longitudinally. Note the striking tan/brown colour of the muscularis propria, compared to its normal grey colour.

Table 19.2 Primary conditions associated with gastrointestinal motility disorders including intestinal pseudo-obstruction

Neuropathies

Absent neurons

Aganglionosis
  Decreased numbers of neurons

Hypoganglionosis

Increased numbers of neurons
  Ganglio-neuromatosis
  Intestinal neuronal dysplasia

Degenerative neuropathy

Inflammatory neuropathies
  Lymphocytic ganglionitis
  Eosinophilic ganglionitis
  Granulomatous neuropathy

Abnormal content in neurons
  Intraneuronal nuclear inclusions

Abnormal neurochemical coding

Relative immaturity of neurons

Abnormal enteric glia

Increased numbers of enteric glia

Myopathies

Muscularis propria malformations

Muscle cell degeneration
  Degenerative leiomyopathy
  Inflammatory leiomyopathy
    Lymphocytic leiomyositis
    Eosinophilic leiomyositis

Muscle hyperplasia / hypertrophy

Muscularis mucosae hyperplasia

Abnormal content in myocytes
  Filament protein abnormalities
    α-Actin myopathy
    Desmin myopathy

Inclusion bodies
  Polyglucosan bodies
  Amphophilic
  Mega-mitochondria

Abnormal supportive tissue
  Atrophic desmosis

Interstitial cell of Cajal (ICC) abnormalities (enteric mesenchymopathy)
  Abnormal ICC networks

Adapted based on Knowles et al. [58].

smooth muscle actin and desmin abnormalities, and polyglucosan bodies [58].

Neurological disorders

Developmental abnormalities of small intestinal innervation are similar to those in the large intestine (see 'Hirschsprung's disease', Chapter 33) and effectively involve an abnormality in the number of neurons. Aganglionosis of the small intestine, which may rarely extend proximally up to the duodenum, is usually associated with colonic involvement [59] whereas hyperganglionosis of the small intestine, characterised by hyperplasia of the submucosal and myenteric plexuses with formation of giant ganglia, can be seen in ganglio-neuromatosis [60]. Both conditions may present with functional small intestinal obstruction, usually in the neonatal period. Intestinal neuronal dysplasia is a more disputed entity but can also be associated with pseudo-obstruction [61].

Familial visceral neuropathies may be inherited as either autosomal dominant [62] or autosomal recessive [63] traits. Although genetic disorders, they rarely present with intestinal symptoms before adult life. The dominant form affects the small intestine almost exclusively and, on histological examination, there is degeneration and loss of argyrophilic neurons in plexuses. Denervation of smooth muscle leads to uncoordinated peristalsis and there may be work hypertrophy of smooth muscle coats [62]. Autosomal recessive visceral neuropathy usually affects the alimentary tract in a more widespread form and frequently has extra-intestinal manifestations [56]. A number of varieties have been described, including one that is associated with abnormalities of the central and peripheral nervous systems, and characterised by the presence of intranuclear eosinophilic inclusions within degenerating neurons [63], and another that is associated with filamin mutations [64]. Mitochondrial disease can affect ganglion cells of both the myenteric plexus and smooth muscle [65]. Isolated cases of chronic intestinal pseudo-obstruction with the features of neuronal degeneration may or may not represent sporadic cases with an underlying genetic cause.

Inflammatory neuropathies can occur with or without neuronal loss. Quantitation of lymphocytic infiltration in and around ganglia can be difficult but, in general, the presence of *any* lymphocyte *within* a ganglion and/or more than five lymphocytes around a ganglion is sufficient for a diagnosis of ganglionitis [58]. Many inflammatory neuropathies are infective in origin and have been reported secondary to Chagas' disease [67] and, rarely, as a result of cytomegalovirus [68] and JC virus [69] infection. Inflammatory neuropathy can also result from autoimmune reactions caused by neoplasms such as small cell carcinoma of the lung [56,70–72]. It has also been reported in association with cystic fibrosis [46]. Granulomatous visceral neuropathy, possibly autoimmune in nature, has been described in a patient with non-small cell bronchial carcinoma [73]. When eosinophilic plexitis is present, and also myositis, it is important to investigate the possibility of parasitic infestation, including unusual agents such as dog hookworm [74].

Other causes of damage to small intestinal innervation include drugs and metabolic disease [40,55,56,66]. Drug-induced visceral neuropathy, though uncommon, is a recognised side effect of tricyclic antidepressants, phenothiazines, anticholinergic drugs and the vinca alkaloids [40, 56]. Metabolic neuropathies can occur secondary to amyloidosis, diabetes mellitus and hypothyroidism [55]. Axonal necrosis of enteric nerves has also been reported in Crohn's disease [75]. Indeed, plexitis in Crohn's disease has been associated with early disease recurrence when it is present at the resection margin of an excision specimen [76].

Disorders of intestinal smooth muscle

Developmental disorders of smooth muscle leading to chronic intestinal pseudo-obstruction chiefly involve additional or absent muscle layers [77]. These include the focal absence of one or both layers of the muscularis propria, the segmental fusion of muscle layers – most commonly fusion of the muscularis mucosae with the two layers of the muscularis propria resulting in a single muscle band – and the presence of additional muscle layers, usually in the circular layer of the muscularis propria. Additional muscle layers should be distinguished from reactive changes which may result in smooth muscle being present in the submucosa and subserosa, e.g. in chronic inflammatory diseases such as Crohn's disease, but this rarely forms discrete layers and is generally associated with a degree of fibrosis.

Familial and sporadic forms of visceral myopathy are recognised, the pathological features of which are similar in both types. Familial visceral myopathy may be inherited as both autosomal dominant and autosomal recessive traits [78–80]. The involvement may be wider than the gut, with the term 'hollow visceral myopathy' being used when both bladder and bowel are involved. Generally speaking, the dominant form of the disease is often localised to the duodenum (although the oesophagus, colon and urinary bladder are also affected), whereas a more severe and widespread involvement of the small intestine is usual in the recessive type, sometimes with the development of intestinal diverticulosis [80]. In rare autosomal recessive variants extra-intestinal involvement has included skeletal myopathy and ophthalmoplegia [80,81]. Hollow visceral myopathy sometimes occurs in familial cases with other characteristic phenotypic features; myopathy with au-

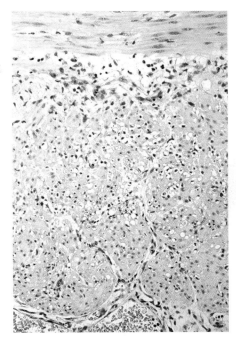

Figure 19.3 Idiopathic hollow visceral myopathy: section of the ileal muscularis propria from a patient with small intestinal pseudo-obstruction. The myocytes of the longitudinal muscle layer (lower three-quarters of field) are vacuolated.

tophagic activity and pink blush myopathy with nuclear crowding are rare variants.

By light microscopy, the pathological features of visceral myopathy reflect degenerative changes and include varying degrees of myofibre atrophy and vacuolar degeneration (Figure 19.3). This is most marked in the muscularis propria but sometimes is seen in the muscularis mucosae, with progressive replacement by fibrosis (Figure 19.4) [56,66,70,78,79]. In some cases, changes are not present on light microscopy and abnormalities are visible only on electron microscopy. Ultrastructural changes include myocyte damage with perinuclear vacuolation, disorientation and dissolution of myofilaments, electron lucency of myocyte cytoplasm and swelling of mitochondria. Variation in the size and staining properties of residual myocytes may be present. The myenteric plexus is, however, normal on both light and electron microscopy. The fundamental smooth muscle abnormality in most cases of visceral myopathy is unknown and, histologically, many of these cases are ill-defined [78]. However, in one sporadic case, in which there was also external ophthalmoplegia, skeletal myopathy and peripheral neuropathy, a generalised defect of mitochondrial cytochrome C oxidase was established [65].

Inflammatory myopathies may be autoimmune in origin [82] or result from infection. In autoimmune myopathy, the

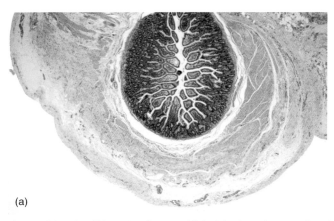

(a)

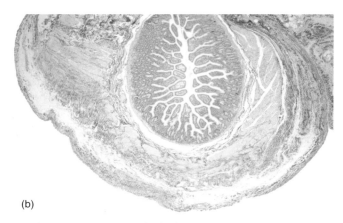

(b)

Figure 19.4 Small intestine from a child with visceral myopathy: the muscularis propria, particularly the longitudinal layer, shows patchy thinning and replacement by pale fibrous tissue, (a) pale on haematoxylin and eosin stain and (b) red in van Gieson's stain.

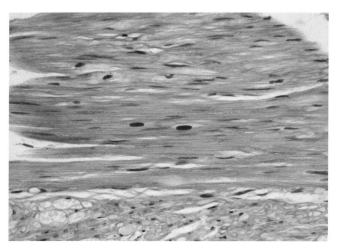

Figure 19.5 Polyglucosan body myopathy: section of muscularis propria showing two polyglucosan bodies. The inclusions are smooth surfaced, oval shaped and stain positively with periodic acid–Schiff.

main pathological abnormality is dense T-cell infiltration of the muscularis propria with or without associated fibrosis. A single case of myopathy due to Epstein–Barr virus infection has been reported [83], as has parasite-associated eosinophilic leiomyositis [76]. Large inflammatory infiltrates are easily identified on routine stains but immunohistochemistry may be required for quantitative assessment of more modest numbers of lymphocytes or for defining lymphocyte subsets.

Myopathies resulting from abnormalities of cytoskeletal filament proteins have been described. These include desmin myopathy, which is usually, but not always, associated with skeletal muscle problems and α-actin deficiency, which may be a secondary response to insult [84] rather than a primary feature. Inclusion bodies may be present in myocytes of the muscularis propria, including two

specific forms: polyglucosan bodies [85], only evident on periodic acid–Schiff staining (Figure 19.5), and amphophilic bodies [86], the latter usually associated with autonomic neuropathy.

So-called 'secondary' smooth muscle disorders leading to chronic intestinal pseudo-obstruction include those associated with connective tissue diseases, especially systemic sclerosis and dermatomyositis [87], polymyositis [88], myotonic dystrophy, desmin myopathy, progressive muscular dystrophy [89] and muscle dysfunction from amyloid infiltration [90]. Although the microscopic appearances of the last are characteristic, the changes in the other conditions are often far from distinct and may be difficult to distinguish from those of primary visceral myopathy. In such cases, clinico-pathological correlation is paramount.

References

1. Gough M. Multiple intussusception and intestinal perforation due to a bezoar. *Br J Surg* 1960;**48**:222.
2. MacMahon B. Data on the etiology of acute intussusception in childhood. *Am J Hum Genet* 1955;**7**:430.
3. Tan N, Teoh YL, Phua KB, et al. An update of paediatric intussusception incidence in Singapore:1997–2007, 11 years of intussusception surveillance. *Ann Acad Med Singapore* 2009;**38**:690.
4. Smith IS, Gillespie C. Adult intussusception in Glasgow. *Br J Surg* 1968;**55**:925.
5. Ein SH. Leading points in childhood intussusception. *J Pediatr Surg* 1976;**11**:209.
6. Wayne E, Campbell J, Burrington J, Davis W. Management of 344 children with intussusception. *Radiology* 1973;**107**:597.
7. Gardner PS, Knox EG, Court SDM, Green CA. Virus infection and intussusception in childhood. *BMJ* 1962;**2**:697.
8. Nicholas JL, Ingrand D, Fortier B, Briscout F. A one year virological survey of acute intussusception in childhood. *J Med Virol* 1982;**9**:267.
9. Knox EC, Court SDM, Gardner PS. Aetiology of intussusception in children. *BMJ* 1962;**2**:692.
10. Abel R, Keen CE, Bingham JB, et al. Heterotopic pancreas as lead point in intussusception: new variant of vitellointestinal tract malformation. *Pediatr Dev Pathol* 1999;**2**:367.

11. Holsclaw D, Rocmans C, Shwachman H. Intussusception in patients with cystic fibrosis. *Pediatrics* 1971;**48**:51.

12. Cornes JS, Dawson IMP. Papillary lymphoid hyperplasia at the ileocaecal valve as a cause of acute intussusception in infancy. *Arch Dis Child* 1963;**38**:89.

13. Burke M. Intussusception in adults. *Ann R Coll Surg Engl* 1977; **59**:150.

14. Marinis A, Yiallourou A, Samanides L, et al. Intussusception of the bowel in adults: a review. *World J Gastroenterol* 2009;**15**:407.

15. Fawaz F, Hill GJ. Adult intussusception due to metastatic tumors. *South Med J* 1983;**76**:522.

16. Chia AY, Chia JK. Intestinal intussusception in adults due to acute enterovirus infection. *J Clin Pathol* 2009;**62**:1026.

17. Riccabono XJ, Haskins RM. Gastroduodenal intussusception: report of 2 cases. *Gastroenterology* 1970;**38**:995.

18. Mock CJ, Moock HE Jr. Strangulated internal hernia associated with trauma. *Arch Surg* 1958;**77**:881.

19. Rooney JA, Carroll JP, Keeley JL. Internal hernias due to defects in the meso-appendix and mesentery of small bowel, and probable Ivemark syndrome. *Ann Surg* 1963;**157**:254.

20. Willwerth BM, Zollinger RM, Izant R. Congenital mesocolic (paraduodenal) hernia. Embryological basis of repair. *Am J Surg* 1974;**128**:358.

21. Cook JL. Bowel herniation through the foramen of Winslow. *Am Surg* 1970;**36**:241.

22. Hansmann GH, Morton SA. Intraabdominal hernia. Report of a case and review of the literature. *Arch Surg* 1939;**39**:973.

23. Janin Y, Stone AM, Wise I. Mesenteric hernia. *Surg Gynecol Obstet* 1980;**150**:747.

24. Stewart JOR. Transepiploic hernia. *Br J Surg* 1962;**49**:649.

25. Kerr WG, Kirkaldy-Willis WH. Volvulus of the small intestine. *BMJ* 1946;**i**:799.

26. Duke JH, Yar MS. Primary small bowel volvulus. *Arch Surg* 1977;**112**:685.

27. Saidi F. The high incidence of intestinal volvulus in Iran. *Gut* 1969;**10**:838.

28. Atamanalp SS, Oren D, Başoğlu M, et al. Ileosigmoidal knotting: outcome in 63 patients. *Dis Colon Rectum* 2004;**47**:906.

29. Murphy FL, Sparnon AL. Long-term complications following intestinal malrotation and the Ladd's procedure: a 15 year review. *Pediatr Surg Int* 2006;**22**:326.

30. Ruiz-Tovar J, Morales V, Sanjuanbenito A, Lobo E, Martinez-Molina E. Volvulus of the small bowel in adults. *Am Surg* 2009; **75**:1179.

31. Bruzoni M, Sudan DL, Cusick RA, Thompson JS. Comparison of short bowel syndrome acquired early in life and during adolescence. *Transplantation.* 2008;**86**:63.

32. Ebert EC, Ruggiero FM, Seibold JR. Intestinal perforation. A common complication of scleroderma. *Dig Dis Sci* 1997;**42**:549.

33. Evans JP. Traumatic rupture of the ileum. *Br J Surg* 1973;**60**:119.

34. Wani I, Parray FQ, Sheikh T, et al. Spectrum of abdominal organ injury in a primary blast type. *World J Emerg Surg* 2009;**21**(4):46.

35. Ellis H, Moran BJ, Thompson JN, et al. Adhesion-related hospital readmissions after abdominal and pelvic surgery: a retrospective cohort study. *Lancet* 1999;**353**:1476.

36. Norberg PB. Food as a cause of intestinal obstruction. *Am J Surg* 1962;**104**:444.

37. Connelly HJ, Del Carmen BV. Intestinal obstruction due to food. *Am Surg* 1969;**35**:820.

38. Koott H, Urca H. Intestinal obstruction after partial gastrectomy due to orange pith. *Arch Surg* 1970;**100**:79.

39. Konvolinka CW, Frederick J. Milk curd syndrome in neonates. *J Pediatr Surg* 1989;**24**:497.

40. George CF. Drugs causing intestinal obstruction: a review. *J R Soc Med* 1980;**73**:200.

41. Hhekwaba EN. Intestinal ascariasis and the acute abdomen in the tropics. *J R Coll Surg Edinb* 1980;**25**:452.

42. Harjola P-T, Scheinin TM. Experimental observations on intestinal obstruction due to foreign bodies. *Acta Chir Scand* 1963; **126**:144.

43. McCarroon MM, Wood JO. The cocaine body packer syndrome. *Diagnosis* and *treatment. JAMA* 1983;**250**:1417.

44. Holsclaw OS, Eckstein HB, Nixon HH. Meconium ileus: a 20-year review of 109 cases. *Am J Dis Child* 1965;**109**:101.

45. Houwen RH, van der Doef HP, Sermet I, et al. Defining DIOS and constipation in cystic fibrosis with a multicentre study on the incidence, characteristics, and treatment of DIOS. *J Pediatr Gastroenterol Nutr* 2010;**50**:38.

46. Smith VV, Schäppi MG, Bisset WM, et al.. Lymphocytic leiomyositis and myenteric ganglionitis are intrinsic features of cystic fibrosis: studies in distal intestinal obstruction syndrome and meconium ileus. *J Pediatr Gastroenterol Nutr* 2009;**49**:42.

47. Brockis JC, Gilbert MC. Intestinal obstruction by gall stones. A record of 179 cases. *Br J Surg* 1957;**44**:461.

48. Clavien PA, Richon J, Burgan S, Rohner A. Gallstone ileus. *Br J Surg* 1990;**77**:737.

49. Newman JH. A case of gall-stone ileus in the absence of a biliary-enteric fistula. *Br J Surg* 1972;**59**:573.

50. Reisner RM, Cohen JR. Gallstone ileus: a review of 1001 reported cases. *Am Surg* 1994;**60**:441.

51. Batke M, Cappell MS. Adynamic ileus and acute colonic pseudo-obstruction. *Med Clin North Am* 2008;**92**:649, ix.

52. Davison JS. Selective damage to cholinergic nerves: possible cause of postoperative ileus. *Lancet* 1979;**i**:1288.

53. The FO, Bennink RJ, Ankum WM, et al. Intestinal handling-induced mast cell activation and inflammation in human postoperative ileus. *Gut* 2008;**57**:33.

54. Boeckxstaens GE, de Jonge WJ. Neuroimmune mechanisms in postoperative ileus. *Gut* 2009;**58**:1300.

55. Faulk DL, Anuras S, Christensen J. Chronic intestinal pseudo-obstruction. *Gastroenterology* 1978;**74**:922.

56. Krishnamurthy S, Schuffler MD. Pathology of neuromuscular disorders of the small intestine and colon. *Gastroenterology* 1987;**93**:610.

57. Mann SD, Debinski HS, Kamm MA. Clinical characteristics of chronic idiopathic intestinal pseudo-obstruction in adults. *Gut* 1997;**41**:675.

58. Knowles CH, De Giorgio R, Kapur RP, et al. Gastrointestinal neuromuscular pathology: guidelines for histological techniques and reporting on behalf of the Gastro 2009 International Working Group. *Acta Neuropathol* 2009;**118**:271.

59. Rudin C, Jenny P, Ohnacker H, Heitz PU. Absence of the enteric nervous system in the newborn: presentation of three patients and review of the literature. *J Pediatr Surg* 1986;**21**:313.

60. Scharli AF, Meier-Ruge W. Localized and disseminated forms of neuronal intestinal dysplasia mimicking Hirschsprung's disease. *J Pediatr Surg* 1981;**16**:835.

61. Martucciello G, Torre M, Pini Prato A, et al Associated anomalies in intestinal neuronal dysplasia. *J Pediatr Surg* 2002;**37**: 219.

62. Mayer EA, Schuffler MD, Rotter JI, Hanna P, Mogard M. Familial visceral neuropathy with autosomal dominant transmission. *Gastroenterology* 1986;**91**:1528.

63. Schuffler MD, Bird TO, Sumi SM, Cook A. A familial neuronal disease presenting as intestinal pseudo-obstruction. *Gastroenterology* 1978;**75**:889.

64. Gargiulo A, Auricchio R, Barone MV, et al. Filamin A is mutated in X-linked chronic idiopathic intestinal pseudo-obstruction with central nervous system involvement. *Am J Hum Genet* 2007;**80**:751.

65. Giordano C, Sebastiani M, De Giorgio R, et al. Gastrointestinal dysmotility in mitochondrial neurogastrointestinal encephalomyopathy is caused by mitochondrial DNA depletion. *Am J Pathol* 2008;**173**:1120.

66. Smith B. The neuropathology of pseudo-obstruction of the intestine. *Scand J Gastroenterol* 1982;**17**(suppl 71):103.

67. Martins-Campos JV, Tafuri WL. Chagas' enteropathy. *Gut* 1973;**14**:910.

68. Sonsino F, Mouy R, Foucaud P, et al. Intestinal pseudo-obstruction related to cytomegalovirus infection of myenteric plexus. *N Engl J Med* 1984;**311**:196.

69. Selgrad M, De Giorgio R, Fini L, et al. JC virus infects the enteric glia of patients with chronic idiopathic intestinal pseudo-obstruction. *Gut* 2009;**58**:25.

70. Roberts PF, Stebbings WS, Kennedy HJ. Granulomatous visceral neuropathy of the colon with non-small cell lung carcinoma. *Histopathology* 1997;**30**:588.

71. Schuffler MD, Baird HW, Fleming CR, et al. Intestinal pseudo-obstruction as the presenting manifestation of small cell carcinoma of the lung: a paraneoplastic neuropathy of the gastrointestinal tract. *Arch Intern Med* 1983;**98**:129.

72. Bell CE Jr, Seetharam S. Identification of the Schwann cell as a peripheral nervous system cell possessing a differentiation antigen expressed by a human lung tumor. *J Immunol* 1977;**118**:826.

73. Lindberg G, Törnblom H, Iwarzon M, et al. Full thickness biopsy findings in chronic intestinal pseudo-obstruction and enteric dysmotility. *Gut* 2009;**58**:1084.

74. Walker NI, Croese J, Clouston AD, Parry M, Loukas A, Prociv P. Eosinophilic enteritis in northeastern Australia. Pathology, association with *Ancylostoma caninum*, and implications. *Am J Surg Pathol* 1995;**19**:328.

75. Dvorak AM, Silen W. Differentiation between Crohn's disease and other inflammatory conditions by electron microscopy. *Ann Surg* 1985;**201**:53.

76. Sokol H, Polin V, Lavergne-Slove A, et al. Plexitis as a predictive factor of early postoperative clinical recurrence in Crohn's disease. *Gut* 2009;**58**:1218.

77. Kapur RP, Correa H. Architectural malformation of the muscularis propria as a cause for intestinal pseudo-obstruction: two cases and a review of the literature. *Pediatr Dev Pathol* 2009;**12**:156.

78. Mitros FA, Schuffler MD, Teja K, Aneiras S. Pathologic features of familial visceral myopathy. *Hum Pathol* 1982;**13**:825.

79. Alstead EM, Murphy MN, Flanagan AM, Bishop AE, Hodgson HJF. Familial autonomic visceral myopathy, with degeneration of the muscularis mucosae. *J Clin Pathol* 1988;**41**:424.

80. Anuras S, Mitros FA, Nowak TV, et al. A familial visceral myopathy with external ophthalmoplegia and autosomal recessive transmission. *Gastroenterology* 1983;**84**:346.

81. Ionasescu VV, Thompson HS, Aschenbrener C, Aneuras S. Late onset oculogastrointestinal muscular dystrophy. *Am J Med Genet* 1984;**18**:781.

82. Ruuska TH, Karikoski R, Smith VV, Milla PJ. Acquired myopathic pseudo-obstruction may be due to auto-immune enteric leiomyositis. *Gastroenterology* 2002;**122**:1133.

83. Debinski HS, Kamm MA, Talbot IC, et al. DNA viruses in the pathogenesis of sporadic chronic idiopathic intestinal pseudo-obstruction. *Gut* 1997;**41**:100.

84. Knowles CH, Silk DBA, Darzi A, et al. Deranged smooth muscle alpha-actin: a biomarker of intestinal pseudo-obstruction. A controlled multinational case series. *Gut* 2004;**53**:1583.

85. Knowles CH, Nickols CD, Feakins R, Martin JE. A systematic analysis of polyglucosan bodies in the human gastrointestinal tract in health and disease. *Acta Neuropathol* 2003;**105**:410.

86. Knowles CH, Nickols CD, Scott SM, et al. Secondary smooth muscle degeneration with inclusion bodies in slow transit constipation. *J Pathol* 2001;**193**:390.

87. Schuffler MD, Beegle RG. Progressive systemic sclerosis of the gastrointestinal tract and hereditary, hollow visceral myopathy: two distinguishable disorders of intestinal smooth muscle. *Gastroenterology* 1979;**77**:664.

88. Boardman P, Nolan DJ. Case report: Small intestinal pseudo-obstruction: an unusual manifestation of polymyositis. *Clin Radiol* 1998;**53**:706.

89. Nowak TV, Ionasescu V, Anuras S. Gastrointestinal manifestations of the muscular dystrophies. *Gastroenterology* 1982;**82**:800.

90. Tada S, Iida M, Yao T, Kitamoto T, Fujishima M. Intestinal pseudo-obstruction in patients with amyloidosis: clinicopathologic differences between chemical types of amyloid protein [see comments]. *Gut* 1993;**34**:1412.

20

Inflammatory disorders of the small intestine

Karel Geboes

University Hospital and Medical School KU Leuven, Leuven, Belgium

Inflammatory pathology of the small bowel is relatively common. Infections are the major cause whereas chronic inflammatory bowel diseases (CIBD) and other conditions are less frequent. Worldwide, enteric infections rank third among all causes of disease burden, being responsible for some 2 million deaths per year, mostly young children in developing countries. The main infectious agents include a variety of viruses and bacterial agents [1]. Infections usually present as acute disease. Chronic enteritis is less common and most notably caused by chronic infections such as tuberculosis, CIBD and drugs. Histology is not the best method for the diagnosis of enteric infections, because stool culture and stool examination have a higher diagnostic yield. Most acute enteritides are non-specific histologically and most patients recover without ever needing a biopsy. Histology is, however, important for chronic conditions and severe acute disease. As endoscopy is more frequently performed, pathologists are more likely to receive small intestinal samples [2].

Inflammation due to identifiable micro-organisms

Viral gastroenteritis

Acute gastroenteritis is a major cause of morbidity and mortality, particularly for children in the developing world. Viruses play a leading part in the aetiology [1,3]. A study of more than 30 000 patients hospitalised for diarrhoea in the USA found that less than 6% had an identified bacterial pathogen, leaving 94% in the diagnostic void. This void was substantially filled in by the introduction of reverse transcription-coupled polymerase chain reaction (rtPCR) for enteric viral pathogens. Among the viruses, rotaviruses remain the leading cause of diarrhoeal disease in the world, whereas human caliciviruses (HuCVs) are the cause of most gastroenteritis outbreaks in industrialised nations. In all age groups, viral gastroenteritis is characteristically associated with outbreaks and epidemics, although isolated cases are also well recognised. The relationship between viral enteritis and the acquired immune deficiency syndrome (AIDS) is less clear than for bacteria and other opportunistic infections. Nevertheless evidence of viral infection can be detected in up to 10% of AIDS patients: the relationship between such viral presence and the production of symptoms such as diarrhoea is less certain [4].

Rotaviruses, so called because of their wheel-like morphology on electron microscopic examination, are the most common cause of infective gastroenteritis in young children in both industrialised and developing countries, but routine immunisation, introduced since 2006, is substantially reducing the number of cases [5]. Rotavirus is a lytic virus that causes diarrhoea primarily by destruction of intestinal villous epithelial cells. Virtually all children have been infected by the time they reach 2–3 years of age. Interestingly, neonates and adults are relatively immune from infection and usually have only mild disease whereas children up to the age of 2 years have more pronounced symptoms. Most symptomatic episodes occur between 7 and 15 months. Large outbreaks and epidemics are well recognised [6].

The pathology of rotavirus infection is not very specific. In a study of 40 infants with acute rotavirus gastroenteritis, only two had abnormal duodenal biopsies [7]. The features include variable shortening of villi, a moderate round cell infiltrate in the lamina propria and elongation of crypts. Early in the infection, supranuclear vacuolation and shedding of enterocytes from the apical portion of the villi may be observed. On routine staining the supranuclear cytoplasmic vacuolation is similar to that seen in abetalipoproteinaemia (and occasionally in juvenile nutritional megaloblastic anaemia) but the distribution of the affected cells is more discontinuous. Lesions are often patchy in nature [8]. Virus particles, demonstrable by electron microscopy, are present in the villi and crypts. Infection with rotavirus may increase the susceptibility of the intestine to other pathogens. In small bowel transplants, infection may mimic acute rejection. In infection, the lamina propria infiltrate looks 'top heavy' or denser towards the lumen. Rotavirus infections are not limited to the gastrointestinal tract and routinely extend beyond the intestine to the blood, and have the potential to cause non-intestinal disease.

Adenoviruses are most commonly associated with respiratory infection but they also cause acute diarrhoea, especially in children [9]. These DNA viruses can also be detected in the stools of asymptomatic children. For the histopathologist, the most important associations are with lymphoid hyperplasia in the terminal ileum and subsequent intussusception in infants [10] and the occurrence of the infection in AIDS diarrhoea and transplants. Infection is associated with mild mixed inflammation and a slight increase in crypt cell apoptosis. A tip-off that adenovirus infection is present is the loss of polarity of surface epithelial cells with dystrophic goblet cells. These goblet cells often contain diagnostic nuclear inclusions, which are readily demonstrable by immunohistochemical techniques (Figure 20.1) [11].

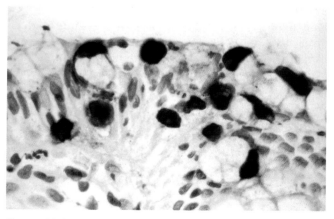

Figure 20.1 Immunohistochemistry demonstrating adenovirus infection in the small intestinal mucosa.

Human caliciviruses, previously called small round structured viruses (SRSVs), are a common cause of mild gastroenteritis in the general population, often after the ingestion of contaminated water and food [12], particularly shellfish [13]. The Norwalk and Hawaii viruses are perhaps the best known members of this family but several others have been described [14–16]. They are particularly associated with outbreaks of diarrhoea in hospitals and residential facilities for elderly people. In one study in the UK, 76% of the total number of infections occurred in these institutions [17]. Many of these viruses are also important causes of travellers' diarrhoea [18] and outbreaks of gastroenteritis in children and infants [19]. In the last several years many outbreaks have occurred on cruise ships, where the combination of buffet dining and close quarters leads to rapid spread of the virus. The disease presents with self-limiting diarrhoea, often accompanied by vomiting and abdominal pain. Histological changes include villous broadening, blunting and irregularity and vacuolation of the surface enterocytes. The villous changes induce a reduction of the surface area by almost 50%. In addition a reactive disarray of surface epithelial cells can be seen. Surface and glandular epithelial cell apoptosis and proliferation of glandular cells are increased. Expression of the tight junctional proteins, occludin, claudin-4 and claudin-5, is reduced. Intra-epithelial lymphocytes are increased (to 60 per 100 enterocytes). In the lamina propria polymorphonuclear and mononuclear cells are increased and correlate with symptomatic illness. In paediatric recipients of small intestinal transplants, HuCVs can produce a prolonged diarrhoeal illness and there is considerable histological overlap between rejection and HuCV infection, as both feature apoptosis [20].

The Picornaviruses (named because they are small and of RNA type) incorporate the Enteroviruses (including polio virus, Coxsackievirus A and B, and echovirus), Astroviruses and Coronaviruses. Enteroviruses are among the first viral agents suggested to cause non-bacterial gastroenteritis in humans. They can cause severe gastroenteritis in immunocompromised patients but they may also be found in asymptomatic carriers. They have been detected, by immunohistochemistry, in the epithelium and lamina propria of the small intestine of patients with type 1 diabetes [21]. Astroviruses are associated with gastroenteritis in children but produce only mild symptoms in adults [22]. Although known as respiratory pathogens, severe acute respiratory syndrome (SARS) and its sister coronaviruses can cause enteric symptoms. The four major serologically distinct groups of Coronaviruses [23] are capable of causing a variety of diseases including gastroenteritis in the tropics and Asia but rarely in Europe. They have been associated with necrotising enterocolitis in infants. Other classically non-enteric viruses such as influenza may also have enteric effects.

Cytomegalovirus in the small intestine

Cytomegalovirus (CMV), a DNA virus, is a member of the herpesvirus family. Approximately 50% of the adult population has acquired CMV antibodies by the fourth decade of life [24]. Persistence of CMV is observed in nasal mucosa, trachea, thyroid, liver and intestine [25]. CMV infection of the gastrointestinal tract is most often seen in patients with AIDS, those who have received a transplant, those with CIBD and in patients receiving immunosuppressive therapy (Figure 20.2) [26]. Primary CMV infection of the small intestine in immunocompetent individuals is rare. It is usually asymptomatic but it can produce non-specific symptoms similar to many acute viral illnesses. It can also cause more serious lesions such as gastrointestinal bleeding and even perforation (probably due to ischaemia) [27]. In the colon, it is seen more often in immunocompetent hosts (although this is still rare), especially when associated with ulcerative colitis [28].

Experimental and clinical data suggest that latent CMV infection can alter mucosal immunity and may be responsible for exacerbation of inflammatory bowel disease activity. Tumour necrosis factor (TNF)-α may be a contributing factor. There is still some doubt as to the virus's primary pathogenicity and it may well be that it is almost always an opportunistic infection, especially involving ulcers and other pathological situations where granulation tissue is a prominent feature. The histological diagnosis depends on recognising the characteristic intranuclear inclusions (Figure 20.2): these are most commonly seen in endothelial cells within small capillary-type blood vessels [29]. They may also be seen in histiocytes and, less commonly, in epithelial cells. When epithelial inclusions are present, Brunner's glands are a common place to find them.

In the small bowel, CMV infection is often evident in otherwise non-specific ulcers and, occasionally, in areas of perforation. (Figure 20.3) [26,30]. Whether it is the primary pathogen in this situation is uncertain [31]. In the context of profound immunosuppression, CMV infection often coexists with other pathogens (Figure 20.2), especially atypical mycobacterial infection, cryptosporidiosis and giardiasis. In such situations, the CMV changes may be striking, often with evidence of a vasculitis [32].

Epstein–Barr virus (EBV), another member of the herpesvirus family, can also induce enteritis with multiple ulcers. This has been reported in the ileum after stem cell transplantation. EBV-positive cells can be detected, usually inflammatory cells. They may surround and involve the glandular epithelium forming lympho-epithelial-like lesions [33]. EBV may also promote opportunistic infections in patients with primary X-linked immunodeficiencies.

HIV and AIDS in the small intestine

Chronic diarrhoea remains a problem in AIDS, notwithstanding the success of antiviral therapy (highly active antiretroviral therapy, HAART) in controlling the disease and its complications [34]. There is now increasing evidence that infection by the virus itself causes both functional and morphological abnormalities in the small bowel, outside the numerous opportunistic infections that complicate the

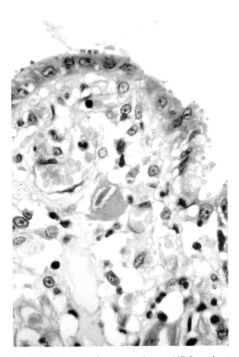

Figure 20.2 Small intestinal mucosa in an AIDS patients. A classic cytomegalovirus inclusion is present centrally whereas the epithelial surface demonstrates innumerable adherent cryptosporidia.

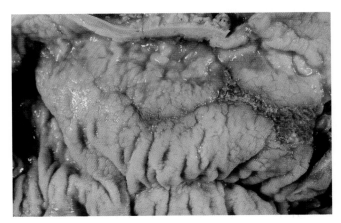

Figure 20.3 Ulceration in cytomegalovirus enteritis: in patients with immune suppression, the ulcers can become very large.

disease [35–37]. The small bowel mucosa, whether in duodenal, jejunal or ileal biopsies, shows various morphological abnormalities, from complete normality to varying chronic inflammation in the lamina propria and partial villous atrophy. Both crypt hyperplastic [38] and crypt hypoplastic atrophy patterns have been described [36]. Crypt stem and transit cell hyperproliferation have been associated with the villous atrophy [37]. Furthermore, HIV antigens and RNA are readily demonstrated in lamina propria inflammatory cells, histiocytes and intra-epithelial lymphocytes (IELs) [39].

Enhanced apoptosis is a characteristic feature of HIV enteropathy. Such increased apoptotic activity is often closely associated with IELs and is typically prominent in crypt bases [40]. The features are similar to those seen in graft-versus-host disease, suggesting an early phase of cell-mediated immunity. Epithelial cells usually appear morphologically and morphometrically normal, despite the villous atrophy and inflammatory changes [35,37]. However there are functional abnormalities: e.g. β-glucosidase activity is greatly reduced, indicating a profound functional immaturity in epithelial cells. The powerful effect of combination therapy in AIDS on gastrointestinal symptoms and on morphological, immunological and virological abnormalities, in terms of decreased apoptotic activity, reduced viral RNA load and raised intraluminal CD4 counts, suggests that the intestinal dysfunction seen in AIDS could well be a direct result of HIV infection [41].

Opportunistic infection of the small intestine has been extremely common in the small bowel in AIDS. Now histopathologists are called upon less often than previously to diagnose such opportunistic infections. This may relate to enhanced detection of these diseases by microbiological techniques but also because of a steady decline in the prevalence of these infections due to the success of combination therapy in AIDS [34,42]. Indeed, the effect of HAART has seen a marked decrease in opportunistic infection in AIDS [43,44].

Nevertheless, infectious diarrhoea remains a considerable problem in HIV/AIDS and histopathological assessment of small bowel biopsies still provides valuable information. Viral, bacterial and protozoal infections are particularly common in AIDS and the pathologist must always be alert to the potential for multiple infections (see Figure 20.2) [20,45]. We have seen cases with no less than six separate infections, including Kaposi's sarcoma and systemic *Pneumocystis jiroveci* infection in a single section from a small intestinal resection specimen. Although the individual infections are more comprehensively covered elsewhere in this chapter, because almost all of them also occur outside AIDS, it is appropriate to outline the infections likely to be detected histopathologically in AIDS.

Chronic diarrhoea in AIDS is most likely to be caused by cryptosporidiosis whereas microsporidiosis, CMV, adeno-virus infection and giardiasis are also common [20,46]. It is important to emphasise that the spectrum of infections may be very different in tropical countries, with their very different spectra of infectious disease in the gut and the less common usage of HAART [42]. CMV infection may be particularly associated with Kaposi's sarcoma in the small bowel and elsewhere. Most of these infections can be demonstrated by simple morphological and immunohistochemical methods, the latter being especially important for viral infection, such as adenovirus and CMV [36]. Electron microscopic assessment is used less often, especially as microsporidiosis and cryptosporidiosis can now by recognised by light microscopy [42,47].

Bacterial infection

Although bacterial infection specific and localised to the small bowel does occur, it is important to realise that, in acute bacterial infection, there is usually evidence of an enterocolitis. The primary presentation is diarrhoea with or without evidence of blood loss. Some infections, such as cholera, and those caused by *Shigella* spp. and *Escherichia coli*, are especially prone to epidemics and this is partly related to the often small inoculum required to produce infection. With some strains of *Shigella*, only about 100 bacteria are required to produce an acute enteritis [47].

Enteric bacterial pathogens can broadly be categorised into three groups:
1. Entero-adherent bacteria, which adhere to and colonise the surface of the intestinal epithelium where they remain for the duration of the infection
2. Entero-toxigenic bacteria, which, in addition to adherence and colonisation, produce potent toxins
3. Entero-invasive bacteria, which are capable of actively crossing the intestinal epithelium.

The entero-invasive group can be subdivided into organisms localised to the mucosa and those that penetrate into deeper tissues and cause systemic infection. The morphology of the lesions observed in bacterial infections depends on the characteristics and the virulence of the pathogens and the host response. Further, the lesions show a variation in time, depending on when the biopsies are obtained early (days) after onset of the infection or late (weeks).

In an early phase, neutrophils may predominate in the inflammatory reaction, whereas lymphocytes and plasma cells are more prominent in a later phase. The pathology of acute enteritides ranges, therefore, from a superficial exudative inflammatory process, as observed in *E. coli* infection, to deeper penetrating pathology, as seen in yersiniosis and amoebiasis [47]. Although bacterial enteritides are extremely common worldwide, histopathologists seldom see such diseases in routine practice. Only occasionally will proximal small bowel biopsies or ileoscopic biopsies demonstrate infectious enteritis. It is much more common for pathologists to see evidence of infections in colonic biopsy series [48]. Furthermore, resection of the small intestine is seldom performed for these diseases. Bacterial enteritides are common in postmortem practice in developing countries but rare post mortem in Europe and North America.

Shigellosis, salmonellosis and campylobacter infection

Bacillary dysentery caused by shigellosis occurs throughout the world. It afflicts about 20 million people each year and kills about three-quarters of a million people every year [49]. *Shigella dysenteriae* type I and *S. flexneri* are the predominant species in developing countries whereas *S. sonnei* is the major isolate in the developed countries. The fourth species, *S. boydii*, is uncommon except in the Indian subcontinent.

Shigellosis is the classical superficial enterocolitis. *Shigella* spp. invade through the M cells in the ileum. Entry into the cells is followed by intracellular multiplication and lysis of the phagosomes. The bacteria are propelled through the cytoplasm, the host cell is killed and bacteria are spread to neighbouring epithelial cells. The process results from the interaction between bacterial proteins IpaA, IpaB and IpaC with cell cytoskeletal components. The bacterial protein IpaB plays an important role in inflammation by directly binding to interleukin-1β-converting enzyme. Macrophages are killed by apoptosis, interleukin-1β (IL-1β) is released and inflammation ensues. Death and sloughing of epithelial cells result in erosions which may extend into the lamina propria, associated with an inflammatory infiltrate that may extend into the submucosa. There is evidence that inflammation increases the pathology of the lesion but decreases the spread of *Shigella* spp. [50].

Evidence of infection starts, clinically, in the small bowel with fever and secretory diarrhoea. In the next few days, bacteria localise to the colon, causing a colitis with ulceration and erosions. Thus, bloody diarrhoea, tenesmus and systemic symptoms supervene. Macroscopic and microscopic damage are most evident in the distal large bowel, becoming progressively milder in the transverse colon. Chronicity is rare. Shigellosis is particularly prevalent in children, especially under-nourished children, and the disease exacerbates under-nourishment by its propensity to enteric protein loss [51]. As a result of the predominant colonic involvement, demonstration of the disease in small bowel biopsies is unusual.

Salmonella infection is the classical food-related enteritis. Enteritis is most commonly caused by *Salmonella enteritidis* and its serotypes (*typhimurium, heidelberg* and *newport*). *S cholera suis* is the other important cause of enteritis. Salmonellae cause an acute gastroenteritis, ileo-colitis or colitis, which is usually short-lived. Seldom is histopathological assessment required, except in longer duration ente-

rocolitis [52]. In severe cases, the changes of acute colitis may be prominent whereas the small bowel mucosa shows more subtle signs [53]. Similar to shigellosis, salmonellosis causes epithelial damage. Entry of cells is followed by interference with normal mechanisms to create a phagolysosome engulfing the salmonellae and alteration of the immune response to favour bacterial survival. Various salmonella proteins have been identified. SipA interacts with actin and is crucial for cytoskeletal changes, SipC interferes with normal intracellular trafficking and SipB promotes chloride secretion. Host inflammatory reactions are mediated, among others, by the production of TNF-α [54].

Campylobacter spp. may be the most common cause of bacterium-mediated, usually food-borne, diarrhoea, being demonstrated in the stools of about 10% of western patients with diarrhoea [55]. Infection occurs in all age groups and results in a syndrome of acute abdominal pain, fever and inflammatory enterocolitis, which ranges from a generally mild secretory diarrhoea to a severe dysentery-like syndrome. Severe post-infectious complications such as Guillain–Barré syndrome may occur. The variable clinical picture is probably more due to the host immune response than to strain virulence factors. Epithelial α-defensins are important for the self-limiting nature of the disease. Campylobacter jejuni causes local acute inflammation in both the small and the large intestine [55]. In cell cultures strains of Campylobacter spp. show different degrees of invasion and transepithelial transfer. Campylobacter spp. contain a single unsheathed flagellum which is necessary to overcome intestinal peristalsis and entry into the mucus layer. Capsular polysaccharides allow epithelial invasion [56].

The enteric fevers: typhoid and paratyphoid

Typhoid fever, caused by *Salmonella enteritidis* serovar *typhi*, remains a serious health problem throughout the world, especially in south and south-east Asia and South America, with an estimated 16–33 million cases and about half a million deaths annually. Its incidence has declined greatly in the western world. This fall and the great improvement in its prognosis are due to improved living conditions and sanitation and the introduction of effective antibiotic therapy. In developed countries, enteric fever can still be seen in travellers. The incidence is estimated to be 3–30 cases per 100 000 travellers to developing countries [57].

The disease is characterised by a sudden onset of fever, headache, nausea, loss of appetite, abdominal discomfort and constipation or diarrhoea in young children. The fever rises in step-wise fashion and remains high for up to 2 weeks. It is important to realise that other *Salmonella* spp., notably the three subtypes of *S. paratyphi*, but also *S. cholerae suis*, yersiniosis and campylobacter infection may mimic enteric fever [58].

S. typhi reaches the small intestine in food or drink contaminated by carriers or polluted by infected excreta. Although salmonellae survive poorly at normal gastric pH (<1.5) they survive well at pH >4.0 and they have an adaptive mechanism for lower pH. After leaving the stomach, they cross the mucus layer of the small intestinal epithelium and interact with enterocytes and M cells overlying Peyer's patches. On contact with these cells they are rapidly internalised and transported into the submucosal lymphoid tissue, where they may enter the bloodstream, without producing any local lesions, and may be isolated by blood culture during the first week or two of the illness. Septicaemia and the accompanying toxaemia are responsible for many of the characteristic clinical features of the disease, such as the 'rose spots' in the skin, the peculiar type of continued fever and the clouded mental state.

After multiplication in the bloodstream, the organisms are excreted by the liver into the bile, and enter the gallbladder and intestinal contents in rapidly increasing numbers; they can be cultured from the faeces in an increasing proportion of cases, the highest incidence of positive stool cultures occurring in the third week of the illness. They are also excreted in the urine. Towards the end of the first week of the illness, specific agglutinating antibodies begin to appear in the patient's blood and the titre rises to its peak by the end of the third week (Widal's reaction). Bacilli are reabsorbed through Peyer's patches in which some degree of local immunity has now developed, leading to a localised immunological reaction with ulceration and necrosis.

There are ulcers over Peyer's patches, particularly in a longitudinal orientation, with more circular ulcers over smaller lymphoid follicles. Occasionally the large bowel and the appendix are also involved [59]. As a result of the marked inflammatory reaction and oedema, the ulcers are often raised above the surrounding mucosa, from which they are sharply demarcated. The base of the ulcer contains black necrotic material: healing begins with shedding of the slough. Healing is complete within a week or so of the subsidence of the acute manifestations of the illness and there is little fibrosis. This accounts for the low frequency of strictures as a result of previous typhoid fever. Local lymph nodes are considerably enlarged, soft and hyperaemic at the height of the disease. Foci of necrosis sometimes form in their substance.

Histologically, enteric fever shows hyperaemia and oedema in the early stages with proliferation of large, often deeply staining mononuclear cells, which are modified phagocytes (containing intracellular organisms) [60]. Moderate numbers of lymphocytes and plasma cells are present but neutrophil polymorphs are strikingly rare, accounting for the typical neutropaenia found in the blood. Later, focal necrosis develops in lymphoid tissue, the necrotic foci becoming confluent and ulceration occurs. Large numbers of typhoid bacilli are present in the intestinal lesions and regional lymph nodes.

Enteric fever is associated with significant local complications such as perforation of the ulcers and haemorrhage. Perforation occurs most frequently in the terminal ileum, in about 5–10% of cases, and it may be that many ulcers perforate or are close to perforation at the same time [61]. At surgery, the small bowel is markedly friable and perforation is a common cause of death from the disease. Haemorrhage from the ulcers is the next most frequent complication and occurs at about the same stage in the course of the disease. Acute typhoid cholecystitis is another frequent complication. Other complications include paralytic ileus, splenomegaly, myocarditis, multifocal necrosis in parenchymatous organs, particularly the liver, kidneys and bone marrow, and Zenker's degeneration of the abdominal muscle. Acute bronchitis, meningitis, nephritis, orchitis, arthritis and osteitis due to the presence of typhoid bacilli in the tissues concerned have all been described. Patients may carry the organism, especially in the biliary tract, for many years.

Paratyphoid is usually a much less serious illness than typhoid. It can be caused by any of the three serotypes of *Salmonella paratyphi*, now named *S. paratyphi A*, *S. schottmulleri* (formerly *paratyphi B*) and *S. hirschfeldii* (formerly *paratyphi C*) [58]. Pathologically the lesions resemble those of typhoid, but they are confined to a smaller area of the terminal ileum. Ulceration is not such a marked feature, and serious complications, comparable with those of typhoid fever, are rare.

Cholera

Cholera is an acutely dehydrating, watery diarrhoeal disease caused by *Vibrio cholerae* serotype O1, a Gram-negative bacterium. Before the advent of an effective rehydration therapy, cholera epidemics were associated with case fatality rates exceeding 40%. Although the disease no longer poses a threat to countries with good standards of hygiene, it remains a challenge to countries where access to safe water and proper sanitation is not guaranteed [1]. Cholera today remains an important threat in almost every developing country. In 2004, 56 countries officially notified the World Health Organization (WHO) of a total of 101 383 cases and 2345 deaths but the true figures are probably higher due to under-reporting and could amount to about 1.8 million cases and 27 000 deaths per year.

After ingestion, *V. cholerae* must pass through the gastric acid barrier of the stomach to colonise the small intestine. There the organism penetrates the mucous gel and adheres to the brush border of intestinal epithelial cells via specific adhesins. Selective adhesion to M cells has been demonstrated. The organism will produce a number of proteins secreted extracellularly, including cholera toxin. This molecule has two important functioning moieties. The first, the β subunit, is responsible for adhesion to the enterocyte surface whereas the second, the α subunit, enters the cytoplasm and activates adenylyl cyclase, which in turn increases intracellular cyclic AMP, stimulating secretion of water and electrolytes from the enterocyte and inhibiting absorption. It has been shown that the genes for this protein are carried by a virus. *V. cholerae* contains two phages required for virulence so that a virus–virus interaction is necessary for pathogenicity.

There is not often cause to seek the histopathological features of cholera because treatment is largely supportive and biopsy adds little to the management of the disease. Clinical and experimental studies have shown villous damage with necrosis of enterocytes, disruption of the underlying basement membrane and necrosis of lymphoid tissue [62]. In the lamina propria there is commonly an increase of lymphocytes and plasma cells but not of eosinophils or neutrophils [63].

Escherichia coli infection

E. coli constitutes a large and diverse group of bacteria, ranging from normal commensals of the human intestinal tract to pathogens with the potential to cause severe diarrhoea. Pathogenic *E. coli* differ from commensal *E. coli* in that the former has acquired groups of virulence genes. Within the versatile species of *E. coli* is practically the entire range of types of microbial enteropathogens, and representative mechanisms by which micro-organisms derange intestinal function to cause secretion and/or inflammation and thus diarrhoea.

There are numerous classes of pathogenic *E. coli*: EPEC, entero-pathogenic *E. coli*; ETEC, entero-toxigenic *E. coli*; STEC, Shiga toxin-secreting *E. coli*; EHEC, entero-haemorrhagic *E. coli*; EIEC, entero-invasive *E. coli*; DHEC, diarrhoea-associated haemolytic *E. coli*; EAAggEC, entero-aggregative *E. coli*; and CDTEC, cytolethal, distending, toxin-secreting *E. coli* [64]. EPEC is an important cause of nosocomial neonatal diarrhoea. EPEC attaches to epithelial cells in a pattern called 'localised adherence', causing loss of microvilli, rearrangement of actin and deformation of the cell. Ultimately the cell is killed but this killing seems slower and less efficient than the killing by invasive bacteria [50]. EPEC has been observed also in the lamina propria and crypt abscesses have been noted in the small intestine. Yet this represents probably the extreme of the pathology. ETEC is the prototype pathogen because the pathogenesis of the disease is dominated by classic enterotoxins: heat-labile and heat-stable toxins. It is the major cause of infantile diarrhoea in developing countries and of travellers' diarrhoea. ETEC attaches to specific receptors on the surface of enterocytes in the small intestine by hair-like fimbriae. More than 25 types of fimbriae, called coli surface

antigens (CSs) or colonisation factor antigens (CFAs), have been described. Once attached, ETEC elaborates the toxins. The heat-labile toxin leads to activation of epithelial adenylyl cyclases whereas the heat-stable toxin activates guanylyl cyclases. Cyclic nucleotides then activate epithelial ion secretion which induces a watery diarrhoea. Microscopic lesions are uncommon. Both EPEC and ETEC may have considerable effects on the small intestine. STEC or EHEC is found more often in the colon.

The nomenclature of STEC is still confusing. Some groups prefer EHEC whereas others use verotoxin-producing *E. coli* (VTEC) (often just O157 or O157:H7) or STEC. These strains have phages encoding the Shiga toxin from *Shigella dysenteriae*. Infection is accompanied by a watery diarrhoea, rapidly progressing to frank haemorrhagic enterocolitis and leads, in up to 20% of children, to serious sequelae including haemolytic–uraemic syndrome. The interaction of STEC and epithelial cells is similar to that of EPEC. The bacterium is able to target the lymphoid tissue of the small bowel and produces a characteristic attaching/effacing lesion on the epithelial surface, by which it instigates an immune reaction that exacerbates the pathological effects [65]. There is evidence that TNF-α is important in this immune reaction [66]. The Shiga toxin is associated with more prominent lesions, typically in the caecum and right colon and sometimes the small intestine. Biopsies may show a pattern of ischaemic injury, sometimes with fibrin thrombi within capillaries.

The EIEC has much in common with shigellosis. As the name implies, it is capable of cell invasion [66]. It causes primarily infections of the colon, described more fully elsewhere (see Chapter 35). EAAggEC is a heterogeneous group that causes persistent diarrhoea in children and in adults with AIDS. It can cause acute diarrhoea in adults. In animal studies, shortening of intestinal villi, haemorrhagic necrosis of the villous tips, and a mild inflammatory response with oedema and mononuclear cells have been reported.

Clostridial infections and pseudo-membranous ileocolitis

The gastrointestinal tract contains an extremely complex ecosystem of microbes which acts as a natural barrier against colonisation by enteropathogens. Once this barrier has been compromised, a person becomes more susceptible to infections. Treatment with antibiotics is one way in which the barrier is altered. Clostridia are part of the normal flora of the large intestine and are also found in the distal part of the small intestine. *Clostridium leptum* may be more abundant in the duodenum in paediatric coeliac disease [67]. *C. difficile*, a spore-forming anaerobe, is potentially pathogenic. It can cause intestinal disease, ranging from mild diarrhoea to fatal pseudo-membranous colitis. It is responsible for pseudo-membranous colitis and causes approximately 25% of all antibiotic-associated diarrhoeas. Antibiotics can substantially reduce the density of anaerobic bacteria in the colon, thereby inhibiting fermentation processes. In these circumstances, osmotically active carbohydrates remain in the colonic lumen and may cause osmotic diarrhoea.

C. difficile disease is mediated by two toxins, A and B, responsible for the diarrhoea, epithelial lesions and inflammation. Multiple mechanisms are involved in the pathogenesis of *C. difficile* toxin-associated intestinal secretion and inflammation, including substance P, enteric nerves, lamina propria macrophages and leukocytes. Although *C. difficile*-mediated disease is primarily colonic, there may also be an accompanying ileitis [67]. This is particularly seen in severe pseudo-membranous colitis, especially in immunosuppressed individuals. In rare cases, genuine pseudo-membranous enteritis can be seen. The macroscopic and microscopic features of pseudo-membranous ileitis are identical to those in the large intestine (see Chapter 35).

After infarction of the bowel, secondary clostridial infection may also occur and contribute to the haemorrhagic and haemolytic appearances frequently seen in infarcts. In fact it is likely that many cases of 'primary clostridial infection' represent secondary effects, with ischaemia as the predominant pathology. Nevertheless, significant primary clostridial infection does occur in the small bowel, although the exact relationship between the bacterial infection and any ischaemic pathology present is often uncertain [68]. The two most common small bowel manifestations of clostridial infection are *C. perfringens* food poisoning and *C. difficile*-mediated pseudo-membranous enterocolitis.

Pigbel (enteritis necroticans) is a focal necrotising and inflammatory disease of the small intestine, especially in poorly nourished children. It is a major cause of morbidity in the highlands of Papua New Guinea where it often follows pig feasting (hence its name) [69]. It is, however, also found elsewhere and has been described in a well-nourished white vegetarian [70]. It seems to be a very similar disease to Darmbrand (meaning 'fire bowels'), a necrotising small bowel disease – epidemic in northern Germany after World War II [71]. Serosal congestion, necrosis, bowel wall thinning and ultimately perforation are the characteristic macroscopic findings of enteritis necroticans, especially occurring in the jejunum. Histologically there is infarction of the mucosa which can be clearly demarcated by a line of inflammatory cells from viable areas [72]. Haemorrhagic infarction and necrosis can extend through the bowel wall. Thrombosis of small vessels may be present and occasionally gas cysts [73]. This describes the most severe acute pattern of disease but there is a complete clinical and pathological spectrum with some patients having more chronic disease and surviving without surgery. Reso-

lution occurs and a subsequent stricture can develop. Both pigbel and *Darmbrand* are the result of *C. perfringens* infection, usually type C.

Staphylococcal enteritis

Staphylococcus aureus is recognised to produce toxins A–E and toxic shock syndrome toxin-1 associated with food poisoning. Outbreaks from ingesting contaminated dairy products, meat or eggs are frequently associated with enterotoxins. Symptoms include nausea, vomiting and abdominal cramps with or without diarrhoea. The organism's role in the production of enterocolitis remains controversial. The variable clinical presentation may be explained by the numerous strains of the pathogen that exist and the different enterotoxins that can be secreted. Cases of necrotising enterocolitis, purported to be due to staphylococci, both *S. aureus* and *S. epidermidis*, are still described in infants, especially after antibiotic administration [73,74] and staphylococcal enterotoxins G and I have been implicated in severe but reversible neonatal enteropathy. Histology shows marked villous atrophy, enterocytes with abnormal brush border and a dense inflammatory infiltrate in the lamina propria. Electron microscopy shows microvillous destruction, dilated mitochondria, lysosomes containing cellular debris and no inclusion bodies [75]. Methicillin-resistant S. aureus (MRSA) may be especially responsible for such necrotising and ulcerating enteritis. Typically transverse linear ulcers occur throughout the small bowel and these may result in perforation [76]. MRSA enteritis causing a high stoma output has also been noted in adults after bowel surgery [77].

In the past staphylococci had also been implicated in the genesis of necrotising enteritis in adults because of the presence of large numbers of cocci lining necrotic ulcers in the small bowel. In many of these cases, it remained uncertain whether the bacteria were a primary cause or a secondary effect of ischaemic ulceration and necrosis. As these organisms can be found in 30% of healthy individuals and 90% of those on antibiotics, with no evidence of diarrhoea, the role of staphylococci in the cause of ulcerating enteritis in patients other than very young children remains uncertain. Many such cases may well represent antibiotic-associated enteritis and are probably caused by bacteria other than staphylococci, such as clostridia and *E. coli*.

Yersiniosis

The genus *Yersinia* includes three human enteric pathogens: *Yersinia enterocolitica, Y. pseudotuberculosis* and *Y. pestis. Y. pestis* is the causative agent of the plague. *Y. enterocolitica* and *Y. pseudotuberculosis* are common causes of diarrhoeal illness in children and adolescents. Pathogenic *Y. enterocolitica* is classified as biogroup 1B (high virulence) and biogroups

2–5 (low virulence). Biogroup 1A was considered non-pathogenic for humans but this may not be correct. Both organisms have invasive properties.

Gastrointestinal disease caused by *Y. enterocolitica* is initiated with binding to intestinal epithelial cells, mediated by different proteins. Subsequently, the organism is internalised through M cells and multiplies in underlying tissues. *Y. enterocolitica* infection causes terminal ileitis, self-limiting colitis, mesenteric lymphadenitis and septicaemia in children and adults. In adults *Y. enterocolitica* is also a frequent cause of post-infectious immune reactions such as polyarthritis, erythema nodosum and Reiter's syndrome. The clinical manifestations of *Y. pseudotuberculosis* resemble those of *Y. enterocolitica* but *Y. pseudotuberculosis* has more invasive characteristics. Human infections with *Y. pseudotuberculosis* are less common than those with *Y. enterocolitica*. Complications of yersinial infection include sepsis and liver abscesses [78,79]. However, it should be noted that *Y. enterocolitica* has been isolated in 2.8–6.7% of stool specimens.

Epidemiological studies have shown that the consumption of (raw) pork and contact with untreated sewage are important risk factors for yersinial infection [80]. Both Y. enterocolitica and Y. pseudotuberculosis cause a terminal ileitis and localised mesenteric adenitis, with thickening of the terminal ileum and local nodes being enlarged and matted together [81–83]. Involvement of the appendix is less common, although, when sequential serological samples were studied in a group of patients presenting with an acute abdomen, 31% of patients with proven Y. pseudotuberculosis were found to have appendicitis [84]. In terminal ileal acute yersiniosis (Figure 20.4), the ileoscopic features may suggest Crohn's disease, especially as aphthoid ulceration, typically over lymphoid aggregates, is a characteristic feature [82–84]. The ulceration may be extensive and involve the adjacent caecum and, in fatal cases, it may involve the whole small and large intestine.

Yersiniosis is characterised by an acute-on-chronic histiocytic and granulomatous inflammation, especially that caused by *Y. pseudotuberculosis* (Figure 20.4). Granulomas are not such a conspicuous feature in Y. enterocolitica infection. Granulomatous inflammation may correlate with low virulence groups and suppurative inflammation with high virulence cases [85]. There appear to be four stages of disease: lymphoid hyperplasia, histiocytic hyperplasia, epithelioid cell granuloma formation and finally central granuloma necrosis (Figure 20.5) [79]. These are best demonstrated in yersinial mesenteric adenitis. First, there is a generalised reactive hyperplasia with preservation of the normal architecture. Histiocytes are conspicuous and may produce a 'starry-sky' appearance. The formation of granulomas, often of geographical shapes and confluent, then supervenes. These often have a central necrotic zone infiltrated by polymorphs and forming a micro-abscess, surrounded by epithelioid cells and histiocytes. This pattern of necrotising granulomatosis is comparable to that seen in other infective lymphadenitides, most notably cat scratch fever and lymphogranuloma venereum. Even giant cells of the Langhans' type may be present. Yet, with immunohistochemistry, it has been shown that the granulomas are composed of numerous histiocytes along with scattered T lymphocytes whereas B cells were rare [86]. The granulomas are predominantly in paracortical zones, particularly in relation to lymphatic sinuses, and the surrounding

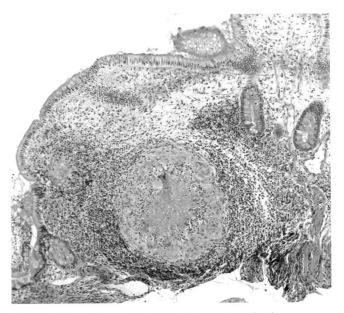

Figure 20.5 Yersiniosis: endoscopic biopsy from the ileum showing a granuloma with central necrosis surrounded by epithelioid cells.

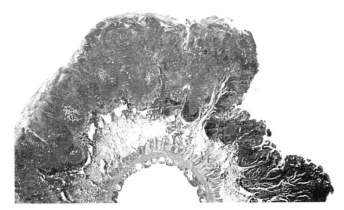

Figure 20.4 A terminal ileal resection for acute-on-chronic yersiniosis. The thickening of the ileal wall is apparent with ulceration of the mucosa over the hyperplastic lymphoid tissue.

capsule usually shows fibrous thickening. Colonies of Gram-negative organisms can be seen [82].

In the ileum and appendix, there is ulceration and focal chronic active inflammation, with or without necrotising granulomas (see Figure 20.4). Evidence of granulomatous pathology is more likely in Y. pseudotuberculosis infection but is less likely to be seen in ileal biopsies than in involved mesenteric lymph nodes. When the disease is more pronounced, there may be evidence of deep ulceration and submucosal oedema, although involvement of the muscularis propria is unusual. When ileitis is seen in ileal biopsies, especially in children and young adults, it is advisable to suggest serology to corroborate the diagnosis of yersiniosis because the histological features are often relatively non-specific and the differential diagnosis from Crohn's disease and, even, tuberculosis may be difficult. In rare instances previous Y. enterocolitica was found in association with collagenous colitis with duodenal and ileal involvement and transient IgG deficiency [87].

Other bacterial causes of enteritis

Acute bacterial enteritis can further be caused by Aeromonads, Gram-negative, oxidase-positive bacteria and *Klebsiella* spp. [88,89]. Aeromonads include Plesiomonas (P. shigelloides), Edwardsiella (E. tarda) and Aeromonas spp. (A. hydrophila) [89]. They are associated with increasing numbers of reports of acute enterocolitis. Infection has been related to the consumption of fresh water. In children, Aeromonads appear to be a relatively common cause of acute self-limiting diarrhoea [90], whereas in older adults it may cause a more chronic enterocolitis [91].

Although strictly not an enteritis, in that it usually presents with an ileo-caecal chronic inflammatory phlegmon, actinomycosis should always be considered in the differential diagnosis of chronic active inflammatory pathology affecting the terminal ileum and proximal colon, especially in women using an intrauterine contraceptive device. Similar to other infections, it can closely mimic Crohn's disease, both clinically and pathologically, and it may also, rarely, complicate Crohn's disease [92]. It is a cause of fistulation and can also cause ileal strictures. A Gram stain will reveal the causative filamentous Gram-positive bacilli, *Actinomyces israelii*, usually demonstrable in large colonies known as 'sulphur granules'.

Bacterial overgrowth in the small intestine

Bacterial overgrowth is a clinical syndrome, presenting with malabsorption, weight loss and diarrhoea [93]. It is primarily a disease of elderly people, in which case it is most often of unknown cause [94]. Previous surgery, especially gastrectomy [95], small intestinal dysmotility including diabetes mellitus [96], jejunal diverticulosis and previous vagotomy are all potential causes [97]. Histopathology is not a primary diagnostic procedure in this disease because the changes are usually mild and non-specific and tend to under-call the severity of the functional abnormality of the small intestinal mucosa. Breath testing, especially for hydrogen, is the preferred diagnostic modality. Nevertheless bacterial overgrowth does cause variable villous atrophy with epithelial lymphocytosis and minor chronic inflammatory changes in the mucosa and has the potential to mimic other causes of malabsorption (see 'Bacterial overgrowth', Chapter 21) [98]. Furthermore small intestinal bacterial overgrowth may cause elevated anti-gliadin antibody levels in small intestinal luminal secretions and therefore has the potential to cause over-diagnosis of coeliac disease.

Tuberculosis and other mycobacterial diseases

Intestinal tuberculosis (TB) is caused mainly by *Mycobacterium tuberculosis* and to a lesser extent by *M. bovis*, the latter being less common in the western hemisphere due to pasteurisation of milk. In western pathological practice, intestinal TB remains rare but there has been a steady increase in the number of recorded cases, in part related to increased immigration from countries where intestinal TB is endemic [99]. Another factor is the development of multidrug-resistant strains of TB. Furthermore AIDS has wrought a dramatic increase in systemic and localised TB in many parts of the world and, together, they are a dangerous combination [99]. In one study in the UK, 84% of cases of intestinal TB were seen in immigrants, especially from the Asian subcontinent [100]. Within the immigrant community, the highest incidence of gastrointestinal involvement occurs in the years soon after arrival in the west.

Both *M. tuberculosis* and *M. bovis* have a predilection for the small bowel, particularly the terminal ileum, although any part of the gastrointestinal tract may be affected. In a large case series, intestinal TB was localised in the small bowel in 33.8%, the large bowel in 22.3%, the peritoneum in 30.7%, the liver in 14.6% and the upper gastrointestinal tract in 8.5% [101]. In a study from Hong Kong, the ileo-caecal region was involved in 86% of patients [102]. Intestinal TB develops when the organism penetrates the mucosa.

It is customary to divide intestinal TB into primary and secondary forms. In the first, ingested bacilli (from contaminated milk) are believed to set up a primary reaction in the intestinal wall or in mesenteric lymph nodes. In the second, the source is swallowed infected sputum from a primary lung lesion or a further oral dose of bacilli establishing a re-infection in an already sensitised individual. The latter used to be the more common form but, in more recent studies, accounts for less than half of all cases [100,103]. A further modality of development is haematogenous spread from active pulmonary disease, whereas direct extension from adjacent organs is very rare. Intestinal TB is more common in younger adults and somewhat more common in females.

Acute intestinal TB usually presents as a severe enterocolitis (so-called dysenteric TB), especially in children. Free perforation is a common complication of acute disease. The macroscopic appearances of intestinal TB vary considerably according to the acuteness and severity of the infection and the stage of disease. Areas of involvement, often multiple, are found with increasing frequency from the jejunum to the ileum, being particularly common in the terminal ileum and ileo-caecal area [104]. This distribution follows the localisation of lymphoid tissue in the small intestine. Ulcerative intestinal TB presents as one or more annular, circular or oval ulcers lying transversely, raised above the normal mucosa and usually producing a stricture (Figure 20.6) [104]. It is a characteristic of intestinal TB that single ulcers are relatively large whereas multiple ulcers are usually much smaller [103,105].

The appearances of the cut surface of the affected bowel depend on the stage of the disease. In acute ulcerating TB, caseation is usually definable and there may be evidence of miliary TB on the peritoneal surface [105]. Regional lymph nodes are enlarged and show caseation on the cut surface [106]. Later stage disease gives rise to dense fibrosis and strictures [104]. It is such strictures with bowel obstruction that predisposes to perforation in chronic intestinal TB [107]. These chronic cases are also prone to fistulae and ileo-caecal inflammatory masses, the pathological features combining to induce mimicry of Crohn's disease [108]. In countries where TB is endemic, notably India, TB is the most common cause of small intestinal stricture.

The microscopic appearances of intestinal TB also vary with the stage of the disease. The morphological features do not differ significantly from those of TB elsewhere. Coalescent and caseating granulomas (Figure 20.7) are seen in all layers of the bowel wall, especially in Peyer's patches

and lymphoid follicles, and in regional nodes [106]. In more chronic disease, caseation may not be a feature and the pathology is dominated by dense fibrosis, with destruction of the normal tissues of the bowel wall, including the muscularis propria. In very chronic lesions, the granulomas become hyalinised and eventually disappear, leaving behind only small aggregates of lymphocytes, an excess of fibrous tissue and, sometimes, 'tombstones' of effete coalescent granulomas. These appearances can closely mimic burnt-out Crohn's disease with the associated mucosal (ulcer-associated cell lineage) and connective tissue changes (including vascular, neural and muscular changes) [109].

The differential diagnosis of Crohn's disease and intestinal TB is very important because treatment is completely different. The differential diagnosis is based on clinical features, although they are not very specific, on the tuberculin skin test, although the value of this test for intestinal TB is not well known, and on imaging studies and histology [109]. The principal microscopic features that separate TB from Crohn's disease are the presence of large granulomas, confluent granulomas, multiple granulomas (10 or more per biopsy site), caseation, ulcers lined by conglomerate epithelioid histiocytes, disproportionate submucosal inflammation, lack of submucosal oedema, the presence of small serosal tubercles and a relative lack of fissuring [99,110]. Clinically, the rarity of anal lesions may be an indication [105]. Examination of regional lymph nodes is particularly important, because they can show better

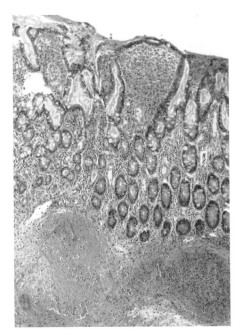

Figure 20.7 Coalescent epithelioid cell granulomas in ileal biopsies in intestinal tuberculosis.

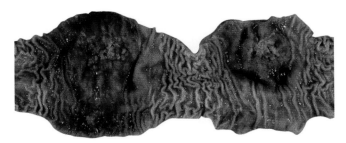

Figure 20.6 Transverse ulceration of the ileum in tuberculosis. (Reproduced with kind permission of Professor Sebastian Lucas, London, UK.)

any evidence of former tuberculous infection. The regional lymph nodes nearly always contain granulomas in intestinal TB, whereas these are relatively infrequent in Crohn's disease.

Acid-fast bacilli can usually be found on Ziehl–Neelsen (ZN) staining when there is caseous necrosis, although their detection may require a prolonged search. However, in chronic fibrosing and stricturing TB, demonstrable mycobacteria may be very scanty or absent. In this situation, it is imperative that ZN stains are performed on involved regional lymph nodes, because these are much more liable to harbour organisms.

TB is a problem in patients receiving immunosuppressive therapy and a major problem in AIDS patients in places where TB is endemic, such as Africa: it is a major cause of death in up to 40% of AIDS patients there [111].

In western countries, atypical mycobacteriosis, predominantly caused by *M. avium-intracellulare* (MAI), is more important as a complication of AIDS. The small bowel is a site of predilection for this opportunistic infection and, overall, the gastrointestinal tract is an early, possibly primary, site of colonisation. The disease is a late manifestation in AIDS, usually occurring when the CD4 count falls below 100/dl [112]. In postmortem studies, evidence of MAI infection is demonstrated in about 50% of cases but only about 10% of AIDS patients with diarrhoea will demonstrate the organism [112]. MAI infection causes a granulomatous reaction in which foamy macrophages predominate (Figure 20.8). These are periodic acid–Schiff (PAS) positive and thus may closely mimic Whipple's disease [113]. Sometimes the changes are very subtle with just scanty collections of foamy histiocytes in the lamina propria. In known AIDS patients with any form of histiocytic infiltrate in small bowel biopsies, a ZN stain is imperative because this will demonstrate the (often large numbers of) mycobacteria and help to refute a diagnosis of Whipple's disease (Figure 20.9) [114]. The importance of a search, in such biopsies, for other infecting organisms in AIDS is once again emphasised: MAI infection often coexists with other infections, especially CMV and cryptosporidiosis. Infection by Rhodococcus equi is another possible mimic of MAI or Whipple's disease in immunocompromised hosts. Electron microscopy may show differences in morphology [115].

Whipple's disease

Whipple's disease, first described in 1907 by George Hoyt Whipple [116], is a multi-systemic chronic disease of bacterial aetiology. The infection is very rare, although the causative bacterium Tropheryma whipplei is ubiquitously present in the environment. The approximate annual incidence is less than 1 per 1 million of the population. The disease mostly affects middle-aged men, with a male:female ratio of 8:1. The typical clinical manifestations are weight

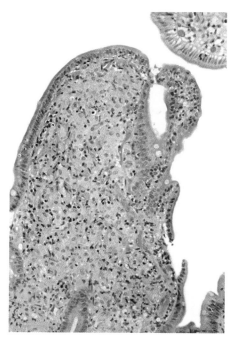

Figure 20.8 The histology of small intestinal *Mycobacteriuum avium-intracellulare* infection in AIDS. There is an ill-defined granulomatous infiltrate with numerous foamy macrophages.

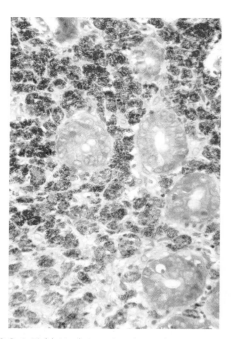

Figure 20.9 A Ziehl–Neelsen stain of *Mycobacterium avium-intracellulare* infection in AIDS demonstrates innumerable acid-fast bacilli.

loss (92% of the cases), diarrhoea (76%), migratory arthralgia of the large joints or, less commonly, non-deforming oligoarthritis or polyarthritis (67%) and abdominal pain (55%). The disease has a propensity to systemic involvement with fever (38%), lymphadenopathy (60%), and cardiac (especially endocarditis), pulmonary and central nervous system involvement all well described. Although arthralgia may precede intestinal symptoms, Whipple's disease, nevertheless, primarily involves the small intestine. Some patients develop severe symptoms of malabsorption, such as ascites and peripheral oedema. The disease is most usually diagnosed by small bowel (either duodenal or jejunal) biopsy. Occasionally the disease can involve the large intestine and colonic and/or rectal biopsies can reveal the characteristic pathological appearances, although the presence of macrophages in the colon is most commonly due to other causes and the diagnosis should be confirmed by electron microscopy or PCR [117,118].

Whipple originally demonstrated rod-shaped structures within the cytoplasm of macrophages [116]. The postulation that these structures were bacteria was supported by the first successful treatment with antibiotics in the 1950s. In 1960, electron microscopic studies showed that the structures had a characteristic bacterial cell wall (Figure 20.10) [119]. Thirty-one years later, PCR enabled the amplification of specific segments of the agent's 16-S ribosomal DNA and, in 1992, it was suggested that the organism should be named *Tropheryma whipplei* (classic Greek: *trophe* = nourishment, *eryma* = barrier) because of the resulting malabsorption [120,121]. After the first successful cultivation the

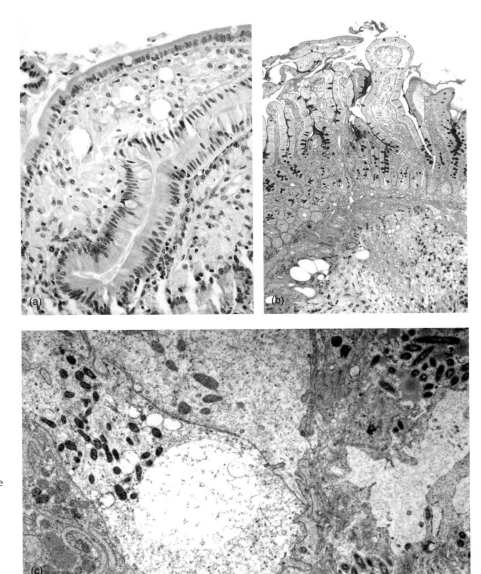

Figure 20.10 Whipple's disease in a duodenal biopsy. (a) Section stained by haematoxylin and eosin (H&E). The villi are expanded by macrophages and large vacuoles. (b) Periodic acid–Schiff (PAS) stain showing PAS-positive macrophages in the submucosa in a case of Whipple's disease presenting with submucosal pathology only. (c) Electron microscopy shows the intracytoplasmic rod-shaped bacteria.

name was officially confirmed as Tropheryma whipplei in 2001 [122]. The sequencing of the complete genome from two different strains elucidated its phylogenetic position as a G–C-rich Gram-positive actinomycete.

Although its natural source has not been defined, *T. whipplei* is found ubiquitously in the environment, including waste water from rural communities and effluxes of sewage plants [123]. Healthy individuals carry *T. whipplei*. The organism has been detected in saliva, subgingival plaque and stool samples [124]. The existence of asymptomatic carriers indicates that not all individuals develop Whipple's disease, supporting the theory that a host immunodeficiency plays a role in the occurrence of the disease. Whether this is an underlying genetic predisposition is not clear. An association between Whipple's disease and the human leukocyte antigen HLA-B27 has been assumed but not confirmed. Rare familial cases have been reported but most studies do not suggest the presence of familial factors [125].

It is, however, clear that the disease can be regarded as an infection caused by a Gram-positive actinomycete, associated with profound immunological defects that allow the survival of the bacteria within macrophages [126]. Although it is not yet known how *T. whipplei* penetrates the human body, the bacteria can be found intracellularly or metabolically active extracellularly in the intestinal mucosa. Macrophages show a persistently diminished ability to degrade the intracellular organisms. This is associated with low production of IL-12 and stimulation of the release of IL-16, which induces macrophage apoptosis. An inappropriate maturation of antigen-presenting cells caused by the presence of IL-16 (and IL-10), and the absence of IL-12 and interferon-γ, might lead to insufficient antigen presentation and inhibit the stimulation of antigen-specific T-helper cells, enabling growth and the spread of *T. whipplei*. These abnormalities correlate with the diminution of immunocompetent B cells, despite the massive histiocytic influx [118,127].

There are also abnormalities of T-cell function, with reduced CD4+ T cells, a shift towards mature T-cell populations, increased T-cell activation and decreased T-cell-mediated responses [128]. However, none of these features provides evidence of a primary immunological abnormality to explain a predilection to infection by *T. whipplei* in Whipple's disease patients. It is still possible to reason that the infection causes secondary immunological abnormalities, in susceptible individuals, which enhance the pathological effects of the infection [119,125]. It has been suggested that glycosylation of the bacterium, an intracellular antigen-masking system, could impair antibody-mediated immune recognition in patients [129].

The small bowel affected by Whipple's disease shows characteristic macroscopic features. Erosions are common but yellow plaques and pale-yellow shaggy mucosa is considered highly suggestive of Whipple's disease [130]. At laparotomy, the affected small bowel serosa is lined by exudate and the intestine appears thickened, dilated and rigid. The mesentery is thickened and there is lymphadenopathy. There may also be peritoneal plaques [131].

Upper gastrointestinal endoscopy of the small intestine is the first diagnostic test of choice. To avoid sampling errors, five biopsies should be taken from various sites of the duodenum. Classic lesions show a degree of villous blunting and villous atrophy with preservation of epithelial cells, whereas the lamina propria is greatly expanded by numerous pale-staining histiocytes. Dilated lymphatics and empty spaces can be present. The empty spaces have been shown to contain fat. The foamy macrophages contain abundant PAS-positive coarse granular material, representing intracellular bacilli (see Figure 20.10). Sarcoid-like granulomas can be observed in samples from other tissues, including lung, stomach and lymph nodes. Although the diagnosis remains primarily a pathological endeavour, PCR is now regarded as a useful confirmatory test [118,132]. When either histology or PCR is positive, the diagnosis of Whipple's disease is confirmed.

In some cases gastrointestinal symptomatology and intestinal involvement is minimal or focal [133]. The histological lesions may be minimal and PAS-positive macrophages can even be limited to the submucosa (Figure 20.10). When PAS staining is negative, PCR and immunohistochemistry should be performed [118]. *T. whipplei* can also be identified in tissues with negative PAS staining and immunohistochemistry using specific antibodies. If only one test, histochemistry or immunohistochemistry, is positive, the diagnosis is tentative. If both tests are negative, but clinical suspicion remains, other samples should be examined. Cases with negative PAS staining underpin the importance of PCR and immunohistochemistry, particularly on other specimens: positive PCR results have been described on analysis of faeces, peripheral blood cells, lymph node biopsies and cerebrospinal fluid (CSF) from patients with Whipple's disease [134–136]. Positive immunohistochemical results have been observed in central nervous system disease. More recently PCR for the *hsp65* gene has been proposed as a suitable target for *T. whipplei* detection [137]. Routine use of electron microscopy as a diagnostic tool is no longer recommended.

The disease has demonstrated an excellent response to antibiotic therapy. Although tetracycline has been the mainstay of treatment, relapse is well described and therefore other antibiotic regimens, usually combination therapies, are now used. These have included penicillin and streptomycin and, more recently, ceftriaxone followed by trimethoprim and sulfamethoxazole, the latter now being the recommended treatment [118,138]. PCR has been advocated as a means of assessing response to treatment and the diagnosis of relapse [139], not least because PAS-positive histiocytes may remain in the small intestinal mucosa for many years after treatment, so histology may not be a useful means for diagnosing relapse, despite the fact that the PAS staining intensity decreases and becomes less granular [140]. Relapses usually occur only a few years after treatment and are accompanied by a re-emergence of viable bacteria. Some patients remain refractory to antibiotic treatment and may require both comprehensive antibiotic regimens and immunomodulatory therapy.

For the pathologist, Whipple's disease provides a striking pathological picture, enhanced by PAS histochemistry, electron microscopy and PCR analysis (see Figure 20.10). Nevertheless it is important to emphasise that other conditions may mimic Whipple's disease. Certainly the most important differential diagnosis is that of mycobacterial infection in AIDS, specifically that by MAI, in which numerous pale-staining histiocytes characteristically pack the distended lamina propria of the intestines. A ZN stain is an important investigation in this situation because it does not stain *T. whipplei*. Other histiocytic accumulations such as storage disorders or lysosomal diseases may also mimic Whipple's disease in colorectal biopsies [141]. Occasionally aggregations of histiocytes in the small intestine may resemble sarcoidosis and Crohn's disease [142].

Fungal infection

Fungal infection of the small intestine is rare: it is virtually never primary and usually occurs in severely immunocompromised individuals. In these patients, candidiasis and aspergillosis are most commonly seen [143]. Candidiasis can occur in the small bowel in AIDS [144] and can result in perforation [145]. Small intestinal infarction due to aspergillosis has been described after chemotherapy (in neutropaenic patients), and in transplant recipients [146–148]. We have observed small bowel infarction with invasive aspergillosis in a young patient with X-linked lymphoproliferative disease, formerly called X-linked recessive, progressive, combined variable immunodeficiency or Duncan's disease [149]. The complication occurred as the result of Epstein–Barr virus infection. Macroscopically fungal infections usually present with ulceration, irregular shaggy mucosal surfaces resembling pseudo-membranous enterocolitis or inflammatory masses [143]. Histologically, *Candida* sp. is usually detectable in the surface ulcer debris whereas *Aspergillus* sp. is more likely to be demonstrated in and around submucosal blood vessels.

The association of ulceration with extensive fungal involvement of intramural blood vessels is also a feature of mucormycosis in the small bowel. Mucormycosis is an often fatal fungal infection, caused by the class Phycomycetes subdivided into the genera *Absidia*, *Mucor* and *Rhizopus*. The infection occurs most frequently in patients with haematological malignancies, transplanted patients receiving immunosuppression and patients with malnutrition or on desferrioxamine treatment for iron overload. It is frequently seen in children [150] and is curiously rare as a complication of AIDS [151]. In the gastrointestinal tract, the stomach is the most frequent site of involvement, followed by the colon and small intestine [150]. The fungal hyphae are characteristically broad and irregular, rarely septate, with right angle branching: these features help to differentiate *Mucor* sp. from *Aspergillus* sp. The Mucorales are usually found in a perivascular or vascular location, inducing arterial thrombosis and subsequent necrosis.

Extra-pulmonary infections with *Pneumocystis jiroveci* are rare and effectively a unique, if rare, complication of profound immunosuppression in AIDS patients. When this involves the small intestine, the bowel wall involvement can be transmural, which can lead to fatal perforation of the small bowel [152].

Histoplasmosis, caused by the dimorphic fungus *Histoplasma capsulatum*, usually involves the colon, whereas the small intestine is affected less often. Small intestinal histoplasmosis is usually seen in its disseminated form [153]. This is mostly associated with immunosuppression and is particularly common in AIDS patients [154]. Occasionally disseminated histoplasmosis can cause malabsorption as a result of small intestinal involvement [155]. Lesions can present as masses, ulcers or polyps, but can also mimic Whipple's disease in the duodenum and Crohn's disease in the ileo-caecal area [156,157]. The histological appearances vary according to the level of immunocompromise present: in advanced AIDS there may be little cellular reaction, extensive necrosis and numerous typical capsulate yeast forms of the fungus. In less severe cases, abnormal villi with numerous macrophages can be seen. Morphologically the fungus measures about $3\,\mu m$ in diameter and resembles *Leishmania* sp. It is often weakly birefringent in polarised light and is well demonstrated with PAS and Grocott's stains.

Protozoal infection

Several species of protozoa infect the small intestine primarily, causing diarrhoea and/or malabsorption. All are particularly associated with immunosuppression but it is increasingly realised that several species also cause enteropathy in immunocompetent individuals. This is particularly the case with cryptosporidiosis, microsporidiosis and cyclosporidiosis [158]. Giardiasis is the most commonly recognised protozoal infection of the small bowel in histopathological practice. Many of the other infections are more likely to be demonstrated by microbiological means: histopathologists are rarely asked to diagnose some of the more esoteric protozoal infections, except in the context of advanced AIDS.

Giardiasis

Giardia lamblia (or *duodenalis*), a motile flagellate protozoan, is the most common small intestinal protozoan enteropathogen worldwide [159]. Antoni van Leeuwenhoek provided the first description in 1681. The infection is most often related to infected water supplies and epidemics are well described. There is pronounced variation in the clinical response to the infection, from an asymptomatic carrier state to debilitating chronic diarrhoea and malabsorption [159–161]. Infection with *Giardia lamblia* is curiously more common in males than females [160]. Giardiasis is a major cause of diarrhoea in children and travellers and it is particularly associated with immunological deficiency, most notably with hypogammaglobulinaemia [162] and AIDS. In these diseases, there is often evidence of extremely heavy colonisation. Although infection is self-limiting in most healthy individuals, a proportion may go on to have persistent diarrhoea.

The host–microbial interactions that govern the outcome of the infection remain incompletely understood. Findings available indicate that the infection causes diarrhoea via a combination of intestinal malabsorption and hypersecretion. Malabsorption and maldigestion mainly result from a diffuse shortening of epithelial microvilli, which is associated with loss of disaccharidase activity. This enterocytic injury is mediated by activated host T lymphocytes. Activation of lymphocytes is secondary to *Giardia*-induced disruption of epithelial tight junctions, which in turn increases permeability. Loss of epithelial barrier function is a result of *Giardia*-induced enterocyte apoptosis. Direct physical injury by the parasite, release of parasite products such as lectins and enzymes and mucosal inflammation due to cytokine release have all been postulated [159,163]. B cells and CD4 T cells are important for anti-giardial host defence but their relative importance is not fully understood. Antigiardial IgA antibodies develop during the infection and CD4 T cells are required for eradication. Nevertheless, an increased intra-epithelial T-cell infiltrate is only occasionally demonstrated in small intestinal biopsies [164].

Giardia spp. exist in two forms: the motile trophozoite that exists exclusively within the intestinal tract and the cyst, which can survive outside the host and transmits the infection. The latter can be identified in stool specimens. Trophozoites are detected in stool specimens, duodenal fluid, mucosal impression smears and biopsies. The trophozoite measures approximately 12–15 μm in length and 5–9 μm in width. It has two nuclei and four symmetrically placed flagella. In biopsies, the parasites are usually demonstrated in clusters in the lumen, on or adjacent to the epithelial surface (Figure 20.11). They appear as sickle shaped, slightly basophilic structures. Flagella may be demonstrable at high power. A Giemsa preparation stains the organism well but, in normal or heavy infestation, special stains are usually not required. It is important not to mistake sickled red blood cells, often present in biopsy material, for the protozoa.

Although varying degrees of villous atrophy, chronic inflammation in the lamina propria and modest intraepithelial lymphocytosis are all seen, it is important to emphasise that, in most cases (96% in one series), the duodenal mucosa appears normal [160]. Thus a search for the parasite should be undertaken in all duodenal biopsies in patients presenting with diarrhoea and malabsorption, whether or not the biopsies are morphologically normal [160]. Furthermore the protozoan may be detected in gastric, jejunal, ileal and colonic mucosa: these mucosae are also usually normal histologically. The presence of giardiasis may presage immunocompromise and a search for other infecting organisms is important in AIDS and hypogammaglobulinaemia. Outside these conditions, there is also strong positive association between giardiasis and gastric helicobacter infection [160].

Coccidiosis

The gut coccidia are obligate intracellular protozoan parasites, four genera of which are human pathogens: *Cryptosporidium, Cyclospora, Isospora* and *Sarcocystis*. The first three are especially associated with enteropathy and diarrhoea in AIDS. Although the incidence of coccidiosis in AIDS patients is declining with the advent of effective antiretroviral therapies, it must be emphasised that coccidiosis is increasingly recognised as a cause of diarrhoea, especially in epidemics and/or as traveller's diarrhoea, in immunocompetent individuals [158].

Cryptosporidiosis

Cryptosporidium parvum is the only type of this genus known to infect humans [165], although a murine *Cryptosporidium* sp. has been detected in otherwise healthy children [166]. The primary site of infection is the upper small bowel, although the disease is most often diagnosed microbiologically in stool samples. Infection occurs through the ingestion of oocysts, which excyst and infect intestinal epithelial cells. Actin-binding proteins play an important role in facilitating the infection. Once *C. parvum* has entered the epithelium, it will mature into infectious forms. The later stages of parasite development are accompanied by apoptosis of host epithelial cells.

Although a characteristic and prevalent feature in AIDS patients, cryptosporidiosis is increasingly associated with outbreaks of diarrhoea in immunocompetent individuals, especially due to contaminated water supplies, and it is also a cause of travellers' diarrhoea [167]. In immunocompetent individuals, the disease is self-limiting, with

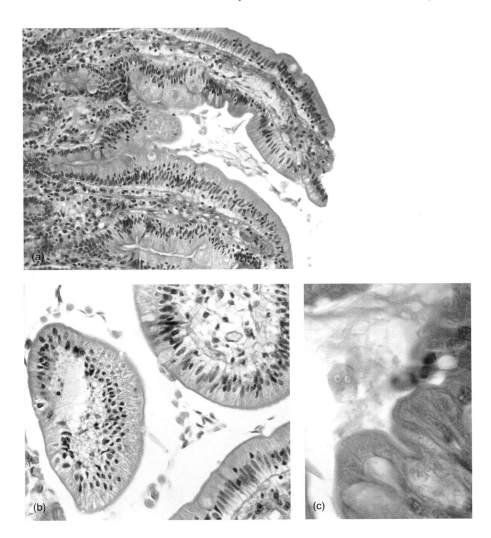

Figure 20.11 (a) A duodenal biopsy showing innumerable *Giardia lamblia* protozoa. (b) They appear as clustered, sickle-shaped, slightly basophilic structures adjacent to the surface of the epithelium. (c) High magnification showing the giardia parasite.

the organisms spontaneously clearing after a few weeks, because the cryptosporidia are, in this situation, minimally invasive mucosal pathogens [165].

In AIDS, cryptosporidiosis is the most common cause of diarrhoea, occurring in about 15–21% of patients, in the UK and the USA [168]. In Haiti and Africa, up to 50% of AIDS patients can be infected. The small bowel mucosa shows strikingly variable changes which correlate with a highly variable clinical picture from minor symptoms, through a cholera-like acute enteritis, to chronic diarrhoea. The symptomatology and morphological changes also correlate with the oocyst concentration in the stool [169]. Although, in most AIDS patients with cryptosporidiosis, the small intestinal mucosa is normal, those with the most severe symptoms show pronounced villous atrophy with an intense neutrophilic infiltration [170]. Such severe cryptosporidial enteritis is often associated with co-infection, particularly with CMV [171]. Extensive involvement of the small and large bowel with heavy oocyst load correlates with the most severe clinical features [171].

The pathogenesis of the enteritis remains poorly understood in both immunocompetent and immunocompromised individuals [172]. In AIDS patients there may also be involvement of the stomach, the biliary tract and, in particular, the colon.

In histological sections the organism is recognised by its proximity to the epithelial surface, being attached to the microvillous border of the epithelial cells (Figures 20.2, 20.12 and 20.13). Cryptosporidia become internalised within the cytoplasm by extension of the cytoplasm around them [173]. In AIDS, the organisms have been shown to enter the lamina propria and may also be found within the cytoplasm of M cells and macrophages [173]. The oocysts measure between 4.5 and 6 μm in diameter and are ZN negative in histological sections (although they are positive in modified ZN stains in stool samples). They are stained by Giemsa. Probably the most useful stains are mucin stains, which help to differentiate the organisms from blobs of mucin, the most likely confounding histopathological feature. Notably, the cryptosporidia are of consistent size

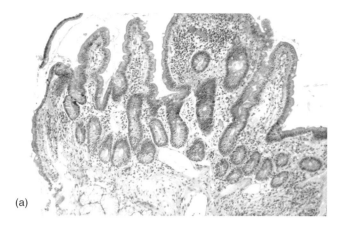

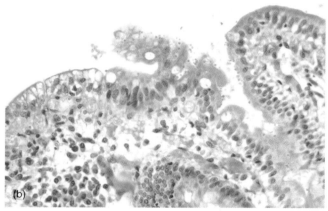

Figure 20.12 Cryptosporidiosis appears as small round structures attached to surface epithelial cells. (a) The villi can be irregular and (b) the surface epithelial cells can show supranuclear vacuolisation.

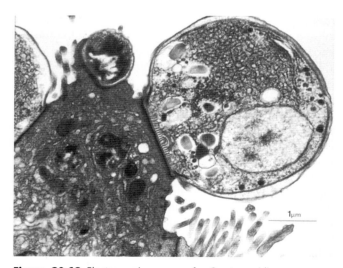

Figure 20.13 Electron microscopy of a *Cryptosporidium parvum* coccidian. It is attached to the microvillous border of the epithelial cell of the duodenum.

whereas mucin blobs are of varying sizes, serving to differentiate the two.

Isosporiasis

Isospora belli is an upper small bowel pathogen that is a relatively common cause of enteropathy in tropical countries. It is an unusual cause of diarrhoea in immunocompetent individuals in western countries, although sporadic outbreaks are described in the USA [174]. It accounts for only about 2% of cases of chronic diarrhoea in AIDS patients in western populations, but up to 15–20% in countries such as Haiti and in Africa. Unlike cryptosporidia, isospora organisms are internalised within the enterocyte cytoplasm and readily detected there by high power light microscopy and electron microscopy. Nevertheless the diagnosis is usually achieved microbiologically by examining stools with a modified ZN stain. In AIDS patients, the coccidian may cause severe diarrhoea and can, on occasion, become systemic [175].

Cyclosporidiosis

Cyclospora cayetanensis is increasingly recognised as cause of diarrhoea, especially in travellers to Nepal, the Caribbean and Central America [176,177]. It primarily involves the proximal small bowel and may be demonstrated in duodenal biopsies [178]. Heavy infection may cause inflammation and epithelial injury with villous blunting [179,180]. The infection results in a cyclical pattern of diarrhoea (hence the name), lasting 6–8 weeks [179], although this is more prolonged in immunosuppressed individuals, especially in AIDS patients [181]. It can be caused by infected water supplies [182] but, in the USA at least, it is particularly associated with infected imported fruit, especially berries [183].

The diagnosis is achieved by parasitological examination of the stool [184]. In histological sections, the parasites are visible, with difficulty, within the cytoplasm of enterocytes, where 2- to 3-µm schizonts and the 5-µm elongated merozoites are visible at high power, with experience, especially in thick sections. They are smaller than *Isospora* spp. and are not PAS positive [185].

Sarcosporidiosis

Sarcocystis hominis is the least common of the human coccidial small intestinal infections, in western countries at least [158]. It is only rarely associated with AIDS and then usually in tropical countries [158].

Microsporidiosis

Microsporidia are obligate, intracellular, spore-forming protozoa of uncertain phylogeny, generally considered closely related to other coccidioses [186]. Among the more than 1000 species, *Enterocytozoon bieneusi* and *Encephalitozoon (Septata) intestinalis* have been associated with diarrhoea, in particular in the context of AIDS and organ transplantation [187–189]. The introduction of HAART has, however, reduced the risk for microsporidiosis dramatically [190]. Overall, the prevalence in HIV-infected patients is low (0.16%) and microsporidiosis is most often diagnosed in patients with very low CD4+ cell counts [191]. Infection, causing diarrhoea, does occur rarely in the immunocompetent patients, sometimes as travellers' diarrhoea, usually from infected water supplies [235]. Sophisticated microbiological methods of diagnosis, including PCR, are now available and pathological examination is less often required [186,192].

The diagnosis formerly relied on electron microscopy, which reveals the phases of the life cycle: a proliferative phase known as merogony and a sporulating phase known as sporogony. The proliferative phase demonstrates small rounded organisms with one to six nuclei found within the cells as electron-lucent structures. The sporulating phase is characterised by electron-dense stacks of discs, which aggregate to form the polar tubule and later the spores. Both phases can be found in the apical portion of enterocytes. *Septata intestinalis* is characterised by numerous intracytoplasmic spores separated by granular material (hence the name *Septata*). Electron microscopic examination has been important for light microscopic diagnosis (Figure 20.14).

By light microscopy, the mucosa shows villous blunting and feathering of the surface epithelium at the tips of the villi. Organisms are concentrated in cells at the villous tips. Jejunal biopsies have the highest diagnostic yield. Semi-thin resin-embedded sections demonstrate the parasite better than routine sections (Figure 20.14). Special stains, including Gram stain (positive), trichrome, Warthin–Starry and Giemsa's stains, help in visualising spores.

In some AIDS cases, *E. bieneusi* spores have been demonstrated within the lamina propria, although this is not commonly associated with systemic infection [193,194]. On the other hand, systemic dissemination is described in *Septata intestinalis* infection [186]. IELs, primed by interferon-γ-producing dendritic cells and antimicrobial peptides, play a role against intracellular parasitic infections and are notably increased in the infection.

Leishmaniasis

Visceral leishmaniasis can involve the small intestine but western pathologists very rarely see the disease at this site except in HIV/AIDS-related disease [185]. There has been a European epidemic of visceral leishmaniasis in AIDS patients, despite the fact that the disease is not endemic there [195]. HIV-associated visceral leishmaniasis presents with fever, diarrhoea and hepatosplenomegaly and is

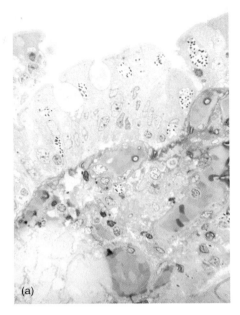

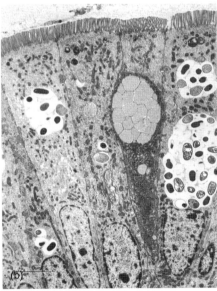

Figure 20.14 Microsporidiosis in the small intestine. This is infection by *Encephalitozoon intestinalis* in an AIDS patient. (a) Semi-thin resin-embedded sections demonstrate the intracellular meronts and sporonts much better than routine sections. (b) Electron microscopy shows the numerous meronts and sporonts.

associated with a high mortality in those untreated [196]. Mucosal biopsies from the small intestine reveal innumerable histiocytes within the lamina propria packed with classic Leishman–Donovan bodies (Figure 20.15), representing the amastigotes of *Leishmania donovani* [185]. Although techniques such as PCR have been successfully applied to the diagnosis of leishmaniasis [185], the diagnosis is usually very straightforward, once the possibility has

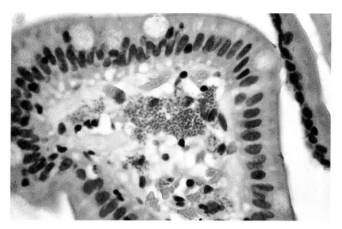

Figure 20.15 *Leishmania donovani* infection in the duodenal mucosa of an AIDS patient. There are numerous Leishman–Donovan bodies within the cytoplasm of intralaminal macrophages.

been entertained, because of the number and characteristic morphology of the parasites. Special stains are not normally required.

Other protozoa

Amoebiasis, caused by *Entamoeba histolytica*, and the ciliate protozoan, *Balantidium coli*, can involve the small intestine, especially the terminal ileum. Nevertheless the colorectum is the primary site of infection and large intestinal biopsies are much more likely to detect these parasites (see 'Amoebiasis' and 'Balantidiasis', Chapter 35). Similarly Chagas' disease, chronic infection with *Trypanosoma cruzi*, can involve the small intestine with enteromegaly, neuropathy, loss of myenteric ganglia and muscle hypertrophy of the small bowel [197]. However, it is doubtful whether small bowel disease ever occurs in the absence of more marked disease in the oesophagus and colon: clinical and pathological features are usually much more marked in these organs (see 'Chagas' disease', in Chapter 4 and see also Chapter 35).

Helminthic infection

A large number of helminthic infections can involve the small intestine. Patients commonly present with lassitude, abdominal pain, diarrhoea and anaemia, the last being a typical presentation of hookworms. The diagnosis of helminthic infection is usually made by microbiological investigation of the stool. Nevertheless some infections may be demonstrated in histological specimens, both duodenal and ileal biopsies, and in resection specimens. Strongyloidiasis and schistosomiasis are perhaps the most commonly encountered, although hookworm larvae and ascariasis may be demonstrated in biopsy specimens. As these diseases are not often encountered in histopathologi-

cal practice, the interested reader should consult specialist texts for more comprehensive descriptions of these helminths, their life cycle and their morphological appearances [199–200].

Hookworms

Hookworm infestation is commonly caused by *Ankylostoma duodenale* in southern Europe, Asia and the Middle East, and by *Necator americanus* in Africa and the American continents, although mixed infections are common [198]. The disease infects around 1.3 billion people worldwide; about 100 million of these have profound long-term morbidity as a result of the infestation [201]. Patients with severe hookworm infestation present with anaemia due to profound blood loss from the small intestine. The blood loss, and subsequent anaemia, appear to be directly proportional to the number of adult worms in the bowel [202]. Most patients do not have true malabsorption and probably have a normal small intestinal mucosa [203]. However, infestation has been associated with a malabsorption syndrome, with shortening and broadening of the villi, many of which have a club-shaped appearance; these morphological changes are said to revert to normal if the disease is successfully treated [204]. The worms have characteristic features [198]: a thick outside cuticle and a wide open mouth buried deep in the mucosa.

Ascariasis

Ascaris lumbricoides is the most common and largest nematode infecting the human gastrointestinal tract [205]. The worms are ingested as ova in infected food or drink. Hatched larvae penetrate the intestinal mucosa and reach the lung via the portal system. Here they develop further before being coughed up and swallowed. The worms then develop in the small intestine and the adult worms, which may be up to 20mm long, can inhabit any part of the small bowel. Usually the anterior part of the worm, and occasionally ova, are found in tissue sections.

The geographical distribution of ascariasis is worldwide, although it is more common in tropical countries [206]. The disease is usually asymptomatic but concentrations of the large worms in the small intestine can cause obstruction, volvulus and even appendicitis [207–209]. More sinister is the worm's ability to migrate into ducts, especially the pancreatic and biliary ducts, where the parasites are a recognised cause of pancreatitis, biliary obstruction and hepatic pathology [205,210].

Anisakiasis

Infection by the helminths *Anisakis* spp. is increasingly recognised in the small intestine and, more particularly, in the stomach [211]. *Anisakis simplex* is most often implicated and this worm has been recognised as a cause of allergic gastroenteritis with or without anaphylaxis, eosinophilic gastroenteritis and intestinal obstruction [212–214]. The disease is particularly associated with the ingestion of raw fish and its gastric manifestations are most readily encountered in Japan [215].

Capillariasis

Infection with the small nematode, *Capillaria philippinensis*, is mainly restricted to south-eastern Asia, especially the Philippines and Thailand, although it is now well recognised in other parts of Asia and in Egypt [202,215]. The disease has also been described in patients from non-endemic areas [216]. A range of symptoms occurs, depending on the parasite population, but severe infection produces diarrhoea, malabsorption with wasting and, sometimes, death. The worm, 3–4 mm long, may be demonstrated embedded in jejunal mucosa. Humans are infected by ingestion of raw freshwater fish [216].

Schistosomiasis

Intestinal schistosomiasis is classically associated with infection with the trematode *Schistosoma mansoni*. However, less commonly *S. haematobium* can involve the intestines, as can *S. japonicum* in eastern Asia. In all forms of schistosomiasis, large bowel involvement is much more common than small bowel pathology (see 'Schistosomiasis', Chapter 35) [217–221]. Small intestinal involvement by schistosomiasis can mimic Crohn's disease, with small bowel stricturing, or TB, with extensive transmural fibrosis and small white serosal nodules resembling milia, or alternatively present with malabsorption [217,222,223]. Schistosomal polyposis does not occur in the small bowel. Microscopically the ova with their characteristic morphology, especially their spines, are surrounded by a granulomatous reaction in which epithelioid cells, lymphocytes and, sometimes, eosinophils predominate [198].

Strongyloidiasis

Strongyloides stercoralis is a small nematode that inhabits the upper small bowel. Its distribution is worldwide and its prevalence rate may reach 80% in lower socio-economic groups of developing countries [224]. Indigenous cases are well described in western countries [225,226]. The helminth is almost unique in its ability to remain dormant in the small intestine for many years and reactivate, often with hyperinfestation, especially in immunocompromised hosts and patients treated for neoplastic disease [224,227,228].

Primary infection presents with abdominal pain and diarrhoea: around 90% of patients will demonstrate a

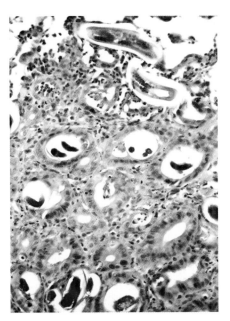

Figure 20.16 Hyperinfestation of the duodenal mucosa with *Strongyloides stercoralis* larvae. They are characteristically seen within the lumina of crypts.

peripheral eosinophilia. The worm is small, measuring 2–3 mm long, and the female is demonstrated in the crypts of the duodenal and jejunal mucosa (Figure 20.16). The male nematode is seldom seen. Biopsy findings are variable but there may be villous atrophy that reverts to normal after therapy. Malabsorption is rare in the primary infection. In hyperinfection, there is massive proliferation of rhabtidiform larvae of *S. stercoralis* and maturation to filariform larvae, which are demonstrable in large numbers embedded in the crypts of the small intestinal mucosa (Figure 20.16). The filariform larvae can invade into the mucosa and soon become systemic, resulting in widespread dissemination. The disease is then rapidly fatal unless detected quickly and treated appropriately [224].

Other helminthic infestations of the small intestine

Many other helminths have life cycles that involve the small intestine and/or may present with symptoms and signs referable to the small bowel. These include *Toxocara canis*, *Trichuris trichuria*, *Trichinella spiralis*, *Angiostrongylus costaricensis*, fluke infections including *Clonorchis sinensis*, *Fasciola hepatica* and *Opisthorchis viverrini*, other trematodes and tapeworm infections. However, seldom, if ever, do any of these infestations present to the histopathologist and a comprehensive account of their pathology is deemed beyond the scope of this book [198,200,229,230].

Crohn's disease

In 1932, Crohn, Ginzberg and Oppenheimer described the condition of regional enteritis, the terminal ileal presentation of Crohn's disease [231]. The condition was recognised earlier, for instance by the Polish physician Lesniowski, and also reported by the Scottish surgeon, Dalziel (in 1913) [232]. Until the 1960s it was believed that Crohn's disease affected only the small intestine. It was then that Lockhart-Mummery and Morson described involvement of the large intestine [233,234]. Subsequently it has become increasingly important to differentiate colorectal Crohn's disease from the other major form of CIBD, ulcerative colitis. This distinction remains a major part of the gastrointestinal pathologist's workload. Later it became clear that Crohn's disease could involve any part of the gut, from mouth to anus, and that there could be extra-intestinal manifestations of the disease [235–239]. Thus Crohn's disease is now accepted as a pan-gastrointestinal pathology with systemic manifestations. It remains an enigmatic condition, not least because it is still uncertain whether it represents one or several different diseases and its aetiopathogenesis is still not fully understood.

Epidemiology

The incidence of CIBD, in general, and of Crohn's disease varies greatly worldwide. Genetic and environmental factors are assumed to play a significant role in the aetiology and these may explain the differences in incidence rates among various geographical areas.

The first assessment of the incidence of CIBD was carried out retrospectively in Rochester, Minnesota. The reported incidence of Crohn's disease was $1.9/10^5$ in 1935–54. The incidence rates began to increase in the late 1930s in the USA and in 1950s in north and western Europe. The increased incidence of Crohn's disease follows the increase in incidence of ulcerative colitis by about 15–20 years. Although the incidence of ulcerative colitis tended to level off to a plateau or even decreased in the late 1990s, the incidence of Crohn's disease continues to increase and is actually in the range 3.1–14.6 cases per 10^5 people [240].

The prevalence of Crohn's disease in North America is in the range 26.0–198.5 cases per 10^5 individuals. In Europe the prevalence is very similar ($144/10^5$). Studies from the UK indicate that the prevalence of Crohn's disease in the population cohort born in 1970 was significantly higher than in the cohort born in 1958. Overall Crohn's disease is becoming more prevalent than ulcerative colitis.

A rising trend in the incidence and prevalence is also noted in Asia. The prevalence of Crohn's disease in Japan increased from 2.9 cases per 10^5 in 1986 to 13.5 cases per 10^5 individuals in 1998. Similar observations have been made in South Korea and Singapore. In contrast to western studies, which generally show an equal gender distribution, Asian data show a male predominance, ranging from 1.67:1 to 2.9:1. The genetic susceptibilities in Asian patients also differ from those of western patients as *NOD2/CARD15* mutations (see below) are much less common.

In western studies, Crohn's disease is diagnosed most frequently in patients in the 20- to 30-year age group. Another peak of incidence has been noted in the 60- to 70-year age group. Several epidemiological studies also suggest that the incidence of Crohn's disease in children has increased since 2000. The data are difficult to assess because of different definitions of childhood, with upper age limits varying between 14 and 17 years of age, but similar rising trends have been observed in Europe and Australia [241,242].

Aetiology and pathogenesis

Although many advances have been made in the understanding of CIBD pathogenesis, the aetiology of Crohn's disease remains a mystery. Prevailing theories suggest that intestinal inflammation is the result of inappropriate and ongoing activation of the mucosal immune system in genetically susceptible persons, triggered by as yet unknown environmental factors. The identification of susceptibility genes for Crohn's disease has demonstrated the importance of the epithelial barrier function and innate and adaptive immunity in the pathogenesis. Studies into the environmental factors have implicated commensal bacteria, rather than conventional pathogens, as drivers of deregulated immunity and Crohn's disease.

Genetic factors

The strongest evidence supporting the contribution of inherited factors to the pathogenesis of Crohn's disease comes from the study of disease concordance rates in twin pairs. These are much higher in monozygotic (20–50%) than in dizygotic twins (0–7%) [243]. As the concordance rates in monozygotic twins are not 100%, environmental factors must play a role as well. The twin data are supplemented by studies of prevalence in patients' relatives showing an increased risk. Reported figures are 2–22%. The risk is greater in siblings than in other family members.

The development of a linkage map of the human genome has enabled scanning of the whole genome for loci associated with susceptibility to monogenic or polygenic diseases [244]. Several studies have identified susceptibility loci with variable degrees of replication and statistical support. Some seem specific for Crohn's disease whereas others seem to infer susceptibility to CIBD overall.

In 2001, two independent groups identified the *CARD15* gene on chromosome 16q as a susceptibility gene in Crohn's disease. The protein product of the *CARD15* gene consists of three functional parts. The C-terminal part contains a leucine-rich repeat (LRR) domain. Most Crohn's disease-associated mutations affect this LRR domain. These LRR domains are also present in toll-like receptors, the most important receptors of the innate immune system. Toll-like receptors are involved in pathogen-associated pattern recognition together with the NOD proteins, to which CARD15 belongs (the older name for CARD15 was NOD2). The CARD15 protein is expressed in cells of monocyte lineage and intestinal epithelial cells. Among the latter, the highest concentration of CARD15 mRNA has been found in Paneth cells. This finding is potentially important because Paneth cells are more abundant in the terminal ileum and CARD15 mutations are associated with ileal Crohn's disease. Furthermore, Paneth cells synthesise and secrete anti-bacterial proteins such as lysozyme and defensins.

NOD2/CARD15 mutations are associated with a decreased activation of NF-κB in mononuclear cells. Loss-of-function mutations may result in altered host–microbe interactions. Mutations of CARD15 are present in about 50% of Crohn's disease patients and in 20% of healthy controls in white (but not in Asian or African) populations. Mutations are therefore neither necessary nor sufficient for disease occurrence.

Further studies have associated the ATG16LI gene with increased risk for Crohn's disease. ATG16LI is a member of a family of genes involved in autophagy, a process contributing to the degradation of intracellular pathogens, antigen processing and regulation of T-cell homoeostasis. It is broadly expressed by intestinal epithelial cells, antigen-presenting cells, CD4+, CD8+ and CD19+ T cells. One of the stronger gene associations observed is in the gene encoding for the IL-23 receptor (IL-23R). IL-23R belongs to the adaptive immune system, and the IL-23R signalling pathway has a key role in mediating end-organ inflammation. The combination of different genetic variants including CARD15, ATG and IL-23R may be used for the prediction of the likelihood of developing the disease [245–250].

Environmental factors, including diet

Smoking is a strong risk factor for the development of Crohn's disease. Appendectomy for an inflammatory condition performed before the age of 20 is associated with a low subsequent risk for ulcerative colitis but with an increased risk for Crohn's disease. The composition of the diet may play a role in development of the disease [251]. Microbes are, however, the most consistently implicated factor in Crohn's disease pathogenesis. This hypothesis is based on epidemiological, clinico-pathological, genetic and experimental evidence. It has been proposed that increased hygiene and the concomitant delayed exposure to enteric pathogens have contributed to the rise in incidence. Chang-

ing dietary practices such as decreased consumption of oats, rye and bran, and drinking well water instead of tap water may further favour a shift from protective to harmful gastrointestinal flora. Another possible factor with sustained alterations in the gut flora may be the increased use of antibiotics. Early appendectomy may also affect the intestinal flora. It has further been observed that Crohn's disease recurrence in the neo-terminal ileum after curative resection depends on the presence of the faecal stream. A possible explanation is that the anastomosis after the resection influences colonisation of the neo-terminal ileum. When compared with control individuals, the neo-terminal ileum in Crohn's disease patients is more heavily colonised by E. coli, enterococci, Bacteroides spp. and fusobacteria.

Experimental evidence supports a role of the flora in the initiation of inflammation. All the genetically engineered animal models require commensal enteric bacteria for the development of intestinal inflammation. Crohn's disease occurs most commonly in the distal ileum and colon, two locations containing high concentrations of intestinal bacteria (10^7–10^8 organisms/g luminal content in the ileum and 10^{11}–10^{12} in the colon). However, despite the abundance of data for the implication of bacteria in the aetiopathogenesis of Crohn's disease, the precise role of bacteria remains elusive.

Three not necessarily mutually exclusive theories have been proposed for the aetiopathogenesis of Crohn's disease:
1. An as yet unidentified persistent pathogen
2. An abnormally permeable mucosal barrier leading to excessive bacterial translocation
3. Breakdown in the balance between putative 'protective' and 'harmful' intestinal bacteria

Numerous specific bacteria have been proposed as candidate causative agents including Mycobacterium avium ss. paratuberculosis, Mycobacterium kansasii and Listeria monocytogenes but for none of these has proof been demonstrated. The variation in results may be partly due to the fastidious culture requirements and the occurrence of some bacteria such as Pseudomonas maltophilia and Mycobacterium kansasii, as cell wall-deficient forms (L-forms). These L-forms may be involved in disease causation or may be a result of the disease process itself. Adherent-invasive E. coli (AIEC) is a special strain that has also been linked to the development of Crohn's disease. The reference strain LF82 is able to adhere to intestinal epithelial cells, invade them, and survive and replicate within macrophages [252–256].

The proportion of surgically treated Crohn's disease patients with bacterial translocation before antibiotics varies between 30% and 50% and is much higher than in control individuals (5–15%). Bacterial material can be recovered from different components of the bowel wall using specific primers and microdissection. Several studies have also shown that the faecal microflora differs between

Crohn's disease patients and healthy control individuals [257,258].

Immunopathology

The pathogenesis of Crohn's disease involves a complex interplay between factors involved in the aetiology of the disease, whether genetic, environmental or immunological. Generally, the intestinal immune response is mounted by the mucosal innate and adaptive immune systems and, similar to systemic immune responses, this reaction is initiated by recognition of targets by the innate immune system, which then mediates the activation of the adaptive immune response. It is commonly hypothesised, although not proven, that, in Crohn's disease, members of the resident flora are targets for the immune activation. A deficiency of the innate intestinal mucosal barrier has been proposed as the primary defect. The hypothesis is based on the analogy between Crohn's disease and genetically defined syndromes of neutrophil and monocyte dysfunction, such as glycogen storage Ib, the identification of *CARD15/NOD2* as a susceptibility variant and the identification of defensin modifications.

In Crohn's colitis tissues, normal epithelial cells show no striking abnormalities, e.g. MUC2 and MUC3 mRNA expression displays a normal pattern, regardless of whether the mucosa manifests active or quiescent disease [259]. However, studies screening for changes in gene expression show changes in barrier genes.

Other alterations include the expression of toll-like receptor (TLR)-4 and TLR-2 which is increased in Crohn's disease, although TLR-2 is also upregulated in diverticulitis and ulcerative colitis, and the expression of Paneth cell α-defensin HD-5. HD-5 is normally found at abundant levels in the small intestine but it is diminished in ileal Crohn's disease. This molecule belongs to the defensins, a group of antimicrobial peptides of the innate immunity with microbicidal activity against Gram-negative and Gram-positive bacteria, viruses, fungi and protozoa. The decreased expression may be responsible for a diminished antimicrobial defence. The findings are supported by differences in the induction of human β-defensin HBD-2 in the colon. Strong HBD-2 induction is observed in ulcerative colitis but not in Crohn's disease [260].

Changes in the gut flora may thus not be contained properly by the innate immune system in Crohn's disease. Subsequently the adaptive immune response would be activated and predominate. This response is composed of a network of cells and can be polarised to secrete a defined set of cytokines. Naïve T cells differentiate to become mature T cells but they may differ depending on the cytokine milieu that they encounter during the differentiation.

Traditionally, T cells have been divided into T-helper (Th) 1-type cells that secrete predominantly IL-2, interferon-γ (INF-γ) and TNF whereas Th2-type cells secrete IL-4, IL-5, IL-10 and IL-13. A predominance of IL-12 favours development of Th1-type cells whereas IL-4 favours Th2-cell differentiation. Differentiation of T cells is, however, more complicated. IL-23, which shares the p40 subunit with IL-12, is a cytokine axis leading to the differentiation of IL-17- and IL-6-secreting cells.

Overall, it appears that expression of Th1 cytokines is dominant in the mucosa of Crohn's disease patients. In the lamina propria, T cells are increased but with a relatively normal CD4:CD8 ratio [261]. However, the number of T cells with an activated phenotype, expressing IL-2 and transferrin receptor, and the levels of TNF-α are increased [262].

There is also a marked increase in total immunoglobulin production within the mucosa, particularly IgG [263]. IgG2, an antibody produced in response to carbohydrate and bacterial antigens, predominates [264]. A significant association between disease activity and the numbers of immunoglobulin-containing cells in the lamina propria has been demonstrated [265] although there is less evidence for autoantibody production in Crohn's disease compared with ulcerative colitis [266].

There is an increase in production of monocytes in patients with Crohn's disease, with increased recruitment into the intestinal wall as macrophages [267,268]. There are two main types of macrophages, mature tissue macrophages (RFD7 antibody positive) and interdigitating dendritic cells, which are antigen presenting and found predominantly in organised lymphoid tissue. The distribution of these subsets is grossly altered in Crohn's disease, especially with clustering of RFD7-positive cells in granulomas [269,270]. In inflamed areas, there is also an overexpression of T-cell co-stimulatory molecules, CD80 and CD86, on monocytes.

Crohn's disease is characterised by a florid neutrophil infiltrate and this produces superoxide radicals and nitric oxide which are thought to be important in the production of epithelial damage [271]. Furthermore, it has been shown that the mucosa in Crohn's disease lacks antioxidant defences [272]. Eosinophils are also elevated in the mucosa: these secrete proteins such as eosinophilic basic protein and IL-5 which may enhance the mucosal damage [273].

Immunohistochemistry has been used for the study of the expression of a large variety of markers including cell-specific markers (subsets of lymphocytes), adhesion molecules, chemokines, cell cycle-related markers and growth factors. Several studies indicate that many different markers are upregulated in active CIBD. Cytokine expression in Crohn's disease has been extensively studied because many of these proteins appear to have a major involvement in the initiation, propagation and recurrence of inflammation. There is increased production of immunostimulatory cytokines, notably IL-1, and the levels of IL-6 and the pro-inflammatory TNF-α are also increased [274–278]. This correlates with the success of monoclonal antibodies to TNF-α in the treatment of Crohn's disease [279,280]. Immunomodulatory cytokines have been less extensively studied: there appears to be overactivity of IL-2 in Crohn's disease whereas, in ulcerative colitis, there is reduced activity [281,282]. There is also evidence of increased activity of IFN-γ [283,284] and possible involvement of IL-4 in early recurrences of Crohn's disease [273].

The local expression of many chemokines is increased and many of these are involved in the destruction of tissue by the recruitment of neutrophils. The chemokine CXCL5 immunoreactivity (mRNA and protein) is increased in tissue sections from inflamed areas. The expression is predominantly situated in crypt epithelial cells. CXCL10, involved in the recruitment of lymphocytes, is observed in mononuclear cells of the lamina propria and its expression is significantly upregulated in inflamed tissue. CXCL8 (IL-8) expression is associated with active lesions. Positively staining cells are focally distributed in samples from patients with Crohn's disease [285].

Several studies have shown that the expression of HLA-DR, major histocompatibility complex (MHC) class II molecules, in stromal cells is increased in ulcerative colitis and Crohn's disease and, in addition, an aberrant expression is noted on colonic epithelial cells. A comparable expression is noted with HLA-G, a non-classic class I molecule [286]. HLA-DR expression is reduced with different types of treatment including 5-acetylsalicylic acid and monoclonal

antibodies directed against TNF-α [287]. The aberrant expression is therefore probably related more to disease activity.

Further evidence for the importance of immunological mechanisms in Crohn's disease has been sought from animal models. There are numerous gene knock-out animal models that show intestinal inflammation, including IL-2- and IL-10-deficient mouse models [288,289]. Other mouse models have demonstrated that intestinal inflammation can be produced when there are abnormalities of the epithelial cell junction complexes, notably N-cadherin expression, suggesting that altered epithelial permeability is an important, and possibly primary, abnormality in CIBD.

Abnormalities are not limited to inflammatory and epithelial cells. There are also substantial changes in the stroma. Aberrant increased expression of tenascin, a component of the extracellular matrix involved in cell migration and healing, is observed underneath the epithelium and in the lamina propria, and correlates with disease activity. In Crohn's disease, the expression of collagen types I, III and IV can be increased and the mucosal distribution becomes irregular. Biochemical analysis demonstrates a quantitative increase in total collagen content and of collagen types I and V in all layers of the bowel wall (Figure 20.17) [290].

Overall, the upregulation of chemokines and other molecules is mostly related with disease activity and does not help to discriminate from Crohn's disease or other inflammatory conditions. The expression of markers may thus help to assess disease activity and response to therapy but

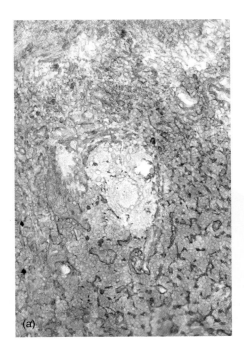 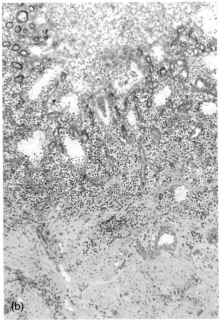

Figure 20.17 Crohn's disease: staining with antibodies directed against (a) collagen type I showing deposition around a granuloma and (b) collagen type V showing stromal deposition in the granulation tissue of an ulcer.

(a)

(b)

it is not useful in routine practice [291]. Immunohistochemistry has, therefore, no current diagnostic value.

Macroscopic appearances

The classic macroscopic manifestations of small intestinal Crohn's disease are ulceration, strictures, fissuring and thickening of the gut wall. The lesions are discontinuous and, in their earliest form, they present as small, aphthous ulcers. They vary in size from tiny, pinpoint haemorrhagic lesions to small, clearly defined, shallow ulcers with a white base, appearing in an otherwise normal mucosa. The white base explains the derivation of the word 'aphtha' from the Greek for a 'white spot'. They can be missed easily if the specimen is not carefully examined (Figure 20.18).

Evidence suggests that these early lesions may take several years to progress sufficiently to give rise to detectable clinical or radiological signs. Serial studies have followed their progression through more extensive linear and serpiginous ulcers to stenosis, the latter developing after at least 3 years (Figure 20.19) [292,293]. Although aphthous ulcers can also occur in infections and drug-related pathology, the larger linear and serpiginous lesions are more characteristic for Crohn's disease and more common on the mesenteric border. More severe ulceration with complete circumferential loss of the mucosa is seen in stenosing areas.

Small bowel strictures in Crohn's disease may be short or long, single or multiple. They are more common in the ileum than in the jejunum (Figure 20.20) and much more common than in the duodenum. The classic, single, long segment, 'hose-pipe' stricture of the terminal ileum is the basis for the 'string sign of Kantor' seen radiologically (Figures 20.17 and 20.21). There is evidence that such extensive stricturing terminal ileal disease is becoming less common [293]. This is possibly because it represents a more advanced form of the disease, less readily seen now because of the relative success of anti-inflammatory treatment.

The classic 'cobblestone' appearance of the mucosal surface in Crohn's disease is seen in about a quarter of all cases. The cobblestones are formed as a result of intercom-

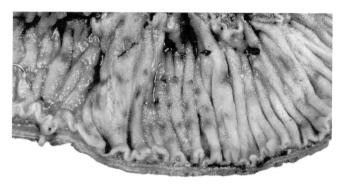

Figure 20.18 Crohn's disease in the ileum: numerous aphthous ulcers are seen in this segment, proximal to a terminal ileal stricture.

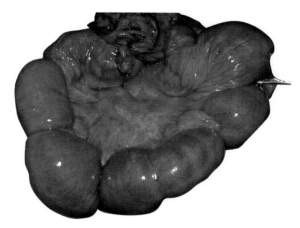

Figure 20.20 Multiple short small intestinal strictures in Crohn's disease.

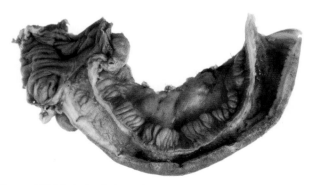

Figure 20.19 A classic hosepipe-type stricture of the terminal ileum with extensive stricturing due to Crohn's disease.

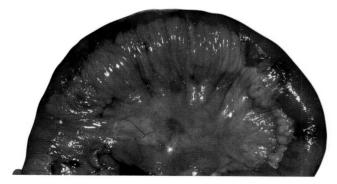

Figure 20.21 Crohn's disease of the ileum: this demonstrates the marked thickening of the bowel wall. The serosal surface shows prominent fat wrapping.

municating crevices or fissures and ulcerations surrounding islands of surviving mucosa, raised up by the underlying inflammation and oedema (Figure 20.22). Considerable oedema of the intestinal mucosa is often a useful sign of active disease. Fissuring is a very important sign of Crohn's disease and must be looked for carefully, at both the macroscopic and microscopic levels. Extensive fissuring and cobblestoning can progress to inflammatory polyp formation, although this feature is much more common in the large bowel [294]. In the small intestine, inflammatory polyps have been reported in approximately 20% of the cases. These are usually small, measuring a few millimetres in length, but giant forms have been described. They are more common in Crohn's disease than in ulcerative colitis and may produce symptoms by themselves.

Fissuring ulcers can give rise to abscesses, sinuses or fistulae between involved segments and adjacent organs or nearby uninvolved loops. Fissuring ulcers often just reach the muscularis propria. Sinuses are lesions that penetrate deep into the mesentery. Fistulae pass through the muscularis propria and are responsible for abnormal communications between the lumen of the gut and the mesentery and another hollow organ, abdominal wall and/or skin. Histologically they are composed of granulation tissue, surrounding a lumen that is mostly filled with debris and inflammatory cells, in particular neutrophils. Occasionally the lumen is lined by flattened intestinal epithelial cells with no goblet cells. Non-epithelialised fistulae are covered by a thin layer of (myo)fibroblasts, focally forming a new basement membrane, as demonstrated by electron micros-

copy. The granulation tissue shows central infiltration by CD45+ T cells, followed by a small band of CD68+ macrophages and dense accumulation of CD20+ B cells. These lesions are observed in about 20–30% of cases. Fistulae are often associated with strictures [294].

Small intestinal Crohn's disease has been divided into three main types according to the Vienna and Montreal classifications: primarily perforating or penetrating; fibro-stenosing or stricturing; and non-stricturing, non-penetrating. The value of this classification remains to be determined. Disease behaviour is dynamic over time. Several studies have demonstrated that patients with predominantly inflammatory disease at diagnosis are very likely to develop either fistulising or stricturing complications within 5–10 years. However, ileal disease and the development of fistulae and strictures seems more commonly associated with mutations in *CARD15* and phenotypes of the disease may well be explained by underlying genetic factors [295–297]. Whether Crohn's disease presents primarily as an ulcerative, stricturing or cobblestone form, or as a combination of these changes, it is almost always a discontinuous pathology. Multiple lesions are common and may be widely separated but, even in extensively diseased intestine, there are almost always small patches of intervening normal bowel (see Figure 20.20).

In small bowel Crohn's disease, the bowel wall is usually considerably thickened and the inflammation is transmural, sometimes with involvement of peri-intestinal fat and serosa by fibrosis and adhesions (Figure 20.23). The connective tissue changes of Crohn's disease include neuronal, vascular, muscular, fibrosing and fat abnormalities [298].

The serosal surface provides useful macroscopic features toward a diagnosis of Crohn's disease (Figure 20.23). These include the presence of tiny 'tubercles' which, when examined microscopically, are seen to be the sarcoid-like

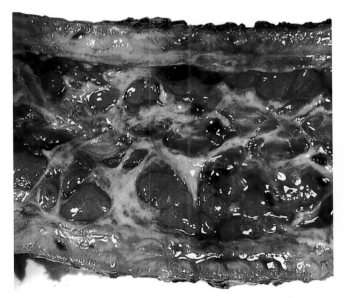

Figure 20.22 Cobblestoning of the mucosa in Crohn's disease: intercommunicating fissures (cleft-like ulcers) and crevices in the mucosa separate islets of mucosa which are raised up by oedema. (Courtesy P. Van Eyken.)

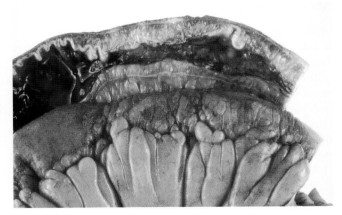

Figure 20.23 A Crohn's disease stricture of the ileum: this demonstrates the marked thickening of the bowel wall. The serosal surface shows prominent fat wrapping, the extent of which correlates directly with the stricture.

granulomas of Crohn's disease, and 'fat wrapping'. The presence of tubercles may be a very prominent feature, resembling the appearance in tuberculosis [299]. Fat wrapping, in which hyperplasia of the subserosal and mesenteric fat extends around the bowel wall to become circumferential on the anti-mesenteric aspect of the bowel, is a characteristic feature of small bowel Crohn's disease (see Figure 20.21) [298,300,301]. It is defined on a transverse section of the intestine and regarded as being present when more than 50% of the intestinal circumference is affected. The corresponding mesentery is usually thickened and retracted. It is observed in 75% of the small intestinal surgical specimens of Crohn's disease. It correlates closely with activity of disease, most notably transmural inflammation, and is used by surgeons to gauge the extent of disease at the time of resection [298,300,302].

In small intestinal Crohn's disease, the regional lymph nodes are often enlarged but, in many cases, they are quite normal histologically. It must be remembered that the ileocaecal lymph nodes are normally relatively large and that the size of nodes varies with age. Mesenteric lymph nodes in Crohn's disease may contain non-caseating epithelioid cell granulomas but only in a minority of cases. Consequently, biopsy of such nodes is not a sensitive method of making the diagnosis. However, it can be useful for distinguishing Crohn's disease from important mimics, notably TB and yersiniosis (see below).

Changes in the proximal small intestine, especially the duodenum, can be much more subtle. Although earlier studies have suggested that duodenal involvement is unusual, only occurring in about 2% of cases [303], it has become clear, from large-scale endoscopic and histopathological studies, that more subtle duodenal pathology is relatively commonplace, changes being demonstrable in about 25% of Crohn's disease patients [304,305].

Microscopic appearances

Small intestinal Crohn's disease exhibits a variable microscopic pattern and some of the more important features may be entirely absent. This may be due to either the natural history of the disease or treatment. A definite diagnosis on endoscopic biopsies may, therefore, be difficult because of the lack of characteristic features. In surgical specimens, however, usually several abnormalities can always be detected, even after treatment, because of the damage in the deep bowel wall, due to transmural inflammation.

The most characteristic microscopic features of the disease are its multifocal involvement and the triumvirate of focal ulceration (which is often fissuring and may result in fistula formation), transmural inflammation in the form of lymphoid aggregates and granulomas. These are essentially observed only in surgical specimens. Endo-

scopic biopsies have to rely on discontinuity of the inflammation, villous architectural abnormalities and granulomas. For the detection of the multifocal involvement, multiple biopsies are indicated [306]. It may, however, be difficult for the endoscopist to obtain multiple biopsies in certain areas of the small intestine. Some lesions are observed with video capsule endoscopy and cannot be biopsied, except during enteroscopy.

Discontinuous involvement, granulomas and transmural inflammation are generally regarded as the hallmarks of intestinal Crohn's disease. Although usually considered a granulomatous disease, it is important to recognise that granulomas may be absent in up to 50% of cases of small intestinal Crohn's disease [307]. Nevertheless, when present, especially in the small bowel, they are a very useful diagnostic pointer.

A granuloma is a circumscribed collection of epithelioid histiocytes, with or without giant cells, which are usually of Langhans' type. Granulomas may be found throughout the bowel wall, including the mucosa and superficial submucosa of duodenal and ileoscopic biopsies (Figure 20.24). They are less common in the small bowel than in the large bowel and anal region [308], are less commonly seen in patients with a long clinical history [308,309] and are more common in younger patients with a shorter duration of disease [307]. Their presence does not influence recurrence rates or prognosis [308,310,311]. Granulomas are often related to areas of ulceration and transmural inflammation but they may be seen in isolation away from areas of active disease [312]. They often have a close relationship to lymphatics [313] whereas a smaller proportion is related to small blood vessels (Figure 20.25) [314,315]. In about 25% of cases, the local lymph nodes in the mesentery will contain granulomas but it is exceptional for granulomas to be present in lymph nodes and not in the bowel wall

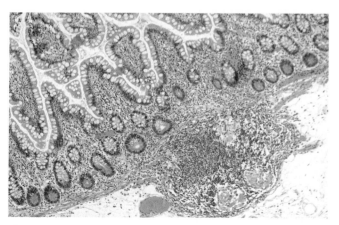

Figure 20.24 An ileoscopic biopsy demonstrating well-formed epithelioid cell granulomas, basally situated in the mucosa and submucosa in the vicinity of a lymphoid aggregate.

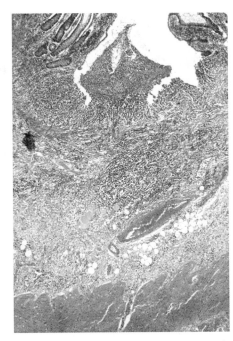

Figure 20.26 An ileal biopsy from a patient with Crohn's disease. It shows an aphthous ulcer with the form of a so-called mountain pike ulcer.

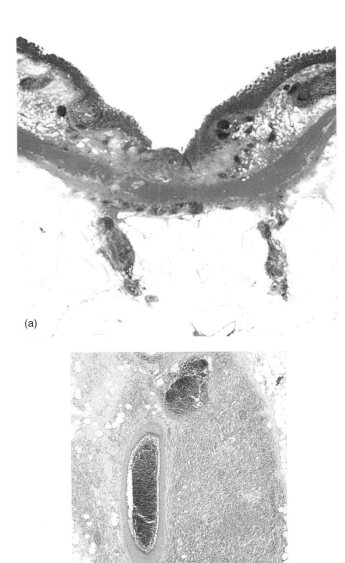

Figure 20.25 (a) A whole-mount section of jejunal Crohn's disease. The transmural inflammation is evident with inflammation extending along two mesenteric blood vessel bundles. (b) A high power view of one of the blood vessel bundles shows prominent chronic inflammation around a vein and artery with a single well-formed granuloma (with giant cell) close to the arterial wall (below).

[307]. Nodes containing granulomas are no larger than those without [316].

Focal inflammation in a background of normal mucosa is a characteristic and highly prevalent feature of small intestinal Crohn's disease. The earliest lesion in the disease is probably a zone of patchy epithelial necrosis including loss of M cells, and inflammation, often superficial to lymphoid aggregates and/or Peyer's patches, which then develops into the characteristic aphthous ulcer (Figure 20.26). Variants of these early lesions are ulcers at the base of crypts with neutrophils streaming into the bowel lumen (leading later to so-called mountain peak ulcers), villous abnormalities and damage of small capillaries [317].

Villous abnormalities include variability in size and shape, the presence of dilated lymphatics and mucin preservation of surface epithelial cells or increased mucin secretion (hypercrinia), even in the presence of inflammation. Distribution of Paneth cells in the crypt base is often irregular. Other mucosal changes may signify previous (or concurrent) ulceration, especially so-called pseudo-pyloric metaplasia. This lesion, which comprises glands of the 'ulcer-associated cell lineage' (UACL), secretes trefoil peptides and growth factors, notably epidermal growth factor (EGF), which may accelerate healing mechanisms subsequent to ulceration [318–320]. UACL is diagnostically useful but is not specific to Crohn's disease: it may be seen in any chronic inflammatory pathology of the small intestine where previous ulceration has occurred, including non-steroidal anti-inflammatory drug (NSAID)-induced lesions, although in the western world Crohn's disease is the most significant causative factor.

Although small aphthous ulcers are a characteristic accompaniment of relatively early Crohn's disease, more extensive ulceration often takes the form of longitudinally orientated or deep crevice-like fissures. These knife-like clefts, sometimes branching, extend deeply into the bowel wall and are the histological basis for the formation of fistulae. Usually lined by granulation tissue, they may demonstrate epithelioid histiocytes and giant cells in their walls. They are particularly useful for the diagnosis of Crohn's disease when granulomas are absent but they are not pathognomonic: similar fissuring ulcers may sometimes occur in other small intestinal conditions including drug-induced ulceration, Behçet's disease and malignant lymphoma. Indeed, fissuring ulceration is also a prominent feature of 'ulcerative jejunitis', which represents early lymphomatous transformation in coeliac disease.

Even when granulomas and fissuring ulceration are absent, there still remain distinctive histological features of Crohn's disease. Perhaps the most prevalent and diagnostically useful feature is transmural inflammation in the form of multiple lymphoid aggregates (Figure 20.29). Often about the size of granulomas or somewhat larger, such well-formed lymphoid collections are scattered throughout the bowel wall but are particularly obvious in the submucosa and subserosa. In the latter, they are usually orientated in a line immediately adjacent to the outer aspect of the muscularis propria, forming the characteristic 'Crohn's rosary' which is readily identifiable in histological slides to the naked eye (Figure 20.27). Associated with the granulomas (Figure 20.28) and the transmural inflammation, there is gross bowel wall thickening, involving all the layers, with oedema and fibrosis being especially prominent in the submucosa. Lymphangiectasia is also a common feature, which is best appreciated in the submucosa and subserosa. It is probably associated with the formation of new lymphatics, a process called lymphangiogenesis.

In more long-standing disease, the 'connective tissue changes' of Crohn's disease become useful diagnostic features [298]. The macroscopic appearance of fat wrapping has already been described. Its microscopic basis is adipose cell hyperplasia, almost certainly related to chronic inflammation (see Figure 20.23) [300,301,302]. Indeed, it may be that the fat hyperplasia perpetuates the inflammation as it has been shown to secrete TNF-α [321]. Histological changes in nerves in Crohn's disease may be pronounced with marked hyperplasia of nerve fibres, especially in the submucosal and myenteric plexuses [298,322]. It could be that the basis of this neuronal hyperplasia is inflammation-induced axonal necrosis, a feature that is readily identifiable at the electron microscopic level [322,323]. Fibromuscular obliteration of the submucosa is another common feature. It may be accompanied by abnormalities of the musculature with splaying of the muscularis mucosae and distortion of the muscularis propria. It is often a major feature in 'burnt-out' disease [109,298].

Remodelling of the wall of arterioles and arteries with medial atrophy is a feature of early and late disease [298, 324]. Vasculitis, including granulomatous vasculitis, is a striking feature of a small number of cases of Crohn's

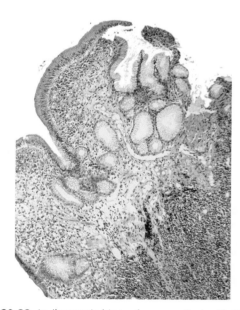

Figure 20.28 An ileoscopic biopsy from a patient with Crohn's disease. Villous architectural abnormalities and focal inflammation are the two most common histological abnormalities seen in ileoscopic biopsies in Crohn's disease. Pseudo-pyloric gland metaplasia or ulcer-associated cell lineage is present but is not specific for Crohn's disease.

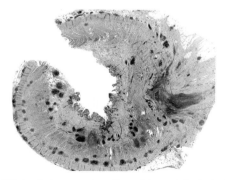

Figure 20.27 A whole-mount section of jejunal Crohn's disease. There is transmural inflammation in the form of lymphoid aggregates, forming the distinctive 'Crohn's rosary'. The subserosal aspect of a fistula is discernible (at right).

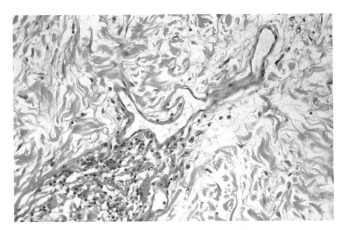

Figure 20.29 Crohn's disease: a granuloma adjacent to a lymphatic.

disease (see Figure 20.25) [325], more often seen in the early stages, but it is more common to find a granulomatous phlebitis. Apart from granulomatous phlebitis, veins in Crohn's disease may show irregular thickening of the media as a result of hyperplasia of fibres and muscle tissue [326]. Finally, lymphatic changes include prominent lymphangiectasia. This feature, along with the submucosal oedema and the close relationship of lymphocytic aggregates and granulomas to intramural and extramural lymphatic channels suggests that lymphatics may play a significant role in the pathogenesis of Crohn's disease [298] (Figure 20.29).

Crohn's disease in the duodenum

There is increasing interest in gastro-duodenal involvement in Crohn's disease, not least because minor abnormalities, easily detectable in mucosal biopsies at the time of upper gastrointestinal endoscopy, appear to be much more common than previously thought. These may provide substantial corroborative evidence for a diagnosis of Crohn's disease, especially when symptoms and signs are caused by more distal occult small intestinal disease which is poorly accessible to conventional diagnostic modalities. In children, upper gastrointestinal endoscopy is considered a standard procedure in the diagnostic work-up of CIBD patients.

About 15% of patients with ileo-colonic Crohn's disease will have histological changes in the duodenum, although gross involvement only affects about 2% of patients [303–305]. The histopathology of gastro-duodenal Crohn's disease includes a wide spectrum of changes, including focally enhanced (active) gastritis and granulomas. Focally enhanced or focal active gastritis is typified by small collections of lymphocytes and histiocytes surrounding a small group of foveolae or gastric glands, often with infiltrates of neutrophils. Focal active gastritis, in the absence of *Helicobacter pylori* involvement, has been said to be characteristic of gastric Crohn's disease with a prevalence ranging from 43% to 76%. Additional studies have found that focally active gastritis is present in up to 20% of children with ulcerative colitis, suggesting that this type of gastritis is a marker of CIBD in general. However, studies that used control groups have reported a prevalence of focally enhanced gastritis in non-CIBD patients in up to 19.4%. Therefore, this type of gastritis may not be such a good marker for the diagnosis of CIBD or CIBD-related gastritis except, probably, in young children [327,328].

Granulomas are clearly useful but are less common in the duodenum than in other parts of the intestines [305]. The frequency varies between 4.6% and 26% depending on the presence of endoscopic lesions, the number of biopsies and the number of sections examined. Microgranulomas are more common, occurring in about a third of cases [329], and are particularly useful in subtyping CIBD [330]. It should be stressed that duodenal Crohn's disease very often demonstrates abnormal histology in the presence of entirely normal endoscopic features [331]. Duodenal involvement is easier to diagnose when it does not involve the first and second parts of the duodenum where *Helicobacter*-associated disease is most prevalent. The morphological differential diagnosis includes duodenitis due to drugs.

Irregular thickening of the duodenal folds, a cobblestone-like appearance, polypoid lesions and focal ulceration are the most common endoscopic abnormalities in duodenal Crohn's disease but the lesions may be limited to oedema or erythema. They represent the macroscopic involvement of the duodenum, which is characterised by three patterns of disease: duodenal stenosis, fistulation and ulcerating disease which often does not evolve into the other two types and often resolves [332]. Fistulae may involve the stomach, other parts of the small bowel and/or the abdominal skin [333]. Duodenal involvement may be complicated by common bile duct obstruction and pancreatitis [334]. Although duodenal Crohn's disease can result in severe pathology, it is often associated with less morbidity and less need for surgical intervention than more distal small bowel disease [303]. Only very rarely is neoplastic change described in duodenal Crohn's disease [335].

The diagnosis of Crohn's disease in ileoscopic biopsies

The value of ileoscopic biopsies in the assessment of inflammatory diarrhoea and for the diagnosis of CIBD is well established [336–338]. Reaching the terminal ileum is now regarded as a prerequisite for adequate colonoscopy; the colonoscope can reach a considerable distance into the terminal ileum and so assess that part of the intestine most likely to be affected in Crohn's disease. Terminal ileal biopsies in CIBD are most useful in two circumstances: the diagnosis of isolated terminal ileal disease and the differential diagnosis of obvious colonic CIBD, both 'pancolitis' and left-sided disease. In combination with clinical data and multiple colonic biopsies, the procedure can provide a final diagnosis in up to 99% of patients [336,337].

Focal active inflammation and disturbed villous architecture are the most common features of terminal ileal Crohn's disease (see Figures 20.26 and 20.28) [336]. Granulomas are less often demonstrated in terminal ileal mucosal biopsies than in the colonic biopsies [307] but they are of great diagnostic value when detected. Other useful pointers include isolated giant cells, an eosinophil infiltrate and the presence of the ulcer-associated cell lineage (pseudopyloric metaplasia) within the mucosa [336]. Isolated terminal ileal chronic inflammatory pathology, in a western population, with some or all of these additional features, is most likely to represent Crohn's disease but caution is always advisable. In a younger age group, yersiniosis is a potential differential diagnosis whereas drugs (especially NSAIDs), other infections, Behçet's disease and the small bowel manifestations of ulcerative colitis should also be considered.

Differential diagnosis

A discussion of the pathological differential diagnosis of small intestinal Crohn's disease depends on the specimens available. In biopsies of the duodenum, the differential diagnosis is primarily *H. pylori*-associated duodenitis, coeliac disease, drug-induced disease and bacterial overgrowth. In biopsies of the ileum, infective enteritis, including infections of limited duration such as *Campylobacter jejuni* and yersiniosis and chronic infections such as TB, drug-induced pathology and small intestinal manifestations of ulcerative colitis are diagnostic alternatives.

TB remains an important differential diagnosis. It can show evidence of active necrotising granulomatous pathology but can also appear effete and closely mimic 'burnt-out' Crohn's disease. Histological features favouring a diagnosis of TB include the number, size and coalescence of granulomas and the presence of caseating necrosis [339]. Small granulomas, confluent granulomas, microgranulomas and focal inflammation with transmural inflammation in the form of lymphoid aggregates favour Crohn's disease [339]. In only about 50% of cases of TB will mycobacteria be detected by ZN staining [48]. Nodal granulomas may be seen in the absence of intramural granulomas in TB, unlike in Crohn's disease [48]. Other infective granulomatous conditions, including schistosomiasis, deep mycoses and larval infestations, are not often confused with Crohn's disease because the causative organisms are usually readily identifiable. Similarly viral enteritis, perhaps most notably caused

by CMV, can be a source of confusion but the cytopathic viral effects are usually evident.

Apart from TB, yersiniosis is the most likely infective enteritis to be confused with Crohn's disease. The most useful differentiating features are the central suppurative necrosis with coalescent granulomatosis, the relative lack of transmural inflammation and the presence of suppurative granulomatosis in local lymph nodes, all of which favour yersiniosis [79]. If there is any doubt, yersinia serology should be recommended.

Ulceration and/or stricturing of the small intestine may be seen as a result of drugs (especially NSAIDs), Behçet's disease, ischaemia, vasculitis and malignant lymphoma [48]. So-called burnt-out Crohn's disease may lack the usual inflammatory pathology and may mimic various hamartomas, ganglio-neuromatous pathology and effete TB [48,298]. Crohn's disease is also an important differential diagnosis of a florid eosinophil infiltrate in the small intestine (see 'Eosinophilic infiltrates in the small intestine' below).

Although granulomas are an important feature of Crohn's disease, it is important not to assume a diagnosis of Crohn's disease just because granulomas are present. They can be observed in metabolic disorders such as glycogen storage Ib, in a variety of infections such as those caused by *Campylobacter* and *Yersinia* spp. and even occasionally in drug-induced disease. In young children, the autosomal recessive disorder, chronic granulomatous disease (CGD), may involve the small intestine [340]. In Hermansky–Pudlak syndrome (HPS), an autosomal recessive multi-system disorder characterised by oculocutaneous albinism, functional platelet disorders and, in some cases, pulmonary fibrosis, a colitis complete with granulomas, which is indistinguishable from Crohn's disease, can be observed. The clinical features are attributable to defects in organelles of lysosomal lineage, particularly melanosomes and platelet-dense granules. The syndrome displays locus heterogeneity: seven different genes cause distinct subtypes (HPS-1 to HPS-7). Of these subtypes, HPS-1 (OMIM 604982) is associated with increased risk for granulomatous colitis and pulmonary fibrosis. The diagnostic feature is the presence of PAS-positive histiocytes in both mucosa and submucosa, related to the multi-systemic deposition of ceroid lipofuscin. In CGD, the granulomas contain lipid vacuoles and lipofuscin-like pigment. If there is any doubt, leukocyte bactericidal activity should be assessed, because this is normal in Crohn's disease [341].

In the pelvic ileal reservoir, granulomas are almost a normal phenomenon, being seen in the lymphoid aggregates of the ileal mucosa in patients with unequivocal ulcerative colitis and familial adenomatous polyposis [341]. Barium granulomas may be present in the small bowel but these granulomas usually contain refractile crystals of barium sulphate [342]. Foreign body-type granulomas containing suture material may mimic Crohn's disease-type granulomas after previous surgery. Finally it is possible for sarcoidosis to affect the small intestine but, in our experience, it is exceptional for sarcoidosis to mimic small intestinal Crohn's disease.

Natural history of Crohn's disease

Only about 10% of patients presenting with 'acute terminal ileitis' subsequently progress to characteristic small bowel Crohn's disease [343]. Most cases of acute ileitis probably have an infectious aetiology. Most patients with symptomatic small intestinal disease present insidiously with recurrent abdominal pain, signs of malabsorption, blood loss and/or change of bowel habit. Investigation, which may include duodenal and/or terminal ileal biopsies, may reveal evidence to support the diagnosis. However, especially in isolated small intestinal disease, the pathological diagnosis may be attained only at the time of surgical resection. Even then, the changes may not be specific and a guarded diagnosis of Crohn's disease may be appropriate.

It has already been indicated that granulomatous inflammation is more characteristic of early than late small intestinal disease. Occasionally, however, resection is carried out in longstanding Crohn's disease or after intensive medical treatment, and then the pathology may reveal the 'healed' or burnt-out phase of the disease. Ulceration may be absent and transmural inflammation minimal. The 'connective tissue changes' of Crohn's disease may predominate with dense fibrosis, muscularisation, neuronal hyperplasia and vascular changes notable [109,298]. In this situation, the late effect of drug-induced enteritis is probably the most important differential diagnosis. In the chronic phase of Crohn's disease, granulomas are often converted into hyalinised tombstones in which Schaumann's bodies may be particularly prominent: this feature is especially seen in Crohn's disease diverted from the faecal stream [344].

Through the years, there has been considerable debate concerning the extent of surgery required in intestinal Crohn's disease and the utility of pathological assessment in predicting recurrence of disease. Initially it was thought that surgery should attempt to remove all disease [345] but it is now clear that relative surgical conservatism (especially in the small bowel) should be practised [346]. Endoscopic and histological studies of patients after previous resection have shown that most (72–84%) will demonstrate endoscopic lesions just proximal to the anastomosis [293,347,348]. In the great majority (approximately 90%) these lesions occur in the neo-terminal ileum just proximal to an ileocolonic anastomosis. Such endoscopic lesions do not themselves predict clinical recurrence [349] and many affected patients will remain asymptomatic [350]. It appears that these changes are induced by exposure to intestinal contents in the first few days after surgery [351,352].

As apparent endoscopic and histological changes at the anastomosis are seen in the most patients and do not predict recurrence, how important is it for the pathologist to assess resection margins in small intestinal resection specimens? Although it was originally thought that the presence of the disease was of importance for the prediction of recurrence [345], it is now clear that the histological demonstration of disease at or close to margins is of no real value [353–357]. Although the observed histological parameters were variable in various studies, none predicted recurrence adequately. An exception to this may be the presence of inflammation at the level of the myenteric plexus but the data are not yet strong enough [358]. Unsurprisingly, it has been shown that frozen section is not contributory in this regard and cannot be recommended [354]. These studies underpin current surgical practice, which is increasingly conservative. Indeed recurrence is also not influenced by the margin of disease-free bowel at the time of primary surgery [359].

Complications

The complications of small intestinal Crohn's disease can be usefully considered as local or systemic. Subacute small intestinal obstruction is a common presentation of the disease relating to its stricturing nature whereas ulceration may cause haemorrhage. The latter usually presents with iron deficiency anaemia but, on occasion, it can be more dramatic. Perforation does occur but only in about 2% of cases [360,361]. Fissuring and fistulation may lead to intra-abdominal abscess formation, especially in the ileo-caecal region. Fistulae are most common, in the disease as a whole, in the terminal ileum: 10% of patients have clinically significant fistulae. Entero-enteric, entero-colic and entero-cutaneous fistulae are the most common types. Extensive small bowel involvement may cause malabsorption, especially of vitamin B_{12}, although malabsorption may also be caused by fistulae, blind loops, strictures and surgical resection.

Neoplastic change in small intestinal Crohn's disease

Adenocarcinomas of the small intestine represent less than 2% of all malignant tumours of the digestive tract. The age-adjusted incidence in the USA is 1.2/100000 per year. As in the large bowel, most adenocarcinomas of the small intestine arise from pre-existing adenomas that occur sporadically or in the context of familial syndromes such as familial adenomatous polyposis (FAP). However, it is now well established that there is also an increased risk of small bowel adenocarcinoma in patients with Crohn's disease. Ratios of observed to expected small bowel adenocarcinoma rates in Crohn's disease cohorts range from 3.4 to

66.7, giving a 27-fold increased overall risk [362–364]. In most cases, small bowel adenocarcinoma in Crohn's disease presents as an ominous surprise, after a median time of 15 years from diagnosis. It occurs in young patients and carries a poor prognosis. About two-thirds of carcinomas occur in the ileum and a third in the jejunum; neoplastic transformation of Crohn's disease is exceptionally rare in the duodenum [365]. The diagnosis is not usually apparent radiologically, at the time of surgery [366] or, necessarily, at the time of macroscopic pathological assessment: the tumour appears similar to adjacent strictures of Crohn's disease. Often neoplastic transformation, in small bowel Crohn's disease, is discovered only at the time of histological assessment [367].

Most Crohn's disease-associated cancers are associated with adjacent dysplasia and there is evidence of a dysplasia–carcinoma sequence (Figure 20.30) [368–370]. Neoplastic transformation is more common in males and typically occurs in patients with extensive disease, evidence of both small and large intestinal involvement and a long history [362,370].

As cancer in small intestinal Crohn's disease is usually 'occult', having not been demonstrated or even suspected by clinical, radiological or surgical means, it is important that the pathologist examines and samples diligently every resection specimen. In 70% of cases, he or she will be the first to identify small intestinal neoplasia in Crohn's disease [367]. Carcinomas in the small bowel are often flat and stricturing and indistinguishable from more 'ordinary' chronic strictures of Crohn's disease [367]. Many are advanced at diagnosis and up to 60% are poorly differentiated [370]. Expression of EGF receptor is frequent [371]. Although much less common, there is evidence of an increased incidence of small intestinal (neuro-)endocrine

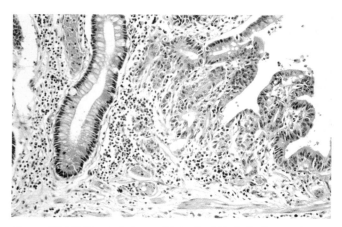

Figure 20.30 Dysplasia in small intestinal Crohn's disease: the dysplasia (at right) contrasts with a prominent non-neoplastic ileal crypt (at left).

tumours in ileal Crohn's disease [372] and rare associations with primary intestinal lymphoma are also recorded [373–375].

Drug-induced enteropathy

A variety of drugs can induce symptoms related to, and/or pathology in, the small bowel but drug-induced changes are less well described in the small bowel than in other parts of the gut because of poor access by endoscopy. The most important drug-related symptoms are diarrhoea and constipation. Malabsorption, haemorrhage, intestinal obstruction (abdominal pain and vomiting), ulceration and ischaemia have been reported. Diarrhoea is a frequent side effect of drugs, accounting for about 7% of all adverse effects [376]. The mechanism by which the diarrhoea is induced can be variable and may involve the small intestine or large intestine or both. Antibiotics such as erythromycin, a motilin agonist, can promote diarrhoea through interference with the enteric nervous system. Slow transit with constipation can be induced by a variety of drugs such as anticholinergics and opiates, and by direct toxicity with vincristine. Transient ileus has been described as an adverse effect of ciclosporin during the first weeks of therapy.

Malabsorption is associated with a variety of drugs. Fat malabsorption is reported with neomycin, p-aminosalicylate, mannitol, calcium carbonate, cholestyramine and clofibrate. Folate and vitamin B_{12} malabsorption is seen with phenytoin, colchicine, methotrexate, oral contraceptives, thiazide diuretics, anti-malarials and metformin. The mechanism is not always clear. From animal work, it appears that cholestyramine produces epithelial damage, resulting in increased lipid accumulation in the mucosa. Thiazide and other diuretics interfere with water and sodium transport and ethacrynic acid inhibits amino acid and glucose transport. Generally these adverse effects are reversible after withdrawal of the medication [377].

Anticoagulants have been implicated in the development of haemorrhage and intramural small bowel haematomas. Haemorrhage due to anti-neoplastic agents is usually the result of low platelet counts.

Drug-induced enteritis can be subdivided into two major types: ischaemic injury and inflammation. Ischaemic injury is frequently multifactorial, one of the factors usually being some form of intrinsic vascular disease in which, when further factors are added, an ischaemic episode may result. The major categories include trauma to vessels after manipulation, vasoconstriction or obstruction, including vasculitis, pump failure or peripheral vasodilatation (see Chapter 22). Radio-embolisation with resin or glass micro-spheres loaded with radioactive isotopes, for instance, produced symptomatic gastroduodenal ulceration in 3.8% of a series of 78 patients. Microspheres can occasionally be recognised in biopsies [378].

The most important inflammatory drug-induced enteritides are those due to NSAIDs, which produce a wide variety of effects in the duodenum, jejunum and ileum [379,380]. Potassium chloride tablets, gold and chemotherapeutic agents have also received some attention because of their effects on the small bowel mucosa.

NSAIDs in the small intestine

NSAIDs are widely used, especially for chronic arthritis, and it is this patient group that is likely to suffer small intestinal complications of their therapy. The major presentations are erosions or ulcers, so-called NSAID enteropathy and strictures. Up to 65% of patients on long-term NSAIDs will develop small intestinal pathology [381] and about 10% show evidence of ulceration in postmortem studies [382]. NSAID-related erosions and ulcers are most commonly seen in the distal ileum. Non-selective cyclo-oxygenase (COX) inhibitors, such as indomethacin, are much more likely to result in small intestinal damage than the more recently introduced specific (COX-2) inhibitor drugs [383]. In the duodenum, erosions and ulcers are common and NSAIDs are likely to increase, relatively, as a cause of duodenitis as *H. pylori*-related duodenitis and peptic ulcer disease become less common [384]. In the more distal small intestine, perforation, ulcers, stricturing and obscure bleeding are the most likely presentations [383,385]. Capsule endoscopy shows that erosions in areas other than the proximal and distal small bowel are also common.

The pathogenesis of mucosal pathology induced by NSAIDs is complex and multifactorial [386,387]. Specific biochemical effects and intracellular organelle damage may be initiating factors [386] but vascular pathology inducing decreased mucosal blood flow, impaired neutrophil function, defective mucosal defence mechanisms and prostaglandin inhibition are all further factors in inducing mucosal damage [386–389]. Loss of prostaglandin biosynthesis may be a promoting factor, as illustrated by reports from patients with chronic recurrent small intestinal ulcers, small bowel perforations and gastrointestinal blood loss. Cytosolic phospholipase A2α (cPLA2α) deficiency may be the underlying genetic defect. Ulceration can occur without use of COX inhibitors [390]. Another mechanism may be the interaction between NSAIDs and bile. The drugs may injure the small intestine by contact irritant effects and the enterohepatic circulation seems to be a key effect. Increased mucosal permeability leads to protein loss whereas ulceration causes obscure haemorrhage, presenting as unexplained anaemia [391,392]. These presentations have been reported as NSAID enteropathy.

Mucosal biopsies from the proximal small intestine of patients on NSAIDs may demonstrate more specific features but often terminal ileal biopsies show non-specific changes and may be unrewarding. Increased epithelial apoptotic activity and mucosal eosinophilia are rare but useful signs of NSAID enteropathy [393] and there may be intra-epithelial lymphocytosis, although this is more often found in colonic mucosal biopsies. In resection specimens, performed because of NSAID therapy complications, the changes of ulceration and stricturing may be non-specific. However, NSAIDs should always be considered as a cause of 'non-specific ulceration' and perforation in the small intestine (Figure 20.31).

Although relatively rare, there is one distinctive pathological feature of chronic NSAID enteropathy. This is so-called diaphragm disease (Figure 20.32) [394]. In this condition, which usually affects the ileum, but is also now increasingly recognised more proximally in the small intestine and the colon, patients present with subacute obstruction due to thin mucosa-lined septa that resemble a perforated diaphragm when seen *en face* (Figure 20.32). They may be single but are usually multiple [395]. It is particularly important for surgeons to know of their existence

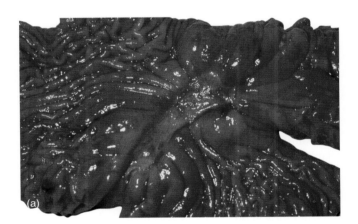

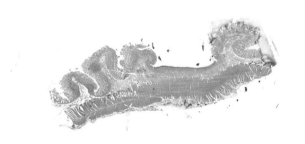

(b)

Figure 20.31 (a) A so-called solitary ulcer of the small intestine as seen on macroscopic examination. (b) A whole mount of the lesion. Once other pathologies have been excluded, the diligent pathologist should seek an accurate drug history because many of these lesions are caused by drugs, especially non-steroidal anti-inflammatory drugs.

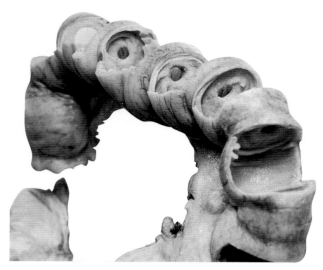

Figure 20.32 A classical black and white picture from the original Price (a former author and editor of this text) studies on this distinctive disease. There are multiple 'diaphragms' compartmentalising the ileum from a patient taking long-term non-steroidal anti-inflammatory drugs. Inflation of the unopened fresh specimen is important to display the lesions to best advantage.

because their involvement of only the mucosa and submucosa means that the small bowel containing diaphragms may appear entirely normal externally. Diaphragms may be associated with ulcers but often the adjacent mucosa is entirely normal [393].

The pathogenesis of diaphragm disease appears to relate to superficial circumferential ulceration, followed by submucosal fibrosis and a high degree of mucosal restitution. Diaphragms show a close resemblance to the normal plicae circulares of the small bowel but have additional characteristic features. Immediately adjacent to the stenotic lumen there is mucosal attenuation and ulceration, often with features of mucosal prolapse in the form of fibromuscular proliferation in the lamina propria in the adjacent intact mucosa (Figure 20.33). There is a well-defined area of underlying submucosal fibrosis, which is more prominent in broad-based lesions (Figure 20.33) [394]. If suspected clinically, diaphragm disease can be diagnosed either radiologically and/or endoscopically and may be treated by enteroscopic means rather than having to resort to surgical resection.

NSAID-induced lesions of the distal small bowel must be distinguished from microscopic lesions similar to Crohn's disease which have been reported in ileal and colonic biopsies from patients with reactive arthritis and ankylosing spondylitis. However, only a minority of these patients developed genuine Crohn's disease [396].

Other drug-induced enteropathies

Enteric-coated potassium supplements and hydrochlorthiazide are both associated with small intestinal ulceration

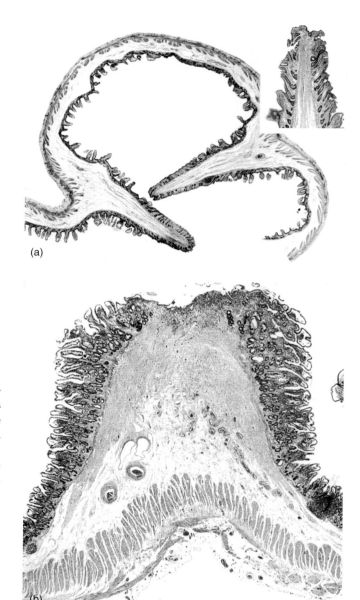

Figure 20.33 Further classical black and white pictures from the original Price studies on this disease. (a) Microscopy of the 'diaphragms' in Figure 20.32 shows a close resemblance to the plicae circulares. At higher power the insert demonstrates submucosal fibrosis at the tip and villous blunting. (b) A broader-based lesion in the same case as (a) showing an increased degree of submucosal fibrosis. There is now some resemblance to the pattern of microscopy in the potassium-induced ulceration.

and haemorrhage [397]. Localised ischaemia is a likely mechanism. As a treatment for hyperkalaemia in uraemic patients, Kayexalate (sodium polystyrene sulphonate in sorbitol) may be given by mouth, via a nasogastric tube or by enema. This can cause localised ulceration and mucosal necrosis in any part of the gut. Small bowel involvement is less common [398]. The characteristic crystalline deposits of Kayexalate, which usually have large, polygonal profiles with angulated contours, and are refractile, basophilic, PAS and ZN positive, are identifiable in the bed of the ulcers [398].

Patients treated for rheumatoid arthritis with gold therapy occasionally develop an eosinophilic enterocolitis with diarrhoea and peripheral eosinophilia usually within 3 months of drug initiation [399,400]. The small and large intestine may be involved. Histopathologically, there is ulceration with diffuse inflammatory changes, including crypt abscesses. Eosinophils are often particularly prominent [399].

Given the rapid cell turnover of the small intestinal mucosa, it is not surprising that chemotherapeutic agents may cause enteropathy. Cyclophosphamide, methotrexate and 5-fluoro-uracil are the agents most associated with, and most widely studied in, this drug-induced enteropathy [401–403]. Acute injury is induced by enhanced apoptotic activity, increased migration of crypt epithelial cells and reduced compensatory mitotic activity leading to a hypoplastic villous atrophy (Figure 20.34) [402,403]. Chemotherapy-induced enteropathy may be exacerbated by radiotherapy [404] although there is some evidence that vitamin A treatment may lessen the effects of methotrexate enteropathy [405]. The immunosuppressive drug mycophenolate mofetil can also damage the small bowel (as well as all other levels of the gastrointestinal tract). This drug-induced injury closely mimics graft-versus-host disease [406].

Another medication known to affect the small bowel is colchicine. Colchicine toxicity, mainly in patients with renal failure, has been linked to increased numbers of metaphase mitoses, epithelial pseudo-stratification and loss of polarity, and an increase in the proliferation zone as demon-

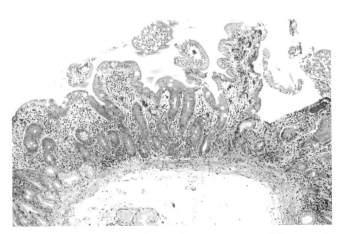

Figure 20.34 A duodenal biopsy from a patient on 5-fluorouracil therapy for metastatic colorectal carcinoma. There is hypoplastic villous atrophy. Enhanced apoptotic activity was prominent in the crypt bases.

strated by Ki67 staining. In patients with therapeutic levels of colchicine, a villous atrophy/hyperplastic crypt pattern has been described in the jejunum. Mitotic arrest with numerous metaphase mitoses in crypt epithelium is also a characteristic feature of recent taxane chemotherapy. Villous atrophy in the ileum or small intestine with lymphocytic ileo-colitis has been reported with ticlodipine and Cyclo 3 Fort (a veinotonic) [407,408]. Finally, successful chemotherapeutic ablation of primary tumours of the small intestine, notably malignant lymphoma, can induce perforation of the intestine through the necrotic tumour and strictures can develop later [409].

Miscellaneous inflammatory conditions of the small intestine

Numerous miscellaneous inflammatory conditions affect the small bowel. Some of these are relatively specific to certain segments. Two more general pathological phenomena not uncommonly presenting to the surgical pathologist and providing a taxing differential diagnosis, often requiring clinical, therapeutic and radiological correlation, are ulceration and/or perforation and tissue eosinophilia of the small intestine.

Ulceration in the small bowel

Small bowel ulcers distal to the duodenum were first described by Baillie in 1795. The incidence is not really known. By 1966 almost 400 cases were reported. Between 1956 and 1979, 59 cases were seen at the Mayo Clinic, which represented approximately 4 cases per 100 000 new patients registered. A steady increase in the number of patients was found in each decade of life from the second to the seventh [410]. Small intestinal resections, performed for penetrating ulceration and perforation are often a source of diagnostic difficulty, usually because characteristic histopathological features indicating a possible aetiology are absent (see Figure 20.31).

The lesions vary from 3 mm to 50 mm in diameter. They are often anti-mesenteric and sometimes have an annular configuration. The edges are often sharply demarcated. Microscopically the ulcer crater is filled with a layer of necrotic and granulation tissue with a variable inflammatory reaction, usually ending at the ulcer edge. Vascular pathological changes such as congestion and narrowing or occlusion of submucosal vessels may or may not be present.

The differential diagnosis of these penetrating small intestinal ulcers, which may be multiple, is broad and includes congenital malformation, inflammation, ingestion of a foreign body, entrapment of a pill, or any other trauma, vascular abnormalities, adhesions, chemical irritation and neoplasia, especially lymphoma and (neuro-)endocrine tumours in the ileum. Congenital absence of the splenic artery and vein has been associated with duodenal ulceration and deformity [411]. Ischaemic duodenal ulcer has been reported as an unusual presentation of sickle cell anaemia [412]. Perforating Crohn's disease is high on the list of differential diagnoses and transmural inflammation with lymphoid hyperplasia, granulomas and the connective tissue changes should be sought. Some of these features may be less pronounced in the more chronic, fibrotic and burnt-out phases of the disease [109,298]. Rarely Behçet's disease (see below) may show similar changes to Crohn's disease and the appropriate clinical setting should be investigated. In young children, obscure ulceration may represent a distinct inherited disease, intractable ulcerating enterocolitis of infancy [413].

Small intestinal ulceration may be infective in origin. Diligent search for cytopathic effects of viruses, particularly CMV, may be rewarding. The pathological features of ulceration related to bacterial infection may be non-specific and microbiological investigation may be required. Especially in AIDS, protozoal infection may cause deep penetrating ulceration and perforation. Ischaemia, whether acute or subacute, causes ulceration and perforation. Nevertheless, the characteristic pathological features of ischaemia should be demonstrable in the adjacent small intestinal mucosa. Jejunal and ileal ulceration may be peptic in origin, especially in Zollinger–Ellison syndrome [414]. Peptic digestion of the ulcer bed and multiplicity of ulcers should prompt investigation of acid secretion and serum gastrin levels. Vascular pathology, including vasculitis and irradiation enteritis, may all cause perforating ulceration in the small bowel. Ulcerative jejunitis, effectively representing an early stage of lymphoma in the small bowel, has been considered elsewhere. Suffice it to say that the features of lymphoma may be very subtle in ulcers of the jejunum and ileum, and evidence of lymphoid malignancy should be diligently sought by morphological, histochemical and, if necessary, molecular biological methodology.

Once all these avenues of investigation have been exhausted, drugs should be strongly considered as the cause of small intestinal ulceration. NSAIDs are available without prescription and are a highly prevalent cause of small intestinal disease. Apart from diaphragm disease due to NSAIDs (see above) and eosinophilic enterocolitis due to gold therapy, the histopathology of drug-induced enteritis and ulceration may be relatively non-specific (see Figure 20.31). Enteric-coated potassium tablets [415] and NSAIDs [416] have a similar pathogenic effect by causing localised mucosal ischaemia or ischaemic-type damage.

Despite comprehensive searching for evidence of drug ingestion, there will remain some cases of small intestinal ulceration that have to be regarded as primary idiopathic disease [417]. Despite regular ileoscopy during colonoscopy and the advent of endoscopic methods, this small patient group remains enigmatic at present.

Eosinophilic infiltrates in the small intestine

Eosinophils are constitutively present in the gastrointestinal mucosa outside the oesophagus. Therefore a diagnosis of eosinophilic (gastro)enteritis is difficult. Eosinophilic disorders can be separated into primary (idiopathic) and secondary diseases, primary having no known cause and secondary being due to other illnesses resulting in tissue eosinophilia. Primary eosinophilic enteritis has been called allergic gastroenteropathy because a subset of patients has an associated allergic component. Although considered idiopathic, an allergic mechanism may be involved because most patients exhibit increased food-specific IgE levels. Secondary disorders include a variety of conditions. Tissue eosinophilia of the small intestine is also seen in malignant lymphoma and in the inflammatory fibroid polyp. In the absence of evidence of secondary disease, a diagnosis of eosinophilic (gastro)enteritis can be considered.

Eosinophilic gastroenteritis

Eosinophilic gastroenteritis is exceedingly rare. Major referral centres may identify one case per 100 000 patients. In the Mayo Clinic 40 patients were identified from 1950 to 1987 from medical records documenting more than 4 million individuals. It can affect any age group but the peak is in the third to fifth decade of life. There is a slight male preponderance. It has been suggested that the clinical features may reflect the extent, location and depth of infiltration of the eosinophils. The Klein classification separates eosinophilic gastroenteritis into mucosal and/or submucosal, muscular or (sub)serosal disease. Approximately 57.5% have mucosal and/or submucosal, 30% muscular and 12.5% (sub)serosal disease.

Patients with mucosal disease present with vomiting, abdominal pain, diarrhoea, gastrointestinal bleeding, iron deficiency anaemia, malabsorption, protein-losing enteropathy or failure to thrive. If muscular layers are involved, obstruction or even acute abdomen has been recorded, whereas serosal involvement may be associated with evidence of ascites.

The diagnosis of eosinophilic gastroenteritis is difficult. Symptoms are non-specific. Peripheral eosinophilia is variable with a normal count in 25% of the patients. Atopy and allergies are present in 25–75% of the cases. Biopsies show increased numbers of eosinophils. Multiple biopsies are required because of the patchy nature of the disease [418]. However, no standards of diagnosis have been established. The normal number of eosinophils has not been defined and may vary between pathology departments, depending on the techniques used but may also show geographical differences, e.g. the normal ileum may show as many as 30 eosinophils per high power field. A suggestive feature is eosinophilic infiltration of intestinal crypts.

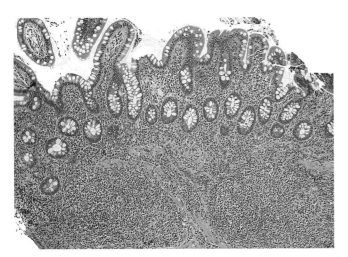

Figure 20.35 Eosinophilic enteritis: although the mucosa is intact, there is a florid eosinophil polymorph infiltrate. In this case, the disease was mucosal and submucosal only, Klein's type 1.

The submucosal type, usually with secondary eosinophilic involvement in the overlying mucosa, is predominant, accounting for about 60% of cases (Figure 20.35) [419]. The striking submucosal eosinophilic infiltrate, often with a distinct paucity of other inflammatory cell types, is accompanied by oedema. Most cases have been diagnosed on surgical full-thickness biopsy or resection performed for obstruction or suspicion of malignancy. The involved small intestine shows thickening and oedema with luminal narrowing and a serosal reaction (Figure 20.35).

In children, allergic or eosinophilic gastroenteritis tends to be a more specific and readily diagnosed condition presenting with anaemia, malabsorption, protein-losing enteropathy, failure to thrive and/or asthma. Unlike adults, it is relatively easily to determine the cause of the allergy, which is usually a dietary antigen. Cows' milk protein is most common [420,421]. Eosinophilic infiltration is only a feature of the immediate post-challenge period. At other times, and usually at the time of biopsy, villous atrophy is the predominant feature with a non-specific increase in chronic inflammatory cells in the lamina propria [420]. The diagnosis is often readily apparent clinically and it is only rarely that biopsies are taken except to exclude other conditions, most notably coeliac disease.

Secondary eosinophilic diseases

Secondary eosinophilic syndromes comprise a variety of disorders. The hypereosinophilic syndromes (HES) represent a heterogeneous group of rare disorders that have been defined by persistent blood eosinophilia for more than 6 months with evidence of organ involvement. The cause is unknown. The spectrum of disorders comprises conditions with familial or genetically based eosinophilia

and neoplastic disorders such as eosinophilic leukaemia. About 25% of cases with HES have eosinophilic infiltration of the gastrointestinal tract. In some cases, this inflammatory reaction is limited to the mucosa of the intestine. In comparison with those with disease localised in non-intestinal sites, involvement of the intestinal tract has been associated with a limited prognosis, lymphoproliferative disorders and, in some, fatal outcome. It is difficult to distinguish HES from primary eosinophilic enteritis.

Other secondary causes of eosinophilia are CIBD, coeliac disease and infections including bacteria (*H. pylori, Clostridium difficile, Shigella* spp.), fungi and parasites. Some cases have been demonstrated to represent a reaction to the herring worm, *Eustoma rotundatum*. Serological evidence has implicated anisakiasis as a cause in up to 40% of cases, particularly in association with gastric involvement and in eastern Asia. Other parasites such as *Toxocara canis* have occasionally been implicated [422].

Rarely, eosinophilic gastroenteritis may be the presentation of systemic disorders such as connective tissue disease or Churg–Strauss syndrome (allergic granulomatosis) [423]. It has also been noted in graft-versus-host disease, systemic mastocytosis (Figure 20.36) and lymphangiectasia. Drugs such as gold, azathioprine, carbamazepine, enalapril, clofazimine and co-trimoxazole have been reported to cause eosinophilia with variable involvement of the gastrointestinal tract.

Radiation enteritis

Radiotherapy used for abdominal and pelvic malignancies continues to provide considerable morbidity and some mortality, despite attempts to minimise damage to the small bowel [424]. The severity of radiation enteritis depends on several factors, anatomical features and host mechanisms, the type of therapy being the most important [424]. The severity of acute radiation enteritis appears to determine the severity of chronic disease: whereas the effects on epithelial cell integrity and kinetics and on vascular epithelium are considerable, host defence responses to intraluminal antigens and pathogens are also of some importance.

Radiation enteritis is most likely to be demonstrated in parts of the small bowel that are fixed, thus allowing a constant maximal dose of radiotherapy to reach them. The duodenum, proximal jejunum and terminal ileum are therefore most likely to show maximal changes but small bowel fixed by adhesions after previous surgery may also be subject to the maximum radiation dose and exhibit marked radiation change [424,425].

Acute radiation enteritis shows predominant mucosal changes with epithelial stem cell damage, leading to villous atrophy and crypt epithelial cell damage with widespread apoptosis. This is accompanied by pronounced

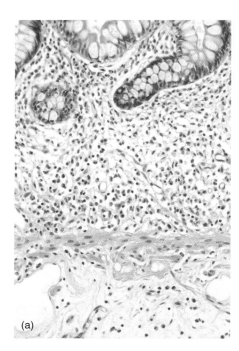
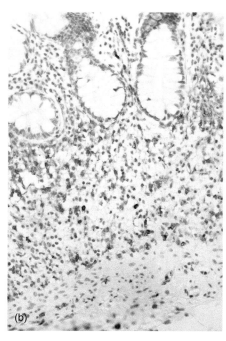

Figure 20.36 Mastocytosis of the ileum (a) showing the presence of numerous large pale cells in the deeper lamina propria, staining positive with antibodies directed against tryptase (b).

regenerative activity in the surviving crypts, which may show marked reactive cytological atypia that can trap the unwary pathologist into a diagnosis of dysplasia. Perforation, adhesions and fistulation (entero-enteric, entero-vesical and entero-vaginal) may all be an early complication [426,427].

The late effects may be seen months or even years (up to 30 years) after radiotherapy. Stricture and malabsorption are common [428] and fistula and perforation less common [426]. Even at this stage there may be mucosal ulceration whereas fibrosing strictures and fine serosal adhesions are the most common macroscopic manifestations. The submucosa is most affected with hyaline sclerosis and 'atypical' or stellate fibroblasts and vascular changes (Figure 20.37) [426]. Enteritis cystica profunda is not uncommon [426]. The mucosa may be ulcerated, show variable villous atrophic changes with chronic inflammation or be relatively normal. Telangiectasia is common and may be a source of gastrointestinal haemorrhage [429]. Vascular changes, particularly in the submucosa and subserosa, include thickening of arteries and arterioles with hyaline fibrosis of the muscularis and foam cells in the intima (Figure 20.37) [430]. The muscularis may be relatively normal or show hyalinising fibrosis. Subserosal fibrosis and fibrous adhesions are common [426].

On occasion, the chronic changes of radiation enteritis can be particularly subtle even though the patient has presented with small intestinal obstruction. The wise pathologist, faced with subtle submucosal changes only, as described above, should always seek a history of previous abdominal or pelvic radiotherapy because this may have been forgotten by the patient and not considered (relevant) by clinicians.

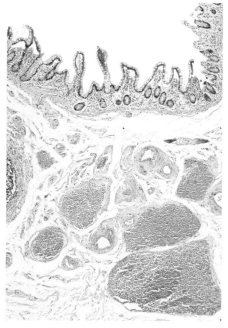

Figure 20.37 Chronic radiation enteritis: this was from an area of stricture. The mucosa is intact but shows architectural distortion. There is gross hyaline thickening of dilated submucosal blood vessels.

Behçet's disease

Behçet's disease is an idiopathic multi-system syndrome characterised by orogenital ulceration and ocular manifestations. It is a disease of young adults that is more severe in males. It has high prevalence rates in the Mediterranean basin, especially Turkey. Neurological involvement, from either direct parenchymal involvement of the brain or major vascular involvement, is one of the most severe manifestations of the disease [431].

Pathologically the disease is characterised by a vasculitis that is usually lymphocytic and affects veins to a greater extent than arteries, although occasionally there may be more necrotising inflammation with leukocytoclasis. Involvement of the gut is relatively unusual. In one series 5% of patients had significant gastrointestinal symptoms [432] whereas only about 1–2% of patients will have small intestinal involvement [433]. Distribution of the disease appears to be geography dependent, ileo-caecal involvement being relatively more common in Japan [434]. The disease is described in children and the differential diagnosis from Crohn's disease and other ulcerating diseases may be particularly difficult in this age group [411,435].

Although it is clear that the disease is primarily a vasculitis, the cause remains uncertain. Familial cases are well described but no specific genetic abnormalities have been discovered [436]. An association with CMV infection has been suggested [437]. Defective T-cell suppressor function, possibly EBV-related, has been described [438]. More recently high levels of truncated actin have been described in the neutrophil polymorphs of patients with Behçet's disease and it has been suggested that this is a specific abnormality [439]. Furthermore, it is clear that the disease represents a vasculitis targeting the vasa vasorum and other small blood vessels [440].

Small intestinal involvement is primarily in the terminal ileum and lymphoid aggregates are a particular site of involvement [441]. Macroscopically the disease is characterised by penetrating ulcers, often with a flask-shaped morphology, and perforation is a relatively common feature (Figure 20.38) [442]. Adjacent to the larger ulcers, there are often smaller aphthous ulcers. Fissuring and linear ulcers up to 5mm long may also be present [434]. Histologically, the ulcers have non-specific appearances. The adjacent ileal mucosa may appear almost entirely normal. A common feature is the presence of a lymphocytic vasculitis, often involving small veins and venules [410], and there may also be fibrinoid necrosis in involved veins and venules.

Perforation and massive gastrointestinal haemorrhage are the most severe complications of intestinal Behçet's disease. As in Crohn's disease, inflammatory masses may involve the ileo-caecal region. Patients with involvement of the small bowel often come to surgery but this is complicated by high rates of recurrence [435]. The vasculitis of Behçet's disease may be difficult to demonstrate histologically and the condition provides diagnostic challenges. Indeed, there remains a considerable overlap between intestinal Behçet's disease and Crohn's disease [443]. A diagnosis of intestinal involvement by Behçet's disease requires the presence of the typical extra-intestinal manifestations, along with pathology in keeping with the diagnosis. Recurrent oral ulceration is a prerequisite for the

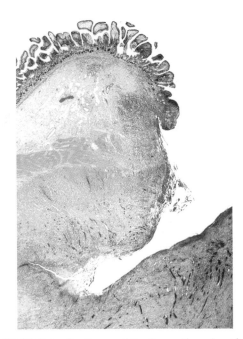

Figure 20.38 Behçet's disease of the ileum: the edge of a deeply penetrating flask-shaped ulcer extending to the subserosa is well seen. There was evidence of a venulitis elsewhere.

diagnosis and additional features such as ocular involvement, arthritis, erythema nodosum and recurrent genital ulceration are helpful corroborative features.

Ileal reservoirs and pouchitis

Pelvic ileal reservoirs were first used for ulcerative colitis and FAP [444] but more recently they have been used for other conditions, such as juvenile polyposis and necrotising colitis, when total colectomy is necessary. Most pouches show a degree of mucosal chronic inflammation and villous architectural abnormality (Figure 20.39) [445,446]. It is likely that these represent a response of the ileal mucosa to the altered environment and probably to changes in the bacterial flora of the ileum.

Studies of serial mucosal biopsies indicate that the changes occur soon after faecal stream exposure and, once present, the mucosa appears to reach a steady state in terms of inflammation, architectural abnormality and proliferation. The chronic changes are particularly concentrated in the posterior and inferior parts of the pouch. Those pouches with the more severe chronic changes are more likely to show so-called colonic metaplasia in the mucosa, demonstrated by the acquisition of morphological, mucin and lectin histochemical and electron microscopic features of large bowel epithelium. However, certain small intestinal characteristics are retained and immunohistochemical evidence suggests that the mucosa does not undergo complete colonic metaplasia [446].

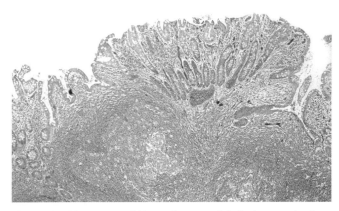

Figure 20.39 A mucosal biopsy from a pelvic ileal reservoir: the biopsy shows villous atrophy and dense chronic inflammation. Within a germinal centre (below) is a small granulomatous focus. This is a common feature of pouch mucosa and should not be taken as evidence, necessarily, for a diagnosis of Crohn's disease.

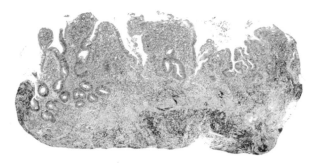

Figure 20.40 Pouchitis in a pelvic ileal reservoir: there is villous atrophy, chronic inflammation and activity in the form of superficial erosions and disruptive crypt abscesses.

The term 'pouchitis' was introduced by Kock to describe inflammation of a continent ileostomy [447]. It also refers to active inflammation of ileal pouch anal anastomosis (IPAA) mucosa. The condition is believed to be a 'non-specific, idiopathic inflammation of the neorectal ileal mucosa'. Various subtypes of pouchitis have been distinguished, the most common form being called 'usual or acute pouchitis'. It responds well to antibiotics. Approximately 5–10% of patients develop 'chronic pouchitis' and a small subset has medically 'refractory pouchitis'. The diagnosis of pouchitis is based on clinical, endoscopic and histological criteria. The term should be restricted to those patients with an acute-on-chronic, relapsing, inflammatory and ulcerating condition with characteristic clinical, endoscopic and pathological features. Symptomatology includes diarrhoea, often bloody, abdominal pain, urgency, discharge, bloating and systemic symptoms. Endoscopic examination reveals increased vascularity, contact bleeding and ulceration, typical features of active chronic inflammatory bowel disease. As a result of the confusion over terminology, many now consider the term 'chronic relapsing pouchitis' to be more appropriate for this disorder [345].

The pathological hallmarks of pouchitis are acute inflammation and focal ulceration, occurring on a background of marked chronic inflammation and villous atrophy (Figure 20.40) [445,448]. The overall histological appearances bear a close similarity to those of ulcerative colitis and are unlike those of Crohn's disease. Histological examination shows neutrophil infiltration with crypt abscesses and chronic inflammatory infiltrate. Ulceration in pouchitis is usually superficial: deep ulceration is unusual and should raise suspicions of a more specific pathology such as ischaemic enteritis. When so defined, the prevalence of pouchitis usually varies between 10% and 20% of ulcerative colitis patients, although striking variation in prevalence rates continues to characterise the ileal reservoir literature. A number of scoring systems are in existence for assessing disease activity [445], which usually combine endoscopic and histopathological characteristics [449,450]. The 'Pouchitis Disease Activity Index (PDAI)' consists of 18 points, calculated from three separate 6-point scores: symptoms, endoscopy and histology. A score of 7 or more indicates active inflammation [448].

Pouchitis should be differentiated from other pathologies that can cause active inflammation in the pouch such as cuffitis, proximal small bowel bacterial overgrowth, pouch stricture, Crohn's disease, NSAID use, infective enteritis, inflammatory polyps, mucosal prolapse and mucosal ischaemia.

The pathophysiology of pouchitis is not known. The fact that pouchitis almost exclusively occurs in patients with ulcerative colitis and not in patients with FAP suggests an underlying genetic predisposition (polymorphisms of IL-1R antagonist, non-carrier status of TNF allele). Alteration in the bowel anatomy with faecal stasis may promote an 'inflammation-prone environment where bacteria could play a critical role'. The existence of pathogens has not been demonstrated consistently but a large body of evidence suggests that alteration of the bacterial community, so-called dysbiosis, could play a role in the initiation and development of chronic inflammation. Alterations of innate and adaptive mucosal immunity in the pouch and in pouchitis have also been reported. Other factors possibly involved include ischaemia and/or microvascular endothelial dysfunction and abnormal angiogenesis, mucosal pathology as a result of a lack of small intestinal nutrients and recurrent ulcerative colitis in a pouch with colonic phenotypic change [345,450]. Although it is clearly possible for Crohn's disease to involve the reservoir, particularly if the pouch was constructed on the basis of an erroneous initial diagnosis or, as an alternative, deliberately in a Crohn's disease patient [451], there is no evidence to implicate Crohn's disease as the cause of chronic relapsing pouchitis [452].

Most accept that pouchitis is essentially a disease of patients with ulcerative colitis. There are interesting associations between an original diagnosis of ulcerative colitis and pouchitis. Ulcerative colitis patients show more inflammatory change in their reservoirs than FAP patients and there are intriguing inter-connections of ulcerative colitis, extra-intestinal manifestations and pouchitis [453]. Similarities in the immunopathology of pouchitis and ulcerative colitis have also been reported [345].

Dysplasia in the ileal pouch is not common and adenocarcinoma of the ileal pouch is definitely rare. The risk for dysplasia or cancer in the anal transitional zone and rectal cuff is also small but real [454–459]. Focal and multifocal low grade dysplasia and DNA aneuploidy were reported in 266 patients with ulcerative colitis with an ileal reservoir. Eight cases of dysplasia in the cuff were noted in a series of 178 ileal pouch patients with a minimum follow-up period of 10 years. Potential neoplastic transformation would seem an argument to ensure that all reservoirs with pouchitis and a remaining inflamed rectal cuff are comprehensively surveyed by endoscopy and biopsy.

Kock's continent ileostomy is performed for the same indications but the pouch is intra-abdominal and continuity is not restored. Unlike the pelvic pouch, Kock's pouches appear to have a different natural history with lower rates of pouchitis: indeed after two decades, the mucosa appears relatively normal in most patients [460]. Nevertheless occasionally cases of neoplasia are described [461].

Ulcerative colitis in the small intestine

Evidence of inflammation in the small bowel, associated with colorectal inflammatory bowel disease, should always raise suspicions of Crohn's disease, although rare enteritides are associated with otherwise classic ulcerative colitis. Clinically the most important are backwash ileitis and chronic pouchitis, but duodenitis has also been recognised. Histologically the duodenitis associated with ulcerative colitis looks very similar to ulcerative colitis (diffuse active chronic inflammation with distortion).

Backwash ileitis

Approximately 10% of total colectomy specimens in ulcerative colitis will show inflammation in the terminal ileum, although the frequency of backwash ileitis in ulcerative colitis has decreased over time [462,463]. The inflammation is usually confined to the terminal 100–150 mm of the ileum. The ileal pathology is usually in continuity with that in the colon. The disease activity level of the ileitis corre-

lates with the level of proximal colonic disease. Macroscopically the mucosa appears diffusely reddened and granular with erosions and ulcers often prominent (Figure 20.41). In its milder form, the disease is superficial but deep ulceration may occur and inflammatory polyp formation is well described. The ileo-caecal valve is usually dilated and incompetent.

The histological hallmarks of backwash ileitis are villous atrophy, chronic active inflammation, ulceration and vascular ectasia (Figure 20.42). There is diffuse chronic inflammation of the mucosa and crypt abscesses are often

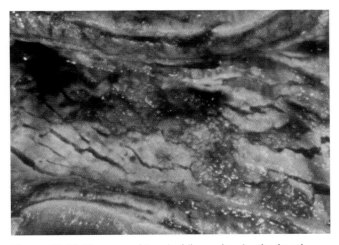

Figure 20.41 The opened terminal ileum showing backwash ileitis from a total colectomy specimen removed for ulcerative colitis. The mucosa is granular and eroded but there is no deep pathology or thickening of the bowel wall.

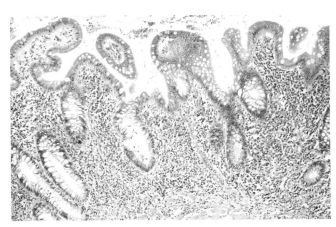

Figure 20.42 The histology of backwash ileitis: there is villous atrophy, diffuse chronic inflammation and activity in the form of small crypt abscesses.

prominent. Deep ulceration may be fissuring. It is important to differentiate backwash ileitis from Crohn's disease. Discontinuity of disease, granulomas, transmural inflammation and connective tissue changes are all features that would make the pathologist suspicious for a diagnosis of Crohn's disease. On ileoscopic biopsy, the same features should be sought, although often only full clinical, radiological and endoscopic correlation will allow the biopsy appearances to be accurately diagnosed [336]. Late-stage backwash ileitis manifests as gross villous atrophy, with epithelial regeneration leading to a flattened mucosa that may closely resemble colonic mucosa. Evidence for true colonic metaplasia due to the long-term presence of colonic contents is currently lacking.

Backwash ileitis has relatively little clinical significance apart from its potential for a misdiagnosis as evidence of Crohn's disease. It is usually associated with severe pancolonic ulcerative colitis and the colonic complications of the disease are usually much more significant than those of the terminal ileum. Perforation of 'backwash ileitis' should raise suspicions of an alternative diagnosis. It remains controversial whether the presence of backwash ileitis predicts the subsequent onset of pouchitis in the pelvic ileal reservoir after proctocolectomy [464]. Given the current theories that the disease is a secondary phenomenon, it would seem more likely that the severity of the colonic disease (which itself determines the presence or absence of backwash ileitis) might predict subsequent pouchitis rather than the presence of backwash ileitis.

The duodenum and jejunum in ulcerative colitis

Evidence of inflammatory pathology in the proximal small bowel in putative ulcerative colitis would usually raise suspicions for an alternative diagnosis, such as Crohn's disease. However, the jejunal mucosa has been shown to harbour chronic inflammation in ulcerative colitis patients and there may also be architectural disturbance [465]. Severe and often fatal panenteritis is also described in ulcerative colitis [466] and diffuse duodenitis is a rare complication [467]. Both before and after colectomy, there may be varying degrees of chronic inflammation and villous architectural disturbance in the duodenal mucosa. Such diffuse duodenitis is also described in children with ulcerative colitis (Figure 20.43) [468].

Post-colectomy small intestinal pathology in ulcerative colitis

Although pelvic ileal reservoir pathology is the most clinically important entity in this category (see above), pathological changes are seen in the small intestinal mucosa as a result of colectomy and proctocolectomy for ulcerative colitis.

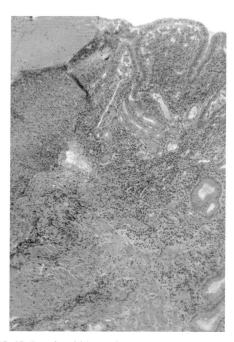

Figure 20.43 Duodenal biopsy from a patient with severe extensive ulcerative colitis, showing ulceration, blunting of the villi and severe inflammation.

Ileorectal anastomosis

Until about 25 years ago, there was a vogue for ileorectal anastomosis in ulcerative colitis before it was appreciated that the rectum was an important site for carcinoma development in ulcerative colitis and before the advent of pelvic pouch surgery. The ileal mucosa proximal to an ileorectal anastomosis shows florid changes on biopsy not unlike those of backwash ileitis. There is villous architectural change, active inflammation, and occasional erosions and ulceration [469]. Eventually, as in backwash ileitis, the mucosa appears relatively atrophic. In this situation, it may well be difficult, on biopsy, to differentiate between ileal and rectal mucosa, both showing architectural distortion and the long-term effects of chronic ulcerative colitis.

Pre-stomal ileitis

Obstructive ileitis is now well recognised proximal to an obstructive lesion in the small bowel but true pre-stomal ileitis is a condition specific to patients who have undergone total proctocolectomy and permanent ileostomy [470]. It is characterised by profuse watery ileostomy discharge with marked systemic symptoms. Perforation is common. The macroscopic features are of deep linear ulceration with normal intervening mucosa. The ulcers may be fissuring and thus there is some resemblance to Crohn's disease. However, the disease lacks the other pathological hallmarks of Crohn's disease such as granulomas, transmural inflammation and the connective changes. The condition is

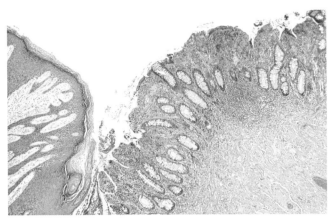

Figure 20.44 Villous atrophy and chronic inflammation are very commonly seen in the ileal mucosa adjacent to an ileostomy. They should not be taken as evidence of Crohn's disease.

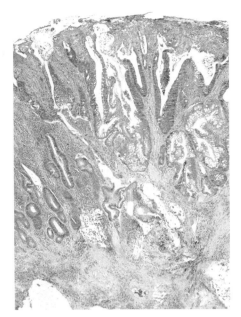

Figure 20.45 Mucosal prolapse changes in the ileal mucosa of an ileostomy: the dramatic epithelial hyperplasia and the enteritis cystica profunda with mucin lakes can trick the unwary into a diagnosis of malignancy.

fortunately rare, because it has a high mortality. Despite its associations with ulcerative colitis, its pathogenesis remains unclear.

Ileostomy pathology and ileal conduits

Various mechanical and ischaemic mechanisms are responsible for villous architectural changes and inflammation that are almost inevitable in the ileostomy mucosa, regardless of the indication for ileostomy (Figure 20.44). Furthermore minor degrees of obstruction are commonplace and these may induce more pronounced inflammation, villous atrophy and ulceration. There may also be the changes of mucosal prolapse (Figure 20.45). Polypoid mucosal prolapse at the site of an ileostomy can lead to enteritis cystica profunda and especial mimicry of malignancy. Obstructive ileitis and pre-stomal ileitis may be seen proximal to an ileostomy. Finally dysplasia and carcinoma are well recognised at ileostomies, especially those performed for IBD and FAP. How important the inflammatory pathology of the stomal mucosa is in carcinogenesis is uncertain [471].

Ileal conduits are urinary reservoirs constructed after bladder resection for malignancy. Varying degrees of mucosal abnormality are described, including villous architectural changes and mucin depletion [472]. There is evidence of some increased malignancy risk, transitional cell carcinomas at the uretero-ileal junction being most commonly described.

Obstructive ileitis

Obstructive ileitis is now well recognised to have characteristic macroscopic and histopathological features [473], but the condition is relatively poorly documented in the

literature [474]. As in the colon, there appears to be a vascular element to the pathogenesis with mural hypoperfusion and secondary localised ischaemia apparently accounting for relatively sharply localised ischaemic-type inflammation and ulceration, often adjacent to relatively normal appearing mucosa. Obstructing endocrine tumours of the small intestine can be associated with proximal ulceration and granulation tissue polyposis, presumably a consequence of obstruction and relative ischaemia due to compromise of blood supply [475]. The latter is putatively induced by a combination of the mechanical effects of the obstructing tumour and vascular spread of the tumour.

Non-specific jejunitis

Isolated jejunitis often has relatively non-specific histological features but it occurs in several specific situations. So-called ulcerative jejunitis is now recognised to be a neoplastic complication of coeliac disease: there is good pathological and molecular evidence that most, if not all, of such cases represent early T-cell lymphoma complicating coeliac disease [476]. Isolated jejunitis is rarely an early manifestation of systemic disorders such as Henoch–Schönlein purpura [477] and microscopic polyarteritis [478]. Severe necrotising jejunitis is an uncommon condition that occurs in children; its potential causes are many but often no cause is found [479]. The disease shows similarities to enteritis necroticans (see above) and may represent a bacterial overgrowth pathology. Corrosive jejunitis due to the ingestion of acids may occur but this is only likely after previous gastroenterostomy allows the undiluted acid to enter the jejunum [480].

Chronic 'non-specific' duodenitis

Inflammation of the duodenum is caused by a large number of pathogenic mechanisms with diverse clinical implications. After prior infections, focal aggregates of T cells may persist in the duodenal mucosa [481]. Epithelial lymphocytosis is observed in a variety of conditions such as food allergy, giardiasis, viral enteritis, NSAID injury, after chemoradiotherapy, autoimmune enteropathy, Crohn's disease and *Helicobacter*-induced duodenitis.

This discussion is divided into two main groups: (1) inflammation maximal in the duodenal bulb and clearly associated with *H. pylori* infection, chronic active gastritis and peptic ulcer disease (variably called chronic non-specific duodenitis, chronic active duodenitis, peptic duodenitis and, even, *H. pylori* bulbitis) [482,483] and (2) that due to other specific causes such as coeliac disease, Crohn's disease, prior infections other than *H. pylori* and drugs. To the practising pathologist, the differentiation of *H. pylori*-related duodenitis, coeliac disease and Crohn's disease is probably the most important. For an account of the pathology of other causes of duodenitis, the reader should seek the appropriate sections elsewhere in this chapter. This account concentrates on the pathology of duodenitis associated with *H. pylori*, maximal in the bulb of the duodenum. Further, for a full account of the pathogenesis of *Helicobacter*-related gastritis and peptic ulcer disease, including that in the duodenum, the interested reader should consult Chapter 11.

Endoscopically, duodenitis may show mucosal swelling, small polyps, erythema, erosions, petechial haemorrhages and ulceration. There is often poor correlation between endoscopy and histology: it is well recognised that the endoscopically normal duodenum will harbour inflammatory changes on biopsy [483]. However, those with detectable macroscopic features are at significant risk for subsequent peptic ulcer disease in the duodenum [484].

The microscopic assessment of duodenitis has not been helped by a lack of uniformity and definition and by the fact that assessment of inflammation is particularly difficult in a mucosa with a considerable mononuclear cell presence in the physiological state. Furthermore, the variation in villous architecture in the normal duodenal bulb is considerable, with leaf and clubbed forms common, and this underpins the importance of well-orientated sections for histological assessment [485]. For these reasons, only gross abnormalities of mononuclear cell numbers and villous

architecture can be regarded as reliable markers for duodenitis (Figure 20.46) [485,486].

Neutrophils are a much more reliable indicator of duodenitis: these are seen in the lamina propria and in crypt and surface epithelium. The infiltrate is often focal, emphasising the importance of examining multiple levels. Surface and crypt epithelial changes are also of importance with degenerative changes in the former and regenerative changes in the latter. Finally, active duodenitis is associated with gastric metaplasia (see Figure 20.40). Although this feature may be seen in duodenal Crohn's disease, and less commonly in coeliac disease [487], it is an important component of *H. pylori*-associated duodenitis and peptic ulcer disease (Figure 20.46) [482,488]. *H. pylori* will not normally

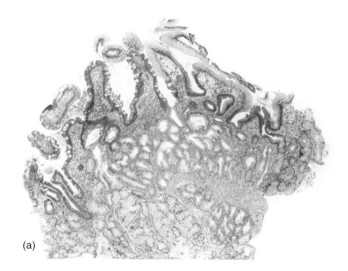

(a)

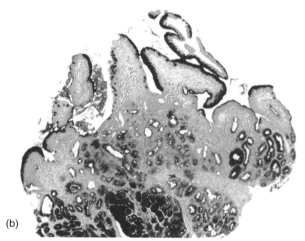

(b)

Figure 20.46 A chronic duodenitis with minor abnormalities of crypt architecture: (a) gastric metaplasia is just discernible at this power. The pathology was *Helicobacter pylori* related. (b) A periodic acid–Schiff (PAS) stain serves to highlight the gastric metaplasia in the biopsy. Many believe that a PAS stain should be a routine procedure for duodenal biopsies.

colonise small intestinal mucosa and gastric metaplasia is an important part of the pathogenesis of *H. pylori*-related duodenitis and duodenal peptic ulceration [489,490].

Other factors known to be important in the genesis of chronic active gastritis are also important in the duodenum, e.g. increased *H. pylori* pathogenicity, determined by cagA and vacuolating toxin positivity, is predictive of duodenitis and ulceration [482,483,491]. *H. pylori* is much more difficult to demonstrate in duodenal mucosal biopsies than in gastric biopsies. They are usually scanty and in coccoid forms [483]. Initial studies suggested that only about 50% of inflamed duodenal biopsies will show identifiable *H. pylori* [490]. Cytology of smears of duodenal biopsies may be more rewarding [492].

References

1. Girard MP, Steele D, Chaignat CL, Kieny MP. A review of vaccine research and development: human enteric infections. *Vaccine* 2006; **24**:2732.
2. O'Mahony S, Morris AJ, Straiton M, Murray L, Mackenzie JF. Push enteroscopy in the investigation of small-intestinal disease. *Q J Med* 1996;**89**:685.
3. Blacklow NR, Greenberg HB. Viral gastroenteritis. *N Engl J Med* 1991;**325**:252.
4. Kaljot KT, Ling JP, Gold JW, et al. Prevalence of acute enteric viral pathogens in acquired immunodeficiency syndrome patients with diarrhea. *Gastroenterology* 1989;**97**:1031.
5. Lieberman JM. Rotavirus and other viral causes of gastroenteritis. *Pediatr Ann* 1994;**23**:529.
6. Hrdy DB. Epidemiology of rotaviral infection in adults. *Rev Infect Dis* 1987;**9**:461.
7. Kohler T, Erben U, Wiedersberg H, Bannert N. Histologische befunde der Dunndarmschleimhaut bei Rotavirusinfektionen im Sauglings-und Kleinkindalter. *Kinderarztl Prax* 1990; **58**:323.
8. Davidson GP, Barnes GL. Structural and functional abnormalities of the small intestine in infants and young children with rotavirus enteritis. *Acta Paediatr Scand* 1979;**68**:181.
9. Jeffries BC, Brandt CD, Kim HW, Rodriguez WJ, Arrobio JO, Parrott RH. Diarrhea-associated adenovirus from the respiratory tract. *J Infect Dis* 1988;**157**:1275.
10. Nicolas JC, Ingrand D, Fortier B, Bricout F. A one-year virological survey of acute intussusception in childhood. *J Med Virol* 1982;**9**:267.
11. Blanshard C, Francis N, Gazzard BG. Investigation of chronic diarrhoea in acquired immunodeficiency syndrome. A prospective study of 155 patients. *Gut* 1996;**39**:824.
12. Luthi TM, Wall PG, Evans HS, Adak GK, Caul EO. Outbreaks of foodborne viral gastroenteritis in England and Wales:1992 to 1994. *Commun Dis Rep CDR Rev* 1996;**6**:R131.
13. Madeley CR. Viruses associated with acute diarrhoeal illness. In: Zuckerman AJ, Banatvala JE, Pattison JR (eds), *Principles and Practice of Clinical Virology*. Chichester: John Wiley & Sons, 1995: 189.
14. Caul EO. Viral gastroenteritis: small round structured viruses, caliciviruses and astroviruses. Part I. The clinical and diagnostic perspective. *J Clin Pathol* 1996;**49**:874.
15. Hale AD, Crawford SE, Ciarlet M, et al. Expression and self-assembly of Grimsby virus: antigenic distinction from Norwalk and Mexico viruses. *Clin Diagn Lab Immunol* 1999;**6**:142.
16. Glass RI, Noel J, Ando T, et al. The epidemiology of enteric caliciviruses from humans: a reassessment using new diagnostics. *J Infect Dis* 2000;**181**(suppl 2):S254.
17. Dedman D, Laurichesse H, Caul EO, Wall PG. Surveillance of small round structured virus (SRSV) infection in England and Wales, 1990–5. *Epidemiol Infect* 1998;**121**:139.
18. Kapikian AZ. Overview of viral gastroenteritis. *Arch Virol Suppl* 1996;**12**:7.
19. Nakata S, Honma S, Numata KK, et al. Members of the family caliciviridae (Norwalk virus and Sapporo virus) are the most prevalent cause of gastroenteritis outbreaks among infants in Japan. *J Infect Dis* 2000;**181**:2029.
20. Morotti RA, Kaufman SS, Fishbein YM, et al. Calicivirus infection in pediatric small intestine transplant recipients: pathological considerations. *Hum Pathol* 2004;**35**:1236.
21. Oikarinen M, Tauriainen S, Honkanen T, et al. Detection of enteroviruses in the intestine of type 1 diabetic patients. *Clin Exp Immunol* 2007;**151**:71.
22. Glass RI, Noel J, Mitchell D, et al. The changing epidemiology of astrovirus-associated gastroenteritis: a review. *Arch Virol Suppl* 1996;**12**:287.
23. Openshaw PJ. Crossing barriers: infections of the lung and the gut. *Mucosal Immunol* 2009;**2**:100.
24. Edert DY, Finance CM, Le Faou AE. Susceptibility of clinical strains of herpes simplex virus to three nucleoside analogues. *Chemotherapy* 2000;**46**:195.
25. Chen T, Hudnall SD. Anatomical mapping of human herpesvirus reservoirs of infection. *Mod Pathol* 2006;**19**:726.
26. Cheung AN, Ng IO. Cytomegalovirus infection of the gastrointestinal tract in non-AIDS patients. *Am J Gastroenterol* 1993; **88**:1882.
27. Petrogiannopoulos CL, Kalogeropoulos SG, Dandakis DC, et al. Cytomegalovirus enteritis in an immunocompetent host. *Chemotherapy* 2004;**50**:276.
28. Cooper HS, Raffensperger EC, Jonas L, Fitts WT. Cytomegalovirus inclusions in patients with ulcerative colitis and toxic dilation requiring colonic resection. *Gastroenterology* 1977;**72**: 1253.
29. Sindre H, Haraldsen G, Beck S, et al. Human intestinal endothelium shows high susceptibility to cytomegalovirus and altered expression of adhesion molecules after infection. *Scand J Immunol* 2000;**51**:354.
30. Genta RM, Bleyzer I, Cate TR, Tandon AK, Yoffe B. In situ hybridization and immunohistochemical analysis of cytomegalovirus-associated ileal perforation. *Gastroenterology* 1993;**104**:1822.
31. Iwasaki T. Alimentary tract lesions in cytomegalovirus infection. *Acta Pathol Jpn* 1987;**37**:549.
32. Shintaku M, Inoue N, Sasaki M, Izuno Y, Ueda Y, Ikehara S. Cytomegalovirus vasculitis accompanied by an exuberant fibroblastic reaction in the intestine of an AIDS patient. *Acta Pathol Jpn* 1991;**41**:900.
33. Tashiro Y, Goto M, Takemoto Y, et al. Epstein–Barr virus-associated enteritis with multiple ulcers after stem cell transplantation: first histologically confirmed case. *Pathol Int* 2006; **56**:530.
34. Plosker GL, Noble S. Indinavir: a review of its use in the management of HIV infection. *Drugs* 1999;**58**:1165.
35. Francis N. Histopathology of the gut in the acquired immune deficiency syndrome. *Eur J Gastroenterol Hepatol* 1992;**4**:449.
36. Bjarnason I, Sharpstone DR, Francis N, et al. Intestinal inflammation, ileal structure and function in HIV. *AIDS* 1996;**10**: 1385.
37. Batman PA, Kotler DP, Kapembwa MS, et al. HIV enteropathy: crypt stem and transit cell hyperproliferation induces villous

atrophy in HIV/Microsporidia-infected jejunal mucosa. *AIDS* 2007;**21**:433.

38. Batman PA, Miller AR, Forster SM, Harris JR, Pinching AJ, Griffin GE. Jejunal enteropathy associated with human immunodeficiency virus infection: quantitative histology. *J Clin Pathol* 1989;**42**:275.

39. Fox CH, Kotler D, Tierney A, Wilson CS, Fauci AS. Detection of HIV-1 RNA in the lamina propria of patients with AIDS and gastrointestinal disease. *J Infect Dis* 1989;**159**:467.

40. Kotler DP, Weaver SC, Terzakis JA. Ultrastructural features of epithelial cell degeneration in rectal crypts of patients with AIDS. *Am J Surg Pathol* 1986;**10**:531.

41. Kotler DP, Shimada T, Snow G, et al. Effect of combination antiretroviral therapy upon rectal mucosal HIV RNA burden and mononuclear cell apoptosis. *AIDS* 1998;**12**:597.

42. Francis N. Infectious complications of HIV disease: a selective review. *Curr Diagn Pathol* 1994;**1**:142.

43. Sepkowitz KA. Effect of HAART on natural history of AIDS-related opportunistic disorders. *Lancet* 1998;**351**:228.

44. Sansone GR, Frengley JD. Impact of HAART on causes of death of persons with late-stage AIDS. *J Urban Health* 2000;**77**:166.

45. Laughon BE, Druckman DA, Vernon A, et al. Prevalence of enteric pathogens in homosexual men with and without acquired immunodeficiency syndrome. *Gastroenterology* 1988;**94**:984.

46. Connolly GM, Forbes A, Gazzard BG. Investigation of seemingly pathogen-negative diarrhoea in patients infected with HIV1. *Gut* 1990;**31**:886.

47. Guerrant RL, Lima AAM. Inflammatory enteritides. In: Mandell GL, Bennett JE, Dolin R (eds), *Principles and Practice of Infectious Diseases*. Philadelphia, PA: Churchill Livingstone, 2000: 1126.

48. Shepherd NA. Pathological mimics of chronic inflammatory bowel disease. *J Clin Pathol* 1991;**44**:726.

49. Lindberg AA, Pal T. Strategies for development of potential candidate Shigella vaccines. *Vaccine* 1993;**11**:168.

50. Wolf MK. Bacterial infections of the small intestine and colon. *Curr Opin Gastroenterol* 2000;**16**:4.

51. Townes JM, Quick R, Gonzales OY, et al. Etiology of bloody diarrhea in Bolivian children: implications for empiric therapy. Bolivian Dysentery Study Group. *J Infect Dis* 1997;**175**:1527.

52. Day DW, Mandal BK, Morson BC. The rectal biopsy appearances in Salmonella colitis. *Histopathology* 1978;**2**:117.

53. Boyd JF. Pathology of the alimentary tract in *Salmonella typhimurium* food poisoning. *Gut* 1985;**26**:935.

54. Arnold JW, Niesel DW, Annable CR, et al. Tumor necrosis factor-alpha mediates the early pathology in Salmonella infection of the gastrointestinal tract. *Microb Pathog* 1993;**14**:217.

55. Blaser MJ, Parsons RB, Wang WL. Acute colitis caused by *Campylobacter fetus* ss. *jejuni. Gastroenterology* 1980;**78**:448.

56. Zilbauer M, Dorrell N, Wren BW, Bajaj-Elliott M. *Campylobacter jejuni*-mediated disease pathogenesis: an update. *Trans R Soc Trop Med Hyg* 2008;**102**:123.

57. Basnyat B, Maskey AP, Zimmerman MD, Murdoch DR. Enteric (typhoid) fever in travellers. *Clin Infect Dis* 2005;**41**:1467.

58. Pearson RD, Guerrant RL. Enteric fever and other causes of abdominal symptoms with fever. In: Mandell GL, Bennett JE, Dolin R (eds), *Principles and Practice of Infectious Diseases*. Philadelphia: Churchill Livingstone, 2000: 1136.

59. Gonzalez A, Vargas V, Guarner L, Accarino A, Guardia J. Toxic megacolon in typhoid fever. *Arch Intern Med* 1985;**145**:2120.

60. Chuttani HK, Jain K, Misra RC. Small bowel in typhoid fever. *Gut* 1971;**12**:709.

61. Noorani MA, Sial I, Mal V. Typhoid perforation of small bowel: a study of 72 cases. *J R Coll Surg Edinb* 1997;**42**:274.

62. Moyenuddin M, Weiss R, Wachsmuth IK, Ahearn DG. Nontoxigenic *Vibrio cholerae* O1 intestinal pathology in adult mice. *Zentralbl Bakteriol* 1995;**283**:43.

63. Asakura H, Morita A, Morishita T, et al. Pathologic findings from intestinal biopsy specimens in human cholera. *Am J Dig Dis* 1973;**18**:271.

64. Clarke SC. Diarrhoeagenic *Escherichia coli* – an emerging problem? *Diagn Microbiol Infect Dis* 2001;**41**:93.

65. Phillips AD, Navabpour S, Hicks S, Dougan G, Wallis T, Frankel G. Enterohaemorrhagic *Escherichia coli* O157:H7 target Peyer's patches in humans and cause attaching/effacing lesions in both human and bovine intestine. *Gut* 2000;**47**:377.

66. Isogai E, Isogai H, Kimura K, et al. Role of tumor necrosis factor alpha in gnotobiotic mice infected with an *Escherichia coli* O157:H7 strain. *Infect Immun* 1998;**66**:197.

67. Borriello SP. Clostridial disease of the gut. *Clin Infect Dis* 1995;**20 Suppl 2**:S242.

68. Tsutaoka B, Hansen J, Johnson D, Holodniy M. Antibiotic-associated pseudomembranous enteritis due to *Clostridium difficile*. *Clin Infect Dis* 1994;**18**:982.

69. Murrell TG, Walker PD. The pigbel story of Papua New Guinea. *Trans R Soc Trop Med Hyg* 1991;**85**:119.

70. Farrant JM, Traill Z, Conlon C, et al. Pigbel-like syndrome in a vegetarian in Oxford. *Gut* 1996;**39**:336.

71. Kreft B, Dalhoff K, Sack K. Necrotizing enterocolitis: a historical and current review. *Med Klin* 2000;**95**:435.

72. Cooke R. The pathology of pig bel. *P N G Med J* 1979;**22**:35.

73. Mintz AC, Applebaum H. Focal gastrointestinal perforations not associated with necrotizing enterocolitis in very low birth weight neonates. *J Pediatr Surg* 1993;**28**:857.

74. Han SJ, Jung PM, Kim H, et al. Multiple intestinal ulcerations and perforations secondary to methicillin-resistant *Staphylococcus aureus* enteritis in infants. *J Pediatr Surg* 1999;**34**:381.

75. Naik S, Smith F, Ho J, et al Staphylococcus enterotoxins G and I, a cause of severe but reversible neonatal enteropathy. *Clin Gastroenterol Hepatol* 2008;**6**:251.

76. Altemeier WA, Hummel RP, Hill EO. Staphylococcal enterocolitis following antibiotic therapy. *Ann Surg* 1963;**157**:847.

77. Haq AI, Cook LJ. MRSA enteritis causing a high stoma output in the early postoperative phase after bowel surgery. *Ann R Coll Surg Engl* 2007;**89**:3003.

78. Bradford WD, Noce PS, Gutman LT. Pathologic features of enteric infection with *Yersinia enterocolitica*. *Arch Pathol* 1974; **98**:17.

79. El Maraghi NR, Mair NS. The histopathology of enteric infection with *Yersinia pseudotuberculosis*. *Am J Clin Pathol* 1979; **71**:631.

80. Tauxe RV, Vandepitte J, Wauters G, et al. *Yersinia enterocolitica* infections and pork: the missing link. *Lancet* 1987;**i**:1129.

81. Vantrappen G, Ponette E, Geboes K, Bertrand P. Yersinia enteritis and enterocolitis: gastroenterological aspects. *Gastroenterology* 1977;**72**:220.

82. Gleason TH, Patterson SD. The pathology of *Yersinia enterocolitica* ileocolitis. *Am J Surg Pathol* 1982;**6**:347.

83. Vantrappen G, Geboes K, Ponette E. Yersinia enteritis. *Med Clin North Am* 1982;**66**:639.

84. Attwood SE, Mealy K, Cafferkey MT, et al. Yersinia infection and acute abdominal pain. *Lancet* 1987;**1**:529.

85. Lamps LW, Havens JM, Gilbrech LJ, Dube PH, Scott MA. Molecular biogrouping of pathogenic *Yersinia enterocolitica*: development of a diagnostic PCR assay with histologic correlation. *Am J Clin Pathol* 2006; **125**:658.

86. Kojima M, Morita Y, Shimizu K, et al Immunohistological findings of suppurative granulomas of *Yersinia enterocolitica* appendicitis: a report of two cases. *Pathol Res Pract* 2007;**203**:115.

87. Navarro-Llavat M, Domènech E, Masnou H, et al. Duodeno-ileo-colitis colagena precedida de infeccion intestinal por *Yersinia enterocolitica*: revision de la literatura a proposito de un caso. *Gastroenterol Hepatol* 2007;**30**:219.

88. Karper CM, Boman I. The significance of Klebsiella enteritis. A study of seven cases. *Am J Clin Pathol* 1966;**46**:632.

89. Janda JM, Abbott SL. Evolving concepts regarding the genus *Aeromonas*: an expanding Panorama of species, disease presentations, and unanswered questions. *Clin Infect Dis* 1998;**27**:332.

90. Alavandi S, Ananthan S, Kang G. Prevalence, in-vitro secretory activity, and cytotoxicity of *Aeromonas* species associated with childhood gastroenteritis in Chennai (Madras), India. *Jpn J Med Sci Biol* 1998;**51**:1.

91. Jones BL, Wilcox MH. Aeromonas infections and their treatment. *J Antimicrob Chemother* 1995;**35**:453.

92. Manley PN, Dhru R. Actinomycosis complicating Crohn's disease. *Gastroenterology* 1980;**79**:934.

93. Kirsch M. Bacterial overgrowth. *Am J Gastroenterol* 1990;**85**:231.

94. Riordan SM, McIver CJ, Wakefield D, Duncombe VM, Bolin TD, Thomas MC. Luminal immunity in small-intestinal bacterial overgrowth and old age. *Scand J Gastroenterol* 1996;**31**:1103.

95. Bragelmann R, Armbrecht U, Rosemeyer D, Schneider B, Zilly W, Stockbrugger RW. Small bowel bacterial overgrowth in patients after total gastrectomy. *Eur J Clin Invest* 1997;**27**:409.

96. Kaye SA, Lim SG, Taylor M, Patel S, Gillespie S, Black CM. Small bowel bacterial overgrowth in systemic sclerosis: detection using direct and indirect methods and treatment outcome. *Br J Rheumatol* 1995;**34**:265.

97. Mathias JR, Clench MH. Review: pathophysiology of diarrhea caused by bacterial overgrowth of the small intestine. *Am J Med Sci* 1985;**289**:243.

98. Haboubi NY, Lee GS, Montgomery RD. Duodenal mucosal morphometry of elderly patients with small intestinal bacterial overgrowth: response to antibiotic treatment. *Age Ageing* 1991;**20**:29.

99. Almadi MJ, Ghosh S, Aljebreen AM. Differentiating intestinal tuberculosis from Crohn's disease: a diagnostic challenge. *Am J Gastroenterol* 2009; **104**:2121.

100. Klimach OE, Ormerod LP. Gastrointestinal tuberculosis: a retrospective review of 109 cases in a district general hospital. *Q J Med* 1985;**56**:569.

101. Al Karawi MA, Mohamed AE, Yasawy MI, et al Protean manifestation of gastrointestinal tuberculosis: report on 130 patients. *J Clin Gastroenterol* 1995; **20**:225.

102. Leung VK, Law ST, Lam CW, et al. Intestinal tuberculosis in a regional hospital in Hong Kong: a 10-year experience. *Hong Kong Med J* 2006;**12**:264.

103. Sherman S, Rohwedder JJ, Ravikrishnan KP, Weg JG. Tuberculous enteritis and peritonitis. Report of 36 general hospital cases. *Arch Intern Med* 1980;**140**:506.

104. Ha HK, Ko GY, Yu ES, Yoon K, et al. Intestinal tuberculosis with abdominal complications: radiologic and pathologic features. *Abdom Imaging* 1999;**24**:32.

105. Tandon HD, Prakash A. Pathology of intestinal tuberculosis and its distinction from Crohn's disease. *Gut* 1972;**13**:260.

106. Gaffney EF, Condell D, Majmudar B, et al. Modification of caecal lymphoid tissue and relationship to granuloma formation in sporadic ileocaecal tuberculosis. *Histopathology* 1987;**11**:691.

107. Talwar S, Talwar R, Prasad P. Tuberculous perforations of the small intestine. *Int J Clin Pract* 1999;**53**:514.

108. Kaushik SP, Bassett ML, McDonald C, Lin BP, Bokey EL. Case report: gastrointestinal tuberculosis simulating Crohn's disease. *J Gastroenterol Hepatol* 1996;**11**:532.

109. Shepherd NA, Jass JR. Neuromuscular and vascular hamartoma of the small intestine: is it Crohn's disease? *Gut* 1987; **28**:1663.

110. Pulimood AB, Ramakrishna BS, Kurion G, et al. Endoscopic mucosal biopsies are useful in distinguishing granulomatous colitis due to Crohn's disease from tuberculosis. *Gut* 1999; **45**:537.

111. Lucas SB, De Cock KM, Hounnou A, et al. Contribution of tuberculosis to slim disease in Africa. *BMJ* 1994;**308**:1531.

112. Hellyer TJ, Brown IN, Taylor MB, Allen BW, Easmon CS. Gastro-intestinal involvement in *Mycobacterium avium-intracellulare* infection of patients with HIV. *J Infect* 1993; **26**:55.

113. Maliha GM, Hepps KS, Maia DM, Gentry KR, Fraire AE, Goodgame RW. Whipple's disease can mimic chronic AIDS enteropathy. *Am J Gastroenterol* 1991;**86**:79.

114. Boylston AW, Cook HT, Francis ND, Goldin RD. Biopsy pathology of acquired immune deficiency syndrome (AIDS). *J Clin Pathol* 1987;**40**:1.

115. Hamrock D, Azmi FH, O'Donnell E, Gunning WT, Philips ER, Zaher A. Infection by *Rhodococcus equi* in a patient with AIDS: histological appearance mimicking Whipple's disease and *Mycobacterium avium-intracellulare* infection. *J Clin Pathol* 1999; **52**:68.

116. Whipple GH. A hitherto undescribed disease characterised anatomically by deposits of fat and fatty acids in the intestinal and mesenteric lymphatic tissues. *Johns Hopkins Hosp Bull* 1907; **18**:382.

117. Lelan C, Dinasquet M, Saum B, et al. Aspect endoscopique et pathologique de l'atteinte intestinale et colique de la maladie de Whipple. *Gastroenterol Clin Biol* 2003;**27**:416.

118. Schneider T, Moos V, Loddenkemper C, Marth T, Fenollar F, Raoult D. Whipple's disease: new aspects of pathogenesis and treatment. *Lancet Infect Dis* 2008;**8**:179.

119. Yardley JH, Hendrix TR. Combined electron and light microscopy in Whipple's disease – demonstration of 'bacillary bodies' in the intestine. *Johns Hopkins Hosp Bull* 1961;**109**:80.

120. Wilson KH, Blitchington R, Frothingham R, Wilson JA. Phylogeny of the Whipple's disease-associated bacterium. *Lancet* 1991;**338**:474.

121. Relman DA, Schmidt TM, MacDermott RP, Falkow S. Identification of the uncultured bacillus of Whipple's disease. *N Engl J Med* 1992;**327**:293.

122. La Scola B, Fenollar F, Fournier PE, Altwegg M, Mallet MN, Raoult D. Description of *Tropheryma whipplei* gen nov, sp nov, the Whipple's disease bacillus. *In J Syst Evol Microbiol* 2001; **51**:1471.

123. Maiwald M, Schuhmacher F, Ditton HJ, von Herbay A. Environmental occurrence of the Whipple's disease bacterium (*Tropheryma whipplei*). *Appl Environ Microbiol* 1998;**64**:760.

124. Amsler P, Bauernfeind P, Nigg C, Maibach RC, Steffen R, Altwegg M. Prevalence of *Tropheryma whipplei* DNA in patients with various gastrointestinal diseases and in healthy controls. *Infection* 2003;**31**:81.

125. Schijf LJ, Becx MCJM, de Bruin PC, Van der Vegt SGL. Whipple's disease: easily diagnosed, if considered. *Neth J Med* 2008; **66**:392.

126. Dobbins WO. Current concepts of Whipple's disease. *J Clin Gastroenterol* 1982;**4**:205.

127. Ectors N, Geboes K, De Vos R, et al. Whipple's disease: a histological, immunocytochemical and electronmicroscopic study of the immune response in the small intestinal mucosa. *Histopathology* 1992;**21**:1.

128. Marth T, Neurath M, Cuccherini BA, Strober W. Defects of monocyte interleukin 12 production and humoral immunity in Whipple's disease. *Gastroenterology* 1997;**113**:442.

129. Bonhomme CJ, Renesto P, Desnues B, et al. *Tropheryma whipplei* glycosylation in the pathophysiologic profile of Whipple's disease. *J Infect Dis.* 2009;**199**:1043.

130. Geboes K, Ectors N, Heidbuchel H, Rutgeerts P, Desmet V, Vantrappen G. Whipple's disease: endoscopic aspects before and after therapy. *Gastrointest Endosc* 1990;**36**:247.

131. Isenberg JI, Gilbert SB, Pitcher JL. Ascites with peritoneal involvement in Whipple's disease. Report of a case. *Gastroenterology* 1971;**60**:305.

132. Von Herbay A, Ditton HJ, Maiwald M. Diagnostic application of a polymerase chain reaction assay for the Whipple's disease bacterium to intestinal biopsies. *Gastroenterology* 1996;**110**:1735.

133. Wilcox GM, Tronic BS, Schecter DJ, Arron MJ, Righi DF, Weiner NJ. Periodic acid–Schiff-negative granulomatous lymphadenopathy in patients with Whipple's disease. Localization of the Whipple bacillus to noncaseating granulomas by electron microscopy. *Am J Med* 1987;**83**:165.

134. Dauga C, Miras I, Grimont PA. Strategy for detection and identification of bacteria based on 16S rRNA genes in suspected cases of Whipple's disease. *J Med Microbiol* 1997;**46**:340.

135. Muller C, Petermann D, Stain C, et al. Whipple's disease: comparison of histology with diagnosis based on polymerase chain reaction in four consecutive cases. *Gut* 1997;**40**:425.

136. Gras E, Matias-Guiu X, Garcia A, et al. PCR analysis in the pathological diagnosis of Whipple's disease: emphasis on extraintestinal involvement or atypical morphological features. *J Pathol* 1999;**188**:318.

137. Morgenegg S, Dutly F, Altwegg M. Cloning and sequencing of a part of the heat shock protein 65 gene (hsp65) of 'Tropheryma whipplei' and its use for detection of 'T. whipplei' in clinical specimens by PCR. *J Clin Microbiol* 2000;**38**:2248.

138. Feurle GE, Marth T. An evaluation of antimicrobial treatment for Whipple's disease. Tetracycline versus trimethoprim–sulfamethoxazole. *Dig Dis Sci* 1994;**39**:1642.

139. Ramzan NN, Loftus E, Burgart LJ, et al. Diagnosis and monitoring of Whipple disease by polymerase chain reaction. *Ann Intern Med* 1997;**126**:520.

140. Geboes K, Ectors N, Heidbuchel H, Rutgeerts P, Desmet V, Vantrappen G. Whipple's disease: the value of upper gastrointestinal endoscopy for the diagnosis and follow-up. *Acta Gastroenterol Belg* 1992;**55**:209.

141. Shepherd NA. What is the significance of muciphages in colorectal biopsies? Muciphages and other mucosal accumulations in the colorectal mucosa. *Histopathology* 2000;**36**:559.

142. Rodarte JR, Garrison CO, Holley KE, Fontana RS. Whipple's disease simulating sarcoidosis. A case with unique clinical and histologic features. *Arch Intern Med* 1972;**129**:479.

143. Prescott RJ, Harris M, Banerjee SS. Fungal infections of the small and large intestine. *J Clin Pathol* 1992;**45**:806.

144. Radin DR, Fong TL, Halls JM, Pontrelli GN. Monilial enteritis in acquired immunodeficiency syndrome. *A J R Am J Roentgenol* 1983;**141**:1289.

145. Fischer D, Labayle D, Versapuech JM, Grange D, Kemeny F. Candidiasis involvement of the small intestine complicated by perforation. A case of favorable course. *Gastroenterol Clin Biol* 1987;**11**:514.

146. Trésalet C, Nguyen-Thanh Q, Aubriot-Lorton MH, et al. Small bowel infarction from disseminated aspergillosis. *Dis Colon Rectum* 2004;**47**:1515.

147. Vianna R, Misra V, Fridell JA, Goldman M, Mangus RS, Tector J. Survival after disseminated invasive aspergillosis in a multivisceral transplant recipient. *Transplant Proc* 2007;**39**:305.

148. Tay MH, Balram C, Foo KF, Busmanis I, Raman S, Khoo KS. Unusual case of bowel infarction with invasive aspergillus in an immunocompromised patient. *Ann Acad Med Singapore* 2003;**32**:122.

149. Halasa NB, Whitlock JA, McCurley TL, et al. Fatal hemophagocytic lymphohistiocytosis associated with Epstein–Barr virus infection in a patient with a novel mutation in the signalling lymphocytic activation molecule-associated protein. *Clin Infect Dis* 2003;**37**:136.

150. Suh W, Park CS, Lee MS, et al. Hepatic and small bowel mucormycosis after chemotherapy in a patient with acute lymphocytic leukaemia. *J Korean Med Sci* 2000;**15**:351.

151. Nagy-Agren SE, Chu P, Smith GJ, Waskin HA, Altice FL. Zygomycosis (mucormycosis) and HIV infection: report of three cases and review. *J AIDS Hum Retrovirol* 1995;**10**:441.

152. Kinchen K, Kinchen TH, Inglesby T Jr. *Pneumocystis carinii* infection of the small intestine. *J Natl Med Assoc* 1998;**90**:625.

153. Haws CC, Long RF, Caplan GE. *Histoplasma capsulatum* as a cause of ileocolitis. *Am J Roentgenol* 1977;**128**:692.

154. Cappell MS, Mandell W, Grimes MM, Neu HC. Gastrointestinal histoplasmosis. *Dig Dis Sci* 1988;**33**:353.

155. Orchard JL, Luparello F, Brunskill D. Malabsorption syndrome occurring in the course of disseminated histoplasmosis: case report and review of gastrointestinal histoplasmosis. *Am J Med* 1979;**66**:331.

156. McCullough K, Damjanov I. Intestinal histoplasmosis mimicking Whipple's disease. *Histopathology* 2005;**48**:306.

157. Alberto-Flor JJ, Granda A. Ileocecal histoplasmosis mimicking Crohn's disease in a patient with Job's syndrome. *Digestion* 1986;**33**:176.

158. Ackers JP. Gut coccidia – *Isospora, Cryptosporidium, Cyclospora* and *Sarcocystis. Semin Gastrointest Dis* 1997;**8**:33.

159. Farthing MJ. Diarrhoeal disease: current concepts and future challenges. Pathogenesis of giardiasis. *Trans R Soc Trop Med Hyg* 1993;**87**(suppl 3):17.

160. Oberhuber G, Kastner N, Stolte M. Giardiasis: a histologic analysis of 567 cases. *Scand J Gastroenterol* 1997;**32**:48.

161. Chester AC, MacMurray FG, Restifo MD, Mann O. Giardiasis as a chronic disease. *Dig Dis Sci* 1985;**30**:215.

162. Ament ME, Rubin CE. Relation of giardiasis to abnormal intestinal structure and function in gastrointestinal immunodeficiency syndromes. *Gastroenterology* 1972;**62**:216.

163. Buret AG. Pathophysiology of enteric infections with *Giardia duodenalis. Parasite* 2008;**15**:261.

164. Oberhuber G, Vogelsang H, Stolte M, Muthenthaler S, Kummer AJ, Radaszkiewicz T. Evidence that intestinal intra-epithelial lymphocytes are activated cytotoxic T cells in celiac disease but not in giardiasis. *Am J Pathol* 1996;**148**:1351.

165. Laurent F, McCole D, Eckmann L, Kagnoff MF. Pathogenesis of *Cryptosporidium parvum* infection. *Microbes Infect* 1999;**1**:141.

166. Katsumata T, Hosea D, Ranuh IG, Uga S, Yanagi T, Kohno S. Short report: possible *Cryptosporidium muris* infection in humans. *Am J Trop Med Hyg* 2000;**62**:70.

167. Jelinek T, Lotze M, Eichenlaub S, Loscher T, Nothdurft HD. Prevalence of infection with *Cryptosporidium parvum* and *Cyclospora cayetanensis* among international travellers. *Gut* 1997;**41**:801.

168. Manabe YC, Clark DP, Moore RD, et al. Cryptosporidiosis in patients with AIDS: correlates of disease and survival. *Clin Infect Dis* 1998;**27**:536.

169. Goodgame RW, Kimball K, Ou CN, et al. Intestinal function and injury in acquired immunodeficiency syndrome- related cryptosporidiosis. *Gastroenterology* 1995;**108**:1075.

170. Genta RM, Chappell CL, White AC, Kimball KT, Goodgame RW. Duodenal morphology and intensity of infection in AIDS-related intestinal cryptosporidiosis. *Gastroenterology* 1993;**105**:1769.

171. Lumadue JA, Manabe YC, Moore RD, Belitsos PC, Sears CL, Clark DP. A clinicopathologic analysis of AIDS-related cryptosporidiosis. *AIDS* 1998;**12**:2459.

172. Kelly P, Thillainayagam AV, Smithson J, et al. Jejunal water and electrolyte transport in human cryptosporidiosis. *Dig Dis Sci* 1996;**41**:2095.

173. Marcial MA, Madara JL. *Cryptosporidium*: cellular localization, structural analysis of absorptive cell-parasite membrane-membrane interactions in guinea pigs, and suggestion of protozoan transport by M cells. *Gastroenterology* 1986;**90**:583.

174. Pape JW, Johnson WD. *Isospora belli* infections. *Prog Clin Parasitol* 1991;**2**:119.

175. Bernard E, Delgiudice P, Carles M, et al. Disseminated isosporiasis in an AIDS patient. *Eur J Clin Microbiol Infect Dis* 1997;**16**:699.

176. Bendall RP, Lucas S, Moody A, Tovey G, Chiodini PL. Diarrhoea associated with cyanobacterium-like bodies: a new coccidian enteritis of man. *Lancet* 1993;**341**:590.

177. Green ST, McKendrick MW, Mohsen AH, Schmid ML, Prakasam SF. Two simultaneous cases of Cyclospora cayatensis enteritis returning from the Dominican Republic. *J Travel Med* 2000;**7**:41.

178. Soave R, Herwaldt BL, Relman DA. Cyclospora. *Infect Dis Clin North Am* 1998;**12**:1.

179. Looney WJ. *Cyclospora* species as a cause of diarrhoea in humans. *Br J Biomed Sci* 1998;**55**:157.

180. Connor BA, Reidy J, Soave R. Cyclosporiasis: clinical and histopathologic correlates. *Clin Infect Dis* 1999;**28**:1216.

181. Verdier RI, Fitzgerald DW, Johnson WD, Pape JW. Trimethoprim-sulfamethoxazole compared with ciprofloxacin for treatment and prophylaxis of *Isospora belli* and *Cyclospora cayetanensis* infection in HIV-infected patients. A randomized, controlled trial. *Ann Intern Med* 2000;**132**:885.

182. Sturbaum GD, Ortega YR, Gilman RH, Sterling CR, Cabrera L, Klein DA. Detection of *Cyclospora cayetanensis* in wastewater. *Appl Environ Microbiol* 1998;**64**:2284.

183. Fleming CA, Caron D, Gunn JE, Barry MA. A foodborne outbreak of *Cyclospora cayetanensis* at a wedding: clinical features and risk factors for illness. *Arch Intern Med* 1998;**158**:1121.

184. Eberhard ML, Pieniazek NJ, Arrowood MJ. Laboratory diagnosis of *Cyclospora* infections. *Arch Pathol Lab Med* 1997;**121**:792.

185. Lucas SB. Imported infectious diseases. In: Lowe DG, Underwood JCE (eds), *Recent Advances in Histopathology*. Edinburgh: Churchill Livingstone, 2000: 23.

186. Franzen C, Muller A. Molecular techniques for detection, species differentiation, and phylogenetic analysis of microsporidia. *Clin Microbiol Rev* 1999;**12**:243.

187. Cali A, Kotler DP, Orenstein JM. *Septata intestinalis* N. G., N. Sp., an intestinal microsporidian associated with chronic diarrhea and dissemination in AIDS patients. *J Eukaryot Microbiol* 1993;**40**:101.

188. Cotte L, Rabodonirina M, Chapuis F, et al. Waterborne outbreak of intestinal microsporidiosis in persons with and without human immunodeficiency virus infection. *J Infect Dis* 1999;**180**:2003.

189. Wichro E, Hoelzl D, Krause R, Bertha G, Reinthaler F, Wenisch C. Microsporidiosis in travel-associated chronic diarrhea in immune competent patients. *Am J Trop Med Hyg* 2005;**73**:285.

190. Van Hal SJ, Muthiath K, Matthews G, et al. Declining incidence of intestinal microsporidiosis and reduction in AIDS-related mortality following introduction of HAART in Sydney, Australia. *Trans R Soc Trop Med Hyg* 2007;**101**:1096.

191. Dworkin MS, Buskin SE, Davidson AJ, et al. Prevalence of intestinal microsporidiosis in human immunodeficiency virus-infected patients with diarrhea in major United States cities. *Rev Inst Med Trop Sao Paulo* 2007;**49**:339.

192. Chabchoub N, Abdelmalek R, Mellouli F, et al. Genetic identification of intestinal microsporidiosis species in immunocompromised patients in Tunisia. *Am J Trop Med Hyg* 2009;**80**:24.

193. Talal AH, Kotler DP, Orenstein JM, Weiss LM. Detection of *Enterocytozoon bieneusi* in fecal specimens by polymerase chain reaction analysis with primers to the small-subunit rRNA. *Clin Infect Dis* 1998;**26**:673.

194. Schwartz DA, Abou-Elella A, Wilcox CM, et al., Enteric Opportunistic Infections Working Group. The presence of *Enterocytozoon bieneusi* spores in the lamina propria of small bowel biopsies with no evidence of disseminated microsporidiosis. *Arch Pathol Lab Med* 1995;**119**:424.

195. Albrecht H, Sobottka I, Emminger C, et al. Visceral leishmaniasis emerging as an important opportunistic infection in HIV-infected persons living in areas nonendemic for *Leishmania donovani*. *Arch Pathol Lab Med* 1996;**120**:189.

196. Alvar J, Canavate C, Gutierrez-Solar B, et al. Leishmania and human immunodeficiency virus coinfection: the first 10 years. *Clin Microbiol Rev* 1997;**10**:298.

197. Koberle F. Enteromegaly and cardiomegaly in Chagas' disease. *Gut* 1963;**4**:42.

198. Binford CH, Connor DH. *Pathology of Tropical and Extraordinary Disease: An atlas*. Washington DC: Armed Forces Institute of Pathology, 1976.

199. Sturchler D. Parasitic diseases of the small intestinal tract. *Baillière's Clin Gastroenterol* 1987;**1**:397.

200. Grencis RK, Cooper ES. *Enterobius, trichuris, capillaria*, and hookworm including *Ancylostoma caninum*. *Gastroenterol Clin North Am* 1996;**25**:579.

201. Albonico M, Savioli L. Hookworm infection and disease: advances for control. *Ann Ist Super Sanita* 1997;**33**:567.

202. Stoltzfus RJ, Dreyfuss ML, Chwaya HM, Albonico M. Hookworm control as a strategy to prevent iron deficiency. *Nutr Rev* 1997;**55**:223.

203. Banwell JG, Marsden PD, Blackman V, Leonard PJ, Hutt MS. Hookworm infection and intestinal absorption amongst Africans in Uganda. *Am J Trop Med Hyg* 1967;**16**:304.

204. Salem SN, Truelove SC. Hookworm disease in immigrants. *BMJ* 1964;**i**:104.

205. Pawlowski ZS. Ascariasis. *Clin Gastroenterol* 1978;**7**:157.

206. Embil JA, Pereira LH, White FM, Garner JB, Manuel FR. Prevalence of *Ascaris lumbricoides* infection in a small Nova Scotian community. *Am J Trop Med Hyg* 1984;**33**:595.

207. Ihekwaba FN. Intestinal ascariasis and the acute abdomen in the tropics. *J R Coll Surg Edinb* 1980; **25**:452.

208. Coskun A, Ozcan N, Durak AC, Tolu I, Gulec M, Turan C. Intestinal ascariasis as a cause of bowel obstruction in two patients: sonographic diagnosis. *J Clin Ultrasound* 1996;**24**:326.

209. de Silva NR, Chan MS, Bundy DA. Morbidity and mortality due to ascariasis: re-estimation and sensitivity analysis of global numbers at risk. *Trop Med Int Health* 1997;**2**:519.

210. Louw JH. Biliary ascariasis in childhood. *S Afr J Surg* 1974; **12**:219.

211. Gomez B, Tabar AI, Tunon T, et al. Eosinophilic gastroenteritis and Anisakis. *Allergy* 1998;**53**:1148.

212. Garcia-Labairu C, Alonso-Martinez JL, Martinez-Echeverria A, Rubio-Vela T, Zozaya-Urmeneta JM. Asymptomatic gastroduodenal anisakiasis as the cause of anaphylaxis. *Eur J Gastroenterol Hepatol* 1999;**11**:785.

213. Cespedes M, Saez A, Rodriguez I, Pinto JM, Rodriguez R. Chronic anisakiasis presenting as a mesenteric mass. *Abdom Imaging* 2000;**25**:548.

214. Kakizoe S, Kakizoe H, Kakizoe K, et al. Endoscopic findings and clinical manifestation of gastric anisakiasis. *Am J Gastroenterol* 1995;**90**:761.

215. Cross JH. Intestinal capillariasis. *Clin Microbiol Rev* 1992;**5**:120.

216. Dronda F, Chaves F, Sanz A, Lopez-Velez R. Human intestinal capillariasis in an area of nonendemicity: case report and review. *Clin Infect Dis* 1993;**17**:909.

217. Al Hanaei A, Hefny AF, El Teraifi H, Abu Zidan FM. Small bowel obstruction due to bilharziasis. *Scand J Gastroenterol* 2008;**43**:382.

218. Rascarachi G, Linares Torres P, Arias Rodriguez L, et al. Intestinal schistosomiasis. *Gastroenterol Hepatol* 2009;**32**:131.

219. Halsted CH, Sheir S, Raasch FO. The small intestine in human schistosomiasis. *Gastroenterology* 1969;**57**:622.

220. Elmasri SH, Boulos PB. Bilharzial granuloma of the gastrointestinal tract. *Br J Surg* 1976;**63**:887.

221. Prata A. Schistosomiasis mansoni. *Clin Gastroenterol* 1978;**7**:49.

222. Sherif SM. Malabsorption and schistosomal involvement of jejunum. *BMJ* 1970;**i**:671.

223. Iyer HV, Abaci IF, Rehnke EC, Enquist IF. Intestinal obstruction due to schistosomiasis. *Am J Surg* 1985;**149**:409.

224. Mahmoud AA. Strongyloidiasis. *Clin Infect Dis* 1996;**23**:949.

225. Berk SL, Verghese A, Alvarez S, Hall K, Smith B. Clinical and epidemiologic features of strongyloidiasis. A prospective study in rural Tennessee. *Arch Intern Med* 1987;**147**:1257.

226. Sprott V, Selby CD, Ispahani P, Toghill PJ. Indigenous strongyloidiasis in Nottingham. *BMJ (Clin Res Ed)* 1987;**294**:741.

227. Gill GV, Bell DR. *Strongyloides stercoralis* infection in Burma Star veterans. *BMJ (Clin Res Ed)* 1987;**294**:1003.

228. Pelletier LL, Baker CB, Gam AA, Nutman TB, Neva FA. Diagnosis and evaluation of treatment of chronic strongyloidiasis in ex-prisoners of war. *J Infect Dis* 1988;**157**:573.

229. Warren KS, Mahmoud AA. Algorithms in the diagnosis and management of exotic diseases. XXI. Liver, intestinal, and lung flukes. *J Infect Dis* 1977;**135**:692.

230. Schantz PM. Tapeworms (cestodiasis). *Gastroenterol Clin North Am* 1996;**25**:637.

231. Crohn BB, Ginzberg L, Oppenheimer GD. Regional ileitis: a pathological and clinical entity. *JAMA* 1932;**99**:1323.

232. Dalziel TK. Chronic interstitial enteritis. *BMJ* 1913;**ii**:1068.

233. Lockhart-Mummery HE, Morson BC. Crohn's disease (regional enteritis) of the large intestine and its distinction from ulcerative colitis. *Gut* 1960;**1**:87.

234. Morson BC, Lockhart-Mummery HE. Anal lesions in Crohn's disease. *Lancet* 1959;**ii**:1122.

235. Fielding JF, Toye DK, Beton DC, Cooke WT. Crohn's disease of the stomach and duodenum. *Gut* 1970;**11**:1001.

236. Basu MK, Asquith P, Thompson RA, Cooke WT. Proceedings: Oral lesions in patients with Crohn's disease. *Gut* 1974;**15**:346.

237. Geboes K, Jansens J, Rutgeerts P, Vantrappen G. Crohn's disease of the esophagus. *J Clin Gastroenterol* 1986;**8**:31.

238. Rankin GB, Watts HD, Melnyk CS, Kelley ML Jr. National Cooperative Crohn's Disease Study: extraintestinal manifestations and perianal complications. *Gastroenterology* 1979;**77**:914.

239. Greenstein AJ, Sachar DB, Smith H, Janowitz HD, Aufses AH Jr. Patterns of neoplasia in Crohn's disease and ulcerative colitis. *Cancer* 1980;**46**:403.

240. Ehlin AG, Montgomery SM, Ekbom A, Pounder RE, Wakefield AJ. Prevalence of gastrointestinal diseases in two British national birth cohorts. *Gut* 2003;**52**:1117.

241. Lakatos PL. Recent trends in the epidemiology of inflammatory bowel diseases: Up or down. *World J Gastroenterol* 2006;**14**:6102.

242. Thia KT, Loftus EV, Sandborn WJ, Yang SK. An update on the epidemiology of inflammatory bowel disease in Asia. *Am J Gastroenterol* 2008;**103**:3167.

243. Orholm M, Binder V, Sorensen TI, Rasmussen LP, Kykvik KO. Concordance of inflammatory bowel disease among Danish twins. Results of a nationwide study. *Scand J Gastroenterol* 2000;**35**:1075.

244. Weissenbach J. The human genome project: from mapping to sequencing. *Clin Chem Lab Med* 1998;**36**:511.

245. Satsangi J, Parkes M, Jewell DP. Molecular genetics of Crohn's disease: recent advances. *Eur J Surg* 1998;**164**:887.

246. Satsangi J, Parkes M, Louis E, et al. Two stage genome-wide search in inflammatory bowel disease provides evidence for susceptibility loci on chromosomes 3, 7 and 12. *Nat Genet* 1996; **14**:199.

247. Hugot JP, Laurent-Puig P, Gower-Rousseau C, et al. Mapping of a susceptibility locus for Crohn's disease on chromosome 16. *Nature* 1996;**379**:821.

248. Hugot J-P, Chamaillard M, Zouali H, et al. Association of NOD2 leucine-rich repeat variants with susceptibility to Crohn's disease. *Nature* 2001;**411**:599.

249. Ogura Y, Bonen DK, Inohara N, et al. A frameshift mutation in *NOD2* associated with susceptibility to Crohn's disease. *Nature* 2001;**411**:603.

250. Cho JH. The genetics and immunopathogenesis of inflammatory bowel disease. *Nat Rev Immunol* 2008;**8**:458.

251. Levine J. Exogenous factors in Crohn's disease. A critical review. *J Clin Gastroenterol* 1992;**14**:216.

252. Prantera C, Scribano ML. Crohn's disease: the case for bacteria. *Ital J Gastroenterol Hepatol* 1999;**31**:244.

253. Moss MT, Sanderson JD, Tizard ML, et al. Polymerase chain reaction detection of *Mycobacterium paratuberculosis* and *Mycobacterium avium* subsp *silvaticum* in long term cultures from Crohn's disease and control tissues. *Gut* 1992;**33**:1209.

254. Frank TS, Cook SM. Analysis of paraffin sections of Crohn's disease for *Mycobacterium paratuberculosis* using polymerase chain reaction. *Mod Pathol* 1996;**9**:32.

255. Chiba M, Fukushima T, Horie Y, Iizuka M, Masamune O. No *Mycobacterium paratuberculosis* detected in intestinal tissue, including Peyer's patches and lymph follicles, of Crohn's disease. *J Gastroenterol* 1998;**33**:482.

256. Van Kruiningen HJ. Lack of support for a common etiology in Johne's disease of animals and Crohn's disease in humans. *Inflamm Bowel Dis* 1999;**5**:183.

257. De Hertogh G, Aerssens J, De Hoogt R, et al Validation of 16S rDNA sequencing in microdissected bowel biopsies from Crohn's disease patients to assess bacterial flora diversity. *J Pathol* 2006;**209**:532.

258. De Hertogh G, Aerssens J, Geboes KP, Geboes K. Evidence for the involvement of infectious agents in the pathogenesis of Crohn's disease. *World J Gastroenterol* 2008;**14**:845.

259. Weiss AA, Babyatsky MW, Ogata S, et al. Expression of MUC2 and MUC3 mRNA in human normal, malignant, and inflammatory intestinal tissues. *J Histochem Cytochem* 1996;**44**:1161.

260. Wehkamp J, Fellermann K, Herrlinger KR, et al. Mechanisms of disease: defensins in gastrointestinal diseases. *Nat Clin Pract Gastroenterol Hepatol* 2005;**2**:406.

261. Selby WS, Janossy G, Bofill M, Jewell DP. Intestinal lymphocyte subpopulations in inflammatory bowel disease: an analysis by immunohistological and cell isolation techniques. *Gut* 1984; **25**:32.

262. Schreiber S, MacDermott RP, Raedler A, Pinnau R, Bertovich MJ, Nash GS. Increased activation of isolated intestinal lamina propria mononuclear cells in inflammatory bowel disease. *Gastroenterology* 1991;**101**:1020.

263. Bookman MA, Bull DM. Characteristics of isolated intestinal mucosal lymphoid cells in inflammatory bowel disease. *Gastroenterology* 1979;**77**:503.

264. MacDermott RP, Bragdon MJ, Thurmond RD. Peripheral blood mononuclear cells from patients with inflammatory bowel disease exhibit normal function in the allogeneic and autologous mixed leukocyte reaction and cell-mediated lympholysis. *Gastroenterology* 1984;**86**:476.

265. Keren DF, Appelman HD, Dobbins III WO, et al. Correlation of histopathologic evidence of disease activity with the presence of immunoglobulin-containing cells in the colons of patients with inflammatory bowel disease. *Hum Pathol*, 1984; **15**:757.

266. Colombel JF, Reumaux D, Duthilleul P, et al. Antineutrophil cytoplasmic autoantibodies in inflammatory bowel diseases. *Gastroenterol Clin Biol* 1992;**16**:656.

267. Meuret G, Bitzi A, Hammer B. Macrophage turnover in Crohn's disease and ulcerative colitis. *Gastroenterology* 1978;**74**:501.

268. Rugtveit J, Brandtzaeg P, Halstensen TS, Fausa O, Scott H. Increased macrophage subset in inflammatory bowel disease: apparent recruitment from peripheral blood monocytes. *Gut* 1994;**35**:669.

269. Allison MC, Cornwall S, Poulter LW, Dhillon AP, Pounder RE. Macrophage heterogeneity in normal colonic mucosa and in inflammatory bowel disease. *Gut* 1988;**29**:1531.

270. Sarsfield P, Jones DB, Wright DH. Accessory cells in Crohn's disease of the terminal ileum. *Histopathology* 1996;**28**:213.

271. Rachmilewitz D, Stamler JS, Bachwich D, Karmeli F, Ackerman Z, Podolsky DK. Enhanced colonic nitric oxide generation and nitric oxide synthase activity in ulcerative colitis and Crohn's disease. *Gut* 1995;**36**:718.

272. Buffinton GD, Doe WF. Depleted mucosal antioxidant defences in inflammatory bowel disease. *Free Radic Biol Med* 1995;**19**:911.

273. Dubucquoi S, Janin A, Klein O, et al. Activated eosinophils and interleukin 5 expression in early recurrence of Crohn's disease. *Gut* 1995;**37**:242.

274. Dinarello CA. Interleukin-1 and its biologically related cytokines. *Adv Immunol* 1989;**44**:153.

275. Nakamura M, Saito H, Kasanuki J, Tamura Y, Yoshida S. Cytokine production in patients with inflammatory bowel disease. *Gut* 1992;**33**:933.

276. Mahida YR, Kurlac L, Gallagher A, Hawkey CJ. High circulating concentrations of interleukin-6 in active Crohn's disease but not ulcerative colitis. *Gut* 1991;**32**:1531.

277. Stevens C, Walz G, Singaram C, et al. Tumor necrosis factor-alpha, interleukin-1 beta, and interleukin-6 expression in inflammatory bowel disease. *Dig Dis Sci* 1992;**37**:818.

278. Braegger CP, Nicholls S, Murch SH, Stephens S, MacDonald TT. Tumour necrosis factor alpha in stool as a marker of intestinal inflammation. *Lancet* 1992;**339**:89.

279. Targan SR, Hanauer SB, van Deventer SJ, et al. A short-term study of chimeric monoclonal antibody cA2 to tumor necrosis factor alpha for Crohn's disease. Crohn's Disease cA2 Study Group. *N Engl J Med* 1997;**337**:1029.

280. Present DH, Rutgeerts P, Targan S, et al. Infliximab for the treatment of fistulas in patients with Crohn's disease. *N Engl J Med* 1999;**340**:1398.

281. Mullin GE, Lazenby AJ, Harris ML, Bayless TM, James SP. Increased interleukin-2 messenger RNA in the intestinal mucosal lesions of Crohn's disease but not ulcerative colitis. *Gastroenterology* 1992;**102**:1620.

282. Sparano JA, Brandt LJ, Dutcher JP, DuBois JS, Atkins MB. Symptomatic exacerbation of Crohn disease after treatment with high-dose interleukin-2. *Ann Intern Med* 1993;**118**:617.

283. Fais S, Capobianchi MR, Pallone F, et al. Spontaneous release of interferon gamma by intestinal lamina propria lymphocytes in Crohn's disease. Kinetics of in vitro response to interferon gamma inducers. *Gut* 1991;**32**:403.

284. Breese E, Braegger CP, Corrigan CJ, Walker-Smith JA, MacDonald TT. Interleukin-2- and interferon-gamma-secreting T cells in normal and diseased human intestinal mucosa. *Immunology* 1993;**78**:127.

285. Gijsbers K, Geboes K, Van Damme J. Chemokines in Gastrointestinal disorders. *Curr Drug Targets* 2006;**7**:47.

286. Torres MI, LeDiscorde M, Lorite P, et al. Expression of HLA-G in inflammatory bowel disease provides a potential way to distinguish between ulcerative colitis and Crohn's disease. *Int Immunol* 2004;**16**:579.

287. Geboes K. Pathology of inflammatory bowel diseases (CIBD): variability with time and treatment. *Colorectal Dis* 2001;**3**:2.

288. Kuhn R, Lohler J, Rennick D, Rajewsky K, Muller W. Interleukin-10-deficient mice develop chronic enterocolitis. *Cell* 1993;**75**:263.

289. Hermiston ML, Gordon JI. Inflammatory bowel disease and adenomas in mice expressing a dominant negative N-cadherin. *Science* 1995;**270**:1203.

290. Geboes K, Yahia El-Zine M, Dalle I, El-Haddad S, Rutgeerts P, Van Eyken P. Tenascin and strictures in inflammatory bowel diseases: an immunohistochemical study. *Int J Surg Pathol* 2001;**9**:281.

291. Geboes K, Rutgeerts P, Opdenakker G, et al. Endoscopic and histologic evidence of persistent mucosal healing and correlation with clinical improvement following sustained infliximab treatment for Crohn's disease. *Curr Med Res Opin* 2005; **21**:1741.

292. Rutgeerts P, Geboes K, Vantrappen G, Kerremans R, Coenegrachts JL, Coremans G. Natural history of recurrent Crohn's disease at the ileocolonic anastomosis after curative surgery. *Gut* 1984;**25**:665.

293. Kelly JK, Sutherland LR. The chronological sequence in the pathology of Crohn's disease. *J Clin Gastroenterol* 1988;**10**:28.

294. Bataille F, Klebl F, Rummele P, Schroeder et al. Morphological characterisation of Crohn's disease fistulae. *Gut* 2004; **53**:1314.

295. Gasche C, Scholmerich J, Brynskow J, et al. A simple classification of Crohn's disease: report of the Working party for the World congress of Gastroenterology, Vienna 1998. *Inflamm Bowel Dis* 2000;**6**:8.

296. Silverberg M; Satsangi J, Ahmad T, et al. Toward an integrated clinical, molecular and serological classification of inflammatory bowel disease: report of a working party of the 2005 Montreal World congress of Gastroenterology. *Can J Gastroenterol* 2005; **19**(suppl A):1A.

297. Satsangi J, Silverberg MS, Vermeire S, Colombel JF. The Montreal classification of inflammatory bowel disease: controversies, consensus, and implications. *Gut* 2006;**55**:749.

298. Shelley-Fraser G, Borley NR, Warren BF, Shepherd NA. The connective tissue changes of Crohn's disease. *Histopathology* 2012;**60**:1034.

299. Heaton KW, McCarthy CF, Horton RE, Cornes JS, Read AE. Miliary Crohn's disease. *Gut* 1967;**8**:4.

300. Sheehan AL, Warren BF, Gear MW, Shepherd NA. Fat-wrapping in Crohn's disease: pathological basis and relevance to surgical practice. *Br J Surg* 1992;**79**:955.

301. Borley NR, Mortensen NJ, Jewell DP, Warren BF. The relationship between inflammatory and serosal connective tissue changes in ileal Crohn's disease: evidence for a possible causative link. *J Pathol* 2000;**190**:196.

302. Desreumaux P, Ernst O, Geboes K, et al. Inflammatory alterations in mesenteric adipose tissue in Crohn's disease. *Gastroenterology* 1999;**117**:73.

303. Nugent FW, Roy MA. Duodenal Crohn's disease: an analysis of 89 cases. *Am J Gastroenterol* 1989;**84**:249.

304. Oberhuber G, Hirsch M, Stolte M. High incidence of upper gastrointestinal tract involvement in Crohn's disease. *Virchows Arch* 1998;**432**:49.

305. Wright CL, Riddell RH. Histology of the stomach and duodenum in Crohn's disease. *Am J Surg Pathol* 1998;**22**:383.

306. Stange EF, Travis SP, Vermeire S, Beglinger C, et al. European evidence based consensus on the diagnosis and management of Crohn's disease: definitions and diagnosis. *Gut* 2006; **55** (suppl 1):i1.

307. Heimann TM, Miller F, Martinelli G, Szporn A, Greenstein AJ, Aufses AH Jr. Correlation of presence of granulomas with clinical and immunologic variables in Crohn's disease. *Arch Surg* 1988;**123**:46.

308. Chambers TJ, Morson BC. The granuloma in Crohn's disease. *Gut* 1979;**20**:269.

309. Schmitz-Moormann P, Pittner PM, Malchow H, Brandes JW. The granuloma in Crohn's disease. A bioptical study. *Pathol Res Pract* 1984;**178**:467.

310. Wolfson DM, Sachar DB, Cohen A, et al. Granulomas do not affect postoperative recurrence rates in Crohn's disease. *Gastroenterology* 1982;**83**:405.

311. Chardavoyne R, Flint GW, Pollack S, Wise L. Factors affecting recurrence following resection for Crohn's disease. *Dis Colon Rectum* 1986;**29**:495.

312. Kuramoto S, Oohara T, Ihara O, Shimazu R, Kondo Y. Granulomas of the gut in Crohn's disease. A step sectioning study. *Dis Colon Rectum* 1987;**30**:6.

313. Mooney EE, Walker J, Hourihane DO. Relation of granulomas to lymphatic vessels in Crohn's disease. *J Clin Pathol* 1995;**48**:335.

314. Wakefield AJ, Sankey EA, Dhillon AP, et al. Granulomatous vasculitis in Crohn's disease. *Gastroenterology* 1991;**100**:1279.

315. Matson AP, Van Kruiningen HJ, West AB, Cartun RW, Colombel JF, Cortot A. The relationship of granulomas to blood vessels in intestinal Crohn's disease. *Mod Pathol* 1995;**8**:680.

316. Cook MG. The size and histological appearances of mesenteric lymph nodes in Crohn's disease. *Gut* 1972;**13**:970.

317. Fujimura Y, Hosobe M, Kihara T. Ultrastructural study of M cells from colonic lymphoid nodules obtained by colonoscopic biopsy. *Dig Dis Sci* 1992; **37**:1089.

318. Wright NA, Pike C, Elia G. Induction of a novel epidermal growth factor-secreting cell lineage by mucosal ulceration in human gastrointestinal stem cells. *Nature* 1990;**343**:82.

319. Hanby AM, Wright NA. The ulcer-associated cell lineage: the gastrointestinal repair kit? *J Pathol* 1993;**171**:3.

320. Poulsom R, Chinery R, Sarraf C, et al. Trefoil peptide gene expression in small intestinal Crohn's disease and dietary adaptation. *J Clin Gastroenterol* 1993;**17**(suppl 1):S78.

321. Belai A, Boulos PB, Robson T, et al. Neurochemical coding in the small intestine of patients with Crohn's disease. *Gut* 1997; **40**:767.

322. Geboes K, Collins S. Structural abnormalities of the nervous system in Crohn's disease and ulcerative colitis. *Neurogastroenterol Motil* 1998;**10**:189.

323. Dvorak AM, Silen W. Differentiation between Crohn's disease and other inflammatory conditions by electron microscopy. *Ann Surg* 1985;**201**:53.

324. Funayama Y, Sasaki I, Naito H, Fukushima K, Matsuno S, Masuda T. Remodeling of vascular wall in Crohn's disease. *Dig Dis Sci* 1999;**44**:2319.

325. Desreumaux P, Huet G, Zerimech F, et al. Acute inflammatory intestinal vascular lesions and in situ abnormalities of the plasminogen activation system in Crohn's disease. *Eur J Gastroenterol Hepatol* 1999;**11**:1113.

326. Knutson H, Lunderquist A, Lunderquist A. Vascular changes in Crohn's disease. *Am J Roentgenol Radium Ther Nucl Med* 1968; **103**:380.

327. Xin W, Greenson JK. The clinical significance of focally enhanced gastritis. *Am J Surg Pathol* 2004; **28**:1347.

328. Yao K, Yao T, Iwashita A, et al. Microaggregate of immunostained macrophages in noninflamed gastroduodenal mucosa: a new useful histological marker for differentiating Crohn's colitis from ulcerative colitis *Am J Gastroenterol* 2000;**95**:1967.

329. Gad A. The diagnosis of gastroduodenal Crohn's disease by endoscopic biopsy. *Scand J Gastroenterol Suppl* 1989;**167**:23.

330. Yao K, Yao T, Iwashita A, Matsui T, Kamachi S. Microaggregate of immunostained macrophages in noninflamed gastroduodenal mucosa: a new useful histological marker for differentiating Crohn's colitis from ulcerative colitis. *Am J Gastroenterol* 2000; **95**:1967.

331. Schmidt-Sommerfeld E, Kirschner BS, Stephens JK. Endoscopic and histologic findings in the upper gastrointestinal tract of children with Crohn's disease. *J Pediatr Gastroenterol Nutr* 1990; **11**:448.

332. Poggioli G, Stocchi L, Laureti S, et al. Duodenal involvement of Crohn's disease: three different clinicopathologic patterns. *Dis Colon Rectum* 1997;**40**:179.

333. Yamamoto T, Bain IM, Connolly AB, Keighley MR. Gastroduodenal fistulas in Crohn's disease: clinical features and management. *Dis Colon Rectum* 1998;**41**:1287.

334. Spiess SE, Braun M, Vogelzang RL, Craig RM. Crohn's disease of the duodenum complicated by pancreatitis and common bile duct obstruction. *Am J Gastroenterol* 1992;**87**:1033.

335. Rubio CA, Befritz R, Poppen B, Svenberg T, Slezak P. Crohn's disease and adenocarcinoma of the intestinal tract. Report of four cases. *Dis Colon Rectum* 1991;**34**:174.

336. Geboes K, Ectors N, d'Haens G, Rutgeerts P. Is ileoscopy with biopsy worthwhile in patients presenting with symptoms of inflammatory bowel disease? *Am J Gastroenterol* 1998;**93**:201.

337. McHugh JB, Appelman HD, McKenna BJ. The diagnostic value of endoscopic terminal ileum biopsies. *Am J Gastroenterol* 2007; **102**:1084.

338. Geboes K. The strategy for biopsies of the terminal ileum should be evidence based. *Am J Gastroenterol* 2007;**102**:1090.

339. Pulimood AB, Ramakrishna BS, Kurian G, et al. Endoscopic mucosal biopsies are useful in distinguishing granulomatous colitis due to Crohn's disease from tuberculosis. *Gut* 1999;**45**:537.

340. Werlin SL, Chusid MJ, Caya J, Oechler HW. Colitis in chronic granulomatous disease. *Gastroenterology* 1982;**82**:328.

341. Shepherd NA. The pelvic ileal reservoir: pathology and pouchitis. *Neth J Med* 1990;**37**(suppl 1):S57.

342. Levison DA, Crocker PR, Smith A, Blackshaw AJ, Bartram CI. Varied light and scanning electron microscopic appearances of barium sulphate in smears and histological sections. *J Clin Pathol* 1984;**37**:481.

343. Kewenter J, Hulten L, Kock NG. The relationship and epidemiology of acute terminal ileitis and Crohn's disease. *Gut* 1974; **15**:801.

344. Warren BF, Shepherd NA. Surgical pathology of the intestines: the pelvic ileal reservoir and diversion proctocolitis. In: Lowe DG, Underwood JCE (eds), *Recent Advances in Histopathology*, 18th edn. Edinburgh: Churchill Livingstone, 2000: 63.

345. Wolff BG, Beart RW Jr, Frydenberg HB, Weiland LH, Agrez MV, Ilstrup DM. The importance of disease-free margins in resections for Crohn's disease. *Dis Colon Rectum* 1983;**26**:239.

346. Fazio VW, Marchetti F. Recurrent Crohn's disease and resection margins: bigger is not better. *Adv Surg* 1999;**32**:135.

347. Tytgat GN, Mulder CJ, Brummelkamp WH. Endoscopic lesions in Crohn's disease early after ileocecal resection. *Endoscopy* 1988;**20**:260.

348. De Jong E, van Dullemen HM, Slors JF, Dekkers P, van Deventer SJ, Tytgat GN. Correlation between early recurrence and reoperation after ileocolonic resection in Crohn's disease: a prospective study. *J Am Coll Surg* 1996;**182**:503.

349. Klein O, Colombel JF, Lescut D, et al. Remaining small bowel endoscopic lesions at surgery have no influence on early anastomotic recurrences in Crohn's disease. *Am J Gastroenterol* 1995;**90**:1949.

350. McLeod RS, Wolff BG, Steinhart AH, et al. Risk and significance of endoscopic/radiological evidence of recurrent Crohn's disease. *Gastroenterology* 1997;**113**:1823.

351. Rutgeerts P, Geboes K, Peeters M, et al. Effect of faecal stream diversion on recurrence of Crohn's disease in the neoterminal ileum. *Lancet* 1991;**338**:771.

352. D'Haens GR, Geboes K, Peeters M, Baert F, Penninckx F, Rutgeerts P. Early lesions of recurrent Crohn's disease caused by infusion of intestinal contents in excluded ileum. *Gastroenterology* 1998;**114**:262.

353. Heuman R, Boeryd B, Bolin T, Sjodahl R. The influence of disease at the margin of resection on the outcome of Crohn's disease. *Br J Surg* 1983;**70**:519.

354. Hamilton SR, Reese J, Pennington L, Boitnott JK, Bayless TM, Cameron JL. The role of resection margin frozen section in the surgical management of Crohn's disease. *Surg Gynecol Obstet* 1985;**160**:57.

355. Cooper JC, Williams NS. The influence of microscopic disease at the margin of resection on recurrence rates in Crohn's disease. *Ann R Coll Surg Engl* 1986;**68**:23.

356. Adloff M, Arnaud JP, Ollier JC. Does the histologic appearance at the margin of resection affect the postoperative recurrence rate in Crohn's disease? *Am Surg* 1987;**53**:543.

357. Kotanagi H, Kramer K, Fazio VW, Petras RE. Do microscopic abnormalities at resection margins correlate with increased anastomotic recurrence in Crohn's disease? Retrospective analysis of 100 cases. *Dis Colon Rectum* 1991;**34**:909.

358. Ferrante M, De Hertogh G, Hlavaty T, et al. The value of myenteric plexitis to predict early postoperative Crohn's disease recurrence. *Gastroenterology* 2006;**130**:1595.

359. Fazio VW, Marchetti F, Church M, et al. Effect of resection margins on the recurrence of Crohn's disease in the small bowel. A randomized controlled trial. *Ann Surg* 1996;**224**:563.

360. Steinberg DM, Cooke WT, Alexander-Williams J. Free perforation in Crohn's disease. *Gut* 1973;**14**:187.

361. Katz S, Schulman N, Levin L. Free perforation in Crohn's disease: a report of 33 cases and review of literature. *Am J Gastroenterol* 1986;**81**:38.

362. Gyde SN, Prior P, Macartney JC, Thompson H, Waterhouse JA, Allan RN. Malignancy in Crohn's disease. *Gut* 1980;**21**:1024.

363. Kvist N, Jacobsen O, Norgaard P, et al. Malignancy in Crohn's disease. *Scand J Gastroenterol* 1986;**21**:82.

364. Piton G, Cosnes J, Monnet E, et al. Risk factors associated with small bowel adenocarcinoma in Crohn's disease: a case–control study. *Am J Gastroenterol* 2008;**103**:1730.

365. Hawker PC, Gyde SN, Thompson H, Allan RN. Adenocarcinoma of the small intestine complicating Crohn's disease. *Gut* 1982;**23**:188.

366. Gillen CD, Wilson CA, Walmsley RS, Sanders DS, O'Dwyer ST, Allan RN. Occult small bowel adenocarcinoma complicating Crohn's disease: a report of three cases. *Postgrad Med J* 1995;**71**:172.

367. Thompson EM, Clayden G, Price AB. Cancer in Crohn's disease – an 'occult' malignancy. *Histopathology* 1983;**7**:365.

368. Simpson S, Traube J, Riddell RH. The histologic appearance of dysplasia (precarcinomatous change) in Crohn's disease of the small and large intestine. *Gastroenterology* 1981;**81**:492.

369. Perzin KH, Peterson M, Castiglione CL, Fenoglio CM, Wolff M. Intramucosal carcinoma of the small intestine arising in regional enteritis (Crohn's disease). Report of a case studied for carcinoembryonic antigen and review of the literature. *Cancer* 1984;**54**:151.

370. Sigel JE, Petras RE, Lashner BA, Fazio VW, Goldblum JR. Intestinal adenocarcinoma in Crohn's disease: a report of 30 cases with a focus on coexisting dysplasia. *Am J Surg Pathol* 1999;**23**:651.

371. Svrcek M, Cosnes J, Tiret E, Bennis M, Parc Y, Fléjou JF. Expression of epidermal growth factor receptor (EGFR) is frequent in inflammatory bowel disease (CIBD)-associated intestinal cancer. *Virchows Arch* 2007;**450**:243.

372. Sigel JE, Goldblum JR. Neuroendocrine neoplasms arising in inflammatory bowel disease: a report of 14 cases. *Mod Pathol* 1998;**11**:537.

373. Perosio PM, Brooks JJ, Saul SH, Haller DG. Primary intestinal lymphoma in Crohn's disease: minute tumor with a fatal outcome. *Am J Gastroenterol* 1992;**87**:894.

374. Brown I, Schofield JB, MacLennan KA, Tagart RE. Primary non-Hodgkin's lymphoma in ileal Crohn's disease. *Eur J Surg Oncol* 1992;**18**:627.

375. Woodley HE, Spencer JA, MacLennan KA. Small bowel lymphoma complicating long-standing Crohn's disease. *AJR Am J Roentgenol* 1997;**169**:1462.

376. Chassany O, Michaux A, Bergmann JF. Drug-induced diarrhoea. *Drug Saf* 2000;**22**:53.

377. Lewis JH. Gastrointestinal injury due to medicinal agents. *Am J Gastroenterol* 1986;**81**:819.

378. Carretero C, Munoz-Navas M, Betes M, et al. Gastroduodenal injury after radioembolization of hepatic tumors. *Am J Gastroenterol* 2007;**102**:1216.

379. Renert WA, Button KF, Fuld SL, Casarella WJ. Mesenteric venous thrombosis and small bowel infarction following infusion of vasopressin into the superior mesenteric artery. *Radiology* 1972;**102**:299.

380. Bjarnason I, Macpherson AJ. Intestinal toxicity of non-steroidal anti-inflammatory drugs. *Pharmacol Ther* 1994;**62**:145.

381. Morris AJ. Nonsteroidal anti-inflammatory drug enteropathy. *Gastrointest Endosc Clin North Am* 1999;**9**:125.

382. Allison MC, Howatson AG, Torrance CJ, Lee FD, Russell RI. Gastrointestinal damage associated with the use of nonsteroidal antiinflammatory drugs. *N Engl J Med* 1992;**327**:749.

383. Davies NM, Saleh JY, Skjodt NM. Detection and prevention of NSAID-induced enteropathy. *J Pharm Pharmaceut Sci* 2000;**3**:137.

384. Taha AS. Histopathological aspects of mucosal injury related to non-steroidal anti-inflammatory drugs. *Ital J Gastroenterol* 1996;**28**(suppl 4):12.

385. Schneider AR, Benz C, Riemann JF. Adverse effects of nonsteroidal anti-inflammatory drugs on the small and large bowel. *Endoscopy* 1999;**31**:761.

386. Bjarnason I, Hayllar J, Macpherson AJ, Russell AS. Side effects of nonsteroidal anti-inflammatory drugs on the small and large intestine in humans. *Gastroenterology* 1993;**104**:1832.

387. Levi S, Shaw-Smith C. Non-steroidal anti-inflammatory drugs: how do they damage the gut? *Br J Rheumatol* 1994;**33**:605–12.

388. Anthony A, Dhillon AP, Thrasivoulou C, Pounder RE, Wakefield AJ. Pre-ulcerative villous contraction and microvascular occlusion induced by indomethacin in the rat jejunum: a detailed morphological study. *Aliment Pharmacol Ther* 1995;**9**:605.

389. Anthony A, Pounder RE, Dhillon AP, Wakefield AJ. Vascular anatomy defines sites of indomethacin induced jejunal ulceration along the mesenteric margin. *Gut* 1997;**41**:763.

390. Adler DH, Cogan JD, Phillips JA 3rd, et al. Inherited human cPLA (2alpha) deficiency is associated with impaired eicosanoid biosynthesis, small intestinal ulceration, and platelet dysfunction. *J Clin Invest* 2008;**118**:2121.

391. Bjarnason I, Fehilly B, Smethurst P, Menzies IS, Levi AJ. Importance of local versus systemic effects of non-steroidal anti-inflammatory drugs in increasing small intestinal permeability in man. *Gut* 1991;**32**:275.

392. Aabakken L. Small bowel side-effects of non-steroidal anti-inflammatory drugs. *Eur J Gastroenterol Hepatol* 1999;**11**:383.

393. Lee FD. Drug-related pathological lesions of the intestinal tract. *Histopathology* 1994;**25**:303.

394. Lang J, Price AB, Levi AJ, Burke M, Gumpel JM, Bjarnason I. Diaphragm disease: pathology of disease of the small intestine induced by non-steroidal anti-inflammatory drugs. *J Clin Pathol* 1988;**41**:516.

395. Levi S, de Lacey G, Price AB, Gumpel MJ, Levi AJ, Bjarnason I. 'Diaphragm-like' strictures of the small bowel in patients treated with non-steroidal anti-inflammatory drugs. *Br J Radiol* 1990;**63**:186.

396. De Vos M, Mielants H, Cuvelier C, et al. Long-term evolution of gut inflammation in patients with spondyloarthropathy. *Gastroenterology* 1996;**110**:1696.

397. Leijonmarck CE, Raf L. Ulceration of the small intestine due to slow-release potassium chloride tablets. *Acta Chir Scand* 1985;**151**:273.

398. Rashid A, Hamilton SR. Necrosis of the gastrointestinal tract in uremic patients as a result of sodium polystyrene sulfonate (Kayexalate) in sorbitol: an underrecognized condition. *Am J Surg Pathol* 1997;**21**:60.

399. Martin DM, Goldman JA, Gilliam J, Nasrallah SM. Gold-induced eosinophilic enterocolitis: response to oral cromolyn sodium. *Gastroenterology* 1981;**80**:1567.

400. Jackson CW, Haboubi NY, Whorwell PJ, Schofield PF. Gold induced enterocolitis. *Gut* 1986;**27**:452.

401. Cunningham D, Morgan RJ, Mills PR, et al. Functional and structural changes of the human proximal small intestine after cytotoxic therapy. *J Clin Pathol* 1985;**38**:265.

402. Smit JM, Mulder NH, Sleijfer DT, et al. Gastrointestinal toxicity of chemotherapy and the influence of hyperalimentation. *Cancer* 1986;**58**:1990.

403. Orazi A, Du X, Yang Z, Kashai M, Williams DA. Interleukin-11 prevents apoptosis and accelerates recovery of small intestinal mucosa in mice treated with combined chemotherapy and radiation. *Lab Invest* 1996;**75**:33.

404. Abratt RP, Pontin AR, Barnes RD. Chemotherapy, radical irradiation plus salvage cystectomy for bladder cancer – severe late small bowel morbidity. *Eur J Surg Oncol* 1993;**19**:279.

405. Nagai Y, Horie T, Awazu S. Vitamin A, a useful biochemical modulator capable of preventing intestinal damage during methotrexate treatment. *Pharmacol Toxicol* 1993;**73**:69.

406. Parfitt JR, Jayakumar S, Driman DK. Mycophenolate mofetil-related gastrointestinal mucosal injury: variable injury patterns, including graft-versus-host disease-like changes. *Am J Surg Pathol* 2008;**32**:1367.

407. Bouvet C, Bellaiche G, Slama R, et al. Colite lymphocytaire et atrophie villositaire après traitement par ticlodipine. *Gastroentérol Clin Biol* 1998;**22**:1117.

408. Dharancy S, Dapuril V, Dupont-Evrard F, Colombel JF. Colite lymphocytaire et atrophie villositaire iléale secondaires à la prise de Cyclo 3 Fort. *Gastroentérol Clin Biol* 2000;**24**:134.

409. Sakakura C, Hagiwara A, Nakanishi M, et al. Bowel perforation during chemotherapy for non-Hodgkin's lymphoma. *Hepato-gastroenterology* 1999;**46**:3175.

410. Boydstun JS, Gaffey T, Bartholomew LG. Clinicopathologic study of nonspecific ulcers of the small intestine. *Dig Dis Sc* 1981;**26**:911.

411. Shin EK, Moon W, Park SJ, et al. Congenital absence of the splenic artery and splenic vein accompanied with a duodenal ulcer and deformity. *World J Gastroenterol* 2009;**15**:1401.

412. Julka RN, Aduli F, Lamps LW, Olden KW. Ischemic duodenal ulcer, an unusual presentation of sickle cell disease. *J Natl Med Assoc* 2008;**100**:339.

413. Sanderson IR, Risdon RA, Walker-Smith JA. Intractable ulcerating enterocolitis of infancy. *Arch Dis Child* 1991;**66**:295.

414. Meko JB, Norton JA. Management of patients with Zollinger–Ellison syndrome. *Annu Rev Med* 1995;**46**:395.

415. Davies DR, Brightmore T. Idiopathic and drug-induced ulceration of the small intestine. *Br J Surg* 1970;**57**:134.

416. Madhok R, MacKenzie JA, Lee FD, Bruckner FE, Terry TR, Sturrock RD. Small bowel ulceration in patients receiving non-steroidal anti- inflammatory drugs for rheumatoid arthritis. *Q J Med* 1986;**58**:53.

417. Thomas WE, Williamson RC. Nonspecific small bowel ulceration. *Postgrad Med J* 1985;**61**:587.

418. Kelly KJ. Eosinophilic gastroenteritis. *J Pediatr Gastroenterol Nutr* 2000;**30**(suppl):S28.

419. Talley NJ, Shorter RG, Phillips SF, Zinsmeister AR. Eosinophilic gastroenteritis: a clinicopathological study of patients with disease of the mucosa, muscle layer, and subserosal tissues. *Gut* 1990;**31**:54.

420. Maluenda C, Phillips AD, Briddon A, Walker-Smith JA. Quantitative analysis of small intestinal mucosa in cow's milk- sensitive enteropathy. *J Pediatr Gastroenterol Nutr* 1984;**3**:349.

421. Jenkins HR, Pincott JR, Soothill JF, Milla PJ, Harries JT. Food allergy: the major cause of infantile colitis. *Arch Dis Child* 1984;**59**:326.

422. Van Laethem JL, Jacobs F, Braude P, Van Gossum A, Deviere J. *Toxocara canis* infection presenting as eosinophilic ascites and gastroenteritis. *Dig Dis Sci* 1994;**39**:1370.

423. Suen KC, Burton JD. The spectrum of eosinophilic infiltration of the gastrointestinal tract and its relationship to other disorders of angiitis and granulomatosis. *Hum Pathol* 1979;**10**:31.

424. MacNaughton WK. Review article: new insights into the pathogenesis of radiation-induced intestinal dysfunction. *Aliment Pharmacol Ther* 2000;**14**:523.

425. Sher ME, Bauer J. Radiation-induced enteropathy. *Am J Gastroenterol* 1990;**85**:121.

426. Oya M, Yao T, Tsuneyoshi M. Chronic irradiation enteritis: its correlation with the elapsed time interval and morphological changes. *Hum Pathol* 1996;**27**:774.

427. Galland RB, Spencer J. Radiation-induced gastrointestinal fistulae. *Ann R Coll Surg Engl* 1986;**68**:5.

428. Galland RB, Spencer J. The natural history of clinically established radiation enteritis. *Lancet* 1985;**i**:1257.

429. Cohen SM. Radiation-induced jejunal mucosal vascular lesions as a cause of significant gastrointestinal hemorrhage. *Gastrointest Endosc* 1997;**46**:183.

430. Hasleton PS, Carr N, Schofield PF. Vascular changes in radiation bowel disease. *Histopathology* 1985;**9**:517.

431. Serdaroglu P. Behcet's disease and the nervous system. *J Neurol* 1998;**245**:197.

432. Yurdakul S, Tuzuner N, Yurdakul I, Hamuryudan V, Yazici H. Gastrointestinal involvement in Behcet's syndrome: a controlled study. *Ann Rheum Dis* 1996;**55**:208.

433. Choi IJ, Kim JS, Cha SD, et al. Long-term clinical course and prognostic factors in intestinal Behcet's disease. *Dis Colon Rectum* 2000;**43**:692.

434. Kasahara Y, Tanaka S, Nishino M, Umemura H, Shiraha S, Kuyama T. Intestinal involvement in Behcet's disease: review of 136 surgical cases in the Japanese literature. *Dis Colon Rectum* 1981;**24**:103.

435. Domizio P. Pathology of chronic inflammatory bowel disease in children. *Baillière's Clin Gastroenterol* 1994;**8**:35.

436. Akpolat T, Koc Y, Yeniay I, et al. Familial Behcet's disease. *Eur J Med* 1992;**1**:391.

437. Sun A, Chang JG, Kao CL, et al. Human cytomegalovirus as a potential etiologic agent in recurrent aphthous ulcers and Behcet's disease. *J Oral Pathol Med* 1996;**25**:212–18.

438. Hamzaoui K, Kahan A, Hamza M, Ayed K. Suppressive T cell function of Epstein-Barr virus induced B cell activation in active Behcet's disease. *Clin Exp Rheumatol* 1991;**9**:131.

439. Yamashita S, Suzuki A, Yanagita T, Hirohata S, Toyoshima S. Characterization of a protease responsible for truncated actin increase in neutrophils of patients with Behcet's disease. *Biol Pharm Bull* 2001;**24**:119.

440. Kobayashi M, Ito M, Nakagawa A, et al. Neutrophil and endothelial cell activation in the vasa vasorum in vasculo-Behcet disease. *Histopathology* 2000;**36**:362.

441. Takada Y, Fujita Y, Igarashi M, et al. Intestinal Behcet's disease – pathognomonic changes in intramucosal lymphoid tissues and effect of a 'rest cure' on intestinal lesions. *J Gastroenterol* 1997;**32**:598.

442. Hamza M, Eleuch M, Kchir N, Zitouna M. [Ileal perforation in 3 cases of Behcet disease.] *Ann Med Interne (Paris)* 1994;**145**:99.

443. Kallinowski B, Noldge G, Stiehl A. Crohn's disease with Behcet's syndrome like appearance: a case report. *Z Gastroenterol* 1994;**32**:642.

444. Parks AG, Nicholls RJ. Proctocolectomy without ileostomy for ulcerative colitis. *BMJ* 1978;**2**:85.

445. Shepherd NA, Jass JR, Duval I, Moskowitz RL, Nicholls RJ, Morson BC. Restorative proctocolectomy with ileal reservoir: pathological and histochemical study of mucosal biopsy specimens. *J Clin Pathol* 1987;**40**:601.

446. de Silva HJ, Millard PR, Kettlewell M, Mortensen NJ, Prince C, Jewell DP. Mucosal characteristics of pelvic ileal pouches. *Gut* 1991;**32**:61.

447. Kock NG, Darle N, Hulten L, et al. Ileostomy. *Curr Probl Surg*, 1977;**14**:18.

448. Gionchetti P, Amadini F, Venturi A, Poggioli G, Campieri M. Diagnosis and treatment of pouchitis. *Best Pract Res Clin Gastroenterol* 2003;**17**:75.

449. Shepherd NA, Hulten L, Tytgat GN, et al. Pouchitis. *Int J Colorectal Dis* 1989;**4**:205.

450. Wu H, Shen B. Pouchitis: lessons for inflammatory bowel disease. *Curr Opin Gastroenterol* 2009;**25**:314.

451. Panis Y, Poupard B, Nemeth J, Lavergne A, Hautefeuille P, Valleur P. Ileal pouch/anal anastomosis for Crohn's disease. *Lancet* 1996;**347**:854.

452. Warren BF, Shepherd NA. The role of pathology in pelvic ileal reservoir surgery. *Int J Colorectal Dis* 1992;**7**:68.

453. Lohmuller JL, Pemberton JH, Dozois RR, Ilstrup D, van Heerden J. Pouchitis and extraintestinal manifestations of inflammatory bowel disease after ileal pouch-anal anastomosis. *Ann Surg* 1990;**211**:622.

454. Shepherd NA. The pelvic ileal reservoir: apocalypse later? *BMJ* 1990;**301**:886.

455. Gullberg K, Stahlberg D, Liljeqvist L, et al. Neoplastic transformation of the pelvic pouch mucosa in patients with ulcerative colitis. *Gastroenterology* 1997;**112**:1487.

456. Bassuini MM, Billings PJ. Carcinoma in an ileoanal pouch after restorative proctocolectomy for familial adenomatous polyposis. *Br J Surg* 1996;**83**:506.

457. Vieth M, Grunewald M, Niemeyer C, Stolte M. Adenocarcinoma in an ileal pouch after prior proctocolectomy for carcinoma in a patient with ulcerative pancolitis. *Virchows Arch* 1998;**433**:281.

458. Thompson-Fawcett MW, Mortensen NJ, Warren BF. 'Cuffitis' and inflammatory changes in the columnar cuff, anal transitional zone, and ileal reservoir after stapled pouch-anal anastomosis. *Dis Colon Rectum* 1999;**42**:348.

459. Sequens R. Cancer in the anal canal (transitional zone) after restorative proctocolectomy with stapled ileal pouch-anal anastomosis. *Int J Colorectal Dis* 1997;**12**:254.

460. Helander KG, Ahren C, Philipson BM, Samuelsson BM, Ojerskog B. Structure of mucosa in continent ileal reservoirs 15 to 19 years after construction. *Hum Pathol* 1990;**21**:1235.

461. Cox CL, Butts DR, Roberts MP, Wessels RA, Bailey HR. Development of invasive adenocarcinoma in a long-standing Kock continent ileostomy: report of a case. *Dis Colon Rectum* 1997;**40**:500.

462. Price AB, Morson BC. Inflammatory bowel disease: the surgical pathology of Crohn's disease and ulcerative colitis. *Hum Pathol* 1975;**6**:7.

463. Goldstein N, Dulai M. Contemporary morphological definition of backwash ileitis in ulcerative colitis and features that distinguish it from Crohn's disease. *Am J Clin Pathol* 2006;**126**:365.

464. Schmidt CM, Lazenby AJ, Hendrickson RJ, Sitzmann JV. Preoperative terminal ileal and colonic resection histopathology predicts risk of pouchitis in patients after ileoanal pull-through procedure. *Ann Surg* 1998;**227**:654.

465. Ferguson R, Allan RN, Cooke WT. A study of the cellular infiltrate of the proximal jejunal mucosa in ulcerative colitis and Crohn's disease. *Gut* 1975;**16**:205.

466. Valdez R, Appelman HD, Bronner MP, Greenson JK. Diffuse duodenitis associated with ulcerative colitis. *Am J Surg Pathol* 2000;**24**:1407.

467. Annese V, Caruso N, Bisceglia M, et al. Fatal ulcerative panenteritis following colectomy in a patient with ulcerative colitis. *Dig Dis Sci* 1999;**44**:1189.

468. Kaufman SS, Vanderhoof JA, Young R, Perry D, Raynor SC, Mack DR. Gastroenteric inflammation in children with ulcerative colitis. *Am J Gastroenterol* 1997;**92**:1209.

469. Bechi P, Romagnoli P, Cortesini C. Ileal mucosal morphology after total colectomy in man. *Histopathology* 1981;**5**:667.

470. Knill-Jones RP, Morson B, Williams R. Prestomal ileitis: clinical and pathological findings in five cases. *Q J Med* 1970;**39**:287.

471. Attanoos R, Billings PJ, Hughes LE, Williams GT. Ileostomy polyps, adenomas, and adenocarcinomas. *Gut* 1995;**37**:840.

472. Deane AM, Woodhouse CR, Parkinson MC. Histological changes in ileal conduits. *J Urol* 1984;**132**:1108.

473. Gratama S, Smedts F, Whitehead R. Obstructive colitis: an analysis of 50 cases and a review of the literature. *Pathology* 1995;**27**:324.

474. Levine TS, Price AB. Obstructive enterocolitis: a clinicopathological discussion. *Histopathology* 1994;**25**:57.

475. Allibone RO, Hoffman J, Gosney JR, Helliwell TR. Granulation tissue polyposis associated with carcinoid tumours of the small intestine. *Histopathology* 1993;**22**:475.

476. Bagdi E, Diss TC, Munson P, Isaacson PG. Mucosal intraepithelial lymphocytes in enteropathy-associated T-cell

lymphoma, ulcerative jejunitis, and refractory celiac disease constitute a neoplastic population. *Blood* 1999;**94**:260.

477. Chesler L, Hwang L, Patton W, Heyman MB. Henoch–Schonlein purpura with severe jejunitis and minimal skin lesions. *J Pediatr Gastroenterol Nutr* 2000;**30**:92.

478. Radaelli F, Meucci G, Spinzi G, et al. Acute self-limiting jejunitis as the first manifestation of microscopic polyangiitis associated with Sjogren's disease: report of one case and review of the literature. *Eur J Gastroenterol Hepatol* 1999;**11**:931.

479. Sharma AK, Shekhawat NS, Behari S, Chandra S, Sogani KC. Nonspecific jejunitis – a challenging problem in children. *Am J Gastroenterol* 1986;**81**:428.

480. Adams JT, Skucas J. Corrosive jejunitis due to ingestion of nitric acid. *Am J Surg* 1980;**139**:282.

481. Kindt S, Tertychnyy A, De Hertogh G, Geboes K, Tack J. Intestinal immune activation in presumed post-infectious functional dyspepsia. *Neurogastroenterol Motil* 2009;**21**:832.

482. Wyatt JI. Histopathology of gastroduodenal inflammation: the impact of *Helicobacter pylori*. *Histopathology* 1995;**26**:1.

483. Walker MM, Crabtree JE. *Helicobacter pylori* infection and the pathogenesis of duodenal ulceration. *Ann N Y Acad Sci* 1998;**859**:96.

484. Sircus W. Duodenitis: a clinical, endoscopic and histopathologic study. *Q J Med* 1985;**56**:593.

485. Kreuning J, Bosman FT, Kuiper G, Wal AM, Lindeman J. Gastric and duodenal mucosa in 'healthy' individuals. An endoscopic and histopathological study of 50 volunteers. *J Clin Pathol* 1978; **31**:69.

486. Jenkins D, Goodall A, Gillet FR, Scott BB. Defining duodenitis: quantitative histological study of mucosal responses and their correlations. *J Clin Pathol* 1985;**38**:1119.

487. Jeffers MD, Hourihane DO. Coeliac disease with histological features of peptic duodenitis: value of assessment of intra-epithelial lymphocytes. *J Clin Pathol* 1993;**46**:420.

488. Walker MM, Dixon MF. Gastric metaplasia: its role in duodenal ulceration. *Aliment Pharmacol Ther* 1996;**10**(suppl 1):119.

489. Wyatt JI, Rathbone BJ, Dixon MF, Heatley RV. *Campylobacter pyloridis* and acid induced gastric metaplasia in the pathogenesis of duodenitis. *J Clin Pathol* 1987;**40**:841.

490. Wyatt JI, Rathbone BJ, Sobala GM, et al. Gastric epithelium in the duodenum: its association with *Helicobacter pylori* and inflammation. *J Clin Pathol* 1990;**43**:981.

491. Hamlet A, Thoreson AC, Nilsson O, Svennerholm AM, Olbe L. Duodenal *Helicobacter pylori* infection differs in cagA genotype between asymptomatic subjects and patients with duodenal ulcers. *Gastroenterology* 1999;**116**:259.

492. Debongnie JC, Mairesse J, Deonnay M, De Koninck X. Touch cytology: a quick, simple, sensitive screening test in the diagnosis of infections of the gastrointestinal mucosa. *Arch Pathol Lab Med* 1994;**118**:1115.

CHAPTER 21

The pathology of malnutrition and malabsorption

Ian Brown

Royal Brisbane and Women's Hospital; Envoi Specialist Pathologists, Brisbane, QLD, Australia

Introduction

Adequate nutrition depends on the ingestion of a suitable diet and its proper digestion, absorption and metabolism. Malnutrition can result from inadequacy of one or more of these functions. In practice, it is helpful to consider differential diagnosis under the following four headings:

1. Malnutrition due to an unsatisfactory diet

2. Malnutrition consequent on maldigestion. The primary disorder may involve the stomach, small bowel, pancreas, liver or biliary system

3. Malnutrition secondary to malabsorption or to faulty intracellular metabolism: there are three principal categories to consider:

- Patients who have an in-born abnormality, often inherited, of either surface enterocytes with their associated enzyme systems, which interferes with the final stages of digestion, absorption or intracellular metabolism, or an abnormality of mucosal immunity, which results in a hypersensitivity to a dietary component
- Patients who sustain sufficient acquired damage to either surface enterocytes, producing interference with normal absorption or metabolism, or the crypt zone sufficient to disturb normal surface enterocyte replacement, or to both
- Patients with disorders usually associated with local organic disease or previous surgery, such as diverticular disease, strictures, fistulae, stagnant loops or short circuits of bowel, which reduce the surface area available for absorption. These patients often have concomitant disturbance of normal small bowel ecology.

4. Malnutrition due to miscellaneous disorders, some of which are of undetermined origin.

Separation of these groups depends on a careful clinical history and use of radiological, laboratory and other techniques, including biopsy. Malabsorption from any cause is usually accompanied by diarrhoea (or steatorrhoea) and anaemia. Clinical investigation should include naked-eye examination of stools which, if fat is present in excess, are characteristically frothy, bulky, offensive and silver-grey in colour: they usually float in water. Laboratory investigations include full blood count, iron studies and vitamin B_{12} and folate levels to assess the presence and cause of any anaemia, liver and thyroid function tests, albumin, calcium and coeliac serology [1]. Selective techniques include: barium meal and follow-through or small bowel barium enema; abdominal computed tomography (CT); measurement of small bowel transit times and carbohydrate absorption by means of hydrogen breath tests; microscopic screening of stools for fat [2]; and faecal fat estimations made over a number of days [1,3]. Upper gastrointestinal endoscopy is now routine in the investigation of malabsorption, potentially providing tissue for histopathology, biochemical samples for disaccharidase levels and jejunal fluid for microbial culture [1]. In a textbook devoted primarily to histopathology only the macroscopic and histological findings in biopsies or resected specimens are considered in detail.

Histopathological diagnosis of malabsorptive states

Intestinal biopsy

The proximal small intestine is the principal site of nutrient absorption so, not surprisingly, most malabsorption

---

Morson and Dawson's Gastrointestinal Pathology, Fifth Edition. Edited by Neil A. Shepherd, Bryan F. Warren, Geraint T. Williams, Joel K. Greenson, Gregory Y. Lauwers and Marco R. Novelli.

disorders result from disease of this site. Many are associated with a morphological abnormality and small bowel biopsy can both establish the presence of disease and exclude disorders that may be in the clinical differential diagnosis [4]. Knowledge of normal appearances and non-significant variations is essential in the assessment of small bowel biopsies and this is reviewed in Chapter 17. The normal duodenum can demonstrate ridge and spade forms of villi, closely resembling those seen in partial flattening caused by disease and a number of adult patients who are symptom-free have a mild cellular infiltration with or without a degree of flattening, usually referred to as 'non-specific duodenitis' [5,6] (see 'Non-specific duodenitis', Chapter 20). These changes are unrelated to malabsorption but they cannot readily be distinguished histologically from the minor degrees of flattening with cellular infiltration sometimes seen in true malabsorption.

Microscopic pathology

Small bowel mucosa can react to injury in only a limited number of ways. In many malabsorption disorders, a common injury pathway is implicated, which results in a reduction in absorptive cell number by a process of enhanced apoptosis [7]. If the damage is mild, increased activity of the crypt replication zone compensates for the increased cell loss and there is little detectable change, although the crypt zone increases in length and in mitotic activity and enterocytes may appear crowded (Figure 21.1).

When cell loss is more severe and more rapid, crypt hyperplasia increases further, enterocytes migrating upwards to cover villi do not have sufficient time to mature and tend to remain crowded together. Goblet cells are fewer. The villi become shorter and broader, probably because the enterocytes can no longer cover them adequately (Figure 21.2), and the basal layer begins to thicken as a direct result of the increased proliferation of the crypt zone. The continued inability of crypt cell proliferation to keep pace with enterocyte loss results in a flattened mucosa with a considerably thickened basal layer (Figure 21.3): there may be complete loss of villi but, because of the thickened basal layer, the total width of the mucosa is little diminished. For this reason many workers, ourselves

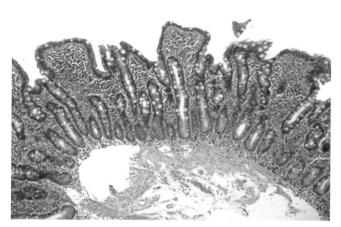

Figure 21.2 Marsh stage 3b lesion of gluten-induced enteropathy characterised by broad, blunted villi, crypt elongation and flattening of enterocytes.

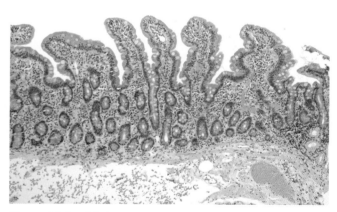

Figure 21.1 Mild abnormality in gluten-induced enteropathy: villi are preserved in length but there is an increase in intra-epithelial lymphocytes and crypt elongation. This is the Marsh type 2 pattern.

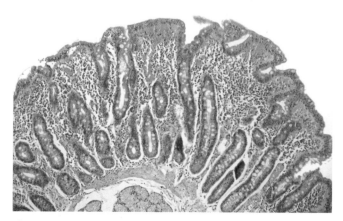

Figure 21.3 Marsh stage 3c lesion of gluten-induced enteropathy: this is the fully developed abnormality characterised by a flat mucosa with compensatory crypt hyperplasia. Persisting intra-epithelial lymphocytes are present and the surface enterocytes have acquired a cuboidal shape.

included, find the term 'mucosal atrophy' as opposed to 'flattening' inappropriate. At the same time there are alterations in the number of both intra-epithelial lymphocytes and lymphocytes and macrophages in the lamina propria; plasma cell numbers also vary and there may be an increase or decrease in the number of cells synthesising particular immunoglobulins. This injury pathway is exemplified by coeliac disease. However, 'all that flattens is not sprue' [8].

Some malabsorption disorders may present normal morphology, the abnormality being at a subcellular level or affecting biochemical or enzyme systems. There are also uncommon disorders, such as microvillous inclusion disease, typified by a unique morphological abnormality, often inherited, which involve a mechanism of cellular injury distinct from that described above.

Malnutrition due to unsatisfactory diet

Protein–calorie malnutrition in children

Protein–calorie malnutrition (usually known as kwashiorkor) results from severe dietary protein deficiency and is found in Asia and in many African tribes, particularly in east Africa and South Africa. It affects children and adults but, in humans and experimental animals, epithelial changes are more severe in the period of growth than in adult life or old age [9]. All layers of the bowel are atrophic. Mucosal changes must be interpreted with care because the 'normal' pattern for the region can be one of complex convolutions and some reduction in villous height, which is probably a manifestation of an almost universal degree of protein deficiency. In severe protein–calorie malnutrition, jejunal and ileal mucosal height, surface area and the total volume of the lamina propria are all reduced. The mucosal flattening can be severe in children, sometimes mimicking gluten-induced enteropathy. The degree of crypt hyperplasia varies [10,11] but is usually mild. There is no constant increase in intra-epithelial lymphocytes or plasma cells in the lamina propria. The mucosa slowly reverts towards normal on an adequate diet [12]. The appearances suggest deficient replacement of the normal enterocyte loss due to failure in crypt cell proliferation, rather than an over-rapid loss of enterocytes [12].

Adult malnutrition

The rare cases of adult malnutrition resemble those of protein calorie malnutrition in children and again crypt cell hyperplasia is not conspicuous. A single case of folate deficiency is reported [13] with flattening which improved and finally disappeared on dietary folate. This was presumably also the result of a failure of crypt zone regeneration.

Malnutrition due to defects in absorption and metabolism

Mechanical defects

Local zones of disease in the small bowel can produce malabsorption in a limited number of ways:
- Sufficient local mucosal damage to impair absorption, particularly in sites where this is specialised, such as the terminal ileum
- Fistula formation with short-circuiting, so that there is too little normal bowel available for absorption and/or the transit time is too short
- Strictures with consequent stagnation of bowel content and disturbance of normal bowel ecology.

The harmless indigenous small intestinal flora may become supplanted by abnormal bacterial colonisation in a large number of circumstances, including stagnant loops and fistulae. Although not necessarily invasive, or causing structural changes visible in haematoxylin and eosin (H&E)-stained sections, such infections damage the glycocalyx, producing a partial loss of disaccharidase enzyme activity, resulting in maldigestion. The surgical resections and anastomoses that local disease may require can themselves produce similar effects.

Local disease is commonly associated with local mucosal ulceration, often with some distortion of the adjacent mucosa. There is rarely any generalised mucosal change and biopsies from uninvolved sites are usually normal. The causes of such localised ulceration are discussed in Chapter 20 (see 'Ulceration in the small intestine') and are not further discussed in this chapter.

Surgical resections

The average length of the small bowel in a live adult is about 2800 mm. As a result of marked individual variation it is difficult to say what length can be resected before malabsorption will occur regularly. Earlier studies suggested that about a third of the upper small bowel could be resected with impunity and half with reasonable safety [14] and that survival is possible after a resection of 90% [15]. Ileal resections are less favourable than jejunal ones because, although the normal ileum can take over the absorptive functions of the jejunum, the reverse is not true. An intact ileo-caecal valve is also important. Children appear to tolerate more extensive resections better than adults, particularly with regard to their long-term effects [16].

Biopsy studies on residual small intestinal mucosa after extensive small bowel resection originally claimed to show that villi were not hypertrophied although there was an increase in the number of absorptive enterocytes per unit length [17]. There is, however, increasing evidence, both from absorption and transit time studies [18] and from experimental studies on rats [19], that adaptive changes certainly occur, with early crypt hyperplasia that may be regulated, at least in part, by endogenous enteroglucagon.

Food intolerance

Up to 20% of the populace of western countries perceive an adverse reaction to one or more foods, and objectively 6% of infants and young children and 3.7% of adults in the USA have genuine food intolerance, although this is less frequent in Europe and rare in Asia [20]. Two main processes account for food intolerance:

1. The development of an immunological reaction to a component of food. A genetic predisposition may exist and the pathogenesis involves a T-cell-mediated immune reaction, for which coeliac disease is the prototypical example, an IgE-mediated (often eosinophil-rich) allergic reaction, such as that induced by shellfish or peanuts or a variable combination of these two, e.g. cows' milk and soy protein intolerance [20]. Cell-mediated immune disorders account for most food intolerance-related malabsorption.

2. A defect in the digestive enzyme systems, particularly those associated with enterocytes, which can be inherited or acquired, the latter by exposure to infection, drugs or other toxic substances. The defect may be transient or permanent and is not usually associated with histological abnormality, although specialised enzyme histochemistry can identify lactase deficiency.

Immunological reaction to gluten (coeliac syndrome; coeliac disease)

The term 'coeliac syndrome' is used here to embrace the conditions alternatively termed 'coeliac disease', 'coeliac sprue', 'non-tropical sprue', 'sprue syndrome', 'gluten-sensitive enteropathy' and 'gluten-induced enteropathy', and also 'refractory' or 'non-responsive coeliac disease'. Coeliac disease is an immunologically mediated inflammatory disorder resulting from intolerance, in genetically susceptible individuals, of structurally related storage proteins, generically termed 'gluten', found in wheat, barley and rye. The important disease manifestation is the development of a characteristic enteropathy. However, coeliac disease may affect other parts of the gastrointestinal system and indeed other organ systems.

It is evident from population-based serotesting that the disease prevalence is much higher than previously appreciated, with seropositivity approximating 1% in people of European ancestry [21,22], although disease appears to be rare in African and east Asian populations. Clinically diagnosed coeliac disease is much less common than the 1% prevalence suggested by serology, leading to speculation

that many gluten-sensitive patients are undiagnosed (and thus representing the underwater base of a coeliac 'iceberg'). Coeliac disease commonly presents in childhood but, in a significant minority, it is first recognised in adult life or, even, in elderly people. In most patients there is a direct relationship between gluten in the diet and disease manifestation, which can be demonstrated by the beneficial effect of gluten withdrawal and conversely by the clinical test of gluten challenge [23]. The condition in these patients can be legitimately described as gluten-induced (or sensitive) enteropathy.

Aetiology and pathogenesis [22,24,25]

The disease involves the complex interaction of an environmental trigger (gluten protein derived from the Triticeae tribe of grains), host factors (genetic predisposition) and environmental co-factors (enteric infection). Gluten is a generic term encompassing grain proteins rich in prolamine and glutamine amino acids that confer pathogenicity for coeliac disease. These proteins include gliadins and glutenins from wheat, hordeins from barley and secalins from rye. Prolamine confers resistance to acid and enzymatic digestion, allowing a high concentration of minimally altered gluten protein to enter the proximal small intestine. Glutamine is the preferred binding substrate for tissue transglutaminase. Avenin protein, derived from oats, shares similar chemical properties, but in low concentration, and is not considered immunologically active. Gluten gains access to the lamina propria via transcellular, paracellular and retrotranscytosis routes, with permeability to gluten peptides enhanced by factors such as enteric infection with adenovirus or rotavirus and upregulation of zonulin, a tight junction regulator [22]. In the lamina propria, gluten peptides trigger both innate and adaptive immune responses.

Genetic factors clearly play a role in initiating the host immune response. Almost all patients carry either HLA-DQ2 (alleles DQA1*05/DQB1*02) or less frequently HLA-DQ8 (alleles DQA1*03/DQB1*0302) encoded by the COELIAC1 locus on chromosome 6p21. Although 90% of patients with coeliac disease are HLA-DQ2, approximately 30–40% of the general population are also HLA-DQ2, so other genetic factors must be important. To date, three further genes with immunomodulatory function are strongly implicated: COELIAC2 (5q31-33), COELIAC3 (2q33) and COELIAC4 (19p13.1). This list is certain to grow.

Initially, the gluten peptides are bound by tissue transglutaminase (TTG), a deamidating enzyme. Both free deamidated gluten and cross-linked gluten–TTG complexes bind strongly to complementary clefts in HLA-DQ2 or -DQ8 proteins on the surface of antigen-presenting cells. Complementary CD4+ T-helper cells induce, via cytokine action, both type 1 and type 2 immune responses. The type 1 response is more significant and leads to upregulation, largely via the action of interferon-γ and interleukin-15 (IL-15), of intra-epithelial cytotoxic CD8+ T cells and less commonly CD8– T cells and natural killer (NK) T cells. These induce enterocyte cell death by Fas–Fas ligand interaction or perforin granzyme process. Matrix metalloproteinase action also contributes and the combination of these factors leads in time to the villous flattening typical of coeliac disease. The type 2 T-helper cell response induces B-lymphocyte expansion and plasma cell differentiation, which produce the anti-TTG antibodies detectable in the serum of coeliac patients. Chemoattractant cytokines are responsible for mast cell, eosinophil and neutrophil infiltration.

Gluten-induced enteropathy

Three components have been necessary for complete certainty in diagnosis; an abnormal pattern on biopsy, improvement in both clinical symptoms and histological mucosal morphology after gluten withdrawal and the reappearance of enteropathy after its re-introduction [21,23]. Histological changes are assessed by way of endoscopic biopsies taken from the duodenum and proximal jejunum. Although jumbo forceps biopsies are preferred, because they provide more tissue and allow better orientation, these do not appear to offer diagnostic advantage over normal-sized pinch biopsies [26]. Histological changes of coeliac disease are often not uniform and varying degrees of damage can be seen in multiple biopsies taken at the same time in up to 25% of adults and 50% of children [27–32]. Diagnostic sensitivity is highest in the duodenal bulb [27,33,34] but this site suffers from being a frequent site for other abnormalities such as peptic duodenitis and ulceration, which may conceal features of gluten enteropathy. The most severe morphological changes are usually found in the distal duodenum [29] and diminish distally in the small intestine. A series of three biopsies, one each from the duodenal bulb, proximal duodenum and distal duodenum, has been shown to have 100% sensitivity for detecting coeliac disease in adults [27], although many advocate examination of at least four biopsies to confidently overcome the problem of disease variability [35,36].

Dissecting microscope appearances

This now plays little role in pathological diagnosis and the villous architectural changes previously appreciated by dissecting microscopy are better identified in vivo via magnification endoscopy. Villous morphology can be classified as normal (cylindrical), finger like (with slightly bulbous tips), leaf like (broad based but tapering to the apex), tongue like (broad base and round top), ridge like (resembling leaf forms but shorter and broader) and flat, producing a mosaic pattern (Figure 21.4). It is potentially important to realise that villous morphology may vary because of geography and age [37]. In general, people who reside in

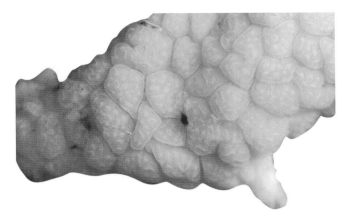

Figure 21.4 A 'flat' mucosa showing a mosaic pattern. The raised mounds of epithelium with crypt openings in their centre are clearly visible (dissecting microscope).

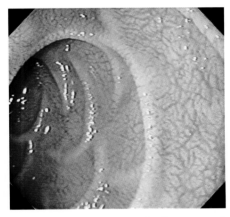

Figure 21.5 Endoscopic appearance of a flat mucosa in gluten-induced enteropathy: there is a mosaic appearance (sometimes described as 'scalloping').

tropical areas tend to have broader, shorter villi (more leaf and ridge forms) than people who reside in temperate climates. Elderly individuals show a similar trend.

Endoscopic appearances

The characteristic features of gluten-induced enteropathy include a reduction in the number of circular (Kerckring) folds, scalloping of folds, mucosal fissures and a mosaic or nodular mucosa [21,38] (Figure 21.5). Although these are sensitive features, they are not specific and may be encountered in other causes of mucosal atrophy [39,40]. New endoscopy techniques hold promise for detection of lesser degrees of abnormality, whereas capsule endoscopy is helpful in documenting the extent of disease and to screen for complications [41].

Serological investigations

The most useful serological test is a serum IgA anti-TTG level that has superseded immunofluorescence testing for IgA anti-endomysial antibody as a screening test for coeliac disease. Anti-TTG is an ELISA (enzyme-linked immuno-sorbent assay) test with published sensitivity ranging from 61% to 100% (mean 87%) and specificity ranging from 86% to 100% (mean 95%) [42]. Sensitivity is lowest when disease is histologically mild [21,43]. IgA deficiency, which is more common in coeliac disease, is problematic and IgG-based tests are substituted but are less sensitive [21,22]. Although still widely performed, current anti-gliadin antibody tests have clinical utility only in patients aged <18 months [25].

Histological appearances

In assessing histological appearances it is important to have correctly orientated specimens and to use step or serial sections. Correct orientation is confirmed by longitu-dinally sectioned crypts. Normal villi are slender, with a length of at least three times the depth of the mucosal crypts. Four consecutive villi with a villous:crypt ratio ≥3:1 indicates normal architecture [37]. It is not uncom-mon for villi to be branched or show fusion of the tips [43] and to appear blunted in the first part of the duodenum or overlying a lymphoid follicle [37].

Increase in intra-epithelial lymphocytes (IELs) is the ear-liest histological abnormality in gluten-induced enteropa-thy and these lymphocytes induce progressive enterocyte loss by triggering apoptosis. Crypt epithelium reacts to enterocyte loss by stem cell differentiation and prolifera-tion with consequent elongation of the crypts. The time taken for epithelial cells to transit from crypt to villus reduces from 3–5 days to 1–2 days [44]. If enterocyte loss exceeds the capacity of crypt proliferation to repopulate the villous epithelium, a reduction in villous height will eventuate. Where the balance between cell loss and regen-eration lies will determine the extent of villous flattening. No matter the degree of villous blunting present, the mucosal thickness is essentially maintained as a conse-quence of compensatory crypt hyperplasia, although this may not occur if there is superimposed protein, vitamin B_{12} or folate deficiency that affects the capacity for crypt epi-thelial cell division.

Traditionally, IEL counts of >40/100 epithelial cells (ECs) have been considered abnormal [45]. However, recent studies have revised the normal range to ≤25/100 IELs:ECs [46,47], with counts 25–29 IELs/100 ECs regarded as bor-derline and ≥30 IELs/100 ECs considered definitely abnor-mal [47]. In gluten-induced enteropathy, IEL density is maximal at the tip of the villus, presumably because of greater exposure to luminal gluten and the term 'decre-scendo sign' refers to the decrease in IEL numbers along villi moving from tip to base [48,49] (Figure 21.6). Assess-ment of IEL density at the villous tip is an easy and sensi-

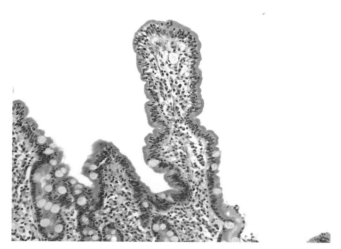

Figure 21.6 Villus in Marsh stage 1 gluten-induced enteropathy demonstrating an increase in intra-epithelial lymphocytes with predominance at the villus tip. This is sensitive but non-specific feature of coeliac disease.

tive method to detect minimal abnormality. In an averaged count of IELs/20 ECs at the tips of five villi, the normal range is ≤5/20 ECs, whereas a density ≥6 IELs/20 ECs is found in gluten sensitivity [48, 50]. Most IELs (>95%) are CD3-positive T cells with 70–90% co-expressing CD8 but not CD4 [51].

IELs may be squeezed between enterocytes or appear surrounded by a pale halo. CD3 immunohistochemistry can help substantiate an increase in cells in subtle cases [52]. In normal mucosa, most IELs bear an αβ T-cell recep-tor (TCR). However, the proportion of IELs expressing a γδ T cell receptor (±CD8) is increased to >10% in gluten enter-opathy [53,54]. The cytotoxic T cells express the cytotoxic markers granzyme, perforin and TIA-1, whereas a propor-tion of IELs have NK cell properties [22,55]. IELs reduce in absolute number as villous flattening progresses but are matched by concomitant enterocyte loss such that the IEL:EC ratio remains elevated at all degrees of architectural disturbance [56].

Depending on the level of injury, small intestinal biopsies may show a normal villous architecture with or without crypt hyperplasia, villous blunting with crypt hyperplasia or complete villous atrophy with a flat mucosa. This vari-ation forms the basis for the commonly used histological classification schemes (Tables 21.1 and 21.2). The architec-ture may vary (by at least one Marsh grade) between biopsy fragments and even within a single fragment, because the reaction in the mucosa is not uniform along the small intestine [28–31]. A histologically normal biopsy is encountered within a series of otherwise abnormal biopsies in up to 36% of cases [28].

Lamina propria inflammation is a characteristic feature and consists principally of lymphocytes and plasma cells

Table 21.1 Grading of gluten-induced enteropathy: modified Oberhuber–Marsh scheme

	0	1	2	3a	3b	3c
IELs	<30	>30	>30	>30	>30	>30
Crypts	Normal	Normal	Hypertrophic	Hypertrophic	Hypertrophic	Hypertrophic
Villi	Normal	Normal	Normal	Atrophy +	Atrophy ++	Absent

IELs, intra-epithelial lymphocytes.

Table 21.2 Corazza classification scheme

Type A: infiltrative, non-atrophic, incorporating type 1 and 2

Type B1: atrophic with shortened but still detectable villi, incorporating types 3a and 3b

Type B2: complete atrophy without detectable villi, corresponding to type 3c

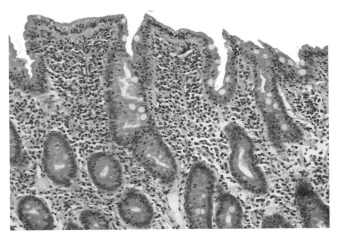

Figure 21.7 Inflammation in the lamina propria, thickening of the subepithelial basement membrane, cuboidal change in surface enterocytes and focal cytoplasmic lipid vacuolation are evident in this example of gluten-induced enteropathy.

[51,56–59]. Lymphocytes are primarily of T-cell type and, in contrast to the intra-epithelial cells, chiefly express CD4, consistent with T-helper cells [22,57]. Small numbers of B lymphocytes and CD8-positive T cells are present. The plasma cell infiltrate is often marked and primarily IgA producing, being responsible for the IgA antibodies to gliadin and TTG that are serological markers of gluten-induced enteropathy [57]. Eosinophils may occasionally be prominent [51,57,58], especially in children, so careful examination for features of gluten-induced enteropathy should be undertaken before rendering a diagnosis of eosinophilic enteritis in a child.

Neutrophils are commonly identified in the mucosa as isolated small collections or irregularly scattered through the lamina propria [51,57,58] or occasionally within the surface and crypt epithelium. The presence of neutrophil crypt abscess formation, especially if accompanied by ulceration, should always prompt consideration of another process such as Crohn's disease, peptic duodenitis or autoimmune enteropathy. Biopsies from the first part of duodenum can show superimposed peptic duodenitis with the predominant histological picture being neutrophil-rich inflammation or erosion and gastric metaplasia. Increased IELs should prompt consideration of gluten enteropathy and typical features should be sought in more distal biopsies [60,61]. Mast cell numbers are increased but are seldom apparent without special stains [62].

Enterocyte damage is evidenced by loss of surface mucin, cytoplasmic basophilia and the acquisition of a flattened, cuboidal appearance to the cells [57,58], at times with cytoplasmic vacuolation due to disturbed lipid processing referred to as the 'lipid hang-up' appearance [63]. Enterocyte nuclei can appear irregular and disorganised and epithelial apoptosis may be identified infrequently. In up to two-thirds of cases, gastric metaplasia is present in the surface epithelium, although never as prominent as seen in peptic duodenitis [64]. Uncommonly, enterocytes may appear normal despite residing in a flat mucosa [51]. The crypt zone undergoes hyperplasia, driven by cytokine factors such as keratinocyte growth factor acting on stem cells [51,57], resulting in increased mitoses that appear higher in the crypts [63].

True thickening of the subepithelial collagen layer, not exceeding 5 µm and sometimes accompanied by epithelial denudation, is encountered in 36–60% of biopsies [65,66]. Fibroblast growth factor, released as part of the inflammatory milieu, might explain this feature. Importantly, this finding does not represent collagenous sprue (discussed below), which is often associated with refractory coeliac disease. Oedema, capillary congestion and serum exudation in the lamina propria are almost universally encountered and, when coupled with the inflammatory cell infiltrate, can expand the mucosal volume by a factor of two compared with normal controls [56] (Figure 21.7).

Paneth cells may appear normal, increased or reduced in number [67,68]. An absence of Paneth cells should prompt consideration of autoimmune enteropathy whereas a noticeable loss has been described in refractory coeliac disease [69]. There are reports that endocrine cell numbers are increased [70,71], although this may simply reflect general crypt hyperplasia. As villous flattening progresses, goblet cells may be less readily identified, particularly at the surface.

Intestinal biopsies allow only a study of the mucosa. At necropsy all coats of the bowel can be assessed but postmortem mucosal autolysis affects morphology. However, carefully performed postmortem studies allow estimation of the extent of the disease and the detection of associated neoplasms [72]. Lesions in the small bowel tend to diminish in severity distally. Within each segment, mucosal changes are patchy and variable. There is often associated thinning of the muscle coats [73] which may have a generalised brown colour due to the presence of lipochrome pigments (see 'The brown bowel syndrome' below).

Histopathological classification

There may be advantages for clinico-pathological liaison and communication between centres in using a grading system for the assessment of duodenal or jejunal biopsies from patients with gluten-induced enteropathy. A modified Marsh classification (see Table 21.1) is useful in characterising the coeliac lesion and allows for good comparison with follow-up biopsies, particularly with a single observer [51]. In practice, type 1 and type 3 patterns are most commonly encountered, type 2 pattern is infrequent and almost never a uniform finding and type 4 pattern is exceedingly rare. Problems exist in the distinction between type 1 and type 2 lesions and in the subclassification of type 3 lesions. To address this, Corazza and colleagues have proposed a simplified, more reproducible grading system (see Table 21.2) [74]. It remains to be seen if either system finds a place in routine pathology reports in favour of descriptive terms such as 'partial', 'subtotal' and 'total' villous atrophy/flattening.

Ultrastructural studies

There are good reports on the scanning and transmission electron microscopic changes in coeliac disease [75,76]. These show a reduction in number and size of microvilli that become short and irregular in shape, and may fuse. Pinocytic vesicles decrease in number and the basement membrane is increased in width and density and becomes disrupted. There is swelling of vascular endothelial cells. Some of these changes, in particular those affecting the microvilli, may be identified before any histological abnormality is appreciated and the term 'microscopic enteritis' has been suggested for this [77].

Histochemical and biochemical studies

Variations on the normal enzyme distribution described in Chapter 18 are well documented in coeliac syndromes [78,79]. Enterocyte content and surface expression of most enzymes are usually reduced [78–80] even in cases with mild or no histological abnormality [81].

Effect of a gluten-free diet

Standard treatment for coeliac disease is removal of the inciting antigen (gluten) by institution of a gluten-free diet. Although symptomatic improvement normally occurs within days, mucosal improvement may be slow and incomplete, especially in adults [82]. Morphological improvement is characterised by a return to normal villous architecture and a decrease in IELs. Villi can take up to 2 years to return to normal, although this is typically more rapid in the distal small intestine [57]. Some patients may not regain normal architecture, generally an indication of a 'refractory' form of disease (see below). Although IELs bearing TCR-αβ reduce quickly, TCR-γσ-bearing IELs remain persistently increased [83], which, when combined with the impossibility of eradicating all dietary gluten, leads to a continual mild elevation of IELs despite a return to a normal villous architecture and good diet compliance [50,84].

Histopathological mimics

Not surprisingly, other antigens, both exogenous and endogenous, induce an immunological reaction that results in a similar morphological appearance to that of gluten-induced enteropathy. In practice, the histological differential diagnosis of coeliac disease is best considered in two situations: conditions leading to an increase in IELs but with preservation of villous architecture (resembling Marsh type 1 lesion) (sometimes called lymphocytic duodenosis) and conditions with increased IELs and villous blunting or flat mucosa (resembling Marsh type 3 or 4 lesions). These are not mutually exclusive because it is the intensity, rather than the cause, of immunoreaction that determines the extent to which villous blunting occurs.

Intra-epithelial lymphocytosis with a normal villous architecture (lymphocytic duodenosis) Between 1.3% and 2.2% of architecturally normal small bowel biopsies display IEL counts of >25/100 ECs [85,86]. Based on serological and clinical follow-up data, 9–40% are ultimately related to gluten sensitivity [85–87]. Excluding gluten sensitivity in the remaining patients is often difficult and there is lingering concern that many patients represent a 'potential' form of coeliac disease that has not become clinically manifest, thus explaining part of the 'coeliac iceberg'. The absence of HLA-DQ2/-DQ8 haplotype in 50% of patients with this morphology provides good evidence that most cases are not due to gluten sensitivity [88].

Table 21.3 lists known associations of proximal small intestinal intra-epithelial lymphocytosis with a normal villous architecture [49,85,89–91]. No doubt further associations exist and drug reactions are an under-reported cause. Common associations are food hypersensitivity due to gluten and other proteins, infection including gastric *Helicobacter pylori* (Figure 21.8), autoimmune disease and drugs, in particular non-steroidal anti-inflammatory drugs (NSAIDs) [90]. The histopathology report should convey to the clinician that this morphological pattern is non-specific. Gluten sensitivity needs to be highlighted as a potential cause because, even in the absence of villous blunting, patients can develop significant nutritional deficiency and are at risk of long-term sequelae such as intestinal lymphoma.

Establishing gluten sensitivity as the cause can be challenging. Positive serology is good evidence for coeliac disease but is often negative when villous architecture is normal [43]. The absence of the HLA-DQ2 haplotype essentially excludes gluten sensitivity. However, as 30–40% of the population carry this haplotype, it is not useful in establishing a positive diagnosis. Gluten challenge with re-biopsy assessment for development of villous blunting has been advocated [87] but is not widely practised. The histopathologist may help by documenting (potentially aided by CD3 immunohistochemistry) the typical villous tip prominence of IELs, although this is not specific for gluten sensitivity [48,52]. In many cases, a diagnosis of coeliac disease is established only by clinical follow-up.

Intra-epithelial lymphocytosis and villous blunting In contradistinction to lymphocytic duodenosis (above), gluten sensitivity accounts for most cases where there is villous blunting and intra-epithelial lymphocytosis. Elevated TTG is good confirmatory evidence for coeliac disease. Many differential diagnostic considerations are considered in detail elsewhere in this chapter and Table 21.4 serves as reminder of these. Childhood presentation is common

---

Table 21.3 Causes of intra-epithelial lymphocytosis with normal architecture

Major:
Gluten sensitivity – including dermatitis herpetiformis and first-degree relatives of patients with coeliac disease

Infection (e.g. viral enteritis, *Giardia* spp., cryptosporidia, *Helicobacter pylori* infection, tropical sprue)

Drugs (e.g. non-steroidal anti-inflammatory drugs, others)

Autoimmune disease (e.g. rheumatoid arthritis, systemic lupus erythematosus, Hashimoto's thyroiditis, Graves' disease, psoriasis, ankylosing spondylitis, type 1 diabetes, scleroderma)

Minor:
Non-gluten food hypersensitivity (e.g. cereals, cows' milk, soy products, fish, rice, chicken)

Autoimmune enteropathy

Immunodeficiency disorders (e.g. IgA deficiency, chronic variable immunodeficiency)

Inflammatory bowel disease

Lymphocytic and collagenous colitis

Morbid obesity

Bacterial overgrowth

Secondary to local inflammation

Idiopathic

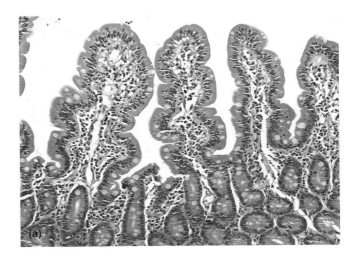

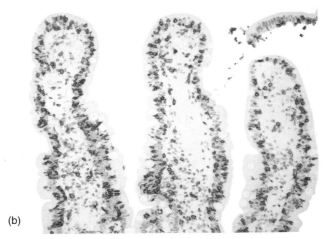

Figure 21.8 (a) Increased intra-epithelial lymphocytes with preserved villous architecture in a patient with gastric *Helicobacter pylori* infection. Lymphocytes returned to normal density after treatment of the gastric infection. (b) CD3 immunohistochemistry highlighting the intra-epithelial T lymphocytes. Unlike gluten-induced enteropathy, there is no villus tip accentuation in this case.

Table 21.4 Causes of villous flattening and intra-epithelial lymphocytosis

Gluten sensitivity (most cases)

Non gluten food hypersensitivity (e.g. cereals, cow's milk, soy products, fish, rice, chicken)

Infection (e.g. viral/bacterial enteritis, tropical sprue, parasitic infection)

Bacterial overgrowth

Autoimmune enteropathy

Immunodeficiency disorders (e.g. IgA deficiency, chronic variable immunodeficiency)

Drugs (e.g. non-steroidal anti-inflammatory drugs)

Inflammatory bowel disease

Collagenous sprue

Graft-versus-host disease

Idiopathic

with non-gluten food hypersensitivity, immunodeficiency disorders and autoimmune enteropathy. In adults, infective enteritis, bacterial overgrowth and tropical sprue are more likely. There are occasional patients who present with symptoms of gluten sensitivity and have typical biopsy morphology but do not manifest positive serology. Moreover, these patients show clinical and histological recovery while on a gluten-containing diet. The cause of this transient morphology is uncertain and may not have a single aetiology, although an infective cause is favoured [92].

Clinical variants of coeliac disease

Symptomatic (or active) disease is usually manifest by diarrhoea and/or abdominal discomfort and normally there is dissipation of symptoms with a return to normal small bowel morphology on a gluten-free diet. The condition is then regarded as treated coeliac disease. Four clinical states not conforming to this normal are appreciated:
1. Silent coeliac disease refers to patients who are asymptomatic but have characteristic enteropathy on duodenal biopsy, often times performed as part of familial screening.
2. Latent coeliac disease, correctly applied, refers to patients who had a fully developed coeliac lesion (Marsh 3 pattern) that recovered on a gluten-free diet but has not re-developed while on a normal diet. However, the term has been broadened to include patients who develop a gluten-induced enteropathy at some time after a normal biopsy while on a normal diet [93].
3. Potential coeliac disease is the appellation when an individual could or should have coeliac disease but has not yet manifested the characteristic enteropathy. Such patients may have a family history, positive serology or duodenal intra-epithelial lymphocytosis.
4. Refractory coeliac disease – discussed below.

Refractory coeliac disease

Usual therapy for coeliac disease is the institution of a gluten-free diet. However, 5–30% of patients show no response either clinically or histologically or have a relapse of symptoms and signs of coeliac disease despite initial treatment success. Although not strictly defined, the term 'refractory coeliac disease' is typically applied to disease not responding after 12 months of gluten-free diet or when further intervention is required earlier because of severe or deteriorating clinical symptoms [22,94–97].

It is important to ensure proper diet compliance and to exclude another cause for persisting symptomatology, such as pancreatic insufficiency, bacterial overgrowth or lymphocytic colitis. In addition, the basis for the initial diagnosis of gluten sensitivity should be reconsidered [97]. Variant morphological features of gluten-induced enteropathy associated with refractory disease include subepithelial collagen deposition (collagenous sprue), basal lymphoid infiltration, crypt atrophy [98] and a reduction in Paneth cell numbers [69]. A syndrome of enlarged, cavitating mesenteric lymph nodes and splenic atrophy may be seen in 30% [96m97,99].

Refractory coeliac disease (RCD) is divided, on the basis of IEL immunophenotype, into type 1 (normal immunophenotype) and type 2 (aberrant IEL immunophenotype with risk of the development of overt enteropathy type T-cell lymphoma [ETTL]) [22]. Distinction relies on a combination of immunohistochemical profiling of the intra-epithelial T cells with CD3 and CD8, flow cytometric analysis of unfixed biopsy tissue and polymerase chain reaction (PCR) TCR clonality studies.

Type 1 RCD typically displays a Marsh type 3 pattern, although infrequently cases with no villous abnormality are encountered [90]. The IEL phenotype is identical to non-refractory disease with expression of surface CD3, CD7, CD8, CD103 and TCR-β [95,97]. Importantly, immunohistochemical expression of CD8 is identified in most IELs. Usually, TCR gene rearrangement is polyclonal. However, a dominant clone can produce a false monoclonal result [94,95], limiting the usefulness of this test as the sole distinction between RCD-1 and RCD-2. Other autoimmune diseases are common in RCD-1 patients [22]. There is, typically, a good clinical response to immunosuppressive therapy, such as corticosteroids and azathioprine, and patients are at no significant risk for developing ETTL [22].

RCD-2 is histologically identical to usual coeliac disease and in particular there is no cytological atypia of IELs. There is, however, immunophenotypic abnormality with loss of multiple surface T-cell markers, including CD3,

CD7 and CD8. CD103 is preserved, as is cytoplasmic CD3 (due to preservation of the immunoreactive ε component), which is detectable by immunohistochemistry but not by flow cytometry [94,95]. Loss of multiple surface markers in more than 20% of IELs determined by flow cytometric analysis [100] and immunohistochemical loss of CD8 in more than 50% of IELs are regarded as abnormal and indicative of RCD-2 [101] (Figure 21.9). Abnormal T-cell immunophenotype can also be found in two-thirds of gastric and colonic biopsies, highlighting that RCD-2 is a diffuse gastrointestinal disease [95,96,102]. Monoclonal TCR is consistently identified and the progression to overt ETTL occurs in 37–50% within 5 years, with an overall survival rate under 50% at 5 years [22]. Immunosuppressant therapy appears to accelerate the development of overt ETTL [94], highlighting the need for accurate classification of RCD.

Ulcerative jejuno-ileitis

Mucosal ulceration in gluten-induced enteropathy may occur as a non-specific phenomenon of uncertain cause or be due to an unrelated process such as peptic or drug injury. Ulcerative jejuno-ileitis (UJ) refers to a clinical syndrome of multiple small intestinal ulcers, particularly involving the proximal jejunum, complicated by haemorrhage, perforation and/or obstruction. Ulceration extends into the submucosa and sometimes deeper and is associated with acute and chronic inflammation, fibrosis and pseudo-pyloric gland metaplasia/ulcer-associated cell lineage. Gluten enteropathy, sometimes with changes of collagenous sprue, is seen in the adjacent mucosa. Intra-epithelial lymphocytes share the aberrant immunophenotype of RCD-2 and TCR monoclonality can usually be documented [94]. It is generally believed that RCD-2, UJ and ETTL represent a continuum in the manifestation of a T-cell neoplastic disorder.

Dermatitis herpetiformis and coeliac disease

It has long been recognised that there is a relationship between coeliac syndromes and dermatitis herpetiformis [103–104]. Two-thirds of patients with dermatitis herpetiformis display villous blunting typical of gluten-induced enteropathy, which improves on gluten withdrawal [105–107] and enteropathy is also more common in their relatives compared with a normal population [108]. However, symptoms of gluten sensitivity are present in less than 10% [107,109] and, in one series, a diagnosis of coeliac disease had only been established in 12.6% of patients with dermatitis herpetiformis [110]. Despite this, approximately 70% of patients have IgA anti-endomysial antibodies and 90% have elevated TTG. Moreover, these can be induced by gluten challenge in the remaining patients [111,112]. The same is true for the development of characteristic enteropathy in patients with initially 'normal' duodenal biopsies [113], which revert back to normal morphology on gluten

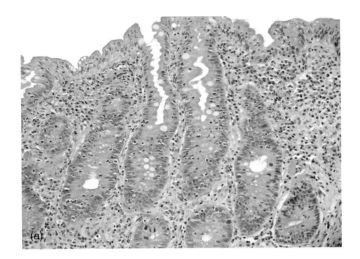

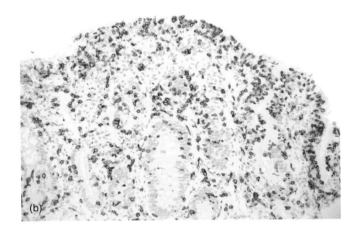

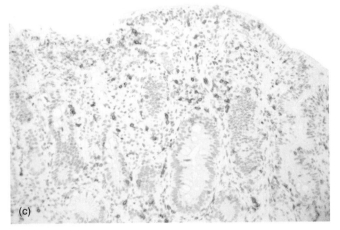

Figure 21.9 (a) Refractory coeliac disease type 2: note the absence of atypia in intra-epithelial lymphocytes. Paneth cells were markedly reduced in this case. (b) CD3 immunohistochemical stain showing preserved cytoplasmic staining. (c) CD8 immunohistochemical stain showing loss of reaction in intra-epithelial lymphocytes.

withdrawal (latent coeliac disease) [114]. The third of dermatitis herpetiformis patients who do not show typical villous blunting will display increased IELs [107] with expansion of γδ-bearing T cells [115].

Disease pathogenesis involves binding of IgA anti-TTG antibodies, formed in the gut, to TTG in the skin [116–118]. At least six isoforms of transglutaminase exist in the skin but most attention has focused on the type 3 isoform which is involved in epidermal stabilisation [118]. Approximately a third of patients with coeliac disease have elevated serum levels of anti-epidermal transglutaminase [119]; despite this the development of characteristic bullous skin lesions is uncommon.

Duodenal and jejunal biopsies have been useful for diagnosis of the often silent enteropathy [120]. There is apparently no correlation between severity of the skin lesions and degree of mucosal flattening [121]. Small bowel disease is often patchy and villous changes vary in degree [107].

Collagenous sprue

This disorder is characterised by prominent collagen deposition beneath the surface epithelium of the small intestinal mucosa, generally accompanied by inflammation in the lamina propria, intra-epithelial lymphocytosis and villous flattening. As mild thickening of the subepithelial collagen is common in gluten enteropathy, a diagnosis of collagenous sprue should not be rendered unless the collagen band is greater than 10-μm thick with capillary entrapment and often an irregular lower border [122] (Figure 21.10). When so defined, this condition is uncommon and often associated with lack of clinical response to gluten-free diet [98]; it may harbour a clonal intra-epithelial T-cell population [122]. A review of 21 refractory coeliac disease cases identified collagenous sprue in a third [123]. Collagenous sprue may develop de novo or arise in preexisting uncomplicated coeliac disease. Importantly, not all collagenous sprue is coeliac disease related. However, the aetiology of other cases is uncertain. Similar to other luminal collagenous disorders, eosinophils are often prominent and this has led to speculation of a drug (e.g. NSAIDs) causation [122].

Other gastrointestinal tract pathology in gluten-induced enteropathy

Gluten sensitivity affecting non-enteric sites is primarily manifest as an intra-epithelial lymphocytosis. Lymphocytic gastritis related to coeliac disease accounts for 10–45% of cases and characteristically has an antral predominance [124–128]. Lymphocytic colitis is associated with coeliac disease in 9–20% of cases [129–134] and patients with coeliac disease display a colonic lymphocytosis in up to 31% of concurrent colonic biopsies [135]. Ileal intra-epithelial lymphocytosis with or without blunting is occasionally encountered and appears to correlate with more clinically severe disease [136–137]. A prominent basal lym-

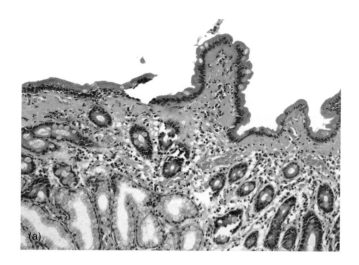

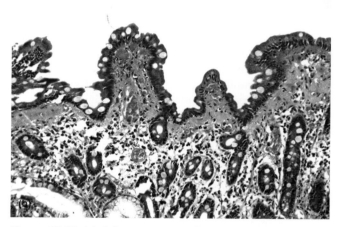

Figure 21.10 (a) Collagenous sprue characterised by deposition of collagen in the subepithelial region. Entrapment and dilatation of capillaries within the collagen is evident. (b) Masson trichrome stain highlights the subepithelial collagen.

phocytic infiltrate in the oesophageal mucosa ('lymphocytic oesophagitis') is a manifestation of coeliac disease in up to 10% of cases [138].

Collagenous disorders of the extra-enteric gut may also be related to coeliac disease, with both collagenous colitis [139] and collagenous gastritis [140] being well-documented associations. Several neoplasms, in addition to UJ/ETTL, are increased in coeliac disease. Up to 13% of small intestinal adenocarcinomas arise in gluten-sensitive patients. Microsatellite instability may play a role in the development of these tumours [142]. However, duodenal adenomas are not significantly more common [141]. Oesophageal squamous cell carcinoma is increased in some studies but not others. The prevalence of Barrett's oesophagus is increased although the risk for oesophageal adenocarcinoma is unknown [143]. Colorectal adenocarcinoma incidence is minimally increased in diet-treated patients [143].

Immunological reactions to other ingested food proteins

Non-IgE, cell-mediated hypersensitivity to ingested proteins and polypeptides is increasingly recognised. The most common antigens are components of cows' milk, soy protein, peanuts, egg, fish, rice and chicken. A failure of oral tolerance to an ingested protein is believed to underlie the process [20]. Clinical symptoms and small intestinal morphology can closely resemble gluten-induced enteropathy. Cessation of symptoms, on avoidance of the inciting food, establishes the diagnosis in most cases [20].

Cows' milk and soy protein intolerance

Symptoms commence in infancy shortly after introduction of cows' milk or soy protein with up to half of patients reacting to both foods [20]. Mucosal abnormality occurs throughout the gastrointestinal tract. However, the proximal duodenum is most prominently affected. Lymphonodular hyperplasia of the duodenal bulb is universal [144] and accompanied by variable villous blunting which is usually milder than in gluten-induced enteropathy [145,146] (Figure 21.11). There is an increase in IEL numbers similar to or quantitatively less numerous than in gluten-sensitive enteropathy but similarly expressing the CD3+/CD8+ cytotoxic immunophenotype and displaying TCR-γσ expansion [144,145]. An increase in CD4+ lymphocytes and plasma cells containing IgE is found. Eosinophil infiltration is almost universal and eosinophils, together with mast cells, may be numerous enough to warrant a designation of eosinophilic enteritis [62,145,146]. Neutrophils are also frequently found. In both conditions, a return to normal mucosal morphology follows the withdrawal of the offending antigen and symptoms subside rapidly, usually within 24–72 hours [20].

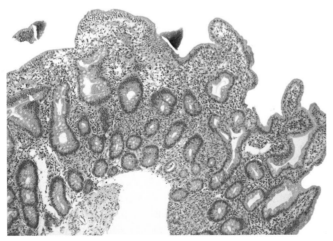

Figure 21.11 Cows' milk protein intolerance characterised by inflammation in the lamina propria, villous shortening and mild intra-epithelial lymphocytosis.

Solid food protein intolerance

Enteropathy identical to that of cows' milk and soy intolerance can be invoked by chicken, turkey, fish, rice, oats, egg white, peanut and green peas [20,147]. Of these, rice protein intolerance is most frequently encountered. Two-thirds of patients who react to a solid food protein have a prior history of cows' milk or soy intolerance [20].

Defects in enzyme systems

Enterocytes possess large numbers of enzyme systems, located in brush borders and cell bodies. Their absence is not, however, usually accompanied by visible histological change. The principal patterns of abnormality are described below.

Disaccharidase deficiency

Disaccharidase deficiency and disaccharide intolerance are not necessarily synonymous, although they commonly coexist. The deficiency can occur in a primary inherited form due to an autosomally inherited recessive gene [148], usually resulting in a specific deficiency in lactase whereas other disaccharidases are present in normal concentrations. At all ages the condition is more commonly secondary to any condition causing epithelial cell injury, e.g. infection, gluten-induced enteropathy and after chemotherapy for cancer [63, 149]. Up to 70% of the world's population may be affected [150,151] by secondary lactase deficiency. Three mechanisms account for clinical symptoms: first, undigested lactose undergoes fermentation by bacterial flora to produce large amounts of gas that cause abdominal discomfort; second, the sugar induces an osmotic diarrhoea; and, third, bacterial overgrowth is favoured with the resultant changes discussed below [63].

Lactase deficiency is not associated with histological abnormality, although changes related to any predisposing condition may be seen. Immunohistochemical stains show a patchy distribution of lactase over the villous surface [152] but these are not used in routine practice. The diagnosis is made by biochemical analysis of disaccharidase concentration in an unfixed duodenal biopsy and/or by administration of an oral lactose (or lactulose) challenge, with measurement of breath hydrogen generated by bacterial fermentation of undigested lactose [150].

Defects in lipid transport

Abetalipoproteinaemia

This rare autosomal recessive disorder is characterised by fat malabsorption, red cell acanthocytosis and hypocholesterolaemia in infancy with the development of retinitis, neuropathy and myopathy in later life [153]. Mutations in the gene encoding for microsomal triglyceride transfer protein lead to absence of plasma apoprotein B-containing lipoproteins, thereby compromising absorption of fat and

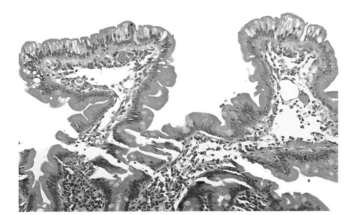

Figure 21.12 Abetalipoproteinaemia: note the clear lipid-filled cytoplasmic vacuoles in the enterocytes covering the upper aspects of the villi.

fat-soluble vitamins from the intestine [153]. Jejunal biopsy shows villi of relatively normal architecture but displaying marked foamy vacuolation of the cytoplasm of enterocytes covering the upper two-thirds of the villus (Figure 21.12) [154]. In cryostat sections of unfixed tissue the vacuoles stain for neutral lipid [155]. Similar cytoplasmic vacuolation has been described in cows' milk sensitivity [156], juvenile nutritional megaloblastic anaemia, coeliac disease ('lipid hang-up' sign), tropical sprue [157] and NSAID injury [158]. More commonly, however, cytoplasmic lipid vacuolation is an incidental finding in patients who have not adequately fasted before endoscopic biopsy, especially if they have recently had a fatty meal.

Other defects in lipid transport

These include homozygous hypobetalipoproteinaemia (a dominantly inherited condition) [159] and Andersen's disease (chylomicron retention disease) [160]. Both are associated with accumulation of esterified lipid in the enterocytes

Autoimmune enteropathy

This rare disorder, originally identified in infants with intractable diarrhoea and weight loss through malabsorption [161], is now known also to affect adults [162–164]. Characteristic of this disease are circulating gut epithelial cell antibodies, predominantly anti-enterocyte type, although anti-goblet cell and anti-Paneth cell antibodies are sometimes encountered [163]. The small bowel is always affected but, in at least a third of patients, the disorder involves the stomach and large intestine causing a pan-gastroenterocolitis [163]. In 80% of patients there is other autoimmune disease [164]. The diagnosis is usually considered in a patient with histological, clinical and sometimes serological features suggestive of gluten-induced enteropathy, but not responding to gluten-free diet or other dietary exclusion [162–164]. Detection of gut epithelial cell antibodies by indirect immunofluorescence on a biopsy sample confirms the diagnosis [163].

The pathogenesis remains unknown. However, potential insight is gained in the subset of autoimmune enteropathy cases with the IPEX syndrome. This disorder usually presents in infancy and is characterised by **i**mmunodysregulation, **p**olyendocrinopathy and **e**nteropathy and is **X**-linked recessive in affected males [165]. In the IPEX syndrome, mutations in the *FOXP3* gene lead to deficiency of CD25+, CD4+ regulatory T cells resulting in loss of self-tolerance, allowing development of autoantibodies targeting self-antigens such as gut enterocytes [165]. Loss of self-tolerance may underlie other cases of autoimmune enteropathy.

Recent attention has also been given to a 75-kilodalton antigen associated with regulation of the gut epithelial cell tight junction, which may allow antigens into the lamina propria, inducing the typical inflammatory reaction [164]. Anti-goblet cell antibodies are found in a subset of patients with inflammatory bowel disease [166] and have been documented in a case of collagenous enterocolitis [167], whereas anti-enterocyte antibodies have been described in HIV infection [168].

The histological features of autoimmune enteropathy in the small intestine can mimic both graft-versus-host disease and coeliac disease [163] (Figure 21.13a). In all cases there is diffuse lamina propria inflammation, mainly comprising lymphocytes with basal lymphoid follicle formation and plasma cells. Enhanced basal crypt apoptosis is always present and can be prominent (Figure 21.13b). Acute inflammation with neutrophil crypt abscess formation is sometimes encountered. In up to 50% there is an increase in CD8+ IELs but, in contrast to gluten-induced enteropathy, the TCR-γσ density is normal [163]. In cases associated with anti-goblet cell and anti-Paneth cell antibodies loss of the corresponding cell type occurs. Gastric and colonic pathology is along similar lines with inflammation, epithelial apoptosis and architectural disturbance. Colonic changes can mimic inflammatory bowel disease. Treatment is with immunosuppressant drugs but prognosis is generally poor [162–164].

Malabsorption related to infections

Temporary malabsorption is common in many patients with small intestinal infections and infestations, particularly giardiasis (see 'Giardiasis', Chapter 20). It usually resolves when the infection is successfully treated. Whipple's disease (*Tropheryma whipplei* infection) may be associated with protracted malabsorption.

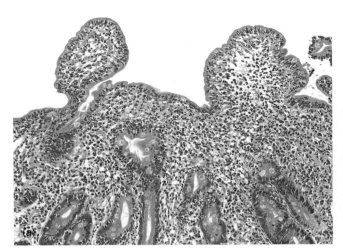

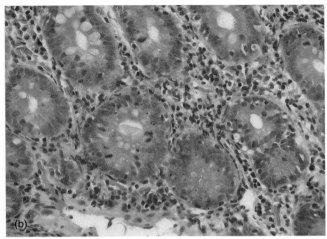

Figure 21.13 (a) Coeliac disease-like pattern of autoimmune enteropathy: there is marked inflammation in the lamina propria and intra-epithelial lymphocytosis is present. Similar inflammatory changes were seen in the stomach and colon. (b) Enhanced basal crypt apoptosis in this case of autoimmune enteropathy.

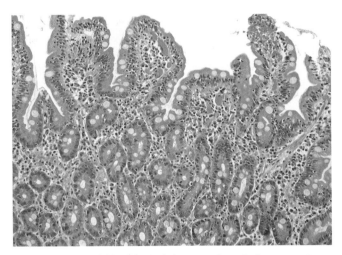

Figure 21.14 Mild histological changes of tropical sprue: note that the intra-epithelial lymphocytosis involves both villous and crypt epithelium. Similar changes were found in the ileum. The patient had recently returned from south-east Asia.

Tropical sprue

Although tropical sprue is now recognised as infective [169], it remains in this chapter because of its histological resemblance to gluten-sensitive enteropathy and its association with malabsorption. It is endemic in Puerto Rica, parts of the Caribbean, northern South America, Nigeria and other countries in west Africa, India, in much of south-east Asia and the Philippines (there is a valuable map in the article by Klipstein [170]) and is acquired by visitors to these regions. The cause is probably a persistent, as opposed to a transitory, contamination, initially of the proximal small bowel, by enteric pathogens, mostly aerobic coliforms, which the individual does not readily expel. This bacterial overgrowth is favoured by relative stasis from reduced peristalsis. These organisms produce enterotoxins that act directly on enterocytes and crypt cells [171–173].

The intriguing suggestion has been made that the trigger for the continuing adverse response to such banal organisms may be a coccidial protozoon [174]. Symptoms may be surprisingly mild despite severe morphological changes. However, diarrhoea and steatorrhoea related to malabsorption frequently result. Ileal involvement leads to vitamin B_{12} malabsorption, which, together with folate deficiency, produces a macrocytic anaemia. Treatment with broad-spectrum antibiotics and vitamin B_{12}/folate replacement produces a good clinical and histological recovery.

The duodenum and jejunum are affected first, followed by involvement of the ileal mucosa, which, distinct from gluten-induced enteropathy, displays a similar severity of disease [175]. Histologically the changes resemble those of gluten enteropathy with crypt hyperplasia, broadening and shortening of villi, enterocyte distortion and crowding, an increase in number of IELs, which usually involves the crypt zone as intensely as the surface epithelium [176], and increased cellularity of the lamina propria, including eosinophils (Figure 21.14). The histological features may be indistinguishable from coeliac disease [177], although villous flattening is rarely complete. Further the changes seen in less severe disease merge with those seen in the indigenous population, so that small intestinal biopsy is not always diagnostic [178].

Tropical sprue must be differentiated from giardiasis (see 'Giardiasis', Chapter 20) and from genuine gluten-induced enteropathy occurring in tropical zones [179,180]. Although the untreated condition is serious in itself, there are few important complications. In particular there is no increased risk of carcinoma or lymphoma, probably because immunological disturbances are not a feature of tropical sprue.

Malabsorption related to bacterial overgrowth

Normal small bowel ecology is discussed in Chapter 17. Although some of the normal indigenous organisms are capable of taking up and metabolising vitamin B_{12} they are not present in sufficient numbers to produce vitamin deficiency or steatorrhoea. When normal ecology is disturbed, non-indigenous organisms, mainly coliforms, colonise spaces normally occupied by indigenous anaerobes. They may then deconjugate sufficient bile acids to produce steatorrhoea and use up enough of the available oxygen to allow overgrowth of anaerobic *Bacteroides* spp. that readily bind and therefore deplete the vitamin B_{12} complex [181,182].

Factors predisposing to bacterial overgrowth include: intestinal stasis related to structural abnormalities, such as strictures in Crohn's disease and radiation enteritis, progressive systemic sclerosis/scleroderma, diverticula, neoplasms and surgical blind loops; abnormal connections between the small and large intestine after surgery or via inflammatory fistula formation; reduced gastric acid production after gastric surgery, atrophic gastritis and prolonged proton pump inhibitor treatment; immunodeficiency states, both primary and acquired; and old age via an unknown mechanism.

Most patients with small bowel bacterial overgrowth are elderly and have diarrhoea and weight loss [183,184]. Anaemia is most often macrocytic due to vitamin B_{12} malabsorption [185]. The condition is under-recognised, particularly in elderly patients, where its prevalence may be as high as 38.5% [186]. The mainstay of diagnosis is the hydrogen breath test, which has good sensitivity. Microbial culture of aspirated small intestinal fluid remains the gold standard investigation [186].

The mucosa may appear histologically normal or can show villous blunting accompanied by crypt hyperplasia and inflammatory changes that typically have a patchy distribution [187]. IELs and neutrophils often accompany the lamina propria inflammation [188,189]. Correction of nutritional deficiencies and antibiotic treatment usually results in dramatic clinical improvement and a return to normal small bowel morphology [184,188].

Malabsorption due to inherited disorders

Microvillous inclusion disease

This very rare disorder, of probable autosomal recessive inheritance, presents in neonates with severe watery diarrhoea from birth, although occasional examples present a little later in infancy [190]. It carries a very poor prognosis because the diffuse abnormality of small intestine enterocytes results in severe intractable malabsorption, controlled only by lifelong total parenteral nutrition or small bowel transplantation.

The abnormality is in brush border assembly and differentiation, such that the normal microvilli of the cell surface become misplaced within the apical cytoplasm to form the micro-inclusions that give the condition its name [191]. These are best identified by electron microscopy as vesicles lined by microvilli which are often structurally unremarkable [192], although, on light microscopy, they are well demonstrated as periodic acid–Schiff (PAS)-positive inclusions in the supranuclear cytoplasm of the enterocytes. The inclusions also stain strongly for carcinoembryonic antigen and alkaline phosphatase [193] and the affected cells display cytoplasmic rather than cell membrane immunostaining for CD10 [194]. At low magnification, the mucosa shows diffuse villous shortening with little or no crypt hyperplasia (so-called crypt hypoplastic atrophy) and normal or even decreased mucosal inflammatory cells. PAS staining reveals the enterocytes to have a poorly staining and discontinuous brush border, especially over the apices of any residual villi, but the other cellular components of the crypt, namely goblet cells, Paneth cells and endocrine cells, are unremarkable [190,191]. Cells in other areas of the gastrointestinal tract that normally harbour microvilli may also be affected, so micro-inclusions may be found in gastric antral and large intestine biopsies, indicating that the defect in brush border assembly is generalised.

Intestinal epithelial dysplasia (tufting enteropathy)

This very rare inherited autosomal recessive disorder presents with intractable watery diarrhoea in infants requiring parenteral nutrition or intestinal transplantation [190,195,196]. A mutation in the gene for Epithelial Cell Adhesion Molecule (EpCAM) is responsible for a basement membrane disturbance leading to abnormal cell–matrix and cell–cell matrix interaction [197]. Secondary loss of mucosal integrity with T-cell activation could explain the lamina propria inflammation seen in this condition [195]. The characteristic histological feature is the presence of widespread enterocyte cell tufts, representing cells that have detached from the basement membrane, affecting the surface epithelium of the small intestine and persisting into the colonic epithelium. Enterocytes within the tufts show apical rounding, inducing a tear-drop shape. Villous atrophy, crypt hyperplasia and normal or increased inflammatory cells in the lamina propria, but no increase in IELs, further characterise the lesion [190,195,196].

Acrodermatitis enteropathica (zinc deficiency)

This rare autosomal recessive condition results from mutations in the *SLC39* gene located at 8q24.3, leading to deficiency of a zinc-specific transporter protein that is normally highly expressed in the mucosa of the proximal small intestine [198]. The resultant inability to absorb zinc produces a syndrome of diarrhoea, dermatitis, alopecia and learning disability that is rapidly corrected by zinc replacement. Similar clinical features can develop in acquired zinc deficiency related to total parenteral nutrition, anorexia nervosa and malabsorptive disorders.

The small intestine can be normal or may show villous blunting of variable degree, crypt hyperplasia and inflammation in the lamina propria. IEL numbers are normal [199]. Ultrastructural studies consistently show distinctive lysosomal inclusions in Paneth cells in affected patients [200,201], a finding due to zinc deficiency of any cause [202] that disappears after zinc replacement.

Intestinal lymphangiectasia

This condition is characterised by dilatation of intestinal lymphatics/lacteals with leakage of protein-rich material into the gut lumen, causing protein-losing enteropathy and malabsorption [202–204]. Most cases are not inherited, being secondary to inflammatory (e.g. Crohn's disease, radiation) or neoplastic conditions (carcinoma, especially pancreatic carcinoma, or lymphoma) affecting the small intestine and associated lymphatic drainage system.

Rare primary intestinal lymphangiectasia results from a congenital defect in lymphatic development and presents in early childhood with signs of hypoproteinaemia [63]. At endoscopy, multiple white spots, representing dilated lacteals in the villi, are found throughout the small intestine, albeit in a patchy distribution in some [205,206]. Histologically, the dilated lymphatics may appear empty, potentially simulating pneumatosis intestinalis, or may contain proteinaceous material and histiocytes, the latter sometimes numerous enough to suggest Whipple's disease or *Mycobacterium avium-intercellulare* infection (Figure 21.15). It is important not to confuse intestinal lymphangiectasia with the focal lymphatic and/or lacteal dilatation that is a relatively common finding in otherwise normal biopsies and has no clinical significance.

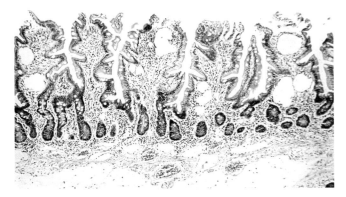

Figure 21.15 Intestinal lymphangiectasia: section of an ileal biopsy, showing numerous dilated lymphatic capillaries in the villi, which are abnormally broad as a consequence.

Malabsorption related to drugs and chemicals

Drugs

Drug-induced malabsorption may be a consequence of direct toxic effects with morphological change in the mucosa, interference with brush border enzyme function, binding and precipitation of bile acids or nutrients, or alterations to the chemical state of nutrients [207]. Commonly implicated medications include antibiotics, antacids, laxatives, NSAIDs, colchicine, cholestyramine, oral hypoglycaemic agents, proton pump inhibitors (by chronic gastric acid suppression), chemotherapeutic drugs and immunosuppressant agents [208–210]. Mucosal inflammation and villous flattening, resembling gluten-induced enteropathy, have been described with methotrexate, azathioprine and NSAID use [158,210] but IEL numbers are normal or only mildly increased.

Alcohol

Malabsorption is common in people with chronic alcohol problems and is consequent on poor dietary nutrient intake, pancreatic insufficiency, a direct toxic effect of alcohol on the enteric mucosa and alterations in small bowel ecology favouring bacterial overgrowth [211,212]. The direct toxic effect, similar to other drugs, is dose related and causes increased static and dynamic membrane fluidity and decreased microvillous membrane cholesterol, leading to impaired absorption [213].

Malabsorption due to organic bowel disease

Secondary malabsorption syndromes can follow a number of organic diseases including Crohn's disease, tuberculosis, neurofibromatosis, vascular insufficiency state, amyloid infiltration, progressive systemic sclerosis, radiation enteritis, and primary or secondary lymphoid neoplasms. The malabsorption and steatorrhoea result from direct damage to the mucosal surface, disturbed peristalsis or the mechanical complications described above.

Miscellaneous causes of malnutrition

Defects in gastric function

The stomach is responsible for mechanical disruption of food, early biochemical breakdown of food, via acid and pepsinogen, and secretion of intrinsic factor required for vitamin B_{12} absorption. Surgical procedures such as gastrectomy, either total or subtotal, bariatric surgery and Nissen's fundoplication may interfere with these functions [63,214,215]. Advanced gastric carcinoma and chronic atrophic gastritis often produce clinically relevant deficiency of acid, pepsinogen and intrinsic factor, particularly when the gastric corpus is diffusely involved. There are also reports of vitamin B_{12} deficiency after long-term proton pump inhibitor therapy [216]. Excess acid production in Zollinger–Ellison syndrome may disrupt small bowel brush border enzyme systems but histological evidence of damage is unusual [217].

Defects in other organs

Normal pancreatic and hepatobiliary function are essential for adequate digestion but disorders of these organs are outside the scope of this book.

Diabetes mellitus and other endocrine disorders

Two groups of patients with diabetes mellitus and steatorrhoea exist: those with diabetic neuropathy, and consequent loss of post-ganglionic sympathetic function with disturbance of peristalsis, and those with associated gluten enteropathy. The former group is not associated with histological abnormality in the small intestine, although dendritic swelling with the presence of giant sympathetic neurons is seen in prevertebral and paravertebral sympathetic ganglia [218]. Patients with type 1 diabetes have overt coeliac disease in 4–9%, with disease risk mediated via the HLA-DR3/-DQ2 haplotype. TTG antibodies may be found in up to a third of patients with type 1 diabetes who are homozygous for this haplotype [219]. Small bowel biopsies in these patients may reveal silent enteropathy or isolated intra-epithelial lymphocytosis.

Other autoimmune endocrine disorders, in particular Addison's disease, type 1 autoimmune polyendocrine syndrome, Graves' disease and Hashimoto's thyroiditis, can be associated with malabsorption, either because of associated gluten-sensitive enteropathy or via a direct effect of the disease process on enteric function [220].

Protein-losing enteropathies

The normal absorption of products of protein digestion is briefly discussed in Chapter 17. The total daily loss of protein from the small bowel in humans is about 84 g, of which some comes from exfoliated cells and the rest from extracellular sources [221]. The small bowel resorbs most of this. In a number of conditions there is excessive loss of protein from the gastrointestinal tract (e.g. intestinal lymphangiectasia, as discussed above) unmatched by an increase in protein synthesis; this leads to hypoproteinaemia in which various proteins are differently affected. 'Protein-losing enteropathy' is, in fact, not a single entity confined to the small intestine but a manifestation of many disorders, some of which (e.g. giant rugal hypertrophy of the stomach, gastric carcinoma and ulcerative colitis) are not primary to the small bowel. The term is now best reserved for a clinical syndrome that includes all those cases where no organic cause can be found for a protein loss.

Malabsorption in immunodeficiency disorders

Immunodeficiency states can be divided into primary disorders, such as IgA deficiency and common variable immunodeficiency, and secondary disorders, such as acquired immune deficiency syndrome (AIDS) and immunoglobulin deficiency in protein-losing enteropathies. Both are associated with malabsorption that is multifactorial but in particular due to the effect of primary disease-related inflammation and superimposed infection. 'Idiopathic AIDS enteropathy' is of unknown cause and is characterised by villous blunting, lamina propria inflammation, a reduction in CD4+ T cells and an increase in CD8+ T cells. By definition an infective agent is not identified [63].

Waldenström's macroglobulinaemia

This is a clinico-pathological disorder characterised by the production and tissue deposition of IgM paraprotein, produced by the neoplastic cells of lymphoplasmacytic lymphoma [222]. In the small intestine the paraprotein deposition, which is brightly eosinophilic, homogeneous and strongly PAS positive, begins within villous lymphatics and between epithelial cells [223] but eventually fills the lamina propria (Figure 21.16). Secondary villous blunting is common as is lymphangiectasia [224], which is responsible for malabsorption and the characteristic diffuse white endoscopic appearance. Absence of Congo red staining but immunoreactivity for IgM, with light chain restriction, aids differentiation from amyloidosis.

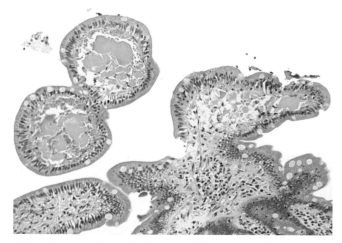

Figure 21.16 Waldenström's macroglobulinaemia: there is deposition of eosinophilic immunoglobulin within the villus lacteals. This material is strongly periodic acid–Schiff positive but negative on Congo red stain.

The 'brown bowel' syndrome

This rare condition develops because of malabsorption, of any cause, of fat-soluble vitamin E, which is essential for stabilising mitochondrial membranes. A smooth muscle 'mitochondrial myopathy' results in lipofuscin deposition within the cytoplasm of cells of the muscularis mucosae, muscularis propria and vascular media, or within histiocytes throughout the gastrointestinal tract [225,226]. The resultant, macroscopically evident, diffuse brown colour gives the condition its name.

Primary bile salt malabsorption [227]

Chronic diarrhoea may be due to excess bile acid loss. In such cases ileal biopsies show hyperplastic villous atrophy, colonisation of the mucosa and increased numbers of plasma cells and lymphocytes in the lamina propria. The diagnosis should be suggested when there is a flat ileal biopsy in the presence of chronic unexplained diarrhoea. Cholestyramine may then produce a dramatic recovery.

References

1. Holbrook I. The British Society of Gastroenterology guidelines for the investigation of chronic diarrhoea, 2nd edition. *Ann Clin Biochem* 2005;**42**(Part 3):170.
2. Ghosh AK, Littlewood JM, Goddard D, Steel WF. Stool microscopy in screening for steatorrhoea. *J Clin Pathol* 1977;**30**:749.
3. Russell RI. Small intestinal investigative tests and techniques. *Curr Opin Gastroenterol* 1985;**1**:266.
4. Thomas AG, Phillips AD, Walker-Smith JA. The value of proximal small intestinal biopsy in the differential diagnosis of chronic diarrhoea. *Arch Dis Child* 1992;**67**:741.
5. Hasan M, Ferguson A. Measurements of intestinal villi in non-specific and ulcer-associated duodenitis – correlation between area of microdissected villus and epithelial cell count. *J Clin Pathol* 1981;**34**:1181.
6. Hasan M, Sircus W, Ferguson A. Duodenal mucosal architecture in non-specific and ulcer-associated duodenitis. *Gut* 1981;**22**:637.
7. Moss SF, Attia L, Scholes JV, Walters JR, Holt PR. Increased small intestinal apoptosis in coeliac disease. *Gut* 1996;**39**:811.
8. Katz AJ, Grand RJ. All that flattens is not 'sprue'. *Gastroenterology* 1979;**76**:375.
9. Rodrigues MAM, De Camargo JLV, Coelho KIR, et al. Morphometric study of the small intestinal mucosa in young adult and old rats submitted to protein deficiency and rehabilitation. *Gut* 1985;**26**:816.
10. Stanfield JP, Hutt MSR, Tunnicliffe R. Intestinal biopsy in kwashiorkor. *Lancet* 1965;**ii**:519.
11. Burman D. The jejunal mucosa in Kwashiorkor. *Arch Dis Child* 1965;**40**:526.
12. Cook GC, Lee FD. The jejunum after kwashiorkor. *Lancet* 1966;**ii**:1263.
13. Dawson DW. Partial atrophy in nutritional megaloblastic anaemia corrected by folic acid therapy. *J Clin Pathol* 1971;**24**:131.
14. Haymond HE. Massive resections of the small intestine: an analysis of 257 collected cases. *Surg Gynecol Obstet* 1935;**61**:693.
15. Pullan JM. Massive intestinal resection. *Proc R Soc Med* 1959;**52**:31.
16. Rickham PP. Massive small intestinal resection in newborn infants. *Ann R Coll Surg* 1967;**41**:480.
17. Porus RL. Epithelial hyperplasia following massive small bowel resection in man. *Gastroenterology* 1965;**48**:753.
18. Curtis KJ, Sleisenger MH, Kim YS. Protein digestion and absorption after massive small bowel resection. *Dig Dis Sci* 1984;**29**:834.
19. Gornacz GE, Al-Mukhtar MYT, Ghatai MA, et al. Pattern of cell proliferation and enteroglucagon response following small bowel resection in the rat. *Digestion* 1984;**29**:65.
20. Mansueto P, Montalto G, Pacor ML, et al. Food allergy in gastroenterologic diseases: Review of literature. *World J Gastroenterol* 2006;**12**:7744.
21. Green PH, Rostami K, Marsh MN. Diagnosis of coeliac disease. *Best Pract Res Clin Gastroenterol* 2005;**19**:389.
22. Di Sabatino A, Corazza GR. Coeliac disease. *Lancet* 2009;**373**:1480.
23. Rubin CF, Eidelman S, Weinstein WM. Sprue by any other name. *Gastroenterology* 1970;**58**:409.
24. Kagnoff MF. Celiac disease: pathogenesis of a model immunogenetic disease. *J Clin Invest* 2007;**117**:41.
25. Green PH, Cellier C. Celiac disease. *N Engl J Med* 2007;**357**:1731.
26. Dandalides SM, Carey WD, Petras R, Achkar E. Endoscopic small bowel mucosal biopsy: a controlled trial evaluating forceps size and biopsy location in the diagnosis of normal and abnormal mucosal architecture. *Gastrointest Endosc* 1989;**35**:197.
27. Yantiss RK, Odze RD. Optimal approach to obtaining mucosal biopsies for assessment of inflammatory disorders of the gastrointestinal tract. *Am J Gastroenterol* 2009;**104**:774.
28. Weir DC, Glickman JN, Roiff T, Valim C, Leichtner AM. Variability of histopathological changes in childhood celiac disease. *Am J Gastroenterol* 2010;**105**:207.
29. Ravelli A, Bolognini S, Gambarotti M, Villanacci V. Variability of histologic lesions in relation to biopsy site in gluten-sensitive enteropathy. *Am J Gastroenterol* 2005;**100**:177.
30. Hopper AD, Cross SS, Sanders DS. Patchy atrophy in adult patients with suspected gluten-sensitive enteropathy: is a multiple duodenal biopsy strategy appropriate? *Endoscopy* 2008;**40**:219.
31. Bonamico M, Mariani P, Thanasi E, et al. Patchy atrophy of the duodenum in childhood celiac disease. *J Pediatr Gastroenterol Nutr* 2004;**38**:204.
32. Bonamico M, Thanasi E, Mariani P, et al. Duodenal bulb biopsies in celiac disease: a multicenter study. *J Pediatr Gastroenterol Nutr* 2008;**47**:618.
33. Brocchi E, Tomassetti P, Volta U, et al. Adult coeliac disease diagnosed by endoscopic biopsies in the duodenal bulb. *Eur J Gastroenterol Hepatol* 2005;**17**:1413.
34. Vogelsang H, Hänel S, Steiner B, Oberhuber G. Diagnostic duodenal bulb biopsy in celiac disease. *Endoscopy* 2001;**33**:336.
35. Rostom A, Murray JA, Kagnoff MF American Gastroenterological Association (AGA) Institute technical review on the diagnosis and management of celiac disease. *Gastroenterology* 2006;**131**:1981.
36. Green PH. Celiac disease: how many biopsies for diagnosis? *Gastrointest Endosc* 2008;**67**:1088.
37. Gramlich TL, Petras RE. Small intestine. In: Mills SE (ed.), *Histology for Pathologists*. Philadelphia, PA: Lippincott, Williams & Wilkins, 2007:3.
38. Brocchi E, Corazza GR, Caletti G, Treggiari EA, Barbara L, Gasbarrini G. Endoscopic demonstration of loss of duodenal folds in the diagnosis of celiac disease. *N Engl J Med* 1988;**319**:741.
39. Bardella MT, Minoli G, Radaelli F, et al. Reevaluation of duodenal endoscopic markers in the diagnosis of celiac disease. *Gastrointest Endosc* 2000;**51**:714.

40. Shah VH, Rotterdam H, Kotler DP, Fasano A, Green PH. All that scallops is not celiac disease. *Gastrointest Endosc* 2000;**51**:717.

41. Spada C, Riccioni ME, Urgesi R, Costamagna G. Capsule endoscopy in celiac disease. *World J Gastroenterol* 2008;**14**:4146.

42. Hill ID. What are the sensitivity and specificity of serologic tests for celiac disease? Do sensitivity and specificity vary in different populations? *Gastroenterology* 2005;**128**:S25.

43. Rostami K, Kerikhaert J. Sensitivity of antiendomysial and antigliadin antibodies in untreated celiac disease: Disappointing in clinical practice. *Am J Gastroenterol* 1999;**94**:888.

44. Rubin CE, Brandborg LL, Phelps PC, Taylor HC Jr. Studies of celiac disease. I. The apparent identical and specific nature of the duodenal and proximal jejunal lesion in celiac disease and idiopathic sprue. *Gastroenterology* 1960;**38**:28.

45. Ferguson A, Murray D. Quantitation of intra-epithelial lymphocytes in human jejunum. *Gut* 1971;**12**:988.

46. Verress B, Franzen L, Bodin L, Borch K. Duodenal intra-epithelial lymphocyte-count revisited. *Scand J Gastroenterol* 2004;**4**:138.

47. Hayat M, Cairns A, Dixon MF, O'Mahony S. Quantitation of intra-epithelial lymphocytes in human duodenum: what is normal? *J Clin Pathol* 2002;**55**:393.

48. Goldstein NS, Underhill J. Morphologic features suggestive of gluten sensitivity lymphocytes in human duodenum: what is normal? *J Clin Pathol* 2002;**55**:393.

49. Goldstein NS. Proximal small-bowel mucosal intra-epithelial lymphocytes. *Histopathology* 2004;**44**:199.

50. Biagi F, Luinetti O, Campanella J, et al. Intra-epithelial lymphocytes in the villous tip: do they indicate potential coeliac disease? *J Clin Pathol* 2004;**57**:835.

51. Oberhuber G, Granditsch G, Vogelsang H. The histopathology of coeliac disease: time for a standardized report scheme for pathologists. *Eur J Gastroenterol Hepatol* 1999;**11**:1185.

52. Mino M, Lauwers GY. Role of lymphocytic immunophenotyping in the diagnosis of gluten-sensitive enteropathy with preserved villous architecture. *Am J Surg Pathol* 2003;**27**:1237.

53. Arató A, Hacsek G, Savilahti E. Immunohistochemical findings in the jejunal mucosa of patients with coeliac disease. *Scand J Gastroenterol Suppl* 1998;**228**:3.

54. Camarero C, Eiras P, Asensio A, et al. Intra-epithelial lymphocytes and coeliac disease: permanent changes in CD3-/CD7+ and T cell receptor gammadelta subsets studied by flow cytometry. *Acta Paediatr* 2000;**89**:285.

55. Augustin MT, Kokkonen J, Karttunen TJ. Duodenal cytotoxic lymphocytes in cow's milk protein sensitive enteropathy and coeliac disease. *Scand J Gastroenterol* 2005;**40**:1398.

56. Marsh MN, Crowe PT. Morphology of the mucosal lesion in gluten sensitivity. *Baillière's Clin Gastroenterol* 1995;**9**:273.

57. Mino-Kenudson M, Brown I, Lauwers GY. Histopathological diagnosis of gluten-sensitive enteropathy. *Curr Diagn Path* 2005;**11**:274.

58. Antonioli DA Celiac Disease: A Progress Report. *Mod Pathol* 2003;**16**:342.

59. Dickson BC, Streutker CJ, Chetty R. Coeliac disease: an update for pathologists. *J Clin Pathol* 2006;**59**:1008.

60. Leonard N, Feighery CF, Hourihane DO. Peptic duodenitis – does it exist in the second part of the duodenum? *J Clin Pathol* 1997;**50**:54.

61. Jeffers MD, Hourihane DO. Coeliac disease with histological features of peptic duodenitis: value of assessment of intra-epithelial lymphocytes. *J Clin Pathol* 1993;**46**:420.

62. Kesuaai I, Kuitonen P, Savilahti E, Sipponen P. Mast cells and eosinophils in the jejunal mucosa of patients with intestinal cows' milk allergy and coeliac disease of childhood. *J Pediatr Gastroenterol Nutr* 1984;**3**:368.

63. Owens SR, Greenson JK. The pathology of malabsorption: current concepts. *Histopathology* 2007;**50**:64.

64. Shaoul R, Marcon MA, Okada Y, Cutz E, Forstner G. Gastric metaplasia: a frequently overlooked feature of duodenal biopsy specimens in untreated celiac disease. *J Pediatr Gastroenterol Nutr* 2000;**30**:397.

65. Bossart R, Henry K, Booth CC, Doe WF. Subepithelial collagen in intestinal malabsorption. *Gut* 1975;**16**:18.

66. Vakiani E, Arguelles-Grande C, Mansukhani MM, et al. Collagenous sprue is not always associated with dismal outcomes: a clinicopathological study of 19 patients. *Mod Pathol* 2010;**23**:12.

67. Scott H, Brandtzaeg P. Enumeration of Paneth cells in coeliac disease: comparison of conventional light microscopy and immunofluorescence staining for lysozyme. *Gut* 1981;**22**:812.

68. Elmes M, Jones JG, Stanton MR. Changes in the Paneth cell population of human small intestine assessed by image analysis of the secretory granule area. *J Clin Pathol* 1983;**36**:867.

69. Di Sabatino A, Miceli E, Dhaliwal W, et al. Distribution, proliferation, and function of Paneth cells in uncomplicated and complicated adult celiac disease. *Am J Clin Pathol* 2008;**130**:34.

70. Challacombe DN, Robertson K. Enterochromaffin cells in the duodenal mucosa of children with coeliac disease. *Gut* 1977;**18**:373.

71. Sjolund K, Alumets J, Berg N-O, et al. Enteropathy of coeliac disease in adults: increased number of enterochromaffin cells in the duodenal mucosa. *Gut* 1982;**23**:42.

72. Thompson H. Necropsy studies on adult coeliac disease. *J Clin Pathol* 1974;**27**:710.

73. Himes HW, Adlersberg D. Pathologic changes in the small bowel in idiopathic sprue: biopsy and autopsy findings. *Gastroenterology* 1958;**35**:142.

74. Corazza GR, Villanacci V. Coeliac disease. *J Clin Pathol* 2005;**58**:573.

75. Shiner M. Electron microscopy of jejunal mucosa in coeliac disease. *Clin Gastroenterol* 1974;**3**:33.

76. Shiner M. Ultrastructural changes suggestive of immune reactions in the jejunal mucosa of coeliac children following gluten challenge. *Gut* 1973;**14**:1.

77. Rostami K, Villanacci V. Microscopic enteritis: novel prospect in coeliac disease clinical and immuno-histogenesis. Evolution in diagnostic and treatment strategies. *Dig Liver Dis* 2009;**41**:245.

78. O'Grady JG, Stevens EM, Keane R, et al. Intestinal lactase, sucrase, and alkaline phosphatase in 373 patients with coeliac disease. *J Clin Pathol* 1984;**37**:298.

79. Prasad KK, Thapa BR, Nain CK, Sharma AK, Singh K. Brush border enzyme activities in relation to histological lesion in pediatric celiac disease. *J Gastroenterol Hepatol* 2008;**23**:e348.

80. Duncan A, Park RP, Lee FD, Russell RI. A retrospective assessment of the clinical value of jejunal disaccharidase analysis. *Scand J Gastroenterol* 1994;**29**:1111.

81. Murray IA, Smith JA, Coupland K, Ansell ID, Long RG. Intestinal disaccharidase deficiency without villous atrophy may represent early celiac disease. *Scand J Gastroenterol* 2001;**36**:163.

82. Ryan BM, Kelleher D. Refractory celiac disease. *Gastroenterology* 2000;**119**:243.

83. Iltanen S, Holm K, Ashorn M, Ruuska T, Laippala P, Mäki M. Changing jejunal gamma delta T cell receptor (TCR)-bearing intra-epithelial lymphocyte density in coeliac disease. *Clin Exp Immunol* 1999;**117**:51.

84. Verkasalo MA, Arató A, Savilahti E, Tainio VM. Effect of diet and age on jejunal and circulating lymphocyte subsets in children with coeliac disease: persistence of CD4–8-intra-epithelial T cells through treatment. *Gut* 1990;**31**:422.

85. Kakar S, Nehra V, Murray JA, Dayharsh GA, Burgart LJ. Significance of intra-epithelial lymphocytosis in small bowel biopsy samples with normal mucosal architecture. *Am J Gastroenterol* 2003;**98**:2027.

86. Mahadeva S, Wyatt JI, Howdle PD. Is a raised intra-epithelial lymphocyte count with normal duodenal villus architecture clinically relevant? *J Clin Pathol* 2002;**55**:424.

87. Wahab PJ, Crusius JB, Meijer JW, Mulder CJ. Gluten challenge in borderline gluten sensitive enteropathy. *Am J Gastroenterol* 2001;**96**:1464.

88. van de Voort JL, Murray JA, Lahr BD, et al. Lymphocytic duodenosis and the spectrum of celiac disease. *Am J Gastroenterol* 2009;**104**:142.

89. Robert ME Gluten sensitive enteropathy and other causes of small intestinal lymphocytosis. *Semin Diagn Pathol* 2005; **22**:284.

90. Brown I, Mino-Kenudson M, Deshpande V, Lauwers GY. Intra-epithelial lymphocytosis in architecturally preserved proximal small intestinal mucosa: an increasing diagnostic problem with a wide differential diagnosis. *Arch Pathol Lab Med* 2006;**130**:1020.

91. Chang F, Mahadeva U, Deere H. Pathological and clinical significance of increased intra-epithelial lymphocytes (IELs) in small bowel mucosa. *APMIS* 2005;**113**:385.

92. Goldstein NS. Non-gluten sensitivity-related small bowel villous flattening with increased intra-epithelial lymphocytes: not all that flattens is celiac sprue. *Am J Clin Pathol* 2004;**121**:546.

93. Ferguson A, Arranz E, O'Mahony S. Clinical and pathological spectrum of coeliac disease – active, silent, latent, potential. *Gut* 1993;**34**:150.

94. Ho-Yen C, Chang F, van der Walt J, Mitchell T, Ciclitira P. Recent advances in refractory coeliac disease: a review. *Histopathology* 2009;**54**:783.

95. Daum S, Cellier C, Mulder CJ. Refractory coeliac disease. *Best Pract Res Clin Gastroenterol* 2005;**19**:413.

96. Al-Toma A, Verbeek WH, Mulder CJ. Update on the management of refractory coeliac disease. *J Gastrointestin Liver Dis* 2007; **16**:57.

97. Freeman HJ. Refractory celiac disease and sprue-like intestinal disease. *World J Gastroenterol* 2008;**14**:828.

98. Robert ME, Ament ME, Weinstein WM. The histologic spectrum and clinical outcome of refractory and unclassified sprue. *Am J Surg Pathol* 2000;**24**:676.

99. Howat AJ, McPhie JL, Smith DA, et al. Cavitation of mesenteric lymph nodes: a rare complication of coeliac disease, associated with a poor outcome. *Histopathology* 1995;**27**:349.

100. Verbeek WH, Goerres MS, von Blomberg BM, et al. Flow cytometric determination of aberrant intra-epithelial lymphocytes predicts T-cell lymphoma development more accurately than T-cell clonality analysis in refractory celiac disease. *Clin Immunol* 2008;**126**:48.

101. Patey-Mariaud De Serre N, Cellier C, et al. Distinction between coeliac disease and refractory sprue: a simple immunohistochemical method. *Histopathology* 2000;**37**:70.

102. Verkarre V, Asnafi V, Lecomte T, et al. Refractory coeliac sprue is a diffuse gastrointestinal disease. *Gut* 2003;**52**:205.

103. Shuster S, Watson A, Marks J. Coeliac syndrome in dermatitis herpetiformis. *Lancet* 1968;**i**:1101.

104. Weinstein WM, Brow JR, Parker F, Rubin CF. The small intestinal mucosa in dermatitis herpetiformis. II. Relationship of the small intestinal lesion to gluten. *Gastroenterology* 1971;**60**:362.

105. Brow JR, Parker F, Weinstein WM, Rubin CE. The small intestinal mucosa in dermatitis herpetiformis. I. Severity and distribution of the small intestinal lesion and associated malabsorption. *Gastroenterology* 1971;**60**:335.

106. Fry L, Seals PP, Harper PG, Hoffbrand AV, McMinn RMH. The small intestine in dermatitis herpetiformis. *J Clin Pathol* 1974;**27**:817.

107. Fry L. Dermatitis herpetiformis. *Baillière's Clin Gastroenterol* 1995;**9**:371.

108. Marks J, Birkell D, Shuster S, Roberts DF. Small intestinal mucosal abnormalities in relatives of patients with dermatitis herpetiformis. *Gut* 1970;**11**:493.

109. Reunala T. Dermatitis herpetiformis: coeliac disease of the skin. *Ann Med* 1998;**30**:416.

110. Alonso-Llamazares J, Gibson LE, Rogers RS 3rd. Clinical, pathologic, and immunopathologic features of dermatitis herpetiformis: review of the Mayo Clinic experience. *Int J Dermatol* 2007;**46**:910.

111. Dieterich W, Laag E, Bruckner-Tuderman L, et al. Antibodies to tissue transglutaminase as serologic markers in patients with dermatitis herpetiformis. *J Invest Dermatol* 1999;**113**:133.

112. Reunala T, Chorzelski TP, Viander M, et al. IgA anti-endomysial antibodies in dermatitis herpetiformis: correlation with jejunal morphology, gluten-free diet and anti-gliadin antibodies. *Br J Dermatol* 1987;**117**:185.

113. Ferguson A. Coeliac disease research and clinical practice: maintaining momentum into the twenty-first century. *Baillière's Clin Gastroenterol* 1995;**9**:395.

114. Weinstein WM. Latent coeliac sprue. *Gastroenterology* 1974; **66**:489.

115. Vecchi M, Crosti L, Berti E, Agape D, Cerri A, De Franchis R. Increased jejunal intra-epithelial lymphocytes bearing gamma/delta T-cell receptor in dermatitis herpetiformis. *Gastroenterology* 1992;**102**:1499.

116. Otley CC, Hall RP 3rd. The pathogenesis of dermatitis herpetiformis. *Clin Dermatol* 1991;**9**:313.

117. Rose C, Armbruster FP, Ruppert J, Igl BW, Zillikens D, Shimanovich I. Autoantibodies against epidermal transglutaminase are a sensitive diagnostic marker in patients with dermatitis herpetiformis on a normal or gluten-free diet. *J Am Acad Dermatol* 2009;**61**:39.

118. Hull CM, Liddle M, Hansen N, et al. Elevation of IgA anti-epidermal transglutaminase antibodies in dermatitis herpetiformis. *Br J Dermatol* 2008;**159**:120.

119. Marietta EV, Camilleri MJ, Castro LA, Krause PK, Pittelkow MR, Murray JA. Transglutaminase autoantibodies in dermatitis herpetiformis and celiac sprue. *J Invest Dermatol* 2008;**128**:332.

120. Gillberg R, Kastnup W, Mobacken H, Stockbrugger R, Ahren C. Endoscopic duodenal biopsy compared with biopsy with the Watson capsule from the upper jejunum in patients with dermatitis herpetiformis. *Scand J Gastroenterol* 1982;**17**:305.

121. Cooney T, Doyle CT, Buckley D, Whelton MJ. Dermatitis herpetiformis: a comparative assessment of skin and bowel abnormality. *J Clin Pathol* 1977;**30**:749.

122. Maguire AA, Greenson JK, Lauwers GY, et al. Collagenous sprue: A clinicopathologic study of 12 cases. *Am J Surg Pathol* 2009;**33**:1440.

123. Cellier C, Delabesse E, Helmer C, et al., French Coeliac Disease Study Group. Refractory sprue, coeliac disease, and enteropathy-associated T-cell lymphoma. *Lancet* 2000;**356**:203.

124. Feeley KM, Heneghan MA, Stevens FM, McCarthy CF. Lymphocytic gastritis and coeliac disease: evidence of a positive association. *J Clin Pathol* 1998;**51**:207.

125. Wolber R, Owen D, DelBuono L, Appelman H, Freeman H. Lymphocytic gastritis in patients with celiac sprue or sprue-like intestinal disease. *Gastroenterology* 1990;**98**:310.

126. De Giacomo C, Gianatti A, Negrini R, et al. Lymphocytic gastritis: a positive relationship with celiac disease. *J Pediatr* 1994;**124**:57.

127. Hayat M, Arora DS, Wyatt JI, O'Mahony S, Dixon MF. The pattern of involvement of the gastric mucosa in lymphocytic gastritis is predictive of the presence of duodenal pathology *J Clin Pathol* 1999;**52**:815.

128. Alsaigh N, Odze R, Goldman H, Antonioli D, Ott MJ, Leichtner A. Gastric and esophageal intra-epithelial lymphocytes in pediatric celiac disease. *Am J Surg Pathol* 1996;**20**:865.

129. Olesen M, Eriksson S, Bohr J, Järnerot G, Tysk C. Lymphocytic colitis: a retrospective clinical study of 199 Swedish patients. *Gut* 2004;**53**:536.

130. Matteoni CA, Goldblum JR, Wang N, Brzezinski A, Achkar E, Soffer EE. Celiac disease is highly prevalent in lymphocytic colitis. *J Clin Gastroenterol* 2001;**32**:225.

131. Baert F, Wouters K, D'Haens G, et al. Lymphocytic colitis: a distinct clinical entity? A clinicopathological confrontation of lymphocytic and collagenous colitis. *Gut* 1999;**45**:375.

132. Wang N, Dumot JA, Achkar E, Easley KA, Petras RE, Goldblum JR. Colonic epithelial lymphocytosis without a thickened subepithelial collagen table: a clinicopathologic study of 40 cases supporting a heterogeneous entity. *Am J Surg Pathol* 1999;**23**:1068.

133. Treanor D, Sheahan K. Microscopic colitis: lymphocytic and collagenous colitis. *Curr Diagn Pathol* 2002;**8**:33.

134. Koskela RM, Niemelä SE, Karttunen TJ, Lehtola JK. Clinical characteristics of collagenous and lymphocytic colitis. *Scand J Gastroenterol* 2004;**39**:837.

135. Wolber R, Owen D, Freeman H. Colonic lymphocytosis in patients with celiac sprue. *Hum Pathol* 1990;**21**:1092.

136. Dickey W, Hughes DF. Histology of the terminal ileum in coeliac disease. *Scand J Gastroenterol* 2004;**39**:665.

137. Hopper AD, Hurlstone DP, Leeds JS, et al. The occurrence of terminal ileal histological abnormalities in patients with coeliac disease. *Dig Liver Dis* 2006;**38**:815.

138. Rubio CA, Sjödahl K, Lagergren J. Lymphocytic esophagitis: a histologic subset of chronic esophagitis. *Am J Clin Pathol* 2006;**125**:432.

139. Freeman HJ. Collagenous colitis as the presenting feature of biopsy-defined celiac disease. *J Clin Gastroenterol* 2004;**38**:664.

140. Leung ST, Chandan VS, Murray JA, Wu TT. Collagenous gastritis: histopathologic features and association with other gastrointestinal diseases. *Am J Surg Pathol* 2009;**33**:788.

141. Howdle PD, Jalal PK, Holmes GK, Houlston RS. Primary small-bowel malignancy in the UK and its association with coeliac disease. *Q J Med* 2003;**96**:345.

142. Potter DD, Murray JA, Donohue JH, et al. The role of defective mismatch repair in small bowel adenocarcinoma in celiac disease. *Cancer Res* 2004;**64**:7073.

143. Freeman HJ. Malignancy in adult celiac disease. *World J Gastroenterol* 2009;**15**:1581.

144. Kokkonen J, Holm K, Karttunen TJ, Mäki M. Children with untreated food allergy express a relative increment in the density of duodenal gammadelta+ T cells. *Scand J Gastroenterol* 2000;**35**:1137.

145. Walker-Smith JA. Gastrointestinal food allergy in childhood. *Ann Allergy* 1987;**59**:166.

146. Ament ME, Rubin CE. Soy protein – another cause of the flat intestinal lesion. *Gastroenterology* 1972;**62**:227.

147. Vitoria JC, Camerero C, Sojo, A, Ruiz, A, Roderiguez-Soriano J. Enteropathy related to fish, rice, and chicken. *Arch Dis Child* 1982;**57**:44.

148. Sahi T. Progress report: dietary lactose and the aetiology of human small intestinal hypolactasia. *Gut* 1978;**19**:1074.

149. Hyams JS, Batrus CL, Grand RJ, Sallan SE. Cancer chemotherapy-induced lactose malabsorption in children. *Cancer* 1982;**49**:646.

150. Lomer MC, Parkes GC, Sanderson JD. Review article: lactose intolerance in clinical practice – myths and realities. *Aliment Pharmacol Ther* 2008;**27**:93.

151. Montalto M, Curigliano V, Santoro L, et al. Management and treatment of lactose malabsorption. *World J Gastroenterol* 2006;**12**:187.

152. Maiuri L, Rossi M, Raia V, et al. Surface staining on the villus of lactase protein and lactase activity in adult-type hypolactasia. *Gastroenterology* 1993;**105**:708.

153. Zamel R, Khan R, Pollex RL, Hegele RA. Abetalipoproteinemia: two case reports and literature review. *Orphanet J Rare Dis* 2008;**3**:19.

154. Anonymous. Case records of the Massachusetts General Hospital. Weekly clinicopathological exercises. Case 35–1992. An eight-month-old boy with diarrhea and failure to thrive. *N Engl J Med* 1992;**327**:628.

155. Greenwood N. The jejunal mucosa in two cases of a-beta-lipoproteinemia. *Am J Gastroenterol* 1976;**65**:160.

156. Variend S, Placzec M, Raafat F, Walker-Smith JA. Small intestinal mucosal fat in childhood enteropathies. *J Clin Pathol* 1984;**37**:373.

157. Joshi M, Hyams J, Treem W, Ricci A Jr. Cytoplasmic vacuolization of enterocytes: an unusual histopathologic finding in juvenile nutritional megaloblastic anemia. *Mod Pathol* 1991;**4**:62.

158. Isaacs PE, Sladen GE, Filipe I. Mefenamic acid enteropathy. *J Clin Pathol* 1987;**40**:1221.

159. Scott BB, Miller JP, Losowsky MS. Hypobetalipoproteinaemia – a variant of the Bassen–Kornzweig syndrome. *Gut* 1979;**20**:163.

160. Bouma ME, Beucler I, Aggerbeck LP, et al. Hypobetalipoproteinemia with accumulation of an apoprotein B-like protein in intestinal cells. Immunoenzymatic and biochemical characterization of seven cases of Anderson's disease. *J Clin Invest* 1986;**78**:398.

161. Walker-Smith JA, Unsworth DJ, Hutchins P, et al. Autoantibodies against gut epithelium in child with small-intestinal enteropathy. *Lancet* 1982;**i**:566.

162. Freeman HJ. Adult auto-immune enteropathy. *World J Gastroenterol* 2008;**14**:1156.

163. Akram S, Murray JA, Pardi DS, et al. Adult auto-immune enteropathy: Mayo Clinic Rochester experience. *Clin Gastroenterol Hepatol* 2007;**5**:1282.

164. Montalto M, D'Onofrio F, Santoro L, et al. Auto-immune enteropathy in children and adults. *Scand J Gastroenterol* 2009;**44**:1029.

165. Patey-Mariaud de Serre N, Canioni D, Ganousse S, et al. Digestive histopathological presentation of IPEX syndrome. *Mod Pathol* 2009;**22**:95.

166. Folwaczny C, Noehl N, Tschöp K, et al. Goblet cell autoantibodies in patients with inflammatory bowel disease and their first-degree relatives. *Gastroenterology* 1997;**113**:101.

167. Hori K, Fukuda Y, Tomita T, et al. Intestinal goblet cell autoantibody associated enteropathy. *J Clin Pathol* 2003;**56**:629.

168. Martín-Villa JM, Camblor S, Costa R, Arnaiz-Villena A. Gut epithelial cell autoantibodies in AIDS pathogenesis. *Lancet* 1993;**342**:380.

169. Haghighi P, Wolf PL. Tropical sprue and subclinical enteropathy: a vision for the nineties. *Crit Rev Clin Lab Sci* 1997;**34**:313.

170. Klipstein FA. Tropical sprue in travellers and ex-patriates living abroad. *Gastroenterology* 1981;**80**:590.

171. Cook GC. Aetiology and pathogenesis of postinfective tropical malabsorption (tropical sprue). *Lancet* 1984;**i**:721.

172. Walker MM. What is tropical sprue? *J Gastroenterol Hepatol* 2003;**18**:887.

173. Ghoshal UC, Ghoshal U, Ayyagari A, et al. Tropical sprue is associated with contamination of small bowel with aerobic

bacteria and reversible prolongation of orocecal transit time. *J Gastroenterol Hepatol* 2003;**18**;540.

174. Cook GC. 'Tropical sprue': some early investigators favoured an infective cause, but was a coccidian protozoan involved? *Gut* 1996;**39**;428.

175. Wheby MS, Swanson VL, Bayless TM. Comparison of the ileal and jejunal biopsies in tropical sprue. *Am J Clin Nutr* 1971;**24**;117.

176. Ross IM, Mathan VI. Immunological changes in tropical sprue. *Q J Med* 1981;**50**;435.

177. Schenk EA, Samloff IM, Klipstein FA. Morphologic characteristics of jejunal biopsies in celiac disease and in tropical sprue. *Am J Pathol* 1965;**47**;765.

178. Brunser O, Eidelman S, Klipstein FA. Intestinal morphology of rural Haitians: a comparison between overt tropical sprue and asymptomatic subjects. *Gastroenterology* 1970;**58**;655.

179. Mongomery RD, Shearer ACI. The cell population of the upper jejunal mucosa in tropical sprue and post infective malabsorption. *Gut* 1974;**15**;387.

180. Misra RC, Kasthuri P, Chuttanni HK. Adult coeliac disease in tropics. *BMJ* 1966;**ii**;1230.

181. Banwell JG, Kistler LA, Gianella RA, et al. Small intestinal bacterial overgrowth syndrome. *Gastroenterology* 1981;**80**;834.

182. Isaacs PFT, Kim YS. Blind loop syndrome and small bowel bacterial contamination. *Clin Gastroenterol* 1983;**12**;395.

183. Mitsui T, Shimaoka K, Goto Y, et al. Small bowel bacterial overgrowth is not seen in healthy adults but is in disabled older adults. *Hepatogastroenterology* 2006;**53**;82.

184. Teo M, Chung S, Chitti L, et al. Small bowel bacterial overgrowth is a common cause of chronic diarrhea. *J Gastroenterol Hepatol* 2004;**19**;904.

185. Elphick HL, Elphick DA, Sanders DS. Small bowel bacterial overgrowth. An underrecognized cause of malnutrition in older adults. *Geriatrics* 2006;**61**(9);21.

186. Stotzer PO, Kilander AF. Comparison of the 1-gram (14)C-D-xylose breath test and the 50-gram hydrogen glucose breath test for diagnosis of small intestinal bacterial overgrowth. *Digestion* 2000;**61**;165.

187. Ament ME, Shimoda SS, Saunders DP, Rubin CE. Pathogenesis of steatorrhea in three cases of small intestinal stasis syndrome. *Gastroenterology* 1972;**63**;728.

188. Haboubi NY, Lee GS, Montgomery RD. Duodenal mucosal morphometry of elderly patients with small intestinal bacterial overgrowth: response to antibiotic treatment. *Age Ageing* 1991;**20**;29.

189. Riordan SM, McIver CJ, Wakefield D, et al. Small intestinal mucosal immunity and morphometry in luminal overgrowth of indigenous gut flora. *Am J Gastroenterol* 2001;**96**;494.

190. Cutz E, Sherman PM, Davidson GP Enteropathies associated with protracted diarrhea of infancy: clinicopathological features, cellular and molecular mechanisms. *Pediatr Pathol Lab Med* 1997;**17**;335.

191. Cutz E, Rhoads JM, Drumm B, et al. Micro inclusion disease: an inherited defect of brush border assembly and differentiation. *N Engl J Med* 1989;**320**;646.

192. Bell SW, Kerner JA Jr, Sibley RK. Microvillous inclusion disease. The importance of electron microscopy for diagnosis. *Am J Surg Pathol* 1991;**15**;1157.

193. Groisman G, Ben-Izhak O, Schwersenz A, et al. The value of polyclonal carcinoembryonic antigen immunostaining in the diagnosis of micro inclusion disease. *Hum Pathol* 1993;**24**;1232.

194. Groisman GM, Amar M, Livne E. CD10: a valuable tool for the light microscopic diagnosis of microvillous inclusion disease (familial microvillous atrophy). *Am J Surg Pathol* 2002;**26**;902.

195. Goulet O, Salomon J, Ruemmele F, et al. Intestinal epithelial dysplasia (tufting enteropathy). *Orphanet J Rare Dis* 2007;**2**;20.

196. Goulet OJ, Brousse N, Canioni D, et al. Syndrome of intractable diarrhoea with persistent villous atrophy in early childhood: a clinicopathological survey of 47 cases. *J Pediatr Gastroenterol Nutr* 1998;**26**;151.

197. Sivagnanam M, Mueller JL, Lee H, et al. Identification of EpCAM as the gene for congenital tufting enteropathy. *Gastroenterology* 2008;**135**;429.

198. Schmitt S, Küry S, Giraud M, et al. An update on mutations of the SLC39A4 gene in acrodermatitis enteropathica. *Hum Mutat* 2009;**30**;926.

199. Kuitunen P, Kosnai I, Savilahti E. Morphometric study of the jejunal mucosa in various childhood enteropathies with special reference to intra-epithelial lymphocytes. *J Pediatr Gastroenterol Nutr* 1982;**1**;525.

200. Bohane TD, Cutz E, Hamilton JR, Gall DG. Acrodermatitis enteropathica, zinc, and the Paneth cell. A case report with family studies. *Gastroenterology* 1977;**73**;587.

201. Kobayashi Y, Suzuki H, Konno T, et al. Ultrastructural alterations of Paneth cells in infants associated with gastrointestinal symptoms. *Tohoku J Exp Med* 1983;**139**;225.

202. Waldmann TA, Steinfeld JL, Dutcher TF, et al. The role of the gastrointestinal system in 'idiopathic hypoproteinemia. *Gastroenterology* 1961;**41**;197.

203. Waldmann TA. Protein-losing enteropathy. *Gastroenterology* 1966;**50**;422.

204. Abramowsky C, Hupertz V, Kilbridge P, et al. Intestinal lymphangiectasia in children: a study of upper gastrointestinal endoscopic biopsies. *Pediatr Pathol* 1989;**9**;289.

205. Aoyagi K, Iida M, Yao T, et al. Characteristic endoscopic features of intestinal lymphangiectasia: correlation with histological findings. *Hepatogastroenterology* 1997;**44**;133.

206. Riemann JF, Schmidt H. Synopsis of endoscopic and other morphological findings in intestinal lymphangiectasia. *Endoscopy* 1981;**13**;60.

207. Longstreth GF, Newcomer AD. Drug-induced malabsorption. *Mayo Clin Proc* 1975;**50**;284.

208. Green PH, Tall AR. Drugs, alcohol and malabsorption. *Am J Med* 1979;**67**;1066.

209. Chassany O, Michaux A, Bergmann JF. Drug-induced diarrhoea. *Drug Saf* 2000;**22**;53.

210. Boscá MM, Añón R, Mayordomo E, et al. Methotrexate induced sprue-like syndrome. *World J Gastroenterol* 2008;**14**;7009.

211. Green PH. Alcohol, nutrition and malabsorption. *Clin Gastroenterol* 1983;**12**;563.

212. Bode JC, Bode C, Heidelbach R, et al. Jejunal microflora in patients with chronic alcohol abuse. *Hepatogastroenterology* 1984;**31**;30.

213. Bjorkman DJ, Jessop LD. Effects of acute and chronic ethanol exposure on intestinal microvillus membrane lipid composition and fluidity. *Alcohol Clin Exp Res* 1994;**18**;560.

214. Connor F. Gastrointestinal complications of fundoplication. *Curr Gastroenterol Rep* 2005;**7**;219.

215. Meyer JH. Nutritional outcomes of gastric operations. *Gastroenterol Clin North Am* 1994;**23**;227.

216. Hirschowitz BI, Worthington J, Mohnen J. Vitamin B_{12} deficiency in hypersecretors during long-term acid suppression with proton pump inhibitors. *Aliment Pharmacol Ther* 2008;**27**;1110.

217. Mansbach CM II, Wilkins RM, Dobbins WO, Tyor MP. Intestinal mucosal function and structure in the steatorrhoea of Zollinger–Ellison syndrome. *Arch Intern Med* 1968;**121**;487.

218. Hensley GT, Soergel KH. Neuropathologic findings in diabetic diarrhoea. *Arch Pathol* 1968;**85**;587.

219. Barker JM. Clinical review: Type 1 diabetes-associated autoimmunity: natural history, genetic associations, and screening. *J Clin Endocrinol Metab* 2006;**91**:1210.

220. Montalto M, Santoro L, D'Onofrio F, et al. Classification of malabsorption syndromes. *Dig Dis* 2008;**26**:104.

221. Da Costa LR, Croft DN, Creamer B. Protein loss and cell loss from the small intestinal mucosa. *Gut* 1971;**12**:179.

222. Lin P, Medeiros LJ. Lymphoplasmacytic lymphoma/Waldenstrom macroglobulinemia: an evolving concept. *Adv Anat Pathol* 2005;**12**:246.

223. Brandt LJ, Davidoff A, Bernstein LH, et al. Small-intestine involvement in Waldenstrom's macroglobulinemia. Case report and review of the literature. *Dig Dis Sci* 1981;**26**:174.

224. Pratz KW, Dingli D, Smyrk TC, Lust JA. Intestinal lymphangiectasia with protein-losing enteropathy in Waldenstrom macroglobulinemia. *Medicine (Baltimore)* 2007;**86**:210.

225. Foster CS. The brown bowel syndrome: a possible smooth muscle mitochondrial myopathy. *Histopathology* 1979;**3**:1.

226. Horn T, Svendsen LB, Nielsen R. Brown-bowel syndrome. Review of the literature and presentation of cases. *Scand J Gastroenterol* 1990;**25**:66.

227. Popovic OS, Milumalavic VB, Milutinovic-Djuric S, et al. Primary bile acid malabsorption. *Gastroenterology* 1987;**92**:1851.

CHAPTER 22

Vascular disorders of the small intestine

Amy E. Noffsinger

Miraca Life Sciences, Camp Dennison, OH, USA

Vascular anatomy of the small intestine

Except for the first part of the duodenum, which is supplied through the coeliac axis, the whole small intestine receives its blood supply from the superior mesenteric artery. This vessel runs along a curved course through the mesentery and branches, the intestinal arteries, arise from its convex aspect, joining together to form arcades. From these arcades, short straight branches, which do not anastomose to a significant extent, supply the jejunum and most of the ileum. Each branch ramifies in the serosa and passes through the muscularis propria to the submucosa; arterioles arise from them to supply the villi. There are free anastomoses between branches from the coeliac and inferior mesenteric arteries around the duodenum, head of the pancreas and the splenic flexure, respectively [1].

Arising from the proximal concave aspect of the superior mesenteric artery is the inferior pancreatico-duodenal artery, and then the middle colic, right colic and ileo-colic arteries distally. The ileo-colic artery supplies the caecum, ascending colon and terminal ileum. It follows from this that occlusion of the superior mesenteric artery at its origin is likely to cause widespread infarction, occlusion of a major branch may be silent or produce infarction according to the state of the collateral circulation in the arcades, and occlusion of a short straight branch is likely to produce local infarction of the whole or part of a segment of bowel.

The venous drainage of the entire small bowel is through the portal system via the superior mesenteric vein. Some portosystemic anastomoses are present around the lower end of the oesophagus, the umbilicus and the anorectal region. Venous obstruction is just as capable of producing infarction as arterial obstruction, but the resultant infarcts develop more slowly and are always haemorrhagic.

Vascular physiology of the small intestine

Approximately 10–15% of cardiac output goes to the small intestine and 5–10% to the large intestine [2]. The measurement of intestinal blood flow is important because up to 50% of all cases of intestinal ischaemia may be the result of reduced flow [3,4]. The splanchnic blood flow at the origin of the main mesenteric vessel does not vary much with alterations of blood pressure within the normal physiological range but, at extremely low pressures, there is a rapid drop in the amount of blood supplied to the gut.

About a fifth of the total cardiac output normally goes to the splanchnic areas. If this has to be redistributed (as, for example, in shock), the splanchnic area contributes significantly because the flow through it can be decreased markedly by vasoconstriction of peripheral vessels, which are very sensitive to pressor amines. If hypotension from any cause produces a marked drop in arterial pressure, particularly across a partial occlusion of a main stem of a mesenteric artery, it is possible for the perfusion pressure to drop below the critical closing pressure of the mesenteric vessels, even if there are no measurable changes in blood flow. This can result in functional closure of arterioles with deprivation of the blood supply to the gut, particularly the mucosa.

Morson and Dawson's Gastrointestinal Pathology, Fifth Edition. Edited by Neil A. Shepherd, Bryan F. Warren, Geraint T. Williams, Joel K. Greenson, Gregory Y. Lauwers and Marco R. Novelli.
© 2013 Blackwell Publishing Ltd. Published 2013 by Blackwell Publishing Ltd.

Of greater importance than the total amount of blood reaching the alimentary tract is the distribution of blood throughout the different layers of the bowel wall. Experimental clearance studies in cats have shown that 75–85% of the blood goes to the mucosa and submucosa, with about 20% of total flow passing through the villi. An increasing proportion of the total flow passes to the villi during arterial hypotension and, under these circumstances, the mean transit time is considerably prolonged [5]. The close association of afferent and efferent vessels running in different directions in the small intestinal villus has led to the proposition that a counter-current exchange mechanism operates [2]. If so, this would play a crucial role in digestive metabolism. In ischaemia, increased shunting of oxygen across the base of the villus, in situations where the transit time is prolonged, would result in necrosis, particularly at the tips of the villi.

The mesenteric circulation is under the control of the autonomic nervous system, and profoundly influenced by the general state of the circulation and the presence of vasoactive agents, such as histamine, 5-hydroxytryptamine (serotonin) and noradrenaline [2]. Disturbances in the normal control of the splanchnic circulation can be used to explain the pathogenesis of some cases of intestinal ischaemia in which no organic vascular block is demonstrated. A finely balanced system of mediators of smooth muscle tone is involved, the final common pathway being nitric oxide, which has a profoundly relaxing effect on both the bowel wall and the vasculature. Injurious stimuli, such as endotoxic shock, result in production of tumour necrosis factor α (TNF-α) which down-regulates nitric oxide synthase (NOS) in vascular endothelial cells, effectively increasing arterial tone and producing inappropriate tissue hypoxia in the small bowel and its mucosa [6]. Direct damage to endothelial cells due, for example, to ischaemia itself, has a similar effect and no doubt explains many of the circumstances in which disproportionate ischaemic damage may occur in the small bowel, with or without overt vascular occlusion.

Pathogenesis of vascular disorders of the small intestine

The essential factor in all forms of intestinal ischaemia is that the affected segment of gut receives less blood than is required to maintain its proper structure and function. The two main causative factors are vascular occlusion and hypotension, which together can result in disturbances in the control of the mesenteric circulation. It is appropriate to mention in this context that tissues have needs other than oxygen, such as proteins, carbohydrates, lipid, water, electrolytes and vitamins. The capacity of cells to obtain these nutrients and to extract oxygen from the blood is intimately associated with their membrane structure and internal metabolism. Ischaemia and inflammation profoundly affect these structures and their function. The mucosal defences weakened by any ischaemic insult will be more susceptible to bacterial invasion, a particular problem in the colon.

The causes of ischaemia (Table 22.1) can be divided into those that are extrinsic to the bowel and those that are intrinsic. Within this division is the important distinction between an occlusive and a non-occlusive aetiology [7].

Table 22.1 Causes of ischaemic bowel disease

Arterial occlusion
Atherosclerosis
Thrombosis
Embolism
Mesenteric vascular compression, e.g. tumours, aneurysm, haematoma
Takayasu's disease
Iatrogenic causes, e.g. ligation at reconstructive vascular surgery, angiography

Venous occlusion
Mesenteric thrombosis
Portal thrombosis, e.g. cirrhosis
Pyothrombosis, e.g. appendicitis
Mesenteric vascular compression (as for arterial occlusion)
Hypercoagulable states, e.g. polycythaemia rubra vera
Oral contraceptives

Increased luminal pressure due to intestinal obstruction
Carcinoma
Faecal impaction
Hirschsprung's disease
Diverticular disease

Low-flow states
Septic shock
Cardiogenic
Haemorrhage
Dehydration
Drugs – functional: vasospasm with hypotension, e.g. ergotamine, digitalis

Small vessel disease
Vasculitis:
   Rheumatoid arthritis
   Systemic lupus erythematosus
   Polyarteritis nodosa
   Progressive systemic sclerosis
   Henoch–Schönlein purpura
   Thrombo-angiitis obliterans (Buerger's disease)
Post irradiation
Ehlers–Danlos syndrome
Kohlmeier–Degos syndrome
Disseminated intravascular coagulation

Non-occlusive or 'low-flow' states operate both at extrinsic and intrinsic levels. It is the balance between the two mechanisms, vessel wall disease versus flow, that determines the clinical presentation and pathology [7,8], e.g. there are patients with two of the three major mesenteric vessels narrowed by over 50% at their origins yet who are without symptoms and signs of ischaemia [9].

Whatever the mechanism that ultimately reduces the mucosal blood flow, the net result is tissue hypoxia and damage. Many variables influence the severity of the insult and the length of time that it acts. For example canine gut can revert to normal after up to 6 hours of severe ischaemia [10]. However, reversal of the ischaemia is unsafe after a more prolonged period, with ensuing haemorrhage and absorption of toxic metabolites [8]. The vascular endothelium becomes damaged, probably more through the local activation of complement than through the effect of oxygen free radicals [11]. This is the condition of 're-perfusion injury' and it explains the high mortality of mesenteric embolectomy in clinical practice. There is, therefore, a complex interaction of events already in motion at the time that the patient clinically presents with ischaemia.

Occlusive ischaemia

Arterial occlusion

About half of all cases of intestinal ischaemia have an associated vascular occlusion, usually due to atheroma [12], thrombus or embolus, although occasionally blockage can be the result of an arteritis or other condition. Arterial narrowing by itself must be extremely severe before symptoms or pathological changes develop [9] and reduction of the blood flow also plays a part in most cases. Careful necropsy studies show that atheromatous lesions are most common and severe in the proximal 20 mm of the superior and inferior mesenteric arteries, leaving the most distal vessels relatively uninvolved [9]. Such narrowing is more common in men than in women, and is usually associated with severe aortic and coronary atherosclerosis, and, often, diabetes mellitus [13].

Attempts to measure the cross-sectional area of the superior mesenteric artery in unselected cases show a remarkable variation in the degree of luminal narrowing from patient to patient [9,14]. Aortography in life and the injection of radio-opaque material into the main arteries at necropsy [15] confirm that narrowing is most common at the ostia and first centimetre of the superior mesenteric artery [16]. These studies suggest that ischaemic symptoms do not occur while two-thirds of the cross-sectional area remain patent and are unlikely until patency is reduced by 50–80% [15,17,18]. Below this, symptoms are to be expected but cross-sectional area always has to be balanced against blood pressure and other extraneous factors. Infarction as opposed to anginal symptoms need not necessarily occur, even when the main stem of the superior mesenteric artery is occluded [19].

Complete occlusion of an artery is usually the result of intravascular thrombosis, embolism or haemorrhage beneath an atheromatous plaque. In the main trunk of the superior mesenteric artery or its major branches, thrombosis, on the basis of pre-existing atheroma, is the most common lesion, particularly in men [12], although in some patients thrombosis follows operation or trauma without significant preceding arterial disease. In smaller arterial branches, where atheroma is less common, thrombosis is rarer but may occur in elderly patients. Thrombosis accounts for about 25% of cases of acute ischaemia [20].

An embolus can effectively block the superior mesenteric artery or its branches, whether or not there is pre-existing arterial disease. Emboli account for 20–33% of cases of acute intestinal ischaemia [12,20]. Common preceding conditions are atrial fibrillation with thrombus formation in the left atrium or myocardial infarction with mural thrombus adherent to the infarcted area.

Although atheroma is the most common cause of arterial narrowing of the superior mesenteric artery, there are other causes. In the controversial 'coeliac axis syndrome' there is said to be stenosis, due to an anomalous origin of the coeliac artery, at or above the level of the lower border of the twelfth thoracic vertebra. This is above the diaphragm rather than opposite the first lumbar vertebra below the diaphragm. When this happens, the artery passes beneath the median arcuate ligament and may be constricted by it.

Venous occlusion

Bowel ischaemia secondary to venous occlusion accounts for approximately 5–15% of cases of mesenteric ischaemia [21] and, unless diagnosed promptly, carries a considerable mortality rate of somewhere between 20% and 50% [22,23]. Among the most common causes are external lesions producing pressure, such as the margins of hernia sacs or large abdominal lymph nodes, intra-abdominal trauma, inflammatory conditions including appendicitis, pelvic inflammation and peritonitis, and prothrombotic states due to inherited or acquired disorders of coagulation. The last include side effects of oral contraceptives and inherited defects of prothrombin and protein C. Mesenteric thrombosis in these disorders begins in small veins and progresses into larger vessels. Cirrhosis or a hepatic tumour may initially cause portal vein thrombosis which can then propagate back to the mesenteric veins.

Non-occlusive ischaemia

The arterial pressure at the origin of the superior mesenteric artery is the same as in the aorta, whereas the portal venous pressure is about 10% of this. Thus there is considerable peripheral resistance in the splanchnic bed [2], the vessels of which are sensitive to pressor amines. In any situation causing hypotension or 'low-flow' states, the splanchnic vessels are likely to constrict in an attempt to maintain normal blood pressure. Thus, both the initial hypotension and the subsequent vascular constriction markedly reduce the effective flow to the bowel.

The most common hypotensive disorders that lead to bowel ischaemia are left ventricular failure, aortic insufficiency and shock. In 25–50% [3,20] of all patients with clinical and pathological evidence of bowel ischaemia, no significant organic vascular block is demonstrated, although minor vascular narrowing is often present. The role of shock has been hotly disputed. Experience from young war casualties who lost blood because of wounds produced no convincing evidence that bowel infarction is an important cause of death [24]. There are, however, reports to show that intestinal necrosis can develop after multiple injuries that do not involve the abdomen and in patients with circulatory depletion [3,25]. Most patients in whom shock is associated with bowel infarction are elderly and they are likely to have accompanying mesenteric vessel atherosclerosis. In such circumstances, any major hypotensive episode may precipitate mucosal damage and allow invasion of intestinal bacteria into the injured tissues. Paracrine mediators of damage to endothelial cells, alluded to earlier, contribute to a vicious cycle. It has been shown that reperfusion injury can be alleviated by transforming growth factor β (TGF-β), through its effect in stimulating NOS [26]. Pure shock, in the absence of any background of mesenteric vascular insufficiency, is probably only rarely a cause of non-occlusive ischaemia.

There is some evidence that haemoconcentration [27] and polycythaemia [28] may predispose to ischaemic lesions, presumably by increasing blood viscosity. Acute small intestinal ischaemia is also a recognised complication of open cardiac surgery in elderly people [29]. In these patients, perioperative dehydration, coupled with atheromatous constriction of the origin of the superior mesenteric artery, appear to be important pathogenic factors. The role of digitalis in the production of non-occlusive mesenteric ischaemia is debatable because any local vasoconstrictive effect that the drug might have is probably counter-balanced by the increased cardiac output resulting from treatment of left ventricular failure [30]. Ischaemia can also be associated with widespread micro-thrombi in other organs as part of disseminated intravascular coagulation [31]. Other factors that may play a crucial or contributory role in the development of intestinal ischaemia include small vessel occlusion due to increased intraluminal pressure and the bacterial content of the gut.

Nomenclature of vascular pathology in the small intestine

When the intestine is deprived of blood, histological changes follow that vary with the acuteness and severity of the ischaemia. The considerable variation in the clinical presentation, as well as the pathological findings, are the main explanations for a confusing nomenclature covering a spectrum ranging from acute infarction, through transient subclinical episodes, to the chronic evolution of a fibrotic stricture. The terms 'gangrene', 'haemorrhagic necrosis', 'necrotising enterocolitis', 'pseudo-membranous enterocolitis' and 'ischaemic enterocolitis' have all been used to describe different clinico-pathological manifestations of acute severe ischaemia. Moreover, some cases reported in the past as segmental enteritis or colitis were probably also due to ischaemic disease. Uraemic enterocolitis is an expression that was used to describe a clinical picture that nowadays might be regarded as having an ischaemic basis. The term 'pseudo-membranous colitis' should not be used diagnostically for ischaemic colitis now that the aetiological role of *Clostridium difficile* in its development is understood.

The chronic variety of ischaemia is best known as ischaemic stricture. However, the histopathology of acute ischaemia and of ischaemic stricture merge into each other and the appearances seen in surgical specimens depend on the stage at which the operation is performed, as well as the severity and duration of the ischaemic episode. Between the clinical emergency of acute infarction and a chronic ischaemic stricture there is an ill-defined stage manifest by transient ischaemic episodes. These may be single, subclinical, reversible thrombotic events, perhaps, for example, due to the contraceptive pill, or they may be attacks of recurrent 'intestinal angina' in patients with chronic arterial obstruction [9].

The clinical patterns of mesenteric vascular disease may be classified as follows [32]:
1. Acute splanchnic ischaemia:
    (a) with occlusion (arterial or venous thrombosis, embolism)
    (b) non-occlusive
2. Chronic splanchnic syndrome (chronic mesenteric ischaemia):
    (a) single vessel disease
    (b) multivessel disease
3. Focal ischaemia:
    (a) of the small bowel
    (b) of the colon.

Acute intestinal ischaemia refers to infarction of major lengths of bowel, chronic obstruction to the controversial subclinical pre-infarctive state of 'intestinal angina' and focal ischaemia to the main local causes of ischaemic bowel disease (see Table 22.1).

Histopathology of intestinal ischaemia

Macroscopic appearances

Infarction requires little explanation. The term derives from the Greek word that literally means 'stuffed with blood'. Thus the small intestine is oedematous and plum-coloured (Figure 22.1). The mucosa is necrotic and has a nodular surface appearance due to extensive submucosal haemorrhage but the deep muscle layers may initially appear well preserved. As necrosis becomes more complete, or gangrene develops, all layers of the intestinal wall are affected. The external surface has a mottled purple or greenish hue and the tissues of the bowel are thin and friable. The mucosal surface becomes covered by patches of white or yellow exudate. Bubbles of gas may be present within mesenteric veins [33,34].

In some cases of acute ischaemic enterocolitis, only the mucosa is affected with quite good preservation of the deeper layers of the bowel wall. This is particularly characteristic of the non-occlusive type of intestinal ischaemia and is due to the muscularis propria being relatively more resistant to acute deprivation of blood than the mucosa and submucosa. The bowel may be a normal colour from the outside, although usually dilated, or it may be reddened and show focal areas of violet discoloration where full-thickness necrosis has occurred. The mucosal surface is haemorrhagic with superficial pinpoint ulcers or deeper longitudinal and serpiginous ulceration. In other cases, necrosis of the mucosa gives rise to diffuse ill-defined yellow (Figure 22.2), greenish or tan-coloured plaques which have sloughed into the bowel lumen or can be easily scraped off the underlying viable tissue. Membranous or pseudo-membranous enterocolitis has been used to describe this appearance of ischaemic mucosal necrosis in the past but the term is now applied to the focal raised creamy-yellow plaques that are seen in the colon due to C.

difficile toxin (see 'Pseudo-membranous colitis/*Clostridium difficile*', Chapter 35).

The distribution and type of lesion in the small intestine and proximal colon will depend on the cause of the ischaemia. If it is due to a vascular obstruction, the pathological changes will have a uniform appearance and segmental distribution that reflect the blood supply of that vessel. In non-occlusive intestinal ischaemia, however, the lesions are often patchy and widespread, and vary in their severity [3].

Microscopic appearances

Early mucosal lesions are usually patchy, with almost normal mucosa separating diseased areas in which crypts show necrosis and there is a surface membrane composed of mucus, fibrin, blood cells and necrotic tissue. Sometimes, only the tips of the intestinal villi are affected (Figure 22.3). There is vascular congestion with oedema and occasional

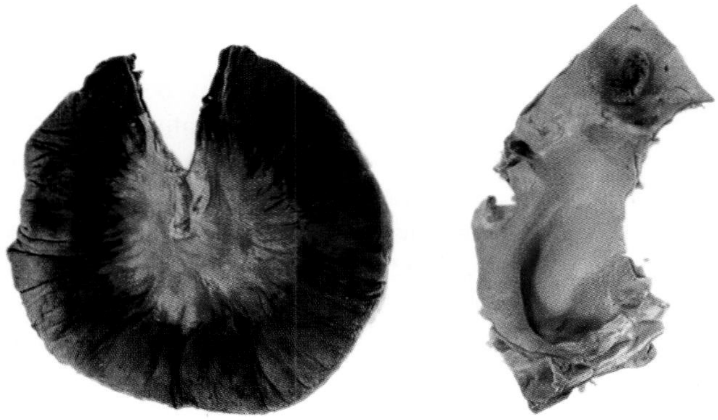

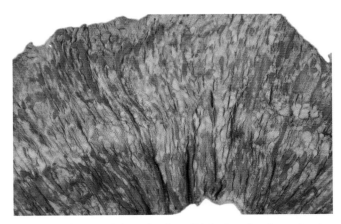

Figure 22.2 Acute ischaemia of small intestine showing extensive yellow plaques of mucosal necrosis.

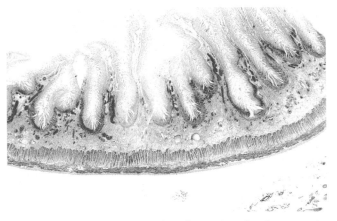

Figure 22.1 Infarction of small bowel following embolism to the superior mesenteric artery from thrombus in the aortic arch (right). The bowel is swollen and haemorrhagic.

Figure 22.3 Acute ischaemia of small intestine, showing necrosis of the upper half of the villi but sparing the basal half of the mucosa.

haemorrhages in the submucosal layer. It is common to see fibrin thrombi within the blood vessels of both the mucosa and the submucosa. In non-occlusive ischaemia, a significant number of patients will also have thrombi in other organs. This pattern might be a manifestation of disseminated intravascular coagulation centred on the gut. A search for minute ischaemic lesions in the mucosa should be made in which the only features are capillary congestion, necrosis of a few crypts and erosions of the surface epithelium.

With increasing severity of ischaemia, the deeper layers of the bowel wall become affected. There should always be a careful inspection of the muscularis propria even when the most obvious changes are mucosal and submucosal because, in the early stages of acute deprivation of blood, the muscle layers show only poor staining with loss of nuclei and little other abnormality. Later, lysis of muscle cells is more obvious, with separation and thinning of fibres by oedema, and the start of an inflammatory infiltrate.

Infarction is manifested by haemorrhage into the bowel wall, particularly the submucosa, with intravascular thrombosis and mucosal ulceration. In cases of intestinal gangrene, widespread necrosis is apparent and accompanied by secondary infection, which often extends through the bowel wall to involve mesenteric tissues and engulf the mesenteric vessels. The latter then show intravascular thrombosis and varying degrees of arteritis. This is more often a secondary rather than a primary cause of ischaemic bowel disease, so it is very important for the pathologist to recognise this superficial vessel thrombosis as a secondary phenomenon and not necessarily the cause of the ischaemic pathology. In fact, in any one case, the histology of the affected gut wall only exceptionally reveals the primary cause(s) of the intestinal ischaemia. More often the underlying diagnosis is determined by consideration of the clinical history and assessment of larger mesenteric blood vessels. It is important to exclude the various types of primary vasculitis that can lead to ischaemic bowel disease (see below). An opinion on whether the vascular changes are the result of venous or arterial occlusion can be useful but this is possible only if the mesenteric vasculature has been carefully examined.

All the features of ischaemic necrosis, however severe, can go through a process of resolution and repair. Granulation tissue replaces the layers of the bowel, often patchily. The whole process is essentially the same for the small intestine and colon (see 'Pathogenesis', Chapter 36) and a stricture is often the end-result. We have observed, in several cases, considerable degrees of mesenteric fat necrosis accompanying major vessel occlusion. One especial feature that helps a pathologist to differentiate chronic ischaemia of the small intestine, in all its forms, from other pathological causes is the dissolution of the muscularis propria and replacement by fibrous connective tissue, which occurs in chronic ischaemia. This may provide a potent clue to the true cause of a chronic fibrous stricture and provides evidence that the muscularis propria may also be severely affected by ischaemic pathology of the small intestine.

Ischaemic strictures and ulcers

Ischaemic strictures occur in the small bowel or colon. Within the small intestine they have been classified into primary and secondary forms. The primary causes are small mesenteric vessel emboli, trauma and the sequelae of herniae or bands. Secondary ischaemic strictures may be due to drugs, in particular potassium chloride tablets [35], the contraceptive pill [36] and non-steroidal anti-inflammatory drugs (NSAIDs) [37], and irradiation [38] but there are a small number whose aetiopathogenesis is unknown.

The strictures can be short or long, single or multiple. Occasionally they present with a malabsorption syndrome (see Chapter 21) but more often they produce signs and symptoms of intestinal obstruction, usually subacute. It is probable that the episodes of acute ischaemia eventually giving rise to a stricture are subclinical. Alternatively, ischaemic strictures may be the result of a slowly developing chronic ischaemic process corresponding to the clinical state of 'intestinal angina' [9]. Partial vascular occlusion and emboli can sometimes be found [39]. They can be produced by specific causes of peripheral arteritis such as polyarteritis nodosa. These are usually obvious on histological examination although there may be difficulty recognising burned-out cases of arteritis. Volvulus of the small intestine and obstruction of the blood supply due to internal hernias are also possible causes. Cholesterol emboli caused by dislodgement of atheromatous plaques are a well-recognised cause of ischaemic small bowel strictures (Figure 22.4), particularly in elderly people [40,41] and especially after major arterial surgery, in particular for abdominal aortic aneurysms.

Ischaemic strictures are usually concentric, with the serosal surface often being whiter than normal due to serosal fibrosis. The mucosal surface may be atrophic or show one or more, small, clearly demarcated ulcers. The cut surface of the stricture will reveal a prominent submucosa that is filled with white fibrous tissue (Figure 22.5). If possible, sections for microscopic examination should be taken from the mesenteric vessels as well as the stricture.

Microscopically, there is mucosal necrosis, commonly with ulceration. The submucosal layer is filled with granulation tissue of a very uniform character, containing many new blood vessels and a sprinkling of inflammatory cells sometimes including haemosiderin-laden macrophages, an indication of former submucosal haemorrhage during the acute phase of the illness. This granulation tissue spreads

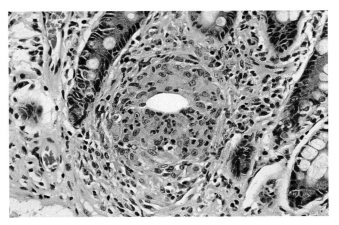

Figure 22.4 Histological section of a duodenal mucosal biopsy from an arteriopathic patient. A cholesterol cleft surrounded by foamy macrophages and inflammatory cells marks the site of embolised material from an atheromatous plaque in a major afferent artery.

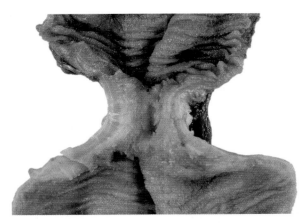

Figure 22.5 Ileum opened through an ischaemic stricture: note the mural thickening, particularly the white fibrous tissue in the submucosa, at the site of the stricture.

beneath intact mucosa beyond the macroscopic limits of the stricture. The deep muscle layers can be normal or show varying degrees of disorganisation by granulation tissue and fibrosis. A useful sign is to see the inner bundles of the circular muscle layer being nipped off by fibrous tissue. The serosa will often contain granulation tissue similar to that seen in the submucosal layer. It is unusual to find vascular changes unless the stricture has been caused by a specific type of arteritis.

Ischaemic stricture of the small bowel has to be distinguished from other causes of intestinal stenosis, including Crohn's disease, tuberculosis, carcinoma and lymphoma. The correct diagnosis is usually apparent from microscopic examination with particular emphasis on the study of the deep muscle layer (see above).

Chronic splanchnic syndrome (intestinal angina)

Chronic splanchnic syndrome is characterised clinically by post-prandial abdominal pain, weight loss and diarrhoea. The term covers what is coming to be accepted as the pre-infarction stage of intestinal ischaemia; the stage when symptoms might occur due to reduction in blood flow, but infarction has not occurred. An attempt to study this problem in an unselected post mortem series found that there was no correlation between degree of stenosis of the main mesenteric vessels and antemortem gastrointestinal symptoms. A 50% reduction in intraluminal diameter, corresponding to an 80% reduction in cross-sectional area, was taken as a critical stenosis but, even then, no clinical correlations could be made [9]. In a clinical study [42], it was possible to identify a small group of patients with symptoms before infarction who had varying degrees of mesenteric vessel stenosis and/or occlusion, in whom surgical reconstruction of the visceral arteries relieved symptoms. Such patients are rare and the relation between symptoms and pathology in chronic ischaemia still remains uncertain [9,17,18].

The relation of symptoms and radiological signs to lesions

It cannot be too strongly emphasised that anoxia must be severe before any symptoms, signs or visible lesions become apparent. In severe anoxia, without complete cessation of blood flow, vague abdominal symptoms appear, of which the most significant is abdominal (visceral) angina. This consists of severe, cramp-like, colicky, upper abdominal pain, weight loss, diarrhoea and, sometimes, vomiting and melaena. It occurs shortly after food and persists for 1–3 hours. Symptoms are much more severe after a large meal [43]. Early barium studies may show either no abnormality or transverse ridging and 'thumb printing'. When present, this corresponds with the fluid transudation and mucosal and submucosal haemorrhage of the early ischaemic lesion. In later lesions, radiology may show one or more solitary ulcers or strictures with proximal bowel dilatation.

When the anoxia is severe enough to produce full-thickness infarction, peristalsis is interrupted with consequent clinical evidence of obstruction and peritonitis. There is usually severe continuous abdominal pain with distension and vomiting. There may also be evidence of shock or hypertension which, on careful enquiry, has usually preceded, rather than followed, abdominal symptoms. The history may suggest a likely source of an embolus. Mesenteric venous thrombosis produces colicky abdominal pain, nausea, vomiting and bloody diarrhoea but the clinical course is usually more gradual [44].

Thus there are two broad clinical patterns of ischaemic enteritis, although neither is clear cut. When the onset is gradual or the anoxia short lasting, as in vascular narrowing and in some patients with hypotensive episodes, symptoms tend to be absent or of an anginal type. Radiology may be negative or demonstrate thumb printing. The lesion is superficial within the mucosa and submucosa, and healing can lead to stricture formation. Occasionally such patients eventually present with painless watery diarrhoea [29]. When anoxia is acute in onset, severe or long lasting, as in patients with complete occlusions or severe hypotension, symptoms include more continuous abdominal pain, severe bloody diarrhoea, intestinal obstruction and collapse with corresponding full-thickness infarction. Many patients in the first group recover spontaneously but may later show evidence of a solitary ulcer or stricture. In the second group, death is common and embolectomy, thrombectomy or resection is the only rational treatment.

Ischaemic enterocolitis and Hirschsprung's disease

The macroscopic and microscopic pathology of the enterocolitis of Hirschsprung's disease seem to be almost identical with that seen in the acute ischaemic enterocolitis of adults [45]. The aetiology of this complication of Hirschsprung's disease is currently unknown but is probably multifactorial [46]. Hirschsprung's disease-associated enterocolitis is considered further elsewhere (see Chapter 33).

Neonatal necrotising enterocolitis

Although this entity may well have an ischaemic element, it develops as a result of immaturity of the intestinal epithelial barrier and the neonatal immune system, which predispose to bacterial invasion and inflammation of the gut [47]. Necrotising enterocolitis is more fully considered elsewhere (see Chapter 35).

'Necrotising' enteritis

Conditions that come under this umbrella term are also considered elsewhere (see 'Clostridial infections', Chapter 20 and Chapter 35). They are necrotising lesions of the small or large bowel most commonly associated with clostridial organisms [48]. As many of the cases occur in children, it is unlikely that they have solely a primary vascular aetiology. An initial infectious insult to the mucosa followed by ischaemic damage, precipitated by the known vasoconstrictive effect of certain clostridial toxins, seems a probable pathogenic mechanism. In the adult it is possible to postulate the reverse: ischaemic damage to the mucosa could be an initial event that allows invasion of necrotic tissue by bacterial organisms. Whether the initial insult is ischaemic or infective cannot currently be resolved by pathological examination because such cases are studied only after surgical excision or death when the bowel is at the 'end-stage'.

Putative drug-induced ischaemic lesions

The small bowel circulation is sensitive to many pharmacological agents and it is not surprising therefore that many drugs have been implicated in ischaemic damage [49]. Cocaine, potassium chloride, non-steroidal anti-inflammatory drugs and oral contraceptives are the best documented. The pathology is difficult, if not impossible, to distinguish from other causes of ischaemic bowel injury.

Cocaine-induced intestinal ischaemia
Cocaine addicts frequently develop vasoconstriction and systemic arterial thrombotic occlusion, which occasionally affect the mesenteric arteries [50]. Ischaemia most often involves the proximal colon but other gastrointestinal sites may also be affected [51]. The small bowel may show sharply demarcated patches of 'pseudo-membranous' enteritis or even extensive regional infarction [52].

Non-steroidal anti-inflammatory drugs
Among the reports of solitary ulcers of the small intestine are cases incriminating NSAIDs [35,37,53]. There are no experimental data to suggest that the lesions are ischaemic, the evidence being based on the morphological similarity with known ischaemic ulceration. A more likely mechanism is via the effects that these drugs have on prostaglandin metabolism which in turn affects mucosal integrity, although ischaemia may have a secondary role. The pathology of NSAID damage to the small bowel is discussed in detail elsewhere (see Chapter 20).

The contraceptive pill
It is well known that oral contraceptive use increases the risk of vascular disease in many systems, although the risk seems to be considerably less with modern low-dose regimens [49]. Ischaemia, both acute and chronic, has been documented in the small intestine and colon [54,55]. Massive infarction of the small bowel may be due to mesenteric arterial or venous thrombosis [56,57]. The patients often have had symptoms before presentation. If the diagnosis is considered, and the oral contraceptive stopped, the ischaemia is reversed [54].

Vasculitis and other primary vascular lesions in the small intestine

The gastrointestinal tract is involved in many conditions in which there is a vasculitis as part of the disease (Table 22.2),

Table 22.2 Vasculitides involving the small bowel

Behçet's disease
Churg–Strauss syndrome
Cytomegalovirus vasculitis
Crohn's disease
Ehlers–Danlos syndrome
Fungal vasculitis
Giant cell arteritis
Henoch–Schönlein syndrome
Hypersensitivity vasculitis
Hypocomplementaemic vasculitis
Kawasaki's disease
Mesenteric inflammatory veno-occlusive disease
Mesenteric phlebosclerosis
Polyarteritis nodosa
Rickettsial vasculitis
Takayasu's arteritis
Thrombo-angiitis obliterans (Buerger's disease)
Vasculitis associated with connective tissue diseases
Wegener's granulomatosis

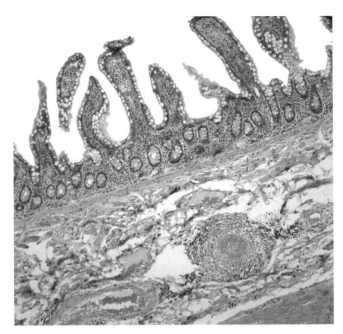

Figure 22.6 Histological section from a resected segment of small bowel from a patient with rheumatoid arthritis. A small submucosal artery is present that shows a necrotising vasculitis and associated thrombosis.

but, overall, vasculitis is an uncommon cause of intestinal ischaemic injury. It results in chronic arterial insufficiency in most cases but sometimes in acute mesenteric ischaemia. The diagnosis of vasculitis is often difficult to make from biopsy material [58], although deep rectal biopsies are said to be helpful in rheumatoid arthritis [59,60]. Surgery is only undertaken for the complications of haemorrhage, perforation, infarction and occasionally a stricture. The distinction between these conditions is usually made based on extra-intestinal findings and serological studies; the vasculitis itself seldom has distinguishing features. Finally, when it is difficult to establish the underlying disease in a patient with mesenteric vasculitis causing small intestinal ischaemia, it should be remembered that occult malignancy can sometimes be responsible [61].

Progressive systemic sclerosis (scleroderma)

In addition to the muscle atrophy and fibrosis commonly seen in scleroderma, a vasculitis can accompany the disease and cause a range of ischaemic pathology in the gut [62]. In the CREST syndrome (calcinosis, Raynaud's phenomenon, oesophageal dysmotility, sclerodactyly and telangiectasia), ectatic vascular lesions can be seen at many sites in the gastrointestinal tract [63,64]. They are similar to the vascular ectasias in the Weber–Osler–Rendu syndrome. Pneumatosis intestinalis has also been documented, perhaps as a result of obstruction and bacterial overgrowth [65].

Rheumatoid arthritis

Approximately 1% of patients with rheumatoid arthritis show a clinical vasculitis and a fifth of these will demonstrate gastrointestinal involvement [66] (Figure 22.6). There have been case reports of gastrointestinal involvement leading to intra-abdominal haemorrhage [67,68], infarction [69] and multiple gastrointestinal ulcers [70]. Involvement is more likely in patients with long-standing disease, a high rheumatoid factor and subcutaneous nodules. Where there is clinical evidence of vasculitis, a deep rectal biopsy may show inflammation involving submucosal vessels in up to 40% of cases [60].

Systemic lupus erythematosus

Gastrointestinal symptoms in systemic lupus erythematosus are common, occurring in from 10% to 34% of patients [71]. The predominant pathology identified is a vasculitis [72], either an arteritis [73] or a venulitis [74,75]. The vasculitis can lead to infarction of the small or large bowel [76], but haemorrhage from ischaemic ulcers may be the presenting feature [74,77]. Immune complexes can be demonstrated within the inflamed vessels and also in the basement membrane beneath the mucosal epithelial cells [74,75].

Henoch–Schönlein purpura

Henoch–Schönlein purpura is a hypersensitivity disease of childhood characterised by immune complex deposition beneath vascular basement membrane, with diverse haemorrhagic leukocytoclastic vasculitic lesions in the skin, kidneys, joints and alimentary tract. Clinically, gut involvement occurs in up to two-thirds of patients [78]. Any bowel segment may be affected but the duodenum, jejunum and ileum are most frequently involved. Endoscopic findings include petechial haemorrhages and multiple irregular areas of ulceration. Haematoma-like mucosal protrusions, which may be associated with the presence of leukocytoclastic vasculitis, may be seen [79]. In patients undergoing resection, the bowel appears oedematous and congested, with mottling, purulent mucosal exudates and superficial erosions. Transmural infarction is rare. Submucosal haematomas are sometimes present and can act as lead points for intussusception [78].

Histologically, variable features of intestinal ischaemia are present. The small vessels show fibrinoid necrosis, and neutrophilic and mononuclear infiltrates in their walls and in the perivascular soft tissues. Fibrin thrombi are often present. If the acute phase of ischaemic injury passes, then a chronic intestinal ischaemic stricture can follow [80]. It is possible to demonstrate IgA and complement (C3) in involved vessels with the use of immunofluorescence.

Polyarteritis nodosa

Polyarteritis nodosa (PAN) is an anti-neutrophil cytoplasmic antibody (ANCA)-unassociated vasculitis affecting medium-sized blood vessels. Up to 30% of cases are associated with hepatitis B infection. An association with hepatitis C has also been described [81]. Of patients with PAN 25–50% have abdominal symptoms [82,83]. Abdominal pain is the most common complaint, followed by diarrhoea and haematochezia. The complete spectrum of ischaemic changes due to an arteriolar or venous vasculitis can be seen, however, including steatorrhoea, perforation, stricture formation, ulcerative enteritis, intussusception and ischaemic necrosis [84,85]. Both the large and small bowel may be affected.

At laparotomy or necropsy, a careful search will usually disclose lesions but some patients have abdominal symptoms with no grossly identifiable disease. Macroscopically, the principal findings are nodules along the course of the mesenteric vessels and localised mucosal ulcers which lie along the anti-mesenteric border and can penetrate deeply and perforate; the bowel is often friable. Localised haemorrhagic infarcts in various stages of resolution may be seen.

Microscopically there is an acute arteritis (Figure 22.7) with fibrinoid necrosis of the vessel wall and often superimposed thrombus formation. The disease may involve

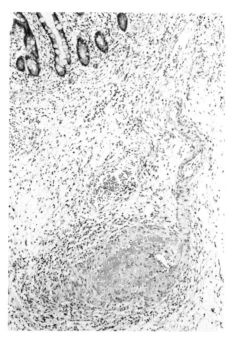

Figure 22.7 Polyarteritis nodosa with involvement of small ileal submucosal arteries. There is fibrinoid necrosis of the vessel wall and periarterial inflammation.

any size of vessel, although small straight arteries are the most commonly affected. Veins can also be involved. Infarction is described with uniform intimal hyperplasia of small arteries that may represent a healing phase [86]. There can be diagnostic difficulty after steroid therapy in which the inflammatory infiltrate has subsided. Here an elastic stain may be helpful to demonstrate destruction of the internal elastic lamina.

Allergic granulomatous vasculitis (Churg–Strauss syndrome)

Churg–Strauss syndrome is a type of small vessel vasculitis associated with granulomatous inflammation of the respiratory tract, asthma and peripheral eosinophilia, which can include gastrointestinal involvement. Discrete nodules are seen along the course of the vessels and the vasculitis is characterised by a heavy eosinophil infiltrate and granuloma formation in relation to small and medium-sized vessels and in extra-vascular positions [87]. The gastrointestinal involvement may resemble that seen in eosinophilic gastroenteritis. Multiple gastric, small intestinal and colonic ulcers may be present [88]. The vasculitis involves both arteries and veins.

Behçet's disease

Behçet's disease is a syndrome of oral, genital and ocular inflammation and ulceration that infrequently involves the gastrointestinal tract. The disease is more common in Japan than in western countries. When the gastrointestinal tract is involved, the terminal ileum and caecum are the most frequently involved sites [89,90]. Grossly and endoscopically, the intestine shows single or multiple, round-to-oval deep ulcers with discrete margins [91]. Histologically, the ulcer base frequently shows either a remnant of an underlying Peyer's patch or a destroyed lymphoid follicle [92]. Mononuclear inflammation around the vessels, intimal thickening, thrombosis and necrotising lymphocytic vasculitis affecting small venules are typical histological features (Figure 22.8). Granulomas are absent. The histological features are not specific, however, and one must rely on clinical information about extra-intestinal manifestations to establish the diagnosis. The disease is considered further in Chapters 20 and 35.

Thrombo-angiitis obliterans (Buerger's disease)

This disease rarely involves the distal branches of the superior mesenteric artery, producing local ischaemia. It may present after the diagnosis of limb disease has been made but cases are described with intestinal ischaemia occurring before any signs of limb claudication [93,94]. Characteristic vascular lesions are present in smaller submucosal and serosal vessels, producing local occlusion of lumina by organising thrombi. There is endothelial proliferation and medial fibrosis but in all vessels the internal elastic lamina is intact. This is characteristic of the disease and distinguishes it from other forms of vasculitis. There can also be perivascular inflammation. Both small and large bowel can be involved.

Kohlmeier–Degos syndrome (progressive arterial occlusive disease)

In this condition, which affects particularly the skin and gastrointestinal tract, the intima of small and medium-sized arteries undergoes progressive occlusive sclerosis, leading to localised zones of infarction [95]. The condition is probably a form of vasculitis and leads to multiple zones of fibrosis throughout the gastrointestinal tract, presumably the end-result of ischaemia with or without infarction.

Ehlers–Danlos syndrome

Patients with Ehlers-Danlos syndrome have hypermobile joints and hyperextensibility of the skin. which are the visible results of a generalised tissue 'fragility', probably itself the result of a defect in collagen metabolism. Vessels are characteristically affected in the type IV variety of the Ehlers–Danlos syndrome, in which they are abnormally fragile, the defect being in type III collagen. Instances have been described of severe intramural haemorrhage and

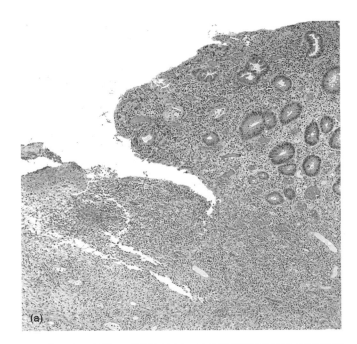

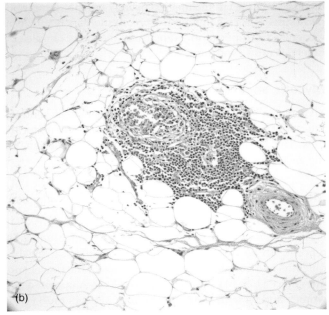

Figure 22.8 Behçet's disease: (a) low power photomicrograph demonstrating an area of non-specific ulceration. The adjacent mucosa shows changes of chronic injury. (b) A submucosal venule is surrounded by a dense mononuclear infiltrate.

spontaneous perforations of the bowel [96]. There are occasional recorded cases of perforation being the presenting illness [97–99]. The correct diagnosis, in one case [97], was made 5 years later when the patient presented with an aortic aneurysm. In the cases where pathology of the gut is documented, the muscle coat is thinned with loss of the submucosa, fibrosis of the circular muscle is apparent and defects in the media of mural arterioles [97–99] can be found.

Intramural haematomas of the small intestine

Bleeding into the wall of the small intestine from any cause is likely to result in swelling and obstruction and to produce a characteristic 'coiled-spring' pattern on a radiograph. In adults such haemorrhage, although occasionally traumatic, more commonly follows the use of anticoagulants [100] and may involve many parts of the small intestine. It can follow endoscopic biopsy [101]. The bleeding associated with the use of NSAIDs is more usually mucosal. In children the haemorrhage is more often duodenal and is the result of 'blunt trauma' without penetrating injury [101]. The duodenum is fixed both at the pylorus and at the end of the fourth part. It is therefore particularly liable to damage in childhood where it crosses an unyielding vertebral column.

Macroscopically the affected bowel is swollen and dark red and may appear gangrenous; on incision, blood and blood clot exude but the mucosa usually remains intact and peritonitis is not a common feature. Acute pancreatitis is a recognised complication. Some cases may be examples of Ehlers–Danlos syndrome.

Mycotic aneurysm

Mycotic aneurysms are rare in the superior mesenteric artery or its branches and are related to bacterial endocarditis. The aneurysm may rupture but secondary lesions in the gastrointestinal tract are rare.

Mesenteric inflammatory veno-occlusive disease

Mesenteric inflammatory veno-occlusive disease (MIVOD) is characterised by subacute intestinal ischaemia which is reported to be associated with, and possibly caused by, phlebitis and venulitis affecting the veins of the bowel and mesentery [102–104]. It occurs twice as often in men as in women and patients range in age from 24 years to 78 years [105]. Arteries are unaffected and, although there was no involvement of extra-intestinal veins in one series of seven cases [103], one of three patients in a second publication had recurrent peripheral thrombophlebitis and pulmonary embolism [102]. The phlebitis is described as lymphocytic, or occasionally necrotising and even granulomatous, and affected veins may show myointimal hyperplasia. Presenting symptoms are most commonly those of abdominal pain and nausea for a period of a few weeks and most make an uneventful recovery after surgical resection of the affected segment. Apart from the phlebitis and venulitis, and the superimposed occlusive venous thrombosis, histological examination of the affected bowel has shown a spectrum of lesions from acute congestion and transmural haemorrhagic infarction to more chronic strictures with intramural fibrosis.

Often it is difficult, in such cases, to be certain that the inflammatory venous changes are not secondary to the bowel ischaemia rather than vice versa. It is not uncommon to find inflammatory infiltration of the walls of mesenteric veins within a segment of infarcted bowel when another primary cause is established (such as entrapment within a hernia). Great care must therefore be taken to exclude other causes before attributing a case to inflammatory veno-occlusive disease.

References

1. Reiner L, Platt L, Rodriguez FL, Jimenez FA. Injection studies on the mesenteric arterial circulation, II: Intestinal infarction. *Gastroenterology* 1960;**39**:747.
2. Lundgren O, Svanvik J. Mucosal hemodynamics in the small intestine of the cat during reduced perfusion pressure. *Acta Physiol Scand* 1973;**88**:551
3. Williams LF, Anastasia LF, Hasiotis C, Bosniak MA, Byrne JJ. Non-occlusive mesenteric infarction. *Am J Surg* 1967;**114**:376.
4. Lundgren O. The regulation and distribution of intestinal blood flow. In: Marston A (ed.), *Vascular Disease of the Gut*. London: Edward Arnold, 1986: 16.
5. Jodal M, Haglund V, Lundgren O. Counter-current exchange mechanisms in the small intestine. In: Shepherd AR, Granger DN (eds), *Physiology of the Intestinal Circulation*. New York: Raven Press, 1984: 83.
6. Marston A. Ischaemia. *Clin Gastroenterol* 1985;**14**:847.
7. Thompson H. Vascular pathology of the splanchnic circulation. *Clin Gastroenterol* 1972;**1**:597.
8. Marston A. Basic structure and function of the intestinal circulation. *Clin Gastroenterol* 1972;**1**:539.
9. Kairaluoma MI, Karkola P, Heikkinen E, Huttunen R, Mokka REM, Larmi TKI. Mesenteric infarction. *Am J Surg* 1977;**133**:188.
10. Kumar PJ, Dawson AM. Vasculitis of the alimentary tract. *Clin Gastroenterol* 1972;**1**:719.
11. May GM, De Weese JA, Rob CG. Haemodynamic effects of arterial stenosis. *Surgery* 1963;**53**:513.
12. Reiner L, Jimenez FA, Rodriguez FL. Atherosclerosis in the mesenteric circulation. Observations and correlations with aortic and coronary atherosclerosis. *Am Heart J* 1963;**66**:200.
13. Jarvinen O, Laurikka J, Salenius JP, Tarkka M. Acute intestinal ischaemia. A review of 214 cases. *Ann Chir Gynaecol* 1994;**83**:22.
14. Dick AP, Gregg D. Chronic occlusions of the visceral arteries. *Clin Gastroenterol* 1972;**1**:689.
15. Reiner L, Rodriguez FL, Jimenez FA, Platt R. Injection studies on mesenteric arterial circulation. III: Occlusions without intestinal infarction. *Arch Pathol* 1962;**73**:461.
16. Wilson C, Gupta R, Gilmour DG, Imrie CW. Acute superior mesenteric ischaemia. *Br J Surg* 1987;**74**:279.
17. Bergan JJ, Yao JS. Acute intestinal ischaemia. In: Rutherford P (ed.), *Vascular Surgery*, 2nd edn. Philadelphia, PA: WB Saunders, 1981: 948.
18. Szilagyi DE, Rian RL, Elliot JP, Smith RF. The coeliac artery compression syndrome: Does it exist? *Surgery* 1972;**72**:849.
19. Dick AP, Graff R, Gregg D, Peters N, Sarner M. An arteriographic study of mesenteric arterial disease. 1. Large vessel changes. *Gut* 1967;**8**:206.

20. Evans W. Long-term evaluation of the coeliac band syndrome. *Surgery* 1974;**76**:867.
21. Civetta JM, Kolodny M. Mesenteric venous thrombosis association with oral contraceptives. *Gastroenterology* 1970;**58**:713.
22. Cotton PB, Thomas ML. Ischaemic colitis and the contraceptive pill. *BMJ* 1971;**3**:27.
23. Schoots IG, Koffeman GI, Legemate DA, Levi M, van Gulik TM. Systematic review of survival after acute mesenteric ischaemia according to disease aetiology. *Br J Surg* 2004;**91**:17.
24. Marston A. The bowel in shock. *Lancet* 1962;**ii**:365.
25. Fogarty TJ, Fletcher WS. Non-occlusive mesenteric ischaemia. *Am J Surg* 1965;**111**:130.
26. Whitehead R. Ischaemic enterocolitis an expression of the intravascular coagulation syndrome. *Gut* 1971;**12**:912.
27. Polansky BJ, Berger RL, Byrne JJ. Massive nonocclusive intestinal infarction associated with digitalis toxicity. *Circulation* 1964;(suppl 30):141.
28. Ming SC. Haemorrhagic necrosis of the gastrointestinal tract and its relation to cardiovascular status. *Circulation* 1965;**32**:332.
29. Drucker WR, Davies JH, Holden WD, Reagan JR. Haemorrhagic necrosis of the intestine. *Arch Surg* 1964;**89**:42.
30. Kay AW, Richards RL, Watson AJ. Acute necrotizing (pseudomembranous) enterocolitis. *Br J Surg* 1958;**46**:45.
31. Freiman DG. Haemorrhagic necrosis of the gastrointestinal tract. *Circulation* 1965;**32**:329.
32. Kolkman JJ, Bargeman M, Huisman AB, Geelkerken RH. Diagnosis and management of splanchnic ischaemia. *World J Gastroenterol* 2008;**14**:7309.
33. van den Hauwe L, Degryse H, Coene L. Portomesenteric vein gas in mesenteric infarction. *JBR-BTR* 2002;**85**:162.
34. Hashimoto A, Fuke H, Shimizu A, Shiraki K. Hepatic portal venous gas caused by non-obstructive mesenteric ischaemia. *J Hepatol* 2002;**37**:870.
35. Brookes VS, Windsor CWO, Howell JS. Ischaemic ulceration with stricture formation in the small bowel. *Br J Surg* 1966;**53**:583.
36. Boydstun JS, Gaffey TA, Bartholomew LG. Clinicopathologic study of non-specific ulcers of the small intestine. *J Am Med Assoc* 1981;**192**:763.
37. Darjee JR. Cholesterol embolism: the great masquerader. *South Med J* 1979;**12**:174.
38. Blundell JW. Small bowel stricture secondary to multiple cholesterol emboli. *Histopathology* 1988;**13**:459.
39. Rob C. Stenosis and thrombosis of the coeliac and mesenteric arteries. *Am J Surg* 1967;**114**:363
40. Jamieson WG, Marchuk S, Rowsom J, Durand D. The early diagnosis of massive intestinal ischaemia. *Br J Surg* 1982;**69**:952.
41. Cokkinis A. Intestinal ischaemia. *Proc R Soc Med* 1961;**54**:354.
42. Kay CR. The Royal College of General Practitioners Oral Contraception Study: some recent observations. *Clin Obstet Gynaecol* 1984;**11**:759.
43. Teich S, Schisgall RM, Anderson KD. Ischaemic enterocolitis as a complication of Hirschsprung's disease. *J Pediatr Surg* 1986;**21**:143.
44. Baker DR, Schradar WH, Hitchcock CR. Small bowel ulceration apparently associated with thiazide and potassium therapy. *JAMA* 1964;**190**:586.
45. Kradjian RM. Ischaemic stenosis of small intestine. *Arch Surg* 1965;**91**:829.
46. Murphy F, Puri P. New insights into the pathogenesis of Hirschsprung's associated enterocolitis. *Pediatr Surg Int* 2005;**21**:773.
47. Petrosyan M, Guner YS, Williams M, Grishin A, Ford HR. Current concepts regarding the pathogenesis of necrotizing enterocolitis. *Pediatr Surg Int* 2009;**25**:309.
48. Lawrason FD, Alpert E, Mohr FL, McMahon FG. Ulcerative obstructive lesions of the small intestine. *JAMA* 1965;**191**:641.
49. Hass DJ, Kozuch P, Brandt LJ. Pharmacologically mediated colon ischaemia. *Am J Gastroenterol* 2007;**102**:1765.
50. Wayte DM, Helwig EB. Small bowel ulceration – iatrogenic or multifactorial origin. *Am J Clin Pathol* 1968;**49**:26.
51. Ellis CN, McAlexander WW. Enterocolitis associated with cocaine use. *Dis Colon Rectum* 2005;**48**:2313.
52. Madhok R, Mackenzie JA, Lee FD, Bruckner FE, Terry TR, Sturrock RD. Small bowel ulceration in patients receiving non-steroidal anti-inflammatory drugs for rheumatoid arthritis. *Q J Med* 1986;**255**:53.
53. Tribe CR, Scott DGI, Bacon PI. Rectal biopsy in the diagnosis of systemic vasculitis. *J Clin Pathol* 1981;**34**:843.
54. Deana DG, Dean PJ. Reversible ischaemic colitis is young women: association with oral contraceptive use. *Am J Surg Pathol* 1995;**19**:454.
55. Preventza OA, Lazarides K, Sawyer MD. Ischaemic colitis in young adults: a single-institution experience. *J Gastrointest Surg* 2001;**5**:388.
56. Carron DB, Douglas AP. Steatorrhoea in vascular insufficiency of the small intestine. *Q J Med* 1965;**34**:331.
57. Roikjaer O. Perforation and necrosis of the colon complicating polyarteritis nodosa. *Acta Chir Scand* 1987;**153**:385.
58. Fisher RS, Myers AR. Progressive systemic sclerosis (scleroderma). In: Bouchier IAD, Allan RN, Hodgson HJF, Keighley MRB (eds), *Textbook of Gastroenterology*. London: Baillière Tindall, 1984: 642.
59. Baron M, Srolovitz. Colonic telangiectasias in a patient with progressive systemic sclerosis. *Arthritis Rheum* 1986;**29**:282.
60. Rosekrans PC, de Rooy DJ, Bosman FT, Eulderink F, Cats A. Gastrointestinal telangiectasia as a cause of severe blood loss in systemic sclerosis. *Endoscopy* 1980;**12**:200.
61. Meihoff WE, Hirschfield JS, Kern F. Small intestinal scleroderma with malabsorption and pneumatosis cystoides intestinalis. *JAMA* 1968;**204**:854.
62. Burt RW, Berenson MM, Samuelson CO, Cathey WJ. Rheumatoid vasculitis of the colon presenting as pancolitis. *Dig Dis Sci* 1983;**28**:183.
63. Lindsay MK, Tavadia HB, Whyte AS, Lee P, Webb J. Acute abdomen in rheumatoid arthritis due to necrotizing arteritis. *BMJ* 1973;**ii**:592.
64. Bienenstock H, Minick R, Rogoff B. Mesenteric arteritis and intestinal infarction in rheumatoid disease. *Arch Intern Med* 1967;**119**:359.
65. Joviasis A, Kraag G. Acute gastrointestinal manifestations of systemic lupus erythematosus. *Can J Surg* 1987;**30**:185.
66. Hoffman BI, Katz WA. The gastrointestinal manifestations of Systemic Lupus Erythematosus: a review of the literature. *Semin Arthritis Rheum* 1980;**9**:237.
67. Jayawardena SA, Sheerin N, Pattison JM, Hartley B, Goldsmith DJ. Spontaneous abdominal haemorrhage with AA-amyloidosis and vasculitis in a patient with rheumatoid arthritis. *J Clin Rheumatol* 2001;**7**:86.
68. Pagnoux C, Mahr A, Cohen P, Guillevin L. Presentation and outcome of gastrointestinal involvement in systemic necrotizing vasculitides. Analysis of 62 patients with polyarteritis nodosa, microscopic polyangiitis, Wegener granulomatosis, Churg–Strauss syndrome, or rheumatoid arthritis-associated vasculitis. *Medicine* 2005;**84**:115.
69. Babain M, Nasef S, Soloway G. Gastrointestinal infarction as a manifestation of rheumatoid vasculitis. *Am J Gastroenterol* 1998;**93**:119.
70. Takeuchi K, Kuroda Y. Rheumatoid vasculitis with multiple intestinal ulcerations: report of a case. *Ryumachi* 2000;**40**:639.
71. Weiser MM, Andres GA, Brentjens JR, Evans JT, Rachlin M. Systemic lupus erythematosus and intestinal venulitis. *Gastroenterology* 1981;**81**:570.

72. Stoddard CJ, Kay PH, Simms JM, Kennedy A, Hugher P. Acute abdominal complications of systemic lupus erythematosus. *Br J Surg* 1978;**65**:625.

73. Papa MZ, Shiloni E, McDonald HD. Total colonic necrosis: a catastrophic complication of systemic lupus erythematosus. *Dis Colon Rectum* 1986;**29**:576.

74. Feldt RH, Sholder GB. The gastrointestinal manifestations of anaphylactoid purpura in children. *Staff Meet Mayo Clin* 1962; **37**:465.

75. Martinez-Frontanilla LA, Haase GM, Ernster JA, Bailey WC. Surgical complications of Henoch–Schonlein purpura. *J Pediatr Surg* 1984;**19**:434.

76. Deitch EA, Sikkema WW. Intestinal manifestations of Buerger's disease: case report and literature review. *Am Surg* 1981;**47**:326.

77. Lombard KA, Shah PC, Thrasher TV, Grill BB. Ileal stricture as a late complication of Henoch–Schonlein purpura. *Paediatrics* 1986;**77**:396.

78. Robson WL, Leung AK. Henoch-Schonlein purpura. *Adv Pediatr* 1994;**41**:163.

79. Esaki M, Matsumoto T, Nakamura S, et al. GI involvement in Henoch–Schonlein purpura. *Gastrointest Endosc* 2002;**56**:920.

80. Beighton PH, Murdoch JL, Votteler T. Gastrointestinal complications of the Ehlers–Danlos syndrome. *Gut* 1969;**10**:1004.

81. Cacoub P, Maisonobe T, Thibault V, et al. Systemic vasculitis in patients with hepatitis C. *J Rheumatol* 2001;**28**:109.

82. Bassel K, Hartford W. Gastrointestinal manifestations of collagen-vascular disease. *Semin Gastrointest Dis* 1995;**6**:228.

83. Krupski W, Selzman C, Whitehall T. Unusual causes of mesenteric ischaemia. *Surg Clin North Am* 1997;**77**:471.

84. Sykes EM Jr. Colon perforation in Ehlers–Danlos syndrome. *Am J Surg* 1984;**147**:410.

85. Silva R, Coghill TH, Hansbrough JF, Zapata-Sirvent RL, Harrington DS. Intestinal perforation and vascular rupture in Ehlers–Danlos syndrome. *Int Surg* 1986;**71**:48.

86. Levine S, Whelan TJ Jr. Small bowel infarction due to intramural haematoma during anticoagulant therapy. *Arch Surg* 1967; **95**:245.

87. Bailey WC, Akers DR. Traumatic intramural hematoma of the duodenum in children: a report of 5 cases. *Am J Surg* 1965;**110**: 695.

88. Memain N, De BM, Guillevin L, Wechsler B, Meyer O. Delayed relapse of Churg-Strauss syndrome manifesting as colon ulcers with mucosal granulomas: 3 cases. *J Rheumatol* 2002;**29**:388.

89. Griffin JW Jr, Harrison HB, Tedesco FJ, Mills LR 4th. Behçet's disease with multiple sites of gastrointestinal involvement. *South Med J* 1982;**75**:1405.

90. Lee RG. The colitis of Behçet's syndrome. *Am J Surg Pathol* 1986;**10**:888.

91. Masugi J, Matsui T, Fujimori T, Maeda S. A case of Behçet's disease with multiple longitudinal ulcers all over the colon. *Am J Gastroenterol* 1994;**89**:778.

92. Takada Y, Fujita Y, Igarashi M, et al. Intestinal Behçet's disease: pathognomonic changes in intramucosal lymphoid tissue and effect of a 'rest cure' on intestinal lesions. *J Gastroenterol* 1997; **32**:598.

93. Moore SW, Erlandson ME. Intramural hematoma of the duodenum. *Ann Surg* 1963;**157**:573.

94. Golding MR, de Jong, Parker JW. Intramural hematoma of the duodenum. *Ann Surg* 1963;**157**:573.

95. DeBakey ME, Cooley DA. Successful resection of mycotic aneurysm of superior mesenteric artery. *Ann Surg* 1953;**19**:202.

96. Stillman AE, Painter R, Hollister DW. Ehlers–Danlos syndrome type IV: diagnosis and therapy of associated bowel perforation. *Am J Gastroenterol* 1991;**86**:360.

97. Anthony A, Dhillon AP, Pounder RE, Wakefield AJ. Ulceration of the ileum in Crohn's disease: correlation with vascular anatomy. *J Clin Pathol* 1997;**50**:1013.

98. Fong YM, Marano MA, Moldawer LL, et al. The acute splanchnic and peripheral tissue metabolic response to endotoxin in humans. *J Clin Invest* 1990;**85**:1896.

99. Spain DA, Fruchterman TM, Matheson PJ, Wilson MA, Martin AW, Garrison RN. Complement activation mediates intestinal injury after resuscitation from hemorrhagic shock. *J Trauma* 1999;**46**:224.

100. Kumar S, Sarr MG, Kamath PS. Mesenteric venous thrombosis. *N Engl J Med* 2001;**345**:1683.

101. Thomas GR, Thibodaux H. Transforming growth factor-beta 1 inhibits postischaemic increases in splanchnic vascular resistance. *Biotechnol Therapeut* 1992;**3**:91.

102. Gross WL. Systemic necrotizing vasculitis. *Baillière's Clin Rheumatol* 1997;**11**:259.

103. Ehrlich GE. Vasculitis in Behçet's disease. *Int Rev Immunol* 1997;**14**:81.

104. Lavu K, Minocha A. Mesenteric inflammatory veno-occlusive disorder: a rare entity mimicking inflammatory bowel disease. *Gastroenterology* 2003;**125**:236.

105. Lie JT. Mesenteric inflammatory veno-occlusive disease (MIVOD): an emerging and unsuspected cause of digestive tract ischaemia. *Vasa* 1997;**26**:91.

CHAPTER 23

Polyps and tumour-like lesions of the small intestine

G. Johan A. Offerhaus,[1] Lodewijk A.A. Brosens[1] and Marnix Jansen[2]

[1]University Medical Centre Utrecht, Utrecht, The Netherlands
[2]Academic Medical Centre, Amsterdam, The Netherlands

Brunner's gland hyperplasia/hamartoma/adenoma

Brunner's gland hyperplasia is commonly encountered in association with peptic duodenitis and it is therefore mostly limited to the duodenal bulb. Endoscopically it presents as a nodular duodenitis. This nodularity should be distinguished from the genuine single polyps that can be encountered in the duodenal bulb, referred to as Brunner's gland hamartoma or adenoma [1]. In view of the nomenclature generally used in the gastrointestinal tract, the term 'adenoma' is considered a misnomer because the lesion is not neoplastic. Therefore the best term for these uncommon lesions is really hamartoma, even though the aetiology is basically unknown.

Brunner's gland hamartomas can present at any age but are most frequently found during the fifth and sixth decades. Both sexes are equally affected. In one series of 27 cases, the lesion was symptomless and found incidentally in 7 cases but 10 cases presented with haemorrhage and there were 10 patients with obstruction [2]. Macroscopically, Brunner's gland hamartomas protrude into the lumen of the duodenum as polyps that are frequently pedunculated. They may measure up to 60 mm in diameter, although most examples are much smaller (Figure 23.1). Histologically they are purely epithelial lesions consisting of groups of Brunner's glands, separated by septa of proliferative smooth muscle derived from and lying deep to the muscularis mucosae [2] (Figure 23.2). Focal cystic change may be seen.

The epithelium of the lesions is of normal Brunner's gland type, with basal nuclei without atypia. Mitoses are very scanty and there is no tendency to neoplastic change. Paneth cells are often present. Brunner's gland hamartomas are not associated with oral pigmentation and there is no known genetic basis, although we have seen a case in a well-established juvenile polyposis patient with a germline mutation of *SMAD4*.

Peri-ampullary myo-epithelial hamartoma/adenomyoma

Small myo-epithelial hamartomas composed of dilated gland elements and surrounded by muscle occur in the duodenum, usually in relation to the ampulla of Vater. They have also been termed 'adenomyomas'. Most cases are asymptomatic and discovered incidentally, although larger pedunculated lesions may cause intermittent biliary or pancreatic obstruction [3]. The sexes appear equally affected.

The macroscopic appearances are usually of an umbilicated sessile polyp. Histological examination reveals a submucosal admixture of hypertrophic smooth muscle bundles and cystic glands lined by cytologically benign low columnar epithelium, Brunner's glands and variable numbers of pancreatic acini and ducts (Figure 23.3). Islets of Langerhans are present in approximately a third of cases and their presence greatly facilitates the diagnosis. Neoplastic change has not been reported.

The complex admixture of epithelial and smooth muscle elements in a peri-ampullary mass may persuade the unwary into a diagnosis of malignancy, especially in frozen sections. Important differentiating features of this lesion are

Morson and Dawson's Gastrointestinal Pathology, Fifth Edition. Edited by Neil A. Shepherd, Bryan F. Warren, Geraint T. Williams, Joel K. Greenson, Gregory Y. Lauwers and Marco R. Novelli.
© 2013 Blackwell Publishing Ltd. Published 2013 by Blackwell Publishing Ltd.

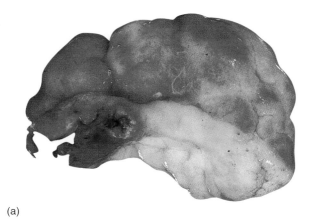

(a)

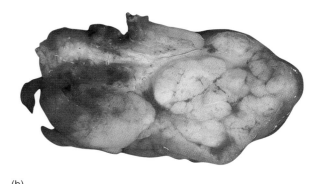

(b)

Figure 23.1 (a) Macroscopic appearance of a Brunner's gland hamartoma. (b) Cut surface.

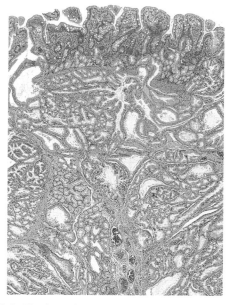

Figure 23.2 Histological section of the Brunner's gland hamartoma in Figure 23.1. There is extensive proliferation of Brunner's glands with thin smooth muscle septa and some cystically dilated glands.

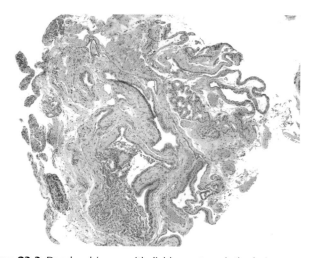

Figure 23.3 Duodenal 'myo-epithelial hamartoma': the lesion consists of dilated gland elements lined by flattened epithelium and surrounded by smooth muscle.

the lack of cytological atypia and the absence of a desmo-plastic reaction in relation to the glandular elements [1].

Peutz–Jeghers polyps

Peutz–Jeghers syndrome

Peutz–Jeghers syndrome classically has three components: gastrointestinal polyposis, perioral pigmentation and an autosomal dominant pattern of inheritance [4,5]. Peutz first recognised the disease in 1921 in a Dutch family; the pedigree of this family continues to be followed [6]. Jeghers described further cases from the USA in the 1940s. Peutz–Jeghers syndrome presents in 1 per 50000 to 1 per 200000 newborns and is caused by a germline mutation in the *LKB1/STK11* gene, which is located on the short arm of chromosome 19 [7]. Penetrance appears to be nearly complete in affected individuals, although the pigmentations may fade after puberty and before the onset of symptoms related to polyp growth. The sex incidence is equal.

Peutz–Jeghers syndrome has a well-established cancer risk and many patients die from malignancies, often at a comparatively young age. Based on large cohort studies, patients are estimated to display an 18-fold increased cancer risk over the normal population [8]. The LKB1 protein functions as serine–threonine kinase and it has been shown to behave as a tumour suppressor. The exact function of the protein remains unclear, because it has now been linked to a plethora of downstream molecules. Current evidence indicates a role for the protein in the regulation of cellular polarity and in cellular energy metabolism through the conserved AMPK module. Studies in animal models have also delineated a role for the protein in the control of stem cell numbers through the regulation of asymmetrical stem cell division [4].

Genetic testing for *LKB1* germline mutations is now available in a number of laboratories. Previously, *LKB1* coding sequence analyses demonstrated disease-causing mutations in only a minor part of families affected by Peutz–Jeghers syndrome. However, with the advent of novel molecular techniques to analyse large genomic deletions such as multiplex ligation probe amplification (MLPA), the majority of families with Peutz–Jeghers syndrome can now be linked to pathogenic germline *LKB1* mutations [9,10].

The distinctive pigmented lesions (melanin spots) in patients are caused by pigment-laden macrophages in the dermis that clinically resemble freckles. These melanin spots are most common in the perioral region, including the buccal mucosa, but may also occur on patients' hands and feet and in the perianal area. Histopathology of these lesions is not specific for Peutz–Jeghers syndrome and malignant transformation does not occur.

Polyps can develop anywhere in the gut but the small bowel appears to be the most common site, with the jejunum predominating, followed by ileum and duodenum. The number of polyps developing in an individual patient appears to vary considerably, even within families, but may run anywhere from solitary polyps to several dozens per segment of bowel. However, counting polyps limited to those that come to clinical attention might misrepresent actual numbers and distribution of polyps. As an example, in one study investigating chemoprophylaxis through cyclo-oxygenase 2 (COX-2) inhibitors in Peutz–Jeghers syndrome patients, hundreds of smaller polyps were described in the stomach of all patients [11]. Potentially novel gastrointestinal imaging techniques such as double-balloon enteroscopy may more accurately define polyp distribution.

Macroscopically, the surface of a Peutz–Jeghers polyp has a coarse lobulation, resembling that of an adenoma but with larger lobules and in marked contrast with the smooth surface of a juvenile polyp (Figure 23.4). The essential diagnostic feature of Peutz–Jeghers polyps microscopically is a branching core of muscle derived from the muscularis mucosae in a strikingly arborising pattern (Figure 23.5); these branches become thinner and eventually disappear

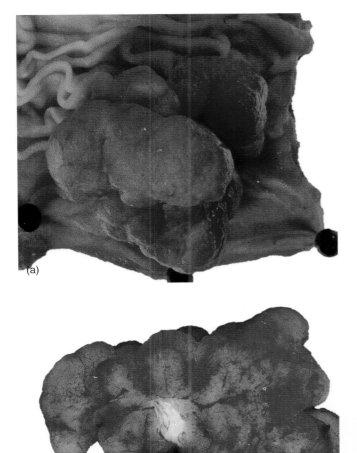

(a)

(b)

Figure 23.4 (a) Peutz–Jeghers polyp in the small intestine of a patient with Peutz–Jeghers syndrome. Note the coarse lobulation. (b) Cut surface of polyp in (a).

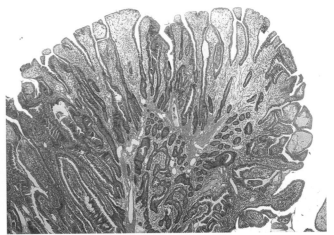

Figure 23.5 Histological section of a Peutz–Jeghers polyp: the lesion is characterised by a branching core of muscle derived from the muscularis mucosae. The polyp is covered by histologically normal epithelium with a normal lamina propria.

as they reach the periphery of the polyp [12]. Each branch is covered by histologically normal epithelium with a normal lamina propria. Paneth and endocrine cells are present in their normal sites at the base of the crypts. Small areas of superficial gastric-type epithelium, gastric mucin cell metaplasia, may be found in small bowel polyps. There is no excess of lamina propria, nuclear hyperchromatism or glandular irregularity as seen in adenomas.

Thus, classic Peutz–Jeghers polyps are covered by non-neoplastic epithelium. Hyperplastic and reactive features can be present and the epithelial crypts and pits are often elongated. In larger polyps one may observe misplacement of epithelial glands and their associated lamina propria within, or even through, the muscularis propria into the stalk of the polyp [13]. This 'pseudo-invasion' is felt to be due to mechanical forces acting on a polyp during gut motility, which may lead to mucosal herniation into the submucosa. To the unwary this may suggest carcinoma. However, the absence of neoplastic cytological features and the presence of features suggesting mucosal trauma, such as deposition of haemosiderin pigment, point to the right diagnosis.

Smaller polyps, <5 mm in size, on the other hand, may only show subtle diagnostic features, e.g. in the aforementioned chemoprophylaxis study, the incipient gastric Peutz–Jeghers syndrome polyps showed foveolar hyperplasia with minimal smooth muscle proliferation but they lacked the prominent smooth muscle stalk typical of larger Peutz–Jeghers syndrome polyps [11]. Thus nascent Peutz–Jeghers syndrome polyps may not yet display the typical arborising smooth muscle core. The differential diagnosis of solitary Peutz–Jeghers polyps is wide and includes other lesions characterised by central areas of proliferating muscle fibres surrounded by normal or reactive mucosa, such as mucosal prolapse, cloacogenic polyp, solitary rectal ulcer syndrome and Brunner's gland hamartoma [12].

The histological precursor for cancer development in patients with Peutz–Jeghers syndrome has not been ascertained with certainty. The classic mature Peutz-Jeghers polyp displaying an arborising core of smooth muscle with overlying non-dysplastic epithelium had previously been thought to contain a potential for malignant change, in spite of its benign histopathological appearance. Sporadic cases of dysplasia or malignant change occurring in classic Peutz–Jeghers polyps supported the view that classic Peutz–Jeghers syndrome polyps would be prone to malignant transformation [14]. However, dysplasia occurring in classic Peutz–Jeghers syndrome polyps appears to be a very uncommon phenomenon: in series of the renowned familial polyposis registry at St Mark's Hospital, a review of 491 polyps showed no evidence of dysplasia in any of them [13] and follow-up over 45 years of 48 patients at the Mayo Clinic also failed to reveal dysplastic change in any polyp [15].

Based on multiple lines of evidence, including the fact that human Peutz–Jeghers syndrome polyps are polyclonal [16], as well as data from murine Peutz–Jeghers models showing that loss of the wild-type *LKB1/STK11* allele is not required for polyp formation [17], it has been suggested that Peutz–Jeghers polyps are in fact not pre-malignant in the strict sense. The classic Peutz–Jeghers polyps are thus a signpost to the malignant condition, not its obligate histological precursor [4]. As microscopic features of mucosal prolapse are regularly observed in conventional adenomatous polyps or carcinomas arisen in an adenomatous polyp, we have proposed that historical accounts of adenomatous transformation and carcinoma occurring in Peutz–Jeghers syndrome polyps might be explained by a blurring of the order of events [12], namely that these lesions might have arisen as a conventional adenoma in a Peutz–Jeghers syndrome patient that secondarily developed a Peutz–Jeghers syndrome-like smooth muscle proliferation due to prolapse.

At this point the risk of adenoma development in Peutz–Jeghers syndrome is unclear, although some reports suggest an increased incidence of adenomatous polyps in these patients [18]. Future studies should be aimed at clarifying this risk with attendant impact on surveillance strategies.

Cancer risk and surveillance

Mechanical problems due to polyp development in Peutz–Jeghers syndrome dominate the first two decades of life [5]. Presenting features in new patients related to polyp growth are gastrointestinal bleeding with consequent anaemia and recurrent attacks of severe colic, sometimes with recurring intussusception. Almost half the patients experience at least one event of intussusception during their life time necessitating surgical intervention, most often in the small intestine [6]. Before this was recognised, multiple resections were often performed, resulting eventually in short bowel and malabsorption syndromes. It has been suggested that a combined endoscopic and laparoscopic approach can be used to treat proximal small bowel intussusception, markedly reducing the need for repeated laparotomies in these patients.

Intestinal and extra-intestinal cancer development become a major clinical concern with advancing age. The cancer spectrum consists mostly of gastrointestinal cancers. However, an increased risk for extra-intestinal cancers has also been noted and the risk of breast cancer in female Peutz–Jeghers syndrome patients is comparable to that associated with either *BRCA-1* or *BRCA-2* mutations [8]. In addition, Peutz–Jeghers syndrome patients are at increased risk for distinctive benign tumours of the genital tract, such as sex cord tumours with annular tubules (SCTATs) of the ovary and feminising Sertoli's cell tumours of the testis [19,20]. Interestingly, SCTATs in female patients with Peutz–

Jeghers syndrome are almost always bilateral, multifocal and benign, and have been described as characteristic for the condition. SCTATs in patients not affected by Peutz–Jeghers syndrome are typically unilateral and often display a malignant clinical course, in contrast to its benign character in Peutz–Jeghers syndrome.

The range of organs affected in Peutz–Jeghers syndrome translates into a cumbersome follow-up strategy and current recommendations include biannual upper endoscopy with polypectomy, colonoscopy with polypectomy and small bowel radiograph series [21]. A rational basis for surveillance strategies in these patients is sorely lacking. A recent analysis of the psychosocial impact of Peutz–Jeghers syndrome in affected patients has shown that a diagnosis of Peutz–Jeghers syndrome affects many important life decisions in these patients, even though physically patients do not feel impacted compared with the general population [22].

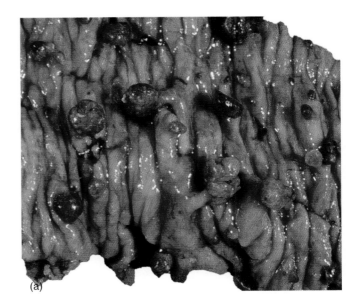
(a)

Juvenile polyps

The first histological description of a juvenile polyp was by Diamond in 1939 [23]. Macroscopically, these polyps vary in size from 5 mm to 50 mm and typically have a spherical, lobulated and pedunculated appearance with surface erosion (Figure 23.6). Histologically, the juvenile polyp is characterised by an abundance of oedematous lamina propria with inflammatory cells and cystically dilated glands lined by cuboidal to columnar epithelium with reactive changes (Figure 23.7).

Solitary colorectal juvenile polyps occur in approximately 2% of children and are not associated with an increased risk of gastrointestinal cancer [24,25]. In contrast, in the setting of juvenile polyposis syndrome, there is an increased risk of gastrointestinal cancer and neoplastic change of the epithelium. Unlike in Peutz–Jeghers polyps, dysplasia is frequently found in the polyps of juvenile polyposis syndrome. In general, juvenile polyps in juvenile polyposis syndrome have a similar appearance to sporadic juvenile polyps, although they often have a frond-like growth pattern with relatively less stroma, fewer dilated glands and more proliferative smaller glands [26]. Importantly, we are not aware of the occurrence of juvenile polyps in the small bowel, outside the context of juvenile polyposis syndrome. So, a juvenile-type polyp detected in the small intestine very likely infers that the patient has juvenile polyposis syndrome.

Juvenile polyposis syndrome

Juvenile polyposis syndrome is an autosomal dominant disorder defined by the presence of five or more juvenile polyps in the colorectum, juvenile polyps throughout the gastrointestinal tract or any number of juvenile polyps and

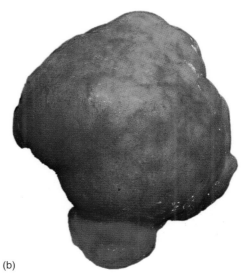
(b)

Figure 23.6 (a) Bowel resection of a patient with juvenile polyposis syndrome and multiple spherical pedunculated polyps with a smooth surface. (b) Gross appearance of a juvenile polyp from a patient with juvenile polyposis syndrome. Note the smooth surface, in contrast with a Peutz–Jeghers polyp.

a positive family history of juvenile polyposis [24,27]. The incidence of juvenile polyposis syndrome is approximately 1/100 000 live births.

In about 50–60% of juvenile polyposis syndrome patients a germline defect in the *SMAD4* or *BMPR1A* gene can be found [28,29]. Both genes are involved in the BMP/TGF-β (bone morphogenetic protein/transforming growth factor β) signalling pathway. Most of these germline defects are point mutations or small base-pair deletions in *SMAD4* or *BMPR1A* that can be identified by conventional sequence

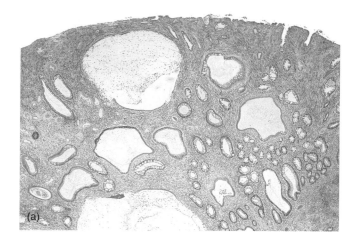

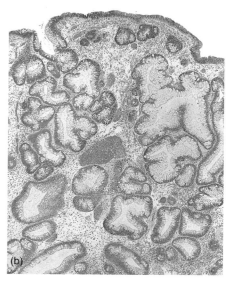

Figure 23.7 (a) Histological section of a juvenile polyp from a juvenile polyposis patient with a germline mutation of *BMPR1A*. Typically juvenile polyps are characterised by a prominent lamina propria with oedema and inflammatory cells and cystically dilated glands lined by cuboidal to columnar epithelium with reactive changes. (b) Histological section of a juvenile polyp from a juvenile polyposis patient with a germline mutation of *SMAD4*. This polyp shows relatively less stroma, fewer dilated glands and more proliferative smaller glands.

analysis. About 15% of the germline genetic defects are deletions of one or more exons or the entire *SMAD4* or *BMPR1A* gene, which can be identified by techniques to analyse large genomic deletions such as MLPA [28,29].

As about half of juvenile polyposis syndrome patients remain without a molecular diagnosis, a number of candidate genes, mostly involved in the TGF-β/BMP pathway, have been investigated for a role in juvenile polyposis syn-

drome pathogenesis. Germline mutation of the TGF-β co-receptor endoglin (*ENG*) has been reported in two juvenile polyposis syndrome patients but the role of *ENG* as a juvenile polyposis syndrome susceptibility gene is under debate because no additional *ENG* mutations have been found in a total of 65 juvenile polyposis syndrome patients [28,30]. In addition, *SMAD1*, *SMAD2*, *SMAD3*, *SMAD5*, *SMAD7*, *BMPR2*, *BMPR1B*, *ACVRL1*, *TGFBRII* and *CDX2* have been investigated but currently no germline mutations have been found in these genes [30]. Also *PTEN*, the gene originally linked to Cowden's syndrome and Bannayan–Riley–Ruvalcaba syndrome, has been suggested as a juvenile polyposis syndrome gene but it is believed that *PTEN* mutations in patients with juvenile polyps probably represent patients with Cowden's or Bannayan–Riley–Ruvalcaba syndrome who have not (yet) developed extra-intestinal clinical features specific to these conditions [31]. A recent study involving a large number of patients with *PTEN* germline, mutation-positive Cowden's syndrome substantiated this notion, showing that both upper and lower gastrointestinal polyps are a common manifestation of this syndrome. Patients afflicted by Cowden's syndrome may develop colorectal juvenile polyps indistinguishable from those in juvenile polyposis syndrome. Therefore, although the exact gastrointestinal manifestations of Cowden's syndrome remain to be clarified, particularly with respect to the upper gastrointestinal tract, Cowden's syndrome should be part of the differential diagnosis in a patient presenting with a small intestinal juvenile polyp [32].

Clinically, juvenile polyposis can present in two forms. One is a generalised form that occurs in infancy, in which polyps are present in the stomach, small bowel and colon. The polyps vary in size from 1 mm to 30 mm, and may be sessile or pedunculated. These infants have diarrhoea, haemorrhage, malnutrition and intussusception, and death is usual at an early age. In addition, many of these patients have congenital abnormalities, including macrocephaly and generalised hypotonia [5]. It has been suggested that this rare form of juvenile polyposis, called juvenile polyposis of infancy, is caused by continuous deletion of *BMPR1A* and *PTEN* genes located on chromosome 10q23.2 and 10q23.3, respectively, although others disagree [33].

The second form, called generalised juvenile polyposis or juvenile polyposis coli, usually presents later in childhood or in adult life and may be sporadic/new or inherited [34]. This form is characterised by the presence of gastrointestinal juvenile polyposis and an increased risk of gastrointestinal cancer [35]. Also, a variety of extra-intestinal manifestations has been reported in about 10–78% of these patients [5]. In about 50% of these colon-restricted or generalised cases of juvenile polyposis syndrome, a heterozygous germline mutation within the *SMAD4* gene or the *BMPR1A* gene can be identified. Differences in the phenotypic expressions between carriers of a *SMAD4* and

BMPR1A mutation may exist, e.g. *SMAD4* mutations have been associated with a more aggressive gastrointestinal phenotype, with higher incidence of colonic adenomas and carcinomas and more frequent upper gastrointestinal polyps than patients with a *BMPR1A* mutation [36]. Also, the combined syndrome of juvenile polyposis syndrome and hereditary hemorrhagic telangiectasia (Osler–Weber–Rendu syndrome) is associated with germline mutations in *SMAD4* [37].

Polyps in juvenile polyposis syndrome predominantly occur in the colorectum, varying in number from five to several hundreds (see Chapter 37). In addition, polyps can be found in the stomach, duodenum, jejunum and ileum, although the incidence of upper gastrointestinal tract polyps in juvenile polyposis syndrome is less well studied (Figure 23.8). A few studies have examined upper gastrointestinal tract involvement in juvenile polyposis more systematically [38–40]. One study found duodenal polyps in 4 of 12 patients with juvenile polyposis syndrome (33%), with two patients having multiple polyps ranging in size from 5 mm to 15 mm and two patients with minute polyps [38]. Other workers have found small intestinal polyps, beyond the range of standard gastroscopy, in 2 of 10 (20%) patients who underwent capsule endoscopy and duodenal polyps in 4 other patients (40%) [40]. Another study reported small bowel polyps in 8 of 56 patients with juvenile polyposis syndrome (14%) [39]. In addition, there are a number of case reports of duodenal, jejunal and ileal polyps in patients with juvenile polyposis syndrome [34,41–44]. Moreover, juvenile polyps are frequently found in the ileal pouch of juvenile polyposis patients who have undergone proctocolectomy [45,46].

Histologically, small intestinal polyps in juvenile polyposis syndrome have been classified as juvenile [39,41], hyperplastic and/or inflammatory polyps [38,42,44] and normal mucosa raised by lymphoid hyperplasia [42,43]. The larger small intestinal polyps resemble those seen in the colon [43]. In addition, juvenile/hamartomatous polyps with dysplastic changes and adenomas have been found in the duodenum, jejunum and ileum of patients with juvenile polyposis syndrome [38,39,44]. Moreover, we have seen a Brunner's gland hamartoma in the duodenum of a juvenile polyposis patient with a *SMAD4* germline mutation. To our knowledge this has not been reported previously.

Juvenile polyposis is associated with an increased risk of gastrointestinal cancer. A recent cancer risk analysis calculated a cumulative life-time risk for colorectal cancer in juvenile polyposis syndrome of 39% and a relative risk of colorectal cancer of 34 [47]. However, this may be a conservative estimate because some patients in this study had undergone prophylactic colectomy. In addition, several cases of stomach, duodenal and pancreatic cancer in juvenile polyposis syndrome have been described in the literature but there is no formal risk analysis for these cancers [35]. One study found small bowel carcinoma in 6 of 56 (11%) patients with juvenile polyposis syndrome but 4 of these cancers occurred in one family [39]. Evaluation of literature reports suggests that gastric and small bowel carcinoma together occur at about a fifth the frequency of colorectal cancers in this patient group [47].

Cancer pathogenesis in juvenile polyposis is still poorly understood. One promulgated theorem is that it develops through the so-called landscaper mechanism. The landscaper model was proposed after the observation that the genetic alterations at chromosome 10q22 (*BMPR1A* locus) occurred predominantly in the stroma of juvenile polyps and postulates that cancer develops as a result of an abnormal stromal environment which can induce carcinogenesis of the adjacent epithelium [48]. More recently, additional evidence in support of the 'landscaper' defect in juvenile polyposis syndrome came from a study where BMP-4 was localised exclusively to the mesenchymal compartment of the intestine in mice and disrupted BMP signalling resulted in development of a juvenile polyposis-like phenotype [49]. In contrast, homozygous *SMAD4* deletions have been found primarily in the epithelium of juvenile polyps from patients with juvenile polyposis syndrome and germline *SMAD4* mutations, and *SMAD4* knockout mice [50]. Although further studies are needed, this suggests that *SMAD4* may act as a 'gatekeeper', rather than a 'landscaper' in the pathogenesis of juvenile polyposis syndrome, which would be in line with the role of *SMAD4* in other cancer types [51].

Management of juvenile polyposis syndrome is mainly based on expert opinion. Patients at risk or with a high

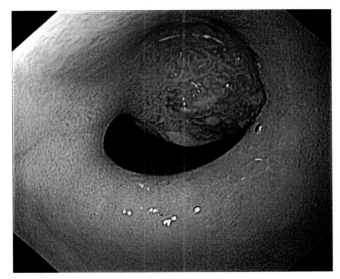

Figure 23.8 Endoscopic picture of a juvenile polyp in the duodenum of a patient with juvenile polyposis syndrome.

suspicion of juvenile polyposis syndrome should have endoscopic screening of the colon and upper gastrointestinal tract at age 15 or at the time of the first symptoms [52]. At the time of diagnosis of juvenile polyposis syndrome, the entire gastrointestinal tract should be examined for the presence of polyps [5]. Genetic testing can be useful for at-risk members from families where germline mutations have been identified. If no germline mutation is found in such an at-risk person, he or she does not have juvenile polyposis syndrome and can be followed in accordance with the guidelines for screening programmes for the general population [52].

Endoscopic examination of the colon and upper gastrointestinal tract is recommended every 2–3 years in patients with juvenile polyposis syndrome. In patients with polyps, endoscopic screening should be performed yearly, until the patient is polyp-free. Patients with mild polyposis can be managed by frequent endoscopic examinations and polypectomy [5,46,52]. Intraoperative enteroscopy to evaluate small intestinal polyps can be considered at the time of colorectal surgery [44]. Endoscopic treatment of gastric polyps is often difficult and patients with symptomatic gastric polyposis (e.g. severe anaemia) eventually need subtotal or total gastrectomy.

Prophylactic surgery needs consideration in patients with polyposis that cannot be managed endoscopically (>50–100 polyps), severe gastrointestinal bleeding or diarrhoea, juvenile polyps with dysplasia and a strong family history of colorectal cancer [45–47]. Surgical options include subtotal colectomy with ileo-rectal anastomosis (IRA) or total proctocolectomy with pouch [45,46]. It is unclear which type of surgery is preferable but, in analogy with familial adenomatous polyposis, it may depend on the extent of the rectal polyposis. Recurrence of rectal polyps in patients with subtotal colectomy is frequent and about half of these individuals require subsequent proctectomy [45,46]. Therefore, total proctocolectomy has been advocated as the initial surgery for patients with massive juvenile polyposis that cannot be managed endoscopically [46]. Although the surgery of choice in juvenile polyposis syndrome remains debatable, patients need frequent postoperative endoscopic surveillance because of high recurrence rates of polyps in the remnant rectum and the pouch [45].

In patients with juvenile polyposis syndrome and a germline *SMAD4* mutation, screening should be considered for arteriovenous malformations using chest radiography, magnetic resonance imaging of the brain and liver sonography [37]. In addition, digital clubbing and pulmonary osteoarthropathy are frequently described in combination with arteriovenous malformations [43].

Recently it has been recognised that COX-2 expression is higher in juvenile polyposis syndrome polyps than in sporadic juvenile polyps and correlates with polyp size and dysplasia [53]. This observation suggests that chemoprevention, using selective or non-selective COX-2 inhibitors, could be beneficial in juvenile polyposis syndrome. Currently, NSAID chemoprevention in juvenile polyposis syndrome has not been studied systematically but two patients with juvenile polyposis syndrome, who had proctocolectomy with a pouch and subsequent polypectomy from the pouch, did not develop further polyps in the pouch while on sulindac [45]. However, the value of NSAID chemoprevention in juvenile polyposis syndrome requires further investigation.

Cronkhite–Canada syndrome

This excessively rare syndrome combines diffuse polypoid thickening of the gastrointestinal mucosa, including the small intestine, with ectodermal changes such as alopecia, hyperpigmentation and atrophy of the nails. There is loss of protein from the gut [54,55]. It was first described in 1955 and occurs primarily in middle-aged patients, aged between 50 and 70 years [56,57]. The mucosa appears grossly to be diffusely inflamed and is carpeted with small rounded polyps (Figure 23.9) which are composed of dilated glands surrounded by an oedematous stroma (Figure 23.10) [58].

There is a histological similarity to juvenile polyps [59] and also to the stomach in Ménétrier's disease [60]. Endocrine and Paneth cells are reduced or absent [61]. Whether the ectodermal changes are the result of the loss of essential amino acids in the excessive secretion of glycoprotein [62], or whether all the manifestations of the syndrome, including the small intestinal changes, are the result of impaired growth, possibly due to a deficiency state [61], is unknown. There is no standard therapy. Limited success has been reported with antibiotics, steroids and partial gastrectomy. The polyps are non-neoplastic but coexisting adenomas and adenocarcinomas have been reported [57,58].

Pyogenic granuloma

Pyogenic granuloma has been described in the small bowel [63]. It resembles pyogenic granuloma at other sites, being a polypoid mass of granulation tissue with a narrow stalk and erosion at the surface (Figure 23.11). The significance of this lesion is unknown. Patients typically present with gastrointestinal bleeding. Kaposi's sarcoma may be in the differential diagnosis. Human herpesvirus 8 (HHV8) immunostaining can reliably distinguish between the two [64]. Very rarely, a condition that is effectively pyogenic granulomatous polyposis of the small intestine, namely multiple polyps composed largely of granulation tissue, occurs as complication of endocrine tumours of the small intestine, the pathogenesis probably resulting from the effect of such tumours on the blood supply of the small intestine [65].

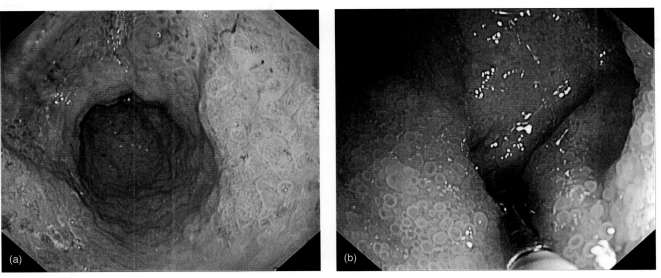

Figure 23.9 Endoscopic picture of (a) the duodenum and (b) the jejunum of a patient with Cronkhite–Canada syndrome. The mucosa appears diffusely inflamed and carpeted with small rounded polyps.

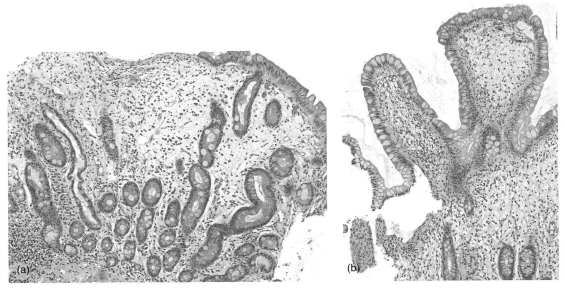

Figure 23.10 Histological section of (a) duodenal and (b) jejunal biopsies from the patient with Cronkhite–Canada syndrome of Figure 23.9, characterised by stromal oedema and reactive epithelial changes.

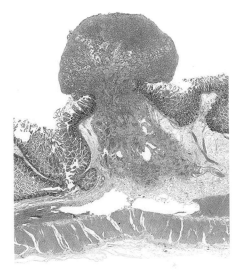

Figure 23.11 Histological section of a pyogenic granuloma in the small bowel.

References

1. Attanoos R, Williams GT. Epithelial and neuroendocrine tumors of the duodenum. *Semin Diagn Pathol* 1991;**8**:149.

2. Levine JA, Burgart LJ, Batts KP, Wang KK. Brunner's gland hamartomas: clinical presentation and pathological features of 27 cases. *Am J Gastroenterol* 1995;**90**:290.

3. Ryan A, Lafnitzegger JR, Lin DH, Jakate S, Staren ED. Myoepithelial hamartoma of the duodenal wall. *Virchows Arch* 1998; **432**:191.

4. Jansen M, Ten Klooster JP, Offerhaus GJ, Clevers H. LKB1 and AMPK family signaling: the intimate link between cell polarity and energy metabolism. *Physiol Rev* 2009;**89**:777.

5. Brosens LA, van Hattem WA, Jansen M, de Leng WW, Giardiello FM, Offerhaus GJ. Gastrointestinal polyposis syndromes. *Curr Mol Med* 2007;**7**:29.

6. Westerman AM, Entius MM, de Baar E, et al. Peutz–Jeghers syndrome: 78-year follow-up of the original family. *Lancet* 1999; **353**:1211.

7. Hemminki A, Tomlinson I, Markie D, et al. Localization of a susceptibility locus for Peutz–Jeghers syndrome to 19p using comparative genomic hybridization and targeted linkage analysis. *Nat Genet* 1997;**15**:87.

8. Hearle N, Schumacher V, Menko FH, et al. Frequency and spectrum of cancers in the Peutz–Jeghers syndrome. *Clin Cancer Res* 2006;**12**:3209.

9. Hearle NC, Rudd MF, Lim W, et al. Exonic *STK11* deletions are not a rare cause of Peutz–Jeghers syndrome. *J Med Genet* 2006; **43**:e15.

10. de Leng WW, Jansen M, Carvalho R, et al. Genetic defects underlying Peutz–Jeghers syndrome (PJS) and exclusion of the polarity-associated *MARK/Par1* gene family as potential PJS candidates. *Clin Genet* 2007;**72**:568.

11. Udd L, Katajisto P, Rossi DJ, et al. Suppression of Peutz–Jeghers polyposis by inhibition of cyclooxygenase-2. *Gastroenterology* 2004;**127**:1030.

12. Jansen M, de Leng WW, Baas AF, et al. Mucosal prolapse in the pathogenesis of Peutz–Jeghers polyposis. *Gut* 2006;**55**:1.

13. Shepherd NA, Bussey HJ, Jass JR. Epithelial misplacement in Peutz–Jeghers polyps. A diagnostic pitfall. *Am J Surg Pathol* 1987; **11**:743.

14. Hizawa K, Iida M, Matsumoto T, Kohrogi N, Yao T, Fujishima M. Neoplastic transformation arising in Peutz–Jeghers polyposis. *Dis Colon Rectum* 1993;**36**:953.

15. Linos DA, Dozois RR, Dahlin DC, Bartholomew LG. Does Peutz–Jeghers syndrome predispose to gastrointestinal malignancy? A later look. *Arch Surg* 1981;**116**:1182.

16. de Leng WW, Jansen M, Keller JJ, et al. Peutz–Jeghers syndrome polyps are polyclonal with expanded progenitor cell compartment. *Gut* 2007;**56**:1475.

17. Rossi DJ, Ylikorkala A, Korsisaari N, et al. Induction of cyclooxygenase-2 in a mouse model of Peutz-Jeghers polyposis. *Proc Natl Acad Sci U S A* 2002;**99**:12327.

18. McGarrity TJ, Amos C. Peutz–Jeghers syndrome: clinicopathology and molecular alterations. *Cell Mol Life Sci* 2006;**63**:2135.

19. Young RH. Sex cord-stromal tumors of the ovary and testis: their similarities and differences with consideration of selected problems. *Mod Pathol* 2005;**18**(suppl 2):S81.

20. Young S, Gooneratne S, Straus FH 2nd, Zeller WP, Bulun SE, Rosenthal IM. Feminizing Sertoli cell tumors in boys with Peutz-Jeghers syndrome. *Am J Surg Pathol* 1995;**19**:50.

21. Giardiello FM, Trimbath JD. Peutz–Jeghers syndrome and management recommendations. *Clin Gastroenterol Hepatol* 2006; **4**:408.

22. Woo A, Sadana A, Mauger DT, Baker MJ, Berk T, McGarrity TJ. Psychosocial impact of Peutz–Jeghers syndrome. *Fam Cancer* 2009;**8**:59.

23. Diamond M. Adenoma of the rectum in children: report of a case in a thirty-year-old girl. *Am J Dis Child* 1939;**57**:360.

24. Giardiello FM, Hamilton SR, Kern SE, et al. Colorectal neoplasia in juvenile polyposis or juvenile polyps. *Arch Dis Child* 1991; **66**:971.

25. Nugent KP, Talbot IC, Hodgson SV, Phillips RK. Solitary juvenile polyps: not a marker for subsequent malignancy. *Gastroenterology* 1993;**105**:698.

26. Aaltonen LA, Jass JR, Howe JR. Juvenile polyposis. In: Hamilton SR, Aaltonen LA (eds), *Pathology and Genetics of Tumours of the Digestive System*. Lyon: IARC Press, 2000: 130.

27. Jass JR, Williams CB, Bussey HJ, Morson BC. Juvenile polyposis – a precancerous condition. *Histopathology* 1988;**13**:619.

28. van Hattem WA, Brosens LA, de Leng WW, et al. Large genomic deletions of *SMAD4*, *BMPR1A* and *PTEN* in juvenile polyposis. *Gut* 2008;**57**:623.

29. Aretz S, Stienen D, Uhlhaas S, et al. High proportion of large genomic deletions and a genotype phenotype update in 80 unrelated families with juvenile polyposis syndrome. *J Med Genet* 2007;**44**:702.

30. Brosens LA, van Hattem WA, Kools MC, et al. No TGFBRII germline mutations in juvenile polyposis patients without SMAD4 or BMPR1A mutation. *Gut* 2009;**58**:154.

31. Eng C, Ji H. Molecular classification of the inherited hamartoma polyposis syndromes: clearing the muddied waters. *Am J Hum Genet* 1998;**62**:1020.

32. Heald B, Mester J, Rybicki L, Orloff MS, Burke CA, Eng C. Frequent gastrointestinal polyps and colorectal adenocarcinomas in a prospective series of *PTEN* mutation carriers. *Gastroenterology* 2010;**139**:1927.

33. Menko FH, Kneepkens CM, de Leeuw N, et al. Variable phenotypes associated with 10q23 microdeletions involving the *PTEN* and *BMPR1A* genes. *Clin Genet* 2008;**74**:145.

34. Sachatello CR, Pickren JW, Grace JT Jr. Generalized juvenile gastrointestinal polyposis. A hereditary syndrome. *Gastroenterology* 1970;**58**:699.

35. Howe JR, Mitros FA, Summers RW. The risk of gastrointestinal carcinoma in familial juvenile polyposis. *Ann Surg Oncol* 1998; **5**:751.

36. Handra-Luca A, Condroyer C, de Moncuit C, et al. Vessels' morphology in *SMAD4* and *BMPR1A*-related juvenile polyposis. *Am J Med Genet A* 2005;**138**:113.

37. Gallione CJ, Repetto GM, Legius E, et al. A combined syndrome of juvenile polyposis and hereditary haemorrhagic telangiectasia associated with mutations in *MADH4* (*SMAD4*). *Lancet* 2004; **363**:852.

38. Jarvinen HJ, Sipponen P. Gastroduodenal polyps in familial adenomatous and juvenile polyposis. *Endoscopy* 1986;**18**:230.

39. Woodford-Richens K, Bevan S, Churchman M, et al. Analysis of genetic and phenotypic heterogeneity in juvenile polyposis. *Gut* 2000;**46**:656.

40. Postgate AJ, Will OC, Fraser CH, Fitzpatrick A, Phillips RK, Clark SK. Capsule endoscopy for the small bowel in juvenile polyposis syndrome: a case series. *Endoscopy* 2009;**41**:1001.

41. Bentley E, Chandrasoma P, Radin R, Cohen H. Generalized juvenile polyposis with carcinoma. *Am J Gastroenterol* 1989;**84**:1456.

42. Sassatelli R, Bertoni G, Serra L, Bedogni G, Ponz de Leon M. Generalized juvenile polyposis with mixed pattern and gastric cancer. *Gastroenterology* 1993;**104**:910.

43. Cox KL, Frates RC J., Wong A, Gandhi G. Hereditary generalized juvenile polyposis associated with pulmonary arteriovenous malformation. *Gastroenterology* 1980;**78**:1566.

44. Rodriguez-Bigas MA, Penetrante RB, Herrera L, Petrelli NJ. Intraoperative small bowel enteroscopy in familial adenomatous and familial juvenile polyposis. *Gastrointest Endosc* 1995;**42**:560.

45. Oncel M, Church JM, Remzi FH, Fazio VW. Colonic surgery in patients with juvenile polyposis syndrome: a case series. *Dis Colon Rectum* 2005;**48**:49; discussion 55.

46. Scott-Conner CE, Hausmann M, Hall TJ, Skelton DS, Anglin BL, Subramony C. Familial juvenile polyposis: patterns of recurrence and implications for surgical management. *J Am Coll Surg* 1995;**181**:407.

47. Brosens LA, van Hattem A, Hylind LM, et al. Risk of colorectal cancer in juvenile polyposis. *Gut* 2007;**56**:965.

48. Kinzler KW, Vogelstein B. Landscaping the cancer terrain. *Science* 1998;**280**:1036.

49. Haramis AP, Begthel H, van den Born M, et al. *De novo* crypt formation and juvenile polyposis on BMP inhibition in mouse intestine. *Science* 2004;**303**:1684.

50. Woodford-Richens K, Williamson J, Bevan S, et al. Allelic loss at *SMAD4* in polyps from juvenile polyposis patients and use of fluorescence in situ hybridization to demonstrate clonal origin of the epithelium. *Cancer Res* 2000;**60**:2477.

51. Schutte M, Hruban RH, Hedrick L, et al. *DPC4* gene in various tumor types. *Cancer Res* 1996;**56**:2527.

52. Howe JR, Ringold JC, Hughes JH, Summers RW. Direct genetic testing for *Smad4* mutations in patients at risk for juvenile polyposis. *Surgery* 1999;**126**:162.

53. van Hattem WA, Brosens LA, Marks SY, et al. Increased cyclooxygenase-2 expression in juvenile polyposis syndrome. *Clin Gastroenterol Hepatol* 2009;**7**:93.

54. Jarnum S, Jensen H. Diffuse gastrointestinal polyposis with ectodermal changes. A case with severe malabsorption and enteric loss of plasma proteins and electrolytes. *Gastroenterology* 1966;**50**:107.

55. Johnston MM, Vosburgh JW, Wiens AT, Walsh GC. Gastrointestinal polyposis associated with alopecia, pigmentation, and atrophy of the fingernails and toenails. *Ann Intern Med* 1962;**56**:935.

56. Cronkhite LW Jr, Canada WJ. Generalized gastrointestinal polyposis; an unusual syndrome of polyposis, pigmentation, alopecia and onychotrophia. *N Engl J Med* 1955;**252**:1011.

57. Daniel ES, Ludwig SL, Lewin KJ, Ruprecht RM, Rajacich GM, Schwabe AD. The Cronkhite–Canada Syndrome. An analysis of clinical and pathologic features and therapy in 55 patients. *Medicine (Baltimore)* 1982;**61**:293.

58. Burke AP, Sobin LH. The pathology of Cronkhite–Canada polyps. A comparison to juvenile polyposis. *Am J Surg Pathol* 1989;**13**:940.

59. Ruymann FB. Juvenile polyps with cachexia. Report of an infant and comparison with Cronkhite–Canada syndrome in adults. *Gastroenterology* 1969;**57**:431.

60. Gill W, Wilken BJ. Diffuse gastrointestinal polyposis associated with hypoproteinaemia. *J R Coll Surg Edinb* 1967;**12**:149.

61. Freeman K, Anthony PP, Miller DS, Warin AP. Cronkhite Canada syndrome: a new hypothesis. *Gut* 1985;**26**:531.

62. Manousos O, Webster CU. Diffuse gastrointestinal polyposis with ectodermal changes. *Gut* 1966;**7**:375.

63. Yao T, Nagai E, Utsunomiya T, Tsuneyoshi M. An intestinal counterpart of pyogenic granuloma of the skin. A newly proposed entity. *Am J Surg Pathol* 1995;**19**:1054.

64. van Eeden S, Offerhaus GJ, Morsink FH, van Rees BP, Busch OR, van Noesel CJ. Pyogenic granuloma: an unrecognized cause of gastrointestinal bleeding. *Virchows Arch* 2004;**444**:590.

65. Allibone RO, Hoffmann J, Gosney JR, Helliwell TR. Granulation tissue polyposis associated with carcinoid tumours of the small intestine. *Histopathology* 1993;**22**:475.

CHAPTER 24

Epithelial tumours of the small intestine

Kieran Sheahan

University College Dublin; St Vincent's University Hospital, Dublin, Ireland

Introduction

Epithelial tumours are rare in the small intestine in comparison with the large bowel. In an analysis of data from multiple tumour registries in the USA [1], small bowel tumours occurred with an average annual incidence rate of $9.9/10^6$ people. Endocrine tumours (ETs), formerly carcinoids and also known as neuro-endocrine tumours (NETs), and adenocarcinomas, were the most common histological subtypes, with average annual incidence rates of 3.8 and $3.7/10^6$ people, respectively, followed by sarcomas ($1.3/10^6$ people) and lymphomas ($1.1/10^6$ people). The incidence of small intestinal malignancies has increased, primarily because of ETs, which are now the most common small bowel cancer [2]. Women are affected slightly more than men [3]. There is elevated risk for ETs of the small intestine with saturated fat intake [4]. Cholecystectomy increases the risk of intestinal cancer, a risk that declines with increasing distance from the common bile duct [5]. The risk of small intestinal adenocarcinoma is higher in patients with familial adenomatous polyposis (FAP), Crohn's disease and coeliac disease [6–9]. There have been two recent reports of small intestinal carcinoma in *MYH* polyposis [10,11]. A family history of cancer is a significant risk factor for all ETs, including carcinoid tumours [3,12].

There is good evidence for an adenoma–carcinoma sequence in the small bowel, as in the large intestine [13]. Although endocrine tumours, lymphomas and sarcomas occur most frequently in the distal small bowel and least frequently in the duodenum, the opposite is true for adenomas and adenocarcinomas [14]. Adenomas are present in the duodenum in over 90% of patients with FAP [9] and there is a high incidence of duodenal adenocarcinomas in these individuals. It is remarkable that the relatively small area of the duodenum is the site for more epithelial neoplasms than the whole of the rest of the small bowel. There is a phenomenon of clustering around the influx of undiluted bile from the ampulla of Vater [15] and it appears that bile salts act as tumour-promoting agents, especially together with acid from the stomach. It has been shown that bile is capable of inducing the formation of DNA adducts in the duodenal epithelium [16]. Despite the influence of bile, DNA adducts are reported to be found far less frequently in the epithelium of the small bowel than in the large bowel, suggesting that the small intestinal epithelium is less susceptible to the effects of environmental carcinogens [17].

Molecular genetics of small intestinal neoplasia

Although small intestinal adenocarcinoma is rare, we are slowly gaining more understanding of the molecular changes that occur in the genesis of these tumours and there is evidence that, despite morphological similarities, these are different to colorectal cancer. Hypermethylation of *hMLH1*, *HPP1*, *p14* (*ARF*), *p16* (*INK4A*) and *APC* is evident in primary adenocarcinomas of the small bowel [18]. There is also evidence that both β-catenin gene mutation [19], abnormal expression of E-cadherin and β-catenin and microsatellite instability may contribute to carcinogenesis of small intestinal tumours [20].

Cell cycle abnormalities are early and important events in the multi-step process of small bowel tumorigenesis, which, in this way, resembles colorectal carcinogenesis [21]. Eighty per cent of primary intestinal adenocarcinomas have deletions of 18q21-q22, which target *SMAD4*, a downstream component of the transforming growth factor β (TGF-β) pathway. Thus disruption of TGF-β signalling may play a role in small intestinal tumorigenesis [22].The frequency of *MSI* and *K-ras* and *p53* mutations appear to be similar to colorectal cancer but *APC* mutations appear to be uncommon [20]. As previously stated, the adenoma–carcinoma sequence model of carcinogenesis, similar to that of the colon, is also postulated to occur in the small intestine, especially in patients with FAP [23,24]. Indeed, the *APC MIN* mouse model, as originally described, produced more adenomas in the mouse small intestine than in the large intestine [25].

Adenomas

Adenomas are found more frequently in the duodenum, especially the peri-ampullary area, than in the more distal small bowel [26]. Although sporadic lesions are rare in the duodenum, in FAP they are found in all adult patients [27]. As in the large bowel, adenomas, within and without FAP, take the form of tubular, tubulovillous or villous adenomas [28]. It is likely that most sporadic small intestinal adenomas are never clinically discovered. Those that have been documented are the ones large enough to cause symptoms by obstructing the lumen [26]. Duodenal villous adenomas arising from the ampulla of Vater have a significant risk of either containing cancer or becoming malignant. Large duodenal villous adenomas usually require pancreatico-duodenectomy. A few studies have examined the role of localised ampullectomy in this setting, with mixed results [29–31]. Ultimately, larger and carpeting adenomas of the duodenum present a difficult management quandary: endoscopic methods of removal, ablative techniques and agents such as non-steroidal anti-inflammatory drugs (NSAIDs, especially sulindac) have all been tried with varying, often disappointing, results.

Most sporadic small bowel adenomas are single, although occasional multiple examples have been described. They can be pedunculated (Figure 24.1) or sessile (when they may be circumferential around the intestine) and can bleed and/or cause obstruction [32]. Macroscopically small bowel adenomas have a coarse lobulated appearance rather like their large bowel counterparts, though some of the duodenal lesions may have a more villous appearance [33].

Microscopically, as in the large bowel, they are classified as tubular, tubulovillous and villous adenomas, and graded as low and high grade. Cells showing absorptive, goblet cell, squamous, endocrine and Paneth cell differentiation can be found [34]. In many adenomas, one can find foci of invasive adenocarcinoma in resected specimens (Figure 24.2).

Adenomas in familial adenomatous polyposis

All adult patients with FAP have the propensity to develop multiple adenomas in the duodenal mucosa [9]. The lesions

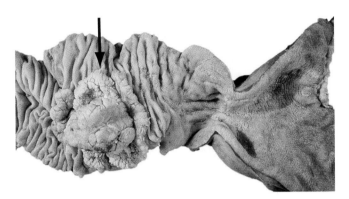

Figure 24.1 An adenomatous polyp (arrow) arising at the duodenal papilla. The lobulated surface is typical.

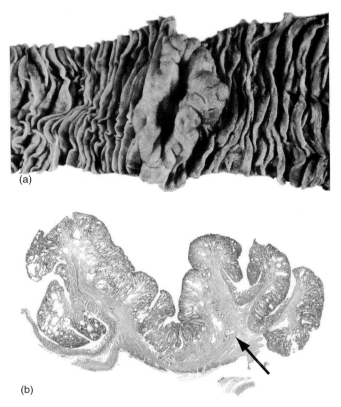

(a)

(b)

Figure 24.2 (a) A tubular adenoma of ileum, with adenocarcinoma arising in its centre, which is depressed. (b) Section of the tubular adenoma in (a), with the focus of adenocarcinoma arrowed.

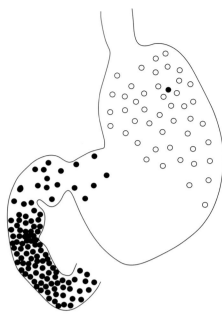

Figure 24.3 Diagram illustrating the frequency of occurrence of duodenal and gastric adenomas (solid circles) in a series of 102 patients with familial adenomatous polyposis. The open circles represent fundic gland polyps. (From Spigelman [37].)

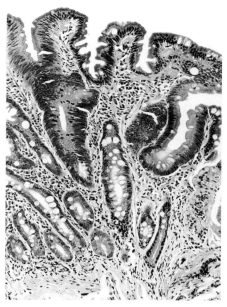

Figure 24.4 A small adenoma of duodenal mucosa from a patient with familial adenomatous polyposis. Although probably tubular, there is ambivalence of structure due to the villous nature of the normal mucosa.

tend to be clustered around the duodenal papilla and frequently involve the ampulla of Vater (Figure 24.3). The mucosa can be carpeted with adenomas but they can also be small and sessile and discovered only as a result of random biopsy of endoscopically normal mucosa. They are usually only a few millimetres in diameter and are composed of dysplastic epithelium, most frequently with a tubular pattern (Figure 24.4). The underlying villous architecture of the duodenal mucosa may confound the tubular nature of small lesions but 10% of these lesions are genuinely villous in structure and 20% are tubulovillous [13]. The dysplasia in most of these lesions is low grade but occasionally there is high grade dysplasia or carcinoma [35], as in adenomas of the large bowel.

Given the evidence for peri-ampullary adenocarcinoma arising as the result of an adenoma–carcinoma sequence [13], duodenal adenomas pose a difficult management problem in patients with FAP. The overall risk of duodenal cancer is, however, 5% of all individuals with FAP [36]. The Spigelman staging scheme for classification of duodenal adenomas in accordance with their malignant potential [37] (Table 24.1) is now the accepted standard [38]. This scheme provides useful guidelines to assist in the clinical management of these patients. Stage IV disease is found in about 10% of patients with FAP [13] but is regarded as a marker of high risk for development of duodenal carcinoma. One study reports a high duodenal polyposis progression rate with an increase in the Spigelman score in

Table 24.1 Staging system for severity of duodenal polyposis in familial adenomatous polyposis

Duodenal disease grading: points

	1	2	3
Polyp number	1–4	5–20	> 20
Polyp size (mm)	1–4	5–10	> 10
Histology	Tubular	Tubulovillous	Villous
Dysplasia	Mild	Moderate	Severe

Stages	
O	0 points
I	1–4 points
II	5–6 points
III	7–8 points
IV	9–12 points

Reproduced from Spigelman AD, Williams CB, Talbot IC, Domizio P, Phillips RK. Upper gastrointestinal cancer in patients with familial adenomatous polyposis. Lancet. 1989; 2: 783.

60% of cases and high grade dysplasia development in 34% [27]. Stage IV patients may need to be considered for prophylactic surgery based on the increased risk of cancer (4 of 11 patients, 36% in this series) and the difficulties in endoscopic surveillance [39]. Patients with FAP also have a high risk of developing adenomas in the ileal pouch [40].

Adenocarcinoma

Incidence

Although the small intestine contributes 75% of the mucosal surface area of the gastrointestinal tract, malignancies of the large bowel are 50 times more numerous [41] and the small bowel is the site of only 1% of all gastrointestinal carcinomas [42]. Conversely, adenocarcinoma is clinically more frequent in the small bowel than symptomatic sporadic adenoma. One study [43] found that only 14% of clinically detected small intestinal tumours were benign. Adenocarcinomas are most frequent in the duodenum and are increasingly less common at more distal sites [14]. They are usually single and reports of multiple small intestinal carcinomas are rare [44]. On the other hand, small intestinal carcinoma is often associated with a second (synchronous or metachronous) primary malignancy at another site, occurring in 20% of cases in one series [45]. The age incidence is similar to large bowel adenocarcinoma, the average age at presentation being 62–68 years [46,47].

Small intestinal adenocarcinoma is increased in gluten enteropathy [48], particularly in refractory coeliac disease, in Crohn's disease [49] and in hereditary non-polyposis colorectal cancer (HNPCC) [50]. Clinical presentations include abdominal pain (71%), an abdominal mass (14%), vomiting (10%), melaena (10%) and/or fever (9%) [51].

Gross appearances

Most small intestinal carcinomas are annular and constricting (Figure 24.5), although a minority are more polypoid.

Histological appearances

Microscopically, small intestinal carcinomas are classified according to the World Health Organization (WHO) classification and comprise adenocarcinoma, mucinous carcinoma, signet-ring carcinoma, small cell carcinoma, squamous cell carcinoma, adenosquamous cell carcinoma, medullary carcinoma and undifferentiated carcinoma [52]. Microscopically, small intestinal adenocarcinomas closely resemble adenocarcinomas of the large bowel (Figure 24.6), most being moderately differentiated. Spread is to regional lymph nodes and intraperitoneal spread to the peritoneal surface of the bowel is not uncommon (Figure 24.7).

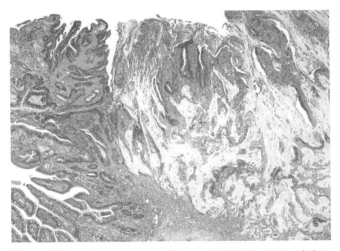

Figure 24.6 Adenocarcinoma of jejunum arising in a pre-existing adenoma. The upper and left hand aspects of the section show an adenoma with a villous pattern. To the right and below, there is carcinomatous change with some mucus secretion, part of which lies deep to the muscularis mucosae.

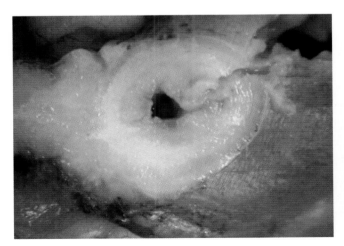

Figure 24.5 A stenosing carcinoma of the jejunum which presented with obstructive symptoms.

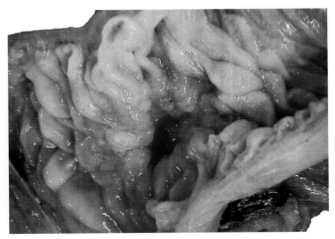

Figure 24.7 Recurrent small bowel adenocarcinoma 2 years post-resection of a pT4, pN1 primary tumour.

Staging

It is important to recognise that small intestinal carcinomas of the ampulla of Vater are staged separately to other small intestinal carcinomas [53]. The seventh edition of the TNM classification has recently updated these staging systems [54] (Tables 24.2 and 24.3). The 5-year survival rates are related to stage at presentation and vary between 20 and 52%, with a trend towards improving rates in recent studies [14,55,56]. In early pT1, pN0 adenocarcinoma of the ampulla of Vater, the prognosis is excellent, unless poorly differentiated [53].

Small bowel carcinoma in Crohn's disease

A recent meta-analysis has demonstrated a 27-fold increased risk of small bowel adenocarcinoma in Crohn's disease [49]. Factors associated with increased risk include duration of disease, fistulous disease, male gender and surgically excluded loops of small intestine. Crohn's disease-associated carcinomas occur at a younger age (46 versus 64 years), are three times more common in males and are more likely to be in the distal jejunum and ileum [57]. Coexisting epithelial dysplasia may be present [58]. As these tumours arise in a background of an abnormal mucosa and can be well differentiated, their diagnosis may also pose a problem for the pathologist.

Small bowel carcinoma in HNPCC

The association between HNPCC and small intestinal adenocarcinoma was first reported in 1985 [50]. The lifetime risk is estimated to be 1–4% with a relative risk of 100 [59]. It is reported to be higher in *MLH1* mutation carriers than in those with *MSH2* [60,61]. One large series reported a younger age of onset (39 years) compared with colorectal cancer, with small bowel cancer often the first manifestation of disease [62]. Of note, 50% of tumours were in the duodenum and accessible to upper endoscopy screening. The histopathological features and the MSI (microsatellite) and MMR (mismatch repair) status were similar to colorectal cancers. The MSI-H phenotype has been found in 5–45% of unselected small bowel carcinomas [20,63–65].

Endocrine tumours

The endocrine cells dispersed within the epithelium of the small intestinal mucosa constitute a major part of the diffuse endocrine system which is distributed throughout the endodermally derived mucosa and together form the largest endocrine organ in the body. The cells contributing

---

Table 24.2 TNM classification of primary small intestinal adenocarcinoma

T: primary tumour
TX: primary tumour cannot be assessed
T0: no evidence of primary tumour
Tis: *carcinoma in situ*
T1: tumour invades lamina propria, or muscularis mucosae, or submucosa
   T1a: tumour invades lamina propria, muscularis mucosae
   T1b: tumour invades submucosa
T2: tumour invades muscularis propria
T3: tumour invades subserosa or non-peritonealised perimuscular tissue (mesentery or retroperitoneum) with extension ≤20 mm
T4: tumour perforates visceral peritoneum or directly invades other organs or structures (including other loops of small intestine, mesentery, or retroperitoneum ≥20 mm and abdominal wall by way of serosa; for duodenum only, invasion of pancreas)

N: regional lymph nodes
NX: regional lymph nodes cannot be assessed
N0: no regional lymph node metastasis
N1: metastasis in one to three regional lymph nodes
N2: metastasis in four or more regional lymph nodes

M: distant metastasis
M0: no distant metastasis
M1: distant metastasis

Reproduced from Sobin LH, Wittekind C. TNM Classification of Malignant Tumours 7th ed.: Wiley-Blackwell; 2010.

Table 24.3 TNM Classification of adenocarcinoma of ampulla of Vater

T: primary tumour
TX: primary tumour cannot be assessed
T0: no evidence of primary tumour
Tis: carcinoma *in situ*
T1: tumour limited to ampulla of Vater or sphincter of Oddi
T2: tumour invades duodenal wall
T3: tumour invades pancreas
T4: tumour invades peri-pancreatic soft tissues, or other adjacent organs or structures

N: regional lymph nodes
NX: regional lymph nodes cannot be assessed
N0: no regional lymph node metastasis
N1: regional lymph node metastasis (splenic and tail of pancreas positive lymph nodes are M1)

M: distant metastasis
M0: no distant metastasis
M1: distant metastasis

Reproduced from Sobin LH, Wittekind C. TNM Classification of Malignant Tumours 7th ed.: Wiley-Blackwell; 2010.

to this system are functionally diverse, synthesising a variety of peptide hormone products. Their features are described in Chapter 17 (see 'Endocrine cells', Chapter 17).

Tumours of the diffuse endocrine system have been termed 'carcinoid tumours', 'neuro-endocrine tumours', 'endocrine tumours', 'endocrine cell tumours' and 'endocrine carcinomas'. Indeed different classifications use different terminology although, in general, there is a move away from the appellation 'carcinoid' because this term does not give an accurate guide to behaviour, the latter being notoriously variable for different sites in the gastrointestinal tract. The small intestine is a prime example, with tumours of the duodenum being either benign or low grade malignant, in general, whereas tumours of the jejunum and ileum tend to more aggressive and more likely to metastasise. Further, in many newer classifications, the prefix 'neuro-' has been dropped because this was initially used to infer that the cell of origin derived from the neural crest: we now understand that all endocrine cells derive locally from stem cells in the intestinal crypt.

So, the generic term 'endocrine tumour' (ET) embraces a heterogeneous collection of tumours defined by their predominantly diffuse endocrine cell differentiation. The most common differentiated tumour within this group is the enterochromaffin cell (EC-cell) tumour, traditionally known as the classic carcinoid tumour. Less common are G-cell tumours (gastrinomas), D-cell tumours (somatostatinomas) and L-cell tumours (tumours that synthesise enteroglucagon, glucagon, glicentin, peptide YY [PYY] and pancreatic polypeptide [PP]), which are mainly found in the mid- and hindgut. Occasionally one of the above tumours will be less well differentiated but the archetypal poorly differentiated endocrine tumour is the small cell ('oat cell') carcinoma. Subdivision according to ontogeny (foregut, midgut and hindgut) [66] provides a theoretical basis for classification. Foregut carcinoids include those of the bronchus, stomach, pancreas and duodenum. Midgut tumours include all other small intestinal endocrine tumours.

Diagnosis and management of endocrine tumours

Clinically, patients present with symptoms of local tumour invasion or tumour-related fibrosis. Carcinoid syndrome represents a minority of clinical presentations. Serum chromogranin A, urinary 5-hydroxyindole acetic acid [5HIAA]) or somatostatin-receptor scintigraphy is invaluable for early diagnosis. Endoscopic techniques using wireless capsule endoscopy are being evaluated for the diagnosis of small intestinal endocrine tumours (ETs) [67]. More advanced ETs, arising in the jejunum and ileum, can be accurately diagnosed on abdominal imaging, especially computed tomography (CT), because of the crab-like contraction of mesenteric connective tissues induced by tumorous involvement of the mesentery.

Surgical resection is the treatment of choice. In patients with liver metastatic disease, resection or local ablation techniques may be considered. Somatostatin analogues are often used to control symptoms due to hypersecretion of functional hormones/peptides (e.g. in the carcinoid syndrome) and has been shown to have an anti-proliferative effect in low-volume, metastatic, well differentiated, midgut ETs [68]. Classic cytotoxic agents are rarely effective in ETs of the small intestine, although novel targeted agents (anti-angiogenic agents, tyrosine kinase inhibitors and mTOR [mammalian target of rapamycin] inhibitors) are currently been tested with some encouraging results. Systemic chemotherapy is usually reserved for poorly differentiated tumours [69].

Classification, grading and staging of small intestinal ETs

According to the WHO classification (Table 24.4), well differentiated ETs with benign or uncertain behaviour account for 10–30% of cases, well differentiated endocrine carcinomas for 50–80% and poorly differentiated endocrine carcinomas for 1–3% [70]. Those endocrine carcinomas >10 mm are more likely to show evidence of local invasion, angio-invasion and/or lymph node metastatic disease. Criteria for staging and grading of ETs of fore-, mid- and hindgut have been proposed by the European Neuro-endocrine Tumour Society (ENETS) [71,72]. The recent TNM classification (seventh edition) is based on these proposals (Table 24.5). It is important to note that high grade endocrine carcinomas are excluded from this staging system. They should be classified using the criteria for their primary site (i.e. small intestinal carcinoma). The use of standard datasets, such as those published by the Royal College of Pathologists in the UK (accessed at www.rcpath.org/resources/pdf/g081dataset giendocrinenov09.pdf) and the College of American Pathologists in the USA (accessed at www.cap.org/apps/docs/committees/cancer/cancer_protocols/2011/Small bowelNET_11protocol.pdf) should ensure more consistency in pathological reporting.

Duodenal endocrine tumours

Only 2% of endocrine tumours arise in the duodenum but those that do are unusual and present diagnostic challenges to the histopathologist. Unusual morphological features and specific clinical syndromes can cause diagnostic confusion. Five types of ETs are reported in the duodenum and upper jejunum [73,74]. These include in decreasing frequency: gastrinomas or G-cell tumours, somatostatin-containing D-cell tumours or somatostatinomas, other

Table 24.4 WHO classification of gastroenteropancreatic endocrine tumours

Site	Well differentiated endocrine tumour (benign behaviour)	Well differentiated endocrine tumour (uncertain behaviour)	Well differentiated endocrine carcinoma (low grade malignant)	Poorly differentiated endocrine carcinoma (high grade malignant)
Duodenum, upper jejunum	Confined to mucosa-submucosa	Confined to mucosa–submucosa	Well to moderately differentiated	Small cell carcinoma
	≤10 mm No vascular invasion	>10 mm or vascular invasion	Invasion to muscularis propria or beyond or metastasis	
Ileum	Confined to mucosa-submucosa, ≤10 mm (small intestine)	Confined to mucosa-submucosa, >10 mm (small intestine)	Well to moderately differentiated Invasion to muscularis propria or beyond or metastasis	Small cell carcinoma

Adapted from Solcia GK, Sobin LH. Histological Typing of Endocrine Tumours (WHO). World Health Organization. International Histological Classification of Tumours. Springer-Verlag; 2000, with kind permission from Springer Science+Business Media.

Table 24.5 TNM classification for small intestinal endocrine tumours of duodenum, ampulla, jejunum and ileum (only well differentiated tumours and carcinomas)

T: primary tumour
TX: primary tumour cannot be assessed
T0: no evidence of primary tumour
T1: tumour invades lamina propria or submucosa and size ≤10 mm[a]
T2: tumour invades muscularis propria or size >10 mm
T3: jejunal or ileal tumour invades subserosa; ampullary or duodenal tumour invades pancreas or retroperitoneum
T4: tumour perforates visceral peritoneum (serosa) or invades other organs or adjacent structures
For any T, add (m) for multiple tumours

N: regional lymph nodes
NX: regional lymph nodes cannot be assessed
N0: no regional lymph node metastasis
N1: regional lymph node metastasis

M: distant metastasis
M0: no distant metastasis
M1: distant metastasis

[a]Note: tumour limited to ampulla of Vater for ampullary gangliocytic paraganglioma.
Reproduced from Sobin LH, Wittekind C. TNM Classification of Malignant Tumours 7th ed.: Wiley-Blackwell; 2010.

well differentiated endocrine tumours, poorly differentiated endocrine carcinomas/small cell carcinomas and the rare gangliocytic paraganglioma. Gangliocytic paragangliomas are usually benign but the behaviour of all the other tumours depends on their size, extent of spread in the duodenal wall, vascular invasion and hormonal function, which may result in a clinical peptide hormone hypersecretion syndrome.

Gastrinomas (G-cell tumours)

The incidence of gastrinomas is 0.5–3/10^6 per year. It is the most common functioning and malignant pancreatic endocrine tumour (30%). However, duodenal tumours account for up to 88% of gastrinomas in sporadic Zollinger–Ellison syndrome and 70–100% of gastrinomas in multiple endocrine neoplasia type 1 (MEN-1) patients [75]. It is important to emphasise that the diagnosis of gastrinoma requires the presence of a gastrin-positive ET with Zollinger–Ellison syndrome. Gastrin-positive ETs without Zollinger–Ellison syndrome are not considered gastrinomas. Gastrinomas have also been rarely described as a primary in other sites (e.g. bile duct, liver and heart).

The diagnosis of duodenal gastrinomas is often difficult, the mean delay from onset of symptoms being 5 years. The mean age of onset is 48–55 years (32–35 years in MEN-1/ Zollinger–Ellison syndrome). Most patients present with peptic ulceration and gastro-oesophageal reflux disease (GORD). The common use of proton pump inhibitors (PPIs) now masks the diagnosis in many cases. Twenty-five per cent of MEN-1 patients lack a family history, so all Zollinger–Ellison syndrome patients should be screened for MEN-1. The diagnosis usually requires a fasting serum gastrin level and is confirmed with a secretin challenge test. Combinations of endoscopic ultrasonography (EUS), duodenal endoscopy, standard axial imaging (CT and magnetic resonance imaging [MRI]) with nuclear imaging (somatostatin receptor scintigraphy, positron emission tomography [PET]/CT using different tracers) are required to identify these often small, indeed very small, lesions. This requires the close cooperation of endoscopists, radiologists and pathologists. Patients with MEN-1/Zollinger–Ellison syndrome (accounting for 30% of Zollinger–Ellison syndrome patients) have predominantly duodenal gastrinomas but usually have additional multi-hormone-secreting pancreatic tumours. At surgery, 80% of gastrinomas are located in the 'gastric triangle' in the duodenal and pancreatic head area.

Gastrinomas are subdivided into four categories by the WHO (see Table 24.4). Multiple small gastrin-producing ETs may be found in the proximal duodenum in up to 90% of patients with MEN-1 [76,77]. Most individuals have hypergastrinaemia and Zollinger–Ellison syndrome. This was previously thought to be the result of gastrin secretion from one or more of the pancreatic endocrine tumours that occur in MEN-1. However, it is now apparent that one or more minute duodenal gastrin-secreting tumours are responsible. These often measure less than 5 mm in diameter (Figure 24.8) [76] and are too small to be identified endoscopically unless random biopsies of the duodenal bulb are taken. At least some appear to arise in a background of duodenal mucosal endocrine cell hyperplasia, allowing a spectrum to be recognised from hyperplasia through multiple intramucosal 'microcarcinoids' to macroscopic infiltrative tumours [77]. Endoscopic or surgical extirpation is important in the clinical management of Zollinger–Ellison syndrome in MEN-1 patients [75].

Microscopically, gastrinomas are infiltrative neoplasms with a trabecular or pseudo-glandular appearance separated by a vascular stroma which allows them to be easily recognised as endocrine tumours (Figure 24.9). The tumour cells have round nuclei containing stippled chromatin and inconspicuous nucleoli, with few or no mitoses, and stain positively for chromogranin, synaptophysin, CD56 and gastrin [77]. Mitotic rate per 10 high power fields (hpf) and Ki67 index should always be reported. The Ki67 index is usually between 2 and 10%.

Liver metastases are the most important prognostic factor. The 10-year survival rate with liver involvement is 10–20%. Other factors associated with a poorer outcome

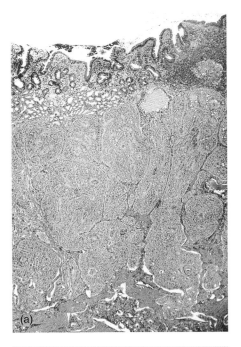

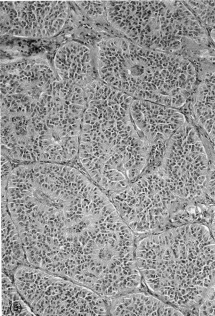

Figure 24.9 A duodenal gastrinoma: (a) low-power view showing a well differentiated endocrine cell neoplasm with a mixed trabecular and acinar architecture. (b) Higher power shows regular tumour cells with granular eosinophilic cytoplasm that is most abundant at the periphery of the cellular aggregates, a typical feature of gastrointestinal endocrine neoplasms.

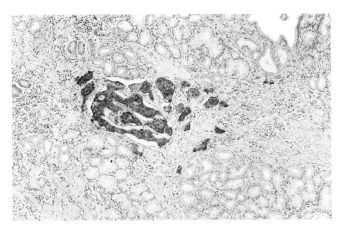

Figure 24.8 Microscopic duodenal gastrinoma in a patient with Zollinger–Ellison syndrome and type 1 multiple endocrine neoplasia. No macroscopic abnormality was visible. Gastrin immunostaining.

are inadequate control of gastric acid hypersecretion, lymph node and/or bone metastatic disease, female gender, absence of MEN-1, short disease history from onset to diagnosis, presence of a large (>30 mm) primary tumour, presence of ectopic Cushing's syndrome, high *HER2* gene expression, 1q loss of heterozygosity (LOH) and adverse histological features [78–82]. Treatment is both medical (control of acid hypersecretion) and surgical. Recommended surgical treatment for duodenal tumours is duodenotomy/enucleation with lymph node dissection. A pancreatico-duodenectomy is not usually recommended [74].

Somatostatin-producing ET (somatostatinoma)

Somatostatinomas are rare tumours with only 105 small intestinal primaries reported in the literature up to 2008, 103 in the duodenum and 2 in the jejunum [83]. In this literature review, 93% of tumours were sporadic and 7% familial [83]. The median age of onset of all somatostatinomas is 54 years. Familial cases are associated with type 1 neurofibromatosis (NF-1) [84], MEN-1 [76], and von Hippel–Lindau syndrome [85]. Phaeochromocytoma has been described in 15% of duodenal somatostatinomas with NF-1, occurring in 6 of 27 cases in one literature review [86]. The coexistence of a duodenal somatostatinoma and duodenal gangliocytic paraganglioma in an NF-1 patient has also been described [87]. There have been reports of a small number of cases of gastrointestinal stromal tumours (GISTs) in association with this tumour, all in association with von Recklinghausen's disease [88].

Somatostatinomas occur almost exclusively around the ampulla of Vater and may be asymptomatic or present with abdominal pain, jaundice or pancreatitis. The classic somatostatinoma syndrome (diarrhoea, cholelithiasis and diabetes) is more common in pancreatic tumours and seen in less than 10% of duodenal cases. Many tumours are incidental findings as duodenal polyps discovered at endoscopy or by imaging. Diagnosis can be confirmed by measuring fasting plasma somatostatin levels. Pathological examination provides the definitive diagnosis.

Macroscopically, duodenal somatostatinomas are small, 20–50 mm, homogeneous, tan-coloured, intramural ampullary or peri-ampullary nodules [89,90], although larger polypoid or ulcerated lesions have been described [91]. Most (90%) cases are solitary. Histologically, glandular structures intermingle with the ducts and smooth muscle of the ampulla of Vater and extend into the mucosa and the wall of the duodenum (Figure 24.10). The neoplastic glands comprise uniform cuboidal or low columnar cells with abundant, finely granular, eosinophilic cytoplasm and small, basally located, vesicular nuclei with small nucleoli. Mitotic figures are scanty. The glandular lumina frequently contain amorphous eosinophilic periodic acid–Schiff (PAS)-positive, diastase-resistant, material. Densely calcified,

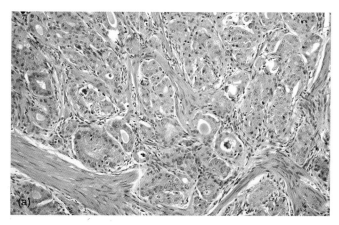

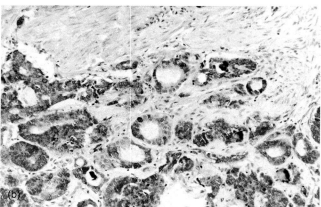

Figure 24.10 Duodenal ampullary somatostatinoma with (a) a prominent glandular architecture and (b) showing strong immunopositivity for somatostatin. Intraluminal calcified psammoma bodies are seen in both images.

concentrically laminated psammoma bodies measuring 5–30 µm in diameter are present in only 50% of cases (Figure 24.10) [77,89].

Confusion with adenocarcinoma, either primary pancreatic/ampullary or metastatic adenocarcinoma (the tumour shows a resemblance to primary prostatic adenocarcinoma), is a distinct possibility unless the focal solid, acinar or trabecular growth patterns, typical of conventional endocrine tumours, are seen. Immunocytochemistry resolves the difficulty, with positive staining for CD56, chromogranin A and synaptophysin and specific staining for somatostatin (see Figure 24.10b). Occasional cells may also be reactive for calcitonin, insulin or gastrin, particularly in tumours not associated with NF-1 [92] but most tumours contain somatostatin alone. Electron microscopy confirms the presence of dense core granules [93].

It is very important that somatostatinomas are distinguished from adenocarcinoma of the peri-ampullary region because the prognosis is completely different. Metastatic disease to regional lymph nodes is present in 30% of tumours [94]), usually from lesions >20 mm [92], and liver metastasis has been described uncommonly [95]. Accordingly, most examples are classified as non-functioning, well differentiated tumours of low grade malignancy (see Table 24.4) and graded and staged according to WHO and TNM criteria.

Differential diagnoses include Brunner's gland hamartoma and metastatic carcinoma. The ampullary location, the infiltrative growth pattern, psammoma bodies and immunocytochemical characteristics allow Brunner's gland hamartoma to be excluded. Metastatic carcinomas should be distinguishable by cytological atypia and mitotic activity. Ovarian metastases containing psammoma bodies usually show a papillary architecture, not seen in glandular endocrine tumours. The psammoma bodies in ovarian cancer are usually stromal rather than intraluminal and endocrine immunohistochemical features are lacking.

Other well differentiated ETs

Rare duodenal endocrine tumours containing immuno-detectable serotonin, calcitonin, cholecystokinin, vasoactive intestinal polypeptide (VIP), bombesin or PP, but, without a significant content of gastrin or somatostatin, may involve the ampulla or elsewhere [96]. Many are multi-hormonal. Those outside the ampulla are usually small and lack infiltrative growth [97], whereas those at the ampulla have produced clinically obstructive effects [96,98]. Another example is the duodenal EC-cell tumour containing serotonin (5-hydroxytryptamine or 5HT), indistinguishable, both pathologically and in its behaviour, from the much more common EC-cell ET of the jejunum and ileum [99].

Gangliocytic paraganglioma

This rare tumour has been the subject of much interest because of its uncertain histogenesis, its peculiar histological appearance and its almost exclusive location in the periampullary portion of the duodenum. The tumour has been reported in patients aged 17–84 years, with a slight female predominance (1.6:1). Gangliocytic paragangliomas are generally solitary, sporadic lesions, although multiple tumours have been recorded [100]. Associations with NF, with [101] or without [102] a somatostatinoma [103], and with duodenal adenocarcinoma [104] have been described. Rare cases of gangliocytic paraganglioma of the jejunum have been reported, one arising in association with pancreatic heterotopia [105].

Macroscopically, gangliocytic paragangliomas are usually polypoid, exophytic lesions that protrude into the lumen of the intestine. They measure up to 70 mm in diameter and present with haemorrhage, anaemia and/or duodenal or biliary obstruction. Grossly, the tumour is centred on the submucosa and there may be focal ulceration.

Although the tumours typically stain for peptide hormones, this does not lead to a clinically overt endocrine hypersecretion syndrome.

Microscopically, gangliocytic paragangliomas are infiltrative lesions composed of an admixture of three cell types: spindle cells, ganglion cells and epithelioid cells with morphological and immunohistochemical features of endocrine differentiation (Figure 24.11) [106–108]. These three components vary in their relative proportions:

- The *spindle cells* usually form the major component of the tumour and have a neural phenotype. They have thin, elongated, wavy nuclei resembling Schwann cells, show strong immunoreactivity for S-100 and neurofilament and are arranged in intertwining fascicles. Sometimes they envelop clusters of the epithelioid cells and ganglion cells, in a manner resembling sustentacular cells.
- The *epithelioid cells* are larger with finely granular eosinophilic cytoplasm and uniform ovoid nuclei with stippled

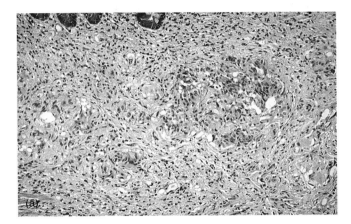

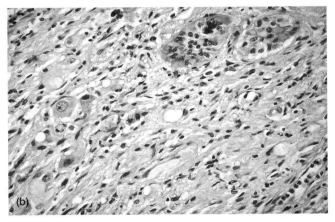

Figure 24.11 Gangliocytic paraganglioma of the duodenum: (a) low-power view showing a spindle cell lesion with loose collections of epithelioid endocrine cells. (b) Higher power shows more compact groups of endocrine cells (top right) and scattered ganglion-like cells (left) in a background of spindle cells of neural type.

chromatin arranged in solid nests and pseudo-glandular or papillary structures (see Figure 24.11). Although endocrine in nature, and typically containing immunoreactive PP and somatostatin (and occasionally 5HT, glucagon, VIP, insulin, gastrin or calcitonin), they are only occasionally positive for chromogranin. They usually stain for low- and intermediate-molecular-weight cytokeratins [109] but they are S-100 protein negative. Amyloid may be found in relation to the epithelioid cells and concentrically laminated psammoma bodies may also be found, especially if the endocrine cells contain somatostatin [109].

• The *ganglion cells* are of two types [110]: some appear as typical ganglion cells surrounded by satellite cells scattered singly in neural tissue and are synaptophysin or glial fibrillary acidic protein positive; others are not so typical, appearing as part of a morphological continuum with the epithelioid cells (although having more vesicular nuclei and more prominent nucleoli). They may contain immunoreactive pancreatic polypeptide or somatostatin. They are often arranged in well-demarcated nests, reminiscent of the *Zellballen* of classic paragangliomas. Mitotic figures and necrosis are virtually never seen, although a moderate degree of pleomorphism may be present.

The three cellular components intermingle with the normal smooth muscle and small pancreatic ducts at the ampulla to produce a complex lesion. Despite their characteristic histological appearance, gangliocytic paragangliomas may be mistaken for other ETs, smooth muscle tumours, gastrointestinal stromal tumours, nerve sheath tumours, adenocarcinomas and extra-adrenal paragangliomas. The triphasic pattern of gangliocytic paraganglioma is the main diagnostic aid but this should be complemented by immunocytochemistry when there is any doubt about the diagnosis.

Two broad theories exist with regard to histogenesis:

The first proposes that they arise because of pancreatic maldevelopment [107]. This is supported by the frequent presence, within the tumour, of misplaced pancreatic tissue and the high incidence of immunoreactivity for pancreatic polypeptide and somatostatin.

The second theory suggests a neoplastic lesion [108], with a complex triphasic growth pattern. Rare reports of local lymph node deposits composed of the endocrine cell component, either alone [111] or with sparse spindle cell or ganglion cell elements [110], support this.

An identical tumour occurs in the cauda equina region [112], the origin of which is difficult to explain on the basis of pancreatic maldevelopment.

Duodenal gangliocytic paragangliomas have an excellent prognosis after complete surgical excision, even if there is lymph node metastatic disease. Although local recurrence has been recorded 11 years after an initial excision [113], there is no published case of distant metastatic disease.

Poorly differentiated endocrine carcinoma/small cell carcinoma

Fewer than 30 cases of this rare and highly aggressive peri-ampullary tumour have been recorded in the literature, most presenting with obstructive jaundice, abdominal pain and weight loss, and followed by a rapidly fatal course [114,115]. The male:female ratio is 3:1 and mean age of onset 70 years. Fifty per cent arise in association with ampullary adenomas [116]. The tumours are small (20–30 mm), ulcerated or protuberant lesions which microscopically reveal sheets or nests of small, mitotically active cells with round or oval hyperchromatic nuclei, scanty cytoplasm and foci of necrosis. Using haematoxylin and eosin (H&E) staining, they resemble either small cell carcinomas or large cell endocrine carcinomas. Malignant lymphoma needs to be excluded by immunocytochemistry and metastatic tumours by clinical examination and radiology. Localised tumours may be resectable and metastatic tumours may respond to chemotherapy [72,117].

Goblet cell carcinoid

A few cases of this rare tumour have been reported within the duodenum, either at the ampulla of Vater [118,119] or within the duodenal bulb [120]. Morphologically, these were small tumours that appeared identical histologically to their more common counterparts in the appendix (see Chapter 30), being composed of small infiltrative nests of cytologically bland goblet cells, signet-ring cells and endocrine cells. By analogy with appendiceal goblet cell carcinoids, their prognosis should be intermediate between those of well differentiated endocrine tumours and adenocarcinomas of the duodenum.

Composite carcinoid–adenocarcinoma

This tumour is sometimes referred to as 'collision' tumour of the ampulla of Vater [121,122], although it has also been reported in the ileum [123]. Microscopically, it is formed of islands of ET cells intermingled with typical adenocarcinoma. Four cases of composite carcinoid–adenocarcinoma of the ileum complicating Crohn's disease have been reported [124]. The neoplasm has an aggressive behaviour and death usually results from widespread metastases [125].

Endocrine tumours of the jejunum and ileum

Endocrine tumours of the jejunum and ileum account for about 30% of all gastrointestinal ETs and for a large proportion of all neoplasms arising in the jejunum and ileum [126,127]. The great majority are EC-cell tumours containing 5HT and substance P with the morphology and immunohistochemical profile of classic 'carcinoids', and may give rise to the carcinoid syndrome after liver metastatic disease. The remainder comprise uncommon well differentiated tumours such as G-cell tumours, L-cell tumours that contain enteroglucagon/PP/PYY and the very rare, poorly differentiated, small cell endocrine carcinoma.

EC-cell tumours (classic carcinoids)

5HT-containing endocrine tumours that show EC-cell differentiation are the tumours traditionally termed 'classic carcinoid tumours' [128]. These tumours arise most commonly in the mid- or distal ileum [129,130] but they also occur more proximally in the ileum, the jejunum, in Meckel's diverticula [131] and even small intestinal duplication cysts. A recent US study has documented a fivefold increase in incidence (from 1.09/100 000 to 5.25/100 000) for all ETs, including small intestinal tumours, over a 30-year period (1973–2004) [12]. This raises the question as to whether this is a true increase in incidence, given the fact that intestinal ETs have been shown to have a much higher frequency at postmortem examination than presenting clinically, stated to be 1.2% in one study [85,132]; 15–29% of cases have an associated non-ET malignancy [133]. A number of cases have been reported arising in ileum in association with Crohn's disease [134,135], including multiple tumours [136] but the pathogenic relationship between these two conditions is uncertain. Although mucosal endocrine cell hyperplasia has been described in some cases of Crohn's disease [137], there is no mention of this in reports of coexisting endocrine cell neoplasia.

Jejuno-ileal EC-cell tumours occur with similar frequency in males and females; the age incidence ranges widely from the third to tenth decades, with a peak in the sixth and seventh decades. Familial clustering of cases has been described [138]. Few molecular/genetic studies have been performed on these tumours. One study showed loss of expression of p14, p15 and p16 in the 9p21 gene cluster [139].

Small tumours are often discovered incidentally post mortem or at laparotomy whereas larger neoplasms present with abdominal pain, intestinal obstruction or ischaemia from the local effects of the tumour. In addition, these tumours frequently result in a dense desmoplastic reaction of the mesentery, often at a distance from the primary tumour; this may cause subacute or frank obstruction. It is this desmoplastic reaction in the mesentery that may lead to radiological colleagues making the diagnosis, on CT of the abdomen, of 'classic carcinoid' of the small intestine because of the characteristic crab-like contraction of mesenteric connective tissues.

Multiple tumours are found in approximately 30% of cases of ileal EC-cell neoplasia [129,130,140] and sometimes dozens of tumours are present, including tiny intra-mucosal tumours. Multiple tumours are associated with a younger age of onset, an increased risk of carcinoid syndrome and

a poorer prognosis [141]. This last finding appears to be consistent with the current view that multiple tumours may represent metastases as opposed to independent primary neoplasms. A recent study [142] showed an identical X-chromosomal inactivation pattern in multiple tumours, implying a common neoplastic clone. Curative surgery consists of segmental bowel resection and lymphadenectomy. Palliative surgery is individualised on a case-by-case basis: resection of an asymptomatic primary tumour, even in the presence of liver metastases, is recommended to prevent small bowel occlusion or local complications at a later stage [143].

Macroscopic appearances

EC-cell tumours usually appear as firm nodules that are embedded in the bowel wall and bulge slightly into the bowel lumen. The overlying mucosa is usually intact but occasionally ulcerated. Some form polypoid masses (Figure 24.12) that may lead to intussusception. The primary lesions in the bowel wall range from barely palpable foci of thickening to nodules measuring up to 35 mms; rarely do the primary tumours exceed this size. Typically, the cut surface is tan, yellow or grey–brown in colour. Extension into the mesentery is often associated with a florid desmoplastic and/or elastotic reaction which causes the adjacent bowel wall to become angulated, kinked or retracted (Figure 24.13), compromises the blood supply to the intestine and promotes the formation of serosal adhesions.

Clinically, patients may present with intestinal obstruction, volvulus or ischaemia. Sometimes there is more widespread ischaemic necrosis of the bowel, due to a peculiar occlusive elastic sclerosis affecting the adventitia and intima of medium-sized mesenteric arteries and veins located away from the tumour (Figure 24.14) [144–146], presumably a paracrine effect of a substance produced by the tumour. Granulation tissue polyposis is an apparently unique manifestation of EC-cell tumours of the ileum and jejunum. It would appear to be a result of the effect on blood vessels by the tumour(s) [147] (see Chapter 23).

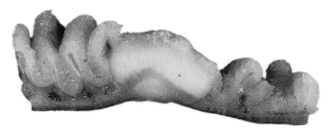

Figure 24.12 Gross appearance of an enterochromaffin-cell tumour (carcinoid) of jejunum. The cut surface typically has a yellow or tan colour.

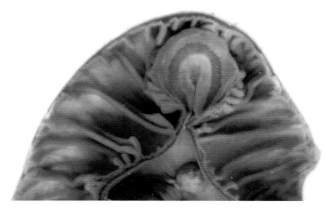

Figure 24.13 Ileal endocrine tumour showing how such tumours often cause retraction and kinking of the bowel wall. There is often thickening of the muscularis propria within them.

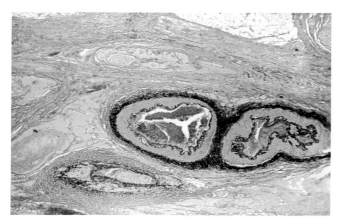

Figure 24.14 Elastic vascular sclerosis associated with an ileal enterochromaffin-cell tumour. Elastic–van Gieson staining reveals adventitial elastic sclerosis of both mesenteric arteries and veins, with luminal venous thrombosis. The patient presented with acute small bowel infarction. Ghosts of necrotic tumour cell islands (yellow) are seen among the perivascular fibrous tissue.

Microscopic appearances

Histologically, these ETs consist of multiple, solid, 'insular' nests of closely packed cells that may show peripheral nuclear palisading, set in a fibrotic or fibrovascular stroma (Figure 24.15). The tumour cells are uniform, with little pleomorphism, nuclear hyperchromasia or mitotic activity. Nuclei are rounded or ovoid with finely stippled chromatin. They have moderate amounts of cytoplasm containing granules that vary from fine and lightly eosinophilic to coarse and bright red (see Figure 24.13). Tumours should be grouped using the WHO criteria (see Table 24.4). A new proposed grading scheme using mitotic count and Ki-67 index offers the possibility of increased prognostic stratification (Table 24.6). It should be noted that grade 3 tumours can belong to both WHO groups 3 and 4. Finding foci of punctuate necrosis may signify a higher grade tumour.

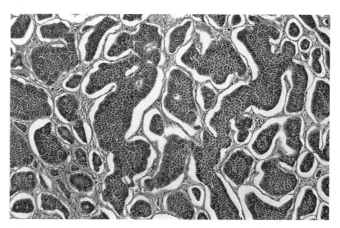

Figure 24.15 Histology of an ET of the ileum: note the insular pattern with solid packets of cells showing deep eosinophilic peripheral staining of the cytoplasm.

Table 24.6 Proposed grading scheme for gastrointestinal endocrine tumours

Grade	Mitotic count (10 hpf)[a]	Ki67 index (%)[b]
G1	<2	≤2
G2	2–20	3–20
G3	>20	>20

[a]10 hpf (high power fields) at $40 \times$ ($2\,mm^2$) magnification examined in areas of highest mitotic density;
[b]Ki67 antibody: percentage of 2000 tumour cells in tumour areas of highest nuclear staining.
Adapted with kind permission from Springer Science+Business Media: Virchows Arch, TNM staging of midgut and hindgut (neuro) endocrine tumors: a consensus proposal including a grading system, vol 451, 2007, p.757, Rindi G, Kloppel G, Couvelard A, Komminoth P, Korner M, Lopes JM, et al, © 2007.

Infiltration of the bowel wall is frequently in the form of distinct masses or cords, which insinuate between undamaged muscle bundles (Figure 24.16). By contrast, in the submucosa and extramural tissues they are often accompanied by dense fibrosis, perineural infiltration and invasion of lymphatics and blood vessels. Erosion of the serosal surface may lead to solitary peritoneal deposits [148] or to a diffuse peritoneal carcinomatosis [149]. Rarely, 5HT release from these, presumably directly into the systemic circulation, may lead to the carcinoid syndrome in the absence of liver metastases [150].

On immunostaining, strong positivity for chromogranin A, synaptophysin and N-CAM (CD56) is seen in grade 1 and 2 tumours. Grade 3 tumours show progressive loss of chromogranin immunopositivity with retention of CD56 and synaptophysin. Tumours are positive for somatostatin receptor subtypes SSTR2A and SSTR5 [151,152]. Nowadays most laboratories do not use silver stains or stain for 5HT.

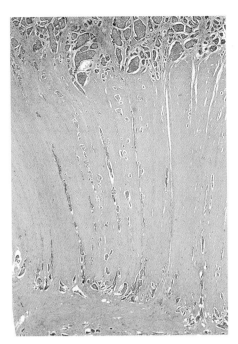

Figure 24.16 Small intestinal ET showing how the neoplastic cells insinuate themselves between undamaged smooth muscle fibres of the muscularis propria.

These tumours also express substance P and infrequently express somatostatin, gastrin, bombesin, PP, calcitonin, cholecystokinin (CCK), adrenocorticotrophic hormone (ACTH), enteroglucagon, motilin and neurotensin [140]. Approximately two-thirds also stain for carcinoembryonic antigen and about 20% for prostatic acid phosphatase (but not prostatic-specific antigen) [140]. Of note, cdx-2 is positive in midgut carcinoids and may be useful in assigning a primary site in cases of an unknown primary [153].

Fibrosis is a common feature of midgut ETs. It may not be localised around the primary tumour and can simulate a desmoplastic response to tumour, leading to mesenteric fibrosis (so-called frozen mesenteric root) and intestinal obstruction. Fibrosis may extend to involve other organs including lungs, skin or cardiac valves [154]. The mechanism of fibrosis is not well understood. Some researchers have linked fibrosis with over-expression of acidic fibroblast growth factor by tumours, which correlates with the amount of fibrous stroma [155], whereas others have highlighted the roles of 5HT and elements of the downstream signalling pathway [153] in fibrosis. Angiogenic polypoid proliferations adjacent to ileal ETs have been described but are also seen in carcinomas and are thought to be a non-specific finding related to mucosal prolapse [156]. On ultrastructural examination, most of these tumours have large, pleomorphic secretory granules, typical of those found in normal EC cells.

Staging of jejuno-ileal endocrine tumours

Surgically resected EC-cell tumours of the jejunum and ileum have frequently metastasised to regional lymph nodes. Involved lymph nodes may become large, measuring up to 60 mm in diameter, and are frequently considerably larger than the primary tumour in the bowel wall. They often become matted together by the fibrosis that is associated with the tumour. Tumours should be staged using the TNM system (see Table 24.5). The Royal College of Pathologists' dataset suggests that the 3-mm rule be used to determine whether an extra-mural nodule of tumour, without evidence of lymph node structure, should be regarded as an involved lymph node.

By far the most common site for distant metastases is the liver, the right lobe being involved more often than the left. The incidence varies greatly in different published series, partly depending on the proportion of symptomatic cases studied [140] but is related to the size of the primary tumour. In one series, 53% of tumours measuring more than 20 mm had liver metastases compared with 20% of smaller tumours [157]. On the other hand, very small (≤5 mm) primaries can be accompanied by liver metastases. Metastatic disease to locations other than the regional lymph nodes and the liver are uncommon but include the ovary, spleen, pleura, heart, breast, skin, uveal tract, cervical lymph nodes and bone marrow [140,158,159].

Carcinoid syndrome

Endocrine tumours of the small intestine can result in a functional syndrome due to the secretion of biologically active substances such as 5HT (and its breakdown product 5HIAA), tachykinins and kallikreins. The carcinoid syndrome results from release of 5HT and other tumour-derived vasoactive substances, usually from liver metastases, directly into the systemic circulation via the hepatic vein. The syndrome does not usually occur if the tumour is confined to the bowel wall or mesentery, because its secretory products drain into the portal venous system and are inactivated in the liver. Consequently, only 5–7% of patients with small intestinal ETs present with the carcinoid syndrome.

The syndrome consists of episodic cutaneous flushing of the face and neck, sweating, diarrhoea, wheezing and hypotension. Right-sided heart disease may develop, due to fibrosis/plaques of the ventricular surface of the tricuspid valve, the pulmonary arterial surface of the pulmonary valve and the subendocardium of the right side of the heart [150]. Such cardiac disease is a major cause of death in affected patients [160]. The frequency of carcinoid heart disease has markedly diminished, probably secondary to the use of somatostatin analogues [154]. Very rarely the left side of the heart can be affected if there is either an anomalous circulation through the heart (e.g. an atrial septal defect) or metastatic disease in the lungs, allowing the vasoactive and fibrogenic substances to reach the systemic circulation. This does not usually happen because the lungs have a 5HT-ase enzyme that metabolises serotonin before it reaches the left side of the heart. The diagnosis of carcinoid syndrome can usually be established by demonstrating elevated levels of the 5HT metabolite 5HIAA in a 24-hour urine sample.

Prognosis of jejuno-ileal endocrine tumours

Despite frequent metastatic disease, small intestinal ETs generally behave in an indolent fashion and their prognosis is much better than conventional adenocarcinomas [129, 130,140,157]. Data from the US SEER programme show a 92% 5-year survival rate for localised ETs: this figure decreases to 86% for those with regional spread [1]. Even in patients with distant metastases, a 5-year survival of 40% compares favourably with the 5% for adenocarcinoma [28]. Overall, the 5-year outcome is also better for ileal tumours (71%) than for jejunal neoplasms [49%]. Small intestinal ETs that infiltrate only the submucosa or extend partly into the muscularis propria are unlikely to metastasise, whereas those that have invaded the subserosal tissues are frequently associated with metastases in regional lymph nodes and at distant sites [161].

Features reported to be of prognostic significance include tumour size, depth of invasion into the bowel wall [161], metastatic disease at the time of surgery, a mitotic rate of more than 4 mitoses per 50 hpf and the presence of the carcinoid syndrome. The last three were found to have independent significance in a multivariate analysis of 167 cases [140]. In that study no patient with an initial tumour <10 mm in diameter, or with no nodal or liver metastases at the time of diagnosis, died of disease. Other adverse prognostic factors include extra-abdominal spread, substantial (>9 kg) weight loss, intestinal ischaemia and carcinoid valvular heart disease [160]. Increased Ki67 index has also been shown to correlate with poor outcome [162]. A recent study suggests that [^{18}F]fluorodeoxyglucose (FDG) PET may be a powerful prognostic indicator [163].

Other well differentiated jejuno-ileal endocrine tumours

Endocrine tumours, other than EC-cell tumours, of the jejuno-ileal region are uncommon. Gastrin-producing G-cell tumours of the jejunum are likely to be functional, giving rise to the Zollinger–Ellison syndrome [164]. Compared with their counterparts in the proximal duodenum, they tend to occur in younger individuals and be larger neoplasms and more aggressive, frequently giving rise to metastases [164]. Small L-cell tumours that contain enteroglucagon and related peptides, morphologically identical to L-cell ETs of the large bowel, may arise rarely in the ileum [165].

Other rarities include a jejunal ET, secreting VIP, that gives rise to severe watery diarrhoea (the Verner–Morrison syndrome) [166], a jejunal tumour in which somatostatin is the major peptide product [167] and an ileal tumour that produces both 5HT and insulin, and gives rise to clinical features of both the carcinoid syndrome and hypoglycaemia [168].

Endocrine tumours in Meckel's diverticula must not be confused histologically with intra-mural or extra-mural nests of heterotopic pancreatic islets of Langerhans. The latter may or may not be accompanied by foci of exocrine pancreas. Langerhans' cell nests are usually small, rounded and unassociated with a desmoplastic stromal reaction. Immunostaining for normal pancreatic islet cell hormones demonstrates the typical islet configuration, with insulin-containing β cells predominating in the central portion of the nests and somatostatin-containing D cells more peripherally.

Poorly differentiated endocrine carcinoma/small cell carcinoma of the jejunum and ileum

Jejuno-ileal, poorly differentiated tumours are exceedingly rare. Toker [169] reported an 'oat cell tumour' of the small bowel that had the histological appearance of a small cell carcinoma. Another biologically aggressive, poorly differentiated, endocrine carcinoma of the jejunum contained scattered, multinucleated, osteoclast-like giant cells [170]. This was described as an 'atypical carcinoid tumour' complicating coeliac disease. The authors suggest that the tumour had arisen in a background of intracryptal endocrine cell hyperplasia, which is reported to occur in some patients with coeliac disease [171]. The differential diagnosis in this setting includes metastatic small cell carcinoma and metastatic malignant melanoma.

Goblet cell carcinoid of the jejunum and ileum

Goblet cell carcinoids, alternatively known as mucinous carcinoid, adenocarcinoid, microglandular goblet cell carcinoma and/or crypt cell carcinoma, arising in the jejunum and ileum, are exceedingly rare [172]. A report details one patient with a 60-mm 'multicentric' goblet cell carcinoid of the ileum and another patient with a 40-mm ileal tumour accompanied by a similar tumour of the appendix. The morphology of the ileal tumours was identical to that described in the appendix (see 'Goblet cell carcinoid', Chapter 30).

Metastatic epithelial tumours

In the small intestine, metastatic tumours are slightly more common than primary malignancies [43,173,174]. Macroscopically, multiple small or seedling deposits must be distinguished from fat necrosis and larger haemorrhagic ones from endometriosis. The primary tumours may be from the breast or can be pulmonary, ovarian, adrenal, uterine,

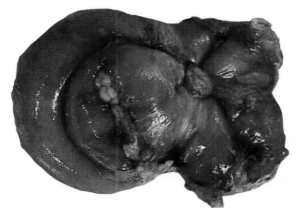

Figure 24.17 Metastatic colonic adenocarcinoma to the small intestine, mimicking a primary tumour.

cervical, renal or testicular in origin. However, recurrent/ metastatic gastrointestinal carcinomas, especially from the stomach and colorectum, are a common presentation in the small intestine and can mimic a primary neoplasm macroscopically (Figure 24.17). In this instance, comparison with the primary tumour is helpful to establish the diagnosis. Immunohistochemistry will usually distinguish between them in difficult cases. The demonstration of an apparent adenomatous component adjacent to adenocarcinoma does not necessarily provide definitive evidence of a primary small intestinal carcinoma. Mimicry of adenomatous change has been described in metastatic adenocarcinoma from the stomach and the colon, by a putative differentiating effect of the intestinal mucosa because of epithelial–stromal interactions [175].

For any unusual tumour in the small bowel, the diligent pathologist should always consider two potential forms of metastatic disease. The first is metastatic lobular carcinoma of the breast which has a particular propensity to spread here and frequently involves the superficial aspects of the bowel wall, diffusely infiltrating the mucosa and mimicking malignant lymphoma and, second, diffuse-type, poorly differentiated adenocarcinoma from, in particular, the stomach. Further, no pathologist should ever forget the potential for malignant melanoma to metastasise to the gut. Although evidently not an epithelial tumour, it can certainly mimic one and, indeed, malignant lymphoma as well. Similar to lobular carcinoma, it has an especial propensity to spread to the small intestinal submucosa, here sometimes resulting in multiple polypoid tumours mimicking a polyposis syndrome macroscopically.

Acknowledgement

The author would like to acknowledge the assistance of Dr Osama Sharaf Eldin with the bibliography.

References

1. Chow JS, Chen CC, Ahsan H, Neugut AI. A population-based study of the incidence of malignant small bowel tumours: SEER 1973–1990. *Int J Epidemiol* 1996;**25**:722.
2. Bilimoria KY, Bentrem DJ, Wayne JD, Ko CY, Bennett CL, Talamonti MS. Small bowel cancer in the United States: changes in epidemiology, treatment, and survival over the last 20 years. *Ann Surg* 2009;**249**:63.
3. Hemminki K, Li X. Incidence trends and risk factors of carcinoid tumors: a nationwide epidemiologic study from Sweden. *Cancer* 2001;**92**:2204.
4. Cross AJ, Leitzmann MF, Subar AF, Thompson FE, Hollenbeck AR, Schatzkin A. A prospective study of meat and fat intake in relation to small intestinal cancer. *Cancer Res* 2008;**68**:9274.
5. Lagergren J, Ye W, Ekbom A. Intestinal cancer after cholecystectomy: is bile involved in carcinogenesis? *Gastroenterology* 2001;**121**:542.
6. Sanders DS, Yousef A, Carr RA, et al. MSI-H 'medullary type' adenocarcinoma complicating ileal Crohn's disease;further molecular insight into Crohn's-related carcinogenesis. *Histopathology* 2008;**52**:519.
7. Howdle PD, Jalal PK, Holmes GK, Houlston RS. Primary small-bowel malignancy in the UK and its association with coeliac disease. *Q J Med* 2003;**96**:345.
8. O'Driscoll BR, Stevens FM, O'Gorman TA, et al. HLA type of patients with coeliac disease and malignancy in the west of Ireland. *Gut* 1982;**23**:662.
9. Domizio P, Talbot IC, Spigelman AD, Williams CB, Phillips RK. Upper gastrointestinal pathology in familial adenomatous polyposis: results from a prospective study of 102 patients. *J Clin Pathol* 1990;**43**:738.
10. Buecher B, Baert-Desurmont S, Leborgne J, Humeau B, Olschwang S, Frebourg T. Duodenal adenocarcinoma and Mut Y human homologue-associated polyposis. *Eur J Gastroenterol Hepatol* 2008;**20**:1024.
11. de Ferro SM, Suspiro A, Fidalgo P, et al. Aggressive phenotype of MYH-associated polyposis with jejunal cancer and intra-abdominal desmoid tumor: report of a case. *Dis Colon Rectum* 2009;**52**:742.
12. Yao JC, Hassan M, Phan A, et al. One hundred years after 'carcinoid': epidemiology of and prognostic factors for neuroendocrine tumors in 35,825 cases in the United States. *J Clin Oncol* 2008;**26**:3063.
13. Spigelman AD, Talbot IC, Penna C, et al. Evidence for adenoma-carcinoma sequence in the duodenum of patients with familial adenomatous polyposis. The Leeds Castle Polyposis Group (Upper Gastrointestinal Committee). *J Clin Pathol* 1994;**47**:709.
14. DiSario JA, Burt RW, Vargas H, McWhorter WP. Small bowel cancer: epidemiological and clinical characteristics from a population-based registry. *Am J Gastroenterol* 1994;**89**:699.
15. Spigelman AD. Familial adenomatous polyposis: recent genetic advances. *Br J Surg* 1994;**81**:321.
16. Scates DK, Spigelman AD, Phillips RK, Venitt S. DNA adducts detected by 32P-postlabelling, in the intestine of rats given bile from patients with familial adenomatous polyposis and from unaffected controls. *Carcinogenesis* 1992;**13**:731.
17. Hamada K, Umemoto A, Kajikawa A, et al. Mucosa-specific DNA adducts in human small intestine: a comparison with the colon. *Carcinogenesis* 1994;**15**:2677.
18. Brucher BL, Geddert H, Langner C, et al. Hypermethylation of *hMLH1*, *HPP1*, *p14* (*ARF*), *p16* (*INK4A*) and *APC* in primary adenocarcinomas of the small bowel. *Int J Cancer* 2006; **119**:1298.

19. Murata M, Iwao K, Miyoshi Y, et al. Molecular and biological analysis of carcinoma of the small intestine: beta-catenin gene mutation by interstitial deletion involving exon 3 and replication error phenotype. *Am J Gastroenterol* 2000;**95**:1576.

20. Wheeler JM, Warren BF, Mortensen NJ, et al. An insight into the genetic pathway of adenocarcinoma of the small intestine. *Gut* 2002;**50**:218.

21. Arber N, Hibshoosh H, Yasui W, et al. Abnormalities in the expression of cell cycle-related proteins in tumors of the small bowel. *Cancer Epidemiol Biomarkers Prev* 1999;**8**:1101.

22. Blaker H, von Herbay A, Penzel R, Gross S, Otto HF. Genetics of adenocarcinomas of the small intestine: frequent deletions at chromosome 18q and mutations of the SMAD4 gene. *Oncogene* 2002;**21**:158.

23. Gassler N, Schneider A, Kopitz J, et al. Impaired expression of acyl-CoA-synthetase 5 in epithelial tumors of the small intestine. *Hum Pathol* 2003;**34**:1048.

24. Kashiwagi H, Kanazawa K, Koizumi M, Shibusawa H, Spigelman AD. Development of duodenal cancer in a patient with familial adenomatous polyposis. *J Gastroenterol* 2000;**35**:856.

25. Moser AR, Pitot HC, Dove WF. A dominant mutation that predisposes to multiple intestinal neoplasia in the mouse. *Science* 1990;**247**:322.

26. Matsuo S, Eto T, Tsunoda T, Kanematsu T, Shinozaki T. Small bowel tumors: an analysis of tumor-like lesions, benign and malignant neoplasms. *Eur J Surg Oncol* 1994;**20**:47.

27. Saurin JC, Gutknecht C, Napoleon B, et al. Surveillance of duodenal adenomas in familial adenomatous polyposis reveals high cumulative risk of advanced disease. *J Clin Oncol* 2004;**22**:493.

28. Perzin KH, Bridge MF. Adenomas of the small intestine: a clinicopathologic review of 51 cases and a study of their relationship to carcinoma. *Cancer* 1981;**48**:799.

29. Bellizzi AM, Kahaleh M, Stelow EB. The assessment of specimens procured by endoscopic ampullectomy. *Am J Clin Pathol* 2009;**132**:506.

30. Grobmyer SR, Stasik CN, Draganov P, et al. Contemporary results with ampullectomy for 29 'benign' neoplasms of the ampulla. *J Am Coll Surg* 2008;**206**:466.

31. Winter JM, Cameron JL, Olino K, et al. Clinicopathologic analysis of ampullary neoplasms in 450 patients: implications for surgical strategy and long-term prognosis. *J Gastrointest Surg* 2009;**14**:379.

32. Delevett AF, Cuello R. True villous adenoma of the jejunum. *Gastroenterology* 1975;**69**:217.

33. Geier GE, Gashti EN, Houin HP, Johnloz D, Madura JA. Villous adenoma of the duodenum. A clinicopathologic study of five cases. *Am Surg* 1984;**50**:617.

34. Mingazzini PL, Malchiodi Albedi F, Blandamura V. Villous adenoma of the duodenum: cellular composition and histochemical findings. *Histopathology* 1982;**6**:235.

35. Boix J, Lorenzo-Zuniga V, Moreno de Vega V, Domenech E, Gassull MA. Endoscopic resection of ampullary tumors: 12-year review of 21 cases. *Surg Endosc* 2009;**23**:45.

36. Vasen HF, Bulow S, Myrhoj T, et al. Decision analysis in the management of duodenal adenomatosis in familial adenomatous polyposis. *Gut* 1997;**40**:716.

37. Spigelman AD, Williams CB, Talbot IC, Domizio P, Phillips RK. Upper gastrointestinal cancer in patients with familial adenomatous polyposis. *Lancet* 1989;**ii**:783.

38. Vasen HF, Moslein G, Alonso A, et al. Guidelines for the clinical management of familial adenomatous polyposis (FAP). *Gut* 2008;**57**:704.

39. Groves CJ, Saunders BP, Spigelman AD, Phillips RK. Duodenal cancer in patients with familial adenomatous polyposis (FAP): results of a 10 year prospective study. *Gut* 2002;**50**:636.

40. Groves CJ, Beveridge G, Swain DJ, et al. Prevalence and morphology of pouch and ileal adenomas in familial adenomatous polyposis. *Dis Colon Rectum* 2005;**48**:816.

41. Chen CC, Neugut AI, Rotterdam H. Risk factors for adenocarcinomas and malignant carcinoids of the small intestine: preliminary findings. *Cancer Epidemiol Biomarkers Prev* 1994;**3**:205.

42. Weiss NS, Yang CP. Incidence of histologic types of cancer of the small intestine. *J Natl Cancer Inst* 1987;**78**:653.

43. Baillie CT, Williams A. Small bowel tumours: a diagnostic challenge. *J R Coll Surg Edinb* 1994;**39**:8.

44. Wagner KM, Thompson J, Herlinger H, Caroline D. Thirteen primary adenocarcinomas of the ileum and appendix: a case report. *Cancer* 1982;**49**:797.

45. Barclay TH, Schapira DV. Malignant tumors of the small intestine. *Cancer* 1983;**51**:878.

46. Hung FC, Kuo CM, Chuah SK, et al. Clinical analysis of primary duodenal adenocarcinoma: an 11-year experience. *J Gastroenterol Hepatol* 2007;**22**:724.

47. Bakaeen FG, Murr MM, Sarr MG, et al. What prognostic factors are important in duodenal adenocarcinoma? *Arch Surg* 2000;**135**:635.

48. Wright DH. The major complications of coeliac disease. *Baillière's Clin Gastroenterol* 1995;**9**:351.

49. Jess T, Gamborg M, Matzen P, Munkholm P, Sorensen TI. Increased risk of intestinal cancer in Crohn's disease: a meta-analysis of population-based cohort studies. *Am J Gastroenterol* 2005;**100**:2724.

50. Love RR. Small bowel cancers, B-cell lymphatic leukemia, and six primary cancers with metastases and prolonged survival in the cancer family syndrome of Lynch. *Cancer* 1985;**55**:499.

51. Zhan J, Xia ZS, Zhong YQ, et al. Clinical analysis of primary small intestinal disease: A report of 309 cases. World *J Gastroenterol* 2004;**10**:2585.

52. Hamilton SR Aaltonen LA. *Pathology and Genetics of Tumours of the Digestive System.* Lyon: IARC Press, 2001.

53. Talbot IC, Neoptolemos JP, Shaw DE, Carr-Locke D. The histopathology and staging of carcinoma of the ampulla of Vater. *Histopathology* 1988;**12**:155.

54. Sobin LH, Wittekind C. *TNM Classification of Malignant Tumours*, 7th edn. Oxford: Wiley-Blackwell, 2010.

55. Zar N, Holmberg L, Wilander E, Rastad J. Survival in small intestinal adenocarcinoma. *Eur J Cancer* 1996;**32A**:2114.

56. Contant CM, Damhuis RA, van Geel AN, van Eijck CH, Wiggers T. Prognostic value of the TNM-classification for small bowel cancer. *Hepatogastroenterology* 1997;**44**:430.

57. Bernstein D, Rogers A. Malignancy in Crohn's disease. *Am J Gastroenterol* 1996;**91**:434.

58. Simpson S, Traube J, Riddell RH. The histologic appearance of dysplasia (precarcinomatous change) in Crohn's disease of the small and large intestine. *Gastroenterology* 1981;**81**:492.

59. Aarnio M, Sankila R, Pukkala E, et al. Cancer risk in mutation carriers of DNA-mismatch-repair genes. *Int J Cancer* 1999;**81**:214.

60. Vasen HF, den Hartog Jager FC, Menko FH, Nagengast FM. Screening for hereditary non-polyposis colorectal cancer: a study of 22 kindreds in The Netherlands. *Am J Med* 1989;**86**:278.

61. Vasen HF, Stormorken A, Menko FH, et al. MSH2 mutation carriers are at higher risk of cancer than MLH1 mutation carriers: a study of hereditary nonpolyposis colorectal cancer families. *J Clin Oncol* 2001;**19**:4074.

62. Schulmann K, Brasch FE, Kunstmann E, et al. HNPCC-associated small bowel cancer: clinical and molecular characteristics. *Gastroenterology* 2005;**128**:590.

63. Achille A, Baron A, Zamboni G, et al. Molecular pathogenesis of sporadic duodenal cancer. *Br J Cancer* 1998;**77**:760.

64. Brueckl WM, Heinze E, Milsmann C, et al. Prognostic significance of microsatellite instability in curatively resected adenocarcinoma of the small intestine. *Cancer Lett* 2004;**203**:181.

65. Planck M, Ericson K, Piotrowska Z, Halvarsson B, Rambech E, Nilbert M. Microsatellite instability and expression of MLH1 and MSH2 in carcinomas of the small intestine. *Cancer* 2003;**97**:1551.

66. Williams ED, Sandler M. The classification of carcinoid tumours. *Lancet* 1963;**i**:238.

67. Yamagishi H, Fukui H, Shirakawa K, et al. Early diagnosis and successful treatment of small-intestinal carcinoid tumor: useful combination of capsule endoscopy and double-balloon endoscopy. *Endoscopy* 2007;**39**(suppl 1):E243.

68. Rinke A, Muller HH, Schade-Brittinger C, et al. Placebo-controlled, double-blind, prospective, randomized study on the effect of octreotide LAR in the control of tumor growth in patients with metastatic neuro-endocrine midgut tumors: a report from the PROMID Study Group. *J Clin Oncol* 2009;**27**:4656.

69. Taal BG. Diagnosis and treatment in intestinal carcinoid tumors. *Curr Gastroenterol Rep* 2005;**7**:1.

70. Solcia GK, Sobin LH. *Histological Typing of Endocrine Tumours (World Health Organization. International Histological Classification of Tumours)*. Berlin: Springer-Verlag, 2000.

71. Rindi G, Kloppel G, Couvelard A, et al. TNM staging of midgut and hindgut (neuro) endocrine tumors: a consensus proposal including a grading system. *Virchows Arch* 2007;**451**:757.

72. Rindi G, Kloppel G, Alhman H, et al. TNM staging of foregut (neuro)endocrine tumors: a consensus proposal including a grading system. *Virchows Arch* 2006;**449**:395.

73. Capella C, Heitz PU, Hofler H, Solcia E, Kloppel G. Revised classification of neuro-endocrine tumours of the lung, pancreas and gut. *Virchows Arch* 1995;**425**:547.

74. Kloppel G, Solcia E, Capella C, Heitz PU. Classification of neuro-endocrine tumours. *Ital J Gastroenterol Hepatol* 1999;**31**(suppl 2):S111.

75. Jensen RT, Niederle B, Mitry E, et al. Gastrinoma (duodenal and pancreatic). *Neuro-endocrinology* 2006;**84**:173.

76. Pipeleers-Marichal M, Somers G, et al. Gastrinomas in the duodenums of patients with multiple endocrine neoplasia type 1 and the Zollinger-Ellison syndrome. *N Engl J Med* 1990;**322**:723.

77. Stamm B, Hedinger CE, Saremaslani P. Duodenal and ampullary carcinoid tumors. A report of 12 cases with pathological characteristics, polypeptide content and relation to the MEN I syndrome and von Recklinghausen's disease (neurofibromatosis). *Virchows Arch A Pathol Anat Histopathol* 1986;**408**:475.

78. Yu F, Venzon DJ, Serrano J, et al. Prospective study of the clinical course, prognostic factors, causes of death, and survival in patients with long-standing Zollinger–Ellison syndrome. *J Clin Oncol* 1999;**17**:615.

79. Weber HC, Venzon DJ, Lin JT, et al. Determinants of metastatic rate and survival in patients with Zollinger-Ellison syndrome: a prospective long-term study. *Gastroenterology* 1995;**108**:1637.

80. Corleto VD, Delle Fave G, Jensen RT. Molecular insights into gastrointestinal neuro-endocrine tumours: importance and recent advances. *Dig Liver Dis* 2002;**34**:668.

81. Maton PN, Frucht H, Vinayek R, Wank SA, Gardner JD, Jensen RT. Medical management of patients with Zollinger-Ellison syndrome who have had previous gastric surgery: a prospective study. *Gastroenterology* 1988;**94**:294.

82. Cadiot G, Vuagnat A, Doukhan I, et al., Groupe d'Etude des Neoplasies Endocriniennes Multiples (GENEM and groupe de Recherche et d'Etude du Syndrome de Zollinger–Ellison (GRESZE). Prognostic factors in patients with Zollinger–Ellison syndrome and multiple endocrine neoplasia type 1. *Gastroenterology* 1999;**116**:286.

83. Nesi G, Marcucci T, Rubio CA, Brandi ML, Tonelli F. Somatostatinoma: clinico-pathological features of three cases and literature reviewed. *J Gastroenterol Hepatol* 2008;**23**:521.

84. Cappelli C, Agosti B, Braga M, et al. Von Recklinghausen's neurofibromatosis associated with duodenal somatostatinoma. A case report and review of the literature. *Minerva Endocrinol* 2004;**29**:19.

85. Karasawa Y, Sakaguchi M, Minami S, et al. Duodenal somatostatinoma and erythrocytosis in a patient with von Hippel-Lindau disease type 2A. *Intern Med* 2001;**40**:38.

86. Griffiths DF, Williams GT, Williams ED. Duodenal carcinoid tumours, phaeochromocytoma and neurofibromatosis: islet cell tumour, phaeochromocytoma and the von Hippel–Lindau complex: two distinctive neuro-endocrine syndromes. *Q J Med* 1987;**64**:769.

87. Stephens M, Williams GT, Jasani B, Williams ED. Synchronous duodenal neuro-endocrine tumours in von Recklinghausen's disease–a case report of co-existing gangliocytic paraganglioma and somatostatin-rich glandular carcinoid. *Histopathology* 1987;**11**:1331.

88. Barahona-Garrido J, Aguirre-Gutierrez R, Gutierrez-Manjarrez JI, et al. Association of GIST and somatostatinoma in a patient with type-1 neurofibromatosis: is there a common pathway? *Am J Gastroenterol* 2009;**104**:797.

89. Dayal Y, Doos WG, O'Brien MJ, Nunnemacher G, DeLellis RA, Wolfe HJ. Psammomatous somatostatinomas of the duodenum. *Am J Surg Pathol* 1983;**7**:653.

90. Griffiths DF, Jasani B, Newman GR, Williams ED, Williams GT. Glandular duodenal carcinoid - a somatostatin rich tumour with neuro-endocrine associations. *J Clin Pathol* 1984;**37**:163.

91. Bornstein-Quevedo L, Gamboa-Dominguez A. Carcinoid tumors of the duodenum and ampulla of Vater: a clinicomorphologic, immunohistochemical, and cell kinetic comparison. *Hum Pathol* 2001;**32**:1252.

92. Juergens KU, Weckesser M, Bettendorf O, Wormanns D. Duodenal somatostatinoma and gastrointestinal stromal tumor associated with neurofibromatosis type 1: diagnosis with PET/CT. *AJR Am J Roentgenol* 2006;**187**: W233.

93. Ranaldi R, Bearzi I, Cinti S, Suraci V. Ampullary somatostatinoma. An immunohistochemical and ultrastructural study. *Pathol Res Pract* 1988;**183**:8.

94. Jensen RT, Rindi G, Arnold R, et al. Well-differentiated duodenal tumor/carcinoma (excluding gastrinomas). *Neuro-endocrinology* 2006;**84**:165.

95. Swinburn BA, Yeong ML, Lane MR, Nicholson GI, Holdaway IM. Neurofibromatosis associated with somatostatinoma: a report of two patients. *Clin Endocrinol (Oxf)* 1988;**28**:353.

96. Sanchez-Sosa S, Angeles A, Orozco H, Larriva-Sahd J. Neuroendocrine carcinoma of the ampulla of vater. A case of absence of somatostatin in a vasoactive intestinal polypeptide-, bombesin-, and cholecystokinin-producing tumor. *Am J Clin Pathol* 1991;**95**:51.

97. Kloppel G, Heitz PU, Capella C, Solcia E. Pathology and nomenclature of human gastrointestinal neuro-endocrine (carcinoid) tumors and related lesions. *World J Surg* 1996;**20**:132.

98. Ricci JL. Carcinoid of the ampulla of Vater. Local resection or pancreaticoduodenectomy. *Cancer* 1993;**71**:686.

99. Warren KW, McDonald WM, Logan JH. Periampullary and duodenal carcinoid tumours. *Gut* 1964;**5**:448.

100. Witkiewicz A, Galler A, Yeo CJ, Gross SD. Gangliocytic paraganglioma: case report and review of the literature. *J Gastrointest Surg* 2007;**11**:1351.

101. Castoldi L, De Rai P, Marini A, Ferrero S, De Luca VM, Tiberio G. Neurofibromatosis-1 and ampullary gangliocytic

paraganglioma causing biliary and pancreatic obstruction. *Int J Pancreatol* 2001;**29**:93.

102. Kheir SM, Halpern NB. Paraganglioma of the duodenum in association with congenital neurofibromatosis. Possible relationship. *Cancer* 1984;**53**:2491.

103. Perrone T. Duodenal gangliocytic paraganglioma and carcinoid. *Am J Surg Pathol* 1986;**10**:147.

104. Anders KH, Glasgow BJ, Lewin KJ. Gangliocytic paraganglioma associated with duodenal adenocarcinoma. Case report with immunohistochemical evaluation. *Arch Pathol Lab Med* 1987;**111**:49.

105. Aung W, Gallagher HJ, Joyce WP, Hayes DB, Leader M. Gastrointestinal haemorrhage from a jejunal gangliocytic paraganglioma. *J Clin Pathol* 1995;**48**:84.

106. Perrone T, Sibley RK, Rosai J. Duodenal gangliocytic paraganglioma. An immunohistochemical and ultrastructural study and a hypothesis concerning its origin. *Am J Surg Pathol* 1985; **9**:31.

107. Reed RJ, Caroca PJ Jr, Harkin JC. Gangliocytic paraganglioma. *Am J Surg Pathol* 1977;**1**:207.

108. Scheithauer BW, Nora FE, LeChago J, et al. Duodenal gangliocytic paraganglioma. Clinicopathologic and immunocytochemical study of 11 cases. *Am J Clin Pathol* 1986;**86**:559.

109. Collina G, Maiorana A, Trentini GP. Duodenal gangliocytic paraganglioma. Case report with immunohistochemical study on the expression of keratin polypeptides. *Histopathology* 1991; **19**:476.

110. Burke AP, Helwig EB. Gangliocytic paraganglioma. *Am J Clin Pathol* 1989;**92**:1.

111. Inai K, Kobuke T, Yonehara S, Tokuoka S. Duodenal gangliocytic paraganglioma with lymph node metastasis in a 17-year-old boy. *Cancer* 1989;**63**:2540.

112. Sonneland PR, Scheithauer BW, LeChago J, Crawford BG, Onofrio BM. Paraganglioma of the cauda equina region. Clinicopathologic study of 31 cases with special reference to immunocytology and ultrastructure. *Cancer* 1986;**58**:1720.

113. Dookhan DB, Miettinen M, Finkel G, Gibas Z. Recurrent duodenal gangliocytic paraganglioma with lymph node metastases. *Histopathology* 1993;**22**:399.

114. Swanson PE, Dykoski D, Wick MR, Snover DC. Primary duodenal small-cell neuro-endocrine carcinoma with production of vasoactive intestinal polypeptide. *Arch Pathol Lab Med* 1986; **110**:317.

115. Zamboni G, Franzin G, Bonetti F, et al. Small-cell neuro-endocrine carcinoma of the ampullary region. A clinicopathologic, immunohistochemical, and ultrastructural study of three cases. *Am J Surg Pathol* 1990;**14**:703.

116. Nassar H, Albores-Saavedra J, Klimstra DS. High-grade neuroendocrine carcinoma of the ampulla of Vater: a clinicopathologic and immunohistochemical analysis of 14 cases. *Am J Surg Pathol* 2005;**29**:588.

117. Sata N, Tsukahara M, Koizumi M, et al. Primary small-cell neuro-endocrine carcinoma of the duodenum – a case report and review of literature. *World J Surg Oncol* 2004;**2**:28.

118. Jones MA, Griffith LM, West AB. Adenocarcinoid tumor of the periampullary region: a novel duodenal neoplasm presenting as biliary tract obstruction. *Hum Pathol* 1989;**20**:198.

119. Kepron C, Kapila V, Hanna S, Khalifa MA. Periampullary carcinoid of the ampulla of Vater presenting as an intraductal papillary mucinous tumour of the pancreas: a sheep in wolf's clothing. *Can J Surg* 2008;**51**:E67.

120. Burke A, Lee YK. Adenocarcinoid (goblet cell carcinoid) of the duodenum presenting as gastric outlet obstruction. *Hum Pathol* 1990;**21**:238.

121. Ferrando Marco J, Pallas Regueira A, Moro Valdezate D, Fernandez Martinez C. [Collision tumor of the ampulla of Vater: carcinoid and adenocarcinoma.] *Rev Esp Enferm Dig* 2007;**99**:235.

122. Williams IM, Williams NW, Stock D, Foster ME. Collision tumour of the ampulla of Vater: carcinoid and adenocarcinoma. *HPB Surg* 1997;**10**:241.

123. Venizelos I, Tamiolakis D, Petrakis G. Primary combined carcinoid and adenocarcinoma of the ileum associated with transitional carcinoma of the bladder. Single case report. *Rev Esp Enferm Dig* 2007;**99**:145.

124. Cioffi U, De Simone M, Ferrero S, Ciulla MM, Lemos A, Avesani EC. Synchronous adenocarcinoma and carcinoid tumor of the terminal ileum in a Crohn's disease patient. *BMC Cancer* 2005; **5**:157.

125. Shah IA, Schlageter MO, Boehm N. Composite carcinoid-adenocarcinoma of ampulla of Vater. *Hum Pathol* 1990;**21**:1188.

126. Rindi G, Kloppel G. Endocrine tumors of the gut and pancreas tumor biology and classification. *Neuro-endocrinology* 2004; **80**(suppl 1):12.

127. Couvelard A, Scoazec JY. [A TNM classification for digestive endocrine tumors of midgut and hindgut: proposals from the European Neuro-endocrine Tumor Society (ENETS).] *Ann Pathol* 2007;**27**:426.

128. Modlin IM, Lye KD, Kidd M. A 5-decade analysis of 13,715 carcinoid tumors. *Cancer* 2003;**97**:934.

129. Wilander E, Scheibenpflug L, Eriksson B, Oberg K. Diagnostic criteria of classical carcinoids. *Acta Oncol* 1991;**30**:469.

130. Moertel CG, Sauer WG, Dockerty MB, Baggenstoss AH. Life history of the carcinoid tumor of the small intestine. *Cancer* 1961;**14**:901.

131. Moyana TN. Carcinoid tumors arising from Meckel's diverticulum. A clinical, morphologic, and immunohistochemical study. *Am J Clin Pathol* 1989;**91**:52.

132. Berge T, Linell F. Carcinoid tumours. Frequency in a defined population during a 12-year period. *Acta Pathol Microbiol Scand A* 1976;**84**:322.

133. Loftus JP, van Heerden JA. Surgical management of gastrointestinal carcinoid tumors. *Adv Surg* 1995;**28**:317.

134. Hsu EY, Feldman JM, Lichtenstein GR. Ileal carcinoid tumors stimulating Crohn's disease: incidence among 176 consecutive cases of ileal carcinoid. *Am J Gastroenterol* 1997;**92**:2062.

135. West NE, Wise PE, Herline AJ, Muldoon RL, Chopp WV, Schwartz DA. Carcinoid tumors are 15 times more common in patients with Crohn's disease. *Inflamm Bowel Dis* 2007; **13**:1129.

136. Kortbeek J, Kelly JK, Preshaw RM. Carcinoid tumors and inflammatory bowel disease. *J Surg Oncol* 1992;**49**:122.

137. Bishop AE, Pietroletti R, Taat CW, Brummelkamp WH, Polak JM. Increased populations of endocrine cells in Crohn's ileitis. *Virchows Arch A Pathol Anat Histopathol* 1987;**410**:391.

138. Hemminki K, Li X. Familial carcinoid tumors and subsequent cancers: a nation-wide epidemiologic study from Sweden. *Int J Cancer* 2001;**94**:444.

139. Lubomierski N, Kersting M, Bert T, et al. Tumor suppressor genes in the 9p21 gene cluster are selective targets of inactivation in neuro-endocrine gastroenteropancreatic tumors. *Cancer Res* 2001;**61**:5905.

140. Burke AP, Thomas RM, Elsayed AM, Sobin LH. Carcinoids of the jejunum and ileum: an immunohistochemical and clinicopathologic study of 167 cases. *Cancer* 1997;**79**:1086.

141. Yantiss RK, Odze RD, Farraye FA, Rosenberg AE. Solitary versus multiple carcinoid tumors of the ileum: a clinical and pathologic review of 68 cases. *Am J Surg Pathol* 2003; **27**:811.

142. Guo Z, Li Q, Wilander E, Ponten J. Clonality analysis of multifocal carcinoid tumours of the small intestine by X-chromosome inactivation analysis. *J Pathol* 2000;**190**:76.

143. Eriksson B, Kloppel G, Krenning E, et al. Consensus guidelines for the management of patients with digestive neuro-endocrine tumors – well-differentiated jejunal-ileal tumor/carcinoma. *Neuro-endocrinology* 2008;**87**:8.

144. Anthony PP, Drury RA. Elastic vascular sclerosis of mesenteric blood vessels in argentaffin carcinoma. *J Clin Pathol* 1970; **23**:110.

145. Eckhauser FE, Argenta LC, Strodel WE, et al. Mesenteric angiopathy, intestinal gangrene, and midgut carcinoids. *Surgery* 1981;**90**:720.

146. Warner TF, O'Reilly G, Lee GA. Mesenteric occlusive lesion and ileal carcinoids. *Cancer* 1979;**44**:758.

147. Allibone RO, Hoffmann J, Gosney JR, Helliwell TR. Granulation tissue polyposis associated with carcinoid tumours of the small intestine. *Histopathology* 1993;**22**:475.

148. Robb JA, Kuster GG, Bordin GM, Unni KK. Polypoid peritoneal metastases from carcinoid neoplasms. *Hum Pathol* 1984; **15**:1002.

149. Vasseur B, Cadiot G, Zins M, et al. Peritoneal carcinomatosis in patients with digestive endocrine tumors. *Cancer* 1996; **78**:1686.

150. Davis Z, Moertel CG, McIlrath DC. The malignant carcinoid syndrome. *Surg Gynecol Obstet* 1973;**137**:637.

151. Kulaksiz H, Eissele R, Rossler D, et al. Identification of somatostatin receptor subtypes 1, 2A, 3, and 5 in neuro-endocrine tumours with subtype specific antibodies. *Gut* 2002;**50**:52.

152. Papotti M, Bongiovanni M, Volante M, et al. Expression of somatostatin receptor types 1–5 in 81 cases of gastrointestinal and pancreatic endocrine tumors. A correlative immunohistochemical and reverse-transcriptase polymerase chain reaction analysis. *Virchows Arch* 2002;**440**:461.

153. Moskaluk CA, Zhang H, Powell SM, Cerilli LA, Hampton GM, Frierson HF Jr. Cdx2 protein expression in normal and malignant human tissues: an immunohistochemical survey using tissue microarrays. *Mod Pathol* 2003;**16**:913.

154. Druce M, Rockall A, Grossman AB. Fibrosis and carcinoid syndrome: from causation to future therapy. *Nat Rev Endocrinol* 2009;**5**:276.

155. La Rosa S, Chiaravalli AM, Capella C, Uccella S, Sessa F. Immunohistochemical localization of acidic fibroblast growth factor in normal human enterochromaffin cells and related gastrointestinal tumours. *Virchows Arch* 1997;**430**:117.

156. Abrahams NA, Vesoulis Z, Petras RE. Angiogenic polypoid proliferation adjacent to ileal carcinoid tumors: a nonspecific finding related to mucosal prolapse. *Mod Pathol* 2001;**14**:821.

157. Strodel WE, Talpos G, Eckhauser F, Thompson N. Surgical therapy for small-bowel carcinoid tumors. *Arch Surg* 1983; **118**:391.

158. Dawes L, Schulte WJ, Condon RE. Carcinoid tumors. *Arch Surg* 1984;**119**:375.

159. Wareing TH, Sawyers JL. Carcinoids and the carcinoid syndrome. *Am J Surg* 1983;**145**:769.

160. Makridis C, Ekbom A, Bring J, et al. Survival and daily physical activity in patients treated for advanced midgut carcinoid tumors. *Surgery* 1997;**122**:1075.

161. Ghevariya V, Malieckal A, Ghevariya N, Mazumder M, Anand S. Carcinoid tumors of the gastrointestinal tract. *South Med J* 2009;**102**:1032.

162. Arnold R, Rinke A, Klose KJ, et al. Octreotide versus octreotide plus interferon-alpha in endocrine gastroenteropancreatic tumors: a randomized trial. *Clin Gastroenterol Hepatol* 2005;**3**:761.

163. Binderup T, Knigge U, Loft A, Federspiel B, Kjaer A. 18F-Fluorodeoxyglucose positron emission tomography predicts survival of patients with neuro-endocrine tumors. *Clin Cancer Res* 2010;**16**:978.

164. Albrecht S, Gardiner GW, Kovacs K, Ilse G, Kaiser U. Duodenal somatostatinoma with psammoma bodies. *Arch Pathol Lab Med* 1989;**113**:517.

165. Wilander E, Grimelius L, Lundqvist G, Skoog V. Polypeptide hormones in argentaffin and argyrophil gastroduodenal endocrine tumors. *Am J Pathol* 1979;**96**:519.

166. Capella C, Polak JM, Buffa R, et al. Morphologic patterns and diagnostic criteria of VIP-producing endocrine tumors. A histologic, histochemical, ultrastructural, and biochemical study of 32 cases. *Cancer* 1983;**52**:1860.

167. Alumets J, Ekelund G, Hakanson R, et al. Jejunal endocrine tumor composed of somatostatin and gastrin cells and associated with duodenal ulcer disease. *Virchows Arch A Pathol Anat Histol* 1978;**378**:17.

168. Pelletier G, Cortot A, Launay JM, et al. Serotonin-secreting and insulin-secreting ileal carcinoid tumor and the use of in vitro culture of tumoral cells. *Cancer* 1984;**54**:319.

169. Toker C. Oat cell tumor of the small bowel. *Am J Gastroenterol* 1974;**61**:481.

170. Gardiner GW, Van Patter T, Murray D. Atypical carcinoid tumor of the small bowel complicating celiac disease. *Cancer* 1985;**56**:2716.

171. Challacombe DN, Robertson K. Enterochromaffin cells in the duodenal mucosa of children with coeliac disease. *Gut* 1977; **18**:373.

172. Hofler H, Kloppel G, Heitz PU. Combined production of mucus, amines and peptides by goblet-cell carcinoids of the appendix and ileum. *Pathol Res Pract* 1984;**178**:555.

173. Kanemoto K, Kurishima K, Ishikawa H, Shiotani S, Satoh H, Ohtsuka M. Small intestinal metastasis from small cell lung cancer. *Intern Med* 2006;**45**:967.

174. Sano F, Kimura R, Fujikawa N, et al. Muscle and small intestinal metastasis of renal cell carcinoma markedly responsive to interferon-alpha therapy: a case report. *Hinyokika Kiyo* 2007; **53**:635.

175. Shepherd NA, Hall PA. Epithelial-mesenchymal interactions can influence the phenotype of carcinoma metastases in the mucosa of the intestine. *J Pathol* 1990;**160**:103.

CHAPTER 25

Stromal tumours of the small intestine

Elizabeth Montgomery

Johns Hopkins Medical Institutions, Baltimore, MD, USA

Gastrointestinal stromal tumours

General features

Gastrointestinal stromal tumours (GISTs) are spindle cell lesions that show differentiation along the lines of interstitial cells of Cajal [1], usually having either a *KIT* (CD117, a receptor tyrosine kinase) or a *PDGFRA* (platelet-derived growth factor α) mutation. Some GISTs exhibit neither of these mutations and are believed to harbour different mutations that affect downstream signalling. The histological appearance of the cells comprising GISTs varies from spindled to epithelioid. Evolving pharmacological treatments, developed through growing understanding of the molecular pathogenesis [2,3], grow increasingly effective, underscoring the importance of accurate identification of GISTs.

GISTs usually arise in adults aged >50 (median age 55–60 years) and are rare in children (<1%) [4]. There is no gender predilection but malignant GISTs are over-represented in men. The classic presentation is gastrointestinal bleeding: both acute bleeding (melaena or haematemesis) and occult bleeding (anaemia) are presenting features [4]. Symptoms of obstruction may be the first sign of the tumour. GISTs are encountered throughout the gastrointestinal tract: about 60% in the stomach, 35% in the small intestine, and less than 5% in the rectum, oesophagus, omentum and mesentery. Most GISTs found in the last site are metastatic rather than primary. About 5% of GISTs occur in patients with neurofibromatosis type 1 (Figure 25.1) (with multiple small intestinal tumours) [5] and the Carney triad (paraganglioma, GIST and pulmonary chondroma, usually in young women) [6]. Familial GISTs occur in patients with inherited germline *KIT* or *PDGFRA* mutations.

Lesions termed 'gastrointestinal autonomic tumour' are now subsumed under the term 'GIST' [7] but were first identified as small bowel 'plexosarcomas' [8]. The term 'gastrointestinal autonomic nerve tumour' was introduced because of ultrastructural evidence of axonal differentiation and the presence of dense core granules [9]. As they are GISTs, lesions described as GANTs (gastrointestinal autonomic nerve tumours) usually express CD117 (c-kit) but they may also express chromogranin, S-100 protein, neuron-specific enolase, synaptophysin and PGP 9.5. CD34 shows variable staining. Underpinning the fact that GANTs are subtypes of GISTs, tumours are found in the small intestine that show predominant GIST differentiation with focal GANT changes.

Small bowel GISTs are more likely to be malignant (40–50%) than gastric GISTs (20–25%) [10,11]. Omental GISTs are probably 'pinched off' gastric tumours and share their favourable prognosis [12] whereas those in the oesophagus, colorectum, mesentery and peritoneum have the aggressive clinical features of small intestinal GISTs. Because of these prognostic differences, the seventh edition TNM staging for GISTs separates them by anatomical location (Figure 25.2) [13,14]. GISTs of other anatomical sites are discussed further in the relevant chapters (see Chapters 7, 14 and 39).

Morson and Dawson's Gastrointestinal Pathology, Fifth Edition. Edited by Neil A. Shepherd, Bryan F. Warren, Geraint T. Williams, Joel K. Greenson, Gregory Y. Lauwers and Marco R. Novelli.
© 2013 Blackwell Publishing Ltd. Published 2013 by Blackwell Publishing Ltd.

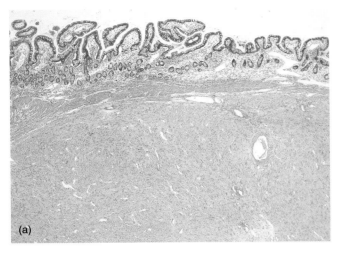

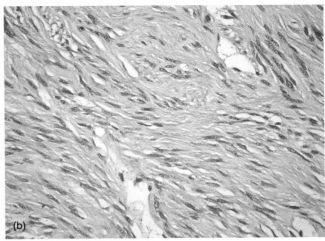

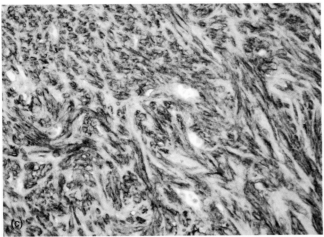

Figure 25.1 Small intestinal gastrointestinal stromal tumour (GIST) in a patient with neurofibromatosis (von Recklinghausen's disease/NF-1]. (a) At low magnification it is a spindle cell neoplasm centred in the muscularis propria. (b) Note the uniform appearance of the spindle cells. Most GISTs have bland cytological features. (c) This lesion is strongly CD117 reactive but lacked *KIT* mutations, a typical profile in NF-1-associated GISTs. The CD117 expression is believed to reflect an interaction between the *NF-1* gene product and the *KIT* gene product.

Ancillary studies

Most GISTs show immunohistochemical labelling for CD117 (see Figure 25.1c) [4]. CD117/KIT immunolabelling was reported in 560 of 571 small intestinal GISTs [98%] [11]. An antibody has been developed to the product of the aptly named gene *DOG1* (discovered on GIST-1) [15] which recognises those GISTs that lack characteristic *KIT* mutations (e.g. *PDGFRA*-mutated GISTs) and thus are negative using CD117 antibodies [16]. DOG1 immunolabelling can complement CD117 antibodies for the identification of GISTs [15–17].

Lack of immunohistochemical labelling for CD117 does not necessarily correspond to a lack of *KIT* or *PDGFRA* mutations, and thus does not mean that the tumour will necessarily show a poor response to imatinib or other tyrosine kinase inhibitors [2], e.g. in one series of GISTs that were negative by CD117/KIT immunohistochemistry (all sites combined), 72% of tumours had *PDGFRA* mutations and 16% had *KIT* mutations [18].

Pathogenesis

The development of GISTs is associated with oncogenic, activating mutations of *KIT* and *PDGFRA* [19]. Both KIT and PDGFRA are tyrosine kinase receptors, the signalling pathways of which act in cell functions such as cell proliferation [20]. Mutations causing inappropriate activation of these receptor tyrosine kinases result in both increased cell proliferation and increased cell survival, leading to

Group	T	N	M	Mitotic rate
Stage IA	T1 or T2	N0	M0	LOW
Stage IB	T3	N0	M0	LOW
Stage II	T1	N0	M0	HIGH
	T2	N0	M0	HIGH
	T4	N0	M0	LOW
Stage IIIA	T3	N0	M0	HIGH
Stage IIIB	T4	N0	M0	HIGH
Stage IV	Any T	N1	M0	Any rate
	AnyT	Any N	M1	Any rate

Gastric and omental GISTS:
T1 = 2 cm or less
T2 = >2 cm, ≤5 cm   Mitoses ≤ 5/50 hpf = low
T3 = >5 cm, ≤10 cm   Mitoses > 5/50 hpf = high
T4 = >10 cm

Group	T	N	M	Mitotic rate
Stage IA	T1 or T2	N0	M0	LOW
Stage II	T3	N0	M0	LOW
Stage IIIA	T1	N0	M0	HIGH
	T4	N0	M0	LOW
Stage IIIB	T2	N0	M0	HIGH
	T3	N0	M0	HIGH
	T4	N0	M0	HIGH
Stage IV	Any T	N1	M0	Any rate
	AnyT	Any N	M1	Any rate

Small intestinal, oesophageal, colorectal, mesenteric and peritoneal GISTS:
T1 = 2 cm or less
T2 = >2 cm, ≤5 cm   Mitoses ≤ 5/50 hpf = low
T3 = >5 cm, ≤10 cm   Mitoses > 5/50 hpf = high
T4 = >10 cm

Figure 25.2 Staging scheme for GISTs: note that the staging underscores the more aggressive behaviour of small intestinal GISTs compared with gastric lesions. The reader is reminded that these data were based on looking at 50 hpf with smaller fields and that today's microscopes have wider fields such that with most modern microscopes only 20 hpf will cover the same area of 5 mm².

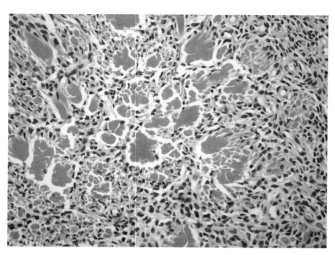

Figure 25.3 Large numbers of eosinophilic skeinoid fibres are seen in this gastrointestinal stromal tumour of the duodenum.

neoplastic growth. *KIT* and *PDGFRA* mutations are mutually exclusive [21].

Specific GIST mutations are associated with the specific tumour locations, likelihood of response to imatinib treatment and degree of aggressiveness. As a general rule, tumours with mutations in exon 11 of *KIT* tend to be gastric and respond to imatinib treatment [2]. However, homozygous *KIT* exon 11 mutations have been shown to associate with a malignant disease course [22]. *KIT* exon 13 and *KIT* exon 17 mutations in gastric GISTs indicate larger and more aggressive tumours [23]. In non-gastric GISTs, *KIT* exon 9 mutations are associated with an unfavourable clinical course [24]. Interestingly, wild-type GISTS (those lacking both *KIT* and *PDGFRA* mutations) typically label strongly with CD117 antibodies on immunohistochemistry but show little response to imatinib treatment [2].

GISTs in the duodenum

GISTs of the duodenum have a slight male predominance and are tumours of adults. About 5–6% of patients with duodenal GISTs have neurofibromatosis (NF-1). In the largest reported series [25], these ranged from small asymptomatic intramural or external nodules to large masses that extended into the retroperitoneum (median size 45 mm). Duodenal GISTs are mostly spindle cell tumours and about half have skeinoid fibres. The latter consist of bundles of collagen arranged between cells in the extracellular stroma (Figure 25.3), so named because of their resemblance to skeins of yarn in early ultrastructural studies [26,27].

Most duodenal GISTs are KIT positive [70%]. The tumours often co-express CD34 and KIT (about 50%), and are variably positive for smooth muscle actin (about 40%) and S-100 protein (about 20%), but never for desmin. On follow-up, 86% of patients with tumours >50 mm, with >5 mitoses/50 high power fields (hpf) (n = 21), died of disease, whereas no tumour <20 mm with <5 mitoses/50 hpf (n = 12) recurred or caused death. Metastases were in the abdominal cavity, liver and, rarely, bones and lungs, but never in the lymph nodes.

GISTs in the jejunum and ileum

GISTs of the jejunum and ileum are more common than duodenal GISTs: there is ample accumulated evidence on their biological characteristics. The largest series of jejunal and ileal cases comprises 906 cases [11] and forms the basis for current staging [13,14]. There is a 55:45 male:female ratio with a median age of 59 years (range 13–94 years). Tumours are rare (<1%) before the age of 21 years and uncommon (13.6%) before the age of 40 years. Jejunal and ileal GISTs range from 3 mm to 400 mm (median 70 mm) and most commonly present with gastrointestinal bleeding or acute abdomen.

Histologically, most are spindle-celled (86%) (Figure 25.4), with fewer epithelioid (5%) or mixed patterns (9%). Skeinoid fibres are present in about 45% of cases and their presence is associated with a favourable course. Most epithelioid tumours are malignant and this morphology sometimes emerges from less cellular and less mitotically active spindle cell tumours, suggesting that it represents malignant transformation. KIT is immunohistochemically detected in nearly all (98%), CD34 in 40%, smooth muscle actin in 34%, desmin in 0.2% and S-100 protein in 14% of the tumours tested (see above).

The outcome is strongly dependent on tumour size and mitotic activity, with an overall 39% tumour-related mortality rate, twice that for gastric GISTs. Less than 3% of tumours <50 mm with a mitotic rate <5/50 hpf metastasise, whereas 86% of tumours >100 mm with a mitotic count in excess of 5/50 hpf metastasise. Tumours >100 mm with mitotic activity <5/50 hpf and those ≤50 mm but with mitotic counts in excess of 5/50 hpf have a high metastatic rate (>50%). Finally tumours between 50 mm and 100 mm with a low mitotic rate have a 24% metastatic rate.

Smooth muscle tumours of the small intestine

True smooth muscle tumours are rare in the small intestine compared with GISTs. The largest series of small intestinal smooth muscle tumours comprises only 25 cases, including 16 leiomyomas and 9 leiomyosarcomas [28]. Small bowel leiomyomas and leiomyosarcomas have the same appearances as those elsewhere, consisting of perpendicularly orientated fascicles of brightly eosinophilic spindle cells (Figure 25.5), with blunt-ended nuclei and paranuclear

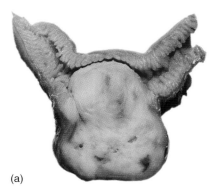

(a)

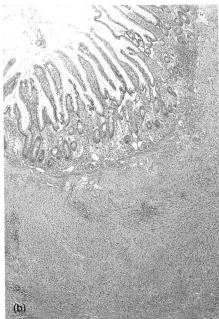

(b)

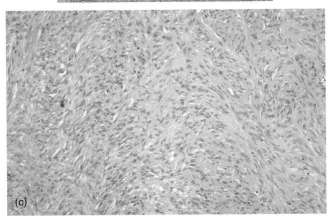

(c)

Figure 25.4 A gastrointestinal stromal tumour (GIST) of the jejunum: (a) macroscopic assessment shows the dumb-bell shape with expansion of the submucosa and subserosa by the tumour, which shows a pale fibroid-like cut surface with some central haemorrhage. (b) As might be expected, the tumour shows early involvement of the overlying mucosa. (c) The GIST shows a spindle cell morphology.

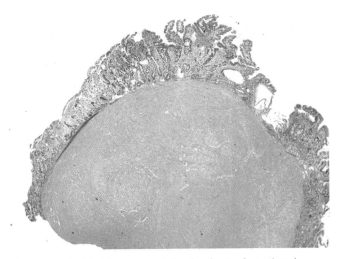

Figure 25.5 This leiomyoma of the duodenum has arisen in association with the muscularis mucosae. Note the brightly eosinophilic cytoplasm.

vacuoles. Leiomyosarcomas have mitoses (which need not be counted – any will do) and atypical nuclei. Smooth muscle neoplasms express smooth muscle actin (SMA) and desmin and lack both CD117 immunolabelling and *KIT* mutations.

Mesenteric fibromatosis

Mesenteric fibromatosis usually presents as a slowly growing mass that involves the small bowel mesentery or retroperitoneum. It is associated with Gardner's syndrome, an autosomal dominant familial disease with a female predilection, consisting of numerous colorectal adenomatous polyps, osteomas, cutaneous cysts, soft tissue masses and other manifestations. Gardner's syndrome is related to familial adenomatous polyposis (FAP), a disorder caused by germline adenomatous polyposis coli (*APC*) gene mutations. It is associated with an 8–12% incidence of developing fibromatosis. Conversely, it has been estimated that FAP patients in general have an 852-fold increased risk of developing desmoids, typically intra-abdominal lesions [29]. There is a unique French Canadian kindred harbouring a germline mutation of codon 2643–2644 of the *APC* gene. These patients have a penetrance of desmoid tumours approaching 100% and cutaneous cysts but few manifest colonic polyposis [30].

Microscopically, the lesion is poorly defined with infiltrative margins consisting of spindled fibroblasts separated by abundant collagen (Figure 25.6). Keloid-like collagen and hyalinisation may be so extensive as to obscure the original pattern of the tumour. Scattered thin-walled, elongated and compressed vessels are usually seen with focal areas of haemorrhage, lymphoid aggregates and, rarely, calcification or chondro-osseous metaplasia. Typically the vessels, though thin walled, appear conspicuous at scanning magnification [31]. The nuclei of the proliferating lesion are typically tinctorially lighter than those of the endothelial cells and the smooth muscle cytoplasm in vessel walls is pinker than the surrounding myofibroblastic cytoplasm of the tumour cells. They have delicate nucleoli and smooth nuclear membranes. Mitotic figures are infrequent.

As mesenteric fibromatoses are myofibroblastic lesions, they sometimes express smooth muscle actin and (less frequently) desmin. They typically lack CD34. Mesenteric fibromatoses can be CD117 immunoreactive in up to 80% of cases [32], resulting in diagnostic confusion between fibromatoses and stromal tumours. Nuclear β-catenin is typically detected in mesenteric fibromatosis [33] (Figure 25.6c) and not in GISTS and other congeners [34], a finding that may occasionally be of diagnostic value.

Mesenteric fibromatoses, particularly familial ones, are prone to local persistence/recurrence, doing so in 90% of Gardner's syndrome cases and in 10–15% of sporadic ones

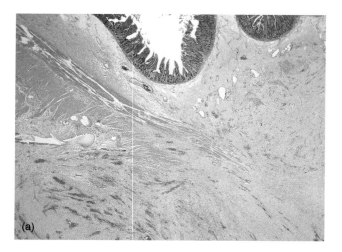

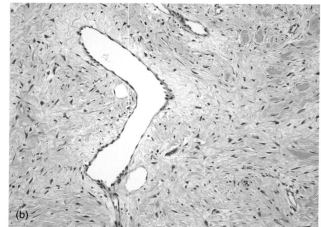

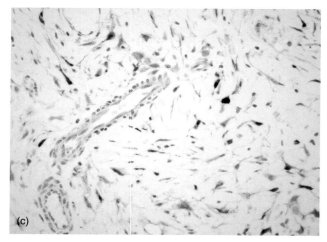

Figure 25.6 Mesenteric fibromatosis (desmoid): (a) at low magnification, the proliferating lesion is paler than the muscularis propria that it invades. The vessels appear prominent against the backdrop of the pale fibromatosis. (b) In mesenteric fibromatosis, gaping vessels appear to be stretched open by the proliferating myofibroblasts. The cells have delicate pale nuclei. (c) There is strong nuclear β-catenin nuclear immunolabelling. The vessel in the left centre of the field provides a negative internal control.

[31]. Fibromatoses do not metastasise. Surgical excision is the mainstay of therapy.

Sclerosing mesenteritis

Sclerosing mesenteritis (also known as mesenteric panniculitis, retractile mesenteritis, liposclerotic mesenteritis, mesenteric Weber–Christian disease, xanthogranulomatous mesenteritis, mesenteric lipogranuloma, systemic nodular panniculitis, inflammatory pseudo-tumour and mesenteric lipodystrophy) most commonly affects the small bowel mesentery (Figure 25.7), presenting as an isolated large mass, although about 20% of patients have multiple lesions. The aetiology remains unknown. The lesion is assumed to reflect a reparative response although the stimulus is not clear; prior trauma/surgery is usually not reported [35].

Lesions consist of fibrous bands infiltrating and encasing fat lobules with an associated admixture of inflammatory cells, typically lymphocytes, plasma cells and eosinophils. Sometimes these lesions have prominent IgG4-reactive plasma cells and they often display a lymphocytic phlebitis pattern [36] akin to that in lymphoplasmacytic pancreatitis and retroperitoneal fibrosis [37]. There seems to be some relationship between sclerosing mesenteritis and the family of so-called 'IgG4-related sclerosing disorders' (Figure

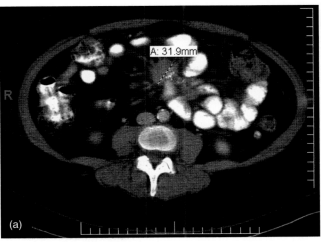

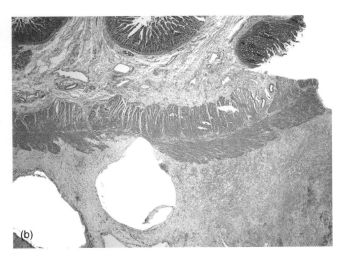

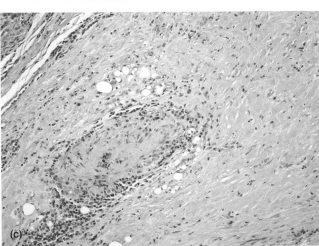

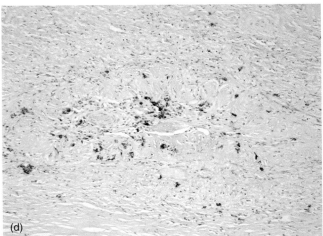

Figure 25.7 Sclerosing mesenteritis: (a) imaging study showing the lesion in the root of the small bowel mesentery. (b) The lesion is a hypocellular mesenteric process. (c) This example is hypocellular. A damaged vein is seen in this field. The inflammation is more prominent than that depicted in Figure 25.6 (fibromatosis) but less prominent than that in inflammatory myofibroblastic tumours (see Figure 25.8). (d) Some examples of sclerosing mesenteritis have prominent IgG4-immunolabelled plasma cells, a feature that suggests that these tumours may be identical to retroperitoneal fibrosis, although they respond poorly to steroid treatment.

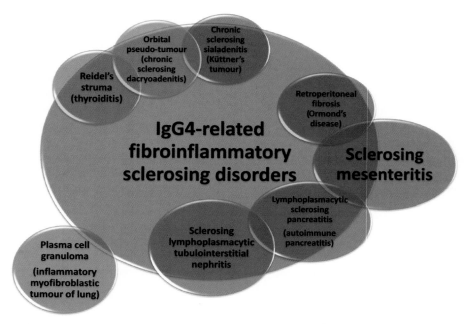

Figure 25.8 Diagram outlining a possible inter-relationship of inflammatory myofibroblastic tumour, sclerosing mesenteritis and retroperitoneal fibrosis.

25.8). However, in contrast to the IgG4-related sclerosing disorders, usually sclerosing mesenteritis does not respond to steroids and is less likely to display prominent IgG4 labelling [38].

This process is benign but a minority or affected patients die of complications such as small bowel obstruction. The disease does not typically progress or recur and the patients' symptoms are usually relieved by resection.

Inflammatory myofibroblastic tumour/inflammatory fibrosarcoma

Although these lesions were originally described as separate entities, they are now recognised as ends of a spectrum of tumours unified by a common molecular profile [39–41] and grouped together by the World Health Organization (WHO) [42]. Gene fusions involving the anaplastic lymphoma kinase (*ALK*) gene at chromosome 2p23 have been described [43–46].

In their original description, these tumours were termed 'inflammatory fibrosarcoma' [47]. They are most common in childhood but with a wide age range. This tumour arises within the abdomen, involving mesentery, omentum and retroperitoneum (in >80% of cases), with occasional cases in the mediastinum, abdominal wall and liver. Sometimes there are associated systemic symptoms. The tumour can be solitary or multi-nodular (30%) and up to 200 mm in diameter. The tumours are composed of myofibroblasts

and fibroblasts in fascicles or whorls and they also contain histiocytoid cells. Pleomorphism is moderate but mitoses are infrequently seen. There is a variable but often marked inflammatory cell infiltrate, predominantly plasmacytic, but with some lymphocytes and occasionally neutrophils or eosinophils as well (Figure 25.9). Fibrosis and calcification can be seen in the stroma. Immunostaining is positive for SMA and many examples express cytokeratin, especially where there is submesothelial extension. By immunohistochemistry, ALK1 has been detected in about 60–70% of cases (Figure 25.9c), a finding that can be exploited for the diagnosis and possibly for prognosis [48]. The tumours invade adjacent viscera. Occasional examples metastasise and are aggressive but most are treated surgically and have indolent behaviour. These lesions are more cellular than sclerosing mesenteritis. Occasionally, a process similar to myositis ossificans can be encountered in the mesentery [49] (Figure 25.10).

Tumours of adipose tissue

Lipomas are relatively common in the colon but are rare in the small bowel. Most are discovered incidentally: occasionally they present with obstruction, haemorrhage and/or intussusception [50]. Macroscopically they are yellowish and histologically they show mature adipose tissue. They are usually submucosal but are on occasion subserosal. There are rare reports of primary liposarcoma of the small intestine [51].

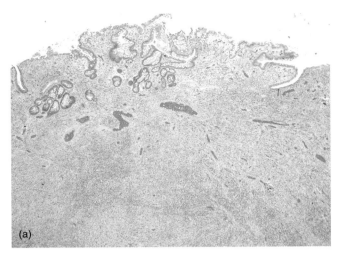

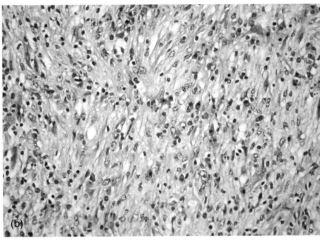

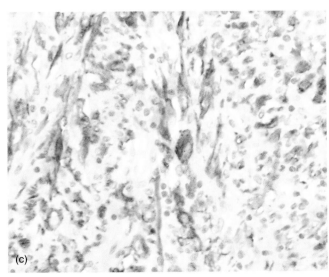

Figure 25.9 Inflammatory myofibroblastic tumour: (a) this inflammatory lesion is centred in the small bowel mesentery, focally extending to the mucosa. (b) Myofibroblastic cells with prominent nucleoli are present in a dense inflammatory background with numerous plasma cells. (c) Note the strong cytoplasmic staining with ALK1.

Vascular tumours

Haemangiomas are rare lesions in the small intestine. They are usually classified into three major types: cavernous, capillary or mixed; the type tends to determine the size of the lesions. Most are small and of capillary type although cavernous tumours may involve long segments of the ileum, in particular, and all layers of the bowel wall (many such tumours may instead be vascular malformations) (Figure 25.11). Most haemangiomas are benign and may be incidental findings at necropsy. However, a significant number present with haemorrhage, which may be covert, and thus presentation is with iron deficiency anaemia or with obstruction or intussusception [52,53]. Protein-losing enteropathy is also a recognised presenting feature of larger haemangiomas [54].

Multiple haemangiomas can be seen in the intestines in several conditions. The blue rubber bleb naevus syndrome [55,56] is associated with cutaneous vascular naevi and, often, life-threatening gastrointestinal haemorrhage. The lesions are small capillary angiomas and have a blue wrinkled surface. The Klippel–Trenaunay–Weber syndrome associates soft tissue and bone hypertrophy, varicose veins and port wine haemangiomas with vascular malformations of the gut. An apparent forme fruste of Peutz–Jeghers syndrome, due to incomplete penetrance of the gene, may result in multiple intestinal haemangiomas [57].

The small bowel is a common site for gastrointestinal involvement by Kaposi's sarcoma in the context of AIDS [58]. Histologically, Kaposi's sarcoma demonstrates spindle cells with clefts in which erythrocytes are entrapped (Figure 25.12). The tumour cells often demonstrate intracytoplasmic hyaline droplets (Figure 25.12b). Primary angiosarcomas of the small bowel are described (Figure 25.13), including some after previous radiotherapy, but such lesions are very rare [59,60]. As they are deep lesions, they are likely to be epithelioid.

Lymphangiomas

These rare anomalies, which are probably hamartomatous and usually solitary, arise in the duodenum [61,62]. They are often incidental findings but they can present with small bowel obstruction or rarely with chronic haemorrhage. The diagnosis of duodenal lymphangioma is usually achieved at the time of endoscopy, when the characteristic elevated yellow–tan lesions are seen, often with satellite lesions, which can be impressed by an endoscopic biopsy forceps [62]. Biopsy results in the exudation of yellow chylous liquid. Histologically lymphangiomas consist of dilated lymphatic channels (Figure 25.14) interspersed with more solid angiomatous-type tissue and some smooth muscle: the presence of lymphocytes helps to differentiate these lesions from true haemangiomas.

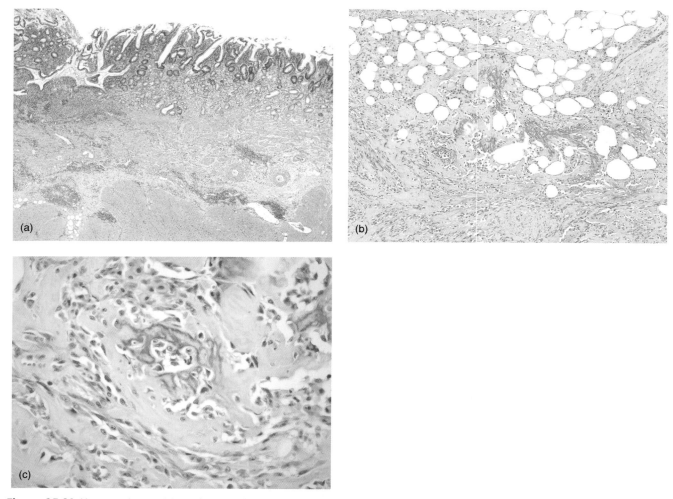

Figure 25.10 Heterotopic myositis ossificans in the mesentery of a patient with Crohn's disease. (a) The overlying small bowel mucosa shows chronic injury with pyloric gland metaplasia (ulcer-associated cell lineage) and a thickened muscularis mucosae. (b) The associated mesentery shows an area of ossification and a cellular zone of reactive-appearing myofibroblasts. (c) Higher magnification of the area seen in (b).

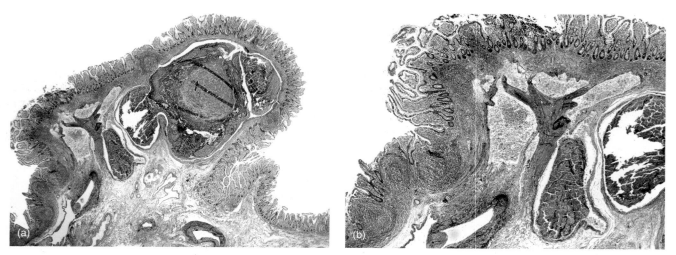

Figure 25.11 Vascular malformation extending into the small bowel: (a) large irregular vascular channels have extended into the submucosa of the small intestine (Movat stain). (b) Higher magnification of image (a). Note the disorganised elastic fibres.

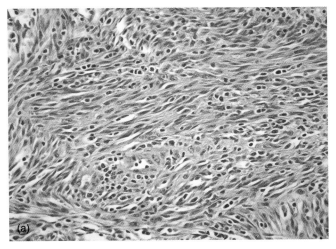

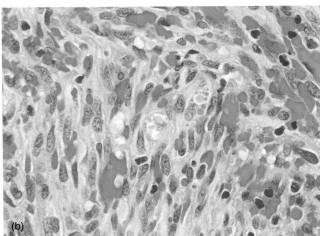

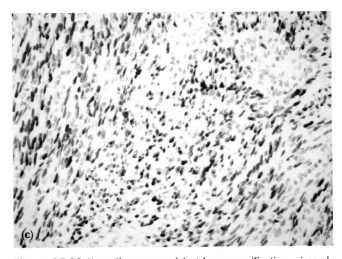

Figure 25.12 Kaposi's sarcoma: (a) at low magnification, visceral Kaposi's sarcoma is a spindle cell lesion with plasma cells and spindle cells. (b) This example of Kaposi's sarcoma shows prominent hyaline globules; these are erythro-phagolysosomes. (c) Note the strong nuclear positivity for human herpesvirus 8 (HHV8) in this case of small intestinal Kaposi's sarcoma. Virtually all cases of Kaposi's sarcoma are associated with HHV8.

Lymphangiectasia

These lesions can be solitary and then tumour-like or the disease can be more diffuse. Solitary lymphangiectasia has considerable overlap with lymphangioma and with lymphatic cysts (see above and below). Furthermore it must be emphasised that localised lymphangiectasia is relatively commonplace in duodenal biopsies and may be considered functional and part of the normal range of appearances in such biopsies. Only if the disease is diffuse throughout the mucosa and pronounced should the condition of diffuse lymphangiectasia be strongly considered.

Diffuse lymphangiectasia was first described by Waldmann [63]. It is a disease of infants, children and young adults; common presentations are malabsorption, protein-losing enteropathy, hypoalbuminaemia, chylous ascites, intermittent diarrhoea and/or steatorrhoea, and failure to thrive [55,64,65]. Histological examination reveals distortion of villi with often grossly dilated lacteals and lymphatics in the lamina propria (Figure 25.15), a finding that can be subtle compared with the dramatic endoscopic appearance. There is associated oedema, attributed to hypoproteinaemia. The dilatation may be restricted to the mucosa and submucosa but usually there is lymphangiectasia in transmural lymphatics with extension to mesenteric vessels and lymph nodes. Although lymphangiectasia can be seen as a consequence of acquired obstruction of the lymphatic system (see Figure 25.14), most cases are congenital in origin and are probably due to failure in the proper formation of lymphatic vessels. Treatment is generally supportive with a medium chain triglyceride (MCT) diet: this may result in normalisation of weight and loss of symptoms [55].

Lymphatic cysts

Lymphatic cysts can occur in the wall of the small intestine or in the mesentery [66,67]. They have been described as lymphangiectatic cysts and thus there is some confusion with intestinal lymphangiectasia. The latter term is best reserved for the diffuse paediatric pathology and other solitary lesions are best termed 'lymphatic (or mesenteric) cysts'. In the wall of the bowel, the cysts present as small, usually symptomless, nodules up to 10mm in diameter; they are commonly in the submucosa and contain thick, creamy fluid [68]. They are most often single but multiple lesions do occur in a small proportion of cases [68]. They are usually unilocular and lined by flattened endothelial cells. There may be some ectasia of afferent lymphatics in the mucosa but this is always localised to the lesion. The condition is not associated with protein-losing enteropathy or malabsorption.

Mesenteric lymphatic cysts are usually multiple, as opposed to their intramural equivalents, and may reach a considerable size, with consequent risk of rupture, small

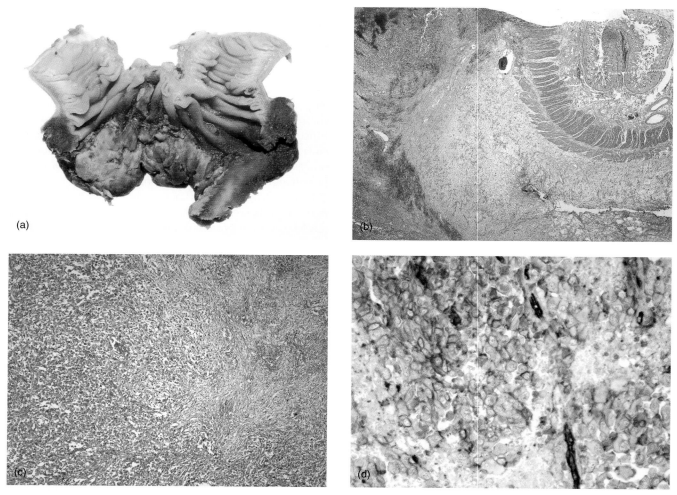

Figure 25.13 Angiosarcoma of the jejunum: (a) a large haemorrhagic tumour replaces much of the wall of the intestine in this resection specimen. These are rare but aggressive tumours. The patient died of metastatic angiosarcoma within 1 year of this resection. (b) This angiosarcoma involving the small bowel is centred in the mesentery and extends nearly to the mucosa in this field. (c) This small bowel angiosarcoma has epithelioid features. (d) CD31 labelling in the angiosarcoma depicted in (c).

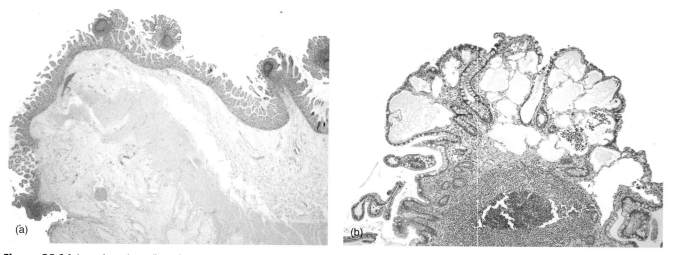

Figure 25.14 Lymphangioma/lymphangiomatosis/lymphatic malformation resected from a child. (a) The lesion courses through all layers of the small bowel. (b) The mucosal component of the large lymphatic lesion seen in (a).

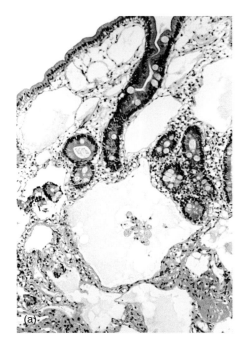

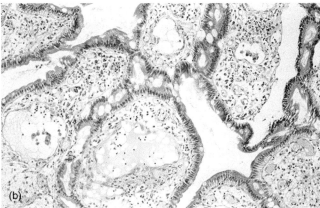

Figure 25.15 Primary and secondary lymphangiectasia of the duodenum: (a) in primary lymphangiectasia, there are grossly dilated lacteals and lymphatics in the lamina propria. (b) Similar changes are seen in secondary lymphangiectasia but, in this case, the cause is discernible. There are papillary groupings of metastatic pancreatic adenocarcinoma within some of the lymphatics.

intestinal volvulus or obstruction (Figure 25.16) [69,70]. Most mesenteric cysts are probably lymphatic in origin, although it is possible that some derive from mesothelial inclusion. The pathogenesis is obscure: the growth and dilatation of embryologically deformed lymphatics, cystic degeneration of mesenteric lymph nodes and dysfunctional fusion of mesenteric leaves have all been proposed as possible pathogenic mechanisms. They may be associated with intramural lymphangiectasia. Microscopically the cyst is lined by flattened cells, which are usually demonstrably endothelial in nature by immunohistochemistry, seemingly confirming the lymphatic nature of the cyst.

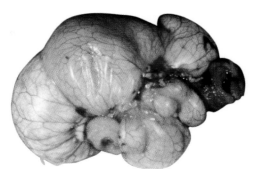

Figure 25.16 A small intestinal mesenteric lymphatic cyst. It is large and multi-loculated. Presentation was with small intestinal obstruction.

Neural tumours of the small intestine

Neural tumours of the small bowel are rare. Occasional examples of neurilemmoma are described, often presenting with haemorrhage [71,72], and there are also reports of primary malignant nerve sheath tumours in the small intestine [73]. Many of the latter may be GISTs. Granular cell tumours, also of nerve sheath origin, are very occasionally described in the small intestine but are much more common in the oesophagus.

Solitary neurofibromas of the small intestine are rare, presenting either incidentally or with obstruction/intussusception [74]. However, small intestinal neurofibromas are more likely to be seen in the context of von Recklinghausen's disease (NF-1): the small intestine is the most common site in the gut for neurofibromas in the syndrome [75]. The neurofibromas of NF-1 present with bleeding or obstruction. Patients with NF-1 may also have other small bowel tumours, including gastrointestinal stromal tumours, ganglioneuromas, gangliocytic paragangliomas (described elsewhere) and endocrine tumours (especially somatostatinomas). Solitary ganglioneuromas and ganglioneuromatosis (Figure 25.17) do arise in the small intestine but these conditions are more fully dealt with in the section on the large intestine (see 'Ganglioneuroma', Chapter 39).

Neuromuscular and vascular hamartoma is a title given to a condition of the small bowel characterised by a haphazard arrangement of neural, muscular and vascular elements. Although it is possible that some of these cases are truly hamartomatous, most cases reflect connective tissue disorganisation as a result of previous inflammatory insults, such as Crohn's disease [76], or as a consequence of non-steroidal anti-inflammatory drug (NSAID)-induced diaphragm disease [77].

Inflammatory fibroid polyp of the small intestine

Inflammatory fibroid polyps were first described in the stomach [78] and are further discussed in Chapter 12 with

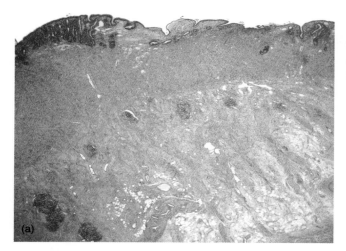
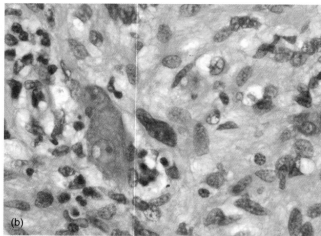

Figure 25.17 Ganglioneuromatosis: (a) this lesion infiltrated all layers of the small intestine. (b) An abnormal appearing ganglion cell in an example of ganglioneuromatosis in a background of Schwann cells.

a fuller account of the possible pathogenesis (see 'Inflammatory fibroid polyps', Chapter 12). Helwig and Ranier coined the current term [79]. The vast majority of these tumours occur in the stomach where they account for about 3–4% of all gastric polyps [80]. Presentation is site specific; small intestinal examples can lead to intussusception (Figure 25.18a) or obstruction. We used to believe that inflammatory fibroid polyps were reactive but have learned that they harbour *PDGFRA* mutations [81], which they share with some GISTs.

Histologically, these tumours are usually non-encapsulated and involve the mucosa and submucosa. One notable difference between the antral and ileal tumours is that the former are almost always small (around 20 mm), very well circumscribed and retained within the mucosa and submucosa. However, their ileal equivalents may be much larger (up to 150 mm), less well circumscribed and may deeply involve the wall of the ileum, including the muscularis propria and subserosa.

They are composed of uniform spindled cells, mixed inflammatory cells and prominent vasculature. The spindle cells have amphophilic elongate cytoplasm and pale ovoid to spindle-shaped nuclei with variable collagen deposition. Most gastric examples display a whorled 'onion-skin' proliferation around vessels but this feature is typically absent in small intestinal lesions (Figure 25.18b,c). All examples are punctuated by abundant background eosinophils, lymphocytes and plasma cells. Mitoses are infrequent.

The immunohistochemical profile of the proliferating cells is that of modified fibroblasts/myofibroblasts, with variable actin positivity but negativity for S100 protein and epithelial markers. They show consistent positivity for CD34. This latter finding raises the differential diagnostic

consideration of gastrointestinal stromal tumours but the morphology is different and inflammatory fibroid polyps lack CD117 and DOG1 positivity.

Translocation sarcomas involving the small intestine

Although synovial sarcoma [82], myxoid liposarcoma [83] and Ewing's sarcoma/primitive neuro-ectodermal tumour (Figure 25.19) [84,85] have all been reported in the small intestine, the most commonly described small bowel translocation-related sarcoma is clear cell sarcoma [86–88]. These are classically encountered in the ileum in young patients, who may present with obstruction or intussusception. They consist of uniform rounded to spindle cells that can be arranged in packets (Figure 25.20). The nuclei are extremely uniform (in contrast to those of melanomas), often with large nucleoli. Pigment is lacking. Some tumours have pseudo-papillary formations.

On immunolabelling, there is consistent S-100 protein expression. Those with the *EWS–CREB1* gene fusion lack melanogenesis and also lack expression of so-called melanoma markers such as HMB45 [86], although some gastrointestinal clear cell sarcomas have the *EWS–ATF1* gene fusion typically found in clear cell sarcomas of the distal extremities. Usually, they can be diagnosed without resorting to molecular techniques by paying attention to the clinical history and the monotonous cytological features but the major differential diagnosis is with metastatic malignant melanoma [87]. As discussed previously (see 'Metastatic tumours', Chapter 24), the small intestine is a relatively common site for metastatic disease from cutaneous and ophthalmic primary malignant melanoma. The latter diagnosis should always be considered

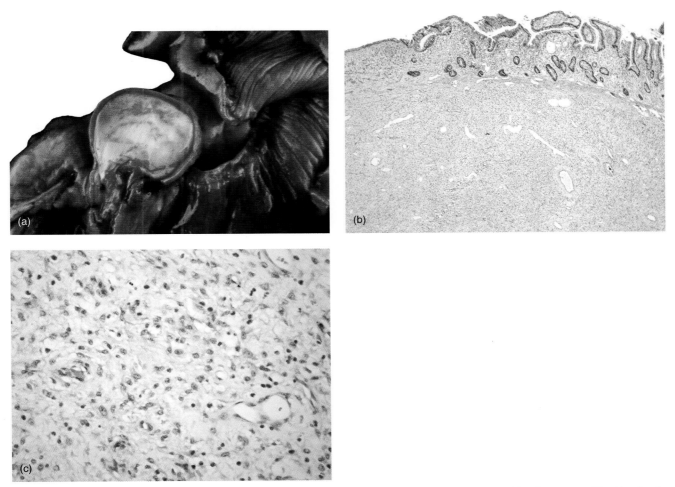

Figure 25.18 Inflammatory fibroid polyp of the small bowel: (a) this lesion resulted in intussusception. (b) Inflammatory fibroid polyp is typically centred on the submucosa. (c) Note the prominent eosinophils and bland cells in this inflammatory fibroid polyp of the small bowel. In contrast to gastric examples, small bowel lesions usually lack a whorled pattern around vessels.

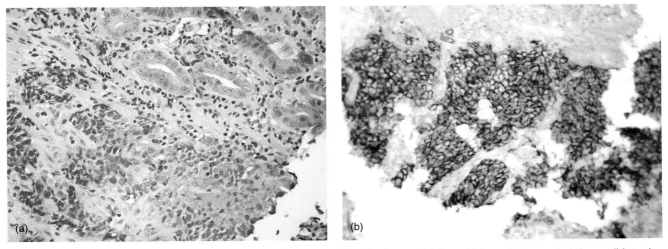

Figure 25.19 Ewing's sarcoma/primitive neuro-ectodermal tumour of the duodenum: (a) 'round blue cell tumours' of the small bowel are rare and often require molecular confirmation. This lesion was shown to harbour an *EWS–FLI1* rearrangement. (b) CD99 immunolabelling in the neoplasm depicted in (a).

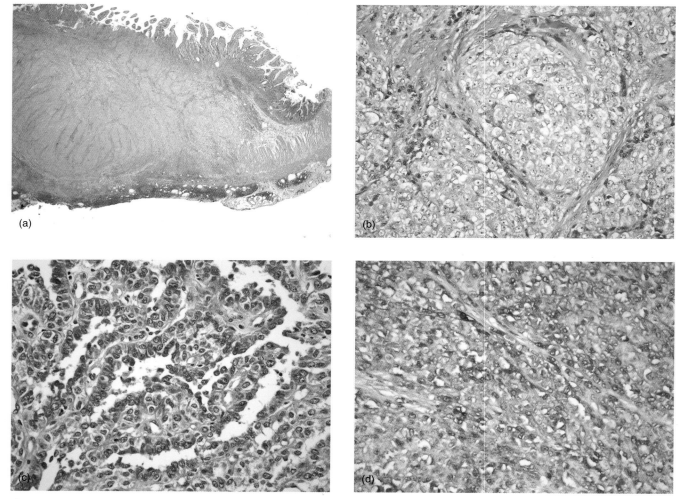

Figure 25.20 Gastrointestinal clear cell sarcoma: (a) at low magnification, the lesion has a 'packeted' appearance. (b) The cells are uniform with prominent nucleoli. (c) Some gastrointestinal clear cell sarcomas have a pseudo-papillary appearance or pseudo-glandular pattern but they are keratin negative. (d) S-100 protein is strongly positive in clear cell sarcoma.

when dealing with an unusual-appearing, high grade, malignant tumour in the small intestine.

References

1. Kindblom LG, Remotti HE, Aldenborg F, Meis-Kindblom JM. Gastrointestinal pacemaker cell tumour (GIPACT): gastrointestinal stromal tumours show phenotypic characteristics of the interstitial cells of Cajal. *Am J Pathol* 1998;**152**:1259.
2. Antonescu C. Targeted therapy of cancer: new roles for pathologists in identifying GISTs and other sarcomas. *Mod Pathol* 2008;**21**(S2):S31.
3. Corless CL, Heinrich MC. Molecular pathobiology of gastrointestinal stromal sarcomas. *Annu Rev Pathol* 2008;**3**:557.
4. Miettinen M, Lasota J. Gastrointestinal stromal tumours: review on morphology, molecular pathology, prognosis, and differential diagnosis. *Arch Pathol Lab Med* 2006;**130**:1466.
5. Miettinen M, Fetsch JF, Sobin LH, Lasota J. Gastrointestinal stromal tumours in patients with neurofibromatosis 1: a clinico-pathologic and molecular genetic study of 45 cases. *Am J Surg Pathol* 2006;**30**:90.
6. Carney JA, Sheps SG, Go VL, Gordon H. The triad of gastric leiomyosarcoma, functioning extra-adrenal paraganglioma and pulmonary chondroma. *N Engl J Med* 1977;**296**:1517.
7. Lee JR, Joshi V, Griffin JW Jr, Lasota J, Miettinen M. Gastrointestinal autonomic nerve tumour: immunohistochemical and molecular identity with gastrointestinal stromal tumour. *Am J Surg Pathol* 2001;**25**:979.
8. Herrera GA, Pinto de Moraes H, Grizzle WE, Han SG. Malignant small bowel neoplasm of enteric plexus derivation (plexosarcoma). Light and electron microscopic study confirming the origin of the neoplasm. *Dig Dis Sci* 1984;**29**:275.
9. Walker P, Dvorak AM. Gastrointestinal autonomic nerve (GAN) tumour. Ultrastructural evidence for a newly recognized entity. *Arch Pathol Lab Med* 1986;**110**:309.
10. Miettinen M, Sobin LH, Lasota J. Gastrointestinal stromal tumours of the stomach: a clinicopathologic, immunohistochemical, and molecular genetic study of 1765 cases with long-term follow-up. *Am J Surg Pathol* 2005;**29**:52.

11. Miettinen M, Makhlouf H, Sobin LH, Lasota J. Gastrointestinal stromal tumours of the jejunum and ileum: a clinicopathologic, immunohistochemical, and molecular genetic study of 906 cases before imatinib with long-term follow-up. *Am J Surg Pathol* 2006;**30**:477.

12. Miettinen M, Sobin LH, Lasota J. Gastrointestinal stromal tumours presenting as omental masses – a clinicopathologic analysis of 95 cases. *Am J Surg Pathol* 2009;**33**:1267.

13. Edge S, Byrd D, Compton C, Fritz A, Greene F, Trotti A. *AJCC Cancer Staging Manual*, 7th edn. New York: Springer, 2010.

14. Sobin L, Gospodarowicz M, Wittenkind C. *TNM Classification of Malignant Tumours*, 7th edn. Singapore: Wiley-Blackwell, 2009.

15. West RB, Corless CL, Chen X, et al. The novel marker, DOG1, is expressed ubiquitously in gastrointestinal stromal tumours irrespective of *KIT* or *PDGFRA* mutation status. *Am J Pathol* 2004; **165**:107.

16. Espinosa I, Lee CH, Kim MK, et al. A novel monoclonal antibody against *DOG1* is a sensitive and specific marker for gastrointestinal stromal tumours. *Am J Surg Pathol* 2008;**32**:210.

17. Miettinen M, Wang ZF, Lasota J. DOG1 antibody in the differential diagnosis of gastrointestinal stromal tumours: a study of 1840 cases. *Am J Surg Pathol* 2009;**33**:1401.

18. Medeiros F, Corless CL, Duensing A, et al. *KIT*-negative gastrointestinal stromal tumours: proof of concept and therapeutic implications. *Am J Surg Pathol* 2004;**28**:889.

19. Isozaki K, Hirota S. Gain-of-function mutations of receptor tyrosine kinases in gastrointestinal stromal tumours. *Curr Genomics* 2006;**7**:469.

20. Steigen SE, Eide TJ, Wasag B, Lasota J, Miettinen M. Mutations in gastrointestinal stromal tumours – a population-based study from Northern Norway. *APMIS* 2007;**115**:289.

21. Heinrich MC, Corless CL, Duensing A, et al. PDGFRA activating mutations in gastrointestinal stromal tumours. *Science* 2003; **299**:708.

22. Lasota J, vel Dobosz AJ, Wasag B, et al. Presence of homozygous KIT exon 11 mutations is strongly associated with malignant clinical behavior in gastrointestinal stromal tumours. *Lab Invest* 2007;**87**:1029.

23. Lasota J, Corless CL, Heinrich MC, et al. Clinicopathologic profile of gastrointestinal stromal tumours (GISTs) with primary KIT exon 13 or exon 17 mutations: a multicenter study on 54 cases. *Mod Pathol* 2008;**21**:476.

24. Antonescu CR, Sommer G, Sarran L, et al. Association of KIT exon 9 mutations with nongastric primary site and aggressive behavior: KIT mutation analysis and clinical correlates of 120 gastrointestinal stromal tumours. *Clin Cancer Res* 2003;**9**:3329.

25. Miettinen M, Kopczynski J, Makhlouf HR, et al. Gastrointestinal stromal tumours, intramural leiomyomas, and leiomyosarcomas in the duodenum: a clinicopathologic, immunohistochemical, and molecular genetic study of 167 cases. *Am J Surg Pathol* 2003; **27**:625.

26. Min KW. Small intestinal stromal tumours with skeinoid fibers. Clinicopathological, immunohistochemical, and ultrastructural investigations. *Am J Surg Pathol* 1992;**16**:145.

27. Min KW. Gastrointestinal autonomic nerve tumours and skeinoid fibers. *Am J Surg Pathol* 1994;**18**:958.

28. Miettinen M, Sobin LH, Lasota J. True smooth muscle tumours of the small intestine: a clinicopathologic, immunohistochemical, and molecular genetic study of 25 cases. *Am J Surg Pathol* 2009;**33**:430.

29. Gurbuz AK, Giardiello FM, Petersen GM, et al. Desmoid tumours in familial adenomatous polyposis. *Gut* 1994;**35**:377.

30. Couture J, Mitri A, Lagace R, et al. A germline mutation at the extreme 3′ end of the *APC* gene results in a severe desmoid phenotype and is associated with overexpression of beta-catenin in the desmoid tumour. *Clin Genet* 2000;**57**:205.

31. Burke AP, Sobin LH, Shekitka KM, Federspiel BH, Helwig EB. Intra-abdominal fibromatosis. A pathologic analysis of 130 tumours with comparison of clinical subgroups. *Am J Surg Pathol* 1990;**14**:335.

32. Yantiss RK, Spiro IJ, Compton CC, Rosenberg AE. Gastrointestinal stromal tumour versus intra-abdominal fibromatosis of the bowel wall: a clinically important differential diagnosis. *Am J Surg Pathol* 2000;**24**:947.

33. Montgomery E, Torbenson MS, Kaushal M, Fisher C, Abraham SC. Beta-catenin immunohistochemistry separates mesenteric fibromatosis from gastrointestinal stromal tumour and sclerosing mesenteritis. *Am J Surg Pathol* 2002;**26**:1296.

34. Bhattacharya B, Dilworth HP, Iacobuzio-Donahue C, et al. Nuclear beta-catenin expression distinguishes deep fibromatosis from other benign and malignant fibroblastic and myofibroblastic lesions. *Am J Surg Pathol* 2005;**29**:653.

35. Emory TS, Monihan JM, Carr NJ, Sobin LH. Sclerosing mesenteritis, mesenteric panniculitis and mesenteric lipodystrophy: a single entity? *Am J Surg Pathol* 1997;**21**:392.

36. Chen TS, Montgomery EA. Are tumefactive lesions classified as sclerosing mesenteritis a subset of IgG4-related sclerosing disorders? *J Clin Pathol* 2008;**61**:1093.

37. Akram S, Pardi DS, Schaffner JA, Smyrk TC. Sclerosing mesenteritis: clinical features, treatment, and outcome in ninety-two patients. *Clin Gastroenterol Hepatol* 2007;**5**:589; quiz 523.

38. Yamamoto H, Yamaguchi H, Aishima S, et al. Inflammatory myofibroblastic tumour versus IgG4-related sclerosing disease and inflammatory pseudotumour: a comparative clinicopathologic study. *Am J Surg Pathol* 2009;**33**:1330.

39. Coffin CM, Watterson J, Priest JR, Dehner LP. Extrapulmonary inflammatory myofibroblastic tumour (inflammatory pseudotumour). A clinicopathologic and immunohistochemical study of 84 cases. *Am J Surg Pathol* 1995;**19**:859.

40. Coffin CM, Dehner LP, Meis-Kindblom JM. Inflammatory myofibroblastic tumour, inflammatory fibrosarcoma, and related lesions: an historical review with differential diagnostic considerations. *Semin Diagn Pathol* 1998;**15**:102.

41. Meis-Kindblom JM, Kjellstrom C, Kindblom LG. Inflammatory fibrosarcoma: update, reappraisal, and perspective on its place in the spectrum of inflammatory myofibroblastic tumours. *Semin Diagn Pathol* 1998;**15**:133.

42. Fletcher C, Unni K, Mertens FE. *World Health Organization Classification of Tumours. Pathology and Genetics of Tumours of Soft Tissue and Bone.* Lyon: IACR Press, 2002.

43. Bridge JA, Kanamori M, Ma Z, et al. Fusion of the *ALK* gene to the clathrin heavy chain gene, CLTC, in inflammatory myofibroblastic tumour. *Am J Pathol* 2001;**159**:411.

44. Cook JR, Dehner LP, Collins MH, et al. Anaplastic lymphoma kinase (ALK) expression in the inflammatory myofibroblastic tumour: a comparative immunohistochemical study. *Am J Surg Pathol* 2001;**25**:1364.

45. Lawrence B, Perez-Atayde A, Hibbard MK, et al. *TPM3-ALK* and *TPM4-ALK* oncogenes in inflammatory myofibroblastic tumours. *Am J Pathol* 2000;**157**:377.

46. Sirvent N, Hawkins AL, Moeglin D, et al. ALK probe rearrangement in a t[2;11;2) (p23;p15;q31) translocation found in a prenatal myofibroblastic fibrous lesion: toward a molecular definition of an inflammatory myofibroblastic tumour family? *Genes Chromosomes Cancer* 2001;**31**:85.

47. Meis JM, Enzinger FM. Inflammatory fibrosarcoma of the mesentery and retroperitoneum. A tumour closely simulating inflammatory pseudotumour. *Am J Surg Pathol* 1991;**15**:1146.

48. Coffin CM, Hornick JL, Fletcher CD. Inflammatory myofibroblastic tumour: comparison of clinicopathologic, histologic, and immunohistochemical features including ALK expression in atypical and aggressive cases. *Am J Surg Pathol* 2007;**31**:509.

49. Wilson JD, Montague CJ, Salcuni P, Bordi C, Rosai J. Heterotopic mesenteric ossification ('intraabdominal myositis ossificans'): report of five cases. *Am J Surg Pathol* 1999;**23**:1464.

50. Baskaran V, Patnaik PK, Seth AK, Dogra R, Chaudhry R. Intestinal lipoma: a rare cause of lower gastrointestinal haemorrhage. *Trop Gastroenterol* 2003;**24**:208.

51. Mohandas D, Chandra RS, Srinivasan V, Bhaskar AG. Liposarcoma of the ileum with secondaries in the liver. *Am J Gastroenterol* 1972;**58**:172.

52. Boyle L, Lack EE. Solitary cavernous hemangioma of small intestine. Case report and literature review. *Arch Pathol Lab Med* 1993;**117**:939.

53. Pradhan DJ, Juanteguy M, Musikabhumma S, Ulfohn A. Gastrointestinal hemangiomas. *Arch Surg* 1972;**104**:704.

54. Jackson AE Jr, Peterson C Jr. Hemangioma of the small intestine causing protein-losing enteropathy. *Ann Intern Med* 1967;**66**:1190.

55. Desai AP, Guvenc BH, Carachi R. Evidence for medium chain triglycerides in the treatment of primary intestinal lymphangiectasia. *Eur J Pediatr Surg* 2009;**19**:241.

56. Bak YT, Oh CH, Kim JH, Lee CH. Blue rubber bleb nevus syndrome: endoscopic removal of the gastrointestinal hemangiomas. *Gastrointest Endosc* 1997;**45**:90.

57. Camilleri M, Chadwick VS, Hodgson HJ. Vascular anomalies of the gastrointestinal tract. *Hepatogastroenterology* 1984;**31**:149.

58. Kahl P, Buettner R, Friedrichs N, Merkelbach-Bruse S, Wenzel J, Carl Heukamp L. Kaposi's sarcoma of the gastrointestinal tract: report of two cases and review of the literature. *Pathol Res Pract* 2007;**203**:227.

59. Fraiman G, Ganti AK, Potti A, Mehdi S. Angiosarcoma of the small intestine: a possible role for thalidomide? *Med Oncol* 2003; **20**:397.

60. Khalil MF, Thomas A, Aassad A, Rubin M, Taub RN. Epithelioid angiosarcoma of the small intestine after occupational exposure to radiation and polyvinyl chloride: a case report and review of literature. *Sarcoma* 2005;**9**:161.

61. Honda K, Ihara E, Ochiai T, et al. Lymphangioma of small intestine. *Gastrointest Endosc* 2003;**58**:574.

62. Shigematsu A, Iida M, Hatanaka M, et al. Endoscopic diagnosis of lymphangioma of the small intestine. *Am J Gastroenterol* 1988; **83**:1289.

63. Waldmann TA, Steinfeld JL, Dutcher TF, Davidson JD, Gordon RS Jr. The role of the gastrointestinal system in 'idiopathic hypoproteinemia'. *Gastroenterology* 1961;**41**:197.

64. Bujanover Y, Liebman WM, Goodman JR, Thaler MM. Primary intestinal lymphangiectasia. Case report with radiological and ultrastructural study. *Digestion* 1981;**21**:107.

65. Donzelli F, Norberto L, Marigo A, et al. Primary intestinal lymphangiectasia. Comparison between endoscopic and radiological findings. *Helv Paediatr Acta* 1980;**35**:169.

66. Moulis H. Duodenal lymphangiectatic cyst. *Gastrointest Endosc* 2003;**57**:97.

67. Shilkin KB, Zerman BJ, Blackwell JB. Lymphangiectatic cysts of the small bowel. *J Pathol Bacteriol* 1968;**96**:353.

68. Aase S, Gundersen R. Submucous lymphatic cysts of the small intestine. An autopsy study. *Acta Pathol Microbiol Immunol Scand A* 1983;**91**:191.

69. Bliss DP, Jr., Coffin CM, Bower RJ, Stockmann PT, Ternberg JL. Mesenteric cysts in children. *Surgery* 1994;**115**:571.

70. Okur H, Kucukaydin M, Ozokutan BH, Durak AC, Kazez A, Kose O. Mesenteric, omental, and retroperitoneal cysts in children. *Eur J Surg* 1997;**163**:673.

71. Gallo SH, Sagatelian MA. Benign schwannoma of the small intestine: an unusual cause of gastrointestinal bleeding. *J Ky Med Assoc* 1995;**93**:291.

72. Hesselfeldt-Nielsen J, Geerdsen JP, Pedersen VM. Bleeding schwannoma of the small intestine: a diagnostic problem. Case report. *Acta Chir Scand* 1987;**153**:623.

73. Mosca F, Stracqualursi A, Lipari G, Latteri F, Palazzo F, Russo G. [Malignant schwannoma of the small intestine: a report of 2 cases.] *G Chir* 2000;**21**:149.

74. Watanuki F, Ohwada S, Hosomura Y, et al. Small ileal neurofibroma causing intussusception in a non-neurofibromatosis patient. *J Gastroenterol* 1995;**30**:113.

75. Fuller CE, Williams GT. Gastrointestinal manifestations of type 1 neurofibromatosis (von Recklinghausen's disease). *Histopathology* 1991;**19**:1.

76. Shepherd NA, Jass JR. Neuromuscular and vascular hamartoma of the small intestine: is it Crohn's disease? *Gut* 1987; **28**:1663.

77. Cortina G, Wren S, Armstrong B, Lewin K, Fajardo L. Clinical and pathologic overlap in nonsteroidal anti-inflammatory drug-related small bowel diaphragm disease and the neuromuscular and vascular hamartoma of the small bowel. *Am J Surg Pathol* 1999;**23**:1414.

78. Vanek J. Gastric submucosal granuloma with eosinophilic infiltration. *Am J Pathol* 1949;**25**:397.

79. Helwig E, Ranier A. Inflammatory fibroid polyps of the stomach. *Surg Gynecol Obstet* 1953;**96**:355.

80. Stolte M, Sticht T, Eidt S, Ebert D, Finkenzeller G. Frequency, location, and age and sex distribution of various types of gastric polyp. *Endoscopy* 1994;**26**:659.

81. Lasota J, Wang ZF, Sobin LH, Miettinen M. Gain-of-function PDGFRA mutations, earlier reported in gastrointestinal stromal tumours, are common in small intestinal inflammatory fibroid polyps. A study of 60 cases. *Mod Pathol* 2009;**22**:1049.

82. Helliwell TR, King AP, Raraty M, et al. Biphasic synovial sarcoma in the small intestinal mesentery. *Cancer* 1995;**75**:2862.

83. Rivkind AI, Admon D, Yarom R, Schreiber L. Myxoid liposarcoma of the small intestine mimicking acute appendicitis. *Eur J Surg* 1994;**160**:251.

84. Batziou C, Stathopoulos GP, Petraki K, et al. Primitive neurectodermal tumours: a case of extraosseous Ewing's sarcoma of the small intestine and review of the literature. *J Buon* 2006; **11**:519.

85. Kim DW, Chang HJ, Jeong JY, et al. Ewing's sarcoma/primitive neuroectodermal tumour (ES/PNET) of the small bowel: a rare cause of intestinal obstruction. *Int J Colorectal Dis* 2007; **22**:1137.

86. Antonescu CR, Nafa K, Segal NH, Dal Cin P, Ladanyi M. *EWS-CREB1*: a recurrent variant fusion in clear cell sarcoma – association with gastrointestinal location and absence of melanocytic differentiation. *Clin Cancer Res* 2006;**12**:5356.

87. Lyle PL, Amato CM, Fitzpatrick JE, Robinson WA. Gastrointestinal melanoma or clear cell sarcoma? Molecular evaluation of 7 cases previously diagnosed as malignant melanoma. *Am J Surg Pathol* 2008;**32**:858.

88. Zambrano E, Reyes-Mugica M, Franchi A, Rosai J. An osteoclast-rich tumour of the gastrointestinal tract with features resembling clear cell sarcoma of soft parts: reports of 6 cases of a GIST simulator. *Int J Surg Pathol* 2003;**11**:75.

Lymphoid and other tumours of the small intestine

Scott R. Owens
University of Pittsburgh Medical Center, Pittsburgh, PA, USA

Benign lymphoid proliferations

The small intestine contains a large amount of lymphoid tissue, organised diffusely within the lamina propria, as well as into discrete aggregates. The latter may be found throughout the intestine but the terminal ileum contains large lymphoid collections known as Peyer's patches, as large as 20 mm in diameter and visible macroscopically, appearing as raised nodules on the mucosal surface. The overlying mucosa contains specialised 'dome' epithelium, which possesses phagocytic columnar cells termed M (microfold or membranous) cells which sample antigen from the intestinal lumen. Antigens are processed and presented to lymphocytes by specialised dendritic cells, eliciting an immune response [1]. In addition to antigen, small particulate matter can be internalised in a process that has been called persorption [2]. This phenomenon may be responsible for the unique appearance of pigmented material commonly found within Peyer's patches, which is thought to be obtained from contents of the small intestine, via soil-contaminated food and/or atmospheric dust [3–5]. When present, this black pigment is useful in the identification of Peyer's patches in intestinal biopsies and thus confirmation that the biopsies derive from the native ileum, especially in ileal pouch mucosal biopsy assessment.

Lymphoid tissue found in mucosal sites throughout the body has been termed 'mucosa-associated lymphoid tissue' (MALT) and the gastrointestinal tract is a major MALT site. MALT is organised into follicles with germinal centres, surrounded by a marginal zone containing cells with ample cytoplasm and a mantle zone composed of cells with smaller, angulated and darkly staining nuclei [6,7]. Pre-existing MALT, such as Peyer's patches, can be considered 'native' MALT, in contrast to that which arises in response to antigenic stimulation ('acquired' MALT). An example of the latter is the lymphoid tissue that develops in the gastric mucosa in response to *Helicobacter pylori* infection. The lamina propria of the small intestine also contains a mixed inflammatory cell population with numerous plasma cells, small lymphocytes and other cell types including mast cells and eosinophils. Intra-epithelial lymphocytes, predominantly cytotoxic T cells, are always present and normally number fewer than 30–40 per 100 epithelial cells [8].

Whether native or acquired, the follicular structures of small intestinal MALT are organised similarly to those seen in the cortex of lymph nodes, although the mantle zone of MALT follicles is located eccentrically, towards the luminal surface. Similarly, the process of antigen presentation followed by B-cell activation and proliferation, aided by T-helper cells, is analogous to that found in lymph nodes. This culminates in the creation of immunoglobulin-producing plasma cells, a high proportion of which manufacture secretory IgA which is transported to the lumen. With this rich background of lymphoid tissue, it is not surprising that a variety of benign lymphoid proliferations, as well as B- and T-cell neoplasms, arise in the small intestine.

Lymphoid hyperplasia in the terminal ileum

Two forms of focal lymphoid hyperplasia are seen in the distal small intestine. The first, seen in very young patients, is rare and presents as a tumour-like appearance in the terminal ileum, sometimes leading to small bowel obstruction, intussusception and/or or haemorrhage [7,9,10]. It has been associated with infectious agents and is thought to be an inappropriately vigorous host response, sometimes shown to be secondary to *Yersinia* spp. or enteric viruses [7,10]. The hyperplastic lymphoid tissue has a striking follicular pattern with germinal centres and expanded Peyer's patches, which protrude into the intestinal lumen. The lymphoid tissue remains normally organised, however, and there is no destruction of the mucosa or intestinal wall unless due to the secondary effects of obstruction or intussusception. This preservation of lymphoid and intestinal tissue architecture helps the pathologist to exclude a malignant process.

The second form of focal hyperplasia in the terminal ileum, also rare, occurs most commonly in older individuals [11]. It may strongly resemble follicular lymphoma or extra-nodal marginal zone lymphoma of MALT lymphoma, extending deeply into the wall and causing mucosal ulcers [11]. Sometimes known as 'florid lymphoid hyperplasia', the process may be very difficult to distinguish from lymphoma. Immunohistochemistry and molecular diagnostic studies are useful, confirming a non-clonal process with preservation of normal lymphoid architecture.

Diffuse nodular lymphoid hyperplasia

Two clinical forms of diffuse lymphoid hyperplasia may involve the small intestine. These typically affect very long segments of the bowel as well as other gastrointestinal tract sites and are associated with an increased risk of the development of lymphoma [12–18]. One form is associated with congenital or acquired immune deficiency syndromes and is most commonly seen in patients with common variable (Swiss-type) immunodeficiency or selective IgA deficiency. Affected individuals are prone to recurrent infections such as bacterial enteritis and giardiasis. The hyperplastic lymphoid nodules measure about 5 mm in diameter and are composed of prominent follicles with germinal centres, although the overlying specialised epithelial features of Peyer's patches are absent (Figure 26.1). When the condition is associated with common variable immunodeficiency, plasma cells may be conspicuously absent from the lymphoid population.

Diffuse nodular lymphoid hyperplasia may also occur in the absence of an accompanying immunodeficiency syndrome [15,19]. It may be an incidental finding, presumably a response to an antigenic stimulus of some sort [7]. This form is more closely associated with an increased lymphoma risk [13,15,20–22]. Most lymphomas arising in association with this condition are MALT lymphomas, with a similar postulated aetiology to MALT lymphomas arising elsewhere in the setting of persistent lymphoid hyperpla-

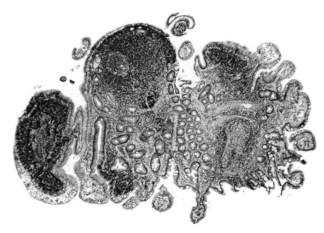

Figure 26.1 Nodular lymphoid hyperplasia: there is follicular hyperplasia with prominent germinal centre formation.

sia [6]. The hyperplastic lymphoid tissue adjacent to the lymphoma may harbour similar clonal lymphoid populations [21].

Primary malignant lymphoma of the small intestine

Primary lymphomas of the small intestine account for only about 2% of all primary gastrointestinal malignancy but the gastrointestinal tract is the most common extra-nodal site of lymphoma, with between 20% and 30% of all gastrointestinal lymphomas originating in the small bowel in western populations [23]. B-cell lymphomas are far more common than T-cell neoplasms and several lymphomas have a distinctive anatomical distribution. Thus, for example, the duodenum is the most common gastrointestinal site for primary follicular lymphoma, most T-cell lymphomas occur in the jejunum and immunoproliferative small intestinal disease (IPSID) typically involves the duodenum or jejunum. Several of the most important entities involving the small intestine are considered here. Rare diseases such as extra-nodal natural killer (NK)/T-cell lymphoma, nasal type, and Hodgkin's lymphoma may also arise in the small intestine but these are exceptionally rare, usually secondary to disease originating elsewhere and not covered in detail here.

Diffuse large B-cell lymphoma

Diffuse large B-cell lymphoma (DLBCL) is the most common lymphoma in the gastrointestinal tract. It accounts for approximately 45% of lymphomas of the small intestine [23–25]. Most DLBCLs arise de novo but there may be a preceding low grade neoplasm, often a MALT lymphoma. Most occur in older individuals, usually presenting as a solitary mass with or without involvement of regional lymph nodes. Stage at presentation is the single most important prognostic feature of DLBCL, necessitating thorough regional lymph node sampling when such lymphomas are resected, although surgical treatment is usually reserved for those cases complicated by intestinal obstruction, intractable bleeding or perforation [7]. Although aggressive, DLBCL is potentially curable using multi-agent chemotherapeutic regimens [7,24].

Macroscopically, DLBCL is an ulcerated, transmurally invasive mass that may perforate the intestine (Figure 26.2) [24]. It exhibits fleshy, tan, often 'fish-flesh', cut surfaces and is composed of intermediate to large cells with inconspicuous nuclei, described as centroblast-like (Figure 26.3). Immunoblast-like cells with prominent central nucleoli may be scattered throughout the tumour and occasional examples are composed predominantly of such cells [25]. The diagnosis is typically straightforward, using a combi-

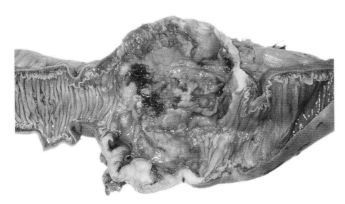

Figure 26.2 A large ulcerating diffuse large B-cell lymphoma of the small intestine. The tumour is transmurally invasive and has a 'fish-flesh' appearance to the cut surface.

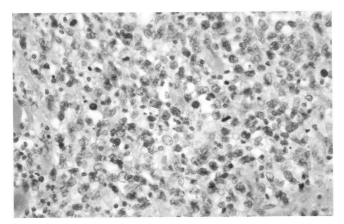

Figure 26.3 Diffuse large B-cell lymphoma: the neoplasm is composed of sheets of large cells, many resembling centroblasts. Individual cell necrosis and apoptosis is prominent, reflecting a high proliferative rate.

nation of morphology on routine sections and immunohistochemical staining with the pan-B-cell marker CD20. Cytogenetic studies may reveal chromosomal translocations involving the *BCL6* gene (3q27), t(14;18) or other abnormalities [26–28]. Gene expression profiling and immunohistochemistry can be used to separate DLBCL into two subgroups: one with a germinal centre B-cell-like phenotype and the other with an activated B-cell-like phenotype [26,29]. Most intestinal DLBCLs seem to be of the germinal centre type, although the prognostic significance of this finding is controversial [24,26,30].

MALT lymphoma

Although the stomach is the site for the vast majority of MALT lymphomas, this disease arises in the small intestine as well. Most patients are middle-aged or older and the distal small intestine, particularly the terminal ileum, is the most common site of involvement. Isolated duodenal MALT lymphoma is rare, duodenal involvement usually occurring together with a gastric primary in the presence of *H. pylori* [31]. Macroscopically, most are localised to the intestine as isolated masses with or without an overlying ulcer, although multiple smaller lesions may be seen and MALT lymphoma is reported to manifest occasionally as so-called 'lymphomatous polyposis' [32]. The process is most often diagnosed at a low stage, although involvement of mesenteric lymph nodes at the time of diagnosis is relatively common (stage II_E). Bone marrow involvement at diagnosis is, however, distinctly uncommon [33]. The clinical behaviour is typically indolent, although the prognosis is not as favourable for intestinal MALT lymphoma as it is for gastric tumours [24,34]. Important indicators suggesting a good prognosis include low stage, lack of perforation and resectability [35]. Duodenal lymphomas may respond to conservative *H. pylori* eradication therapy [36].

Histologically, intestinal MALT lymphomas are identical to their gastric counterparts (see 'MALT lymphoma', Chapter 15). Reactive follicular structures are surrounded by small neoplastic B cells with ample cytoplasm and indented nuclei, imparting a 'monocytoid' appearance. These neoplastic cells classically expand the marginal zone surrounding the reactive follicles but can so widely infiltrate the mucosa and underlying wall that the marginal zone pattern becomes impossible to discern. The neoplastic lymphocytes also infiltrate and destroy the crypt epithelium, creating so-called 'lympho-epithelial lesions' which can be highlighted using cytokeratin immunostains. Lymphocytes infiltrating epithelial structures are not specific to MALT lymphoma, however, particularly in the vicinity of Peyer's patches, where intra-epithelial lymphocytes are common (Figure 26.4). Plasmacytic differentiation of the lymphoma cells is present in about a third of cases and some MALT lymphomas are composed almost entirely of

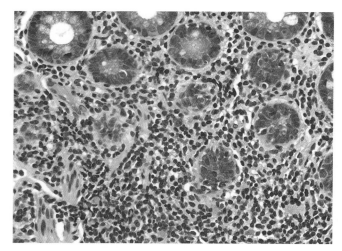

Figure 26.4 Several 'pseudo-lympho-epithelial lesions' in the vicinity of an intestinal lymphoid aggregate. Intra-epithelial lymphocytes are common near such aggregates, particularly near Peyer's patches, and are not specific to MALT lymphoma.

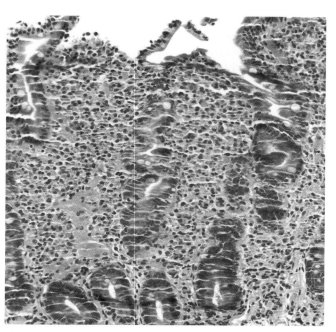

Figure 26.5 Immunoproliferative small intestinal disease: neoplastic plasma cells expand the lamina propria, causing broadened villi and the appearance of crypt loss. The plasma cells were all immunohistochemically positive for IgA heavy chain.

clonal plasma cells [33]. Immunostains for κ and λ light chains are very helpful in establishing the diagnosis in this setting. Scattered, large, transformed-appearing or immunoblast-like cells may also be found. If sheets of such cells are present, however, or if they are the predominant cell type, the appropriate diagnosis is DLBCL, because the diagnosis of so-called 'transformed' or high grade MALT lymphoma is no longer advocated [33]. A low grade component in such a lymphoma should be mentioned in the report, however, if present.

In addition to the light chain immunostains mentioned above, other ancillary tests may be useful. CD43 is aberrantly co-expressed by the neoplastic B cells in a subset of MALT lymphomas and can be helpful when present. Its absence does not, however, argue against lymphoma and it is normally expressed by many cells, including plasma cells. Identical cytogenetic abnormalities to those found in gastric MALT lymphomas can be seen in intestinal cases. These include the translocations t(11;18) and t(1;14) and trisomies of chromosomes 3 and 18. The first of these results in a fusion of the *API2* and *MALT1* genes and has been reported to be associated with higher tumour stage [37]. Aberrations found in MALT lymphomas from other sites, including t(14;18) and t(3;14), have not been reported in intestinal cases [33].

Immunoproliferative small intestinal disease

IPSID is now considered a subtype of MALT lymphoma and, although it has been reported from several continents, it is most common in the eastern Mediterranean, the Middle East and the Cape region of South Africa [33]. The disease was first described in the Middle East in 1962 [38] and further characterised from Israel in 1965 [39]. It usually occurs in young adults and may present with malabsorption or alternatively with the symptoms and signs of lymphoma, and a history of diarrhoea, steatorrhoea, weight loss and clubbing of the fingers [40–42].

The most unique feature of IPSID is its prominent plasma cell differentiation with production of abnormal, truncated Ig α heavy chains in the absence of light chains [43,44]. In a large proportion of cases, the α heavy chain proteins are detectable in the serum, saliva, small intestinal secretions or elsewhere [42,45]. In the remainder the immunoglobulin is detectable in the neoplastic plasma cells but not secreted [42,46,47]. This unique protein production distinguishes IPSID from other MALT lymphomas with extensive plasmacytic differentiation and led early observers to coin the term 'α-chain disease'. It has also been called 'Mediterranean lymphoma' [41].

IPSID primarily affects the duodenum and jejunum, although the ileum or the entire organ may be involved. There is a characteristic diffuse mural thickening, involving long, contiguous segments, which may be circumferential and cause obstruction due to stricturing [44,47,48]. There is also usually mesenteric lymphadenopathy. Histologically the disease has features of MALT lymphoma but with extensive plasmacytic differentiation; the mucosa is expanded by a predominant plasmacytic or lymphoplasmacytic infiltrate, resulting in broadening of the villi and the appearance of crypt loss due to expansion of the lamina propria (Figure 26.5) [6,42,48]. Other features of

MALT lymphoma may also be seen, including sheets of centrocyte-like cells, lympho-epithelial lesions and colonisation of reactive lymphoid follicles [6,42,49].

Immunohistochemistry reveals the neoplastic small lymphocytes to be CD20+. The plasmacytic component is negative for CD20 but can be highlighted with CD79a and CD138. Cytokeratin stains can emphasise lympho-epithelial lesions. Both the neoplastic small lymphocytes and plasma cells can be demonstrated to express the truncated α heavy chain proteins using immunohistochemistry, whereas κ and λ light chain stains are negative [49,50]. Although the neoplastic nature of the disease in its early phases has been questioned in the past, molecular genetic analysis confirms the clonality of the process even in the early stage [51]. Various cytogenetic abnormalities have also been reported, including chromosomal translocations [44,52].

Three disease stages have been described, correlating with clinical features and macroscopic appearance [6,42,53]. Initially the disease is mucosal and associated with malabsorption. Later, there is expansion into the submucosa by lymphomatous nodules with follicular colonisation of reactive lymphoid aggregates by the neoplastic cells. Finally high grade transformation results in large tumour masses with deep (often transmural) involvement of the intestinal wall. Mesenteric lymph nodes are involved early, initially by a plasmacytic infiltrate in sinuses with preservation of nodal architecture. As the disease progresses, the lymph nodes are overrun and nodal architecture completely effaced. Disease progression is accompanied by increased numbers of large, immunoblast-like cells and progression to frank DLBCL is possible [42]. Advanced tumours may have bizarre cytological features, although more typical immunoblastic and plasmacytoid morphology is also seen.

Although there is a dearth of large therapeutic trials, IPSID is reported to have a capacity for clinical remission, and possibly cure, when treated in its early stages with broad-spectrum antibiotics [44,53,54]. A possible pathogenic association with *Campylobacter jejuni* infection has been reported, allowing comparison with the chronic inflammatory response to helicobacter antigens and the development of gastric MALT lymphoma [55]. Whatever the cause(s), IPSID has a long, relapsing and remitting course [44,53,54]. Although early stage disease may respond to conservative therapy with antibiotics, chemotherapy is the treatment of choice for advanced disease. Resection is generally reserved for cases with symptomatic intestinal obstruction, haemorrhage and/or perforation [44].

Burkitt's lymphoma

Burkitt's lymphoma is an aggressive B-cell neoplasm with three clinical variants: endemic, sporadic and immunodeficiency-associated [56]. All may affect the small intestine but the sporadic form most commonly involves the ileo-caecal region, mainly affecting children and young adults, and leading to bulky disease with overlying mucosal ulceration and frequent obstruction [7,24,56]. Histologically, there is a monotonous infiltrate of medium-sized transformed cells with fine chromatin and multiple nucleoli that do not touch the nuclear membrane. A deeply basophilic cytoplasm containing lipid droplets may be seen on touch imprints [6]. The tumour's extremely rapid turnover rate is reflected in the presence of numerous tingible-body macrophages, imparting a classic 'starry-sky' pattern at low magnification. Some cases, previously termed 'atypical Burkitt's lymphoma', contain more pleomorphic cells with single prominent nucleoli, although these possess the same molecular profile as typical cases and are no longer considered separately [56].

Immunohistochemical studies reveal the neoplastic lymphocytes to express B-cell antigens such as CD20, along with markers of follicle centre differentiation, including CD10 and bcl-6 [57]. They are TdT−, allowing distinction from B-lymphoblastic leukaemia/lymphoma, and are usually negative (or only weakly positive) for bcl-2. Epstein–Barr virus (EBV), although aetiologically implicated and demonstrable in essentially all endemic cases, is present in only about 30% of sporadic cases [56]. There is essentially 100% nuclear positivity using immunohistochemistry for the proliferation marker Ki-67 (MIB-1) and the diagnosis should be questioned in the absence of this finding. Cytogenetic analysis in most cases reveals translocations involving the c-*MYC* gene on chromosome 8q24, usually to the Ig heavy chain region on 14q32, resulting in the classic t(8;14) translocation [58,59]. Alternative translocations, t(2;8) and t(8;22), involve the κ and λ light chain genes, respectively [56,60].

Although highly aggressive, Burkitt's lymphoma is potentially curable with combination chemotherapy [61,62]. With its rapid doubling time, tumour lysis syndrome may be encountered during therapy, risking intestinal perforation and possibly systemic symptoms as the tumour cells become necrotic [63]. Outcomes are less favourable in adults compared with children [64].

Primary intestinal follicular lymphoma

The small intestine is the most common site of primary gastrointestinal follicular lymphoma and primary intestinal follicular lymphoma occurs most commonly in the duodenum [65–67]. This form of the disease seems to be a distinct entity with different epidemiology and behaviour from its extra-intestinal counterpart, specifically tending to occur in middle-aged women [68,69]. The lymphoma preferentially involves the second portion of the duodenum in the vicinity of the ampulla of Vater and may present as multiple small polyps or as a large mass mimicking ampullary carcinoma [65]. The histological and immunohistochemical features are similar to lymphomas occurring in lymph nodes. A nodular/follicular pattern is prominent and the neoplastic cells stain positively with CD20, CD10 and bcl-6. Positive bcl-2 staining in the follicular structures distinguishes the neoplasm from reactive follicular hyperplasia. The lymphoma is usually of low grade (grade 1), the neoplastic follicles being composed predominantly of small cells with cleaved nuclei. The prognosis is reported to be very good, perhaps even without aggressive treatment [70].

Enteropathy-associated T-cell lymphoma

First described in 1978 and then termed 'malignant histiocytosis of the intestine', enteropathy-associated T-cell lymphoma (EATL) is a rare neoplasm of intra-epithelial T lymphocytes that accounts for fewer than 5% of gastrointestinal lymphomas, usually arising in association with coeliac disease (also known as gluten-sensitive enteropathy or coeliac sprue) (see 'Complications of coeliac disease', Chapter 21) [71–75]. Recent classification has separated the disease into two types: classic EATL and so-called monomorphic or 'type II EATL'; the latter is less common, less strongly associated with coeliac disease and composed of a more monomorphic population of medium-sized cells [72,75,76].

The proximal jejunum is the most common site of origin for EATL; the remainder of the small intestine gives rise to the disease less frequently, and the colon, stomach and other sites are rarely involved. The association of coeliac disease and classic EATL was the subject of earlier controversy but the relationship is now well established, with strong evidence of HLA haplotypes (HLA-DQ2 and -DQ8) and other associated conditions such as dermatitis herpetiformis being shared between the two diseases (see 'Complications of coeliac disease', Chapter 21) [77]. Type II EATL patients possess the HLA-DQ2 and -DQ8 haplotypes in the frequency of the general white population.

The clinical presentation is variable. The classic form of the lymphoma, accounting for 80–90% of cases, presents in the setting of coeliac disease, with associated malabsorption and diarrhoeal symptoms. Most patients are diagnosed with coeliac disease as adults but a few have a history of the disorder since childhood and the diagnoses of coeliac disease and lymphoma are occasionally made concurrently. Some patients may have a prodrome of 'refractory sprue', wherein the patient's diarrhoea fails to respond to a gluten-free diet (see 'Refractory coeliac disease', Chapter 21) [78]. Abdominal pain is a frequent presenting complaint and diagnostic investigations may reveal a large, solitary mass (Figure 26.6) or, more often, multiple ulcerating lesions. Indeed, most cases of so-called 'ulcerative jejunitis' or 'ulcerating sprue' are probably EATL [8]. Intestinal obstruction and perforation are possible, with attendant peritonitis and haemorrhage [72,75,79].

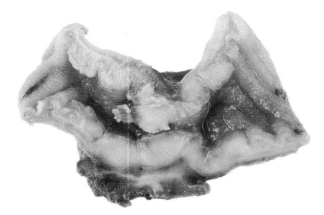

Figure 26.6 A stricturing jejunal lymphoma occurring in the setting of coeliac disease and presenting clinically with small bowel obstruction. The tumour was confirmed histologically to be enteropathy-associated T-cell lymphoma.

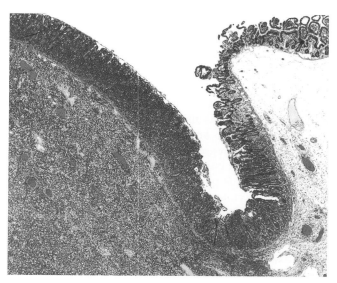

Figure 26.7 Enteropathy-associated T-cell lymphoma, classic type: the lymphoma is composed of medium-sized and large cells centred on the mucosa with diffuse infiltration of the underlying wall.

The clinical presentation of type II EATL is similar, although usually unaccompanied by the signs and symptoms of coeliac disease.

Classic EATL is typically composed of medium-to-large cells with vesicular nuclei and prominent nucleoli (Figure 26.7). Necrosis is common and this form of the disease may strongly resemble DLBCL, although it may be accompanied by a striking infiltrate of mixed inflammatory cells including eosinophils, sometimes almost obscuring the lymphoma cells [80]. Occasional cases have pleomorphic cells mimicking anaplastic large cell lymphoma. In the intact mucosa, the intra-epithelial population of neoplastic cells is prominent, with infiltration and destruction of both crypt and surface epithelium. While centred on the mucosa, the infiltrate spreads deeply into the wall and can cause penetrating ulcers. The adjacent mucosa as well as that in the duodenum contains evidence of the precursor coeliac disease, with increased intra-epithelial lymphocytes and variable villous blunting. The monomorphic variant exhibits similar epitheliotropism by smaller and more monotonous cells. There may be villous blunting and crypt hyperplasia similar to that seen in the classic form but the striking mixed inflammatory background is typically absent [75].

The neoplastic cells in the classic form of EATL are most often 'double-negative' (CD4–, CD8–) T cells that aberrantly lack CD5 and express cytotoxic proteins such as TIA-1 and granzyme B [75,81–83]. Molecular assays for clonal T-cell receptor (TCR)-β or TCR-γ gene rearrangement are positive. Commonly, the intra-epithelial lymphocytes in the adjacent uninvolved mucosa exhibit an identical antigen expression and gene rearrangement pattern [72,75,84]. In contrast to the classic form, type II EATL cells usually express CD8 and CD56, further highlighting the distinction between the two forms. Despite their distinguishing features, both forms have a dismal prognosis, particularly in those patients whose course is complicated by abdominal catastrophes such as perforation and sepsis. Patients with underlying coeliac disease are often further debilitated by chronic malabsorption.

Immunodeficiency-related lymphoproliferative disease

In addition to lymphomas arising in the background of immunodeficiency associated with diffuse nodular lymphoid hyperplasia, as described earlier, other immunodeficient states have known predispositions to lymphoma. Human immunodeficiency virus (HIV) infection is associated with a markedly increased lymphoma risk, with a predilection for involvement of the gastrointestinal tract [85,86]. Most lymphomas arising in this setting are aggressive diseases, such as DLBCL, Burkitt's lymphoma and plasmablastic lymphoma.

The gastrointestinal tract, particularly the small intestine, is a common site of involvement by post-transplantation lymphoproliferative disorders (PTLD). These conditions are associated with immunosuppressive therapy and most, but not all, are driven by EBV infection [87–90]. So-called 'early lesions' strongly resemble reactive conditions such as plasmacytic hyperplasia or infectious mononucleosis, are not associated with destruction of the native tissue architecture and may be very responsive to a reduction of immunosuppression. More advanced lesions cause tissue destruction and may require more aggressive therapy.

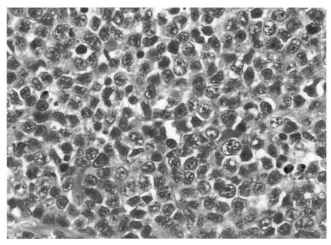

Figure 26.8 Monomorphic post-transplantation lymphoproliferative disorder: the histological features are indistinguishable from diffuse large B-cell lymphoma and scattered immunoblast-like cells with prominent central nucleoli are visible. This case occurred in a solid-organ transplant recipient but was Epstein–Barr virus negative.

They may be polymorphic or monomorphic; the former is composed of a mixture of cell types including plasma cells, immunoblasts and lymphocytes, whereas the latter is often composed of neoplastic cells that fulfil the diagnostic criteria for non-Hodgkin's lymphoma such as DLBCL or Burkitt's lymphoma (Figure 26.8). Monomorphic lesions may also be identical to a plasmacytoma and less commonly may take the form of a T/NK-cell neoplasm. When encountered, the diagnosis of monomorphic PTLD should be made in the diagnostic summary, followed by a subclassification of the process based on the corresponding type of lymphoma occurring in an immunocompetent host. Very rarely, PTLD may take the form of classic Hodgkin's lymphoma [90].

Leukaemic and secondary lymphomatous involvement of the small intestine

Secondary involvement of the small intestine by systemic haemato-lymphoid neoplasms is common and may be incidentally discovered during endoscopic examination for non-specific symptoms such as diarrhoea or bleeding or at post mortem. Some of the aforementioned conditions, such as DLBCL and follicular lymphoma, may be primarily centred outside the intestine and an unequivocal distinction between primary and secondary involvement can be difficult. Acute myeloid leukaemia (AML), particularly cases with monocytic differentiation, can present as myeloid sarcoma in the small intestine. This diagnosis may precede or coincide with the presentation of leukaemia and should

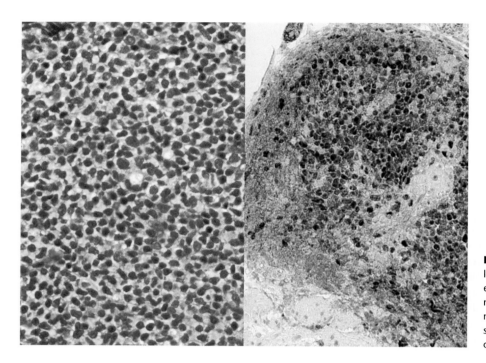

Figure 26.9 Mantle cell lymphoma: the left panel shows the haematoxylin and eosin (H&E) appearance, composed of monotonous small cells with angulated nuclei, whereas the left panel shows the strong nuclear cyclin-D1 expression characteristic of this lymphoma.

be considered an equivalent diagnosis to AML [91–93]. The process can mimic primary lymphoma, with a diffuse infiltrate of blasts that can resemble high grade lymphoma cells. The presence of eosinophilic myelocytes and/or megakaryocytes within the tumour may be helpful and immunohistochemistry for CD68, myeloperoxidase and/or lysozyme in combination with markers of immaturity such as CD117 or CD34 can be useful [93].

Mantle cell lymphoma (MCL) is a B-cell neoplasm composed of small neoplastic lymphocytes with angulated nuclei that almost always express cyclin D1 by immunohistochemistry (Figure 26.9) [94]. The disease has classically been associated with the appearance of so-called 'multiple (or malignant) lymphomatous polyposis' in the gastrointestinal tract, characterised by multiple polypoid tumours composed of monotonous neoplastic mantle cells, which may mimic adenomatous polyposis syndromes macroscopically [94–96]. However, several other types of primary gastrointestinal lymphoma, including MALT lymphoma and primary follicular lymphoma, have been reported to present as 'lymphomatous polyposis' [97–99], although MCL remains the most likely cause of this presentation. Although primary gastrointestinal MCL is possible, the disease is usually widely disseminated at presentation, with bone marrow, lymph nodes, liver and spleen commonly involved [94]. Conversely, gastrointestinal involvement is reported to be extremely common even when the disease is centred outside the gut [100]. Chronic lymphocytic leukaemia/small lymphocytic lymphoma (CLL/SLL) is another important entity that may involve the intes-

tine and can mimic MALT lymphoma or MCL. Both CLL/SLL and MCL typically express CD5 aberrantly but cyclin-D1 expression by MCL is helpful in distinguishing the two.

Metastatic disease to the small intestine

Any malignant tumour can metastasise to the small intestine and metastatic disease in this location is much more common than primary adenocarcinoma [101]. Tumours may spread via a lymphovascular route or may arrive on the serosa of the intestine after disseminating through the peritoneal cavity. Two malignancies have a propensity for small intestinal metastasis and merit specific mention. First, carcinoma of the breast may present with strictures or polypoid masses of the small bowel. Most such tumours have the histological appearance of lobular carcinoma [102]. Second, malignant melanoma has predilection for metastasis to the small intestine (Figure 26.10) [103]. Although 'primary' malignant melanomas have been described in the small intestine without history of an antecedent cutaneous primary, metastatic disease is much more likely [104,105]. Importantly, metastatic malignant melanoma may be amelanotic, tends to produce multiple tumours and can histologically mimic many epithelial and mesenchymal neoplasms. Thus, the possibility of metastatic melanoma should always be considered in the differential diagnosis of small intestinal neoplasms. Immunohistochemistry for S-100, melan-A/MART-1 and HMB-

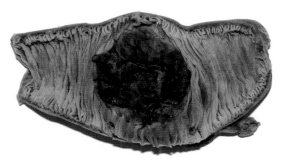

Figure 26.10 Metastatic malignant melanoma in the ileum: this tumour is clearly pigmented but amelanotic examples, in particular, can be easily mistaken for primary tumours, including lymphoma.

45 is extremely useful in this setting. Non-small cell carcinomas of the lung will also occasionally spread to the small intestine, often with more extensive involvement of the serosal aspects of the bowel wall.

References

1. Owen RL, Jones AL. Epithelial cell specialization within human Peyer's patches: an ultrastructural study of intestinal lymphoid follicles. *Gastroenterology* 1974;**66**:189.
2. Volkheimer G. Persorption of particles: physiology and pharmacology. *Adv Pharmacol Chemother* 1977;**14**:163.
3. Shepherd NA, Crocker PR, Smith AP, Levison DA. Exogenous pigment in Peyer's patches. *Hum Pathol* 1987;**18**:50.
4. Urbanski SJ, Arsenault AL, Green FH, Haber G. Pigment resembling atmospheric dust in Peyer's patches. *Mod Pathol* 1989; **2**:222.
5. Ghadially FN, Boone SA, Walley VM. A comparison of the ultrastructure of pigment granules in melanosis ilei and pulmonary lymph nodes. *Histopathology* 1998;**23**:167.
6. Isaacson PG, Norton AJ. *Extranodal Lymphomas.* Edinburgh: Churchill Livingstone 1994: 15.
7. Banks PM. Gastro-intestinal lymphoproliferative disorders. *Histopathology* 2007;**50**:42.
8. Owens SR, Greenson JK. The pathology of malabsorption: current concepts. *Histopathology* 2007;**50**:64.
9. Fieber SS, Schaefer HJ. Lymphoid hyperplasia of the terminal ileum – a clinical entity? *Gastroenterology* 1966;**50**:83.
10. Atwell JD, Burge D, Wright D. Nodular lymphoid hyperplasia of the intestinal tract in infancy and childhood. *J Pediatr Surg* 1985;**20**:25.
11. Rubin A, Isaacson PG. Florid reactive lymphoid hyperplasia of the terminal ileum in adults: a condition bearing a close resemblance to low-grade malignant lymphoma. *Histopathology* 1990;**17**:19.
12. Hermans PE, Huizenga KA, Hoffman HN, Brown AL Jr, Markowitz H. Dysgammaglobulinemia associated with nodular lymphoid hyperplasia of the small intestine. *Am J Med* 1966;**40**:78.
13. Rambaud JC, Saint-Louvent P, Marti R, et al. Diffuse follicular lymphoid hyperplasia of the small intestine without primary immunoglobulin deficiency. *Am J Med* 1982;**73**:125.
14. Hermans PE, Diaz-Buxo JA, Stobo JD. Idiopathic late-onset immunoglobulin deficiency: clinical observations in **50** patients. *Am J Med* 1976;**61**:221.
15. Matuchansky C, Touchard G, Lemaire M, et al. Malignant lymphoma of the small bowel associated with diffuse nodular lymphoid hyperplasia. *N Engl J Med* 1985;**313**:166.
16. Webster AD, Kenwright S, Ballard J, et al. Nodular lymphoid hyperplasia of the bowel in primary hypogammaglobulinaemia: study of in vivo and in vitro lymphocyte function. *Gut* 1977;**18**:364.
17. Lamers CB, Wagener T, Assmann KJ, van Tongeren JH. Jejunal lymphoma in a patient with primary adult-onset hypogammaglobulinemia and nodular lymphoid hyperplasia of the small intestine. *Dig Dis Sci* 1980;**25**:553.
18. Rubio-Tapia A, Hernandez-Calleros J, Trinidad-Hernandez S, et al. Clinical characteristics of a group of adults with nodular lymphoid hyperplasia: a single center experience. *World J Gastroenterol* 2006;**12**:1945.
19. Kahn LB, Novis BH. Nodular lymphoid hyperplasia of the small bowel associated with primary small bowel reticulum cell lymphoma. *Cancer* 1974;**33**:837.
20. Matuchansky C, Morichau-Beauchant M, Touchard G, et al. Nodular lymphoid hyperplasia of the small bowel associated with primary jejunal malignant lymphoma. Evidence favoring a cytogenetic relationship. *Gastroenterology* 1980;**78**:1587.
21. Harris M, Blewitt RW, Davies VJ, Steward WP. High-grade non-Hodgkin's lymphoma complicating polypoid nodular lymphoid hyperplasia and multiple lymphomatous polyposis of the intestine. *Histopathology* 1989;**15**:339.
22. Otter R, Bieger R, Kluin PM, Hermans J, Willemze R. Primary gastro-intestinal non-Hodgkin's lymphoma in a population-based registry. *Br J Cancer* 1989;**60**:745.
23. Andrews CN, Gill MJ, Urbanski SJ, Stewart D, Perini R, Beck P. Changing epidemiology and risk factors for gastro-intestinal non-Hodgkin's lymphoma in a North American population: population-based study. *Am J Gastroenterol* 2008;**103**:1762.
24. Domizio P, Owen RA, Shepherd NA, Talbot IC, Norton AJ. Primary lymphoma of the small intestine. A clinicopathological study of 119 cases. *Am J Surg Pathol* 1993;**17**:429.
25. Mitchell KA, Finn WG, Owens SR. Differences in germinal centre and non-germinal centre phenotype in gastric and intestinal diffuse large B-cell lymphoma. *Leuk Lymphoma* 2008;**49**:1717.
26. Stein H, Warnke RA, Chan WC, Jaffe ES. *Diffuse large B-cell lymphoma, not otherwise specified.* In: Swerdlow SH, Campo E, Harris NL, et al. (eds), *WHO Classification of Tumours of Haematopoietic and Lymphoid Tissues.* IARC: Lyon, 2008: 233.
27. Offit K, Lo CF, Louie DC, et al. Rearrangement of the bcl-6 gene as a prognostic marker in diffuse large-cell lymphoma. *N Engl J Med* 1994;**331**:74.
28. Weiss LM, Warnke RA, Sklar J, Cleary ML. Molecular analysis of the t(14;18) chromosomal translocation in malignant lymphomas. *N Engl J Med* 1987;**317**:1185.
29. Alizadeh AA, Eisen MG, Davis RE, et al. Distinct types of diffuse large B-cell lymphoma identified by gene expression profiling. *Nature* 2000;**403**:503.
30. Connor J, Ashton-Key M. Gastric and intestinal diffuse large B-cell lymphomas are clinically and immunophenotypically different. An immunohistochemical and clinical study. *Histopathology* 2007;**51**:697.
31. Toshima M, Aikawa K, Soga K, Shibasaki K, Yoshida K, Emura I. Primary duodenal MALT lymphoma. *Intern Med* 1999;**38**:957.
32. Breslin NP, Urbanski SJ, Shaffer EA. Mucosa-associated lymphoid tissue (MALT) lymphoma manifesting as multiple lymphomatous polyposis of the gastro-intestinal tract. *Am J Gastroenterol* 1999;**94**:2540.
33. Isaacson PG, Chott A, Nakamura S, Müller-Hermelink HK, Harris NL, Swerdlow SH. Extranodal marginal zone lymphoma of mucosa-associated lymphoid tissue (MALT lymphoma). In:

Swerdlow SH, Campo E, Harris NL, et al. (eds), *WHO Classification of Tumours of Haematopoietic and Lymphoid Tissues*. IARC: Lyon, 2008: 214.

34. Nakamura S, Matsumoto T, Takashita M, et al. A clinicopathologic study of primary small intestine lymphoma: prognostic significance of mucosa-associated lymphoid tissue-derived lymphoma. *Cancer* 2000;**88**:286.

35. Radaszkiewicz T, Dragosics B, Bauer P. Gastro-intestinal malignant lymphomas of the mucosa-associated lymphoid tissue: factors relevant to prognosis. *Gastroenterology* 1992;**102**:1628.

36. Nagashima R, Takeda H, Maeda K, et al. Regression of duodenal mucosa-associated lymphoid tissue lymphoma after eradication of *Helicobacter pylori*. *Gastroenterology* 1996;**111**:1674.

37. Streubel B, Seitz G, Stolte M, Birner P, Chott A, Raderer M. MALT lymphoma associated genetic aberrations occur at different frequencies in primary and secondary intestinal MALT lymphomas. *Gut* 2006;**55**:1581.

38. Azar HA. Cancer in Lebanon and the Near East. *Cancer* 1962; **15**:16.

39. Ramot B, Shahin N, Bubis JJ. Malabsorption syndrome in lymphoma of the small intestine. A study of 13 cases. *Isr J Med Sci* 1965;**1**:221.

40. Doe WF, Henry K, Hobbs JR, Jones FA, Dent CE, Booth CC. Five cases of alpha chain disease. *Gut* 1972;**13**:947.

41. Lewin KJ, Kahn LB, Novis BH. Primary intestinal lymphoma of 'Western' and 'Mediterranean' type, alpha chain disease and massive plasma cell infiltration: a comparative study of 37 cases. *Cancer* 1976;**38**:2511.

42. Salem PA, Estephan FF. Immunoproliferative small intestinal disease: current concepts. *Cancer J* 2005;**11**:374.

43. Seligmann M. Alpha chain disease: immunoglobulin abnormalities, pathogenesis and current concepts. *Br J Cancer* 1975; **31**(suppl 2):356.

44. Al-Saleem T, Al-Mondhiry H. Immunoproliferative small intestinal disease (IPSID): a model for mature B-cell neoplasms. *Blood* 2005;**105**:2274.

45. Seligmann M, Danon F, Hurez D, Mihaesco E, Preud'homme, JL. Alpha-chain disease: a new immunoglobulin abnormality. *Science* 1968;**162**:1396.

46. Rambaud JC. Small intestinal lymphomas and alpha-chain disease. *Clin Gastroenterol* 1983;**12**:743.

47. Nassar VH, Salem PA, Shahid MJ, et al. 'Mediterranean abdominal lymphoma' or immunoproliferative small intestinal disease. Part II: pathological aspects. *Cancer* 1978;**41**:1340.

48. Fine K, Stone M. Alpha-heavy chain disease, Mediterranean lymphoma, and immunoproliferative small intestinal disease. *Am J Gastroenterol* 1999;**94**:1139.

49. Isaacson PG, Dogan A, Price SK, Spencer J. Immunoproliferative small-intestinal disease. An immunohistochemical study. *Am J Surg Pathol* 1989;**13**:1023.

50. Isaacson PG, Price SK. Light chains in Mediterranean lymphoma. *J Clin Pathol* 1985;**38**:601.

51. Smith WJ, Price SK, Isaacson PG. Immunoglobulin gene rearrangement in immunoproliferative small intestinal disease (IPSID). *J Clin Pathol* 1987;**40**:1291.

52. Berger R, Bernheim A, Tsapis A, Brouet JC, Seligmann M. Cytogenetic studies in four cases of alpha chain disease. *Cancer Genet Cytogenet* 1986;**22**:219.

53. Gilinsky NH, Novis BH, Wright JP, Dent DM, King H, Marks IN. Immunoproliferative small-intestinal disease: clinical features and outcome in 30 cases. *Medicine* 1987;**66**:438.

54. Ben Ayed F, Halphen M, Najjar T, et al. Treatment of alpha chain disease. Results of a prospective study in 21 Tunisian patients by the Tunisian-French Intestinal Lymphoma Study Group. *Cancer* 1989;**63**:1251.

55. Lecuit M, Abachin E, Martin A, et al. Immunoproliferative small intestinal disease associated with *Campylobacter jejuni*. *N Engl J Med* 2004;**350**:239.

56. Leoncini L, Raphaël M, Stein H, Harris NL, Jaffe ES, Kluin PM. Burkitt lymphoma. In: Swerdlow SH, Campo E, Harris NL, et al. (eds), *WHO Classification of Tumours of Haematopoietic and Lymphoid Tissues*. IARC: Lyon 2008: 262.

57. Payne CM, Grogan TM, Cromey DW, Bjore CG, Kerrigan DP. An ultrastructural morphometric and immunophenotypic evaluation of Burkitt's and Burkitt's-like lymphomas. *Lab Invest* 1987;**57**:200.

58. Lenoir GM, Land H, Parada LF, Cunningham JM, Weinberg RA. Activated oncogenes in Burkitt's lymphoma. *Curr Top Microbiol Immunol* 1984;**113**:6.

59. Zimber-Strobl U, Strobl L, Hofelmayr H, et al. EBNA2 and c-myc in B cell immortalization by Epstein–Barr virus and in the pathogenesis of Burkitt's lymphoma. *Curr Top Microbiol Immunol* 1999;**246**:315.

60. Glassman AB, Hopwood V, Hayes KJ. Cytogenetics as an aid in the diagnosis of lymphomas. *Ann Clin Lab Sci* 2000;**30**:72.

61. Patte C, Michon J, Frappaz D, et al. Therapy of Burkitt and other B-cell acute lymphoblastic leukaemia and lymphoma: experience with the LMB protocols of the SFOP (French Paediatric Oncology Society) in children and adults. *Baillière's Clin Haematol* 1994;**7**:339.

62. Patte C, Auperin A, Gerrard M, et al. Results of the randomized international FAB/LMB96 trial for intermediate risk B-cell non-Hodgkin lymphoma in children and adolescents: it is possible to reduce treatment for the early responding patients. *Blood* 2007;**109**:2773.

63. Veenstra J, Krediet RT, Somers R, Arisz L. Tumour lysis syndrome and acute renal failure in Burkitt's lymphoma. Description of 2 cases and a review of the literature on prevention and management. *Neth J Med* 1994;**45**:211.

64. Divine M, Casassus P, Koscielny S, et al. Burkitt lymphoma in adults: a prospective study of 72 patients treated with an adapted pediatric LMB protocol. *Ann Oncol* 2005;**16**:1928.

65. Misdraji J, Fernandez del Castillo C, Ferry J. Follicle center lymphoma of the ampulla of Vater presenting with jaundice. *Am J Surg Pathol* 1997;**21**:484.

66. Yoshino T, Miyake K, Ichimura A, et al. Increased incidence of follicular lymphoma in the duodenum. *Am J Surg Pathol* 2000;**24**:688.

67. Shia J, Teruya-Feldstein J, Pan D, et al. Primary follicular lymphoma of the gastrointestinal tract: a clinical and pathologic study of 26 cases. *Am J Surg Pathol* 2002;**26**:216.

68. Damaj G, Verkarre V, Delmer A, et al. Primary follicular lymphoma of the gastrointestinal tract: a study of 25 cases and a literature review. *Ann Oncol* 2003;**14**:623.

69. Poggi MM, Cong PJ, Coleman CN, et al. Low-grade follicular lymphoma of the small intestine. *J Clin Gastroenterol* 2002;**34**:155.

70. Harris NL, Swerdlow SH, Jaffe ES, et al. Follicular lymphoma. In: Swerdlow SH, Campo E, Harris NL, et al. (eds), *WHO Classification of Tumours of Haematopoietic and Lymphoid Tissues*. IARC: Lyon, 2008: 220.

71. Isaacson P, Wright DH. Malignant histiocytosis of the intestine. Its relationship to malabsorption and ulcerative jejunitis. *Hum Pathol* 1978;**9**:661.

72. Zettl A, deLeew R, Haralambieva E, Mueller-Hermelink H-K. Enteropathy-type T-cell lymphoma. *Am J Clin Pathol* 2007; **127**:701.

73. Isaacson PG, O'Connor NT, Spencer J, et al. Malignant histiocytosis of the intestine: a T-cell lymphoma. *Lancet* 1985;**ii**:688.

74. Ashton-Key M, Diss TC, Du Pan LMQ, Isaacson PG. Molecular analysis of T-cell clonality in ulcerative jejunitis and enteropathy-associated T-cell lymphoma. *Am J Pathol* 1997;**151**:493.

75. Isaacson PG, Chott A, Ott G, Stein H. Enteropathy-associated T-cell lymphoma. In: Swerdlow SH, Campo E, Harris NL, Jaffe ES, et al. (eds), *WHO Classification of Tumours of Haematopoietic and Lymphoid Tissues.* IARC: Lyon, 2008: 289.

76. deLeeuw RJ, Zettl A, Klinker E, et al. Whole-genome analysis and HLA genotyping of enteropathy-type T-cell lymphoma reveals 2 distinct lymphoma subtypes. *Gastroenterology* 2007; **132**:1902.

77. Howell WM, Leung ST, Jones DB et al. HLA-DRB, -DQA, and -DQB polymorphism in celiac disease and enteropathy-associated T-cell lymphoma. Common features and additional risk factors for malignancy. *Hum Immunol* 1995;**43**:29.

78. Mulder CJ, Wahab PJ, Moshaver B, Meijer JW. Refractory coeliac disease: a window between coeliac disease and enteropathy associated T cell lymphoma. *Scand J Gastroenterol Suppl* 2000;**232**:32.

79. Isaacson P, Wright DH. Intestinal lymphoma associated with malabsorption. *Lancet* 1978;i:67.

80. Shepherd NA, Blackshaw AJ, Hall PA, et al. Malignant lymphoma with eosinophilia of the gastro-intestinal tract. *Histopathology* 1987;**11**:115.

81. Isaacson PG, Du MQ. Gastro-intestinal lymphoma: where morphology meets molecular biology. *J Pathol* 2005;**205**:255.

82. Murray A, Cuevas EC, Jones DB, Wright DH. Study of the immunohistochemistry and T cell clonality of enteropathy-associated T cell lymphoma. *Am J Pathol* 1995;**146**:509.

83. de Bruin PC, Connolly CE, Oudejans JJ, et al. Enteropathy-associated T-cell lymphomas have a cytotoxic T-cell phenotype. *Histopathology* 1997;**31**:313.

84. Bagdi E, Diss TC, Munson P, Isaacson PG. Mucosal intra-epithelial lymphocytes in enteropathy-associated T-cell lymphoma, ulcerative jejunitis, and refractory celiac disease constitute a neoplastic population. *Blood* 1999;**94**:260.

85. Levine AM. AIDS-associated malignant lymphoma. *Med Clin North Am* 1992;**76**:253.

86. Raphaël M, Said J, Borish B, Cesarman E, Harris NL. Lymphomas associated with HIV infection. In: Swerdlow SH, *Campo E, Harris NL,* et al. (eds), *WHO Classification of Tumours of Haematopoietic and Lymphoid Tissues.* IARC: Lyon, 2008: 340.

87. Nalesnik MA. Involvement of the gastro-intestinal tract by Epstein–Barr virus-associated posttransplant lymphoproliferative disorders. *Am J Surg Pathol* 1990;**14**(suppl 1):92.

88. Craig FE, Gulley ML, Banks PM. Posttransplantation lymphoproliferative disorders. *Am J Clin Pathol* 1993;**99**:265.

89. Nalesnik MA. Clinical and pathological features of posttransplant lymphoproliferative disorders (PTLD). *Semin Immunopathol* 1998;**20**:325.

90. Swerdlow SH, Webber SA, Chadburn A, Ferry JA. Posttransplant lymphoproliferative disorders. In Swerdlow SH, Campo E, Harris NL, et al. (eds), *WHO Classification of Tumours of Haematopoietic and Lymphoid Tissues.* IARC: Lyon, 2008: 343.

91. Brugo EA, Larkin E, Molina-Escobar J, Contanzi J. Primary granulocytic sarcoma of the small bowel. *Cancer* 1975;**35**:1333.

92. Brugo EA, Marshall RB, Riberi AM, Pautasso OE. Preleukemic granulocytic sarcomas of the gastro-intestinal tract. Report of two cases. *Am J Clin Pathol* 1977;**68**:616.

93. Pileri SA, Orazi A, Falini B. Myeloid sarcoma. In: Swerdlow SH, Campo E, Harris NL, et al. (eds), *WHO Classification of Tumours of Haematopoietic and Lymphoid Tissues.* IARC: Lyon, 2008: 140.

94. Swerdlow SH, Campo E, Seto M, Muller-Hermelink HK. Mantle cell lymphoma. In: Swerdlow SH, Campo E, Harris NL, et al. (eds), *WHO Classification of Tumours of Haematopoietic and Lymphoid Tissues.* IARC: Lyon, 2008: 229.

95. Isaacson PG, MacLennan KA, Subbuswamy SG. Multiple lymphomatous polyposis of the gastro-intestinal tract. *Histopathology* 1984;**8**:641.

96. Moynihan MJ, Bast MA, Chan WC, et al. Lymphomatous polyposis. A neoplasm of either follicular mantle or germinal center cell origin. *Am J Surg Pathol* 1996;**20**:442.

97. Kodama T, Ohshima K, Nomura K, et al. Lymphomatous polyposis of the gastro-intestinal tract, including mantle cell lymphoma, follicular lymphoma and mucosa-associated lymphoid tissue lymphoma. *Histopathology* 2005;**47**:467.

98. Hokama A, Tomoyose T, Yamamoto Y, et al. Adult T-cell leukemia/lymphoma presenting multiple lymphomatous polyposis. *World J Gastroenterol* 2008;**14**:6584.

99. Yang SF, Liao YL, Kuo SY, et al. Primary intestinal diffuse large B-cell lymphoma presenting as multiple lymphomatous polyposis. *Leuk Lymphoma* 2009;**50**:1219.

100. Salar A, Juanpere N, Bellosillo B, et al. Gastro-intestinal involvement in mantle cell lymphoma: a prospective clinic, endoscopic and pathologic study. *Am J Surg Pathol* 2006;**30**:1274.

101. Idelevich E, Kashtan H, Mavor E, et al. Small bowel obstruction caused by secondary tumors. *Surg Oncol* 2006;**15**:29.

102. McLemore EC, Pockaj BA, Reynolds C, et al. Breast cancer: presentation and intervention in women with gastro-intestinal metastasis and carcinomatosis. *Ann Surg Oncol* 2006;**12**:886.

103. Blecker D, Abraham S, Furth EE, Kochman ML. Melanoma in the gastro-intestinal tract. *Am J Gastroenterol* 1999;**94**:3427.

104. Elsayed AM, Albahra M, Nzeako UC, Sobin LH. Malignant melanomas in the small intestine: a study of **103** patients. *Am J Gastroenterol* 1996;**91**:1001.

105. Schuchter LM, Green R, Fraker D. Primary and metastatic diseases in malignant melanoma of the gastro-intestinal tract. *Curr Opin Oncol* 2000;**12**:181.

CHAPTER 27

Miscellaneous disorders of the small intestine

Joel K. Greenson

University of Michigan Medical School, Ann Arbor, MI, USA

Amyloidosis

Amyloid in the small bowel may be predominantly mucosal and subepithelial in distribution, confined to the vasculature or deposited in the muscularis mucosae and muscularis propria (Figure 27.1). The distribution is partly related to the nature of the underlying systemic amyloidosis. Clinical effects depend on the pattern of involvement and include malabsorption, ischaemia and motility disorders. Gastrointestinal amyloidosis is discussed more fully in Chapter 40 (see 'Amyloidosis', Chapter 40).

Deposits of immunoglobulin secondary to Waldenström's macroglobulinaemia may mimic amyloidosis in the small intestine, especially in duodenal biopsies (see 'Waldenström's macroglobulinaemia', Chapter 21). These deposits will stain with periodic acid–Schiff (PAS) but not with Congo red. In Waldenström's macroglobulinaemia, the eosinophilic deposits may be found within dilated lymphatics and lacteals [1–3]. The deposits will also stain with IgM and will be light chain restricted, although these stains are generally not needed to make the diagnosis of Waldenström's macroglobulinaemia in the small intestine.

Bypass operations

Obesity surgery with bypass of small bowel segments is performed rarely now but there are still many individuals who have had this surgery performed in the past. The non-bypassed functioning segments of ileum show a gradual increase in length and diameter. In both the functioning and excluded or diverted segments there is an increase in mucosal height due to lengthening and broadening of the villi and an increase in the number of mucosal folds [4,5]. These changes are considered to be adaptive and may explain the failure of many patients to continue to lose weight after satisfactory initial weight loss. We have seen one case in which the excluded segment not only developed hyperplastic villous changes but also increased numbers of lymphoid follicles and mild diffuse chronic mucosal inflammation, reminiscent of the changes seen in diverted colonic segments (see 'Diversion colitis', Chapter 35), although there was also an intra-epithelial lymphocytosis (but no evidence of gluten sensitivity).

Complications of intestinal bypass surgery may occur both within the excluded segment and outside the gastrointestinal tract. Enteric hyperoxaluria may produce acute renal failure [6]. Other complications include electrolyte imbalance, malnutrition, diarrhoea, liver disease including cirrhosis, nephrolithiasis, arthritis and pathological fractures. Of these complications, the electrolyte imbalance, malnutrition and diarrhoea usually improve after reversal [7]. A dermal leukocytoclastic vasculitis that is responsive to tetracycline may also occur as part of the so-called 'bowel bypass arthritis dermatitis syndrome' [8]. Within the bypassed segment itself pneumatosis cystoides intestinalis, severe blood loss, localised ulceration, intussusception, adhesions and bacterial overgrowth have all been observed [9,10].

Cholesterol ester storage disease

This is a very rare inherited disorder of lipid metabolism in which the liver and spleen are enlarged, serum cholesterol is raised and cholesterol esters are stored in various

---

Morson and Dawson's Gastrointestinal Pathology, Fifth Edition. Edited by Neil A. Shepherd, Bryan F. Warren, Geraint T. Williams, Joel K. Greenson, Gregory Y. Lauwers and Marco R. Novelli.

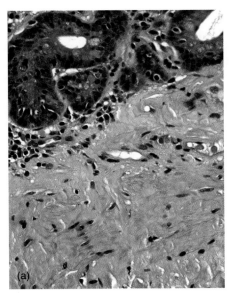

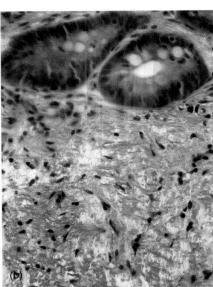

Figure 27.1 Amyloidosis in the small intestine. (a) A medium-power view of the submucosa showing amorphous eosinophilic material admixed with fibres of smooth muscle. (b) Same area as part (a) stained with Congo red. Note the apple-green birefringence with polarised light.

body tissues. Macroscopically the small bowel mucosa has a yellow tinge. Microscopically the epithelium is normal but foamy macrophages may be seen in considerable numbers in the lamina propria at the tips of villi [11]. This may mimic atypical mycobacterial infection or Whipple's disease and appropriate special stains may be necessary to exclude these possibilities.

Endometriosis

The small bowel is much less commonly affected by endometriosis than the large bowel (see 'Endometriosis', Chapter 40). Lesions are recognised on finding endometrial glands and stroma, most frequently in the serosa but occasionally intramurally, and sometimes in association with haemosiderin-laden macrophages. Dense stromal fibrosis may lead to multiple complex adhesions, especially after laparoscopic surgery for endometriosis. In postmenopausal women inactive endometriotic foci composed of glands but little stroma should not be confused with deposits of adenocarcinoma. Immunostains for oestrogen receptor and CD10 may be helpful in establishing the diagnosis of endometriosis in problematic cases. Pregnancy causes especial consternation with intestinal endometriosis because the stroma becomes decidualised and the glands cystically dilated.

Pneumatosis cystoides intestinalis

Pneumatosis cystoides intestinalis of the small bowel occurs in two forms [12–14]. The first, in patients with chronic obstructive pulmonary disease, is the result of gaseous dissection through the perivascular space of intra-abdominal blood vessels. The second occurs in infants with necrotising enterocolitis and in adults with ischaemic bowel and is the result of intramural gas-forming organisms (especially *Clostridium perfringens*, *Enterobacter aerogenes* and *Escherichia coli*). More recently this condition has been associated with immunosuppressive drug therapies, collagen vascular diseases and a variety of gastrointestinal pathologies [15,16]. The cysts are found in the mucosa, submucosa and subserosa. They may be single or multiple and give rise to sessile or even pedunculated mucosal polyps (Figure 27.2a). They are usually lined by mixed inflammatory cells, macrophages or foreign body giant cells (Figure 27.2b) but occasionally those associated with lung disease have an apparent lining of endothelial cells. In mucosal biopsies they are recognised as incomplete cysts surrounded by macrophages in the submucosa. Eosinophils are often prominent. Care must be taken not to misinterpret the changes as Crohn's disease, because a biopsy may crush the cyst and demonstrate only macrophages, giant cells and eosinophils.

Malakoplakia

Malakoplakia is rarer in the small intestine than in the large bowel (see 'Malakoplakia', Chapter 40). It may be seen complicating pre-existing chronic inflammatory bowel disease or arising in isolation in adults, often in association with *E. coli* infection [17]. Infections with *Klebsiella* and *Yersinia* spp. have also been associated with malakoplakia.

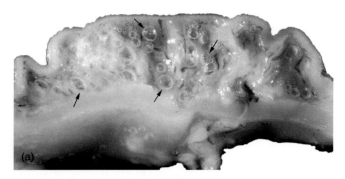

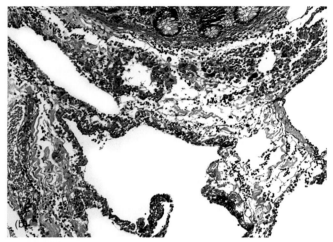

Figure 27.2 Pneumatosis cystoides intestinalis: (a) gross photograph of the small intestine cut in cross-section showing numerous cysts in the submucosa (arrows), muscularis propria and serosa. (Photo courtesy of Jason Carvalho, MD.) (b) Medium-power view of small bowel submucosa showing numerous gas-filled cysts lined by multinucleated giant cells and eosinophils.

Systemic mastocytosis

Steatorrhoea may occasionally complicate urticaria pigmentosa and systemic mastocytosis. Some cases show small intestinal mucosal flattening with infiltration by mast cells, accompanied by eosinophils and neutrophils [18]. Mast cells may be identified by metachromatic staining with toluidine blue or with immunohistochemistry using antibodies to mast cell tryptase, CD68 and CD117 [19]. Positive staining of mast cells with CD25 appears to be a specific marker of systemic mastocytosis [20].

Melanosis and pseudo-melanosis

Melanosis (or more accurately pseudo-melanosis), due to lipofuscin deposition in mucosal macrophages, which is commonly seen in the large bowel (see 'Melanosis coli', Chapter 40) of patients taking anthraquinone laxatives,

virtually never occurs in the small bowel. However, a melanin-like pigmentation of the duodenal mucosa has been described rarely in association with peptic ulceration and folate deficiency [21] and in patients with AIDS or those receiving haemodialysis [22]. This appears to start with iron deposition and the pigment later stains with the Masson–Fontana reaction. These rare cases of mucosal pigmentation should be distinguished from the brown bowel syndrome which is seen in association with severe malabsorption, in which the lipofuscin pigmentation occurs within the intramural musculature (see 'The brown bowel syndrome', Chapter 21).

Zinc deficiency

A rare autosomal recessive disorder, acrodermatitis enteropathica, results in zinc malabsorption [23] and morphological effects on the small bowel mucosa, including focal villous atrophy with crypt hyperplasia, reduced brush border enzymes and mild focal chronic inflammation in the lamina propria. Electron microscopy shows that Paneth cells contain characteristic pleomorphic cytoplasmic inclusions [24].

Pseudo-lipomatosis

This is another condition that is common in the colorectum but rarely reported in the duodenum [25]. There are numerous tiny gas bubbles, usually measuring $<50\,\mu m$ in diameter, in the lamina propria of the mucosa. On superficial examination they resemble adipocytes, hence the term 'pseudo-lipomatosis'. They may cause expansion of the villous cores, and separation of the crypts, and must be distinguished from lymphangiectasia and Whipple's disease, if necessary, by immunostaining. Pseudo-lipomatosis is now considered to be an artefact of mucosal biopsies that results from penetration of gas into the mucosa because of gas insufflation during endoscopy (see 'Pseudo-lipomatosis', Chapter 40).

Graft-versus-host disease

The small intestine, similar to other parts of the gastrointestinal tract, may be involved in graft-versus-host disease (GVHD) after bone marrow/stem cell transplantation. The duodenum is easily biopsied and the changes seen here typically mirror those seen in the large intestine [26] (see Graft-versus-host disease', Chapter 40). Increased apoptotic bodies within the crypt proliferative zones are the hallmark of GVHD (Figure 27.3). Mild forms may demonstrate only occasional apoptotic bodies in crypt epithelium whereas severe cases will show complete denudation of the mucosa. In such severe cases, all one may find in the lamina propria are nests of endocrine cells [27], the tombstones of

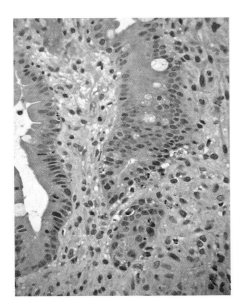

Figure 27.3 High power view of duodenal mucosa in graft-versus-host disease. Note the numerous apoptotic bodies and the empty appearing lamina propria, devoid of plasma cells.

epithelial crypts in which all the other cells have been destroyed by programmed cell death/apoptosis.

Although enhanced apoptosis is characteristic of GVHD, it is in no way specific. Many infectious pathogens (cytomegalovirus, adenovirus, HIV, cryptosporidia) will induce increased apoptosis, as will the drug mycophenolate mofetil, which is ironically used to treat GVHD in many cases [28,29]. Non-steroidal anti-inflammatory drugs and chemotherapy can also cause enhanced apoptosis that mimics GVHD. The latter is important in the early bone marrow transplant period because it generally takes 3 weeks for the effects of conditioning chemotherapy to resolve [29]. The healing phase of GVHD may show marked architectural distortion, reminiscent of inflammatory bowel disease.

Small intestinal transplantation

The number of small bowel and multi-visceral organ transplantations has steadily increased since the first successful transplantations back in 1989 [30]. As one might expect with any allogeneic transplant, problems with rejection are quite common, with most patients having acute cellular rejection, especially early in their postoperative course [31,32]. The histology of acute cellular rejection in the small intestine typically shows increased apoptosis in the bases of the crypts (more than 2 per 10 crypts) and increased mononuclear lymphoid cells in the lamina propria [31]. The lamina propria mononuclear cells often contain blastic or transformed lymphocytes. Acute cellular rejection is most often found in the ileum [31]. Cases of acute antibody-

mediated rejection have also been reported [30]. The use of C4d immunohistochemistry can be used to confirm this diagnosis [30]. Chronic rejection with foam cell arteriopathy may also occur [30].

Patients who receive small bowel transplants are also at risk from the same opportunistic infections that chronically immunosuppressed patients are prone to [30]. Early on, the incidence of post-transplantation lymphoproliferative disorder was quite high in small bowel transplant recipients but decreased immunosuppression and prophylaxis against EBV infections has resulted in a marked decrease in this problem [32]. GVHD is also a problem in small bowel and multi-visceral transplant recipients, owing to the large amount of donor lymphoid tissue present within the graft [32,33]. Recipients of other solid organ transplants rarely get GVHD (only about 1–2%), whereas those who receive small bowel transplants have a prevalence of GVHD of between 5% and 10% [33,34]. Furthermore, the histological changes of GVHD in the small bowel are quite similar to those of acute cellular rejection. Hence histological confirmation of GVHD is most often to be found in biopsies of the skin.

References

1. Bedine MS, Yardley JH, Elliott HL, Banwell JG, Hendrix TR. Intestinal involvement in Waldenström's macroglobulinemia. *Gastroenterology* 1973;**65**:308.
2. Harris M, Burton IE, Scarffe JH. Macroglobulinaemia and intestinal lymphangiectasia: a rare association. *J Clin Pathol* 1983;**36**:30.
3. Pratz KW, Dingli D, Smyrk TC, Lust JA. Intestinal lymphangiectasia with protein-losing enteropathy in Waldenström macroglobulinemia. *Medicine* 2007;**86**:210.
4. Solhaug JH, Tvelte S. Adaptive changes in the small intestine following bypass operation for obesity: a radiological and histological study. *Scand J Gastroenterol* 1978;**13**:401.
5. Asp N-G, Gudmand-Hoyer E, Andersen B, Berg NO. Enzyme activities and morphological appearance in functioning and excluded segments of the small intestine after shunt operation for obesity. *Gut* 1979;**20**:553.
6. Wharton R, D'Agati V, Magun AM, Whitlock R, Kunis CL, Appel GB. Acute deterioration of renal function associated with enteric hyperoxaluria. *Clin Nephrol* 1990;**34**:116.
7. Dean P, Joshi S, Kaminski DL. Long term outcome of reversal of small intestinal bypass operations. *Am J Surg* 1990;**159**:118.
8. Sandbank M, Weltfriend S, Wolf R. Bowel bypass arthritis dermatitis syndrome: a histological and electron microscopical study. *Acta Derm Venereol* 1984;**64**:79.
9. Leung FW, Drenick EJ, Stanley TM. Intestinal bypass complications involving the excluded small bowel segment. *Am J Gastroenterol* 1982;**77**:67.
10. Ikard RW. Pneumatosis cystoides intestinalis following intestinal bypass. *Am J Surg* 1977; **43**:467.
11. Partin JC, Schubert WK. Small intestinal mucosa in cholesterol ester storage disease: a light and electron microscopic study. *Gastroenterology* 1969;**57**:542.
12. Galandiuk S, Fazio VW. Pneumatosis cystoides intestinalis. *Dis Colon Rectum* 1986;**29**:358.

13. Koss LK. Abdominal gas cysts (Pneumatosis cystoides intestinalis hominis): an analysis with a report of a case and a critical review of the literature. *Arch Pathol* 1952;**53**:523.
14. Hughes DTD, Gordon KCD, Swann JC, Bolt GL. Pneumatosis cystoides intestinalis. *Gut* 1966;**7**:553.
15. Gagliardi G, Thompson IW, Hershman MJ, Forbes A, Hawley PR, Talbot IC. Pneumatosis coli: a proposed pathogenesis based on study of 25 cases and review of the literature. *Int J Colorect Dis* 1996;**11**:111.
16. Matsumoto A, Isomoto H, Shikuwa S, et al. Pneumatosis intestinalis in ulcerative colitis. *Med Sci Monit* 2009;**15**:139.
17. McClure J. Malakoplakia of the gastrointestinal tract. *Postgrad Med J* 1981;**57**:95.
18. Braverman DZ, Dollbergh L, Shiner M. Clinical, histological and electron microscopic study of mast cell disease of the small bowel. *Am J Gastroenterol* 1985;**80**:30.
19. Li W, Kapadia S, Sonmez-Alpan E, et al. Immunohistochemical characterisation of mast cell disease in paraffin sections using tryptase, CD68, myeloperoxidase, lysozyme, and CD20 antibodies. *Mod Pathol* 1996;**9**:982.
20. Hahn HP, Hornick JL. Immunoreactivity for CD25 in gastrointestinal mucosal mast cells is specific for systemic mastocytosis. *Am J Surg Pathol* 2007;**31**:1669.
21. Sharp JR, Insalaco DJ, Johnson LJ. Melanosis of the duodenum associated with a gastric ulcer and folic acid deficiency. *Gastroenterology* 1980;**78**:366.
22. Kang JY, Wu AYT, Chia JLS, et al. Clinical and ultrastructural studies in duodenal pseudomelanosis. *Gut* 1987;**8**:1673.
23. Danbolt N, Closs K. Acrodermatitis enteropathica. *Acta Derm Venereol* 1942;**3**:127.
24. Bohane TD, Cutz E, Hamilton JR, et al. Acrodermatitis enteropathica, zinc and the Paneth cell. *Gastroenterology* 1977;**73**:587.
25. Cook DS, Williams GT. Duodenal 'pseudolipomatosis'. *Histopathology* 1998;**33**:394.
26. Ponec RJ, Hackman RC, McDonald GB. Endoscopic and histologic diagnosis of intestinal graft-versus-host disease after marrow transplantation. *Gastrointest Endosc* 1999;**49**:612.
27. Bryan RL, Antonakopoulos GN, Newman J, Milligan DW. Intestinal graft versus host disease. *J Clin Pathol* 1991;**44**:866.
28. Shulman HM, Kleiner D, Lee SJ, et al. Histopathological diagnosis of chronic graft-versus-host disease: National Institutes of Health Consensus Development Project on criteria for clinical trials in chronic graft-versus-host disease: II. Pathology Working Group Report. *Biol Blood Marrow Transplant* 2006;**12**:31.
29. Washington K, Jagasia M. Pathology of graft-versus-host disease in the gastrointestinal tract. *Hum Pathol* 2009;**40**:909.
30. Nayyar N, Mazariegos G, Ranganathan S, et al. Pediatric small bowel transplantation. *Semin Pediatr Surg* 2010;**19**:68.
31. Lee RG, Nakamura K, Tsamandas AC, et al. Pathology of human intestinal transplantation. *Gastroenterology* 1996;**110**:1820.
32. Ueno T, Fukuzawa M. Current status of intestinal transplantation. *Surg Today* 2010;**40**:1112.
33. Mazariegos GV, Abu-Elmagd K, Jaffe R, et al. Graft versus host disease in intestinal transplantation. *Am J Transplant* 2004;**4**:1459.
34. Shin CR, Nathan J, Alonso M, et al. Incidence of acute and chronic graft-versus-host disease and donor T-cell chimerism after small bowel or combined organ transplantation. *J Pediatr Surg* 2011;**46**:1732.

PART 4

Appendix

PART

Appendix

Normal appendix: anatomy, specimen dissection and histology relevant to pathological practice

Nadine Ectors

Translational Cell and Tissue Research, AC Biobanking, University Hospitals and University Leuven, Leuven, Belgium

Historical texts indicate that the vermiform appendix has been recognised as an organ in its own right since the beginning of the sixteenth century, and probably earlier by Egyptian and Arabic anatomists. The name appendix originates from Latin and means 'appendage' (of the caecum). The term 'vermiform', also of Latin derivation, means 'worm shaped'. Previously, the appendix was referred to in Arabic as 'ear' (*orecchio*) [1].

Anatomy

The appendix is a diverticulum of the posteromedial wall of the caecum, into which it opens approximately 25 mm below the ileocaecal valve [2]. It normally lies behind the caecum and the ascending colon but may be situated on the psoas muscle near to or overhanging the pelvic brim, behind or in front of the terminal ileum, or beside the ascending colon [3]. Its size varies considerably from person to person, partly depending on age, but averages 100 mm in length in the unfixed state, ranging from 20 mm to 200 mm, and between 3 and 8 mm in external diameter [4,5]. The diameter is maximal at the age of 4 years and diminishes thereafter [6]. The lumen usually measures 1–2 mm in diameter and changes from triangular/stellate to round/oval in transverse contour between adolescence and adulthood, as a consequence of involution of the lymphoid tissue. A short meso-appendix, which is a prolongation of the mesentery of the terminal ileum, attaches the base of the appendix to the retroperitoneum of the posterior abdominal wall. The remainder of the organ lies free in the peritoneal cavity and is covered by a serosal surface.

The blood supply to the appendix is mainly from the appendicular branch of the ileo-colic artery [2], which enters the meso-appendix at a short distance from the base of the appendix and runs along the free border, giving repeated branches that form a prominent submucosal plexus and a network underneath the mucosal surface. An accessory appendicular artery, a branch of the posterior caecal artery, often anastomoses with the main appendicular vessel. The venous drainage occurs along the ileocaecal vein into the superior mesenteric vein and thence into the portal venous system. The lymphatics from the base of the appendix drain first into the nodes of the meso-appendix and then towards the anterior ileo-colic nodes and the upper and lower nodes of the ileo-colic chain, whereas the lymphatic drainage from the body and tip of the appendix drain posteriorly into the lower and upper ileo-colic nodes.

The appendix is innervated by the autonomic nervous system. The sympathetic supply arises from the superior mesenteric plexus and the parasympathetic from the vagus nerve.

Histology

The histological structure of the appendix is similar to that of the remainder of the large intestine (see Chapter 32), apart from a marked excess of lymphoid tissue, predominantly in the form of B-cell-rich lymphoid follicles that expand the mucosa and submucosa and distort the overall architecture [7]. These follicles become prominent soon after birth, persist until early adulthood, and regress in late middle age, with corresponding changes in the overall diameter of the appendix.

The epithelium of the appendix is organised into crypts that are lined predominantly by a single layer of mucus-secreting goblet cells and tall columnar absorptive cells with a brush border [5]. These open on to the luminal surface, which is lined by a single layer of absorptive epithelium alternating with M (microfold) cells overlying the lymphoid follicles [8]. Scattered intra-epithelial T-lymphocytes are present within the surface epithelium. The lower third of the crypt represents the mitotically active proliferative zone and includes the stem cell niche, the progeny of which undergo maturation into goblet cells and absorptive cells as they migrate towards the luminal surface. Occasional differentiated Paneth cells and endocrine cells remain anchored in the crypt bases, the latter comprising mostly argentaffin, chromogranin A-containing enterochromaffin (EC) cells that produce serotonin (5-hydroxtryptamine, 5HT) but also a range of argyrophil cells, some of which are chromogranin A negative (but synaptophysin positive), that contain a range of peptide hormones [9]. Although the crypts are generally straight, without significant branching, they are often distorted by abundant lymphoid tissue in children and young adults.

The lamina propria of the appendiceal mucosa is composed of loose connective tissue and separated from the crypt epithelium by the pericryptal fibroblast sheath. In addition to fibroblasts and capillary-sized blood vessels, it contains endocrine cells that are similar to those within the crypts, either scattered or forming small groups that associate with occasional ganglion cells, S-100-positive Schwann cells and a meshwork of fine non-myelinated nerve fibrils to form 'EC-cell–nerve fibre complexes' or 'neuro-endocrine complexes' [4,9–12]. These intriguing structures, which appear to be almost unique to the appendix in the gastrointestinal tract, are of unknown significance but have generated numerous theories as to their role in the pathogenesis of appendicitis [13], so-called appendicular colic [9,11] and appendiceal endocrine tumours [14]. The lamina propria also contains a significant component of B and T lymphocytes, plasma cells and macrophages that along with the lymphoid follicles and the intraepithelial lymphocytes are organised into 'mucosa-associated lymphoid tissue' (MALT) which resembles that of the small intestine [7]. The deepest component of the mucosa, the muscularis mucosae, is a discontinuous structure composed of smooth muscle fibres that are frequently interrupted by the lymphoid follicles.

In addition to hosting the deeper aspects of the lymphoid follicles, the appendiceal submucosa consists of loose connective tissue that includes variable amounts of mature adipose tissue. Atrophy or involution of the lymphoid tissue frequently results in the connective tissue appearing more compact: this should not necessarily be interpreted as fibrosis, with the implication of some previous pathological process [6].

In contrast to the colon, the muscularis propria of the entire circumference of the appendix consists of two distinct layers – an outer longitudinal and an inner circular layer – albeit with some structural irregularities. The outer layer develops from a convergence of the three taeniae coli towards the tip of the caecum. Periodic acid–Schiff (PAS)-positive 'granular cells' have occasionally been described in the muscularis propria, spilling into the submucosa [15,16]. Based on electron microscopic studies they may be degenerative myocytes. Knowledge of their existence should prevent any misdiagnosis of epithelial malignancy.

Although submucosal (Meissner's) and myenteric (Auerbach's) plexuses do exist in the appendix, they form rather indistinct networks that are intermingled within the muscularis propria [17]. Similarly, the distribution of interstitial cells of Cajal appears to be less well organised than in the remainder of the gastrointestinal tract [18,19].

Specimen dissection

Despite the benefits and cost-effectiveness of routine histopathological examination of macroscopically normal-appearing appendixes being debated on many occasions, it remains the practice of most surgical gastroenterology centres in the western world. Apart from having the potential to audit surgical services, a number of studies have found that it identifies clinically significant unsuspected findings in 2–3% of such 'normal' specimens [20–22].

The pathological examination of the appendix should follow the classic general principles of macroscopic and microscopic examination, in the context of the clinical picture and the surgical findings. Accordingly, it is important to know all of the relevant clinical and intraoperative information before embarking. Both the Royal College of Pathologists [23–25] and the College of American Pathologists [26–28] have published useful guidelines.

Appendicectomy specimens can be received fixed or unfixed. Depending on the size of the specimen it might be necessary to incise it to ensure optimal fixation. If this is done, care must be taken to preserve the identification of important landmarks, especially the caecal and the non-peritonealised resection margins, in case an unsuspected tumour is identified on subsequent examination, e.g. in a resected 'appendix mass'.

The initial macroscopic examination of the fixed appendix should address and record the specimen type (whether or not any caecal wall is included), its integrity, its maximum length and external diameter, and the size of any attached meso-appendix. Any externally overt abnormalities should then be described, such as localised or generalised enlargement, tumour-like masses, serosal abnormalities such as congestion, exudates, perforation or mucus deposits, abscesses and any mesenteric nodules or enlarged lymph nodes.

Before embarking on slicing the fixed appendix, it is prudent to mark the resection margin at the base with coloured ink or gelatine. For large, distorted appendixes that may contain occult tumours, it is also important to mark similarly any non-peritonealised surgical resection margin but not the serosal surface. The specimen can then be sliced in one of two ways. The first involves slicing transversely at 3- to 4-mm intervals from the base towards the tip, leaving the last 15 mm of the tip to be bisected longitudinally. The alternative is to bisect both the proximal and the distal 15 mm of the appendix longitudinally, such that the former includes the surgical margin at the base of the appendix, and to serially slice the remainder transversely. The two methods have their proponents and detractors, based on which is perceived to give the best assessment of the resection margin but, because specimens vary both in their size and in the degree of crush or heat artefact from intraoperative manipulation, it is best to tailor the approach to the individual specimen.

Once the appendix is sliced, any macroscopic abnormalities are recorded, such as pus, faecoliths, worms or foreign bodies in the lumen, haemorrhage or thickening of the wall, diverticula, localised mass lesions, and any mucus in the lumen or within the wall. Routinely, the slice (transverse or longitudinal) that contains the surgical margin at the base, marked with ink or by some other distinguishing means, is submitted for histology, along with at least half of the tip and one more transverse section. Representative slices of any focal lesions or other abnormal areas are also embedded. If there is any hint of a neoplastic lesion macroscopically or clinically, including the presence of mucus within the wall, on the serosal surface or distending the appendiceal lumen, it is important to sample the whole of the appendix and the meso-appendix adjacent to the tumour, along with the nearest serosal surface and non-peritonealised resection margin, in order to undertake comprehensive tumour staging. Needless to say, any meso-appendiceal nodules or lymph nodes are also blocked for histology. Any region of unexplained dilatation of the appendiceal lumen should be sampled, as well as the junction with the segment of normal calibre.

It is important that all appendiceal slices that have not been embedded for processing and microscopy are retained until histological examination is complete. It is recommended that the entire appendix is embedded for histological examination if any unsuspected epithelial or endocrine tumour is discovered, if there is serosal inflammation in the absence of overt intramural appendicitis, or if the initial routine histological examination is normal in the face of clinically suspected appendicitis.

References

1. McMurrich JP. The organs of digestion. In: *Leonardo da Vinci – the Anatomist 1452–1519*. Baltimore, MA: Williams & Wilkins, 1930.
2. Strandring S, ed. *Gray's Anatomy: the Anatomical Basis of Clinical Practice*. 40th edn. Oxford: Elsevier, 2008.
3. Wakeley CPG, Gladstone RJ. The relative frequency of the various positions of the vermiform appendix, as ascertained by an analysis of 5000 cases. *Lancet* 1928;**i**:178.
4. Dhillon AP, Williams RA, Rode J. Age, site and distribution of subepithelial neuroendocrine cells in the appendix. *Pathology* 1992;**24**:56.
5. Segal GH, Petras RE. Vermiform appendix. In: Sternberg SS (ed.), *Histology for Pathologists*. New York: Raven Press Ltd, 1992.
6. Andreou P, Blain S, Du Boulay CEH. A histopathological study of the appendix at autopsy and after surgical resection. *Histopathology* 1990;**17**:427.
7. Spencer J, Finn T, Isaacson PG. Gut-associated lymphoid tissue: a morphological and immunocytochemical study of the human appendix. *Gut* 1985;**26**:672.
8. Bockman DE, Cooper MD. Early lymphoepithelial relationships in human appendix. A combined light and electron microscope study. *Gastroenterology* 1975;**68**:1160.
9. Hofler H, Kasper M, Heitz PU. The neuroendocrine system of the normal human appendix, ileum and colon and in neurogenic appendicopathy. *Virchows Arch Pathol Anat* 1983;**399**:127.
10. Millikin PD. Extra-epithelial enterochromaffin cells and Schwann cells in the human appendix. *Arch Pathol Lab Med* 1983;**107**:189.
11. Aubock L, Ratzenhofer M. 'Extra-epithelial enterochromaffin cell–nerve fibre complexes' in the normal human appendix and in neurogenic appendicopathy. *J Pathol* 1982;**136**:217.
12. Papadaki L, Rode J, Dhillon AP, Dische FE. Fine structure of a neuroendocrine complex in the mucosa of the appendix. *Gastroenterology* 1983;**84**:490.
13. Vasei M, Zakeri Z, Azarpira N, Hosseini SV, Solaymani-Dodaran M. Serotonin content of normal and inflamed appendix: a possible role of serotonin in acute appendicitis. *APMIS* 2008;**116**:947.
14. Rode J, Dhillon AP, Papadaki L, Griffiths D. Neurosecretory cells of the lamina propria of the appendix and their possible relationship to carcinoid. *Histopathology* 1982;**6**:69.
15. Husman R. Granular cells in musculature of the appendix. *Arch Pathol* 1963;**75**:360.
16. Sobel HJ, Marquet E, Schwarz R. Granular degeneration of appendiceal smooth muscle. *Arch Pathol* 1971;**92**:427.
17. Emery JL, Underwood J. The neurological junction between the appendix and ascending colon. *Gut* 1970;**11**:118.
18. Miller SM, Narasimhan RA, Schmalz PF, et al. Distribution of interstitial cells of Cajal and nitrergic neurons in normal and diabetic human appendix. *Neurogastroenterol Motil* 2008;**20**:349.
19. Richter A, Wit C, Vanderwinden JM, Wit J, Barthlen W. Interstitial cells of Cajal in the vermiform appendix in childhood. *Eur J Pediatr Surg* 2009;**19**:30.
20. Cross SS, Stone JL. Proactive management of histopathological workloads: analysis of the UK Royal College of Pathologists' recommendations on specimens of limited or no clinical value on the workload of a teaching hospital gastrointestinal pathology service. *J Clin Pathol* 2002;**55**:850.
21. Jones AE, Phillips AW, Jarvis JR, Sargen K. The value of routine histopathological examination of appendicectomy specimens. *BMC Surg* 2007;**7**:17.
22. Swank H, Eshuis E, Ubbink D, Bemelman W. Is routine histopathological examination of appendectomy specimens useful? A systematic review of the literature. *Colorectal Dis* 2011;**13**:1214.

23. Feakins R, Campbell F, Mears L, Moffat C, Scott N, Allen D. *Tissue Pathways for Gastrointestinal and Pancreatobiliary Pathology.* London: Royal College of Pathologists, 2009.

24. Williams GT, Quirke P, Shepherd NA. *Standards and Datasets for Reporting Cancers. Dataset for colorectal cancer,* 2nd edition. London: Royal College of Pathologists, 2007.

25. Stephenson TJ, Cross SS, Williams GT. *Standards and Datasets for Reporting Cancers. Dataset for endocrine tumours of the gastrointestinal tract including pancreas.* London: Royal College of Pathologists, 2009.

26. Compton CC. Updated protocol for the examination of specimens from patients with carcinomas of the colon and rectum, excluding carcinoid tumors, lymphomas, sarcomas, and tumors of the vermiform appendix: a basis for checklists. *Arch Pathol Lab Med* 2000;**124**:1016.

27. Misdraji J, Oliva E, Goldblum JR, et al. Protocol for the Examination of Specimens From Patients With Invasive Carcinomas of the Appendix. *Arch Pathol Lab Med* 2006;**130**:1433.

28. Washington MK, Tang LH, Berlin J, et al. Protocol for the examination of specimens from patients with neuroendocrine tumors (carcinoid tumors) of the appendix. *Arch Pathol Lab Med* 2010;**134**:171.

Inflammatory disorders of the appendix

Fiona Campbell

Royal Liverpool University Hospital, Liverpool, UK

Acute non-specific appendicitis

Acute appendicitis is the most common abdominal emergency in childhood, adolescence and young adult life, but the cause is still not fully known.

Incidence

Acute appendicitis is common in western Europe, North America and Australia but is rare in tropical Africa [1] and India, suggesting that dietary differences may play an important role. The incidence of acute appendicitis in the developed world continues to fall, with crude incidence rates of 180/100 000 in the 1970s and 120/100 000 in the 1990s [2–4], now falling to approximately 60/100 000 in the early twenty-first century [5]. Acute appendicitis is rare before the age of 5 years and has its peak incidence in the second and third decades; it is slightly more common in males and this sex difference is accentuated in early childhood. The lifetime risk of developing acute appendicitis is 9% for males and 7% for females [2]. A recent study has shown that acute appendicitis occurs more frequently in HIV-infected patients than the general population and is not related to opportunistic pathogens [6]. Deaths from appendicitis are very rare and usually occur in elderly people, in whom the symptoms are less striking in relation to the severity of the disease and in whom 'silent' perforation of the appendix with peritonitis is more common.

Aetiology and pathogenesis

Acute appendicitis is not thought to be regularly associated with any specific bacterial, viral or protozoal invader, although a number of claims for particular organisms have been made. Outbreaks of dysentery are not normally associated with an increased incidence of appendicitis, although there is good evidence that a few cases may be so precipitated [7,8]. Bacteriological studies usually show a wide variety of aerobic and anaerobic organisms drawn from those normally present in the caecum, which suggests that these are secondary invaders into already damaged tissues.

The most likely precipitating factor is obstruction of the appendiceal lumen. There are a number of possible causes for this [9]: the mucosa can undergo inflammatory changes with oedema; lymphoid tissues in the lamina propria and submucosa may hypertrophy; foreign material, particularly food residues, can lodge in the lumen and become surrounded by faecal material, forming a slow-growing laminated faecolith, which can subsequently calcify to form a stone; kinks and adhesions may angulate the organ upon itself; a low-residue diet may predispose to exaggerated muscle activity and muscle spasm in the wall of the appendix or at its base; and tumours in the caecum or appendix may block the lumen of the appendix. Appendicitis has also followed barium enema examinations [10] and colonoscopy, including endoscopic mucosal resection [11]. All these factors have in common the single feature that they obstruct the lumen and so interfere with normal peristaltic

Morson and Dawson's Gastrointestinal Pathology, Fifth Edition. Edited by Neil A. Shepherd, Bryan F. Warren,
Geraint T. Williams, Joel K. Greenson, Gregory Y. Lauwers and Marco R. Novelli.
© 2013 Blackwell Publishing Ltd. Published 2013 by Blackwell Publishing Ltd.

drainage. The role of some of them is fairly readily assessable, e.g. faecoliths are commonly present in appendices removed for proven acute appendicitis. The presence of faecoliths is geographically distributed and appears to correlate with the incidence of appendicitis in a population [12]. However, in one study their prevalence was greater in a postmortem population when compared with a younger, surgically resected group, implying that they were not a major cause of appendicitis [13]. It is well known that the age of greatest liability to acute appendicitis coincides with the age of maximal development of appendiceal lymphoid tissue, which tends to bulge into and narrow the lumen [14]. Lymphoid hyperplasia may occur with viral infection. It is more difficult to assess the degree of mucosal oedema present in a resected specimen, and oedema at the caeco-appendiceal junction cannot be assessed at all, because this part of the appendix is invaginated into the caecum at operation and is not available for examination.

Bacterial infection is probably important as a concomitant factor. There is good experimental evidence that, in dogs, rabbits, apes and humans, bacterial infection will not by itself cause acute appendicitis. Artificially produced obstruction also rarely does so when the appendix has previously been washed free of faecal material. Combined obstruction and bacterial infection, however, nearly always result in lesions [15,16]. The likely course of events is obstruction, damming up of normal mucus secretions, distension of the lumen with ischaemic damage of the mucosa, access into the tissues of bacteria normally confined to the lumen, and secondary bacterial infection leading first to non-suppurative and then to suppurative appendicitis. Enterobius infestation is probably not a causative factor [17] and there is little positive evidence to support a primary blood-borne infection [18]. Once an infection has become established, microangiographic studies suggest that the occlusion of arterioles, either by intravascular thrombus or by pressure from inflammatory oedema, may increase the liability to rapid perforation and gangrene [19].

Macroscopic appearances

The earliest visible external macroscopic change is dilatation and congestion of the small vessels on the serosal surface, which gives rise to a localised or generalised hyperaemia. The distal part may be swollen and, if the appendix is opened longitudinally, particularly after fixation, the distal lumen is often dilated and contains purulent material. A patchy purulent exudate commonly forms on the serosal surface, dulling it. Later the tip, and sometimes the whole organ, becomes soft, purplish and haemorrhagic as necrosis supervenes. The lumen becomes more markedly distended with pus, often blood stained, and suppurative foci are often visible in the wall. There is visible thrombosis in the veins of the meso-appendix [20]. It is

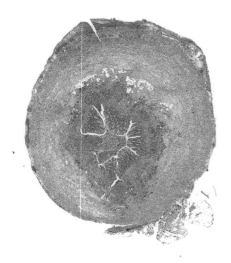

Figure 29.1 Acute appendicitis with ulceration and transmural inflammation.

difficult to give an accurate time scale for these events. It is well known that gangrenous changes can be present within a few hours of the onset of symptoms, but these may be related to concomitant ischaemia.

Microscopic appearances

Acute appendicitis is characterised by oedema and congestion of the wall, transmural infiltration of neutrophil polymorphs, often forming small intramural abscesses, ulceration of the mucosa and local fibrinopurulent peritonitis (Figure 29.1). Vascular thrombosis is often present and, in the most florid examples, the combination of suppurative inflammation and ischaemia leads to gangrenous appendicitis with necrosis of the wall and perforation [21]. Intravascular lymphocytosis within the wall of the appendix and the meso-appendix occurs frequently (Figure 29.2) and should not be confused with chronic lymphocytic leukaemia [22]. Acute inflammation in older patients may be secondary to a ruptured appendiceal diverticulum (see Chapter 31).

Although the histological diagnosis of established appendicitis is easy, difficulties may arise when an appendix, removed from a patient with the clinical features of acute appendicitis, shows only mild acute inflammation confined to the mucosa. Although it is tempting to regard this as early appendicitis, a number of studies have shown that up to 35% of appendices removed electively show small collections of neutrophil polymorphs in the lumen, focal ulceration of the surface epithelium with pus cells in the adjacent lamina propria and even a few crypt abscesses [23]. On the other hand, studies of experimental appendi-

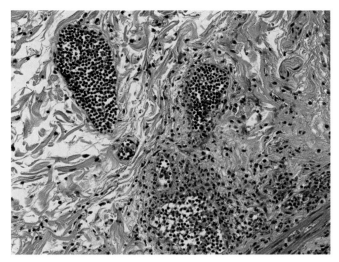

Figure 29.2 Intravascular lymphocytosis in acute appendicitis.

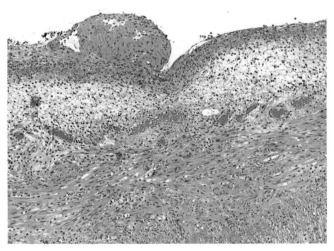

Figure 29.3 Peri-appendicular fibrin and acute inflammation found to be related to acute appendicitis on taking further sections.

citis have shown that identical mucosal lesions can progress rapidly to established acute appendicitis with gangrene and perforation [16]. It is obviously not possible to dismiss acute inflammation, even if confined to the mucosa, in patients with clinical features of appendicitis, but in such cases it is prudent to exclude other causes for acute abdominal pain. To confound the issue further, one study has shown that a significant proportion of histologically normal appendices from patients with a clinical diagnosis of acute appendicitis have expressed abnormal amounts of cytokines (tumour necrosis factor α [TNF-α] and interleukin-2), sensitive markers of inflammation, when examined using *in situ* hybridisation [24].

Luminal or peri-appendiceal neutrophil polymorphs, without acute inflammation in the appendix wall, should not be called acute appendicitis. When initial sections of appendix show only peri-appendiceal acute inflammation, then the whole appendix should be examined microscopically (Figure 29.3). If acute appendicitis is excluded as the cause of the peri-appendiceal inflammation, the surgeon should be informed of the need to consider other sources of intra-abdominal sepsis.

On occasion, examination of appendicectomy specimens shows the features of an infective colitis with diffuse active inflammation confined to the mucosa (see Chapter 35). Causative agents include organisms of *Salmonella*, *Shigella* and *Campylobacter* spp. [7,25,26].

Complications and sequelae

Perforation, peritonitis and abscess formation

It is probable that resolution occurs in some cases of early acute appendicitis but, once any significant amount of pus has formed, there are likely to be complications if the appendix is not removed quickly. Perforation is the most common and serious. It occurs most frequently in children under the age of 5 years, in whom appendicitis itself is uncommon [27], and in elderly people, thought to be due to delayed presentation. However, a recent analysis of the American National Hospital Discharge Survey database from 1970–2006 has suggested that perforating and non-perforating appendicitis may be different entities and not related to delayed treatment [28].

When associated with fulminating inflammation and gangrene, acute appendicitis commonly leads to peritonitis; if the patient survives, pus tends to localise in the pelvis or beneath the diaphragm. When the inflammation is less acute or the appendix is retrocaecal, retrocolic or subhepatic, in maldescent of the caecum [29], localised adhesions form and wall off the perforation, leading to a localised appendix abscess. Once formed, such an abscess may persist after appendicectomy; it can localise in the pelvis and secondarily involve the bladder [30] or the caecum, where it gives rise to so-called appendicular granuloma (see below). Pelvic abscesses can 'point' and perforate into the rectum or vagina with subsequent resolution, but peri-appendicular abscesses and subdiaphragmatic collections of pus tend to remain localised and become walled off by fibrous tissue. Fistula formation can occur between the appendix and the gastrointestinal tract, bladder or skin [31]. Appendicitis with perforation in women is associated with an increased risk of tubal infertility [32] or ectopic pregnancy due to peritubal adhesions [33]. Appendicitis and its complications may also occur in appendices sited in hernial sacs [34,35]. Acute appendicitis in neutropaenic patients is associated with a high risk of perforation and peritonitis [36].

Suppurative pylephlebitis

Infected thrombi in the small vessels of the serosa and meso-appendix are common in acute appendicitis. Rarely, the thrombus extends into larger vessels, which may lead to hepatic metastatic abscesses [37]. This complication is rare since the advent of efficient antibiotics.

Ileo-colic intussusception

Rare examples of ileo-colic intussusception have been reported after inversion of the appendiceal stump into the caecum at appendicectomy [38].

The development of 'chronic appendicitis'

There has been considerable doubt and controversy about whether acute appendicitis can progress to a chronic form and whether some of the vague abdominal symptoms that go to make the diagnosis of a 'grumbling appendix' have any pathological basis. There is no doubt that many appendices seen at necropsy [13] or removed electively are small, shrunken and without lumina, and on histological examination show atrophy of the mucosa and lymphoid tissue and virtual replacement of the submucosa by fibrous tissue and fat. The difficulty is to decide whether these changes are the result of physiological atrophy or previous acute inflammation. Studies comparing the appendices from patients with symptoms suggesting appendicitis with electively removed appendices from patients without symptoms have shown little difference in pathology [39]. There must be evidence of active chronic inflammation, with infiltration of the muscle coats and serosa by lymphocytes and plasma cells, before one can diagnose chronic appendicitis. There is one report to suggest that the presence of stainable iron is a reliable indication of inflammation within the previous 6 months [40]. Interval appendicectomy may be associated with granulomatous inflammation or xanthogranulomatous inflammation [41].

The presence of other sequelae of previous acute appendicitis, such as old adhesions, is evidence of previous inflammation, whether or not the appendix is histologically normal [42]. These adhesions can predispose to volvulus and obstruction, but such a condition should not be called chronic appendicitis.

Obstructive appendicopathy

It is common for an appendicectomy specimen to be histologically normal when there have undoubtedly been symptoms and signs of 'appendicitis' or 'appendicular colic'. In such cases, evidence of obstruction or narrowing of the lumen by fibrosis, a faecolith or a foreign body should be sought. In some specimens, the lumen is slightly dilated and packed with soft faeces. Whether this is the cause of the obstructive symptoms is uncertain.

Simple mucocele

Mucocele is defined as distension of part, or all, of the appendix by accumulation of mucus within the lumen. It is not a specific diagnosis but merely a description of a gross appearance that is common to simple mucocele, mucinous cystadenoma and mucinous cystadenocarcinoma of the appendix.

About 0.2% of all appendices examined at operation or necropsy have a dilated distal lumen that is distended with mucus [43,44]. This dilatation or simple mucocele, which is most common in middle-aged individuals and has an equal sex incidence, is thought by many to follow attacks of acute appendicitis with obstruction of the lumen. Postinflammatory fibrosis and faecolith are mentioned in the literature as the most common causes. Most mucoceles are small and symptomless but occasionally they are larger, containing thick, gelatinous mucin which occasionally forms numerous, small discrete globules, similar to fish eggs, so-called myxoglobulosis [45].

The microscopic appearances of simple mucocele have to be distinguished from mucinous cystadenoma and this is not always straightforward. The diagnosis of simple mucocele is restricted to those cases in which there is no evidence of any epithelial abnormality in the mucosal lining of the appendix, other than flattening. If there is any evidence of epithelial dysplasia, papillary infoldings or a multiloculated appearance, then the diagnosis of mucinous cystadenoma should be made.

Mucoceles can become secondarily infected, producing an empyema. Uncommonly, they rupture, discharging mucin to form a local collection of mucus around the appendix, sometimes referred to as localised pseudomyxoma peritonei. Removal of the appendix leads to regression of this localised (non-neoplastic) pseudomyxoma peritonei.

Prognosis

The overall mortality rate for acute appendicitis is extremely low (0.24%) and has remained fairly constant over the last 20 years [4, 46–48]. Most deaths occur in elderly people and are related to perforation.

Other forms of appendicitis

Tuberculous appendicitis

Tuberculosis (TB) of the appendix is described in association with local tuberculous disease in the ileo-caecal region and secondary to pulmonary TB [49,50]. Examples of apparent primary lesions have also been described. Macroscopically, the appendix can form part of a mass of granulomatous tissue, which also involves the caecum and meso-appendix [51], or can be indistinguishable from acute purulent appendicitis. Histology reveals characteristic tuberculoid granulomas that may also be present in mesenteric lymph nodes.

The appendix in Crohn's disease

Involvement of the appendix is found in about a quarter of all cases of Crohn's disease of the terminal ileum, but is also found synchronously with disease at a considerable distance from the ileo-caecal region, e.g. in the rectum or upper small intestine. The histology of Crohn's disease of the appendix (Figure 29.4) in no way differs from the appearances in other parts of the intestinal tract, with acute inflammatory changes of the mucosa, including cryptitis, erosion and ulceration, which may be fissuring, and transmural inflammation with scattered aggregates of lymphoid tissue. Granulomas are seen in a minority of cases. Secondary adhesion formation is common.

Identical histological features, often associated with prominent numbers of granulomas, are occasionally seen in appendicectomy specimens from patients without a history of Crohn's disease. Many have presented with the typical symptoms of acute appendicitis and the postoperative course has usually been uneventful, but granulomatous appendicitis appears to be particularly common in so-called interval (delayed) appendicectomy specimens [41]. Although Crohn's disease may appear at a later date elsewhere in the gastrointestinal tract, in a minority [52–54], follow-up studies have shown that this sequence is distinctly unusual [55,56]. The term 'idiopathic granulomatous appendicitis' has been used in this context when other causes of granulomatous inflammation, such as yersiniosis, TB and coexistent Crohn's disease, have been excluded [57].

Acute suppurative (non-granulomatous) appendicitis can occur in patients with Crohn's disease but appears to be rare [58].

Sarcoid lesions in the appendix

There are occasional case reports of sarcoid granulomas in the appendix in patients with other stigmata of sarcoidosis [59].

The appendix in ulcerative colitis

Involvement of the appendix has been variably reported in 28–86% of patients with pancolitis, although this is seldom obvious macroscopically [60–62]. The microscopic features are no different from those seen in the colon (Figure 29.5) and, as they are confined to the mucosa, do not result in any of the complications associated with ordinary appendicitis. Appendiceal inflammation may be present as a discontinuous 'skip' lesion in patients with colitis in the absence of either active or quiescent changes of ulcerative colitis in the caecum [63–65]. It may even be present in patients with colitis restricted to the distal colon and rectum, and be apparent at endoscopic examination as small erosions or ulcers identified at the mouth of the appendix [66]. Case–control studies suggest that previous appendicectomy is rare in patients with ulcerative colitis [67–69], raising the possibility that the appendix may play an initiating role in the subsequent development of colorectal inflammation in this disease. In contrast, appendicectomy may increase the risk of Crohn's disease [70], but other studies have shown a protective effect in Crohn's disease [71].

Actinomycosis

True acute actinomycotic inflammation of the appendix must be distinguished from ileo-caecal actinomycosis and the presence of *Actinomyces* spp. in the appendiceal lumen.

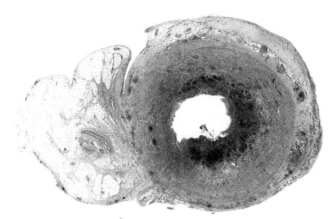

Figure 29.4 Crohn's disease: there is complete mucosal ulceration and transmural inflammation with many prominent lymphoid aggregates in the submucosa.

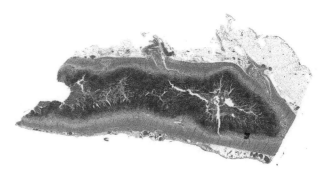

Figure 29.5 Ulcerative colitis: inflammation is confined to the mucosa.

It is sometimes seen in stained sections of normal appendices, and even when present in acute appendicitis it cannot be identified as the causative organism, unless it is actually present in the inflamed tissues. True acute actinomycotic appendicitis is extremely rare but it is important to diagnose it because failure to treat it adequately may result in protracted illness with extensive local spread and the risk of metastatic abscesses.

Chronic suppurative appendicitis can follow the acute condition and, although rare, is the form most often seen. Chronic abscesses, in which colonies of organisms can readily be identified, develop in the coats of the appendix and become surrounded by dense fibrous tissue, in which the organisms and consequent inflammation spread to produce sinus tracks and fistulae between the appendix, adjacent bowel and other organs and skin surfaces. The possibility of actinomycosis should be considered in all patients who develop faecal fistulae after appendicectomy. The infection may spread into veins and give rise to metastatic abscesses in the liver.

Yersiniosis

The appendix is not infrequently involved in ileal and mesenteric lymph nodal yersiniosis but disease may be confined to the appendix [57]. Lesions are similar to those described in the ileum (Chapter 20) and are usually confined to the mucosa and submucosa (Figure 29.6).

Schistosomiasis

In endemic areas, schistosomes have been found in 1–2% of appendicectomy specimens [72,73], although not necessarily from symptomatic individuals. Results of a study from Saudi Arabia [73] suggested that the clinical picture of acute appendicitis could result from schistosomal infection via one of two possible pathogenic pathways. Granulomatous appendicitis occurs in younger patients during the early phase of egg laying in the appendix and is associated with acute granulomatous inflammation around viable ova, with tissue necrosis and eosinophilia, although neutrophil exudation is not a feature. So-called obstructive appendicitis, which tended to occur in an older age group, was a secondary suppurative bacterial inflammation consequent upon fibrosis of a portion of the wall of the appendix as a result of long-standing inflammation to schistosomal ova, which appear calcified in tissue sections.

Enterobius infestation

Infestation of the appendix by *Enterobius vermicularis* (*Oxyuris vermicularis*, pinworms, threadworms) is quite common in temperate or cold climates, especially in children [17]. Adult worms in the lumen of the appendix are best recognised by the paired, narrow, lateral, barb-like alae that protrude from the cuticle (Figure 29.7). Infestation produces no symptoms attributable to the appendix and it is generally considered to play no part in the pathogenesis of acute appendicitis. Nevertheless, on rare occasions invasion of the wall of the appendix may occur, resulting in a florid granulomatous reaction with abundant eosinophils.

Spirochaetosis

Spirochaetosis of the appendix has not been associated with histological evidence of acute appendicitis, although its prevalence is greater in non-inflamed appendices from

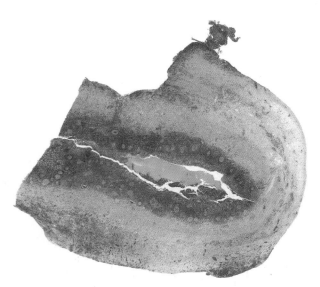

Figure 29.6 *Yersinia* sp.: granulomatous inflammation and micro-abscesses within hyperplastic lymphoid tissue.

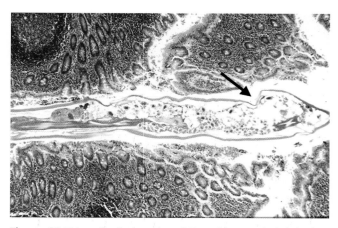

Figure 29.7 Longitudinal section of *Enterobius vermicularis* in the appendiceal lumen: one of the characteristic lateral barbed alae is arrowed.

individuals clinically suspected of appendicitis, compared with incidentally removed organs [74].

Viral appendicitis

Viral appendicitis may account for the appendicectomy with lymphoid hyperplasia and no acute inflammation. However, viral infection may lead to erosion, secondary bacterial infection and acute appendicitis [28]. Implicated viruses include adenovirus, Coxsackievirus, measles virus and cytomegalovirus [75], the last being described in immunocompetent, as well as immunocompromised, patients with acute appendicitis [76].

'Appendicular granuloma' (ligneous caecitis, pseudo-neoplastic appendicitis)

In this unusual form of inflammatory disease, which presents clinically as carcinoma of the caecum, usually in patients aged >70 years [77–79], the appendix is either incorporated into, or replaced by, a large mass of granulation or fibrous tissue, which also grows around the adjacent caecum or ileum, binding the appendix to them so that separation by dissection is impossible. There is no specific causative factor and it is probable that the condition results from incomplete resolution of an abscess in a retrocaecal appendix.

Miscellaneous forms of appendicitis

Polyarteritis nodosa can occasionally present as acute appendicitis without specific histological lesions in the appendix [80]. However, a similar focal necrotising arteritis of the appendix also occurs as an incidental finding, usually in young women, unrelated to appendicitis or any systemic disease [81]. Isolated cases of appendicitis secondary to metastatic carcinoma, lymphoma [82] and Kaposi's sarcoma in HIV-1-positive patients have been described [83,84]. Other causes of appendicitis include amoebiasis [85,86], balantidial infection [87], strongyloidiasis [88], mucormycosis [89], aspergillosis [90] and histoplasmosis [91]. The appendix may be involved in cases of pseudo-membranous colitis [92].

References

1. Walker AR, Segal I. Appendicitis: an African perspective. *J R Soc Med* 1995;**88**:616.
2. Addiss DG, Shaffer N, Fowler BS, Tauxe RT. The epidemiology of appendicitis and appendectomy in the United States. *Am J Epidemiol* 1990;**132**:910.
3. Williams NMA, Jackson D, Everson NW, Johnstone JM. Is the incidence of acute appendicitis really falling? *Ann R Coll Surg Engl* 1998;**80**:122.
4. Kang JY, Hoare J, Majeed A, Williamson RCN, Maxwell JD. Decline in admission rates for acute appendicitis in England. *Br J Surg* 2003;**90**:1586.
5. Paterson HM, Qadan M, de Luca SM, Nixon SJ, Paterson-Brown S. Changing trends in surgery for acute appendicitis. *Br J Surg* 2008;**95**:1188.
6. Crum-Cianflone N, Weekes J, Bavaro M. Appendicitis in HIV-infected patients during the era of highly active antiretroviral therapy. *HIV Med* 2008;**9**:421.
7. White MEE, Lord MD, Rogers KB. Bowel infection and acute appendicitis. *Arch Dis Child* 1961;**36**:394.
8. Thompson RG, Harper IA. Acute appendicitis and salmonella infections. *BMJ* 1973;**ii**:300.
9. Burkitt DP. The aetiology of appendicitis. *Br J Surg* 1971;**58**:695.
10. Sisley JF, Wagner CW. Barium appendicitis. *South Med J* 1982;**75**:498.
11. Horimatsu T, Fu K-I, Sano Y, et al. Acute appendicitis as a rare complication after endoscopic mucosal resection. *Dig Dis Sci* 2007;**52**:1741.
12. Jones BA, Demetriades D, Segal I, Burkitt DP. The prevalence of appendiceal faecoliths in patients with and without appendicitis. *Ann Surg* 1985;**202**:80.
13. Andreou P, Blain S, du Boulay CEH. A histopathological study of the appendix at autopsy and after surgical resection. *Histopathology* 1990;**17**:427.
14. Bohrod MG. The pathogenesis of acute appendicitis. *Am J Clin Pathol* 1946;**16**:752.
15. Wangensteen OH, Bowers WF. Significance of the obstructive factor in the genesis of acute appendicitis. An experimental study. *Arch Surg* 1937;**34**:496.
16. Buirge RE, Dennis C, Varco RL, Wangensteen OH. Histology of experimental appendiceal obstruction (rabbit, ape and man). *Arch Pathol* 1940;**30**:481.
17. Arca MJ, Gates RL, Groner J, Hammond S, Caniano DA. Clinical manifestations of appendiceal pinworms in children: an institutional experience and a review of the literature. *Pediatr Surg Int* 2004;**20**:372.
18. Wakeley C, Childs P. Appendicitis. *BMJ* 1950;**ii**:1347.
19. Lindgren I, Aho AJ. Microangiographic investigations on acute appendicitis. *Acta Chir Scand* 1969;**135**:77.
20. Remington JH, MacDonald JR. Vascular thrombosis in acute appendicitis. *Surgery* 1948;**24**:787.
21. Butler C. Surgical pathology of acute appendicitis. *Hum Pathol* 1981;**12**:870.
22. Lee S, Ogilvie RT, Dupre M, Gao Z-H. Intravascular lymphocytosis in acute appendicitis: potential mimicry of chronic lymphocytic leukaemia. *Histopathology* 2009;**55**:660.
23. Pieper R, Kager L, Nasman P. Clinical significance of mucosal inflammation of the vermiform appendix. *Ann Surg* 1983;**197**:368.
24. Wang Y, Reen DJ, Puri P. Is a histologically normal appendix following emergency appendicectomy always normal? *Lancet* 1996;**347**:1076.
25. Sanders DY, Cort CR, Stubbs AJ. Shigellosis associated with appendicitis. *J Pediatr Surg* 1972;**7**:315.
26. van Spreeuwel JP, Lindeman J, Bax R, Elbers HJR, Sybrandy R, Meijer CJLM. *Campylobacter*-associated appendicitis: prevalence and clinicopathologic features. *Pathol Annu* 1987;**22**:55.
27. Gilbert SR, Emmens RW, Putman TC. Appendicitis in children. *Surg Gynecol Obstet* 1985;**161**:261.
28. Alder AC, Fomby TB, Woodward WA, Haley RW, Sarosi G, Livingston EH. Association of viral infection and appendicitis. *Arch Surg* 2010;**145**:63.
29. Scott KJ, Sacks AJ, Goldschmidt RP. Subhepatic appendicitis. *Am J Gastroenterol* 1993;**88**:1773.

30. Fox M. Appendix abscess with stone formation and traction diverticulum of bladder. *BMJ* 1962;**ii**:1731.

31. Walker LG Jr, Rhame DW, Smith RB III. Enteric and cutaneous appendiceal fistulae. *Arch Surg* 1969;**99**:585.

32. Mueller BA, Daling JR, Moore DE, et al. Appendectomy and the risk of tubal infertility. *N Engl J Med* 1986;**315**:1506.

33. Lehmann WE, Mecke H, Riedel HH. Sequelae of appendectomy, with special reference to intra-abdominal adhesions, chronic abdominal pain, and infertility. *Gynecol Obstet Invest* 1990; **29**:241.

34. Thomas WEG, Vowles KDJ, Williamson RCN. Appendicitis in external herniae. *Ann R Coll Surg Engl* 1982;**64**:121.

35. Lyass S, Kim A, Bauer J. Perforated appendicitis within an inguinal hernia: case report and review of the literature. *Am J Gastroenterol* 1997;**92**:700.

36. Forghieri F, Luppi M, Narni F, et al. Acute appendicitis in adult neutropenic patients with haematological malignancies. *Bone Marrow Transplant* 2008;**42**:701.

37. Milliken NT, Stryker HB Jr. Suppurative pylethrombophlebitis and multiple liver abscesses following acute appendicitis. Report of case with recovery. *N Engl J Med* 1951;**244**:52.

38. Harson EL, Goodkin L, Pfeffer RB. Ileocolic intussusception in an adult caused by a granuloma of the appendiceal stump. *Ann Surg* 1967;**166**:150.

39. Thackray AC. 'Chronic appendicitis' – some pathological observations. *Br J Radiol* 1959;**32**:180.

40. Howie JGR. The Prussian-Blue reaction in the diagnosis of previous appendicitis. *J Pathol Bacteriol* 1966;**91**:85.

41. Guo G, Greenson JK. Histopathology of interval (delayed) appendectomy specimens: strong association with granulomatous and xanthogranulomatous appendicitis. *Am J Surg Pathol* 2003;**27**:1147.

42. Muller S. Macroscopic changes in so-called 'chronic appendicitis'. *Acta Chir Scand* 1959;**118**:146.

43. Carleton CC. Mucoceles of appendix and peritoneal pseudomyxoma. *Arch Pathol* 1955;**60**:39.

44. Wesser DR, Edelman S. Experiences with mucoceles of the appendix. *Ann Surg* 1961;**153**:272.

45. Gonzalez JEG, Hann SE, Trujillo YP. Myxoglobulosis of the appendix. *Am J Surg Pathol* 1988;**12**:962.

46. Baigrie RJ, Dehn TCB, Fowler SM, Dunn DC. Analysis of 8651 appendicectomies in England and Wales during 1992. *Br J Surg* 1995;**82**:933.

47. Guller U, Hervey S, Purves H, et al. Laparoscopic versus open appendectomy. Outcomes comparison based on a large administrative database. *Ann Surg* 2004;**239**:43.

48. Faiz O, Clark J, Brown T, et al. Traditional and laparoscopic appendectomy in adults. Outcomes in English NHS hospitals between 1996 and 2006. *Ann Surg* 2008;**248**:800.

49. Carson WJ. Tuberculosis of appendix. *Am J Surg* 1936;**34**:379.

50. Bobrow ML, Friedman S. Tuberculosis appendicitis. *Am J Surg* 1956;**91**:389.

51. Patkin M, Robinson BL. Tuberculosis of the appendix. *Br J Clin Pract* 1964;**18**:741.

52. Ewen SWB, Anderson J, Galloway JMD, Miller JDB, Kyle J. Crohn's disease confined to the appendix. *Gastroenterology* 1971; **60**:853.

53. Yang SS, Gibson P, McCaughey RS, Arcari FA, Bernstein J. Primary Crohn's disease of the appendix: report of 14 cases and review of the literature. *Ann Surg* 1979;**189**:384.

54. Allen DC, Biggart JD. Granulomatous disease in the vermiform appendix. *J Clin Pathol* 1983;**36**:632.

55. Ariel I, Vinograd I, Hershlag A, et al. Crohn's disease isolated to the appendix: truths and fallacies. *Hum Pathol* 1986;**17**:1116.

56. Dudley TH Jr, Dean PJ. Idiopathic granulomatous appendicitis, or Crohn's disease of the appendix revisited. *Hum Pathol* 1993; **24**:595.

57. Lamps LW, Madhusudhan KT, Greenson JK, et al. The role of *Yersinia enterocolitica* and *Yersinia pseudotuberculosis* in granulomatous appendicitis. *Am J Surg Pathol* 2001;**25**:508.

58. Rawlinson J, Hughes RG. Acute suppurative appendicitis – a rare associate of Crohn's disease. *Dis Colon Rectum* 1985;**28**:608.

59. Cullinane DC, Schultz SC, Zellos L, Holt RW. Sarcoidosis manifesting as acute appendicitis. *Dis Colon Rectum* 1997;**40**:109.

60. Saltzstein SL, Rosenberg BP. Ulcerative colitis of the ileum, and regional enteritis of the colon: a comparative histopathologic study. *Am J Clin Pathol* 1963;**40**:60.

61. Davison AM, Dixon MF. The appendix as a 'skip lesion' in ulcerative colitis. *Histopathology* 1990;**16**:93.

62. Groisman GM, George J, Harpaz N. Ulcerative appendicitis in universal and nonuniversal ulcerative colitis. *Mod Pathol* 1994;**7**:322.

63. Cohen T, Pfeffer RB, Valensi O. 'Ulcerative appendicitis' occurring as a skip lesion in ulcerative colitis: report of a case. *Am J Gastroenterol* 1974;**62**:151.

64. Kroff SH, Stryker SJ, Rao MS. Appendiceal involvement as a skip lesion in ulcerative colitis. *Mod Pathol* 1994;**7**:912.

65. Scott IS, Sheaff M, Coumbe A, Feakins RM, Rampton DS. Appendiceal inflammation in ulcerative colitis. *Histopathology* 1998;**33**:168.

66. Okawa K, Aoki T, Sano K, Harihara S, Kitano A, Kuroki T. Ulcerative colitis with skip lesions at the mouth of the appendix: a clinical study. *Am J Gastroenterol* 1998;**93**:2405.

67. Gilat T, Hacohen D, Lilos P, Langman MJ. Childhood factors in ulcerative colitis and Crohn's disease. An international cooperative study. *Scand J Gastroenterol* 1987;**22**:1009.

68. Rutgeerts P, D'Haens G, Hiele M, Geboes K, Vantrappen G. Appendectomy protects against ulcerative colitis. *Gastroenterology* 1994;**106**:1251.

69. Cosnes J, Carbonnel F, Beaugerie L, Blain A, Reijasse D, Gendre J-P. Effects of appendicectomy on the course of ulcerative colitis. *Gut* 2002;**51**:803.

70. Andersson RE, Olaison G, Tysk C, Ekbom A. Appendectomy is followed by increased risk of Crohn's disease. *Gastroenterology* 2003;**124**:40.

71. Radford Smith GL, Edwards JE, Purdie DM, et al. Protective role of appendicectomy in onset and severity of ulcerative colitis and Crohn's disease. *Gut* 2002;**51**:808.

72. Onuigbo WIB. Appendiceal schistosomiasis – method of classifying oviposition and inflammation. *Dis Colon Rectum* 1985; **28**:397.

73. Satti MB, Tamimi DB, Al Sohaibani MO, Al Quorain A. Appendicular schistosomiasis: a cause of clinical acute appendicitis? *J Clin Pathol* 1987;**40**:424.

74. Henrik-Nielsen R, Lundbeck FA, Teglbjaerg PS, Ginnerup P, Hovind-Hougen K. Intestinal spirochetosis of the vermiform appendix. *Gastroenterology* 1985;**88**:971.

75. Katzoli P, Sakellaris G, Ergazaki M, Charissis G, Spandidos DA, Sourvinos G. Detection of herpes viruses in children with acute appendicitis. *J Clin Virol* 2009;**44**:282.

76. Dzabic M, Bostrom L, Rahbar A. High prevalence of an active cytomegalovirus infection in the appendix of immunocompetent patients with acute appendicitis. *Inflamm Bowel Dis* 2008;**14**:236.

77. Le Brun HI. Appendicular granuloma. *Br J Surg* 1958;**46**:32.

78. Gruhn J, Tetlow F. Granulomatous pseudoneoplastic appendicitis. *Am J Surg* 1960;**99**:358.

79. Rex JC, Harrison EG, Priestley JT. Appendicitis and ligneous perityphlitis. *Arch Surg* 1961;**82**:735.

80. Gallagher HW, Hanna WA. Polyarteritis presenting as acute appendicitis. *J R Coll Surg Edinb* 1964;**9**:294.

81. Plaut A. Asymptomatic focal arteritis of the appendix (88 cases). *Am J Pathol* 1951;**27**:247.

82. Misdraji J, Graeme-Cook FM. Miscellaneous conditions of the appendix. *Semin Diagn Pathol* 2004;**21**:151.

83. Ravalli S, Vincent RA, Beaton H. Primary Kaposi's sarcoma of the gastrointestinal tract presenting as acute appendicitis. *Am J Gastroenterol* 1990;**85**:772.

84. Chetty R, Slavin JL, Miller RA. Kaposi's sarcoma presenting as acute appendicitis in an HIV-1 positive patient. *Histopathology* 1993;**23**:590.

85. Malik AK, Hanum N, Yip CH. Acute isolated amoebic appendicitis. *Histopathology* 1994;**24**:87.

86. Guzman-Vadivia G. Acute amebic appendicitis. *World J Surg* 2006;**30**:1038.

87. Dorfman S, Rangelo O, Bravo LG. Balantidiasis: report of a fatal case with appendicular and pulmonary involvement. *Trans R Soc Trop Med Hyg* 1984;**78**:833.

88. Noodleman JS. Eosinophilic appendicitis – demonstration of *Strongyloides stercoralis* as a causative agent. *Arch Pathol* 1981; **105**:148.

89. ter Borg F, Kuijper EJ, van der Lelie H. Fatal mucormycosis presenting as an appendiceal mass with metastatic spread to the liver during chemotherapy-induced granulocytopenia. *Scand J Infect Dis* 1990;**22**:499.

90. Rogers S, Potter MN, Slade RR. Aspergillus appendicitis in acute myeloid leukaemia. *Clin Lab Haematol* 1990;**12**:471.

91. Lamps LW, Molina CP, West AB, Haggitt RC, Scott MA. The pathologic spectrum of gastrointestinal and hepatic histoplasmosis. *Am J Clin Pathol* 2000;**113**:64.

92. Coyne JD, Dervan PA, Haboubi NY. Involvement of the appendix in pseudomembranous colitis. *J Clin Pathol* 1997;**50**:70.

CHAPTER 30

Tumours of the appendix

Joseph Misdraji

Massachusetts General Hospital, Harvard Medical School, Boston, MA, USA

Despite its small size, the appendix is associated with several neoplasms, some of which have been the subject of intense controversy in the literature. This chapter reviews appendiceal mucinous tumours, adenocarcinomas, endocrine tumours, goblet cell carcinoids, lymphomas and mesenchymal tumours, and ends with a brief discussion of metastatic tumours to the appendix.

Low grade appendiceal mucinous neoplasms

Low grade appendiceal mucinous neoplasms (LAMNs) are epithelial neoplasms of the appendix that have gone by a variety of names, including villous adenoma, cystadenoma, mucinous tumour of uncertain malignant potential and borderline tumour of the appendix [1–3]. These tumours occasionally spread to the peritoneal cavity, a phenomenon that, when grossly apparent, carries the descriptive term 'pseudomyxoma peritonei' (PP). The nomenclature of these tumours has been inconsistent in the literature, particularly when they are associated with PP, because the appendiceal tumour lacks the usual features of an invasive neoplasm yet manages to spread to the peritoneum and, in women, the ovaries. Some authors refer to these lesions as 'ruptured adenomas' and consider the epithelium in the peritoneum adenomatous in nature [4–7], whereas others contend that epithelium proliferating in the peritoneum must be considered adenocarcinoma and any tumour that produced it must be an invasive adenocarcinoma, despite the lack of consensus criteria for invasion in these tumours [1,3,8].

LAMNs typically occur in patients in their sixth decade [1]. Abdominal pain that mimics acute appendicitis or an abdominal mass (sometimes ovarian) is the most common presentation [3,6,7,9], but a significant number are discovered incidentally. Appendices with LAMNs may appear grossly unremarkable, or be cystically dilated and filled with tenacious mucin. The wall is variably fibrotic and calcified. Gross rupture may be evident with mucin extruding on to the serosal surface (Figure 30.1). On microscopic examination, the appendiceal mucosa is replaced by a villous or flat mucinous epithelial proliferation (Figure 30.2) [1,5,9]. The mucinous epithelial cells are columnar and mucin rich and have elongated, mildly hyperchromatic nuclei, nuclear pseudo-stratification, rare mitoses and apoptotic nuclear debris [3,9,10]. Cystic tumours are lined by mucinous epithelium that can be partly villous, flat or attenuated. Many LAMNs demonstrate herniation of the neoplastic epithelium through the muscularis propria, and these diverticula may be a route by which these tumours disseminate to the peritoneal cavity [11].

The prognosis of low grade appendiceal mucinous neoplasms is dependent on the presence or absence of epithelial cells outside the appendix. Tumours that are confined to the appendix and have not ruptured have an excellent prognosis. Tumours that have ruptured may be associated with mucin spillage into the peritoneal cavity. If that mucin is acellular, there is a low risk of recurrence [1,9,12,13]. The presence of epithelial cells in the extra-appendiceal mucin, even if limited and confined to the right lower quadrant, increases the risk of recurrence [12,13]. Tumours that have spread beyond the right lower quadrant or to the ovaries

Morson and Dawson's Gastrointestinal Pathology, Fifth Edition. Edited by Neil A. Shepherd, Bryan F. Warren, Geraint T. Williams, Joel K. Greenson, Gregory Y. Lauwers and Marco R. Novelli.

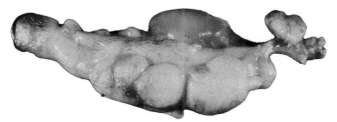

Figure 30.1 Gross photograph of an appendix with extrusion of mucus on the serosa due to a mucinous neoplasm.

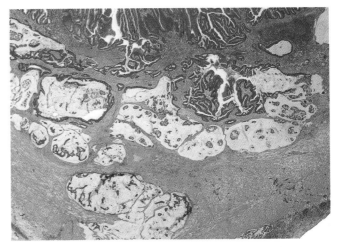

Figure 30.3 Invasive mucinous adenocarcinoma: irregular infiltration of the appendiceal wall by glands and pools of mucin containing strips and clusters of epithelial cells.

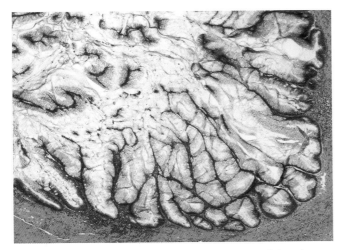

Figure 30.2 Low grade appendiceal mucinous neoplasm: the appendiceal mucosa is replaced by a villous mucinous proliferation. The villi are slender and lined by low grade mucinous epithelium.

often pursue an indolent but progressive course (see 'Pseudomyxoma peritonei' below). Colonoscopy is usually advised in patients found to have appendiceal mucinous tumours, because of a significant association with synchronous and metachronous colorectal neoplasia.

Adenocarcinoma

Adenocarcinoma of the appendix is rare; Collins found an incidence of 0.082% among 50000 appendectomy specimens [14]. Patients are usually in their fifth to seventh decades [15–18] and have symptoms of appendicitis, although they may present with a palpable mass, obstruction, gastrointestinal bleeding or symptoms referable to metastases [7,16–20]. In general, appendiceal adenocarcinomas manifest as either cystic mucinous tumours that are prone to rupture and spread to the ovaries and peritoneum

or intestinal-type carcinomas that infiltrate the appendiceal wall and metastasise to lymph nodes and the liver.

Mucinous adenocarcinoma accounts for approximately 40% of appendiceal adenocarcinomas [18]. The histology of invasive mucinous carcinoma in the appendix is similar to mucinous carcinoma elsewhere in the colon (see Chapter 38), with infiltrating pools of mucin harbouring cytologically malignant glandular epithelium arranged as strips, clusters or complex glands (Figure 30.3). Appendiceal non-mucinous carcinomas show a range of morphology of the invasive component. In some cases, the tumour has an appearance identical to colonic adenocarcinoma with malignant glands lined by columnar epithelium. In other cases, the malignant glands are tubular in shape, lined by cuboidal epithelium and associated with modest amounts of extracellular mucin. Signet-ring cell carcinoma is rare in the appendix and has a poor prognosis due to rapid dissemination within the peritoneal cavity [21]. The histology is similar to signet ring cell carcinoma of other sites.

The reported 5-year survival rate for patients with appendiceal adenocarcinoma ranges from 18.7% [22] to 55% [17]. Patients with mucinous adenocarcinomas fare better than those with non-mucinous adenocarcinomas [17,19]. Several studies have shown that histological grade and Dukes' stage correlate with prognosis [7,17,19,23]. Patients with peritoneal carcinomatosis carry a poor prognosis [15,18,19,24].

Virtually all authors agree that right hemicolectomy is indicated for invasive adenocarcinoma, both to achieve complete tumour resection and to stage the tumour by examining the right colic lymph nodes [17,19,20]. Furthermore, hemicolectomy offers improved 5-year survival rates relative to appendectomy [10,17,20]. Some authors advocate oophorectomy in women both for staging purposes and to remove a site where tumour frequently recurs [17,19].

Pseudomyxoma peritonei

Pseudomyxoma peritonei refers to the accumulation of mucin and mucinous epithelial cells within the peritoneal cavity, secondary to peritoneal spread of a mucinous neoplasm. Peritoneal spread occurs most often in association with appendiceal LAMNs and mucinous adenocarcinomas. The peritoneal tumours in patients with LAMNs demonstrate abundant mucin dissecting hyalinised, fibrotic stroma and harbouring scant strips of low grade mucinous epithelium (Figure 30.4) [9]. This is the classic morphology in the clinical syndrome known as PP. Peritoneal mucinous tumours with high grade cytological atypia and more cellular, complex, epithelial proliferations are usually associated with either severely atypical mucinous neoplasms or frankly invasive mucinous carcinomas [4,9]. The mucinous peritoneal deposits accumulate in the greater omentum, undersurface of the right hemidiaphragm, pelvis, right retrohepatic space, left abdominal gutter and ligament of Treitz [25]. This 'redistribution' phenomenon is the result of tumour accumulating at sites where ascitic fluid is resorbed from the abdomen and in dependent areas due to puddling [26].

Ronnett et al. [4] proposed a classification of PP that separated peritoneal mucinous tumours into two categories based on cytological and architectural features. They proposed the term 'disseminated peritoneal adenomucino-

sis' (DPAM) for mucinous implants derived from an appendiceal adenoma and containing scant strips of mucinous epithelium with mild atypia and no significant mitotic activity. In contrast, peritoneal tumours characterised by more abundant proliferative epithelium, arranged as glands, nests or individual cells, were classified as peritoneal mucinous carcinomatosis (PMCA). These peritoneal tumours derived from an appendiceal or intestinal mucinous adenocarcinoma and were characterised by parenchymal organ invasion and lymph node metastases. The 5- and 10-year survival rates were significantly better for patients with DPAM (75% and 68% respectively) as opposed to those with PMCA (14% and 3%).

Bradley et al. also found that PP can be separated into low and high grade categories that have prognostic significance; however, they maintain that epithelial cells growing outside the appendix are unequivocally malignant. They propose that all PP be classified as mucinous carcinoma peritonei, either low or high grade [8].

The treatment for pseudomyxoma peritonei has not been standardised. Historically, treatment was considered palliative and consisted of serial surgical tumour debulking until abdominal adhesions precluded further debulking and the patient died of bowel obstruction. Sugarbaker and colleagues [27] advocate an approach that aims for cure and consists of peritonectomy procedures to achieve complete cytoreduction, coupled with intra-peritoneal chemotherapy. Treated in this manner, patients with low grade peritoneal disease (DPAM) have a reported 5-year survival rate of 86% and those with peritoneal carcinomatosis of 50% [27]. However, these protocols are associated with significant morbidity and others have reported similar results with more conservative approaches [28].

Hyperplastic polyp, diffuse mucosal hyperplasia and sessile serrated adenoma

Hyperplastic polyps occur rarely in the appendix and are similar to hyperplastic polyps elsewhere in the colon. They are small, localised areas in which the crypts are elongated and lined by mucinous epithelium, which contains a mixture of goblet cells interspersed among mucinous cells with smaller mucin vacuoles. The crypt lumens appear serrated, predominantly toward the luminal surface of the lesion. Hyperplastic polyps of the appendix are frequently incidental findings but may occur in patients with symptoms of appendicitis. Diffuse mucosal hyperplasia uncommonly affects the appendix and is usually an incidental finding [3]. The histology is similar to hyperplastic polyp, but a large segment of the appendix or even the entire circumference is involved (Figure 30.5) [3].

Sessile serrated adenoma (SSA), sometimes termed 'sessile serrated polyp' or 'sessile serrated lesion', is a

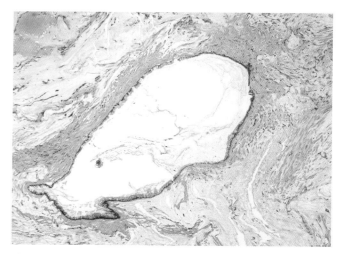

Figure 30.4 Peritoneal involvement by low grade appendiceal mucinous neoplasm: the characteristic pathological appearance in the 'pseudomyxoma peritonei' syndrome consists of abundant extracellular mucin dissecting variably hyalinised fibrous tissue and containing scant, relatively bland mucinous epithelial cells arranged in strips and glands, such as the one pictured here.

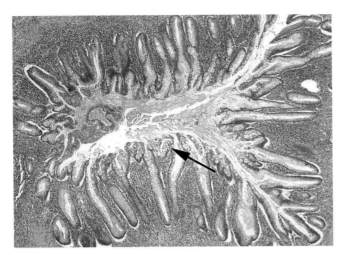

Figure 30.5 Mucosal hyperplasia of the appendix: the appendiceal mucosa in this case is expanded with tall crypts that show epithelial tufting at the surface (arrow). The remainder of the crypt is tubular without serration. The appendix appears to be inflamed.

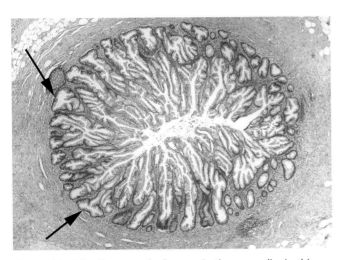

Figure 30.6 Sessile serrated adenoma in the appendix: in this example, the crypts show complex serration that begins at the crypt base, resulting in dilated, horizontally orientated crypts (arrows).

recently described lesion in the colon that resembles a hyperplastic polyp, but has subtle architectural and cytological features that are considered evidence of maturation disarray of crypt epithelial cells (Figure 30.6) [29]. In the colon, these lesions have been implicated in the serrated pathway of colorectal tumorigenesis characterised by *BRAF* mutations, methylation of CpG islands in promoter regions of DNA-mismatch repair genes and microsatellite instability (see Chapter 37). Similar proliferations are often seen in the appendix and a recent molecular study of serrated

lesions in the appendix found *BRAF* mutations in almost half of SSAs in the appendix [30]. However, four cancers adjacent to serrated lesions lacked *BRAF* mutations, raising questions about the biological potential of polyps with *BRAF* mutations in the appendix.

Traditional serrated adenoma

Traditional serrated adenomas (TSA) show complex serrated crypt lumina but, unlike SSAs, the epithelium is overtly dysplastic. In the colon, TSAs have also been implicated in the serrated pathway of colorectal tumorigenesis (see Chapter 37) and are presumably more advanced than SSAs. A series of 10 serrated adenomas in the appendix [31] found invasive carcinoma in 4 cases, suggesting a high likelihood of progression in these lesions. In the series by Yantiss et al. [30] serrated adenomas harboured *KRAS* (38%) or *BRAF* (25%) mutations at a rate similar to colonic serrated adenomas. They did not corroborate aggressive behaviour in their series.

Colonic-type tubular adenomas

Localised polypoid adenomas of the type seen in the colon (see Chapter 37) are rare in the appendix [32]. They may occur in patients with familial adenomatous polyposis [1,26]. The histological appearance of these polyps is identical to tubular adenomas in the colon.

Endocrine (carcinoid) tumours

Appendiceal endocrine (carcinoid) tumours account for approximately 18.9% of all carcinoids and 25.7% of gastrointestinal endocrine neoplasms [33]. They are found in approximately 0.32–0.6% of surgically removed appendices [34,35]. They occur with greatest frequency in the fourth to fifth decades of life [33,35,36], although they can occur at any age, including childhood [37–39]. Most are found incidentally [36,40], although occasional tumours present with appendicitis or recurrent abdominal pain [34,41], particularly in children [37,38]. Presentation with the carcinoid syndrome is exceptional.

At gross examination, appendiceal endocrine tumours appear as yellow–tan firm nodules usually located at the appendiceal tip (Figure 30.7) [34-36]. Approximately 75% of them are <10mm in diameter and approximately 5% are >20mm [34,36,42]. Most tumours are enterochromaffin (EC) cell tumours that microscopically demonstrate a nested or insular pattern (Figure 30.8) [34]. Less common are L-cell tumours that demonstrate a trabecular architecture. Tumour cells are uniform, with modest amounts of eosinophilic, finely granular cytoplasm. Tumour cell nuclei show the classic endocrine 'salt-and-pepper' chromatin pattern (Figure 30.9) [34]. The tumour often extends deeply

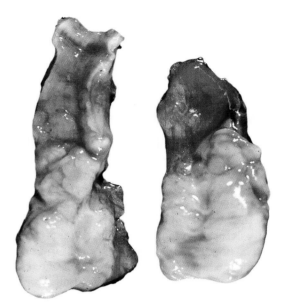

Figure 30.7 Gross photograph of an endocrine (carcinoid) tumour in the appendix: a white–tan fleshy tumour is present at the appendiceal tip.

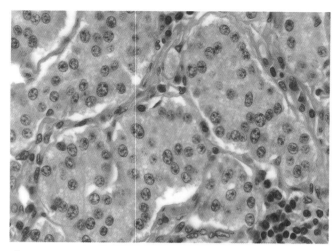

Figure 30.9 High power view of a classical appendiceal carcinoid tumour: the tumour cells are uniform with round, bland nuclei, mildly course chromatin with small nucleoli and abundant granular eosinophilic cytoplasm.

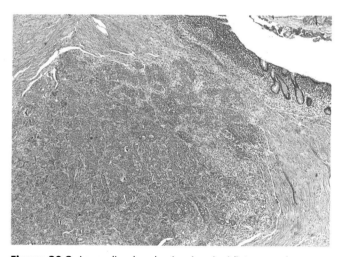

Figure 30.8 Appendiceal endocrine (carcinoid) tumour: low power view shows a neoplasm with a nested and solid pattern (lower left); the appendiceal mucosa is at upper right.

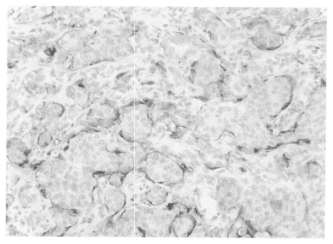

Figure 30.10 S-100 immunohistochemical stain shows staining of cells at the periphery of tumour cell clusters, presumably Schwann cells.

into the wall and even to the peritoneal surface [34,42]. Lymphatic invasion and perineural invasion are common [34,35,42]. Infiltration of the meso-appendix occurs in up to 27% of cases [35,41,42], although this is proportionate to tumour size.

Immunohistochemically, EC-cell carcinoids stain positively with endocrine markers, including chromogranin, synaptophysin and neuron-specific enolase. They also express serotonin and substance P [43]. Staining for S-100 protein demonstrates positive cells (presumably Schwann cells) surrounding tumour islands (Figure 30.10) [44,45]. EC-cell tumours are negative for carcinoembryonic antigen (CEA) [45] and L-cell carcinoids stain for enteroglucagon, pancreatic polypeptide (PP/PYY) and CEA [43,46]. These tumours stain unreliably for chromogranin A but express chromogranin B and synaptophysin [45,46].

Classical appendiceal carcinoids have an excellent prognosis. Lymph node metastases are uncommon and liver metastases are rare [34–36,47]. The frequency of metastasis is highly dependent on tumour size, with 0% for tumours <10 mm, 3–6.7% for tumours 10–20 mm and 21–30% for tumours >20 mm [48]. Patients with local disease have a 5-year survival rate of 92–100%, those with regional metastasis 81% and those with distant metastasis 31% [36,49,50]. Investigators attempting to define which features of appendiceal carcinoid tumours predict behaviour have found only tumour size to be relevant: tumours <20 mm infrequently metastasise and those <10 mm are essentially benign [34,51]. Factors that have been dismissed as prognostic factors are depth of invasion, location of the tumour in the appendix, perineural invasion, lymphatic invasion and the presence of serosal tumour [42,51]. Studies examining the significance of invasion of the meso-appendix have yielded conflicting results. Some authors report an increased likelihood of metastatic disease in patients with meso-appendiceal infiltration independent of tumour size [52], whereas others report that meso-appendiceal invasion has no effect on prognosis in tumours <20 mm [35,53].

Simple appendectomy is curative for lesions <10 mm if the margin of resection is negative for tumour. Tumours >20 mm in diameter carry an increased risk of metastatic disease, so right hemicolectomy is recommended for these tumours, particularly if there is involvement of the meso-appendix or vascular invasion [51]. The management of tumours measuring between 10 and 20 mm is not standardised and other factors must be considered, including meso-appendix invasion, serosal extension, angiolymphatic invasion, gross evidence of regional lymph node metastases at appendicectomy, patient age and co-morbidities.

Tubular carcinoid

Tubular carcinoids are small endocrine tumours composed of discrete tubules lined by bland, cuboidal epithelial cells compressed in a fibrotic stoma (Figure 30.11) [54,55]. The lesions are typically located in the submucosa and muscularis propria of the appendiceal tip, span a few millimetres and are virtually always an incidental finding discovered on microscopic examination. Unlike classic carcinoid tumours, tubular carcinoids stain with antibodies to CEA and glucagon but not serotonin [45]. Chromogranin immunohistochemistry is variable and weak [45,54,55] but the tumours are usually positive for synaptophysin.

Goblet cell carcinoid

Goblet cell carcinoids (GCCs) are distinctive appendiceal tumours with both mucinous and endocrine differentiation. They most often affect patients in their fifth decade with an equal sex distribution [56]. The tumours most often present as appendicitis [57,58], although they can be an incidental finding or in women present with ovarian metastases [59–62].

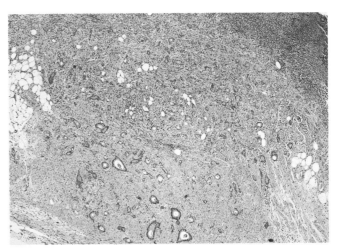

Figure 30.11 Tubular carcinoid of the appendix: a proliferation of relatively uniform tubules is present in the submucosa and muscularis propria of the appendix.

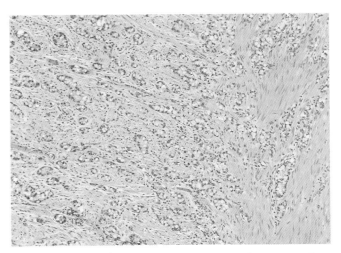

Figure 30.12 Goblet cell carcinoid tumour: medium power view shows infiltration of the muscularis propria by uniform clusters of tumour cells that resemble goblet cells.

Grossly, these tumours usually appear as circumferential thickening of the appendix and are only recognised on microscopic examination. Tumour size is, therefore, difficult to determine in many cases but averages 20 mm [56]. Histological examination shows circumferential infiltration of the appendix by a tumour that seems to arise from the base of crypts with no recognisable precursor lesion. The tumour is composed of discrete clusters of goblet cells admixed with cells with eosinophilic cytoplasm and occasionally cells with eosinophilic granules (Figures 30.12 and 30.13) [54,63–65]. Most tumour cell clusters lack lumina [63]; those with lumina resemble intestinal crypts. Nuclear pleomorphism and mitoses are exceptional. Perineural and lymphatic vessel invasion may be present [63].

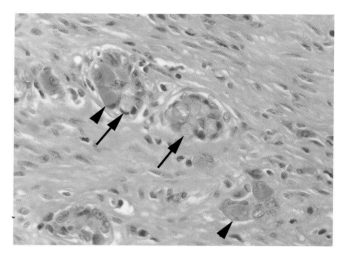

Figure 30.13 Goblet cell carcinoid tumour: high power view of the tumour clusters shows a mixture of goblet-like cells (arrows) admixed with cells that contain brightly eosinophilic cytoplasmic granules (arrowheads).

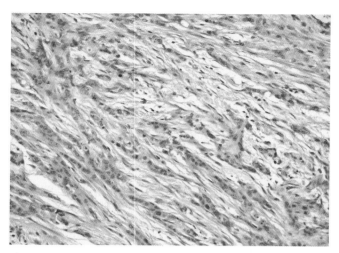

Figure 30.14 Mixed adenocarcinoma–carcinoid: tumour cells in ribbons and single file structures infiltrate the appendix, inducing a cellular desmoplastic stroma, in this example of carcinomatous growth pattern.

Extracellular mucin pools harbouring tumour clusters are not an uncommon finding but, unlike mucinous carcinoma, the glands in the mucin lakes have preserved central lumina and remain separate. Immunohistochemically, GCCs express CEA and keratin 20 and most co-express keratin 7 [66,67]. Immunohistochemistry for chromogranin and synaptophysin shows staining of occasional endocrine cells in the tumour clusters [67].

Although historically goblet cell carcinoids were considered to be a form of carcinoid (hence the name), they are now considered to be a type of adenocarcinoma. Isaacson demonstrated that many tumours show staining for IgA, secretory component and lysozyme, typical of intestinal crypt cells. He concluded that GCCs are carcinomas that derive from crypt cells and proposed the name crypt cell carcinoma [65]. Electron microscopic studies have shown evidence of both mucin production and electron-dense granules in GCCs [68,69].

Features that predict a worse prognosis include tumour extension beyond the appendix at presentation, atypical histological features and more than two mitoses per 10 high power fields [70]. In 1990, Burke et al. defined carcinomatous growth patterns in GCCs as fused or cribriform glands, single file structures, diffusely infiltrating signet ring cells or sheets of tumour cells (Figure 30.14) [54]. Tumours lacking significant amounts of carcinomatous growth patterns (<25%) were designated GCC and had a benign course. Tumours composed of >50% carcinomatous growth pattern were classified as mixed carcinoid–adenocarcinoma and were highly likely to have spread outside the appendix at presentation and to behave aggressively. Recently, Tang et al. [71] proposed a three-tiered histological classification of GCCs that correlated with

prognosis: typical GCC was reserved for tumours with well defined goblet cells in cohesive clusters with minimal cytological atypia; 'adenocarcinoma ex GCC, signet ring cell type' was applied to tumours with goblet cells arranged in irregular large clusters, single file infiltration or discohesion; and 'adenocarcinoma ex GCC, poorly differentiated carcinoma type' was applied to tumours with a component (at least $1 mm^2$) indistinguishable from poorly differentiated adenocarcinoma.

The treatment for goblet cell carcinoid is controversial. Although some authors recommend right hemicolectomy for all patients [57,68], others recommend hemicolectomy only for tumours with atypical histological features such as high mitotic rates or carcinomatous growth patterns, or extension beyond the appendix [72,73]. The European Neuroendocrine Tumour Society Consensus Guidelines also recommend bilateral salpingo-oophorectomy, because of the high risk of metastases to the ovaries [74]. Metastatic goblet cell carcinoid has limited response to chemotherapy.

Mesenchymal tumours

Of the mesenchymal tumours that occur in the appendix, the most common is leiomyoma, but even that is rare: Collins found 1214 in a series of 71 000 appendices (1.712%) [75]. They are usually found incidentally during surgery or post mortem. However, they can present with abdominal symptoms that can be mistaken for appendicitis [76,77] or as a pelvic mass [78]. About half the leiomyomas arise from the tip of the appendix and the appendix is frequently described as being partially embedded in the tumour [78,79]. The size of the tumour varies from a few millimetres to 150 mm. The histological features are identical to leiomyoma elsewhere in the body, with interlacing fascicles of smooth muscle cells continuous with the muscularis propria, particularly the outer longitudinal layer.

Gastrointestinal stromal tumours (GISTs) have been rarely reported in the appendix [80,81]. The tumour appears to have a predilection for males and the mean age of patients is 67 years. Some tumours present as appendicitis, whereas others are discovered incidentally. Histologically, they are composed of uniform spindle cells and some have skeinoid fibres. As with GISTs elsewhere, the spindle cells stain with antibodies to c-KIT and molecular analysis in two cases demonstrated *KIT* exon 11 mutations [81]. Appendiceal GISTs reported so far have been small and biologically benign.

Appendiceal granular cell tumour is rare and can present as appendicitis or incidentally [82,83]. The histological appearance is characteristic, with sheets and nests of polygonal cells with granular cytoplasm infiltrating the appendix (Figure 30.15), sometimes mimicking endocrine tumours, neural tumours or leiomyomas [83]. Periodic acid–Schiff (PAS) stain highlights granules in the cytoplasm. The tumour cells are positive for S-100 and neuron-specific enolase by immunohistochemistry, and demonstrate numerous lysosomes on electron microscopy.

Appendiceal Kaposi's sarcoma occurs mainly in patients with AIDS. More often cutaneous and multifocal gastrointestinal involvement is present; rarely, no skin disease is apparent [84–86]. Although gastrointestinal Kaposi's sarcoma is often asymptomatic, appendiceal Kaposi's sarcoma often presents as acute appendicitis or appendiceal rupture [84–86]. Grossly, the tumours may be grey and firm, or haemorrhagic and spongy [84,85]. Histologically,

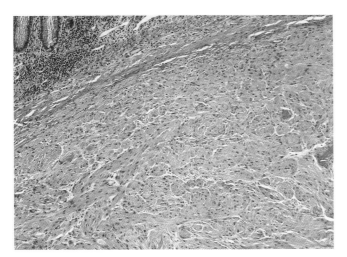

Figure 30.15 Granular cell tumour of the appendix: in this low power view, the appendiceal mucosa (upper left) is undermined by a neoplasm composed of sheets and intersecting bundles of bland, granular eosinophilic cells.

the lesions are composed of spindle cells forming slit-like vascular channels.

Neural proliferations have rarely been described in the appendix in association with von Recklinghausen's neurofibromatosis (NF-1) [87,88]. Marked thickening of the appendiceal wall with nodular masses extending into the mesentery characterised these cases. Microscopic examination demonstrated plexiform neurofibromas in the appendix and meso-appendix associated with proliferations of ganglion cells. A case of giant neurofibroma not associated with NF-1 has also been reported [89]. A thickened appendix with infiltration of large areas of the wall, submucosa and mucosa by a neural proliferation was described in this case.

Malignant lymphoma

Primary lymphoma of the appendix is rare. Most patients are in their second to fourth decades but the age range is broad, with reports of some as young as 3 years [90] and as old as 84 years [91]. Most patients present with symptoms of acute appendicitis with abdominal pain [90,92–98]. Less common presentations include a palpable mass, intussusception and lower gastrointestinal bleeding [92,99].

Gross examination of the appendix in cases of lymphoma often shows a circumferential soft, white to yellowish homogeneous tumour similar to lymphoma elsewhere [98]. Occasionally, the tumour occludes the lumen. Appendiceal perforation is not uncommon [90].

Age is a major determinant of the lymphoma type. Burkitt's lymphoma is the histological diagnosis in virtually all reported cases occurring in children and young adults [90,96,100,101]. Although serology for Epstein–Barr virus (EBV) has not established an association between EBV and appendiceal Burkitt's lymphoma [90,96] in none of the reported cases was *in situ* hybridisation for EBV-encoded nuclear RNA (EBER) or immunohistochemistry for EBV nuclear antigen (EBNA) performed on tumour tissue. Among adults, diffuse large B-cell lymphoma is the most common subtype of lymphoma [92–95]. Other reported subtypes include small lymphocytic lymphoma/chronic lymphocytic leukaemia (Figure 30.16) [102], extranodal marginal zone B-cell lymphoma of MALT (mucosa-associated lymphoid tissue) type [103], mantle cell lymphoma [93], follicular lymphoma [104] and peripheral T-cell lymphoma [91]; Hodgkin's lymphoma has been reported rarely [105].

The prognosis and management of appendiceal malignant lymphoma depend on the histological subtype of the tumour and its stage. Some reports advocate appendicectomy alone for patients whose tumour is confined to the appendix, with right hemicolectomy and adjuvant chemotherapy and/or radiotherapy reserved for patients whose tumour has spread beyond the appendix [102]. In the case of Burkitt's lymphoma of the appendix, adjuvant

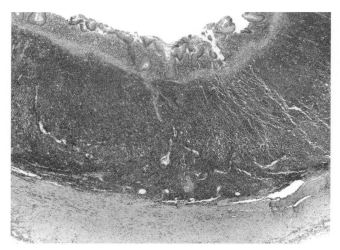

Figure 30.16 Small lymphocytic lymphoma/chronic lymphocytic leukaemia involving the appendix. The appendiceal mucosa lies above a dense and diffuse lymphocytic neoplasm that has effaced the normal follicular structures of the appendiceal mucosal lymphoid tissue.

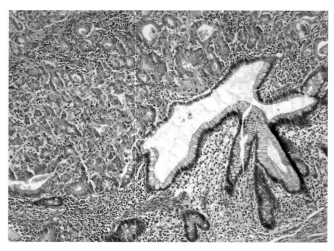

Figure 30.17 Metastatic pancreatic acinar cell carcinoma to the appendix: the appendiceal mucosa shows a proliferation of tubules that are lined by uniform cells with granular cytoplasm. This tumour might easily have been mistaken for an endocrine tumour of the appendix.

chemotherapy and radiotherapy have often been incorporated into the treatment regimen, with good result [90].

Secondary involvement of the appendix by malignant lymphoma has also been described. The appendix has been reported as the site of relapse of diffuse large B-cell lymphoma [106], NK/T-cell lymphoma of nasal type [107] and T-cell acute lymphoblastic leukaemia [108].

Secondary tumours (other than lymphoma)

In women the most common secondary neoplasia in the appendix is metastatic ovarian carcinoma, particularly serous ovarian adenocarcinoma, and peritoneal serous carcinoma. The usual setting is involvement of the appendix in a woman with advanced stage ovarian carcinoma [109–111]. However, patients with apparently early disease may rarely be found to have appendiceal serosal involvement on microscopic examination, so some authors advocate appendicectomy as part of the primary staging procedure for ovarian carcinoma [112].

Other tumours metastatic to the appendix are occasionally encountered (Figure 30.17) and several have been the subject of case reports, including breast carcinoma [113], bronchogenic adenocarcinoma and pulmonary small cell carcinoma [114,115], nasopharyngeal carcinoma [116], cholangiocarcinoma [117], transitional cell carcinoma [118] and prostatic adenocarcinoma [119]. The metastatic tumour often obstructs the appendiceal lumen, resulting in acute appendicitis, which can be the initial manifestation of a malignant neoplasm elsewhere.

References

1. Carr NJ, McCarthy WF, Sobin LH. Epithelial noncarcinoid tumours and like-like lesions of the appendix. A clinicopathologic study of 184 patients with a multivariate analysis of prognostic factors. *Cancer* 1995;**75**:757.
2. Young RH, Gilks CB, Scully RE. Mucinous tumours of the appendix associated with mucinous tumours of the ovary and pseudomyxoma peritonei. A clinicopathological analysis of 22 cases supporting an origin in the appendix. *Am J Surg Pathol* 1991;**15**:415.
3. Higa E, Rosai J, Pizzimbono CA, et al. Mucosal hyperplasia, mucinous cystadenoma, and mucinous cystadenocarcinoma of the appendix. A re-evaluation of appendiceal 'mucocele'. *Cancer* 1973;**32**:1525.
4. Ronnett BM, Kajdacsy-Balla A, Gilks CB, et al. Pseudomyxoma peritonei in women: a clinicopathologic analysis of 30 cases with emphasis on site of origin, prognosis, and relationship to ovarian mucinous tumours of low malignant potential. *Hum Pathol* 1995;**26**:509.
5. Qizilbash AH. Mucoceles of the appendix. Their relationship to hyperplastic polyps, mucinous cystadenomas, and cystadenocarcinomas. *Arch Pathol Lab Med* 1975;**99**:548.
6. Wolff M, Ahmed N. Epithelial neoplasms of the vermiform appendix (exclusive of carcinoid). II. Cystadenomas, papillary adenomas, and adenomatous polyps of the appendix. *Cancer* 1976;**37**:2511.
7. Wolff M, Ahmed N. Epithelial neoplasms of the vermiform appendix (exclusive of carcinoid). I. Adenocarcinoma of the appendix. *Cancer* 1976;**37**:2493.
8. Bradley RF, Stewart JH, Russell GB, et al. Pseudomyxoma peritonei of appendiceal origin: a clinicopathologic analysis of 101 patients uniformly treated at a single institution, with literature review. *Am J Surg Pathol* 2006;**30**:551.
9. Misdraji J, Yantiss RK, Graeme-Cook FM, et al. Appendiceal mucinous neoplasms: a clinicopathologic analysis of 107 cases. *Am J Surg Pathol* 2003;**27**:1089.

10. Appelman HD. Epithelial neoplasia of the appendix. In: Norris H (ed.), *Pathology of the Colon, Small Intestine, and Anus.* New York: Churchill Livingstone, 1991: 263.

11. Lamps LW, Gray GF Jr, Dilday BR, Washington MK. The coexistence of low-grade mucinous neoplasms of the appendix and appendiceal diverticula: a possible role in the pathogenesis of pseudomyxoma peritonei. *Mod Pathol* 2000;**13**:495.

12. Yantiss RK, Shia J, Klimstra DS, et al. Prognostic significance of localized extra-appendiceal mucin deposition in appendiceal mucinous neoplasms. *Am J Surg Pathol* 2009;**33**:248.

13. Pai RK, Beck AH, Norton JA, et al. Appendiceal mucinous neoplasms: Clinicopathologic study of 116 cases with analysis of factors predicting recurrence. *Am J Surg Pathol* 2009;**33**:1425.

14. Collins DC. A study of 50,000 specimens of the human vermiform appendix. *Surg Gynecol Obstet* 1955;**101**:437.

15. Proulx GM, Willett CG, Daley W, et al. Appendiceal carcinoma: patterns of failure following surgery and implications for adjuvant therapy. *J Surg Oncol* 1997;**66**:51.

16. Harris GJ, Urdaneta LF, Mitros FA. Adenocarcinoma of the vermiform appendix. *J Surg Oncol* 1990;**44**:218.

17. Nitecki SS, Wolff BG, Shclinkert R, et al. The natural history of surgically treated primary adenocarcinoma of the appendix. *Ann Surg* 1994;**219**:51.

18. Cerame MA. A 25-year review of adenocarcinoma of the appendix. A frequently perforating carcinoma. *Dis Colon Rectum* 1988;**31**:145.

19. Cortina R, McCormick J, Kolm P, et al. Management and prognosis of adenocarcinoma of the appendix. *Dis Colon Rectum* 1995;**38**:848.

20. Conte CC, Petrelli NJ, Stulc J, Herrera L, Mittelman A. Adenocarcinoma of the appendix. *Surg Gynecol Obstet* 1988;**166**:451.

21. Qizilbash AH. Primary adenocarcinoma of the appendix. A clinicopathological study of 11 cases. *Arch Pathol Lab Med* 1975;**99**:556.

22. Chang P, Attiyeh FF. Adenocarcinoma of the appendix. *Dis Colon Rectum* 1981;**24**:176.

23. Gilhome RW, Johnstone DH, Clark J, Kyle J. Primary adenocarcinoma of the vermiform appendix: report of a series of ten cases, and review of the literature. *Br J Surg* 1984;**71**:553.

24. Ronnett BM, Zahn CM, Kurman RJ, et al. Disseminated peritoneal adenomucinosis and peritoneal mucinous carcinomatosis. A clinicopathologic analysis of 109 cases with emphasis on distinguishing pathologic features, site of origin, prognosis, and relationship to 'pseudomyxoma peritonei'. *Am J Surg Pathol* 1995;**19**:1390.

25. Sugarbaker PH. Pseudomyxoma peritonei. A cancer whose biology is characterized by a redistribution phenomenon. *Ann Surg* 1994;**219**:109.

26. Carr NJ, Sobin LH. Unusual tumours of the appendix and pseudomyxoma peritonei. *Semin Diagn Pathol* 1996;**13**:314.

27. Sugarbaker PH, Chang D. Results of treatment of 385 patients with peritoneal surface spread of appendiceal malignancy. *Ann Surg Oncol* 1999;**6**:727.

28. Miner TJ, Shia J, Jacques DP, et al. Long-term survival following treatment of pseudomyxoma peritonei: an analysis of surgical therapy. *Ann Surg* 2005;**241**:300.

29. Torlakovic E, Skovlund E, Snover D, Torlakovic G, Nesland JM. Morphologic reappraisal of serrated colorectal polyps. *Am J Surg Pathol* 2003;**27**:65.

30. Yantiss RK, Panczykowski A, Misdraji J, et al. A comprehensive study of nondysplastic and dysplastic serrated polyps of the vermiform appendix. *Am J Surg Pathol* 2007;**31**:1742.

31. Rubio CA. Serrated adenomas of the appendix. *J Clin Pathol* 2004;**57**:946.

32. Collins DC. Adenomatous polyps of the vermiform appendix. *Surg Clinics North Am* 1932;**12**:1063.

33. Modlin IM, Sandor A. An analysis of 8305 cases of carcinoid tumours. *Cancer* 1997;**79**:813.

34. Moertel CG, Dockerty MB, Judd ES. Carcinoid tumours of the vermiform appendix. *Cancer* 1968;**21**:270.

35. Glasser CM, Bhagavan BS. Carcinoid tumours of the appendix. *Arch Pathol Lab Med* 1980;**104**:272.

36. Roggo A, Wood WC, Ottinger LW. Carcinoid tumours of the appendix. *Ann Surg* 1993;**217**:385.

37. Pelizzo G, La Riccia A, Bouvier R, Chappuis JP, Franchella A. Carcinoid tumours of the appendix in children. *Pediatr Surg Int* 2001;**17**:399.

38. Moertel CL, Weiland LH, Telander RL. Carcinoid tumour of the appendix in the first two decades of life. *J Pediatr Surg* 1990;**25**:1073.

39. Doede T, Foss HD, Waldschmidt J. Carcinoid tumours of the appendix in children – epidemiology, clinical aspects and procedure. *Eur J Pediatr Surg* 2000;**10**:372.

40. Syracuse DC, Perzin KH, Price JB, et al. Carcinoid tumours of the appendix. Mesoappendiceal extension and nodal metastases. *Ann Surg* 1979;**190**:58.

41. Anderson JR, Wilson BG. Carcinoid tumours of the appendix. *Br J Surg* 1985;**72**:545.

42. Gouzi JL, Laigneau P, Delalande JP, et al., The French Associations for Surgical Research. Indications for right hemicolectomy in carcinoid tumours of the appendix. *Surg Gynecol Obstet* 1993;**176**:543.

43. Iwafuchi M, Watanabe H, Ajioka Y, et al. Immunohistochemical and ultrastructural studies of twelve argentaffin and six argyrophil carcinoids of the appendix vermiformis. *Hum Pathol* 1990;**21**:773.

44. Moyana TN, Satkunam N. A comparative immunohistochemical study of jejunoileal and appendiceal carcinoids. Implications for histogenesis and pathogenesis. *Cancer* 1992;**70**:1081.

45. Burke AP, Sobin LH, Federspiel BH, et al. Appendiceal carcinoids: correlation of histology and immunohistochemistry. *Mod Pathol* 1989;**2**:630.

46. Nash SV, Said JW. Gastroenteropancreatic neuroendocrine tumours. A histochemical and immunohistochemical study of epithelial (keratin proteins, carcinoembryonic antigen) and neuroendocrine (neuron-specific enolase, bombesin and chromogranin) markers in foregut, midgut, and hindgut tumours. *Am J Clin Pathol* 1986;**86**:415.

47. Goede AC, Caplin ME, Winslet MC. Carcinoid tumour of the appendix. *Br J Surg* 2003;**90**:1317.

48. Stinner B, Kisker O, Ziele A, et al. Surgical management for carcinoid tumours of small bowel, appendix, colon, and rectum. *World J Surg* 1996;**20**:183.

49. Modlin IM, Lye KD, Kidd M. A 5-decade analysis of 13,715 carcinoid tumours. *Cancer* 2003;**97**:934.

50. Godwin JD 2nd. Carcinoid tumours. An analysis of 2,837 cases. *Cancer* 1975;**36**:560.

51. Moertel CG, Weiland LH, Nagorney DM, Dockerty MB. Carcinoid tumour of the appendix: treatment and prognosis. *N Engl J Med* 1987;**317**:1699.

52. MacGillivray DC, et al. Distant metastasis from a carcinoid tumour of the appendix less than one centimetre in size. *Surgery* 1992;**111**:466.

53. Rossi G, et al. Does mesoappendix infiltration predict a worse prognosis in incidental neuroendocrine tumours of the appendix? A clinicopathologic and immunohistochemical study of 15 cases. *Am J Clin Pathol* 2003;**120**:706.

54. Burke AP, Sobin LH, Federspiel BH, et al. Goblet cell carcinoids and related tumors of the vermiform appendix. *Am J Clin Pathol* 1990;**94**:27.

55. Goddard MJ, Lonsdale RN. The histogenesis of appendiceal carcinoid tumours. *Histopathology* 1992;**20**:345.

56. Stancu M, Wu TT, Wallace C, et al. Genetic alterations in goblet cell carcinoids of the vermiform appendix and comparison with gastrointestinal carcinoid tumours. *Mod Pathol* 2003;**16**:1189.

57. Park K, Blessing K, Kerr K, et al. Goblet cell carcinoid of the appendix. *Gut* 1990;**31**:322.

58. Berardi RS, Lee SS, Chen HP. Goblet cell carcinoids of the appendix. *Surg Gynecol Obstet* 1988;**167**:81.

59. Hood IC, Jones BA, Watts JC. Mucinous carcinoid tumour of the appendix presenting as bilateral ovarian tumours. *Arch Pathol Lab Med* 1986;**110**:336.

60. Klein EA, Rosen MH. Bilateral Krukenberg tumours due to appendiceal mucinous carcinoid. *Int J Gynecol Pathol* 1996;**15**:85.

61. Hirschfield LS, Kahn LB, Winkler B, et al. Adenocarcinoid of the appendix presenting as bilateral Krukenberg's tumour of the ovaries. Immunohistochemical and ultrastructural studies and literature review. *Arch Pathol Lab Med* 1985;**109**:930.

62. Hristov AC, Young RH, Vang R, Yemelyanova AV, Seidman JD, Ronnett BM. Ovarian metastases of appendiceal tumours with goblet cell carcinoid like and signet ring cell patterns: a report of 30 cases. *Am J Surg Pathol* 2007;**31**:1502.

63. Klein HZ. Mucinous carcinoid tumour of the vermiform appendix. *Cancer* 1974;**33**:770.

64. Watson PH, Alguacil-Garcia A. Mixed crypt cell carcinoma. A clinicopathological study of the so-called 'goblet cell carcinoid'. *Virchows Archiv A Pathol Anat Histopathol* 1987;**412**:175.

65. Isaacson P. Crypt cell carcinoma of the appendix (so-called adenocarcinoid tumour). *Am J Surg Pathol* 1981;**5**:213.

66. van Eeden S, Offerhaus GJ, Hart AA, et al. Goblet cell carcinoid of the appendix: a specific type of carcinoma. *Histopathology* 2007;**51**:763.

67. Alsaad KO, Serra S, Schmitt A, et al. Cytokeratins 7 and 20 immunoexpression profile in goblet cell and classical carcinoids of appendix. *Endocr Pathol* 2007;**18**:16.

68. Edmonds P, Merino M J, LiVolsi VA, Duray PH. Adenocarcinoid (mucinous carcinoid) of the appendix. *Gastroenterology* 1984;**86**:302.

69. Warner TF, Seo IS. Goblet cell carcinoid of appendix: ultrastructural features and histogenetic aspects. *Cancer* 1979;**44**:1700.

70. Bak M, Asschenfeldt P. Adenocarcinoid of the vermiform appendix. A clinicopathologic study of 20 cases. *Dis Colon Rectum* 1988;**31**:605.

71. Ferrone CR, Tang LH, Tomlinson J, et al. Pathologic classification and clinical behavior of the spectrum of goblet cell carcinoid tumours of the appendix. *Am J Surg Pathol* 2008;**32**:1429.

72. Bucher P, Gervais P, Ris F, Oulhachi W, Egger J-F, Morel P. Surgical treatment of appendiceal adenocarcinoid (goblet cell carcinoid). *World J Surg* 2005;**29**:1436.

73. Varisco B, McAlvin B, Dias J, Franga D. Adenocarcinoid of the appendix: is right hemicolectomy necessary? A meta-analysis of retrospective chart reviews. *Am Surg* 2004;**70**:593.

74. Plockinger U, Couvelard A, Falconi M, et al. Consensus guidelines for the management of patients with digestive neuroendocrine tumours: well-differentiated tumour/carcinoma of the appendix and goblet cell carcinoma. *Neuroendocrinology* 2008;**87**:20.

75. Collins DC. 71,000 Human appendix specimens. A final report, summarizing forty years' study. *Am J Proctol* 1963;**14**:265.

76. Iovetz-Tereshchenko NN. Myomata of the vermiform appendix. *Lancet* 1950;**i**:903.

77. Koontz AR. Myoma of the appendix. *Ann Surg* 1929;**89**:272.

78. Powell JL, Fuerst JF, Tapia RA. Leiomyoma of the appendix. *South Med J* 1980;**73**:1298.

79. Cullen TH, Voss HJ. Leiomyoma of the appendix. *Br J Surg* 1972;**59**:579.

80. Miettinen M, Sobin LH. Gastrointestinal stromal tumours in the appendix: a clinicopathologic and immunohistochemical study of four cases. *Am J Surg Pathol* 2001;**25**:1433.

81. Agaimy A, Pelz AF, Wieacker P, et al. Gastrointestinal stromal tumours of the vermiform appendix: clinicopathologic, immunohistochemical, and molecular study of 2 cases with literature review. *Hum Pathol* 2008;**39**:1252.

82. Pipeleers-Marichal M, Goossens A, De Waele B, Kloppel G. Granular cell tumour of the appendix in a patient irradiated for a rectal carcinoma. *Virchows Arch A Pathol Anat Histopathol* 1990;**417**:177.

83. Johnston J, Helwig EB. Granular cell tumours of the gastrointestinal tract and perianal region: a study of 74 cases. *Dig Dis Sci* 1981;**26**:807.

84. Deziel DJ, Saclarides TJ, Marshall JS, et al. Appendiceal Kaposi's sarcoma: a cause of right lower quadrant pain in the acquired immune deficiency syndrome. *Am J Gastroenterol* 1991;**86**:901.

85. Chetty R, Arendse MP. Gastro-intestinal Kaposi's sarcoma, with special reference to the appendix. *S Afr J Surg* 1999;**37**:9.

86. Ravalli S, Vincent RA, Beaton H. Primary Kaposi's sarcoma of the gastrointestinal tract presenting as acute appendicitis. *Am J Gastroenterol* 1990;**85**:772.

87. Lie KA, Lindboe CF, Kolmannskog SV, et al. Giant appendix with diffuse ganglioneuromatosis. An unusual presentation of von Recklinghausen's disease. *Eur J Surg* 1992;**158**:127.

88. Merck C, Kindblom LG. Neurofibromatosis of the appendix in von Recklinghausen's disease. A report of a case. *Acta Pathol Microbiol Scand A* 1975;**83**:623.

89. Olsen BS. Giant appendicular neurofibroma. A light and immunohistochemical study. *Histopathology* 1987;**11**:851.

90. Caine YG, Peylan-Ramu N, Livoff AF, Schiller M. Primary Burkitt's lymphoma of the appendix. *Z Kinderchir* 1990;**45**:251.

91. Kitamura Y, Ohta T, Terada T. Primary T-cell non-Hodgkin's malignant lymphoma of the appendix. *Pathol Int* 2000;**50**:313.

92. Uncu H, Erdem E, Tuzuner A. Primary malignant lymphoma of the appendix (a case report and review of the literature). *Acta Chir Hung* 1998;**37**:11.

93. Pickhardt PJ, Levy AD, Rohrmann CA Jr, et al. Non-Hodgkin's lymphoma of the appendix: clinical and CT findings with pathologic correlation. *AJR Am J Roentgenol* 2002;**178**:1123.

94. Chuang SS, Li CY. Clinicopathological features of primary intestinal lymphoma in Taiwan: a study of 21 resected cases. *Pathol Res Pract* 2002;**198**:381.

95. Hanna GB, Frizelle FA, Santoro GA. Lymphoma of the appendix. A case report. *G Chir* 1997;**18**:219.

96. Ghani SA, Syed N, Tan PE. A rare cause of acute appendicitis: Burkitt's lymphoma of the appendix. *Med J Malaysia* 1984;**39**:311.

97. Lewin KJ, Ranchod M, Dorfman RF. Lymphomas of the gastrointestinal tract: a study of 117 cases presenting with gastrointestinal disease. *Cancer* 1978;**42**:693.

98. Muller G, Dargent JL, Duwel V, et al. Leukaemia and lymphoma of the appendix presenting as acute appendicitis or acute abdomen. Four case reports with a review of the literature. *J Cancer Res Clin Oncol* 1997;**123**:560.

99. Mori M, Kusunoi T, Kikuchi M, Motoori T, Sugimachi K. Primary malignant lymphoma of the appendix. *Jpn J Surg* 1985;**15**:230.

100. Sin IC, Ling ET, Prentice RS. Burkitt's lymphoma of the appendix: report of two cases. *Hum Pathol* 1980;**11**:465.

101. Bambery P, Vasishta RK, Das DK, et al. Acute tumour lysis syndrome: clinicomorphological correlations in adult primary appendicular Burkitt's lymphoma – a case report. *Indian J Cancer* 1986;**23**:117.

102. Pasquale MD, Shabahang M, Bitterman P, Lack EE, Evans SR. Primary lymphoma of the appendix. Case report and review of the literature. *Surg Oncol* 1994;**3**:243.

103. Radha S, Afroz T, Satyanarayana G. Primary marginal zone B-cell lymphoma of appendix. *Indian J Pathol Microbiol* 2008; **51**:392.

104. Furuse M, Aoyagi KE, Saki M, et al. Endoscopic appearance of primary appendiceal lymphoma. *Gastrointest Endosc* 1998; **48**:86.

105. Umer MA, Date RS, Mellor S, et al. Hodgkin's disease of appendix: report of a case. *Colorectal Dis* 2009;**11**:985.

106. Katz DS, Stein LB, Mazzie JP. Recurrent non-Hodgkin's lymphoma of the appendix. *AJR Am J Roentgenol* 2002;**179**:1443.

107. Tsujimura H, Takagi T, Tamaru JI, Sakai C. Involvement of the appendix in a relapsed case of primary nasal NK/T-cell lymphoma. *Leuk Lymphoma* 2000;**37**:633.

108. Lyman MD, Neuhauser TS. Precursor T-cell acute lymphoblastic leukemia/lymphoma involving the uterine cervix, myometrium, endometrium, and appendix. *Ann Diagn Pathol* 2002;**6**:125.

109. Sonnendecker EW, Margolius KA, Sonnendecker HE. Involvement of the appendix in ovarian epithelial cancer – an update. *S Afr Med J* 1989;**76**:667.

110. Fontanelli R, Paladini D, Raspagliesi F, di Re E. The role of appendectomy in surgical procedures for ovarian cancer. *Gynecol Oncol* 1992;**46**:42.

111. Bese T, Kosebay D, Kaleli S, et al. Appendectomy in the surgical staging of ovarian carcinoma. *Int J Gynecol Obstet* 1996;**53**:249.

112. Rose PG, Abdul-Karim FW. Isolated appendiceal metastasis in early ovarian carcinoma. *J Surg Oncol* 1997;**64**:246.

113. Maddox PR. Acute appendicitis secondary to metastatic carcinoma of the breast. *Br J Clin Pract* 1990;**44**:376.

114. Goldstein EB, Savel RH, Walter KL, et al. Extensive stage small cell lung cancer presenting as an acute perforated appendix: case report and review of the literature. *Am Surg* 2004;**70**:706.

115. Gopez EV, Mourelatos Z, Rosato EF, Livolsi VA. Acute appendicitis secondary to metastatic bronchogenic adenocarcinoma. *Am Surg* 1997;**63**:778.

116. Hsu KL, Wang KS, Chen L, Chou FF. Acute appendicitis secondary to metastatic nasopharyngeal carcinoma. *J Surg Oncol* 1995;**60**:131.

117. Man KM, Keeffe EB, Garcia-Kennedy R, et al. Acute appendicitis secondary to metastatic cholangiocarcinoma. *Am J Gastroenterol* 1993;**88**:1966.

118. Stein A, Sova Y, Almalah I, Lurie A. The appendix as a metastatic target for male urogenital tumours. *Br J Urol* 1996;**78**:647.

119. Ansari MA, Pintozzi RL, Choi YS, et al. Diagnosis of carcinoid-like metastatic prostatic carcinoma by an immunoperoxidase method. *Am J Clin Pathol* 1981;**76**:94.

Miscellaneous conditions of the appendix

Robert P. Eckstein

Pacific Laboratory Medicine Services, Royal North Shore Hospital, St Leonards, NSW, Australia

Normal embryology and fetal development

The appendix is a derivative of the caecum. The caecum appears as an outgrowth from the wall of the primitive midgut at the end of week 5, before the latter differentiates into small and large intestines [1]. The distal three-quarters of this outgrowth elongate rapidly to form a conical caecum, the tip of which extends further to form a narrow, tubular primitive appendix. This arrangement persists throughout fetal life and is often present at birth. At term and subsequently, the lateral wall of the caecum grows faster than the medial, so that the appendix is 'pushed' round to approach the ileo-caecal valve, in relation to which it can adopt a number of positions. At the same time it narrows and becomes a more definitely separate, thin, tube-like structure.

A little lymphoid tissue is present in the lamina propria in the fetus at 17–20 weeks but there are no germinal centres present at birth. These develop rapidly between weeks 3 and 6 of postnatal life, presumably after the introduction of foreign proteins into the gut in ingested food and milk.

Developmental abnormalities

Duplications

Appendiceal duplication is very rare, but clinically important because of the possibility of occurrence of acute appendicitis despite prior appendicectomy. The patterns of appendiceal duplication are generally classified according to the Cave–Wallbridge classification system [2]. In type A, there is a single caecum, a single appendiceal base and a partially duplicated appendix. In type B, there is a single caecum with two separate appendiceal bases and two separate appendixes. This may take the form of either two symmetrically placed appendixes, one on either side of the ileo-caecal valve, or one appendix present in the usual position and a rudimentary second appendix arising separately from the caecum, usually in relation to one of the taeniae. In type C, there is a double caecum each with an appendix. Double- and triple-barrelled appendixes have also been described, in which a single muscle coat surrounds multiple lumina, each surrounded by a separate mucosal layer [3]. Triplication of the appendix [4] and a horseshoe anomaly with two separate openings of the appendix into the caecal lumen [5] have also been described.

Absence of the appendix

Agenesis with congenital absence of the appendix is rare with an incidence of about 1 in 100000 laparotomies for appendicitis [6,7]; some cases appeared to represent a thalidomide-induced anomaly [8]. Agenesis must be separated from hypoplasia in which, although the caecum is fully developed, only rudimentary appendiceal tissue is present. Agenesis can be associated with a normal caecum or caecal dysgenesis, and other congenital anomalies may

Morson and Dawson's Gastrointestinal Pathology, Fifth Edition. Edited by Neil A. Shepherd, Bryan F. Warren, Geraint T. Williams, Joel K. Greenson, Gregory Y. Lauwers and Marco R. Novelli.
© 2013 Blackwell Publishing Ltd. Published 2013 by Blackwell Publishing Ltd.

be present [9]. Agenesis has to be distinguished from autoamputation secondary to inflammation, intussusception or volvulus.

Malpositions

Occasional examples of acute appendicitis have been described in which the appendix is subhepatic. These are associated with maldescent of the caecum [10]. Other forms of malposition can occur, related to intestinal malrotation.

Congenital appendico-umbilical fistula

Although the omphalo-mesenteric (vitelline) duct normally connects to the ileum, on occasion it may connect to the caecum or appendix. There have been six reported cases of appendico-umbilical fistulae, resulting from failure of closure of the omphalo-mesenteric duct [11].

Heterotopias in the appendix

Heterotopic epithelium is rare in the appendix but gastric, oesophageal and pancreatic tissue have been reported [12,13].

Appendiceal septa

Single or multiple, complete or incomplete septa, consisting of mucosa and submucosa, have been described in appendixes showing acute inflammation [26]. When complete septa were present the inflammatory process was frequently confined to one compartment. Most cases occurred in the 15- to 19-year age group and there was a clear male predominance. Whether this is a congenital or post-inflammatory abnormality is not clear.

Diverticular disease

Diverticula are found within surgically removed appendixes in about 2% of specimens [14]. Appendiceal diverticula are acquired in the great majority of cases [15].

Congenital diverticula

In congenital diverticula the muscularis propria is continuous around the diverticulum. They are apparently more common in males and the diverticula are usually solitary [16,17]. Congenital appendiceal diverticula have been reported in association with the trisomy 13 syndrome [18].

Acquired diverticula

These are outpouchings of mucosa through the appendiceal wall, which are typically not invested by muscularis

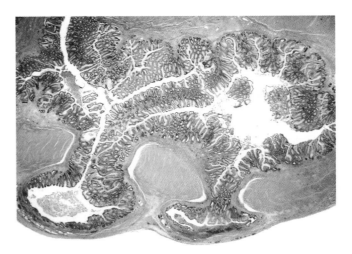

Figure 31.1 Diverticulosis: the muscular wall of the appendix is thick and penetrated by two diverticula of acquired type.

propria, although occasionally a few strands of the longitudinal muscle coat may be present (Figure 31.1). They may occur on the mesenteric or the anti-mesenteric border of the appendix, usually in the distal third, and are more often multiple than single, giving the appendix a distinctive beaded appearance externally. They may contain faecoliths. Microscopically they are lined by appendiceal mucosa. They may be asymptomatic or associated with recurrent abdominal pain [19]. They can be recognised preoperatively by computed tomography [20].

Acquired diverticula probably result from increased intraluminal pressure due to distension combined with muscular contraction. They are typically found in adults. In children an association with cystic fibrosis has been recorded [21]. Inflammation in the past may weaken the appendiceal wall. The diverticula subsequently develop at sites of deficient muscle associated with penetrating arteries. There has been recent emphasis on the importance of neoplasms in the pathogenesis of some cases [22]. A tumour may raise intraluminal pressure either by obstruction or, in the case of mucinous tumours, by mucin hypersecretion. In the latter case, perforation of diverticula may result in pseudomyxoma peritonei [23].

Appendiceal diverticulitis

Histological examination of some appendicectomy specimens reveals diverticulitis and peri-diverticulitis at the appendiceal tip, and the thin wall of an acquired diverticulum means that there is little in the way of a barrier to perforation and consequent peritonitis or peri-diverticular abscess formation. Compared with typical acute appendicitis, diverticulitis of the appendix generally occurs in older patients and is more likely to be associated with pre-existing, often intermittent, symptoms and to present with perforation. [19,24,25].

Intussusception

Appendiceal intussusception is uncommon. It may involve either a normal [27] or an abnormal appendix [28] and its recognition in right hemicolectomy specimens can be difficult unless it is suspected. Clinical presentation is usually with abdominal pain, vomiting or blood per rectum and symptoms are often present intermittently for some weeks or months before diagnosis. Sometimes a preoperative diagnosis can be made by imaging or at colonoscopy. At colonoscopy, an erythematous mushroom-like lesion with a central dimple is seen, which may be mistaken for a polyp or tumour, and biopsy has occasionally led to bowel perforation [29].

McSwain classified appendiceal intussusception into four types [30]:
1. Type 1: there is intussusception of the distal appendix into the proximal appendix
2. Type 2: there is intussusception of the distal appendix into the caeco-appendiceal valvular opening
3. Type 3: there is intussusception of the proximal appendix into the distal appendix
4. Type 4: there is complete inversion of the appendix, usually as part of ileo-caecal intussusception.

Appendiceal intussusception occurs in young children and adults. It is likely that a wide proximal appendix lumen and a mobile meso-appendix, along with abnormal peristalsis, are predisposing factors. In children, lymphoid hyperplasia may act as a 'lead point'. This has been linked to adenovirus and other viral infections [31] and very occasionally to bacterial infection such as *Yersinia enterocolitica* infection [32]. In adults there is a high incidence of mass lesions [33], including endometriosis [34–36] and benign and malignant tumours [37–39]. In resections for appendiceal intussusception it is important for the pathologist to exclude these (Figure 31.2).

Torsion

Torsion of the appendix is rare, with fewer than 30 reported cases. The twist occurs at or near the base of the appendix. Although usually presenting clinically as acute appendicitis, it characteristically leads to sharply demarcated ischaemic necrosis (Figure 31.3) with little suppuration [40]. It is found in children and, less commonly, in adults. It is said to be more common in long appendixes and appendixes with a long or misshapen mesentery. In adults, the twist may occur proximal to tumours, most often mucinous cystadenomas [41].

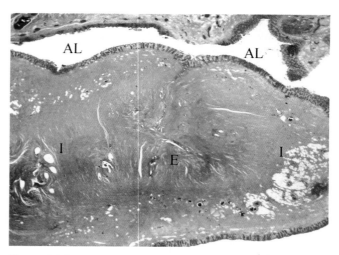

Figure 31.2 Intussusception due to endometriosis: lying within the dilated appendiceal lumen (AL) is the intussusceptum (I). Islands containing endometrial glands and stroma (E) are present in the intussuscepted appendiceal muscularis.

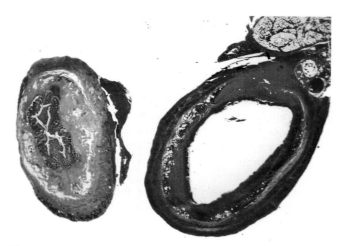

Figure 31.3 Torsion: a section of the proximal appendix (left) is normal, contrasting with ischaemic necrosis in the distal appendix (right).

Endometriosis and conditions related to pregnancy

Endometriosis

The appendix is involved in approximately 1% of cases of pelvic endometriosis and usually represents an incidental finding at laparotomy [42]. Patients may present with acute appendicitis, in some cases related to intramural haemorrhage that has occluded the appendiceal lumen [43]. Decidualisation of endometriosis may result in the onset of appendicitis during pregnancy [44]. Severe haemorrhage leading to massive lower gastrointestinal haemorrhage has been reported [45]. A number of cases have presented with intussusception [34–36]. Most endometriotic deposits are subserosal or intramuscular and, as elsewhere in the large bowel, they are associated with reactive thickening of the muscularis propria (see Figure 31.2).

Endosalpingiosis

Very rarely endosalpingiosis affects the appendix. It presents without symptoms but may form a multicystic mass mimicking a neoplasm. The cysts are lined by tubal type epithelial cells, which show positive staining for oestrogen receptors. They are negative for markers of mesothelial cells, in contrast with mesothelial inclusion cysts. The absence of endometrial stroma excludes endometriosis [46].

Decidual reaction

In pregnant women, during laparoscopy or laparotomy, decidual nodules may be seen involving the appendix and other sites within the peritoneal cavity. They may be confused with tumour, both at the time of surgery and at subsequent microscopic examination. Decidual nodules are thought to arise through metaplasia of submesothelial stromal cells under the influence of progesterone. The nodules are composed of cells that are usually plump with plentiful eosinophilic cytoplasm, but which may also be vacuolated or spindle shaped (Figure 31.4). They can be distinguished from carcinoma and mesothelioma by the lack of nuclear atypia, negative staining for keratins in most cases and positive staining for progesterone receptors [47].

Vernix caseosa

Spillage of vernix caseosa at the time of a caesarean section may, in the immediate postpartum period, result in peritonitis. The appendix may be resected in the belief that appendicitis is present. Grossly the appendix is covered with a cheesy exudate. Microscopically, the appendix is covered with aggregates of anucleate squamous cells, often accompanied by a foreign body giant cell reaction [48] (Figure 31.5).

Cystic fibrosis

In this condition, the appendix is typically distended with inspissated mucus and, microscopically, the goblet cells are enlarged and the crypts dilated. There is an increased incidence of diverticulosis and ileo-colic intussusception [21,49].

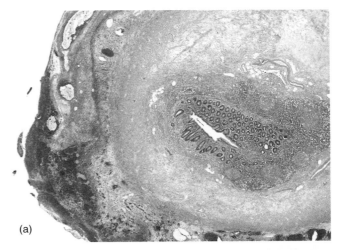

(a)

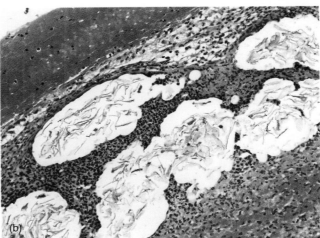

(b)

Figure 31.5 Vernix caseosa: (a) the appendix shows a serosal acute inflammatory exudate on low power examination.
(b) Admixed aggregates of squamous cells are seen at high power.

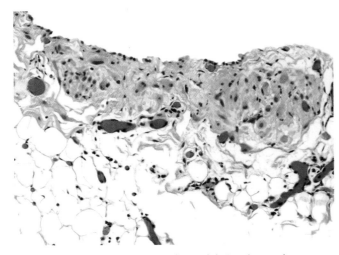

Figure 31.4 Decidual reaction: the nodule is subserosal.

Foreign bodies

The appendix may be prone to lodgement of foreign bodies because its orifice is located in a dependent position in the caecum [50].

The incidence of appendicitis due to foreign bodies has decreased since the nineteenth century, in part due to less frequent ingestion of sewing needles and gunshot (the latter derived from the ingestion of wild game). The range of objects seen is wide, including tongue studs, prosthetic teeth, a dental drill bit, pills, nails, bullets, bones and hair, as well as seeds and other vegetable matter, parasites and barium [50,51] (Figure 31.6).

Appendicitis may occur from days to years after ingestion of the object. Sharp, pointed or long objects are more likely to cause perforation [51].

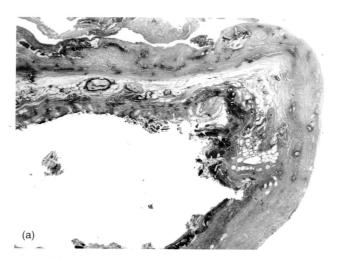

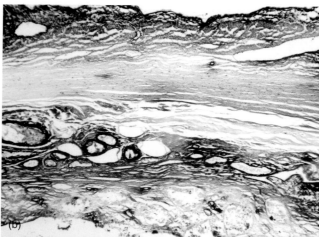

Figure 31.6 Foreign body: (a) in this case an iron tablet impacted in the base of the appendix has resulted in ischaemic necrosis with brown pigmentation. (b) Perls' stain confirms massive deposition of iron. The tablet was found lying free in the specimen jar.

Melanosis

Melanosis of the appendix, histologically similar to that seen in the colon, has been described in 7.4% of appendixes in a series of adults and 46% in a series of children [52,53]. In adults about half the cases have concomitant melanosis coli. In both age groups the base of the appendix is more affected than the tip. The generation and deposition of lipofuscin pigment are probably related to increased epithelial cell turnover, with a multiplicity of poorly defined underlying causes (see Chapter 40).

References

1. Malas MA, Sulak O, Gokcimen A, Sari A. Development of the vermiform appendix during the fetal period. *Surg Radiol Anat* 2004;**26**:202.
2. Travis RJ, Weppner JL, Paugh JC. Duplex vermiform appendix: case report of a ruptured second appendix. *J Pediatr Surg* 2008;**43**:1726.
3. Uriev L, Maslovsky I, Mnouskin Y, Ben-Dora D. Triple-barreled type of appendiceal triplication. *Ann Diagn Pathol* 2006;**10**:160.
4. Tinckler LF. Triple appendix vermiformis – a unique case. *Br J Surg* 1968;**55**:79.
5. Mesko TW, Lugo R, Breitholtz T. Horseshoe anomaly of the appendix: a previously undescribed entity. *Surgery* 1989;**106**:563.
6. Collins DC. Agenesis of vermiform appendix. *Am J Surg* 1951; **82**:689.
7. Greenberg SLL, Eyers AA, MacKay S. Congenital absence of the appendix. *ANZ J Surg* 2003;**73**:166.
8. Bremner DM, Mooney G. Agenesis of appendix: a further thalidomide anomaly (letter). *Lancet* 1978;**i**:826.
9. Cserni T, Magyar A, Tamás Nemeth T, Paran TS, Csízy I, Józsa T. Atresia of the ileocecal junction with agenesis of the ileocecal valve and vermiform appendix: report of a case. *Surg Today* 2006;**36**:1126.
10. Scott KJ, Sacks AJ, Goldschmidt RP. Subhepatic appendicitis. *Am J Gastroenterol* 1993;**88**:1773.
11. Crankson SJ, Ahmed GS, Palkar V. Patent omphalomesenteric duct of the vermiform appendix in a neonate: congenital appendicoumbilical fistula. *Pediatr Surg Int* 1998;**14**:229.
12. Droga BW, Levine S, Baber JJ. Heterotopic gastric and esophageal tissue in the vermiform appendix. *Am J Clin Pathol* 1963; **40**:190.
13. Aubrey DA. Gastric mucosa in the vermiform appendix. *Arch Surg* 1970;**101**:628.
14. Lipton S, Estrin J, Glasser I. Diverticular disease of the appendix. *Surg Gynecol Obstet* 1989;**168**:13.
15. AbdullGaffar B. Diverticulosis and diverticulitis of the appendix. *Int J Surg Pathol* 2009;**17**:231.
16. Beswick JS, Desai S. Diverticular disease of the vermiform appendix and its clinical relevance. *Australas Radiol* 1994;**38**:260.
17. Trollope ML, Lindenauer SM. Diverticulosis of the appendix: a collective review. *Dis Colon Rectum* 1974;**17**:200.
18. Favara BE. Multiple congenital diverticula of the vermiform appendix. *Am J Clin Pathol* 1968;**49**:60.
19. Majeski J. Diverticulum of the vermiform appendix is associated with chronic abdominal pain. *Am J Surg* 2003;**186**:129.
20. Lee KH, Lee HS, Park SH, et al. Appendiceal diverticulitis: diagnosis and differentiation from usual acute appendicitis using computed tomography. *J Comput Assist Tomogr* 2007;**31**:763.
21. George DH. Diverticulosis of the vermiform appendix in patients with cystic fibrosis. *Hum Pathol* 1987;**18**:75.

22. Dupre MP, Jadavji I, Matshes E, Urbanski SJ. Diverticular disease of the vermiform appendix: a diagnostic clue to underlying appendiceal neoplasm. *Hum Pathol* 2008;**39**:1823.

23. Lamps LW, Gray GF, Dilday BR, Washington MK. The coexistence of low-grade mucinous neoplasms of the appendix and appendiceal diverticula: a possible role in the pathogenesis of pseudomyxoma peritonei. *Mod Pathol* 2000;**13**:495.

24. Delikaris P, Teglbjaerg PS, Fisker-Sorensen P, Balslev I. Diverticula of the vermiform appendix. *Dis Colon Rectum* 1983; **26**:374.

25. Place RJ, Simmang CI, Huber PJ. Appendiceal diverticulitis. *South Med J* 2000;**93**:76.

26. De la Fuente AA. Septa in the appendix: a previously undescribed condition. *Histopathology* 1985;**9**:1329.

27. Patton KR, Ferrera PC. Intussusception of a normal appendix. *Am J Emerg Med* 2000;**18**:115.

28. Desai N, Wayne MG, Taub PJ, Levitt MA, Spiegel R, Kim U. Intussusception in adults. *Mt Sinai J Med* 1999;**66**:336.

29. Ozuner G, Davidson P, Church J. Intussusception of the vermiform appendix: preoperative colonoscopic diagnosis of two cases and review of the literature. *Int J Colorectal Dis* 2000;**15**:185.

30. McSwain B. Intussusception of the appendix. Review of the literature and report of a case. *South Med J* 1941;**34**:263.

31. Porter HJ, Padfield CJH, Peres LC, et al. Adenovirus and intranuclear inclusions in appendices in intussusception. *J Clin Pathol* 1993;**46**:154.

32. Winesett MP, Pietsch JB, Barnard JA. *Yersinia enterocolitica* in a child with intussusception. *J Pediatr Gastroenterol Nutr* 1996;**23**:77.

33. Chaar CIO, Wexelman B, Zuckerman K, Longo W. Intussusception of the appendix: comprehensive review of the literature. *Am J Surg* 2009;**198**:122.

34. Nycum LR, Moss H, Adams JQ, Macri CI. Asymptomatic intussusception of the appendix due to endometriosis. *South Med J* 1999;**92**:524.

35. Liang H-H, Ming-Te Huang M-T, Wei P-L, et al. Endometriosis-induced appendiceal intussusception. *Am J Surg* 2009;**197**:66.

36. Moradi P, Barakate M, Gill A, Farrow G. Intussusception of the vermiform appendix due to endometriosis presenting as acute appendicitis. *ANZ J Surg* 2007;**77**:758.

37. Ohno M, Nakamura T, Hori H, Tabuchi Y, Kuroda Y. Appendiceal intussusception induced by a villous adenoma with carcinoma: report of a case. *Surg Today* 2000;**30**:441.

38. Yoshikawa A, Kuramoto S, Mimura T, et al. Peutz–Jeghers syndrome manifesting complete intussusception of the appendix associated with a focal cancer of the duodenum and a cystadeno-carcinoma of the pancreas: report of a case. *Dis Colon Rectum* 1998;**41**:517.

39. Karabulut R, Sonmez K, Turkyilmaz Z, et al. Mucosa associated lymphoid tissue lymphoma in the appendix, a lead point for intussusception. *J Pediatr Surg* 2005;**40**:872.

40. Merrett ND, Lubowski DZ, King DW. Torsion of the vermiform appendix: a case report and review of literature. *ANZ J Surg* 1992;**62**:981.

41. Bowling CB, Lipscomb GH. Torsion of the appendix mimicking ovarian torsion. *Obstet Gynecol* 2006;**107**:466.

42. Ortiz-Hidalgo C, Cortes-Aguilar D, Ortiz de la Pena J. Endometriosis of the vermiform appendix (EVA) is an uncommon lesion with a frequency <1% of all cases of pelvic endometriosis. *World J Surg* 1999;**23**:427.

43. Mittal VK, Choudhury SP, Cortez JA. Endometriosis of the appendix presenting as acute appendicitis. *Am J Surg* 1981; **142**:519.

44. Perez CM, C. Minimo C, Margolin G, Orris J. Appendiceal endometriosis presenting as acute appendicitis during pregnancy *Int J Gynecol Obstet* 2007;**98**:164.

45. Shome GP, Nagaraju M, Munis A, Wiese D. Appendiceal endometriosis presenting as massive lower intestinal haemorrhage. *Am J Gastroenterol* 1995;**90**:1881.

46. Pollheimer MJ, Leibl S, Pollheimer VS, Ratschek M, Langner C. Cystic endosalpingiosis of the appendix. *Virchows Arch* 2007; **450**:239.

47. Rodriguez FJ, Abraham SC, Sendelbach KM, Nascimento AG. Florid decidual reaction mimicking gastrointestinal malignancy in a primipara woman. *Histopathology* 2006;**49**:82.

48. Selo-Ojeme D. Vernix caseosa peritonitis. *J Obstet Gynaecol* 2007; **27**:660.

49. Coughlin PJ, Gauderer MWL, Stern RC, Doershuk CF, Izant RJ, Zollinger RM. The spectrum of appendiceal disease in cystic fibrosis. *J Pediatr Surg* 1990;**25**:835.

50. Hartin CW, Lau ST, Caty MG. Metallic foreign body in the appendix of 3-year-old boy. *J Pediatr Surg* 2008;**43**:2106.

51. Klingler PJ, Smith SL, Abendstein BJ, Brenner E, Hinder RA. Management of ingested foreign bodies within the appendix: a case report with review of the literature. *Am J Gastroenterol* 1997; **92**:2295.

52. Rutty GN, Shaw PAV. Melanosis of the appendix: prevalence, distribution and review of the pathogenesis of 47 cases. *Histopathology* 1997;**30**:319.

53. Graf NS, Arbuckle S. Melanosis of the appendix: common in the paediatric age group. *Histopathology* 2001;**39**:243.

Large Intestine

Normal large intestine: anatomy, specimen dissection and histology relevant to pathological practice

Gordon Hutchins, Nicholas P. West and Phil Quirke

Leeds Institute of Molecular Medicine, University of Leeds, Leeds, UK

Anatomy

Anatomical relationships and gross appearance

The large intestine is the penultimate portion of the gastrointestinal tract lying between the small bowel and the anal canal. It measures approximately 1500 mm in length from the caecal pole to the anorectal junction, although a degree of variation may be observed. The large bowel can be differentiated from small bowel by its wider diameter, three thickened longitudinal muscle bands (taeniae coli), sacculations of the wall (haustra) and presence of omental appendages (appendices epiploicae). Its transverse diameter diminishes continually towards the distal end, except for the rectal dilatation known as the ampulla.

The large bowel and its mesentery are invested by a layer of peritoneum to a variable degree and can be divided into specific anatomical regions. The pouch-like caecum is usually completely invested by peritoneum and measures approximately 50–70 mm in length. It is located below the ileo-caecal valve, where the terminal ileum opens into the large bowel. The vermiform appendix opens into the posteromedial aspect of the caecum. The ascending colon measures 120–200 mm in length and extends from the caecum to the hepatic flexure. It has a broad attachment at its posterior aspect that is of variable size and shape, forming the retro-peritoneal surgical margin in a right hemicolectomy specimen. Running between the hepatic and splenic flexures lies the transverse colon, which is approximately 450 mm in length. The transverse colon has a true mesentery, although this is often not resected in its entirety. Beyond the splenic flexure, the descending colon drops down towards the pelvis for 220–300 mm, becoming the sigmoid colon as it crosses the pelvic brim. The descending colon is predominantly retroperitoneal with a broad posterior attachment. The sigmoid colon is an 'S'-shaped piece of bowel with a true mesentery located within the pelvis, measuring approximately 400 mm in length. Adequate removal of the mesentery of the colon (the mesocolon) and its lymphatics and vascular supply is of crucial importance in colonic cancer surgery.

The rectum is the fixed terminal portion of the large intestine that lies largely within the posterior pelvis. It begins at the level of the third sacral vertebra and feeds into the anal canal, measuring approximately 120–150 mm in length. The wall of the rectum has a uniform distribution of longitudinal muscle, unlike the colon, and is surrounded by a layer of fat, the mesorectum, which contains the blood supply and lymphatics. The mesorectum varies markedly in size between individuals but is generally much larger posteriorly with less fat anteriorly. It increases in volume towards the peritoneal reflection, after which it rapidly reduces to a point of maximal 'waisting' 35–42 mm above the anal verge at the level of the puborectalis muscle (Figure 32.1) [1]. The anterior two-thirds of the rectum are covered by peritoneum as far down as the peritoneal reflection, where the remainder continues as an infra-peritoneal organ. The non-peritonealised aspect of the mesorectum is invested by a layer of fascia, the mesorectal fascia, which may be apparent on the surface of good quality resection specimens; above the peritoneal reflection it abuts the lateral aspects of the incised peritoneum. At the anterior

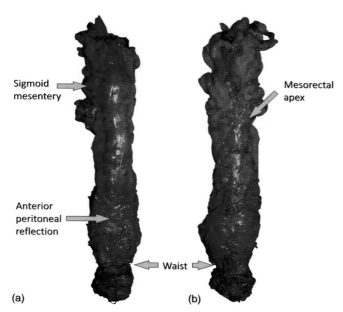

Figure 32.1 (a) Anterior and (b) posterior views of a fresh abdomino-perineal excision of the rectum and anus. The surgically created mesorectal margin is seen below the peritoneal reflection anteriorly and the mesorectal apex posteriorly. The surgical 'waist' is also clearly visible.

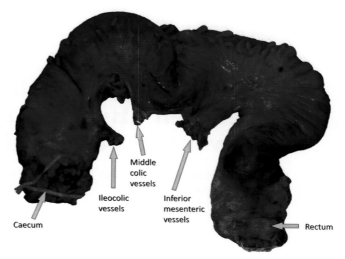

Figure 32.2 Fresh subtotal colectomy specimen for multiple colonic tumours: the mesentery has been removed intact and all three major vascular ties are seen.

aspect, between the rectum and the prostate, lies the fascia of Denonvilliers that should be apparent in an optimal cancer resection specimen [2]. An appreciation of the anatomy of the anal sphincter and levator ani muscles is important when assessing resection specimens for low rectal cancer, because they may be removed en bloc with the mesorectum and anal canal. The internal anal sphincter is composed of thickened smooth muscle and is formed by a continuation of the inner circular layer of the rectal muscularis propria and to a more variable extent the longitudinal muscle. The external anal sphincter is composed of striated muscle fibres, some of which fuse with the levator ani muscles that form the pelvic floor lying above the sphincters. The puborectalis muscle is anatomically part of the pelvic floor and forms a sling around the lower rectum to aid the sphincter muscles in maintaining continence.

Transverse sectioning of the large bowel reveals five distinct layers: the mucosa, submucosa, muscularis propria, subserosa and serosa. The mucosa lines the inner surface of the bowel and has a smooth appearance on gross examination with the innominate grooves being visible on closer inspection. The submucosa appears as a thin layer of loose connective tissue. The muscularis propria is made up of two layers of smooth muscle: the continuous inner circular and the band-like outer longitudinal (taeniae coli). Both become gradually thicker towards the rectosigmoid junction where the taeniae coli fuse. The taeniae coli act to shorten the colon, puckering the circular muscle into sac-

culations and haustral clefts. This throws the mucosa into transverse folds, the plicae semilunares, gathered along three longitudinal parallel lines, representing the midpoints of the taeniae that are typically the sites of ulceration in ulcerative colitis. The circular and longitudinal muscles form complete layers in the rectum, although anterior and posterior thickenings of the longitudinal layer cause some shortening. This gives rise to the three lateral flexures with their corresponding crescentic shelves, composed of circular muscle and mucous membrane and known as the valves of Houston. The subserosa is located outside the main muscle coats and appears as a band of fat in which blood vessels and lymph nodes may be seen. The serosa refers to the shiny layer of peritoneum covering the surface of the bowel and its mesentery. Non-peritonealised surfaces may be covered with a layer of fascia if resected in an embryological tissue plane.

Blood supply

There is considerable variation in large intestinal vasculature that must be appreciated by the pathologist in order to understand the type of resection performed and the location of the vascular ties. The large bowel is mainly supplied by branches of the superior and inferior mesenteric arteries (Figure 32.2) [3]. The supplying blood vessels pierce the muscularis propria and enter the submucosal layer to form a network of capillaries, which ramify in the mucosa. In diverticular disease the mucosa herniates through these points of weakness formed where the blood vessels penetrate the muscular wall.

The colon from the caecum to the splenic flexure is supplied by branches of the superior mesenteric artery, which arises at the anterior aspect of the aorta beneath the coeliac trunk. The caecum and ascending colon are supplied by the ileo-colic and right colic branches, and the transverse colon is predominantly supplied by the middle colic branch. Extensive collaterals provide a continuous network among the ileo-colic, right colic, middle colic and left colic arteries, giving rise to the continuous marginal artery of Drummond along the mesenteric border of the colon.

The left side of the colon and the upper rectum are supplied by branches of the inferior mesenteric artery, which also arises anteriorly from the aorta, approximately 30–40 mm above the bifurcation. The left colic artery originates from the inferior mesenteric artery and supplies the left colon through its ascending branch, which heads upwards towards the transverse colon, and the descending branch, which heads downwards to supply the descending and sigmoid colon. Several sigmoid branches arise from the inferior mesenteric artery, which continues as the superior rectal artery, splitting into two branches descending on either side of the mesorectum. The middle rectal arteries, which are not always present, arise from the internal iliac arteries to supply the middle and lower rectum along with the inferior rectal arteries that arise from the internal pudendal arteries.

The arteries are accompanied, as components of neurovascular bundles, by veins, lymphatics and nerves. The veins are tributaries of the portal system forming a well-developed submucosal plexus and another less well-developed plexus outside the muscularis propria. The territory supplied by the superior mesenteric artery is drained by the superior mesenteric vein, which runs just to the right of the artery. Similarly the territory supplied by the inferior mesenteric artery is drained by the inferior mesenteric vein and its tributaries. The venous tributaries correspond to and run with the arterial branches. The rectum is drained by the superior and middle rectal veins that communicate to form a site of portosystemic anastomosis.

Lymphatic drainage

The regional lymph nodes can be classified into those that lie close to the bowel wall (paracolic and pararectal nodes), those that follow the course of the blood supply (intermediate nodes) and those at the origin of the main supplying vessels (central nodes) [4]. The paracolic/pararectal nodes are situated along the marginal arteries and include the mesorectal lymph nodes. The lymphatic vessels pass through nodes along the relevant colic artery to the central vessels at the colic artery root. Proximal to this the lymphatics drain along either the superior mesenteric artery (superior mesenteric nodes) or the inferior mesenteric artery (inferior mesenteric nodes) to the aorta/inferior vena cava (para-aortic nodes). The para-aortic lymphatics

drain into the cisterna chyli, which continue as the thoracic duct and ascend into the thorax. The lymphatics of the rectum may also drain along the middle rectal artery to the internal iliac, common iliac, obturator and external iliac nodes, or inferiorly to the inguinal region (inguinal nodes).

Cancers of the colon spread through the lymphatics in an upward fashion along the supplying arterial chain [5], hence the optimal oncological specimen should include the pericolic, intermediate and central nodes in an intact peritoneum-lined package. Surgeons utilising this type of operation report higher lymph node yields and better outcomes when compared with less radical surgery [6,7]. Although central spread along the main lymphatic trunks is most important, occasionally lateral spread along pericolic lymphatics can be quite considerable [8].

Nerve supply

The nerve supply may be divided into extrinsic and intrinsic components [9], with the intrinsic enteric nervous system providing most of the control. The two arms of the autonomic nervous system, sympathetic and parasympathetic, provide the extrinsic supply. Parasympathetics arrive via the vagus nerve for the proximal colon and via the sacral spinal nerves for the distal colon and rectum, terminating in the myenteric plexus between the muscle layers of the muscularis propria. Sympathetic fibres from the thoracic and lumbar spinal nerves end in the superior and inferior mesenteric ganglia, from which postganglionic fibres terminate in the myenteric (Auerbach's) or submucosal (Meissner's) plexus. Most of the direct innervation of the smooth muscle of the bowel wall is through the intrinsic neurons of the two plexuses. These neurons are in turn driven, inhibited or modulated by intrinsic interneurons or extrinsic parasympathetic fibres.

Specimen handling

Consistent handling of large intestinal specimens for both neoplastic and non-neoplastic disease is crucial in order to make a correct diagnosis and identify all the relevant prognostic information. The dissection should be appropriate to the likely diagnosis as indicated on the surgical request form.

Types of specimen

There are a wide variety of specimens, ranging from tiny biopsies through to removal of the entire large intestine. Endoscopic biopsies are usually embedded whole and hence are not considered in any more detail. Most major colorectal resections can be performed either open or laparoscopically, including robotic surgery that has recently been introduced. The resulting specimen and long-term outcomes for the patient should not differ whichever technique is used [10].

Major colonic resections

Right hemicolectomy/ileo-colic resection
The caecum and ascending colon may be removed with a portion of terminal ileum for either right colonic tumours or terminal ileal Crohn's disease.

Transverse colectomy
Transverse colonic tumours may be removed either by a wedge resection or by extending a right or left hemicolectomy to include the transverse colon.

Left hemicolectomy/sigmoid colectomy
The descending and/or sigmoid colon may be removed for cancer or diverticular disease.

Subtotal colectomy/total colectomy/panproctocolectomy
In cases of multiple tumours, hereditary polyposis or inflammatory bowel disease, surgeons may remove most of or the entire large bowel with or without the anal canal.

Major rectal resections

Anterior resection
Anterior resection may be used to remove rectosigmoid or rectal tumours. The infra-peritoneal part of the rectum should be resected in the mesorectal fascial plane as described by Heald (total mesorectal excision) [11]. This can be extended to remove part of the internal sphincter in very low tumours (intersphincteric dissection). The sigmoid colon can be anastomosed to the distal rectum or anal canal to restore intestinal continuity. Occasionally for anterior tumours where the margin is threatened, a cuff of vaginal wall or prostate may be taken with the specimen.

Hartmann's operation
This is similar to anterior resection but is more commonly used for emergency operations or in elderly patients. The rectal stump is oversewn and the distal colon brought out as a colostomy.

Abdomino-perineal excision
Abdomino-perineal excision of the rectum and anus is used for low rectal tumours close to the dentate line or those that involve the sphincters. The sphincters, with or without the levator ani muscles, are removed en bloc with the mesorectum and anal canal: hence the patient requires a permanent colostomy. Occasionally, for large advanced tumours involving multiple organs, a total pelvic exenteration may be needed, where all the pelvic organs, and sometimes the sacrum and coccyx too, are removed in continuity with the bowel.

Local colorectal excisions

Polypectomy
Colorectal polyps can be excised during colonoscopy by the use of a diathermy snare passed around the stalk (if pedunculated) or sessile base. Preferably the specimen is removed whole; however, larger polyps or sessile lesions may be removed piecemeal. Intact small polyps may be embedded whole or bisected through the stalk. Larger lesions should be serially sliced at 2- to 3-mm intervals and ideally embedded in their entirety. The polyp base should be inked if identifiable to confirm the completeness of excision.

Endoscopic mucosal/submucosal resection
These excisions may be used for more sessile or flat adenomas, or for early cancers. The lesion is elevated by submucosal fluid injection and dissected off the submucosa with a small rim of normal mucosa. In the rectum, larger lesions may be removed by transanal endoscopic mucosal resection. This approach can also remove deeper muscle and even mesorectal fat. The specimen should be pinned out to prevent shrinkage and rolling of the edges during fixation. After inking the deep and lateral margins, the specimen should be serially sliced and embedded in separate cassettes. Cruciate sectioning may be useful to determine accurate distances to the lateral resection margin.

Specimen handling and dissection

Ideally, resection specimens should be received in the fresh state directly from the operating theatre, along with a request form confirming the patient identity and full clinical and specimen details. If the pathologist is not immediately available, the specimen can be refrigerated at 4°C for up to 24 hours without any danger of significant autolytic destruction. If a longer delay is anticipated or in the case of small biopsies, the specimen should be placed directly into an adequate amount of formalin fixative, at least 10 times greater than the tissue volume.

Examination of the fresh specimen can be very useful before fixation, particularly in the case of large or complex excisions. For non-neoplastic disease, the bowel can be opened before fixation through the anterior peritoneal surface along the anterior taeniae coli. For cancer specimens, it is important that the tumour segment is left intact for 20–50 mm either side in order to preserve the peritoneum and surgical margins. For rectal cancers, the area distal to the tumour should usually be left unopened so that assessment of the circumferential resection margin is not compromised. If the tumour is of a sufficient size it can be everted through the proximal incision to take fresh material for tissue banking if desired. The specimen should then be loosely pinned on to a corkboard to inhibit shrinkage and floated in an adequate volume of formalin fixative for at least 48 hours. If the luminal aspect of the tumour can be traversed, a piece of foam or tissue soaked in formalin can be inserted to aid fixation. Specimens may be unpinned and free floated after 24 hours to avoid suboptimal fixation.

After fixation, the specimen should be accurately described before the dissection takes place. The location and extent of any gross abnormalities should be carefully documented. In the case of inflammatory bowel disease, the specimen should be inspected for the presence of any potentially neoplastic lesions, which should be sampled in addition to areas of inflammation. A full list of all core and non-core items along with the evidence for their inclusion in cancer specimen reports is provided in the dataset for colorectal cancer of the Royal College of Pathologists (RCPath) [12]. Important areas of confusion relate to the presence of perforations and a description of the plane of dissection.

Perforations

It is important that the specimen is carefully inspected for perforations, which should be correctly described. Perforations carry a very poor prognosis for the patient, particularly if in the region of a tumour [13]. They are defined as any defect in the bowel wall that communicates with the exterior surface of the specimen. For cancer excisions there are two types of perforation that each carry different potential consequences: first, perforations can occur through the peritoneum, which can allow intra-peritoneal spread if it involves the tumour (staged as pT4). Even if outside the tumour segment, these perforations can be fatal due to faecal peritonitis. Second, non-peritoneal tumour perforations can occur below the peritoneal reflection of the rectum, into the mesorectum or retroperitoneum, which can potentially give rise to local disease recurrence. Although under TNM rules this does not denote a pT4 stage, it carries an equivalent prognosis and therefore must be reported.

Plane of dissection

Surgical removal of the large intestine creates a resection margin at the mesocolic attachments of the colon, the non-peritonealised areas in the ascending and descending colon, and very importantly the mesorectal surface of the rectum. The latter is entirely circumferential below the peritoneal reflection. Pathologists have recognised the significance of the mesorectal circumferential resection margin in rectal cancer surgery over many years [14], although the retroperitoneal margin in the right colon appears less important [15].

For all major cancer resections, pathologists should record and feed back to the surgical team their assessment of the plane of dissection. The assessment in anterior resection specimens has been mandatory in the UK since the introduction of the second RCPath minimum dataset in 2007 [12]. Poorer planes in rectal cancer are strongly related to local disease recurrence [16], and there is a developing body of evidence to suggest that a similar assessment in abdomino-perineal excisions [17] and colonic resections [18] may be useful.

Anterior resection specimens

The quality of the mesorectal resection plane should be graded into one of three levels: mesorectal, intra-mesorectal or muscularis propria (Figure 32.3). A *mesorectal* excision

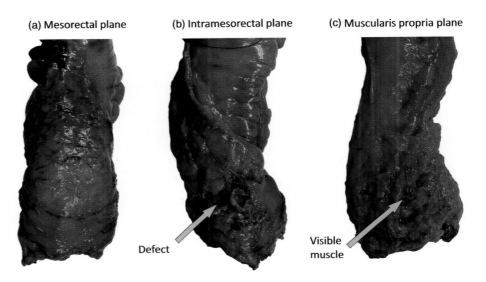

(a) Mesorectal plane   **(b) Intramesorectal plane**   **(c) Muscularis propria plane**

Defect

Visible muscle

Figure 32.3 Grading the plane of surgery for the mesorectum: note the intact mesorectal envelope lined by shiny mesorectal fascia in the mesorectal plane (a); significant defects should be graded as intra-mesorectal (b) or muscularis propria (c) if they extend down to the muscle layer.

follows the mesorectal fascial plane with an intact bulky mesorectum showing only minor surface irregularity. An *intra-mesorectal* excision shows some significant surface defects, although none should be so deep as to reach the muscularis propria. A *muscularis propria* excision is a very deficient mesorectum with extensive defects extending deep into the muscle layer.

Abdomino-perineal excision specimens

In addition to grading the mesorectum, the plane of dissection around the anal sphincters should be graded (Figure 32.4). A *levator* excision requires the levator ani muscles to be left attached to the mesorectum and anal canal, with or without the coccyx, in order to create a more cylindrical specimen as described by Miles [19]. This type of resection removes more tissue around the tumour, reduces incomplete tumour removal and perforations [20], and appears to improve clinical outcomes for the patient [21–23]. A

sphincteric excision follows the mesorectal plane down on to the sphincters with no levator attached, giving the classic waist/apple core appearance. An *intersphincteric/submucosal* excision occurs if the surgeon enters the sphincter muscles or submucosa, or perforates the specimen at any point.

Colonic specimens

Grading the plane of colonic dissection follows a similar system to that used in rectal cancer surgery (Figure 32.5). A *mesocolic* excision has an intact mesentery covered by peritoneum and fascia where appropriate, with only minor irregularity. An *intra-mesocolic* excision has defects in the mesentery, and a *muscularis propria* excision has extensive defects reaching the colonic muscularis propria. In addition, it is useful to measure the distance between the main vascular ties and the tumour or the nearest bowel wall, which indicates how radical the resection has been. Although the value of a 'high-tie' resection has been

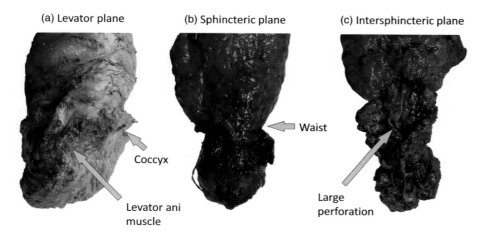

(a) Levator plane (b) Sphincteric plane (c) Intersphincteric plane

Coccyx

Levator ani muscle

Waist

Large perforation

Figure 32.4 Grading the plane of surgery around the anal sphincters in abdomino-perineal excisions of the rectum and anus. (a) Note the adherent levator muscle in the levator excision that prevents the waisting seen (b) when following the sphincteric plane. (c) Any defects into the sphincter muscles, submucosa or lumen should be classed as an intersphincteric excision.

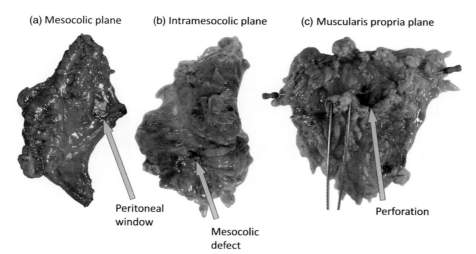

(a) Mesocolic plane (b) Intramesocolic plane (c) Muscularis propria plane

Peritoneal window

Mesocolic defect

Perforation

Figure 32.5 Grading the plane of colonic cancer surgery: (a) note the intact peritoneal lining of the mesocolon, even in the physiological 'windows' that are devoid of fat, in a mesocolic excision. (b) A defect not involving the muscle layer is seen in an intra-mesocolic excision. (c) Any extensive defects down to the muscle, or intraoperative perforations, indicate a muscularis propria excision.

Proximal

Anterior

Posterior

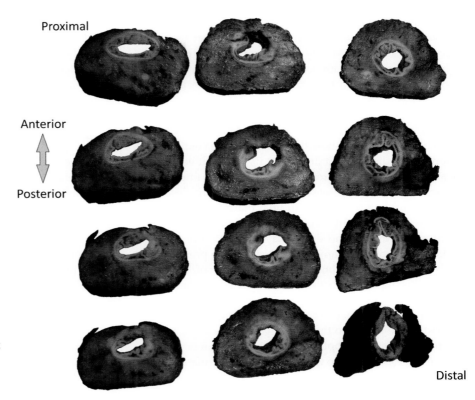

Distal

Figure 32.6 Cross-sectional slices from an anterior resection specimen for rectal cancer. Ink has been applied to the mesorectal surface before slicing at 3- to 4-mm intervals. Note the reduction in fat at the anterior aspect and in the distal slices as the mesorectum reduces in volume.

debated for decades, surgeons using a combination of mesocolic plane surgery with central vascular ligation remove more tissue and lymph nodes [24] and report better outcomes [7].

Inking and slicing

For cancer specimens, any surgically created margin should be marked with ink so that an accurate distance can be given from the tumour to the closest surface. For rectal cancers, the infra-peritoneal circumferential resection margin can be substantial, particularly posteriorly where it extends to the apex of the mesorectal triangle. The peritoneal surface must be differentiated from the fascia-lined, non-peritonealised margin, because tumour involvement of these two structures has markedly different implications for the patient. Peritoneal involvement (staged as pT4) risks intra-peritoneal spread, whereas an involved surgical margin risks tumour being left behind in the operative bed and the potential for local disease recurrence. We prefer to use India ink subsequently fixed with acetic acid, although a variety of other products are available. The ink can be applied to the fresh specimen, although we recommend application after fixation, particularly if the specimen is complex. The ink must be dried on the surface of the specimen before cross-sectional slicing to stop leakage on to other areas of the specimen. After inking, the specimen

should be transversely cross-sectioned at the level of the tumour and the slices laid out, so that block selection can be directed at areas of specific interest (Figure 32.6). The slices should be as thin as possible with 3- to 4-mm slices being easily obtainable after adequate fixation provided that a sharp knife is used.

Block selection

For cancer specimens, the ideal pathological processing would include embedding the whole tumour segment in large mount blocks. However, we recognise that in most laboratories a more pragmatic approach is required. A minimum of five standard-sized tumour blocks should be taken to include areas of prognostic importance, e.g. the closest inked surgical margin [25] and areas suspicious of peritoneal involvement [26] or extramural vascular invasion. It is important to remember that failure to find poor prognostic indicators may deny patients access to the adjuvant therapy that they require to increase their chances of cure. It is not necessary to sample the longitudinal margins of the specimen if they are >30 mm from the tumour, although often the closest margin will provide an adequate block of background mucosa. All lymph nodes should be carefully searched for and embedded, remembering that they are most frequently encountered around the arterial vascular supply. The highest node should be blocked separately. More than one highest node may be present in colonic specimens if the tumour lies between separate vascular arcades. There is no minimum number of nodes to be examined, and pathologists are strongly encouraged to regularly audit their lymph node yields and ensure that they always exceed a mean of at least 12 [12].

Resections for non-neoplastic disease should be sampled according to the most likely diagnosis. It is necessary to select blocks that will allow the pathologist to confirm the nature of the disease and document its extent. It is recommended that every 100 mm of intestine be sampled in inflammatory bowel disease, in addition to any discrete lesions. Sampling of the longitudinal margins is useful in such cases to document involvement by inflammation and confirm that there is no dysplasia. A selection of lymph nodes should also be sampled to look for the presence of granulomas or other abnormalities. In cases of vascular disease it is important that the mesenteric vessels are identified and sampled.

It is very important that an accurate block list is kept within the text of the report so that a case can be reviewed in the future. This may be supplemented by a diagram or indication on photographs as to where the blocks originated from if the specimen is complex.

Photography

Photography forms an important part of the pathological audit of both the underlying disease and the surgery used to treat it. It provides a permanent record of the specimen that can be used at multidisciplinary team meetings, and provides a very useful adjunct to lengthy complex macroscopic descriptions. The whole specimen should be photographed, preferably in the fresh state but otherwise after fixation, from both the anterior and the posterior aspects. Inclusion of a metric scale can be useful. Areas of particular interest, e.g. the site of a tumour, perforations or mesorectal/sphincter defects, should be highlighted and photographs of the cross-sectional tumour slices also taken. 'Photocopying' the specimen can be used if a digital camera is not available.

Histology

The colon serves two major purposes: the storage and delivery of faecal matter and the absorption of salt and water [27]. Additional metabolic [28] and immunological functionality [29] are also attributable to this region of the gastrointestinal tract.

Although formerly regarded as a single functional organ, insights into gene expression [30], physiology [31], disease manifestation [32] and relative cellular morphometry [33] augment the concept of the colon being composed of two separate regional functional units: the right and left colon.

This notion is perhaps unsurprising given the embryological derivation of the aforementioned regions, the right colon (the caecum, ascending colon and proximal transverse colon) being derived from the midgut whereas the left colon (distal transverse colon, the descending and sigmoid colon and rectum) is of hindgut derivation [34].

General organisation of the colonic wall

Under the scrutiny of light microscopy, colonic wall architecture recapitulates the general organisation of the entire gastrointestinal tract as observed from proximal oesophagus to anus: *mucosa* overlying *submucosa* that in turn is bounded by distinct inner circular and outer longitudinal smooth muscle layers (collectively known as the muscularis propria), the antagonistic actions of which serve to propel ingested material through proximal and distal regions. Deep to this, a connective tissue sheath envelopes the muscularis (Figure 32.7). Where the colon is bounded by visceral peritoneum, a loose connective tissue zone termed the 'subserosa', is covered by a thin layer of mesothelium, the serosa. In partially or fully non-peritonealised colonic segments, such as the ascending colon and rectum, tissue identical to the subserosa is bounded by deeper fascial planes such as the anterior renal fascia of Gerota and the mesorectal fascia, respectively. Knowledge of such fascial planes is of critical importance, to both surgeons and pathologists, to ensure effective operative/postoperative patient management.

The mucosa
Contrasting the small intestine, colonic mucosa represents a relatively smooth surface due to the absence of villi or

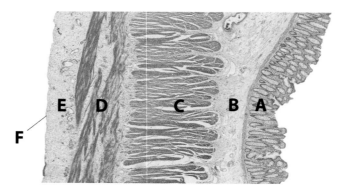

Figure 32.7 Low power haematoxylin and eosin (H&E) view of colonic wall. (A) Colonic mucosa is separated from (B) submucosa by muscularis mucosae. The muscularis propria consists of (C) an inner layer of circular muscle and (D) an outer layer of longitudinal muscle. (E) Underlying connective tissues are covered in (F) serosa in peritonealised colonic segments. In the non-peritonealised colonic segments, the connective tissue layer merges with pericolic tissue planes.

plicae circulares. The colorectal glands (crypts) are tubular and composed of a simple columnar epithelium that hosts a variety of cell types such as goblet cells, absorptive colonocytes and endocrine cells; their relative cellular composition depends on the location within the large bowel [33]. The crypts are surrounded by a pericryptal myofibroblast sheath, beyond which is a loose connective tissue matrix (the lamina propria) that contains myofibroblasts, a mixed immune cell population, capillaries and lymphatic arcades immediately above the muscularis mucosae [35], the last being the lower limit of the mucosal layer. Immune cells are also aggregated into highly organised lymphoid follicles with germinal centres that lie astride the muscularis mucosae and form dome-shaped lymphoglandular complexes with the crypt and surface epithelium.

Epithelium

Spatial orientation of epithelial cells results in the formation of both surface epithelium and epithelium contained within colonic crypts. The histological appearance of these crypts is characteristic and specific for the colon as manifested by the classic 'rack of test-tubes' appearance.

The epithelial layer is maintained by an extensively studied, yet still poorly defined, stem cell population postulated to be contained within the base of the colonic crypt in the so-called stem cell niche [36]. Through asymmetrical cell division both the stem cell and epithelial cell populations are simultaneously maintained, the latter through terminal differentiation of progenitor cells into multiple cell phenotypes that collectively form the colonic epithelium, with the overwhelming majority of cells being absorptive colonocytes or goblet cells (Figure 32.8).

Goblet cells

Goblet cells, a name derived from the 'goblet' shape imparted as a result of apical mucin accumulation, form a conspicuous population within the colonic epithelium in standard haematoxylin and eosin (H&E) sections. The accumulated mucin is observed as a large, clear, luminal cytoplasmic region overlying an irregular, hyperchromatic, basally located nucleus. Glycoprotein-specific tinctorial stains such as mucicarmine, Alcian blue and periodic acid–Schiff emphasise mucin and thus enhance visualisation of goblet cells [37]. They, along with antibodies directed against specific mucin gene products, allow further characterisation of complex mucin subtypes that vary between different zones of the crypt, between different parts of the large intestine, and between individuals and populations.

Absorptive colonocytes

Absorptive colonocytes are the principal cellular constituent of the colonic epithelium and are mainly responsible for colonic ion and water transportation [38]. The cytoplasm of the colonocyte is relatively eosinophilic due to a paucity of mucin, with only small apical mucin granules identifiable on tinctorial stains. Colonocyte nuclei are positioned basally and oriented perpendicular to the crypt lumen, with cytoplasm expanding towards the apical surface of the cell, where it almost completely covers the apical aspect of adjacent goblet cells. The apical surfaces of colonocytes display striate borders that are faintly visible on light microscopy, a feature that corresponds to both microvilli and glycocalyx [38]. The colonocytes (and goblet cells) show expression of several antigens that are used in diagnostic applications. These include cytoplasmic markers cytokeratin 20, mono-/polyclonal carcinoembryonic antigen, villin and nuclear CDX2. Colonocytes also have an important role in mucosal immunity, in that they elaborate secretory component that is essential for the epithelial translocation of IgA.

Endocrine cells

Endocrine cells of the colon are predominantly confined within colonic crypts, with only occasional cells localised

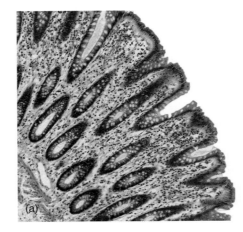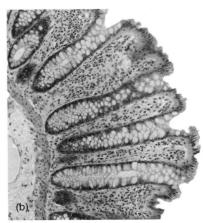

Figure 32.8 Low power haematoxylin and eosin (H&E) view of colonic mucosa taken from both (a) right and (b) left colon. Note the variation in goblet cell numbers.

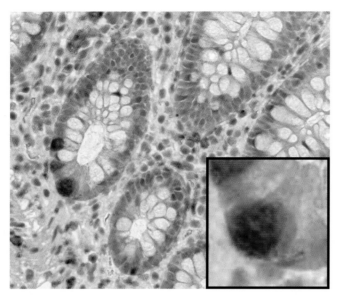

Figure 32.9 Endocrine cells in the colonic crypt stained with synaptophysin: note the 'inverse polarity' with the apical nuclei overlying the cytoplasm.

within the lamina propria. In contrast to both goblet cells and absorptive colonocytes, the wedge-shaped endocrine cell population displays 'inverse polarity', with rounded apical nuclei localised to a narrow cytoplasmic apical tip that overlies basal cytoplasm (Figure 32.9). It is within this cytoplasm that numerous peptide hormone products are contained within eosinophilic granules that historically were visualised using argentaffin and argyrophil reactions [39]. Nowadays, immunohistochemical markers such as synaptophysin and chromogranin are used. The peptide hormones secreted vary in different parts of the colon, with serotonin and neurotensin predominating on the right side and the enteroglucagon or glicentin group of peptides, which includes peptide YY, most abundant in the distal colon and rectum.

Paneth cells

Paneth cells are pyramidal shaped cells that unlike endocrine cells retain basal–luminal polarity in a similar manner to colonocytes and goblet cells. The cytoplasm, located apically above an oval nucleus, contains eosinophilic apical granules that are easily visualised on H&E. These granules hold numerous mediators of innate immunity, such as lysozyme and tumour necrosis factor α (TNF-α), indicating immunological functionality [40]. Paneth cells represent a physiological feature of midgut derivation and are thus normally found within the right colon [37]. Paneth cells within the left colon represent a pathological manifestation of metaplasia, typically as a result of inflammation [41]. Although not normally required diagnostically, Paneth

cells stain with tinctorial stains [42]; immunohistochemical markers include pancytokeratins.

Intra-epithelial inflammatory cells

Intra-epithelial lymphocytes (IELs) are a normal component of both the right and left colon. Typically located in either a paracellular location between colonocytes or epithelium overlying lymphoid follicles, IELs show both morphological and numerical variation depending on their epithelial location. IELs confined to paracellular spaces are T cells that possess indistinct cytoplasm and display nuclear moulding [37]. In such locations, the proportion of IELs to colonocytes approximates between 1 and 5%, with numbers decreasing from the right colon to the rectum [43]. Irrespective of location, the presence of IELs in excess of 20 per 100 colonocytes in an epithelial location distant to lymphoid aggregates is considered pathological [44].

In contrast, IELs associated with lymphoid follicles are B cells that possess rounded nuclei and a small rim of cytoplasm, and may be present in great numbers [37]. In such locations, IELs may be associated with specialised epithelial cells that overly lymphoid follicles, so-called membranous or M cells. Such cells possess an 'intraepithelial pocket' visible on ultrastructural examination that serves as a receptacle for IELs, allowing M cells to interact with intra-luminal antigen and the transfer of antigen to adjacent antigen-presenting cells [45].

Colonic stem cells and early progenitor cells

Colonocytes/goblet cells constitute most of the cells within the colonic crypt and represent a dual cell population that is replenished approximately every 4 days [46] by the progeny of a putative multipotent stem cell niche localised to the colonic crypt base [36]. These stem cells are thought to undergo specialised asymmetrical cell division that yields both a daughter progenitor cell and a replacement stem cell to replenish the niche. The resultant progenitor cells or transit amplifying cells (TACs) are readily identifiable by means of proliferative markers such as Ki67 and are located immediately above the colonic crypt base. They replicate rapidly but with limited replicative potential, and serve to replenish most of the overlying epithelial component. As a result, the stem cell population remains relatively quiescent, thus protecting genomic integrity together with the retention of original genetic material after asymmetrical division. Gastrointestinal stem cells are phenotypically hard to define [47], and many putative stem cell markers such as CD133 fail to identify them reliably [48]. More recently, *in situ* hybridisation assays for genes such as *lgr5* [49] has been postulated to identify colonic stem cells, yet experimental consistency using these and other methodologies remains elusive, as do reliable immunohistochemical markers of the stem cell population.

Basement membrane

The basement membrane is a thin, lightly eosinophilic, collagen plate that interlocks the colonic epithelial component to the underlying lamina propria and facilitates physiological interaction between these two compartments. The normal thickness of this plate is approximately 3 μm. Thickening beyond 10 μm is considered pathological [50].

Lamina propria

The lamina propria, the connective tissue bed surrounding colonic crypts, contains a multitude of cell types that are maintained within a loose connective tissue matrix. Fibroblasts and myofibroblasts constitute a significant multifunctional cell population within this region but immune cells predominate.

The normal immune cell gradient observed is of higher density at the luminal surface, decreasing towards the muscularis mucosae, reflecting increased antigenic load within the gut lumen. It comprises principally lymphocytes (mostly T cells) and plasma cells (most secreting IgA) [51]. Other cell types including macrophages, eosinophils and mast cells are less frequently observed. Extra-vascular neutrophils are not seen within the normal lamina propria except as occasional single cells [38].

Both capillaries and lymphatics are found within the lamina propria. In contrast to capillaries and associated venules, the branches of which extend throughout the mucosal compartment, lymphatics are restricted to a region immediately superficial to the muscularis mucosae [35] (Figure 32.10).

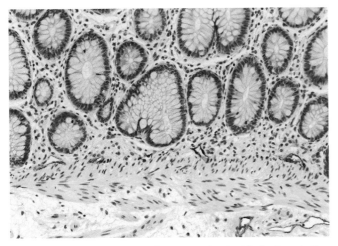

Figure 32.10 Colon mucosa immunostained with the lymphatic endothelial marker D2-40. Note the small lymphatic channels immediately above the muscularis mucosae. Lymphatic channels can also be seen in the submucosa in the bottom right corner of the picture.

Muscularis mucosae

The muscularis mucosae represents the lower border of the mucosa and consists of a thin layer of smooth muscle fibres of mixed orientation, which interact with neuronal fibres from the submucosal plexus. This muscle layer is traversed by various vascular and lymphatic structures in addition to neural branches [38]. The muscularis mucosae represents an important structure in diagnostic pathology, because its penetration by neoplastic colonic epithelium is defined currently as carcinoma. Increased awareness of the presence of lymphatic channels above the level of the muscularis mucosae has heightened interest in the introduction of the concept of intra-mucosal carcinoma, a highly controversial term that is currently not recommended.

The submucosa

Underlying the muscularis mucosae, the submucosa consists of a loose arrangement of connective tissue components including collagen, smooth muscle and mature adipose tissue. Embedded within it lie blood vessels, lymphatics and cells of the enteric nervous system. A physiologically important component of the submucosa, the enteric nervous system, serves to relay central, parasympathetic and sympathetic signalling to the colon in order to regulate function. The two neural plexuses of the submucosa, the submucosal plexus below the muscularis mucosae (Meissner's) and the deeper submucosal plexus above the muscularis propria (Henle's), consist of various interacting cell types such as interstitial cells of Cajal and ganglion cells [38]. Interstitial cells of Cajal represent modified myofibroblasts that are believed to regulate gut motor activity and are easily identified using immunohistochemical markers such as CD117 (c-kit) [52]. Ganglion cells tend to be more conspicuous with a large oval nucleus harbouring a prominent eosinophilic nucleolus. Distributional and morphological abnormalities of cells of the enteric nervous system may be assessed using both enzyme histochemistry and immunohistochemistry and thus aid the in diagnosis of Hirschsprung's disease and other colonic neuropathies [53].

The muscularis propria

Also known as the muscularis externa, this muscular layer is composed of an inner circular smooth muscle layer bounded by an outer longitudinal layer. A third plexus of the enteric nervous system (Auerbach's) lies between these two muscle layers and is seen alongside interstitial cells of Cajal, which can be identified throughout the muscularis [38]. In addition to this neuronal component, the muscularis also harbours many blood vessels and lymphatics.

The subserosa/serosa

As mentioned earlier, the subserosa is connective tissue that immediately underlies the muscularis. Confusion often exists in use of the terms 'subserosa' and 'serosa': the latter represents *only* the mesothelial connective tissue layer located on the outer aspect of peritonealised colonic segments.

Regional variations in histological appearances

As stated previously, the colorectum can be regarded as two separate functional units, each with particular physiological and pathological manifestations. This regional variation is reflected in terms of histological variation with several features seen to vary from proximal to distal colon.

The ratio of absorptive colonocytes to goblet cells is elevated in the right colon when compared with the left. This reflects the absorptive function of the right colon, compared with the conductive nature of the left colon where increased goblet cells facilitate enhanced secretion of lubricating mucin. An associated increase of muciphages is noted within the lamina propria of left colon.

The right colon also serves to process luminal antigen arriving within highly immunoreactive ileal contents. Accordingly, it harbours more immunoregulatory cells in the form of IELs and lymphoid follicles. Paneth cells are also found at much higher density in the right colon when compared with the left.

Other regional variations, such as differential secretory mucin composition [33], are of academic interest but are of limited diagnostic value to the practising pathologist.

References

1. Salerno G, Chandler I, Wotherspoon A, et al. Sites of surgical waisting in the abdominoperineal specimen. *Br J Surg* 2008; **95**:1147.
2. Heald RJ, Moran BJ, Brown G, Daniels IR. Optimal total mesorectal excision for rectal cancer is by dissection in front of Denonvilliers' fascia. *Br J Surg* 2004;**91**:12.
3. Griffiths JD. Extramural and intramural blood-supply of colon. *BMJ* 1961;**i**:323.
4. Japanese Society for Cancer of the Colon and Rectum. *Japanese Classification of Colorectal Carcinoma*, 2nd edn. Tokyo: Kanehara & Co., 2009.
5. Jamieson JK, Dobson JF VII. Lymphatics of the colon: with special reference to the operative treatment of cancer of the colon. *Ann Surg* 1909;**50**:107.
6. Enker WE, Laffer UT, Block GE. Enhanced survival of patients with colon and rectal cancer is based upon wide anatomic resection. *Ann Surg* 1979;**190**:350.
7. Hohenberger W, Weber K, Matzel1K, Papadopoulos T, Merkel S. Standardized surgery for colonic cancer: complete mesocolic excision and central ligation – technical notes and outcome. *Colorectal Dis* 2009;**11**:354.
8. Grinnell RS. Lymphatic block with atypical and retrograde lymphatic metastasis and spread in carcinoma of the colon and rectum. *Ann Surg* 1966;**163**:272.
9. Baumgarten HG. Morphological basis of gastrointestinal motility: structure and innervation of gastrointestinal tract. In: Bertaccini G (ed.), *Mediators and Drugs in Gastrointestinal Motility I.*

10. Guillou PJ, Quirke P, Thorpe H, et al. Short-term endpoints of conventional versus laparoscopic-assisted surgery in patients with colorectal cancer (MRC CLASICC trial): multicentre, randomised controlled trial. *Lancet* 2005;**365**:1718.
11. Heald RJ, Husband EM, Ryall RD. The mesorectum in rectal cancer surgery – the clue to pelvic recurrence? *Br J Surg* 1982; **69**:613.
12. Williams GT, Quirke P, Shepherd NA. *Standards and Datasets for Reporting Cancers. Dataset for Colorectal Cancer*, 2nd edn, London: Royal College of Pathologists, 2007.
13. Eriksen MT, Wibe A, Syse A, Haffner J, Wiig JN. Inadvertent perforation during rectal cancer resection in Norway. *Br J Surg* 2004;**91**:210.
14. Quirke P, Durdey P, Dixon MF, et al. Local recurrence of rectal adenocarcinoma due to inadequate surgical resection. Histopathological study of lateral tumour spread and surgical excision. *Lancet* 1986;**ii**:996.
15. Scott N, Jamali A, Verbeke C, Ambrose NS, Botterill ID, Jayne DG. Retroperitoneal margin involvement by adenocarcinoma of the caecum and ascending colon: what does it mean? *Colorectal Dis* 2008;**10**:289.
16. Quirke P, Copeland J, Smith AM, et al. Effect of the plane of surgery achieved on local recurrence in patients with operable rectal cancer: a prospective study using data from the MRC CR07 and NCIC-CTG CO16 randomised clinical trial. *Lancet* 2009;**373**:821.
17. Nagtegaal ID, van de Velde CJH, Marijnen CAM, et al. Low rectal cancer: a call for a change of approach in abdominoperineal resection. *J Clin Oncol* 2005;**23**:9257.
18. West NP, Morris EJA, Rotimi O, et al. Pathology grading of colon cancer surgical resection and its association with survival: a retrospective observational study. *Lancet Oncol* 2008;**9**:857.
19. Miles WE. A method of performing abdomino-perineal excision for carcinoma of the rectum and of the terminal portion of the pelvic colon. *Lancet* 1908;**ii**:1812.
20. West NP, Finan PJ, Anderin C, et al. Evidence of the oncologic superiority of cylindrical abdominoperineal excision for low rectal cancer. *J Clin Oncol* 2008;**26**:3517.
21. Dehni N, Tiret E, Singland J, et al. Oncologic results following abdominoperineal resection for adenocarcinoma of the low rectum. *Dis Colon Rectum* 2003;**46**:867.
22. Holm T, Ljung A, Haggmark T, et al. Extended abdominoperineal resection with gluteus maximus flap reconstruction of the pelvic floor for rectal cancer. *Br J Surg* 2007;**94**:232.
23. Bebenek M, Pudelko M, Cisarz K, et al. Therapeutic results in low-rectal cancer patients treated with abdominosacral resection are similar to those obtained by means of anterior resection in mid- and upper-rectal cancer cases. *Eur J Surg Oncol* 2007; **33**:320.
24. West NP, Hohenberger W, Weber K, Perrakis A, Finan PJ, Quirke P. Complete mesocolic excision with central vascular ligation produces an oncologically superior specimen compared with standard surgery for carcinoma of the colon. *J Clin Oncol* 2010; **28**:272.
25. Adam IJ, Mohamdee MO, Martin IG, et al. Role of circumferential margin involvement in the local recurrence of rectal cancer. *Lancet* 1994;**344**:707.
26. Shepherd NA, Baxter KJ, Love SB. The prognostic importance of peritoneal involvement in colonic cancer: a prospective evaluation. *Gastroenterology* 1997;**112**:1096.
27. Guyton AC, Hall JE. Transport and mixing of food in the alimentary tract. In: Guyton AC, Hall JE (eds), *Textbook of Medical Physiology*. Philadelphia, PA: WB Saunders, 1996: 803.

28. Cani PD, Delzenne NM. The role of the gut microbiota in energy metabolism and metabolic disease. *Curr Pharm Des* 2009;**15**:1546.

29. Elson CO, Cong Y. Understanding immune-microbial homeostasis in intestine. *Immunol Res* 2002;**26**:87.

30. Noble CL, Abbas AR, Cornelius J, et al. Regional variation in gene expression in the healthy colon is dysregulated in ulcerative colitis. *Gut* 2008;**57**:1398.

31. Macfarlane GT, Gibson GR, Cummings JH. Comparison of fermentation reactions in different regions of the human colon. *J Appl Bacteriol* 1992;**72**:57.

32. Benedix F, Kube R, Meyer F, et al. Comparison of 17,641 patients with right- and left-sided colon cancer: differences in epidemiology, perioperative course, histology, and survival. *Dis Colon Rectum* 2010;**53**:57.

33. Arai T, Kino I. Morphometrical and cell kinetic studies of normal human colorectal mucosa. Comparison between the proximal and the distal large intestine. *Acta Pathol Jpn* 1989;**39**:725.

34. Sadler TW. Digestive system. In: Sadler TW (ed.), *Langman's Medical Embryology*. Baltimore, MA: Williams & Wilkins, 1995: 242.

35. Fenoglio CM, Kaye GI, Lane N. Distribution of human colonic lymphatics in normal, hyperplastic, and adenomatous tissue. Its relationship to metastasis from small carcinomas in pedunculated adenomas, with two case reports. *Gastroenterology* 1973; **64**:51.

36. Kim KM, Shibata D. Methylation reveals a niche: stem cell succession in human colon crypts. *Oncogene* 2002;**21**:5441.

37. Dahl J, Greenson JK. Colon. In: Mills SE (ed.), *Histology for Pathologists*. Philadelphia, PA: Lippincott Williams & Wilkins, 2007: 627.

38. Levine DS, Haggitt RC. Normal histology of the colon. *Am J Surg Pathol* 1989;**13**:966.

39. Grimelius L. Silver stains demonstrating neuroendocrine cells. *Biotech Histochem* 2004;**79**:37.

40. Ayabe T, Ashida T, Kohgo Y, Kono T. The role of Paneth cells and their antimicrobial peptides in innate host defense. *Trends Microbiol* 2004;**12**:394.

41. Symonds DA. Paneth cell metaplasia in diseases of the colon and rectum. *Arch Pathol* 1974;**97**:343.

42. Porter EM, Bevins CL, Ghosh D, Ganz T. The multifaceted Paneth cell. *Cell Mol Life Sci* 2002;**59**:156.

43. Kirby JA, Bone M, Robertson H, et al. The number of intraepithelial T cells decreases from ascending colon to rectum. *J Clin Pathol* 2003;**56**:158.

44. Kingham JG, Levinson DA, Ball JA, Dawson AM. Microscopic colitis – a cause of chronic watery diarrhoea. *BMJ* 1982; **285**:1601.

45. Neutra MR, Mantis NJ, Kraehenbuhl JP. Collaboration of epithelial cells with organized mucosal lymphoid tissues. *Nat Immunol* 2001;**2**:1004.

46. Lipkin M. Proliferation and differentiation of normal and diseased gastrointestinal cells. In: Johnson LR (ed.), *Physiology of the Gastrointestinal Tract*. New York: Raven, 1987: 255.

47. Potten CS, Gandara R, Mahida YR, et al. The stem cells of small intestinal crypts: where are they? *Cell Prolif* 2009;**42**:731.

48. Shmelkov SV, Butler JM, Hooper AT, et al. CD133 expression is not restricted to stem cells, and both CD133+ and CD133– metastatic colon cancer cells initiate tumors. *J Clin Invest* 2008; **118**:2111.

49. Barker N, van Es JH, Kuipers J, et al. Identification of stem cells in small intestine and colon by marker gene *Lgr5*. *Nature* 2007; **449**:1003.

50. Gledhill A, Cole FM. Significance of basement membrane thickening in the human colon. *Gut* 1984;**25**:1085.

51. Medina F, Segundo C, Campos-Caro A, et al. Isolation, maturational level, and functional capacity of human colon lamina propria plasma cells. *Gut* 2003;**52**:383.

52. Sanders KM. A case for interstitial cells of Cajal as pacemakers and mediators of neurotransmission in the gastrointestinal tract. *Gastroenterology* 1996;**111**:492.

53. Di Nardo G, Blandizzi C, Volta U, et al. Review article: molecular, pathological and therapeutic features of human enteric neuropathies. *Aliment Pharmacol Ther* 2008;**28**:25.

CHAPTER 33

Embryogenesis and developmental abnormalities (including the anal region)

Adrian C. Bateman

Southampton General Hospital, Southampton, UK

Normal development

Overview

Formation of the gut tube occurs during week 4 of embryological development and, by the end of week 12, the stomach and small and large intestines are present and situated in their final positions. Further details of this process are given at the start of Chapter 18. Of particular note are the physiological herniation of the midgut during week 6 and the two episodes of rotation of the gut tube (90° and then 180°) that occur, resulting in the correct positioning of the small and large intestine within the abdominal cavity. The gut tube is initially blind ending at both ends due to the presence of the *buccopharyngeal* and *cloacal membranes*; within both of these, endoderm and ectoderm are in direct contact [1,2].

Proximal large intestine

The caecum, appendix, ascending colon and a variable length of the transverse colon are of *midgut* origin. Originally they share a mesentery with the small intestine, derive their blood supply from the superior mesenteric artery, and are included in the physiological herniation and return of the midgut between weeks 6 and 10. The further development of the appendix is described in Chapter 31. The mesentery attached to the caecum and the ascending colon is normally absorbed after they return to the abdomen, anchoring them to the posterior abdominal wall, although the transverse colon retains its mesentery.

Distal large intestine

The descending and sigmoid colons, the rectum and the upper two-thirds of the anal canal are derived from the *hindgut* and are supplied by the inferior mesenteric artery. Anastomoses between the superior and inferior mesenteric arteries are not well developed and the splenic flexure can be a relatively poorly vascularised zone – hence it is susceptible to ischaemic damage.

Anorectal region

During weeks 4–5 the hindgut, allantois and urogenital tract end in a common *cloaca* lined by endoderm. The ventral cloacal wall is formed by the cloacal membrane, which is bounded on its external (ectodermal) aspect by the genital swellings and folds. A vertical partition, the *urorectal septum*, develops in the angle between the allantois and the hindgut and grows transversely and caudally, separating a *urogenital sinus* ventrally from the developing rectum dorsally; it fuses caudally with the cloacal membrane, thus dividing it into dorsal and ventral parts (Figure 33.1). Two *anal tubercles* develop beneath the ectoderm posterior to the ventral cloaca and fuse with the urorectal septum to form the *proctodeum*; here the ectoderm and the endoderm are in direct contact. The proctodeum is later invaded by mesoderm that will form the external anal sphincter. The whole mass then moves backwards and grows inwards to fuse with the rectum as a solid plug, the future anus; it canalises during the third month.

Morson and Dawson's Gastrointestinal Pathology, Fifth Edition. Edited by Neil A. Shepherd, Bryan F. Warren, Geraint T. Williams, Joel K. Greenson, Gregory Y. Lauwers and Marco R. Novelli.

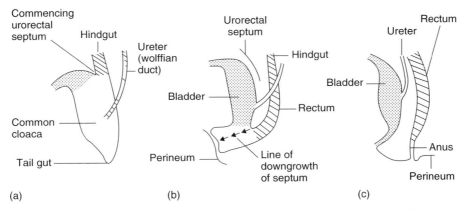

Figure 33.1 Figures (a) to (c) depict the progressive embryological development of the rectum and bladder from the cloaca.

Microscopic appearances

At the 20-mm stage, villous structures resembling those in the developing small bowel are found throughout the large bowel; as growth proceeds they thicken, shorten and gradually disappear with the development of the mucosal crypts. Brush border enzyme systems begin to develop at about 8 weeks in oral–anal direction [3]. Tubular glands grow outwards from the cloacogenic zone of the anal canal and penetrate through the submucosa into the internal anal sphincter.

Malpositions

Most malpositions of the large intestine are consequent on malrotation of the small bowel occurring at the time when the contents of the physiological hernia return to the alimentary cavity in weeks 10–11. The small bowel may come to lie superficial to the transverse colon, which then usually passes through an aperture in the mesentery; the caecum and ascending colon often retain their mesentery and are not anchored to the posterior abdominal wall. If the small bowel fails to rotate, the caecum may lie in the left iliac fossa or the midline, in which case both it and the ascending colon retain a mesentery and the ascending colon is connected to a normal descending colon by a shortened transverse length; the whole bowel from duodenum to splenic flexure is then supported by a single mesentery with a narrow base, prone to volvulus [1,4]. Among the more common minor anomalies is failure of absorption of the caecal and ascending colonic mesentery, with development of fibrous bands between the colon and the abdominal wall; these can cross and compress the duodenum or upper jejunum, leading to high intestinal obstruction, the cause of which may not be obvious at laparotomy. A useful general review is available [5].

Vestigial remnants

At the 4- to 6-mm stage, the embryo possesses a definite tail that has totally regressed by the 30- to 35-mm stage. During the formation of the cloacal septum, a small part of the distal hindgut becomes separated and lies isolated as the *tailgut*; it has normally disappeared by the 8-mm stage. Microscopically a number of types of epithelium can be recognised, including mucin-containing cells, but muscle coats are not present, although there may be clumps of smooth muscle cells [6]. A number of post-anal cysts without muscle coats and lined by a variety of epithelial, including squamous and columnar cells, sometimes ciliated, have been described [6] and carcinomatous epithelial changes have been reported in them [6]. They are probably of tailgut origin.

Maldevelopments

Atresias and stenoses

Atresia (absence of bowel lumen) and stenosis (narrowing of bowel lumen) are extremely rare in the caecum, colon and upper rectum; we know of one example in the colon [7] and of a congenital diaphragm in the upper rectum [8].

Atresia and stenosis of the lower rectum and anal canal occur about once in every 5000 births. A number of different classifications exist [9,10] and an international one has been suggested and is reproduced in Table 33.1; the important differentiation appears to be between 'high' and 'low' anomalies, i.e. those above and below the pelvic floor [9,10]. In the high anomalies there is often a considerable gap between the lower end of the rectum and the anal canal, which is normally formed, and fistulae between the rectum and some part of the urogenital apparatus are relatively common. In males these are usually recto-urethral or recto-urethral and recto-vesical, and the anus is usually

Table 33.1 Anorectal anomalies: a suggested international classification

Male	Female
Low (trans-levator)	
a. At normal site	All the same
i. Anal stenosis	
ii. Covered anus – complete	
b. At perineal site	All the same
i. Anocutaneous fistula (covered anus – incomplete)	
ii. Anterior perineal anus	
	c. At vulvar site
	i. Anovulvar fistula
	ii. Anovestibular fistula
	iii Vestibular anus
Intermediate	
a. Anal agenesis	Same apart from:
i. Without fistula	ii. With fistula (recto-vestibular, recto-vaginal, low)
ii. With fistula (rectobulbar)	
High (supralevator)	
a. Anorectal agenesis	Same apart from:
i. Without fistula	ii. With fistula (recto-vaginal
ii. With fistula (recto-urethral, recto-vesical)	– high, recto-cloacal, recto-vesical)
b. Rectal atresia	Same
Miscellaneous	
Imperforate anal membrane	All same
Cloacal exstrophy	
Others	

Reproduced from Santulli TV, Keisewetter WB, Bill AH, Jr. (1970). Anorectal anomalies: a suggested international classification. J Pediatr Surg 5: 281.

normal; in females they are recto-vaginal, recto-vestibular or recto-perineal and anal stenosis is not uncommon [11]. Occasional cases of persistent cloaca occur in association with multiple anomalies, which are usually inoperable [12,13].

Duplications, diverticula and cysts

Duplications

These are extremely uncommon in the large bowel. There is compete or partial formation of a second tube with its own mucosa and submucosa but often with incomplete separation of muscle coats; the duplicated segment is always on the mesenteric aspect of the normal bowel. Examples are described in the caecum, transverse colon, rectum and anus [14], and there are more complex examples associated with duplications in the urinary and genital

tracts [15]. Triplications have been described [16]. Squamous cell carcinoma [17] and adenocarcinoma [18] have been recorded as complications, and it is possible that some of the anorectal 'fistulae' in which adenocarcinomas have occurred may in fact represent duplications [19].

Diverticula

Congenital diverticula are very rare in the large bowel [20] and, when present in the rectum, can be associated with vertebral anomalies. They commonly have a more or less complete covering of all bowel coats.

Cysts

Developmental cysts localised within the bowel wall are extremely rare [21]; many of them almost certainly represent remnants of the tailgut [22] (see above).

Heterotopias and metaplasias

Heterotopic tissue is rare in the large bowel and is usually associated with malformations such as duplications, diverticula or cysts. Every example that we have seen has been in the rectum, which agrees with the findings of others [23–25], although occasional examples are reported in the colon [26,27]. Virtually all the epithelia described are gastric in type and the difficulty is to know whether this is heterotopic or metaplastic. Points in favour of a heterotopia are the presence of more than one type of epithelium, or full-thickness and perfectly structured fundic mucosa; the presence of appreciable pyloric-type mucosa suggests an acquired lesion [23]. Pancreatic elements are occasionally seen [28]. Gastric mucosa in the rectum presents endoscopically as a well demarcated area of granularity or as a polypoid lesion.

Disturbances of innervation

New insight into the innervation of the gut has broadened our understanding of Hirschsprung's disease and many related disorders.

In the complete absence of a nerve supply, bowel muscle will still contract, but not in a coordinated fashion; an intact nervous system is needed for coordinated peristalsis. This system has three components: a sympathetic and a parasympathetic inflow, and a widespread intrinsic peptidergic system that allows much more local control of bowel movement than earlier workers appreciated [29]. Within the bowel wall there are two plexuses of ganglion cells and neurons, a submucosal and a myenteric, which are more independent of each other than has sometimes been realised. The myenteric plexus contains ganglia in which there are two types of neuron: argyrophil cells that have well-stained nerve processes, many of which are multi-axonal and branch frequently, terminate on other argyrophil and on argyrophobe cells, but do not supply muscle fibres directly; and argyrophobe cells that are acetylcholinesterase (AChE) positive and have axons, some of which appear to end directly on muscle fibres. The myenteric nerve trunks are made up of axons from the argyrophil cells and extrinsic nerve fibres. These are of two kinds: sympathetic (which show catecholamine fluorescence and end around neurons) and parasympathetic (which end on intrinsic neurons and are probably all argyrophilic) [30]. All the intrinsic neurons and nerve fibres are probably peptidergic, non-adrenergic and non-cholinergic, and this system can function autonomously; substance P and enkephalin probably act as excitatory factors in the myenteric plexus whereas vasoactive intestinal polypeptide (VIP), which is mainly located in the submucosal plexus, is probably inhibitory. It appears that nerve cells and fibres that are cholinergic are actually responsible for muscle contraction, and cells and fibres that are adrenergic and sympathetic or peptidergic and intrinsic exert a controlling influence [31].

It is clear that, if the account given above is correct, any factors that damage these nerve cells or fibres or interfere with their development can disturb gut motility and lead to chronic constipation or diarrhoea. A number of syndromes are being recognised in which different components of the systems are damaged; they are discussed below.

Hirschsprung's disease

Over 100 years ago Hirschsprung first described a condition in children, in which a widely dilated and hypertrophied colon ended in a narrowed segment of rectum that extended to the anus [32]. It occurs once in every 20 000–30 000 live births [33] and is 6–9 times more common in boys than in girls. There is evidence for a familial incidence but most cases are sporadic [34]. At least three genes have been implicated, including the tyrosine kinase receptor Ret [35], endothelin receptor B and its ligand endothelin 3 [36]. Ten per cent of all cases occur in children with Down's syndrome and 5% are associated with other congenital abnormalities [37]. The most common time of presentation is during the neonatal period (first 4 weeks of life) with symptoms such as delayed passage of meconium, abdominal distension and vomiting [38,39], but patients may present in infancy with constipation, gaseous abdominal distension and repeated episodes of intestinal obstruction. There may be an accompanying colitis that can be severe, leading to perforation. Others present with persistent constipation in later childhood or even adulthood, although this is relatively unusual [40]. On clinical examination the anus is normal whereas the anal canal and a variable length

of affected rectum are small and empty. The most commonly encountered form of the condition is short segment disease, in which the aganglionic segment extends proximally from the anus but not beyond the sigmoid colon. However, the condition can extend more proximally than this and may affect the entire colon. At the junction of the diseased and unaffected bowel, the enormously dilated proximal part empties into the contracted lower segment in a funnel-shaped manner (Figure 33.2). In virtually all cases the narrowed segment extends proximally from the anus. Its length varies. In one large series of 1560 cases [41], 53.8% involved rectum and sigmoid, 25.6% had ultra-short segments and 20.6% were so-called 'long segment' in that they extended proximal to the sigmoid, and some involved the whole large and sometimes the small bowel.

Microscopically, in the classic disease and using conventionally stained sections, there are two principal abnormalities in the affected bowel. The first is a total absence of ganglion cells in both the submucosal and myenteric plexuses. The second is the presence of increased numbers of enlarged wavy nerve trunks, most conspicuous in the myenteric plexus but also present in the submucosa (Figure 33.3). Muscle coats are essentially normal and inflammatory changes, if present, are secondary. Some children show a form of arteritis that may present as intimal or adventitial fibroplasia or medial fibromuscular dysplasia [41]. At the junction of the narrowed affected bowel with the normal is a transitional zone of variable length, in which occasional ganglion cells are present and in which the nerve fibres have a more normal appearance, although some thickening and waviness persist [42]. The advent of immunohistochemical techniques for demonstrating peptidergic nerves and nerve cells [43] has shown that in Hirschsprung's disease substance P and VIP are both diminished. The number of enteroglucagon- and somatostatin-containing

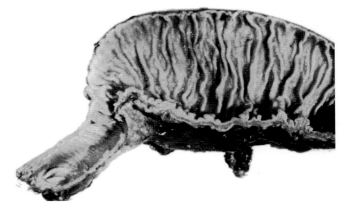

Figure 33.2 Resected rectum and sigmoid colon in Hirschsprung's disease, showing the narrowed aganglionic distal segment on the left and the dilated normally innervated proximal bowel on the right.

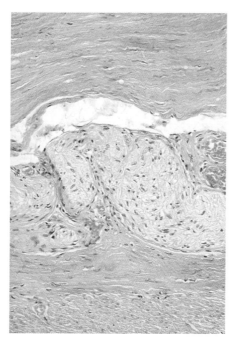

Figure 33.3 Myenteric plexus in Hirschsprung's disease: the enlarged wavy nerve trunks without ganglion cells are well shown.

cells in the mucosa is also reduced [43]; this may be a secondary effect.

The pathogenesis of Hirschsprung's disease is not fully understood. There is a failure of migration of neurons from the neural crest that would normally form the intrinsic nervous system [41,42]. Possible explanations could be a primary shortage of neuroblasts, failure of neuroblast survival during the process of migration or a defect in microenvironment sensing after successful migration. A number of nerve growth factors are critical for this process including glial cell line-derived neurotrophic factor (GDNF), which is the ligand for Ret, and endothelin 3 (EDN3). Disruption of these genes, or genes implicated in the associated cell signalling pathways, could result in apoptotic deletion of the neuroblasts [36]. Whatever the mechanism, the loss of neuroblasts results in secondary hyperplasia and ingrowth of preganglionic fibres, which can be visualised through the AChE histochemical technique (see below) [42].

Allied Hirschsprung's disorders

This term covers a number of conditions in which patients have had all or some of the clinical features of Hirschsprung's disease but in whom at least some ganglion cells have been found on biopsy and abnormal nerve trunks are not always present. The nature of some of them is becoming clearer and their classification is now possible [44].

Hypoganglionosis

A number of neonates with symptoms suggestive of Hirschsprung's disease have a reduction in the number of ganglion cells immediately above the dentate line; there are no abnormal AChE-positive fibres in the lamina propria in early biopsies, although these appear in some patients by the age of 9 months [44,45]. Appearances closely resemble those seen in the transitional zone of Hirschsprung's disease and hypoganglionosis may represent a form of Hirschsprung's disease. A deficiency of c-kit-positive pacemaker cells of Cajal has been described in hypoganglionosis, neuronal intestinal dysplasia (see below) and individuals with immature ganglia [46].

Zonal aganglionosis

Patients have been described in whom there are zones of aganglionosis, usually narrow, with normal ganglion cells above and below the zones [41,47–49]; in these zones abnormal nerve trunks can also be present [49,50]. This contrasts with classic Hirschsprung's disease in which the aganglionic zone extends in a confluent fashion proximally from the anus for a variable distance.

Ultra-short segment Hirschsprung's disease

Ultra-short segment Hirschsprung's disease (also known as achalasia of the internal sphincter) is a term that has been used to describe a very localised segment of aganglionosis in the region of the internal anal sphincter, which shows neuronal hyperplasia on AChE histochemistry, in contrast to biopsies from the physiological aganglionic zone of the low rectum that do not show this feature [51]. The histological features on rectal biopsy may be subtle and manometry may be the only way to diagnose this condition with confidence.

Other forms

Hirschsprung's disease-like syndromes have also been described in patients who, on investigation, have hyperplasia of ganglion cells in submucosal and muscle coats [49], along with the formation of giant ganglia and the presence of occasional ganglion cells in the lamina propria [52]. Occasional patients with apparently immature ganglion cells are also described [44]. This rare condition is described as neuronal intestinal dysplasia or hyperganglionosis [53].

Diagnostic techniques for Hirschsprung's disease and allied disorders

Ideally, the maximum information would be gained from a full-thickness biopsy, with tissue processed for both 'routine' (i.e. formalin-fixed and paraffin-embedded tissue) histology and sent fresh for AChE histochemistry. The latter reveals the presence of fine cholinergic nerve fibres

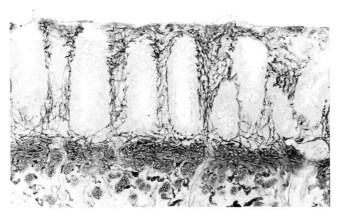

Figure 33.4 Acetylcholinesterase preparation from a fresh rectal biopsy in Hirschsprung's disease, showing prominent nerve fibres extending into the mucosa.

extending through the muscularis mucosae into the lamina propria [42,54–56]; these fibres are greatly increased in number, thicker and more tortuous in Hirschsprung's disease and in many workers' opinion are sufficiently characteristic to allow diagnosis even on mucosal punch biopsy (Figure 33.4). If these prominent nerve fibres are present, the diagnosis is reasonably certain, but if they are absent and the clinical picture is suggestive, a submucosal biopsy should be taken – ideally with a suction biopsy technique that can be performed in an outpatient setting. A positive result on mucosal or submucosal biopsy can confirm the diagnosis but a negative result does not exclude it and, in some circumstances, a full-thickness biopsy may be necessary [54,57,58]. When examining the 'routine' sections, it is usually necessary to examine multiple levels to confirm the presence or absence of ganglion cells. Immunohistochemistry (e.g. for PGP 9.5 or S-100) can be performed on formalin-fixed and paraffin-embedded material to highlight the enlarged nerve fibres characteristic of Hirschsprung's disease, but AChE histochemistry performed on fresh tissue is usually the favoured technique [59]. Recently, immunostaining for microtubule-associated protein-2 (MAP-2) has been recommended as a sensitive and specific marker for the identification of submucosal ganglion cells in formalin-fixed, paraffin-embedded suction biopsies, when haematoxylin and eosin-stained sections are equivocal [60].

Biopsies taken from very low within the rectum (e.g. within 10 mm of the dentate line) often contain no ganglion cells in normal individuals and are therefore not suitable for examination during the investigation of possible Hirschsprung's disease. Biopsies from the very low rectum usually contain prominent thick-walled blood vessels within the submucosa, which should alert the histopathologist to the possibility that they are derived from a segment that is physiologically (i.e. normally) aganglionic. These

techniques may fail in the case of ultra-short segment Hirschsprung's disease, when one may need to rely on manometry and clinical history. Intraoperative frozen section biopsies may be taken to confirm the presence of ganglion cells. Again, it will usually be necessary to examine multiple levels.

References

1. Synder WH. The embryology of the alimentary tract with special emphasis on the colon and rectum. *Surg Gynecol Obstet* 1958; **106**:311.
2. Willis RA. *The Borderland of Embryology and Pathology*, 2nd edn. London: Butterworths, 1962.
3. Lacroix B, Kedinger M, Simon-Assman P, et al. Developmental patterns of brush border enzymes in the human fetal colon. Correlation with some morphological events. *Early Hum Dev* 1984;**9**:95.
4. Thorlakson PHT, Monie IW, Thorlakson TK. Anomalous peritoneal encapsulation of small intestine; report of 3 cases. *Br J Surg* 1953;**40**:490.
5. Filston HC, Kirk DR. Malrotation: the ubiquitous anomaly. *J Pediatr Surg* 1981;**16**:614.
6. Marco V, Autonell J, Farre J, Fernandez-Layos M, Doncel F. Retrorectal cyst hamartomas. Report of two cases with adenocarcinoma developing in one. *Am J Surg Pathol* 1982;**6**:707.
7. Peck DA, Lynn HB, Harris LE. Congenital atresia and stenosis of the colon. *Arch Surg* 1963;**87**:428.
8. Cole GJ. Congenital diaphragm in the upper rectum. *Br J Surg* 1963;**50**:523.
9. Partridge JP, Gough MH. Congenital abnormalities of the anus and rectum. *Br J Surg* 1961;**49**:37.
10. Santulli TV, Keisewetter WB, Bill AH Jr. Anorectal anomalies: a suggested international classification. *J Pediatr Surg* 1970;**5**:281.
11. Chatterjee SK. Double termination of the alimentary tract – a second look. *J Pediatr Surg* 1980;**15**:623.
12. Koffler H, Aase JM, Papile LuA, Coen RW. Persistent cloaca with absent penis and anal atresia in one of identical twins. *J Pediatr* 1978;**93**:821.
13. Williams DA, Weiss T, Wade E, Dignan P. Prune perineum syndrome: report of a second case. *Teratology* 1983;**28**:145.
14. Teja K, Geissinger WT, Shaw A. Duplication of the transverse colon. Report of a case. *Dis Colon Rectum* 1975;**18**:430.
15. Beach PD, Brascho DJ, Hein WR, Nichol WW, Geppert LJ. Duplications of the primitive hindgut of the human being. *Surgery* 1961;**49**:779.
16. Ravitch MM. Hindgut duplication – doubling of colon and of genital and lower urinary tracts. *Ann Surg* 1953;**137**:588.
17. Hickey WF, Corson JM. Squamous cell carcinoma arising in a duplication of the colon; case report and literature review of malignancy complicating colonic duplication. *Cancer* 1981;**47**:602.
18. Weitzel RA, Breed JR. Carcinoma arising in a rectal duplication (enterocystoma). *Ann Surg* 1963;**157**:476.
19. Jones EA, Morson BC. Mucinous adenocarcinoma in anorectal fistulae. *Histopathology* 1984;**8**:279.
20. Morison JE. Giant congenital diverticula and neonatal rupture of colon: a case associated with true congenital partial hypertrophy of the crossed type. *Arch Dis Child* 1944;**19**:135.
21. Singh S, Minor CL. Cystic duplication of the rectum. A case report. *J Pediatr Surg* 1980;**15**:205.
22. Caropreso PR, Wengert PA Jr, Milford HE. Tailgut cyst – a rare retrorectal tumour. Report of a case and review. *Dis Colon Rectum* 1975;**18**:597.

23. Wolf M. Heterotopic gastric epithelium in the rectum. *Am J Clin Pathol* 1971;**55**:604.

24. Picard EJ, Picard JJ, Jorissen J, Jardon M. Heterotopic gastric mucosa in the epiglottis and rectum. *Am J Dig Dis* 1978;**23**:217.

25. Debas HT, Chaun H, Thomson FB, Soon-Shiong P. Functioning heterotopic oxyntic mucosa in the rectum. *Gastroenterology* 1980;**79**:1300.

26. Dubilier LD, Caffrey PR, Hyde GL. Multifocal gastric heterotopia in a malformation of the colon presenting as a megacolon. *Am J Clin Pathol* 1969;**51**:646.

27. Taylor FM, Swank RI. Epithelial heterotopia in the colon of a child; a case presentation and review of the literature. *J Fla Med Assoc* 1982;**69**:788.

28. Willis RA. Some unusual developmental heterotopias. *BMJ* 1968;**iii**:627.

29. Bishop AE, Ferri G-L, Probert L, Bloom SR, Polak JM. Peptidergic nerves. *Scand J Gastroenterol* 1982;**17**:43.

30. Smith B. The neuropathology of pseudo-obstruction of the intestine. *Scand J Gastroenterol* 1982;**17**:103.

31. Goyal RK, Hirano I. The enteric nervous system. *N Engl J Med* 1996;**334**:1106.

32. Hirschsprung H. Stuhltragheit Neugeborener in Folge von Dilatation und Hypertrophic des Colons. *J Kinderheilk* 1888;**27**:1.

33. Bodian M, Carter CO, Ward BCH. Hirschsprung's disease. *Lancet* 1951;**i**:302.

34. Bodian M, Carter CO. A family study of Hirschsprung's disease. *Ann Hum Gen* 1963;**26**:261.

35. Edery P, Lyonnet S, Mulligan LM, et al. Mutations of the RET proto-oncogene in Hirschsprung's disease. *Nature* 1994;**367**:378.

36. Wartiovaara K, Salo M, Sariola H. Hirschprung's disease genes and the development of the enteric nervous system. *Ann Med* 1998;**30**:66.

37. Blisard KS, Kleinman R. Hirschsprung's disease: a clinical and pathological overview. *Hum Pathol* 1986;**17**:1189.

38. Ghosh A, Griffiths DM. Rectal biopsy in the investigation of constipation. *Arch Dis Child* 1998;**79**:266.

39. Lewis NA, Levitt MA, Zallen GS, et al. Diagnosing Hirschsprung's disease: increasing the odds of a positive rectal biopsy result. *J Pediatr Surg* 2003;**38**:412.

40. Wu JS, Schoetz DJ Jr, Coller JA, Veidenheimer MC. Treatment of Hirschsprung's disease in the adult. Report of five cases. *Dis Colon Rectum* 1995;**38**:655.

41. Taguchi T, Tanaka K, Ikeda K. Fibromuscular dysplasia of arteries in Hirschsprung's disease. *Gastroenterology* 1985;**88**:1099.

42. Meier-Ruge W. Hirschsprung's disease: its aetiology, pathogenesis and differential diagnosis. *Curr Top Pathol* 1974;**59**:131.

43. Bishop AE, Polak JM, Lake BD, Bryant MG, Bloom SR. Abnormalities of the colonic regulatory peptides in Hirschsprung's disease. *Histopathology* 1981;**5**:679.

44. Munakata K, Okabe I, Morita K. Histologic studies of rectocolic aganglionosis and allied diseases. *J Pediatr Surg* 1978;**13**:67.

45. Scharli AF, Sossai R. Hypoganglionosis. *Semin Pediatr Surg* 1998;**7**:187.

46. Yamataka A, Ohshiro K, Kobayashi H, et al. Intestinal pacemaker C-KIT+ cells and synapses in allied Hirschsprung's disorders. *J Pediatr Surg* 1997;**32**:1069.

47. MacIver AG, Whitehead R. Zonal colonic aganglionosis, a variant of Hirschsprung's disease. *Arch Dis Child* 1972;**47**:233.

48. Kadair RG, Sims JE, Critchfield CF. Zonal colonic hypoganglionosis. *JAMA* 1977;**238**:1838.

49. MacMahon RA, Moore CCM, Cussen LJ. Hirschsprung-like syndromes in patients with normal ganglion cells on suction rectal biopsy. *J Pediatr Surg* 1981;**16**:835.

50. Fu CG, Muto T, Masaki T, Nagawa H. Zonal adult Hirschsprung's disease. *Gut* 1996;**39**:765.

51. Meier-Ruge WA, Bruder E, Holschneider AM, et al. Diagnosis and therapy of ultrashort Hirschsprung's Disease. *Eur J Pediatric Surg* 2004;**14**:392.

52. Scharli AF, Meier-Ruge W. Localized and disseminated forms of neuronal intestinal dysplasia mimicking Hirschsprung's disease. *J Pediatr Surg* 1981;**16**:164.

53. Meier-Ruge WA, Bronnimann PB, Gambazzi F, et al. Histopathological criteria for intestinal neuronal dysplasia of the submucosal plexus (type B). *Virchows Archiv* 1995;**426**:549.

54. Trigg PH, Belin R, Haberkorn S, et al. Experience with a cholinesterase histochemical technique for rectal suction biopsies in the diagnosis of Hirschsprung's disease. *J Clin Pathol* 1974;**27**:207.

55. Lake BD, Puri P, Nixon HH, Claireaux AE. Hirschsprung's disease. An appraisal of histochemically demonstrated acetyl cholinesterase activity in suction rectal biopsy specimens as an aid to diagnosis. *Arch Pathol Lab Med* 1978;**102**:244.

56. Patrick WJA, Besley GTN, Smith II. Histochemical diagnosis of Hirschsprung's disease and a comparison of the histochemical and biochemical activity of acetylcholine. *J Clin Pathol* 1980;**33**:336.

57. Chow CW, Chan WC, Yue PCK. Histochemical criteria for the diagnosis of Hirschsprung's disease in rectal suction biopsies by acetylcholinesterase activity. *J Pediatr Surg* 1977;**12**:675.

58. Venugopal S, Mancer K, Shandling B. The validity of rectal biopsy in relation to morphology and distribution of ganglion cells. *J Pediatr Surg* 1981;**16**:433.

59. Robey SS, Kuhajda FP, Yardley JH. Immunoperoxidase stains of ganglion cells and abnormal mucosal nerve proliferations in Hirschsprung's disease. *Hum Pathol* 1988;**19**:432.

60. Burtelow MA, Longacre TA. Utility of microtubule associated protein-2 (MAP-2) immunohistochemistry for identification of ganglion cells in paraffin-embedded rectal suction biopsies. *Am J Surg Pathol* 2009;**33**:1025.

CHAPTER 34

Neuromuscular and mechanical disorders of the large intestine

Paola Domizio and Joanne E. Martin

Barts and the London School of Medicine and Dentistry, Queen Mary University of London; The Royal London Hospital, London, UK

Diverticular disease of the colon

This is a common and important condition in most western countries where it causes considerable morbidity and has a low, but significant, mortality in older members of the population.

Terminology

Terminology has been a cause of much confusion. The name diverticulosis is used merely to indicate the presence of multiple diverticula in the large intestine, with or without the accompanying muscle abnormality found in classic diverticular disease and irrespective of aetiology or symptomatology. Consequently it has no clinical connotations. Diverticular disease, on the other hand, is used to describe a specific clinical disorder with defined radiological and pathological appearances, in which there is a characteristic muscle abnormality, usually, but not invariably, accompanied by the presence of diverticula that may or may not be inflamed. When this muscular abnormality occurs in the absence of established diverticula the term 'pre-diverticular disease' is sometimes used. Diverticulitis is applied when one or more diverticula are the source of visible macroscopic inflammation. It is often accompanied by pericolic abscess formation.

Epidemiology

The prevalence of diverticular disease has been calculated from radiological studies [1–4], colonoscopy [5] and at necropsy [6–9]. Several studies have been published looking at admissions to hospital, hospital-related episodes and mortality [10–14]. In most studies from western nations, the incidence of diverticular disease rises steadily with increasing age, up to approximately 30% over the age of 60. There are no or only minor differences in incidence between males and females, with some studies showing a small excess in females [3–9,12].

Diverticular disease is common in northern Europe, North America and Australia [7,13,14], but is less common in southern Europe and South America, where the population is mainly of Latin origin. It is rare in the Middle East, Africa, India and the Orient [8,12,13,15,16]. There are also variations, both racial and socio-economic, within national boundaries [4,5]. Diverticulosis is eight times more common in white people than among the black population of Johannesburg, where the condition is much more common in urban communities than in rural areas [17]. In Israel it is much more common among the Ashkenazim than in Sephardic and Oriental Jews and Arabs; the incidence is increasing in the latter groups but is stable in the Ashkenazi population [18]. Patients of Indian subcontinent Asian origin were less likely to have diverticular disease (6%) than non-Asian patients (23%) in a large metropolitan population undergoing endoscopy in the UK, even after sex and age differences were taken into account [5]. The differences between the lower rates in non-western immigrants and the native western population appears to diminish with time in the country, as noted in a large population study in Sweden [12].

Population studies show that not only has the prevalence of diverticular disease increased over the last 20 years, but

Morson and Dawson's Gastrointestinal Pathology, Fifth Edition. Edited by Neil A. Shepherd, Bryan F. Warren, Geraint T. Williams, Joel K. Greenson, Gregory Y. Lauwers and Marco R. Novelli.
© 2013 Blackwell Publishing Ltd. Published 2013 by Blackwell Publishing Ltd.

also the rate of perforation has doubled in the same period [14]. Although only 1–2% of affected individuals ever develop symptoms, most commonly diverticulitis, and only about 0.5% require surgery [10,14], the increased prevalence means that diverticular disease is responsible for a significant proportion of health-care spending in the western world. A recent population based study has shown an overall 10-year mortality rate of 0.003% [12], but this increases significantly to approximately 3% after admission for complications [11].

Macroscopic and microscopic appearances

From an anatomical point of view diverticula of the colon are of typical pulsion type, consisting of a pouch of mucous membrane (including muscularis mucosae) projecting through and beyond the circular muscle layers of the bowel wall, so that the diverticula come to lie in the pericolic fat and appendices epiploicae. They remain covered by the investing layer of longitudinal muscle, but this is extremely thin. It has been confirmed that most diverticula pass through the bowel wall at weak points in the circular muscle layer, through which the main blood vessels pass to supply the colonic mucosa [19]. This important anatomical fact explains the complication of diverticular haemorrhage, discussed later. It is usual to find two rows of diverticula, one on each side of the bowel wall between the mesenteric and anti-mesenteric taeniae [19] (Figure 34.1). In about 50% of cases a third row of very small diverticula can be found between the two anti-mesenteric taeniae [20].

In western populations, diverticula are most common in the sigmoid colon; indeed they are confined to this segment in most patients. In classic diverticular disease, the proximal colon is affected only when the sigmoid is also diseased and involved in continuity; total colonic diverticulosis is not so very uncommon. The rectum is never involved.

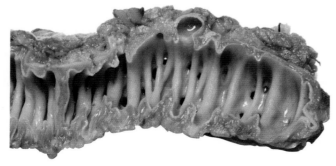

Figure 34.1 Diverticular disease of colon: note the concertina-like appearance produced by hypertrophy of the circular muscle coat. The mouths of diverticula lie between the corrugations, reaching the pericolic fat.

Regardless of the length of colon affected, the number of diverticula is variable, ranging from 1 or 2 to over 100. We have seen a few examples of diverticulosis confined to the right colon, but this seems to be a separate condition (see below). So-called diverticula of the rectum are congenital duplications and unrelated to diverticular disease of the colon.

The muscle

The muscle abnormality is the most striking and consistent abnormality in diverticular disease of the sigmoid colon [9,21,22]. The taeniae coli appear thick, assuming an almost cartilaginous consistency in some cases. The circular muscle is also much thicker than normal and has a corrugated or concertina-like appearance (the so-called saw-tooth sign on barium enema radiographs). In between these muscular corrugations, the mouths of the diverticula are found penetrating the bowel wall to reach the pericolic fat. Sometimes, the bowel wall between the corrugations shows no diverticulum formation but rather a tendency to sacculation. These sacs are outbulgings that retain the circular muscle coat in their walls. In some specimens the mucosal surface between the corrugations appears trabeculated and looks very similar to the trabeculation of the bladder seen in chronic prostatic obstruction. The corrugations are inter-digitating processes of circular muscle. If the structure of the bowel is studied in transverse section or by opening longitudinally without bisection it can be seen that these inter-digitating processes are not continuous around the circumference of the bowel wall. They are, in fact, semilunar arcs of muscle confined to the zone between the mesenteric and anti-mesenteric taeniae. Each consists of two layers of circular muscle in apposition. In some specimens of long-standing disease the number of arcs of circular muscle is so great that they appear fused. The circular muscle between the anti-mesenteric taeniae of the sigmoid shows only small muscle ridges projecting into the lumen of the bowel. The degree of muscular thickening is variable, being particularly obvious in specimens from the sigmoid. It has been suggested that a ridge width of 1.8 mm might be regarded as the dividing line between normal and abnormal [22]. Corrugation is never present to the same degree in other parts of the colon containing diverticula, although slight muscle thickening with an increase in the number of haustral clefts can be seen in the ascending and transverse colon of otherwise normal specimens.

Excess fat around the sigmoid colon has been described in many patients with diverticular disease. It has been suggested that this results from a local response to chronic inflammation. It is also possible, however, that this observation merely reflects the fact that overweight middle-aged people (who have more intra-abdominal fat) are more susceptible to the disease. This 'fat excess' is probably more apparent than real and is due to bunching of the pericolic and mesenteric tissues, consequent on shortening of the bowel by muscle contraction.

The muscle abnormality of diverticular disease is recognisable in surgical specimens and at autopsy [7,23]. It is not well demonstrated, however, unless the colon is fixed by distension with formalin under pressure and then cut longitudinally (Figure 34.2). When this is done, the abnormality correlates very well with the appearance in barium enema radiographs [24,25]. Occasionally, the muscle abnormality is seen in the absence of diverticula [26,27], a fact that is important in explaining the pathogenesis of diverticular disease. Histologically, the muscle in diverticular disease shows thickening but no evidence of hyperplasia or hypertrophy of muscle cells [28,29]. The circular muscle is broken up into well demarcated fasciculi separated from each other by loose connective tissue that is probably only an exaggeration of the normal structure. In the longitudinal taeniae, however, there is a significant increase in both

coarse and fine elastic fibres that distorts the normal fascicular pattern [29]. This elastosis of the taeniae appears to be an early manifestation of diverticular disease, being consistently found in uncomplicated cases and may, through shortening, be responsible for the concertina-like corrugation of the circular muscle [29]. There does not seem to be any abnormality of the submucosal and myenteric nerve plexuses in diverticular disease. Although there may appear to be some excess of nervous tissue, this is likely to be due to shortening of the bowel rather than to any true thickening of nerve trunks or an increase in neuronal numbers.

The mucosa

In the absence of complications, particularly inflammation, the diverticula themselves are lined by colonic mucosa that is entirely normal apart from an increase in size and number of lymphoid follicles. These follicles are especially prominent when a faecolith is present and probably represent a response to faecal stasis within the diverticulum, analogous to the effects of a faecolith in the appendix. Sometimes diverticula can become everted, the result being nipple-like tags of redundant but otherwise normal mucosa protruding into the colonic lumen. These tags, which can be mistaken for polyps at colonoscopy, could be described as true 'pseudo-polyps' (Figure 34.3). In some cases of sigmoid diverticular disease, and to a lesser extent pre-diverticular disease, a distinctive feature is filling of the bowel lumen with redundant folds of mucosa, gathered as a result of shortening of the bowel by muscle contraction. The lumen may be so obliterated by these mucosal folds that it is difficult to pass even a narrow probe from one end of the specimen to the other. The luminal narrowing cannot be described as a stricture but the folds add to the stenosis caused by the muscle thickening. Hence, diverticular disease can cause intestinal obstruction, and features of obstructive colitis (see Chapter 35) are frequently found in the proximal mucosa.

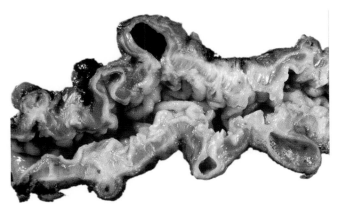

Figure 34.2 Diverticular disease of sigmoid colon showing mucosal redundancy, thickened circular muscle coat and extramural diverticula, some still bounded by the longitudinal muscle coat.

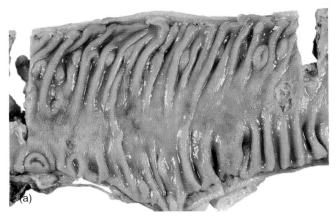
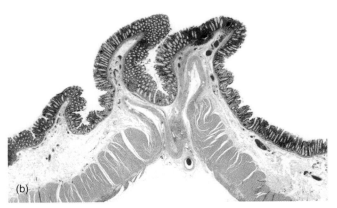

Figure 34.3 (a) Nipple-like tags of mucosa formed by everted colonic mucosal diverticula. (b) Histological appearances of everted diverticulum (a 'pseudo-polyp').

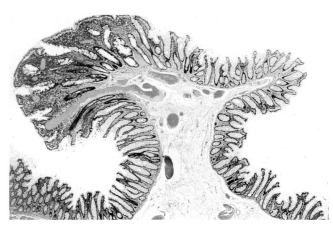

Figure 34.4 A redundant tag of mucosa in sigmoid diverticular disease showing features of mucosal prolapse and forming an inflammatory myoglandular polyp.

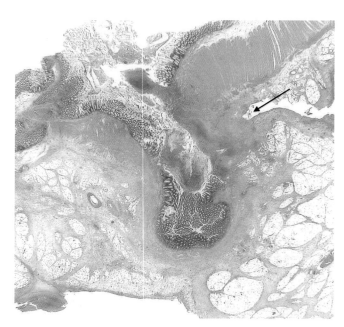

Figure 34.5 Diverticular disease with diverticulitis: part of the wall of the diverticulum is eroded, with inflammation extending into the extramural tissues and a local peritonitis (arrow).

The mucosa of the gathered folds may be subjected to mechanical stress from peristalsis, particularly when the stool is firm, and localised mucosal ischaemia may develop. The folds may then become congested or haemorrhagic and even ulcerated, a condition for which the term 'crescentic fold colitis' has been coined [30]. More diffuse inflammation, involving the whole segment of bowel affected by diverticular disease, is the condition of 'segmental' or diverticular colitis (see Chapter 35) [31,32]. This must be distinguished from ulcerative colitis by its relatively mild distortion of mucosal architecture and mild activity, but particularly by its segmental distribution.

Chronic mechanical stress to the redundant folds leads to the state of mucosal prolapse and polypoid tags of prolapsed mucosa are frequently found in bowel affected by diverticular disease [33,34]. These show histological features indistinguishable from so-called inflammatory 'myoglandular' polyps [35] (Figure 34.4).

Complications

Inflammation (diverticulitis)

Diverticula are mainly extramural structures and, as inflammation commonly starts at the apex and rarely involves the mucosa proximal to the neck of the sac, the inflammatory process usually affects only the pericolic and mesenteric fat. Diverticula become inflamed because faecal matter is not discharged through the narrow neck, becomes inspissated to produce a faecolith and abrades the mucosal lining of the sac to produce low grade, chronic inflammation. The mucosal lymphoid tissue undergoes hyperplasia and the earliest signs of inflammation are often found in lymphoid tissue at the apices of diverticula [21]. Usually only one diverticulum becomes inflamed; it is uncommon for more than three or four to be affected. As the coats of

the sac are thin there is early involvement of pericolic fat and local peritonitis is common [36] (Figure 34.5); free perforation into the peritoneal cavity is a recognised complication [14,37] and there may be adherence of the colon to other intra-abdominal structures such as small intestine or bladder with subsequent fistula formation.

The inflammation often spreads longitudinally from the apex of the diverticulum parallel to the outer aspect of the deep muscle layers to form a dissecting abscess (Figure 34.6). With its source in only one diverticulum, inflammation may thus spread widely up and down immediately outside the bowel wall, ensheathing it with inflammatory and later fibrous tissue and forming a large mass around the colon.

The clinical, surgical or radiological diagnosis of 'diverticulitis' implies the presence of both diverticula and inflammation, but the latter is often absent in resected specimens of sigmoid colon [38]. This could be explained by resolution of former inflammation, but it is likely that the pain and diarrhoea in diverticular disease are produced by the muscle abnormality rather than any inflammatory change. It is most important when examining surgical or postmortem specimens of diverticular disease to examine every diverticulum for signs of pericolic abscess formation because these can be very small and hidden in fatty tissue.

Haemorrhage

Some degree of overt or occult bleeding is common in diverticular disease. In most patients the bleeding is con-

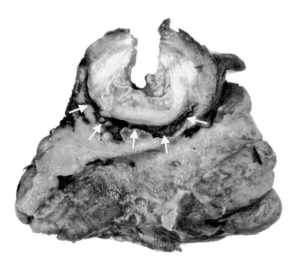

Figure 34.6 Diverticular disease of sigmoid colon with a pericolic abscess that is tracking in the subserosal space immediately outside the bowel wall (arrows). Perforation has led to a florid fibrinopurulent peritonitis that is most obvious in the lower half of the image.

tinuous, with loss of relatively small amounts of blood, but it may occasionally be sudden and massive. The cause of the haemorrhage is usually erosion of mucosa inside a diverticulum with exposure of an adjacent artery [19,38]. As diverticula arise at the sites of vascular entry into the colonic wall, the arteries involved may be of considerable size. Sometimes the bleeding originates from vascular granulation tissue either within an infected diverticulum or at the site of mucosal prolapse at the neck of a diverticulum [21,33]. It is often stated that massive haemorrhage usually comes from a diverticulum of the right side of the colon [39,40], but in such cases there can be confusion over whether the bleeding arises within the diverticulum itself or from coexisting angiodysplasia [41,42]. Often the amount of inflammation is minimal in patients who have bleeding from diverticula [40,41] and this makes it all the more difficult to pinpoint the source of the haemorrhage. Rupture of an ectatic vascular channel, which happens to lie at the neck of diverticulum, is a hypothetical possibility that is very difficult to prove or disprove.

Fistulae

The formation of a pericolic abscess and local peritonitis can cause adhesions to the abdominal wall or to organs within the abdominal cavity, with subsequent formation of a fistulous track. Colo-vesical fistula is the most common [43,44] but colo-vaginal, colo-colic, colo-ileal, colo-cutaneous and colo-anal fistulae have all been described. Fistulae may occur as a complication in patients operated on for diverticulitis [44].

Intestinal obstruction

Chronic obstructive symptoms are a common manifestation of diverticular disease because, as described above, there is always some luminal narrowing [36]. Acute intestinal obstruction is rare and seems always to occur in the presence of very extensive inflammation.

Perforation

Free perforation in an infected diverticulum is an uncommon but dangerous complication, with a high mortality from generalised peritonitis, usually faecal [36,37]. Patients being treated with non-steroidal anti-inflammatory drugs (NSAIDs) are particularly vulnerable, probably due to mucosal damage induced by the inhibition of prostanoid synthesis, together with a reduced awareness of warning pain due to the analgesic effect of these drugs. In one study of mode of presentation of patients with diverticular disease in general practice, 19 (61%) of 31 patients taking NSAIDs presented with a perforation or peritonitis, compared with only 8 (13%) of 61 patients not taking NSAIDs [45]. Purulent peritonitis may also follow rupture of a pericolic abscess.

Differential diagnosis

The diagnosis of diverticular disease of the colon, with or without muscle abnormality, is usually obvious. The most important distinctions are from duplication of the colon (see Chapter 33) and from solitary or few diverticula of the caecum and ascending colon, which are likely to be unrelated. When examining surgical specimens of diverticular disease of the sigmoid, it is not uncommon to find adenomatous polyps or a small carcinoma hidden between the muscular corrugations. It is sometimes these, rather than the diverticular disease, that are the cause of symptoms, particularly bleeding [46]. On clinical and radiological grounds diverticular disease of the sigmoid colon often mimics Crohn's disease. The induction of lymphoid follicle development in and around the mucosa of diverticula, the presence of fistulae and pericolic abscesses, particularly a granulomatous inflammatory reaction within the diverticular segment, can present a diagnostic dilemma [32,47]. Studies have described granulomatous vasculitis within the bowel wall, and small granulomas in the regional lymph nodes, of patients with diverticulitis who did not develop any other features of Crohn's disease on follow-up [48]. Critical evaluation of all aspects of the patient's clinical picture is therefore required to avoid inappropriate overdiagnosis of Crohn's disease [49]. Indeed, it is questionable whether a diagnosis of Crohn's disease can be made at all in the absence of inflammatory disease elsewhere in the bowel or the anus. When the two conditions do coexist, involvement of diverticula by Crohn's disease may result in an increased incidence of diverticulitis [50] and there is often extensive fistula formation.

Aetiology and pathogenesis

As the diverticula of classic diverticular disease are of pulsion type, at least two factors must be involved in their pathogenesis: raised intraluminal pressure and foci of weakness of the colonic wall. There is an increase in both incidence and complications of diverticular disease in obese patients, particularly diverticulitis and diverticular bleeding [51]. The sites of penetration of blood vessels through the circular muscle coats are undoubtedly predetermined areas of weakness, enhanced by expansion of perivascular adipose tissue in obese individuals, but additional factors must be involved, if only to explain the propensity for involvement of the sigmoid colon. Changes in the connective tissues of the bowel wall influence its tensile strength and elasticity. Defective collagen probably plays a part in the development of diverticula in patients with Marfan's or Ehlers–Danlos syndrome [52], and the increasing frequency of diverticular disease with age in western societies may well be related to the fact that the ageing colon loses its tensile properties, probably as a result of alterations in the structure and arrangement of collagen molecules [53,54]. There is also evidence that the thickened colonic wall of diverticular disease has an increased compliance [55].

Many studies have found an increase in both colonic intraluminal pressure [55–57] and the frequency of colonic contractions [58] in diverticular disease, although others suggest that these changes are confined to those with abdominal symptoms [59]. Simultaneous cine-radiology and pressure recordings have shown that the high intraluminal pressures are produced by segmenting, which effectively converts the affected segment of colon into a series of small compartments [60]. These are partially sealed off from each other by a valvular mechanism produced by alternation and overlap of the semicircular arcs of thickened circular muscle. Although muscular thickening of the colonic wall in diverticular disease may be a response to increased intraluminal pressure or work hypertrophy after repeated contraction, there is no morphological evidence of hypertrophy of individual fibres or of hyperplasia [28,29,56]. The alternative – supported by radiological evidence of failure of the muscle to elongate causing a permanent state of 'contracture' and the finding of normal colonic pressures in asymptomatic patients [59] – is that a primary overactivity of colonic muscle is responsible for the increased intraluminal pressure, occurring intermittently at first but becoming persistent later.

One group demonstrated increased density of cholinergic (excitatory) nerves in right-sided diverticular disease and reduced nitrergic (inhibitory) nerves, whereas studies of the sigmoid colon have shown the possibility of cholinergic denervation hypersensitivity in smooth muscle of the bowel wall and a reduced nitric oxide relaxation response [61–63]. The thickening of muscle might then be a manifestation of prolonged contraction. Elastosis of the taeniae may be important in maintenance of the muscular thickening; contraction of the elastic fibres producing shortening of the colon and widening of the circular muscle until it eventually becomes corrugated like a concertina. It could even be the primary cause of the muscle abnormality in diverticular disease [29,63].

In recent years, a number of geographical and population studies have implicated low dietary fibre in the aetiology of diverticular disease [64]. Conversely, a diet high in cellulose fibre seems to be particularly protective [65]. Individuals with diverticular disease consume fewer vegetables, brown bread and potatoes, and more meat and dairy products than control individuals [66]; vegetarians have less than half the expected prevalence of asymptomatic diverticulosis [67]. In Japan an increase in the prevalence of the disease has coincided with a decline in the consumption of dietary fibre [68], whereas rats fed a diet low in bran develop lesions similar to colonic diverticula, although lacking taeniae coli [69]. Dietary fibre derived from plant cell walls binds salt and water within the colon, giving bulky, moist faeces that are easily propelled along the colon by peristalsis. It is postulated that propulsion of the low-volume faeces resulting from fibre-deficient diets requires increased muscular effort, leading to muscular thickening, hypersegmentation and increased intraluminal pressure, and ultimately the formation of diverticula [64]. Clinical studies indicate that symptomatic diverticular disease is improved by a high-fibre diet [70], with a concomitant lowering of sigmoid intraluminal pressure [71] and the frequency of colonic contractions [58].

Although numerous studies have concentrated on fibre and pressure, other investigators have studied microflora and mitochondria and have also improved our understanding of the pathogenesis of diverticular disease. Many changes reported in diverticular disease are also seen in ageing, such as changes in connective tissue, neuronal loss and mitochondrial dysfunction, and some insight may be gained from studies of these normal processes [72]. Despite a large volume of research there remain many areas of uncertainty and many contradictory studies. It seems likely that different mechanisms operate in different patients, the parts played by abnormalities of motility and colonic wall strength varying considerably from case to case. The fact that diverticulosis itself, without any morphological evidence of thickened muscle, is commonly seen by pathologists at post mortem and by radiologists during barium enema examinations suggests that either the muscle abnormality in such patients is reversible, the diverticula representing 'scars' of previous episodes of muscular dysfunction, or the diverticula are the result of a primary weakness of the colonic wall.

Diverticulosis of the right colon

Diverticulosis of the caecum and ascending colon seems to be an entirely different condition from diverticular disease of the sigmoid colon or from generalised diverticulosis. Although it occurs worldwide, it is particularly common in Hawaii, Japan and the Orient [8,12,16,73,74] where its prevalence overshadows that of sigmoid diverticulosis and appears to be increasing. Right-sided diverticula may be single or few in number – it is uncommon to find more than 15 – and affected individuals are younger than those with sigmoid diverticulosis. In Japan solitary diverticula account for about a third of cases of right-sided diverticulosis [74] but this proportion is much higher in western countries, where solitary diverticulum of the caecum or ascending colon is not an uncommon incidental finding at laparotomy or post mortem, but multiple right-sided diverticulosis is rare [75]. Histological examination of the diverticula shows that a few are true diverticula surrounded by attenuated fibres of the colonic muscularis propria, suggesting a congenital maldevelopment, but most appear to be pulsion-type diverticula composed of mucosal herniations through the muscle coat of the colonic wall. Thickening of the muscularis propria of the colon, the cardinal feature of sigmoid diverticular disease, is not prominent in right-sided cases, but intraluminal pressure studies suggest that abnormal colonic motility might play an important pathogenic role [75,76]. It is interesting to note that the adoption of a western-type lifestyle in Japan during recent years has been accompanied by an increase in both right- and left-sided colonic diverticular disease [74], suggesting that the two conditions may have predisposing factors in common, but that the underlying differences in location of the lesions may reflect underlying anatomical differences in the populations [75].

Most diverticula of the right colon are asymptomatic, but diverticulitis, which usually mimics acute appendicitis, may lead to haemorrhage, pericolic abscess or peritonitis [73–75] (Figure 34.7). Some so-called 'solitary ulcers' of the caecum or ascending colon are probably the result of inflammation in or around a solitary diverticulum [77]. A proportion of patients with right-sided diverticulosis have recurrent attacks of right lower quadrant abdominal pain, possibly related to abnormal colonic motility.

The irritable bowel syndrome

Approximately half of patients referred to hospital gastro-enterology clinics in the UK with symptoms of recurrent abdominal pain or bowel disturbance have no demonstrable pathological abnormality of the intestinal tract despite

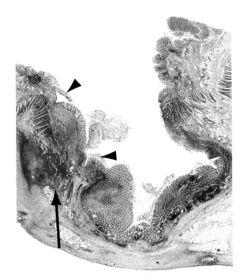

Figure 34.7 Isolated diverticulum of right colon: there is mucosal ulceration (arrowheads) with early abscess formation in the pericolic fat (arrowed). This may be the pathogenesis of some cases of 'solitary ulcer' of the right colon.

intensive investigation. In most of these patients the clinical features have a characteristic symptom complex defined as the irritable bowel syndrome (IBS). Three subtypes are recognised: diarrhoea predominant, constipation predominant and mixed [78,79].

IBS affects women more than men and has a peak incidence in the third and fourth decades of life. Acute bacterial gastroenteritis, including that caused by *Salmonella*, *Campylobacter* and *Shigella* spp., has been reported as a risk factor for the development of IBS [80–82]. Up to a quarter of patients, more commonly women, report persistent altered bowel habit after infection and 7–10% go on to develop IBS [81,82]. It has been suggested that the greater the duration and severity of the infection, the higher the risk of developing IBS [82,83].

The role of personality factors has also been considered with regard to the aetiology of IBS [85]. In many patients there is evidence of an enhanced visceral sensation, with the intestine unusually sensitive to luminal distension, and there is a balance between biological and psychological factors [86]. Fibre intake may also be important; indeed, diarrhoea-predominant IBS has been associated with diverticular disease [87].

Although most biopsies from IBS patients show no significant histological abnormality, several lines of evidence point to the presence of low grade inflammation and activation of the mucosal immune system in the pathogenesis of IBS. Raised levels of interleukins have been reported [82], as have an increased number of mast cells in the mucosa and muscularis propria, an increased number of mucosal T lymphocytes and endocrine cells, inflammatory cells around enteric nerves and nerve fibres staining for substance P and serotonin (5-hydroxytryptamine or 5HT [84,88]. In practice, however, when reporting routine biopsies, the literature is difficult to apply, because most of the observed changes have been described as part of detailed morphometric and quantitative studies, which are hardly practical or informative in giving a diagnostic opinion on an individual specimen.

Idiopathic constipation, megacolon, megarectum and pseudo-obstruction

Disorders of colonic motility resulting in impairment or failure of propulsion of faecal contents are not uncommon and result in a spectrum of clinical effects ranging from chronic constipation to acute functional colonic obstruction, so-called pseudo-obstruction. This may be indistinguishable clinically from mechanical or organic obstruction due to inflammation or neoplasia. As in the small intestine (see Chapter 19), this group of disorders may be neuropathic in origin, myopathic or both. An example of a neuropathic disorder that can cause significant constipation is aganglionosis of the large intestine, commonly known as Hirschsprung's disease (see Chapter 33). Although congenital in origin, this disorder may not present clinically until adolescence or even adult life [89], so its diagnosis is not solely in the realm of paediatric pathologists. Other causes of neuropathy include inflammation, infection, metabolic disorders and toxins, all of which can damage the colorectal nerve supply. Some cases are associated with disorders of the central nervous system, including psychiatric illnesses. In a minority of patients, a primary myopathy of the colonic smooth muscle or a primary neuropathy is present. (For detailed classification see Tables 34.1 and 34.2.)

Idiopathic constipation

Unexplained constipation, with a frequency of bowel motion of fewer than three a week, is common in western society. Approximately 2–27% of the population are affected, the greatest prevalence being in young women [90,91]. Three main categories of disorder are recognised: normal transit constipation, seen in approximately 59% of patients; failure of defecation mechanisms in 25%; and slow transit in 13%: a combination of patterns may be present in the remaining 3% [92]. The severity of the symptoms is variable but in those worst affected there may be less than one bowel action a week (even with the help of laxatives), abdominal pain, bloating and nausea.

In patients with normal transit constipation, the frequency of bowel movement is normal, but abdominal pain and discomfort, together with straining at stool, are common. Investigations often show increased rectal compliance and decreased rectal sensation. The condition usually resolves with increased fibre intake and laxatives [90].

Table 34.1 Classification of enteric myopathies

Primary myopathies

Abnormal developmental (morphogenic) phenotypes
  Focal absence of enteric muscle coats
  Segmental fusion of enteric muscle coats
  Presence of additional muscle coats
  Colonic desmosis (absent connective tissue scaffold)

Myopathies with vacuolation, atrophy and fibrosis
  Hollow visceral myopathies: sporadic and familial
  Degenerative leiomyopathy
  Myopathy with autophagic activity
  Pink blush myopathy with nuclear crowding

Myopathies with inflammation
  Lymphocytic leiomyositis
  Eosinophilic leiomyositis

Inclusion body myopathies
  Polyglucosan body myopathy
  Mitochondrial leiomyopathy

Other smooth muscle findings
  Contractile protein abnormality
  Amphophilic inclusion bodies

Secondary myopathies

Systemic disorders
  Desmin myopathy
  Muscular dystrophies
  Mitochondrial cytopathies
  Metabolic storage disorders
  Amyloidosis
  Progressive systemic sclerosis
  Other collagen vascular disorders
  Cystic fibrosis

Local disorders
  Obstructive/post-irradiation muscle failure

Reproduced from Knowles CH, De Giorgio R, Kapur RP et al. The London Classification of gastrointestinal neuromuscular pathology: report on behalf of the Gastro 2009 International Working Group. Gut, 2010; 59: 882, with permission from BMJ Publishing Group Ltd.

In defecatory disorders there may be local rectal or anal pathology, including anal sphincter dysfunction, or dysfunction of the muscles of the pelvic floor, with poorly coordinated contraction leading to inability to evacuate the rectum. The presenting features of this group of disorders include constipation, overflow incontinence and pain. Rarely, anorectal dysfunction may be associated with rectocele, previous anal trauma and myopathy of the internal anal sphincter with polyglucosan inclusions [90,93]. More

Table 34.2 Classification of enteric neuropathies

Primary neuropathies

Abnormal developmental phenotypes

Aganglionosis: Hirschsprung's disease

Hypoganglionosis

Intestinal neuronal dysplasia

Retarded neuronal maturation

Hyperganglionosis including ganglio-neuromatous hyperplasia

Degenerative neuropathies

Degenerative neuropathy without neuronal loss

Degenerative neuropathy with neuronal loss, e.g. Shy–Drager syndrome

Neuropathies with inflammation

Lymphocytic ganglionitis

Eosinophilic ganglionitis

Inclusion body neuropathies

Intraneuronal inclusion disease

Mega-mitochondria in mitochondrial neuro-gastrointestinal encephalomyopathy

Other neuronal findings

Axonal degeneration

Secondary neuropathies

Systemic disorders

Para-neoplastic inflammatory neuropathy

Diabetic neuropathy

Chagasic neuropathy

Connective tissue disorder-associated neuropathy

Storage disease

Amyloidosis

Local disorders

Crohn's disease

Reproduced from Knowles CH, De Giorgio R, Kapur RP et al. The London Classification of gastrointestinal neuromuscular pathology: report on behalf of the Gastro 2009 International Working Group. Gut, 2010; 59: 882, with permission from BMJ Publishing Group Ltd.

commonly, however, there is incoordination of the anorectal muscle, leading to contraction rather than relaxation, obstructing defecation [94].

In slow transit constipation the flow of faeces through the colon is slowed and the colon remains of normal diameter. The symptoms include abdominal pain, bloating and a diminished urge to defecate [90,91]. The response to pharmacological stimulation on physiological testing is reduced, so the term 'colonic inertia' has also been used. A high-fibre diet, laxatives, prokinetics and biofeedback therapy have all shown therapeutic benefit [90], although some patients

are very resistant to therapy and require colonic resection. The results of surgery are usually good [92], although in patients with associated small bowel dysfunction [95] the outcome is not so positive.

The pathophysiology of this disorder is not entirely clear. Histological studies have demonstrated abnormalities in the myenteric plexus with damage or loss of neurons, including argyrophilic neurons, changes in glial cells and reduction in the interstitial cells of Cajal. Alteration in the neurochemical coding of neurons has been reported, as have changes in levels of the vasoactive intestinal polypeptide (VIP) and substance P [96–100]. It has been suggested that some of these changes could be the result of extrinsic damage to the myenteric plexus, as might occur (for example) during pelvic surgery or childbirth. Usually, however, the intestinal symptoms predate these events and their aetiological significance is at present unclear. It seems likely that many of the features associated with idiopathic constipation, such as disorders of micturition and symptoms of Raynaud's phenomenon [91], may also be the result of malfunctioning central nervous and autonomic reflexes.

Megacolon and megarectum

Megacolon and megarectum are characterised by constipation and irreversible dilatation of the large bowel in the absence of underlying organic disease. Both disorders are slightly more common in men than in women. Megarectum, in which the proximal colon is of normal diameter, typically presents with faecal impaction in childhood or adolescence. Megacolon, in contrast, tends to present with constipation in later childhood or adulthood. Spinal dysraphism is associated with both conditions, suggesting that extrinsic nerve control may be abnormal [101]. The histological features of both conditions are similar. There is thickening of the muscularis mucosae and of both the circular and longitudinal layers of the muscularis propria, together with patchy fibrosis. A reduction in ganglion cells with relative preservation of enteric neural architecture has also been reported [100,102].

Colonic pseudo-obstruction

Colonic pseudo-obstruction describes a clinical syndrome in which the symptoms and signs of colonic obstruction occur in the absence of any recognisable mechanical obstructing lesion. Other parts of the gastrointestinal tract, notably the small intestine, can also be affected, in which case the term 'chronic intestinal pseudo-obstruction' is used (see Chapter 19). Colonic pseudo-obstruction can be acute or chronic.

Acute colonic pseudo-obstruction

Acute colonic pseudo-obstruction (Ogilvie's syndrome) nearly always occurs in elderly, hospitalised, bedridden patients who have from a wide range of conditions, including chronic neurological diseases, cardiac failure, chronic alcoholism and malignancy. In a significant proportion of patients, the condition develops after abdominal surgery, in which case the term 'paralytic ileus of the colon' is sometimes used. The symptoms are of rapidly progressive colonic obstruction mimicking acute mechanical obstruction. The disorder is usually transient and reversible, and cases managed by colonoscopic deflation or surgical decompression usually have no further symptoms, especially if the underlying disease process is also controlled and the patient is mobilised [103]. In patients who are not decompressed, there is a risk of intestinal perforation, usually of the caecum. The aetiology of acute colonic pseudo-obstruction is unknown. Postoperative cases probably have a similar aetiology to postoperative small intestinal ileus (see Chapter 19) but, in patients who have not undergone surgery, it seems that chronic immobility somehow leads to an acute functional failure of colonic transit.

Chronic colonic pseudo-obstruction

Chronic colonic pseudo-obstruction is characterised by chronic constipation. In many patients this leads to megacolon, although, unlike acute colonic pseudo-obstruction, perforation of the colon is extremely rare. The abnormal motility is usually secondary to an underlying systemic disease, although in some patients there is a primary disorder of the colon itself. The causes of chronic colonic pseudo-obstruction can be classified into two main groups: disorders of colonic smooth muscle and neurological disorders (see Tables 34.1 and 34.2).

Disorders of colonic smooth muscle (see Table 34.1)

Disorders of smooth muscle can be inherited or acquired. Inherited (familial) visceral myopathy can be autosomal dominant or autosomal recessive. In some patients with this disorder, there is selective involvement of the large bowel [104], but more commonly the whole gastrointestinal tract, especially the small intestine, is involved [104,105]. Atrophy of the muscularis propria leads to a failure of motility, eventually resulting in a dilated, atonic, thin-walled megacolon. Histopathological examination reveals degeneration of intestinal smooth muscle with myocytes showing nuclear enlargement and hyperchromasia with cytoplasmic vacuolation (Figure 34.8). Progressive interstitial fibrosis culminates in the complete fibrous replacement [104] of both the muscularis mucosae and muscularis propria [105]. In visceral leiomyopathy and mitochondrial neuro-gastrointestinal encephalomyopathy (MNGIE) the longitudinal layer of the muscularis propria is often more affected than the circular layer [99,100]. Unlike other conditions that cause fibrosis, such as ischaemia and radiotherapy, the fibrosis of acquired or inherited degenerative leiomyopathy tends to be continuous and associated with variation in the size and staining of myocytes [100].

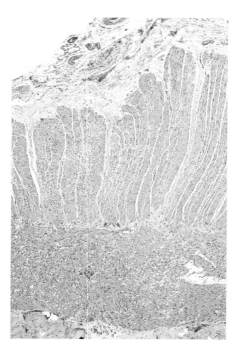

Figure 34.8 Familial visceral myopathy of autosomal recessive type. There is vacuolar degeneration of myocytes in the longitudinal layer of the muscularis propria and patchy fibrosis of the circular muscle layer.

Lymphocytic and eosinophilic leiomyositis have both been reported in association with colonic pseudo-obstruction. In patients with lymphocytic leiomyositis, associated vasculitis or other autoimmune conditions should be excluded carefully. In patients with eosinophilic leiomyositis, parasitic infection should be considered [100,106].

Acquired damage to colonic smooth muscle occurs in the collagen diseases including dermatomyositis [107] and scleroderma (systemic sclerosis) [108]. Involvement of the large intestine is particularly common in scleroderma, and symptoms of colonic pseudo-obstruction may even precede other manifestations of the disease. Replacement of the smooth muscle coats of the intestinal wall by collagen and elastic fibres is the main histological abnormality. This occurs patchily at first, but in advanced cases the circular muscle coat becomes obliterated by fibrosis. The taeniae coli are relatively spared. This muscular fibrosis closely mimics that found in familial visceral myopathy (Figure 34.9). Vacuolar degeneration of the surviving smooth muscle fibres in visceral myopathy is said to be useful in distinguishing between the two [109]. Examination of the arterial supply to the bowel wall, particularly the marginal vessels, will sometimes show intimal proliferation with elastosis and luminal narrowing. Scattered haemosiderin-laden macrophages in the colonic wall suggest that the

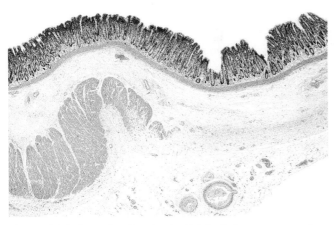

Figure 34.9 Systemic sclerosis: the histological appearances of the transverse colon in a patient with pseudo-obstruction. There is severe patchy replacement of the muscularis propria by relatively acellular fibrous tissue.

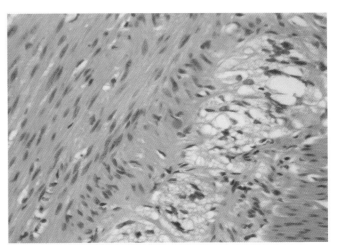

Figure 34.10 A single amphophilic inclusion body within a myocyte lies close to the myenteric plexus in a case of neuropathic pseudo-obstruction. The inclusion is smooth-surfaced, round and stains dark pink with haematoxylin and eosin.

changes are at least in part due to ischaemia. Patchy fibrosis of the muscle coats accounts for the characteristic macroscopic appearances of scleroderma affecting the colon. Large, multiple sacculations appear that are confined to the anti-mesenteric border, presumably because the tissues of the mesenteric side continue to give support to the weakened bowel wall, or possibly because the blood supply is more precarious at the anti-mesenteric border. In some specimens there are no sacculations, only a dilated, thin-walled colon.

Abnormal colonic motility, especially constipation, is common in patients with myotonic dystrophy [110] and progressive muscular dystrophy [111], in whom atrophy of the colonic smooth muscle fibres without fibrosis may be found. There may be a surprising degree of lymphocytic infiltration in the muscularis propria, not to be confused with a myositis. Colonic motor dysfunction also occurs rarely in systemic amyloidosis, possibly due to a combination of smooth muscle infiltration, autonomic neuropathy and vascular insufficiency [112].

Neurological disorders (see Table 34.2)

Neurological disorders leading to chronic colonic pseudo-obstruction can affect either the intrinsic intramural nerve plexuses or the extramural components of the sympathetic and parasympathetic nervous system. Our understanding of the changes that occur in neuronal neurochemistry as a result of these diseases is advancing rapidly, although for most motility disorders it is not yet known whether such changes are primary or secondary [100].

Defects of colonic innervation may produce a number of different clinical and pathological effects. Denervation of intestinal smooth muscle usually results in peristaltic activity that is increased in rate but uncoordinated. This occasionally causes diarrhoea, but far more commonly results in constipation with colicky abdominal pain due to a failure of colonic transit. The functional obstruction leads to luminal dilatation that along with the 'overwork' of denervation stimulates hypertrophy of the colonic smooth muscle [113]. The end-result is a dilated colon with prominent muscular thickening. Not all causes of colonic neuropathy lead to muscular hypertrophy, however. Some neuropathies, notably those caused by drugs or toxins, are accompanied by atrophy rather than hypertrophy of smooth muscle, resulting in a colon that is thin walled, inert and adynamic. In many cases of acquired neuropathic pseudo-obstruction amphophilic ovoid cytoplasmic inclusion bodies are present in scattered myocytes within the muscularis propria (Figure 34.10) [114]. These inconspicuous bodies seem to be markers of denervation, rather than specific products of a degenerative myopathy.

Neurological disorders that lead to chronic colonic pseudo-obstruction can be congenital or acquired. By far the most common congenital disorder is classic Hirschsprung's disease in which there is aganglionosis of the large intestine that starts in the anorectum and extends proximally for a variable distance (see Chapter 33). Almost all cases of Hirschsprung's disease present in infancy or childhood. On rare occasions, however, the diagnosis can be delayed and so should be considered in any adolescent or adult presenting with chronic constipation and megacolon [89]. Developmental abnormalities related to Hirschsprung's disease include aganglionosis of the entire colon, zonal aganglionosis, hypoganglionosis and hyperganglionosis (colonic neuronal dysplasia). Unusually for diseases causing colonic pseudo-obstruction, these disorders are can be diagnosed on rectal suction biopsy, without the need for sophisticated neuropathological techniques. They are considered fully with developmental disorders in Chapter 33. Ganglio-neuromatosis is a diffuse pattern of neuronal hyperplasia that can be associated with disordered colonic motility with or without megacolon. Histologically, it is characterised by neurons embedded in an expanded plexus and expanded nerve tracts with spindly glial and neurofibrillary stroma. As well as occurring sporadically, ganglioneuromatosis can also be associated with neurofibromatosis [115] and type 2b multiple endocrine neoplasia (medullary thyroid carcinoma, phaeochromocytoma and mucosal neuromas) [116] (Figure 34.11). In a small number of individuals with mucosal ganglio-neuromatosis, the diffuse hyperplastic process involves the lamina propria and so is visible in mucosal biopsy specimens. Mucosal ganglioneuromatosis has also been associated with the neoplasia syndromes listed above [117].

Though rare, at least two forms of familial visceral neuropathy (FVN) have been described, an autosomal recessive (OMIM 243180) form and an autosomal dominant (OMIM 609629) form. Both disorders lead to abnormal colonic motility accompanied by a spectrum of central and peripheral nervous system abnormalities [118]. Histologically, both varieties are characterised by neuronal loss and eosinophilic intranuclear inclusions within the neurons of both myenteric and submucosal plexuses. The inclusions, which appear to consist of non-viral filamentous proteins, may also be found in the brain, spinal cord, autonomic ganglia and peripheral nerves, where they are presumed to cause the variety of neurological symptoms that accompanies the intestinal abnormality. Other forms of FVN are recognised, including an X-linked form in which the filamin A gene is aberrant. This results in abnormal layering of the small bowel wall and multinucleate small and large bowel myocytes [119]. In most cases of FVN, routine histology of the colon fails to demonstrate an abnormality, the exception being the X-linked form. Detailed neuropathological examination, however, will usually reveal the degeneration of intramural neurons and the intraneuronal inclusions. Rare cases of sporadic visceral neuropathy affecting the colon and other parts of the gastrointestinal tract, without extra-intestinal pathology, have also been described [100]. Such cases appear to be degenerative disorders of the intestinal plexuses but their precise aetiology is unknown.

Acquired disorders of visceral innervation leading to chronic colonic pseudo-obstruction can have a number of different aetiologies. By far the most common cause worldwide is Chagas' disease, which results from infection with the parasite *Trypanosoma cruzi*. It is estimated that approximately seven million people, almost all in South America, are affected. The parasite has a specific affinity for the myenteric plexus (see Chapter 4) and causes a prominent chronic inflammatory reaction comprising lymphocytes and plasma cells. The consequence of this inflammatory reaction is destruction of the myenteric plexus with marked neuronal loss and Schwann cell hyperplasia. Smooth muscle hypertrophy resulting from denervation is common, as is megacolon [120,121]. A similar inflammatory destruction of the myenteric plexus has been described as a consequence of cytomegalovirus infection [122] and Epstein–Barr virus infection [123]. It has also been reported in patients with small cell carcinoma of the lung [100,113,124] (Figure 34.12), possibly

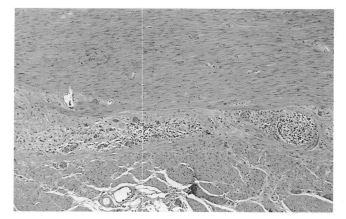

Figure 34.12 Autonomic plexitis: the colonic myenteric plexus is infiltrated by lymphocytes and plasma cells in this patient with pseudo-obstruction. Many of the neurons show degenerative changes. The condition was idiopathic in this man aged 28, who had progressive constipation. However, similar features can be seen in Chagas' disease or as a result of cytomegalovirus or Epstein–Barr virus infection, and also as a para-neoplastic effect in, for example, small cell carcinoma of the lung.

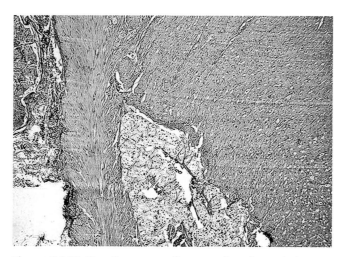

Figure 34.11 Ganglio-neuroma-like expansion of myenteric plexus in the colon of a young woman with multiple endocrine neoplasia type 2b.

due to an immunological reaction elicited by antigens on the neoplastic cells that cross-react with neural tissue in the myenteric plexus. Similar lesions in the posterior root ganglia have been found in other para-neoplastic neurological syndromes.

Autonomic neuronal damage leading to chronic colonic pseudo-obstruction is sometimes part of a more widespread chronic autonomic neuropathy. This is classically seen in the Shy–Drager syndrome, where colonic symptoms are frequently overshadowed by other manifestations of autonomic failure, notably orthostatic hypotension. In this condition the nerve cells both in the myenteric plexus and in the extramural sympathetic chain show a distinctive vacuolar change [113]. Colonic symptoms, may also occur when autonomic neuropathy occurs in metabolic disorders, notably diabetes mellitus [125] and myxoedema [126], although in these conditions the primary pathology may occur in the Schwann cells rather than in the neurons themselves [113].

In recent years it has been recognised that drugs are an important cause of damage to the colonic autonomic innervation. Those implicated include psychotropic drugs, especially phenothiazines and tricyclic antidepressants, anticholinergic drugs and anti-neoplastic drugs, used in cancer chemotherapy, notably the vinca alkaloids and daunorubicin. It has been postulated that the high frequency of severe constipation and megacolon in psychotic patients [127] may be due to the toxic effects of large doses of phenothiazines used in their management. Similar problems in patients with Parkinson's disease may be related to the use of anticholinergic drugs.

The condition of cathartic colon, in which the colon is thin, dilated and atonic with marked melanosis coli, was attributed by Smith [128] to a toxic neuropathy of the submucosal and myenteric plexuses induced by chronic ingestion of laxatives, especially of anthraquinone type. It is widely accepted that anthraquinone drugs cause melanosis coli (see Chapter 40) but since the original description of cathartic colon, there have been no acceptable reported cases of atonic, dilated colon directly attributable to such drugs, leading some authors to question the existence of this entity [129,130]. It seems likely that the features originally described were the end-stage of one or more neuromuscular problems unrelated to any laxatives the patients may have taken.

There have been several reports of functional colonic obstruction associated with eosinophilic [131] and lymphocytic plexitis [132] of the colon. In some cases, the plexitis is accompanied by circulating anti-neuronal antibodies, including anti-Hu antibodies [132]. It is unclear, however, whether or not such antibodies are primarily pathogenic. It may be that they arise as a consequence of the neurological damage to the large bowel. In Chagas' disease, they may even attenuate the disease process [133].

Complications

Despite the sometimes huge dilatation of the colon in idiopathic constipation, pseudo-obstruction and megacolon, perforation is actually very unusual. Most complications result from faecal overloading or impaction, which often lead to non-specific mucosal inflammation, sometimes with crypt abscesses. Stercoral ulceration (see Chapter 40), with consequent pain and rectal bleeding, can arise from faecal impaction, in which case perforation is a possibility. Melanosis coli (see Chapter 40) is common in these conditions. It is usually mild, but can be very conspicuous if purgatives have been used long term.

Volvulus

A volvulus is a twisting of the bowel in such a way as to obstruct its lumen; many of the effects are secondary to interruption of the venous return. The classic sites of large bowel volvulus are the caecum and the sigmoid colon, although there are reports of volvulus of the transverse colon and splenic flexure [134].

Caecum

Volvulus of the caecum accounts for 25–45% of cases of intestinal volvulus. In the western world it rarely leads to intestinal obstruction, but does so more frequently in India, Africa and Scandinavian countries. The essential predisposing factor is an abnormally mobile caecum [135], although colonic distension, chronic constipation, previous abdominal surgery and pregnancy may also play a part. The caecum twists axially, except in the 10% of cases that are of caecal bascule type (when the distended caecum is situated in the pelvis), when it folds upwards and anteriorly [136]. Twisting of the mesentery with obstruction of the blood supply leads to infarction, gangrene and other manifestations of ischaemia. The prognosis of caecal volvulus may be better than that of sigmoid volvulus [134].

Sigmoid colon

Sigmoid volvulus is due to twisting of a large redundant sigmoid loop on an elongated mesentery [137]. An uncommon disease in the western world, it is more frequent in countries such as Iran, Africa, India, Scandinavia, Russia and Peru [134,135,138,139]. It is interesting that the condition is rare in those countries where diverticular disease of the colon is common. The geographical distribution has been explained by dietary factors leading to bowel distension – in those countries where volvulus is prevalent the population eats a high-residue or cereal diet which is often taken as one large meal during the day [140]. Sigmoid volvulus in such high-incidence areas is usually seen in those aged <50 years whereas in western countries affected individuals are often elderly, give a history of constipation and frequently have mental illness [141]. There are also differences in the gross appearances of the distended sigmoid loop between sigmoid volvulus in 'high-risk' areas and that in the west. In the former the affected bowel is long and thin walled and has a narrow mesentery, whereas in the western world the sigmoid loop shows marked muscular thickening of its wall and a broader mesentery that contains thick-walled blood vessels and shows fibrous scarring due to repeated attacks of volvulus [142]. The exception to this may be the colon in those living in the high-altitude Andes, which appears thicker than normal [139]. Twisting sufficient to cause infarction and gangrene of the bowel wall is rare in the western type of volvulus but is common in high-incidence areas. Paradoxically, the affected segment shows marked faecal loading in low-incidence areas whereas in countries with a high-residue diet the sigmoid loop is distended, mainly with gas. Melanosis coli is sometimes present if the patient comes from the western world, and occasionally there is pneumatosis coli in the affected segment [143]. Although most reports stress the importance of diet in the aetiology of sigmoid volvulus, congenital factors, such as a long sigmoid loop, also play a part, as indicated by one report of sigmoid volvulus in three members of a family [144]. Another rarer variety of sigmoid volvulus is so-called ileo-sigmoid knotting. In this condition, a loop of ileum knots around the base of a sigmoid volvulus in a complex manner, often resulting in gangrene of both bowel loops [145]. This condition is virtually unknown in the western world but better recognised in Africa, Asia and Middle Eastern countries.

Mucosal prolapse and the solitary ulcer syndrome

Prolapse of large intestinal mucosa may be found in a number of situations [146]. It occurs at the margin of a colostomy [147], at the apex of a prolapsing haemorrhoid, alongside any polypoid lesion of the large bowel and at the margins of colonic diverticula. However, the best recognised site of mucosal prolapse is the anterior wall of the rectum, where it gives rise to the so-called solitary ulcer syndrome [148], a fairly common but poorly recognised benign condition that is important because it may be confused both clinically and histologically with carcinoma of the rectum – we have knowledge of patients in whom such a mistaken diagnosis has led to unnecessary major excision. The name 'solitary ulcer' itself is misleading because sometimes there is more than one ulcer and there seems to be a stage of the disease when no ulceration is present.

Solitary ulcer of the rectum is quite unrelated to so-called solitary ulcer of the small intestine (see Chapter 22) or right colon (see 'Diverticulosis of the right colon' above). It

occurs predominantly in young adults of either sex who may present with any of the diverse symptoms of anorectal disease. Rectal bleeding is most common and may be severe enough to require transfusion; other symptoms include the passage of mucus, perineal pain and tenesmus. There may be associated complete rectal prolapse. Macroscopically, solitary ulcers are distinctive. They are situated on the anterior or anterolateral walls of the rectum and are usually flat, well demarcated lesions with an irregular shape, often covered by a white slough (Figure 34.13). They vary in size from 5 mm to 50 mm in diameter. The surrounding mucosa shows a mild proctitis and may appear lumpy. In cases in which no ulcer is present the anterior rectal mucosa shows a localised, roughened, inflamed area. Although the solitary ulcer syndrome is benign in its behaviour, it is notorious for its chronicity. No treatment is entirely satisfactory and often patients have to adjust to their symptoms.

Biopsy of the abnormal mucosa in solitary ulcer syndrome reveals characteristic appearances [148,149] now recognised to be distinctive of mucosal prolapse [146]. The earliest and most significant change is a curious obliteration of the lamina propria by fibrosis and smooth muscle fibres extending towards the lumen from a thickened muscularis mucosae (Figure 34.14). In a tangentially cut biopsy the appearance of mucosal glands surrounded by muscle

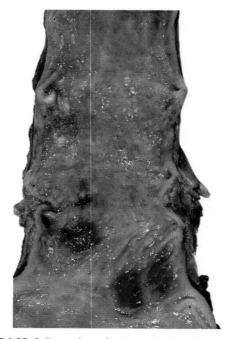

Figure 34.13 Solitary ulcer of rectum: despite the name, these lesions are often multiple. They are typically covered by granulation tissue and slough. The ulcers are shallow but have an indurated texture and irregular thickening of mucosa at the edges is a potential cause of clinical confusion with carcinoma.

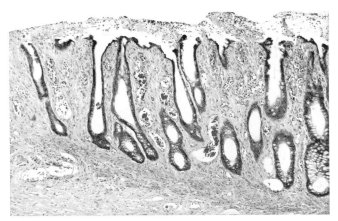

Figure 34.14 Histology of the edge of a solitary rectal ulcer (proctectomy specimen): there is surface erosion and the crypt epithelium shows regenerative hyperplasia. The lamina propria is fibrosed and contains ectatic blood capillaries. Smooth muscle fibres extend upwards from the muscularis mucosae between the bases of the crypts, which tend to be pinched and pointed.

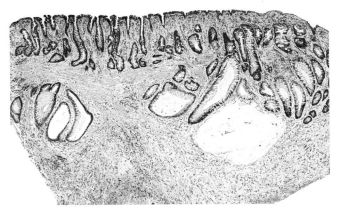

Figure 34.15 Solitary rectal ulcer syndrome: in this case there is misplacement of mucus-containing glands into the submucosa with the formation of cysts. The appearance is sometimes called 'colitis cystica profunda'.

can give the false impression of invasive carcinoma. Additional features include superficial mucosal erosion, irregularity of the crypts with serrated changes in the epithelium [150] and depletion of goblet cells. Occasionally the lesion becomes covered by a mass of exuberant granulation tissue, giving rise to a 'cap' polyp or, rarely, multiple polyps [151] (see Chapter 37).

When an ulcer is present it is invariably superficial and never penetrates beyond the submucosa. Its floor is covered by necrotic cells overlying organising granulation tissue. In some cases there is misplacement of mucus-filled glands lined by normal colonic epithelium into the submucosa at the edge of the ulcer, another feature that may be mistaken for adenocarcinoma (Figure 34.15). This appearance

has been described under a variety of names such as 'localised colitis cystica profunda' (not to be confused with the diffuse condition also given this name – see Chapter 35) [152], hamartomatous inverted polyp of the rectum [153] and enterogenous cyst [154]. Thickening of the media and even fibrinoid necrosis of submucosal blood vessels have been reported in occasional biopsies [146]. Finally, in resection specimens, histological examination may reveal fibrosis of the submucosa and thickening of the muscularis propria [155].

The pathogenesis of the solitary ulcer syndrome has become clearer in recent years. There is now little doubt that mucosal prolapse during excessive straining at stool is the primary abnormality, with superadded trauma and ischaemia eventually leading to ulceration [146,150]. The excessive straining that results in the mucosal prolapse is seen as an attempted response to overcome an abnormality of the pelvic floor musculature during defecation, notably in the puborectalis muscle and the external anal sphincter, which undergo inappropriate contraction rather than relaxation during straining [156]. Repeated trauma of the prolapsing mucosa against the contracting puborectalis muscle and mucosal ischaemia, caused by the high intrarectal pressures necessary for voiding, act synergistically to cause mucosal damage and eventually lead to ulceration [157, 158]. Similar prolapse of the anterior rectal mucosa, but usually without ulceration, occurs in the so-called descending perineum syndrome, a condition in which there is 'descent' of the perineum with loss of the normal anorectal angle during straining at stool [159]. There may also be incontinence. Affected patients, women more commonly than men, give a long history of abnormal straining. The descending perineum syndrome differs from the solitary ulcer syndrome in that, instead of overactivity of the puborectalis muscle or the anal sphincter, there is denervation of the pelvic floor musculature that can often be demonstrated histochemically. This may be due to a traction neuropathy of the pudendal or perineal nerves secondary to the excessive straining, or it may result from damage at childbirth or some other pelvic injury.

Intussusception and complete rectal prolapse

Colonic intussusception is a relatively uncommon condition that is most frequent in the early years of life. In adults it is usually secondary to a polypoid tumour, either benign or malignant [160,161]; in the neonatal period no cause is usually found whereas in older children there is frequently a coexisting viral-type illness that may lead to mesenteric lymphadenopathy (see Chapter 19). There are three main varieties: caeco-colic, colo-colic and sigmoido-rectal. When intussusception occurs it is usually in a distal direction, although retrograde intussusception of the colon has been described [162].

Caeco-colic intussusception is very rare, except in areas of Africa where it is the most common type of all intussusceptions and often lacks a demonstrable underlying cause [163,164]. Caeco-colic intussusception has also been reported after an appendicectomy due to oedema and inflammation of the appendix stump [165].

Colo-colic intussusception and sigmoido-rectal intussusception are almost always caused by a tumour [166]. Of the benign tumours, lipoma is the most common but smooth muscle tumours and villous adenomas have also been reported. Of the malignant tumours, adenocarcinoma is the usual cause. Sigmoido-rectal intussusception is less common than the colo-colic variety.

Complete rectal prolapse through the anal sphincter is essentially an anterograde intussusception of the rectal wall that usually begins at a circular fold 60–80mm above the dentate line [167,168]. It is seen mainly in young children aged up to 3 years and in elderly nulliparous women. In children it is usually precipitated by alteration in bowel habit, either diarrhoea or constipation, and resolves without any specific treatment [169]. The aetiology in elderly women is, however, quite different. Affected patients often give a long history of straining at stool, mucous diarrhoea and anal incontinence. Laxity of the external anal sphincter and pelvic floor musculature is thought to be an important predisposing factor. In some patients there is histochemical evidence of denervation of the external sphincter [170]. The condition appears to be related to the descending perineum syndrome (see above), and it would appear that sometimes an initial mucosal prolapse leads first to rectal intussusception (internal procidentia) and later to prolapse of the full thickness of the rectal wall through the anal sphincter, to produce complete rectal prolapse.

Trauma

Traumatic perforation of the colon or rectum is caused by knife and bullet wounds as well as blast injury and blunt trauma to the abdominal wall, pelvis or perineum [171,172]. Large intestinal perforation, especially of the rectosigmoid region, is a well recognised complication of endoscopy, barium enema and CT colonography [173,174]. In addition, there are rare reports of diathermy for colonoscopic polypectomy leading to explosive rupture of the colon due to the ignition of flammable gases, chiefly hydrogen, which are produced by the bacterial fermentation of non-absorbed carbohydrates [175]. For this reason mannitol, itself a non-absorbed carbohydrate, is no longer recommended for bowel preparation for colonoscopy if electrosurgery is to be used. Impalement injury to the rectum and perineum is uncommon, but is most frequently reported after a fall, especially in farm labourers, building workers and children [176–178]. The placing of fireworks in the region of the anus can also have dramatic effects. There is one bizarre report of a patient who exploded a firework in his own rectum, causing laceration of the rectal wall [179]. There are reports of colonic perforation after seat-belt injury at road traffic accidents [180], and of severe perineal, anal and rectal lacerations after the insertion of a hand, fist or even the whole forearm into the rectum [181].

Spontaneous rupture of the colon in adults and children can occur. In adults it appears to be largely in the setting of pre-existing constipation or stercoral ulceration, excessive straining at stool and the taking of alkalis [182,183]. The sigmoid colon is the most common site; perforation of the right colon is rare [184]. Cases have been reported in association with Ehlers–Danlos syndrome [185]. In children with cystic fibrosis, the meconium plug syndrome (see 'Mucoviscidosis', Chapter 18) is a possible cause [186]. Gross pneumo-peritoneum with extensive surgical emphysema is a rare complication of colonic perforation [187].

Foreign bodies

Most swallowed foreign bodies pass through the gastrointestinal tract without complications but fish, chicken and meat bones seem to be particularly dangerous [188]. Metallic foreign bodies such as coins, safety pins and nails are relatively harmless. There is experimental evidence that soft, malleable objects are more likely to give rise to complications than hard objects [189]. When foreign bodies are found in surgical specimens or in the faeces they are often surrounded by a globular mass of mucus.

The two main complications caused by foreign bodies are perforation and obstruction, both of which occur more frequently in the small bowel than in the colon and rectum. Symptoms are most common when the foreign body becomes impacted in a segment of diseased bowel, usually in patients with diverticulosis [190] or carcinoma [191]. Pericolic abscess formation due to foreign body perforation can be the mode of presentation. Recent advances in endoscopic stenting have given rise to cases where colonic stents used for the palliation of colonic cancer or biliary stents, which have migrated to the colon, have produced complications, notably in the rectosigmoid region, including perforation [192].

Obstruction due to food is not uncommon in the small intestine, but we have never seen this in the large bowel. Calculi of varying types may occasionally become impacted in the colon. These may be gallstones, true enteric stones composed of bile salts or minerals formed within the small intestine when there is stasis (as in diverticula), or false stones such as bezoars or calcified faecoliths [190,193]. Faecal masses may become so large and hard that they cause obstruction of the distal large bowel [194].

There are numerous case reports describing a wide variety of objects that have been inserted into the rectum accidentally or deliberately [195,196,197–200]. When insertion is deliberate, the array of causes includes sexual gratification, underlying mental health problems and smuggling drugs such as cocaine ('back-packing') [201]. Occasionally an individual may be driven to introduce a foreign body in order to obtain relief of severe symptoms referable to the anus or rectum. The variety of objects inserted is almost equalled by the ingenious methods that have been devised for their removal [200]. Complications include intestinal obstruction, laceration, pressure necrosis of the bowel wall and perforation, sometimes with fatal consequences. The discharge of fetal bones per rectum has been reported on a number of occasions [202].

References

1. Pemberton JJ, Black BM, Maino CR. Progress in the surgical management of diverticulitis of the sigmoid colon. *Surg Gynecol Obstet* 1947;**85**:523.
2. Smith CC, Christensen WR. The incidence of colonic diverticulosis. *Am J Roentgenol Radium Ther Nucl Med* 1959;**82**:996.
3. Manousos ON, Truelove SC, Lumsden K. Prevalence of colonic diverticulosis in general population of the Oxford area. *BMJ* 1967;**3i**:762.
4. Eastwood MA, Sanderson J, Pocock SJ, Mitchel WD. Variation in the incidence of diverticular disease within the City of Edinburgh. *Gut* 1977;**18**:571.
5. Kang JY, Dhar A, Pollock R, et al. Diverticular disease of the colon : ethnic differences in frequency. *Aliment Pharmacol Ther* 2004;**19**:765.
6. Kocour EJ. Diverticulosis of the colon: its incidence in 7000 consecutive autopsies with reference to its complications. *Am J Surg* 1937;**37**:433.
7. Hughes LE. Post-mortem survey of diverticular disease of the colon. Part 1. Diverticulosis and diverticulitis. *Gut* 1969;**10**:336.
8. Lee YS. Diverticular disease of the large bowel in Singapore. An autopsy survey. *Dis Colon Rectum* 1986;**29**:330.
9. Eide TJ, Stalsberg H. Diverticular disease of the large intestine in Northern Norway. *Gut* 1979;**20**:609.
10. Kyle J, Davidson AI. The changing pattern of hospital admission for diverticular disease of the colon. *Br J Surg* 1975;**62**:537.
11. Kang JY, Hoare J, Tinto A, et al. Diverticular disease of the colon – on the rise: a study of hospital admissions in England between 1989/1990 and 1999/2000. *Aliment Pharmacol Ther* 2003;**17**:1189.
12. Hjern F, Johansson C, Mellgren A, Baxter NN, Hjern A. Diverticular disease and migration – the influence of acculturation to a Western lifestyle on diverticular disease. *Aliment Pharmacol Ther* 2007;**23**:797.
13. Kyle J, Adesola AO, Tinckler LF, de Baeux J. Incidence of diverticulitis. *Scand J Gastroenterol* 1967;**2**:77.
14. Humes DJ, Solaymani-Dodaran M, Fleming KM, Simpson J, Spiller RC, West J. A population-based study of perforated diverticular disease incidence and associated mortality. *Gastroenterology* 2009;**136**:1198.
15. Kim EH. Hiatus hernia and diverticulosis of the colon: their low incidence in Korea. *N Engl J Med* 1964;**271**:764.
16. Pan C-Z, Liu TH, Chen MZ, Chang HC. Diverticular disease of colon in China: a 60-year retrospective study. *Chinese Med J* 1984;**97**:391.
17. Segal I, Solomon A, Hunt JA. Emergence of diverticular disease in the urban South African black. *Gastroenterology* 1977;**72**:215.
18. Levy N, Stermer E, Simon J. The changing epidemiology of diverticular disease in Israel. *Dis Colon Rectum* 1985;**28**:477.
19. Slack WW. The anatomy, pathology and some clinical features of diverticulosis of the colon. *Br J Surg* 1962;**50**:185.
20. Watt J, Marcus R. The pathology of diverticulosis of the intertaenial area of the pelvic colon. *J Pathol Bacteriol* 1964;**88**:97.
21. Morson BC. The muscle abnormality in diverticular disease of the sigmoid colon. *Br J Radiol* 1963;**36**:385.
22. Hughes LE. Post-mortem survey of diverticular disease of the colon. Part II. The muscle abnormality in the sigmoid colon. *Gut* 1969;**10**:344.
23. Parks TG. Post-mortem studies of the colon with special reference to diverticular disease. *Proc R Soc Med* 1968;**61**:932.
24. Williams I. Changing emphasis in diverticular disease of the colon. *Br J Radiol* 1963;**36**:393.
25. Fleischner FG, Ming SC, Henken EM. Revised concepts on diverticular disease of the colon. *Radiology* 1964;**83**:859;**84**:599.
26. Williams I. Diverticular disease of the colon without diverticula. *Radiology* 1967;**89**:401.
27. Cassano C, Torsoli A. Idiopathic muscular strictures of the colon. *Gut* 1968;**9**:325.
28. Slack WW. Bowel muscle in diverticular disease. *Gut* 1966;**7**:668.
29. Whiteway J, Morson BC. Elastosis in diverticular disease of the sigmoid colon. *Gut* 1985;**26**:258.
30. Gore S, Shepherd NA, et al. Endoscopic crescentic fold disease of the sigmoid colon: the clinical and histopathological spectrum of a distinctive endoscopic appearance. *Int J Colorectal Dis* 1992;**7**:76.
31. Makapugay LM, Dean PJ. Diverticular disease-associated chronic colitis. *Am J Surg Pathol* 1996;**20**:94.
32. Mulhall AM, Mahid SS, Petras RE, Galandiuk S. Diverticular disease associated with inflammatory bowel disease-like colitis: a systematic review. *Dis Colon Rectum* 2009;**52**:1072.
33. Kelly JK. Polypoid prolapsing mucosal folds in diverticular disease. *Am J Surg Pathol* 1991;**15**:871.
34. Tendler DA, Aboudola S, Zacks JF, O'Brien MJ, Kelly CP. Prolapsing mucosal polyps: an under recognized form of colonic polyp – a clinicopathological study of 15 cases. *Am J Gastroenterol* 2002;**97**:370.
35. Nakamura S, Kino I, Akagi T. Inflammatory myoglandular polyps of the colon and rectum. A clinicopathological study of 32 pedunculated polyps, distinct from other types of polyps. *Am J Surg Pathol* 1992;**16**:772.
36. Hughes LE. Complications of diverticular disease: inflammation, obstruction, and haemorrhage. *Clin Gastroenterol* 1975;**4**:147.
37. Hart AR, Kennedy HJ, Stebbings WS, Day NE. How frequently do large bowel diverticula perforate? An incidence and cross-sectional study. *Eur J Gastroenterol Hepatol* 2000;**12**:661.
38. Morson BC. The muscle abnormality in diverticular disease of the colon. *Proc R Soc Med* 1963;**56**:798.
39. Meyers MA, Alonso DR, Gray GF, Baer JW. Pathogenesis of bleeding diverticulosis. *Gastroenterology* 1976;**71**:577.
40. Casarella WJ, Kanter IE, Seaman WB. Right-sided colonic diverticula as a cause of acute rectal haemorrhage. *N Engl J Med* 1972;**286**:450.
41. Barnert J, Messmann H. Diagnosis and management of lower gastrointestinal bleeding. *Nat Rev Gastroenterol Hepatol* 2009;**6**:637.
42. Welch CE, Athanasoulis CA, Galdabini JJ. Haemorrhage from the large bowel with special reference to angiodysplasia and diverticular disease. *World J Surg* 1978;**2**:73.
43. Melchior S, Cudovic D, Jones J, Thomas C, Gillitzer R, Thüroff J. Diagnosis and surgical management of colovesical fistulas due to sigmoid diverticulitis. *J Urol* 2009;**182**:978.

44. Colcock BP, Stahman FD. Fistulas complicating diverticular disease of the sigmoid colon. *Ann Surg* 1972;**175**:838.

45. Wilson RG, Smith AN, Macintyre IM. Complications of diverticular disease and non-steroidal anti-inflammatory drugs: a prospective study. *Br J Surg* 1990;**77**:1103.

46. Teague RH, Thornton JR, Manning AP, Salmon PR, Read AE. Colonoscopy for investigation of unexplained rectal bleeding. *Lancet* 1978;**i**:1350.

47. Gledhill A, Dixon MF. Crohn's-like reaction in diverticular disease. *Gut* 1998;**42**:392.

48. Burroughs S, Bowrey DJ, Morris-Stiff GJ, Williams GT. Granulomatous inflammation in sigmoid diverticulitis: two diseases or one? *Histopathology* 1998;**33**:349.

49. Shepherd NA. Diverticular disease and chronic idiopathic inflammatory bowel disease: associations and masquerades. *Gut* 1996;**38**:801.

50. Meyers MA, Alonso DR, Morson BC, Bartram C. Pathogenesis of diverticulitis complicating granulomatous colitis. *Gastroenterology* 1978;**74**:24.

51. Strate LL, Liu YL, Aldoori WH, Syngal S, Giovannucci EL. Obesity increases the risks of diverticulitis and diverticular bleeding. *Gastroenterology* 2009;**136**:115.

52. Beighton PH, Murdoch JL, Votteler T. Gastrointestinal complications of the Ehlers–Danlos syndrome. *Gut* 1969;**10**:1004.

53. Wess L, Eastwood MA, Wess TJ, Busuttil A, Miller A. Cross linking of collagen is increased in colonic diverticulosis. *Gut* 1995;**37**:91.

54. Smith AN. Colonic muscle in diverticular disease. *Clin Gastroenterol* 1986;**15**:917.

55. Parks TG, Connell AM. Motility studies in diverticular disease of the colon. *Gut* 1969;**10**:538.

56. Arfwidsson S. Pathogenesis of multiple diverticula of the sigmoid colon in diverticular disease. *Arch Chir Scand Suppl* 1964;**342**:5.

57. Painter NS, Truelove SC. The intraluminal pressure patterns in diverticulosis. *Gut* 1964;**5**:201.

58. Taylor I, Duthie HL. Bran tablets and diverticular disease. *BMJ* 1976;**i**:988.

59. Weinreich J, Andersen D. Intraluminal pressure in the sigmoid colon. II. Patients with sigmoid diverticula and related conditions. *Scand J Gastroenterol* 1976;**11**:581.

60. Painter NS, Truelove SC, Ardran GM, Tuckery M. Segmentation and the localization of intraluminal pressures in the human colon, with special reference to the pathogenesis of colonic diverticula. *Gastroenterology* 1965;**49**:169.

61. Golder M, Burleigh DE, Belai A, et al. Smooth muscle cholinergic denervation hypersensitivity in diverticular disease. *Lancet* 2003;**361**:1945.

62. Tomita R, Tanjoh K, Fujisaki S, Fukuzawa M. Physiological studies on nitric oxide in the right sided colon of patients with diverticular disease. *Hepatogastroenterology* 1999;**46**:2839.

63. Golder M, Burleigh DE, Ghali L, et al. Longitudinal muscle shows abnormal relaxation responses to nitric oxide and contains altered levels of NOS1 and elastin in uncomplicated diverticular disease. *Colorectal Dis* 2007;**9**:218.

64. Painter NS, Burkitt DP. Diverticular disease of the colon: a deficiency disease of Western civilization. *BMJ* 1971;**2**:450

65. Aldoori WH, Giovannucci EL, et al. A prospective study of dietary fiber types and symptomatic diverticular disease in men. *J Nutr* 1998;**128**:714.

66. Manousos O, Day NE, Tzonou A, et al. Diet and other factors in the aetiology of diverticulosis: an epidemiological study in Greece. *Gut* 1985;**26**:544.

67. Gear JSS, Ware A, Fursdon P, et al. Symptomless diverticular disease and intake of dietary fibre. *Lancet* 1979;**i**:511.

68. Ohi G, Minowa K, Oyama T, et al. Changes in dietary fiber intake among Japanese in the 20th century: a relationship to the prevalence of diverticular disease. *Am J Clin Nutr* 1983;**38**:115.

69. Berry CS, Fearn T, Fisher N, Gregory JA, Hardy J. Dietary fibre and prevention of diverticular disease of the colon: evidence from rats. *Lancet* 1984;**ii**:294.

70. Painter NS, Almeida AZ, Colebourne KW. Unprocessed bran in treatment of diverticular disease of the colon. *BMJ* 1972;**ii**:137.

71. Findlay JM, Smith AN, Mitchell WD, Anderson JB, Eastwood MA. Effect of unprocessed bran on colon function in normal subjects and in diverticular disease. *Lancet* 1974;**i**:146.

72. Commane DM, Arasaradnam RP, Mills S, Mathers JC, Bradburn M. Diet, ageing and genetic factors in the pathogenesis of diverticular disease. *World J Gastroenterol* 2009;**15**:2479.

73. Peck DA, Labat R, Waite VC. Diverticular disease of the right colon. *Dis Colon Rectum* 1968;**11**:49.

74. Sugihara K, Muto T, Morioka Y, Asano A, Yamamoto T. Diverticular disease of the colon in Japan. *Dis Colon Rectum* 1984;**27**:531.

75. Nakaji S, Danjo K, Munakata A, et al. Comparison of etiology of right-sided diverticula in Japan with that of left-sided diverticula in the West. *Int J Colorectal Dis* 2002;**17**:365.

76. Sugihara K, Muto T, Morioka Y. Motility study in right-sided diverticular disease of the colon. *Gut* 1983;**24**:1130.

77. Williams KL. Acute solitary ulcers and acute diverticulitis of the caecum and ascending colon. *Br J Surg* 1960;**47**:351.

78. Chaudhary NA, Truelove SC. The irritable bowel syndrome. A study of the clinical features, predisposing causes and prognosis in 130 cases. *Q J Med* 1962;**31**:307.

79. Olden KW. Diagnosis of irritable bowel syndrome. *Gastroenterology* 2002;**122**:1701.

80. McKendrick MW, Read NW. Irritable bowel syndrome – post salmonella infection. *J Infection* 1994;**29**:1.

81. Rodriguez LAG, Ruigomez A. Increased risk of irritable bowel syndrome after bacterial gastroenteritis: cohort study. *BMJ* 1999;**318**:565.

82. Wang L-H, Fang X-C, Pan G-Z. Bacillary dysentery as a causative factor of irritable bowel syndrome and its pathogenesis. *Gut* 2004;**53**:1096.

83. Neal KR, Hebden J, Spiller R. Prevalence of gastrointestinal symptoms six months after bacterial gastroenteritis and risk factors for development of the irritable bowel syndrome: postal survey of patients. *BMJ* 1997;**314**:779.

84. Spiller RC, Jenkins D, Thornley JP, et al. Increased rectal mucosal enteroendocrine cells, T lymphocytes, and increased gut permeability following acute *Campylobacter* enteritis and in post-dysenteric irritable bowel syndrome. *Gut* 2000;**47**:804.

85. Harvey RF, Mauad EC, Brown AM. Prognosis in the irritable bowel syndrome: a 5-year prospective study. *Lancet* 1987;**i**:963.

86. Gwee KA, Leong YL, Graham C, et al. The role of psychological and biological factors in postinfective gut dysfunction. *Gut* 1999;**44**:400.

87. Jung H, Choung RS, Locke GR III, Schleck CD, Zinsmeister AR, Talley NJ. Diarrhea-predominant irritable bowel syndrome is associated with diverticular disease: a population-based study. *Am J Gastroenterol* 2010 ;**105**:652.

88. Kirsch RH, Riddell R. Histopathological alterations in irritable bowel syndrome. *Mod Pathol* 2006;**19**:1638.

89. Barnes PRH, Lennard-Jones JE, Hawley PR, Todd IP. Hirschsprung's disease and idiopathic megacolon in adults and adolescents. *Gut* 1986;**27**:534.

90. Lembo A, Camilleri M. Chronic constipation. *N Engl J Med* 2003;**349**:1360.

91. Preston DM, Lennard-Jones JE. Severe chronic constipation of young women: 'idiopathic slow transit constipation'. *Gut* 1986;**27**:41.

92. Knowles CH, Scott M, Lunniss PJ. Outcome of colectomy for slow transit constipation. *Ann Surg* 1999;**230**:627.

93. Kamm MA, Hoyle CHV, Burleigh DE, et al. Hereditary internal anal sphincter myopathy causing proctalgia fugax and constipation: a newly identified condition. *Gastroenterology* 1991;**100**:805.

94. Turnbull GK, Lennard-Jones JE, Bartram CI. Failure of rectal expulsion as a cause of constipation: why fibre and laxatives sometimes fail. *Lancet* 1986;**i**:767.

95. Glia A, Akerlund JE, Lindberg G. Outcome of colectomy for slow-transit constipation in relation to presence of small-bowel dysmotility. *Dis Colon Rectum* 2004;**47**:96.

96. Krishnamurthy S, Schuffler MD, Rohrmann CA, Pope CE. Severe idiopathic constipation is associated with a distinctive abnormality of the colonic myenteric plexus. *Gastroenterology* 1985;**88**:26.

97. Wedel T, Spiegler J, Söllner S, et al. Interstitial cells of Cajal and the enteric nervous system are concomitantly altered in patients with slow transit constipation and megacolon. *Gastroenterology* 2002;**123**:1459.

98. Bassotti G, Villanacci V, Maurer CA, et al. The role of glial cells and apoptosis of enteric neurons in the neuropathology of intractable slow transit constipation. *Gut* 2006;**55**:41.

99. Krishnamurthy S, Schuffler MD. Pathology of neuromuscular disorders of the small intestine and colon. *Gastroenterology* 1987;**93**:610.

100. Knowles CH, De Giorgio R, Kapur RP, et al. The London Classification of gastrointestinal neuromuscular pathology: report on behalf of the Gastro 2009 International Working Group. *Gut* 2010;**59**:882.

101. Gattuso JM, Kamm MA. Clinical features of idiopathic megarectum and idiopathic megacolon. *Gut* 1997;**41**:93.

102. Gattuso JM, Kamm MA, Talbot IC. Pathology of idiopathic megarectum and megacolon. *Gut* 1997;**41**:252.

103. De Giorgio R, Knowles CH. Acute colonic pseudo-obstruction. *Br J Surg* 2009;**96**:229.

104. Mitros FA, Schuffler MD, Teja K, Anuras S. Pathologic features of familial visceral myopathy. *Hum Pathol* 1982;**13**:825.

105. Fitzgibbons PL, Chandrasoma PT. Familial visceral myopathy. Evidence of diffuse involvement of intestinal smooth muscle. *Am J Surg Pathol* 1987;**11**:846.

106. Ruuska TH, Karikoski R, Smith VV, Milla PJ. Acquired myopathic pseudo-obstruction may be due to an autoimmune enteric leiomyositis. *Gastroenterology* 2002;**122**:1133.

107. Kleckner FS. Dermatomyositis and its manifestations in the gastrointestinal tract. *Am J Gastroenterol* 1970;**53**:141.

108. Poirier TJ, Rankin GB. Gastrointestinal manifestations of progressive systemic scleroderma based on a review of 364 cases. *Am J Gastroenterol* 1972;**58**:30.

109. Schuffler MD, Beegle RG. Progressive systemic sclerosis of the gastrointestinal tract and hereditary hollow visceral myopathy: two distinguishable disorders of intestinal smooth muscle. *Gastroenterology* 1979;**77**:664.

110. Pruzanski W, Huvos AG. Smooth muscle involvement in primary muscle disease. I. Myotonic dystrophy. *Arch Pathol* 1967;**83**:229.

111. Huvos AG, Pruzanski W. Smooth muscle involvement in primary muscle disease. II. Progressive muscular dystrophy. *Arch Pathol* 1967;**82**:234.

112. Ebert EC, Nagar M. Gastrointestinal manifestations of amyloidosis. *Am J Gastroenterol* 2008;**103**:776.

113. Smith B. The neuropathology of pseudo-obstruction of the intestine. *Scand J Gastroenterol* 1982;**17**(suppl 71):103.

114. Knowles CH, Nickols CD, Feakins R, et al. Smooth muscle denervation in humans is associated with inclusion body formation in the gastrointestinal tract. *J Pathol* 2001;**193**:390.

115. Feinstat T, Tesluk H, Schuffler MD, et al. Megacolon and neurofibromatosis: a neuronal intestinal dysplasia. *Gastroenterology* 1984;**86**:1573.

116. Carney JA, Go VLW, Sizemore GW, Hayles AB. Alimentary-tract ganglioneuromatosis: a major component of the syndrome of multiple endocrine neoplasia, Type 2b. *N Engl J Med* 1976;**295**:1287.

117. Shekitka KM, Sobin LH. Ganglioneuromas of the gastrointestinal tract. Relation to von Recklinghausen disease and other multiple tumor syndromes. *Am J Surg Pathol* 1994;**18**:250.

118. Schuffler MD, Bird TD, Sumi SM, Cook A. A familial neuronal disease presenting as intestinal pseudoobstruction. *Gastroenterology* 1978;**75**:889.

119. Kapur RP, Robertson SP, Hannibal MC, et al. Diffuse abnormal layering of small intestinal smooth muscle is present in patients with *FLNA* mutations and X-linked intestinal pseudo-obstruction. *Am J Surg Pathol* 2010;**34**:1528.

120. Todd IP, Porter NH, Morson BC, Smith B, Friedmann CA, Neal RA. Chagas' disease of the colon and rectum. *Gut* 1969;**10**:1009.

121. Martins-Campos IV, Tafuri WL. Chagas' enteropathy. *Gut* 1973;**14**:910.

122. Sonsino E, Mouy R, Foucaud P, et al. Intestinal pseudoobstruction related to cytomegalovirus infection of myenteric plexus. *N Engl J Med* 1984;**311**:196.

123. Debinski HS, Kamm MA, Talbot IC, Khan G, Kangro HO, Jeffries DJ. DNA viruses in the pathogenesis of sporadic chronic idiopathic intestinal pseudo-obstruction. *Gut* 1997;**41**:100.

124. Schuffler MD, Baird HW, Fleming CR, et al. Intestinal pseudo-obstruction as the presenting manifestation of small cell carcinoma of the lung: a paraneoplastic neuropathy of the gastrointestinal tract. *Ann Intern Med* 1983;**98**:129.

125. Berenyi MR, Schwartz GS. Megasigmoid syndrome in diabetes and neurologic disease. *Am J Gastroenterol* 1967;**47**:311.

126. Bacharach T, Evans JR. Enlargement of the colon secondary to hypothyroidism. *Ann Intern Med* 1957;**47**:121.

127. Watkins GL, Oliver GA, Rosenberg BF. Giant megacolon in the insane. *Ann Surg* 1961;**153**:409.

128. Smith B. Pathology of cathartic colon. *Proc R Soc Med* 1972;**65**:288.

129. Gattuso JM, Kamm MA. Adverse effects of drugs used in the management of constipation and diarrhoea. *Drug Saf* 1994;**10**:47.

130. Muller-Lissner S. What has happened to the cathartic colon? *Gut* 1996;**39**:486.

131. Schäppi MG, Smith VV, Milla PJ, Lindley KJ. Eosinophilic myenteric ganglionitis is associated with functional intestinal obstruction. *Gut* 2003;**52**:752.

132. Smith VV, Gregson N, Foggensteiner L, Neale G, Milla PJ. Acquired intestinal aganglionosis and circulating autoantibodies without neoplasia or other neural involvement. *Gastroenterology* 1997;**112**:1366.

133. Lu B, Luquetti AO, Rassi A, Pereira Perrin M. Autoantibodies to neurotrophic receptors TrkA, TrkB and TrkC in patients with acute Chagas' disease. *Scand J Immunol* 2010;**71**:220.

134. Ballantyne GH, Brandner MD, Beart RW, Ilstrup DM. Volvulus of the colon: Incidence and mortality. *Ann Surg* 1985;**202**:83.

135. Dowling BL, Gunning AJ. Caecal volvulus. *Br J Surg* 1969;**56**:124.

136. Consorti ET, Liu TH. Diagnosis and treatment of caecal volvulus. *Postgrad Med J* 2005;**81**:772.

137. Sutcliffe MML. Volvulus of the sigmoid colon. *Br J Surg* 1968;**55**:903.

138. Nuhu A, Jah A. Acute sigmoid volvulus in a West African population. *Ann Afr Med* 2010;**9**:86.

139. Frisancho O. Dolichomegacolon of the Andes and intestinal volvulus due to altitude. *Rev Gastroenterol Peru* 2008;**28**:248.

140. Delafield RH, Hellreigel K, Meza A, Urteaga O. Sigmoid volvulus. *Rev Gastroenterol* 1953;**20**:29.

141. Khoury GA, Pickard R, Knight M. Volvulus of the sigmoid colon. *Br J Surg* 1977;**64**:587.

142. Hughes LE. Sigmoid volvulus. *J R Soc Med* 1980;**73**:78.

143. Gillon J, Holt S, Sircus W. Pneumatosis coli and sigmoid volvulus: a report of four cases. *Br J Surg* 1979;**66**:802.

144. Northeast ADR, Dennison AR, Lee EG. Sigmoid volvulus: new thoughts on the epidemiology. *Dis Colon Rectum* 1984;**27**:260.

145. Machado NO. Ileosigmoid knot: A case report and literature review of 280 cases. *Ann Saudi Med* 2009;**29**:402.

146. DuBoulay CEH, Fairbrother J, Isaacson PG. Mucosal prolapse syndrome – a unifying concept for solitary ulcer syndrome and related disorders. *J Clin Pathol* 1983;**36**:1264.

147. Rosen Y, Vaillant JG, Yermakov V. Submucosal mucous cysts at a colostomy site: relationship to colitis cystica profunda and report of a case. *Dis Colon Rectum* 1976;**19**:453.

148. Rutter KRP, Riddell RH. The solitary ulcer syndrome of the rectum. *Clin Gastroenterol* 1975;**4**:505.

149. Madigan MR, Morson BC. Solitary ulcer of the rectum. *Gut* 1969;**10**:871.

150. Franzin G, Scarpa A, Dina R, Novelli P. 'Transitional' and hyperplastic-metaplastic mucosa occurring in solitary ulcer of the rectum. *Histopathology* 1981;**5**:527.

151. Brosens LAA, Montgomery EA, Bhagavan BS, Offerhaus GJA, Giardello FM. Mucosal prolapse syndrome presenting as rectal polyps. *J Clin Pathol* 2009;**62**:1034.

152. Epstein SE, Ascari WQ, Ablow RC, Seaman WB, Lattes R. Colitis cystica profunda. *Am J Clin Pathol* 1966;**45**:186.

153. Allen MS. Hamartomatous inverted polyps of the rectum. *Cancer* 1954;**19**:257.

154. Talerman A. Enterogenous cysts of the rectum. *Br J Surg* 1971;**58**:643.

155. Kang YS, Kamm MA, Engel AF, et al. Pathology of the rectal wall in solitary rectal ulcer syndrome and complete rectal prolapse. *Gut* 1996;**38**:587.

156. Rutter KRP. Electromyographic changes in certain pelvic floor abnormalities. *Proc R Soc Med* 1974;**67**:53.

157. Womack NR, Williams NS, Holmfield JHM, Morrison JFB. Pressure and prolapse – the cause of solitary rectal ulceration. *Gut* 1987;**28**:1228.

158. Rutter KRP. Solitary rectal ulcer syndrome. *Proc R Soc Med* 1975;**68**:22.

159. Parks AG, Porter NH, Hardcastle JD. The syndrome of the descending perineum. *Proc R Soc Med* 1966;**59**:477.

160. Dick A, Green GJ. Large bowel intussusception in adults. *Br J Radiol* 1961;**34**:769.

161. Bond MR, Roberts JBM. Intussusception in the adult. *Br J Surg* 1964;**51**:818.

162. Joseph T, Desai AL. Retrograde intussusception of sigmoid colon. *J R Soc Med* 2004;**97**:127.

163. Cole GJ. Caeco-colic intussusception in Ibadan. *Br J Surg* 1966;**53**:415.

164. Richards RC, Richards RC. Idiopathic caeco-caecal intussusception. *Am J Surg* 1966;**112**:641.

165. Levis CD. Caeco-colic intussusception following appendicectomy. *BMJ* 1958;**ii**:550.

166. Davidson JRM. Sigmoido-rectal intussusception. *Aust N Z J Surg* 1966;**36**:13.

167. Broden B, Snellman B. Procidentia of the rectum studied with cineradiography: a contribution to the discussion of causative mechanisms. *Dis Colon Rectum* 1968;**11**:330.

168. Ihre T, Seligson U. Intussusception of the rectum – internal procidentia: treatment and results in 90 patients. *Dis Colon Rectum* 1975;**18**:391.

169. Corman ML. Rectal prolapse in children. *Dis Colon Rectum* 1985;**28**:535.

170. Parks AG, Swash M, Urich H. Sphincter denervation in anorectal incontinence and rectal prolapse. *Gut* 1977;**18**:656.

171. Roof WR, Morris GC, DeBakey ME. Management of perforating injuries to the colon in civilian practice. *Am J Surg* 1960;**99**:641.

172. Vertrees A, Wakefield M, Pickett C, Greer L, Wilson A, Gillern. S. Outcomes of primary repair and primary anastomosis in war-related colon injuries. *J Trauma* 2009;**66**:1286.

173. Lüning TH, Keemers-Gels ME, Barendregt WB, Tan AC, Rosman C. Colonoscopic perforations: a review of 30366 patients. *Surg Endosc* 2007;**21**:994.

174. Sosna J, Blachar A, Amitai M, et al. Colonic perforation at CT colonography: assessment of risk in a multicenter large cohort. *Radiology* 2006;**239**:457.

175. Bigard MA, Gaucher P, Lasalle C. Fatal colonic explosion during colonoscopic polypectomy. *Gastroenterology* 1979;**77**:1307.

176. Thomas LP. Impalement of the rectum. *Lancet* 1953;**i**:704.

177. Kaufer N, Shein S, Levowitz BS. Impalement injury of the rectum. *Dis Colon Rectum* 1967;**10**:394.

178. Beiler HA, Zachariou Z, Daum R. Impalement and anorectal injuries in childhood: a retrospective study of 12 cases. *J Pediatr Surg* 1998;**33**:1287.

179. Butters AG. An unusual rectal injury. *BMJ* 1955;**i**:602.

180. Shennan J. Seat-belt injuries of the left colon. *Br J Surg* 1973;**60**:673.

181. Shook LL, Whittle R, Rose EF. Rectal fist insertion. An unusual form of sexual behaviour. *Am J Forensic Med Pathol* 1985;**6**:319.

182. Berger PL, Shaw RE. Spontaneous rupture of the colon. *BMJ* 1961;**i**:1422.

183. Dickinson PH, Gilmour J. Spontaneous rupture of the distal large bowel. *Br J Surg* 1961;**49**:157.

184. Shanon DP. Spontaneous rupture of the ascending colon. *Br J Surg* 1962;**50**:199.

185. Sykes EM Jr. Colon perforation in Ehlers–Danlos syndrome. Report of two cases and review of the literature. *Am J Surg* 1984;**147**:410.

186. Thomas CS, Brockman SK. Idiopathic perforation of the colon in infancy. *Ann Surg* 1966;**164**:853.

187. Maw AR. Perforation of the sigmoid colon. *Br J Surg* 1968;**55**:712.

188. Ashby S, Hunter-Craig D. Foreign body perforation of the gut. *Br J Surg* 1967;**54**:382.

189. Harjola PT, Scheinin TM. Experimental observations on intestinal obstruction due to foreign bodies. *Acta Chir Scand* 1963;**126**:144.

190. Pryor JH. Gall-stone obstruction of the sigmoid colon with particular reference to aetiology. *Br J Surg* 1959;**47**:259.

191. Persky L, Frank ED. Foreign body perforation of the gastrointestinal tract. *N Engl J Med* 1952;**246**:223.

192. Namdar T, Raffel AM, Topp SA, et al. Complications and treatment of migrated biliary endoprostheses : a review of the literature. *World J Gastroenterol* 2007;**13**:5397.

193. Atwell JD, Pollock AV. Intestinal calculi. *Br J Surg* 1960;**47**:367.

194. Kaufman SA, Karlin H. Faecaloma of the sigmoid flexure. *Dis Colon Rectum* 1966;**9**:133.

195. Israel GI. An unusual foreign body in the rectum. *Dis Colon Rectum* 1961;**4**:139.

196. Lowicki EM. Accidental introduction of giant foreign body into the rectum. *Ann Surg* 1966;**163**:395.

197. Lockhart-Mummery JP. *Diseases of the Rectum and Colon.* London: Ballière, Tindall & Cox, 1937: 377.

198. Vaughn AM, White MS. Foreign body (drinking glass) in the rectum. *JAMA* 1959;**171**:2307.

199. Fuller RC. Foreign bodies in the rectum and colon. *Dis Colon Rectum* 1965;**8**:123.

200. Eftaiha M, Hambrick E, Abcarian H. Principles of management of colorectal foreign bodies. *Arch Surg* 1977;**112**:691.

201. Beerman R, Nunez D, et al. Radiographic evaluation of the cocaine smuggler. *Gastrointest Radiol* 1986;**11**:351.

202. Barnett VH. Discharge of foetal bones by the rectum. *BMJ* 1951;**ii**:1385.

Inflammatory disorders of the large intestine

Dhanpat Jain,[1] Bryan F. Warren[2] and Robert H. Riddell[3]

[1]Yale University School of Medicine, New Haven, CT, USA
[2]John Radcliffe Hospital, Oxford, UK
[3]Mount Sinai Hospital, Toronto, ON, Canada

Inflammatory disorders are common in the large bowel, sometimes in association with small intestinal disease but more often as primary pathology of the large intestine. The large bowel can be affected focally or diffusely and for varying lengths. Diseased mucosa can usually be visualised and biopsied using rigid procto-sigmoidoscopy, the flexible sigmoidoscope or the colonoscope. Most infections of the large intestine are diagnosed clinically or by microbiological methods and often do not require histological assessment. Bacterial culture of faeces is easy, although not always sensitive, and various parasites can be demonstrated in faeces or mucus on direct microscopy. Nevertheless it is important for pathologists to recognise the histological appearances of these infective colitides, primarily because they can closely mimic the pathology of chronic inflammatory bowel disease. Erroneous treatment with immunosuppressive therapy, e.g. in amoebiasis or strongyloidiasis, can have grave consequences for the patient.

It is therefore important for the histopathologist to be able to differentiate between the histological appearances of infective causes of colitis and those of Crohn's disease and ulcerative colitis. Bacterial infections that mimic chronic inflammatory bowel disease clinically are those that invade the mucosa. The most common of these are those caused by *Clostridium difficile* and *Salmonella*, *Shigella* and *Campylobacter* spp. The pathology of these organisms is often referred to as 'acute self-limiting colitis'. In practice many of the diagnostic difficulties concerning large intestinal inflammatory disorders relate to the distinction between Crohn's disease and ulcerative colitis. To maintain a perspective on the size of this problem, it should be remembered that only in 20–25% of cases of Crohn's disease is the disease limited to the large intestine, although the assessment of the differential diagnosis of chronic inflammatory bowel disease inevitably forms a large part of the workload in a specialised gastrointestinal pathology practice.

Histologically, we try to avoid the use of 'non-specific' when applied to inflammation, because all inflammation is non-specific, and it tends to be a shield to hide behind. 'There is a chronic colitis present' gains nothing if 'non-specific' is added to the statement. In all inflammatory conditions of the colorectum, the art is in the interpretation of the lesions.

Inflammation due to viruses

Although acute gastrointestinal infection is a major cause of morbidity throughout the world and viruses play a leading part in its aetiology, viral infection of the colorectum rarely comes to the attention of the practising histopathologist. In fact, in most acute viral infections of the intestines, the small intestine is the primary seat of infection. For a fuller description of viral infection in the intestines, the interested reader is referred to Chapter 20. In this chapter, only those viral infections with cytopathic effects demonstrable in histopathological sections of colorectal mucosal biopsies are considered.

Adenoviruses

Adenoviruses are most commonly associated with respiratory infection but are also a common cause acute diar-

Morson and Dawson's Gastrointestinal Pathology, Fifth Edition. Edited by Neil A. Shepherd, Bryan F. Warren, Geraint T. Williams, Joel K. Greenson, Gregory Y. Lauwers and Marco R. Novelli.
© 2013 Blackwell Publishing Ltd. Published 2013 by Blackwell Publishing Ltd.

rhoea, especially in outbreaks in children where they are second only as a cause to rotavirus [1]. The incidence has increased due to its occurrence in AIDS and transplant recipients. Among transplant recipients its incidence is highest in bone marrow transplant recipients occurring in about 5–20% of patients, children being more susceptible [2]. For the histopathologist, probably the most important associations are causing lymphoid hyperplasia in the terminal ileum and subsequent intussusception in infants [3]. The virus is also identified in some patients with acute appendicitis. However, its aetiological role in this setting remains unclear [4]. The adenovirus inclusions are intranuclear and eosinophilic with perinuclear halo, similar to herpes virus, and are readily demonstrable in colorectal epithelium by immunohistochemical techniques. The presence of intranuclear inclusions can often be seen on haematoxylin and eosin (H&E) staining, although they are more subtle than herpetic inclusions [5,6]. Sometimes the nuclei appear hyperchromatic and smudgy without obvious inclusions.

Cytomegalovirus

The role of this herpes group virus as a primary colonic pathogen is disputed. Infection is usually subclinical and it is uncertain whether the virus can initiate infection. Apparent documented examples of primary cytomegalovirus (CMV) infection affecting the large bowel are described [7–9] but appear to be rare. In some examples CMV infection appears to have preceded the onset of ulcerative colitis, which raises the suspicion that subclinical disease was already present [10,11], but these cases appear genuine. In patients with pre-existing ulcerative colitis, CMV infection may prevent healing of established ulcers [12].

Most infection is reactivation of latent virus, especially in the setting of immunosuppression or severe ulcerative colitis. Overt CMV disease can develop in patients who are immunologically suppressed, especially in those with AIDS [13,14], or following transplantation. In the colon, the endoscopic or gross appearance is variable and ranges from normal ('incidental') to severe inflammation and ulceration. The most typical presentation is in inflammatory bowel disease, especially ulcerative colitis [15,16], and is associated with ulceration. Ulcers may be minute or up to several centimetres across. The ulcers are discrete and punched out with oedematous margins, in contrast to the usual diffuse appearance of ulcerative colitis.

The diagnosis of CMV infection depends on demonstrating the characteristic nuclear, and sometimes cytoplasmic, inclusions within macrophages or in capillary endothelial cells (Figure 35.1). Less commonly the inclusions can be seen in the colorectal epithelium and other stromal cells including smooth muscle cells. The infected cells are large;

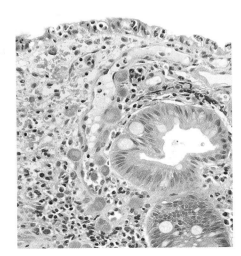

Figure 35.1 Rectal mucosal biopsy from a patient with chronic ulcerative colitis, showing multiple cytomegalovirus inclusions within vascular endothelial cells and some within the lamina propria.

the nuclear inclusion is dark and amphophilic with a perinuclear halo. Basophilic granular cytoplasmic inclusions that are much smaller are seen more often than nuclear inclusions in sections and are diagnostically equally characteristic. CMV inclusions are easily overlooked and the diagnosis should be borne in mind when confronted by large atypical cells in the floor of an ulcer. Immunohistochemical staining with anti-CMV antibody demonstrates clear staining of the inclusions and is a very useful routine stain in patients in whom no definite or occasional smudgy doubtful inclusions are seen in routine sections. *In situ* hybridisation and polymerase chain reaction (PCR)-based assays are also available for routine diagnostic use. However, when complicating severe chronic inflammatory bowel disease, inclusions are usually florid and the significance of occasional inclusions only less clear.

Herpes simplex virus

This DNA virus most often causes a proctitis restricted to the distal 100 mm of the rectum, although primary herpes colitis has also been rarely reported [17]. It is a consequence of unprotected anal intercourse and oral–faecal contact [18]. It is therefore more common in homosexuals and immunosuppressed individuals, including patients with AIDS. Anal fissures may coexist with herpes proctitis [18]. The rectal mucosa may be friable and ulcerated. On microscopy the rectal mucosa shows multinucleate giant cells, intranuclear inclusions and a perivascular lymphocytic infiltrate [19]. Immunohistochemical staining is useful to confirm the diagnosis.

HIV and AIDS in the large intestine

Although enterocolic infection with human immunodeficiency virus (HIV) and AIDS has been covered in Chapter 20, some comments on the disease are appropriate here. Notwithstanding the success of antiviral therapy, notably HAART (highly active anti-retroviral therapy) in controlling the disease and its complications [19,20], the complications of AIDS are still regularly seen by the histopathologist analysing biopsies of the colorectum. HIV infection itself is associated with a characteristic enhanced apoptosis [21]. Such increased apoptotic activity is often closely associated with intra-epithelial T lymphocytes and is typically prominent in crypt bases [5,21]. The features are similar to those seen in graft-versus-host disease. Despite these changes, the colorectal epithelial cells usually appear morphologically and morphometrically normal.

It is the infective complications of HIV infection, especially AIDS, that most often come to the attention of the practising histopathologist. Although the individual infections will be dealt with in the appropriate sections, it is important to note that evidence of viral infection (particularly CMV, herpes simplex virus and adenovirus), bacterial infection (including sexually transmitted bacteria, bacteria causing bacillary colitis and atypical mycobacterial infection), protozoal infection and infections caused by larger organisms may all be seen as a colorectal complication of AIDS [6]. Furthermore, multiplicity of infections is a characteristic feature of AIDS. Identification of one opportunistic infection should always alert the pathologist to the possibility of identifying other organisms in biopsy and resection material [22].

Bacterial infection

Shigellosis

All four *Shigella* spp. (*S. dysenteriae*, *S. flexneri*, *S. boydii* and *S. sonnei*) are pathogenic and only a small number of organisms are required as an infecting dose. Epidemics of bacillary dysentery are a major problem in many developing countries, where there is an association with a high population density as well as conditions of bad sanitation, poor personal hygiene and contaminated food. Shigellosis is seen more commonly in AIDS patients, where the condition may behave somewhat differently from that in the non-immunocompromised host. Along with *Salmonella* and *Campylobacter* spp., *Shigella* spp. may be more difficult to eradicate in the AIDS patient and result in bacteraemia. Due to the higher recurrence rate in AIDS patients, they may require long-term treatment.

The shigella bacterium is a non-motile Gram-negative bacillus. Person-to-person transmission and ingestion of infected food and water are responsible for the infection.

S. sonnei generally causes a more severe colitis than the other species and the mildest colitis is usually seen with *S. dysenteriae*. Toxins are released in the bowel lumen and there is bacterial invasion of colonic mucosa, both of which contribute to shigellosis. The organism's virulence depends on its ability to invade cells [23]. A toxin is produced and a cross-reactivity exists between this toxin and toxins of certain *Escherichia coli* strains, salmonella strains and *Vibrio cholerae*. The toxin and the Shiga-like toxin of these other bacteria probably have a role in the pathogenesis of diarrhoea [24,25].

The shigella cytotoxin reduces protein synthesis in epithelial cells, whereas an endotoxin causes mitochondrial damage, leading to cell death and formation of ulcers. Further absorption of the endotoxin leads to thrombosis in small vessels, with consequent haemorrhage and ischaemia, causing further epithelial damage. Consequently transmural inflammation may be seen [23]. The inflammation is most severe in the rectum and sigmoid colon but colonoscopy may disclose a pancolitis [24,26], and occasionally the terminal ileum can be involved. The affected mucosa shows friability, adherent mucopurulent exudate, mimicking pseudo-membranes, and occasionally aphthous ulcers. Deep ulceration of the colon has been demonstrated radiologically in severe infection [27] but normally inflammation is superficial and, although perforation is rare, it is known to occur in the setting of fulminant colitis with or without toxic megacolon. The regional lymph nodes are usually enlarged.

Histologically, the initial inflammation is seen in the lymphoid follicles of the mucosa, which breaks down to form ulcers. It has been shown that, in experimental peroral infection in the guinea-pig, dysenteric bacilli penetrate the intact epithelium of the intestine and pass through the mucosa in a matter of hours [28]. Inflammatory changes follow and include the formation of crypt abscesses, focal haemorrhages and goblet cell depletion. Sometimes volcano-like eruptions of the crypts with pseudo-membrane formation can be seen. The inflammatory response diminishes from the surface down through the mucosa, with virtually no reaction in the submucosa [26]. Electron microscopic studies on rectal biopsy material have failed to reveal any specific change that might differentiate shigellosis from other inflammatory disorders of the large intestine [27,28].

The colorectal biopsy appearances in shigellosis are similar to those of other bacterial infections of the large intestine, notably salmonellosis (see below) and campylobacter infection (see 'Campylobacter colitis' below). The histology in human rectal biopsy material has a notable resemblance to that reported for experimental shigellosis in rhesus monkeys [29]. Finally, it should be noted that chronic shigellosis may result in chronic inflammatory changes and significant crypt architectural distortion, thereby being a potential mimic of chronic ulcerative colitis.

Salmonella colitis

Food poisoning by salmonella organisms is a common problem worldwide [30,31]. *S. typhi*, *S. paratyphi*, *S. argona*, *S. javiana* and *S. oranienburg* all cause salmonella gastroenteritis [32]. *S. enteritidis* has been increasing as a cause of food poisoning in recent years, usually from infected eggs and poultry [33]. Whereas the organisms *S. typhi* and *S. paratyphi* cause septicaemic illnesses, salmonella infection of food poisoning type (salmonellosis) is generally confined to the gastrointestinal tract. In some patients this results in vomiting and profuse watery diarrhoea, usually with colicky peri-umbilical abdominal pains that suggest predominantly gastric and small intestinal involvement. In others, dysenteric features such as frequent small-volume bloody motions, tenesmus and tenderness of the sigmoid colon are present. The appreciation of colonic involvement and its frequency in salmonellosis has gained acceptance over the last two decades [31,34,35].

The pathology of salmonella colitis has been appreciated from necropsy and biopsy studies. Fatal infection is mostly a disease of young or elderly individuals [36]. A postmortem series of 68 children who died with salmonella enteritis, mostly aged <1 year and many with nutritional deficiencies, showed bowel lesions in 46 cases with colitis more prominent than enteritis [37]. In another necropsy study of nine patients, despite fatalities, the lack of gross abnormalities with only minimal mucosal reddening was emphasised [36]. Others have described more severe abnormalities with gross oedema and transverse ulceration. The left colon was most affected in these series [38–40], but we have also seen predominantly right-sided disease and pseudo-membranes, primarily in children. In these postmortem studies, the histology was of a subtle diffuse colitis with prominent crypt abscesses and crypt epithelial damage [36]. Signs of healing were frequent. Superficial mucosal necrosis is common, with haemorrhage and occasional fibrin thrombi [35]. In clinical practice, the colonoscopic appearances are of mucosal hyperaemia, friability and inflammation, which may be patchy or diffuse. It is important to remember that salmonellosis is a cause of patchy inflammation at colonoscopy; it should not be expected always to be a diffuse colitis. The biopsy pathology of the rectal mucosa in salmonella infection [38,41] is described along with the other forms of infective colitis below.

The concurrence of salmonellosis and chronic idiopathic inflammatory bowel disease suggests that this association is not a rarity and it can present problems in diagnosis and management [39,40]. The appearances in rectal biopsies in such patients are of chronic inflammatory bowel disease with active inflammation [41]. It is probable that, in ulcerative colitis and Crohn's disease, there is a predisposition to supervening salmonella infection and this would be more likely to occur with prolonged steroid therapy [42]. The possibility that some of these cases, in which no antecedent bowel disturbance was present, represent chronic post-dysenteric colitis [42–44] seems less likely as, in countries where bacillary dysentery is prevalent, this is very unusual. In contrast, persistent diarrhoea with or without ulceration of the colon is not uncommon in amoebic dysentery [45,46]. It is now possible to analyse food by PCR to detect both *Salmonella* and *Shigella* spp.

Rectal mucosal prolapse in association with massive diarrhoea may sometimes occur in salmonellosis, and appendicitis or ileitis may be seen, complicated occasionally by toxic megacolon and/or perforation. Patients with salmonellosis may also develop extra-intestinal manifestations, including erythema nodosum and reactive arthropathy. Infection with *Salmonella* spp. may be particularly problematic in those with HIV infection or with sickle cell disease.

Campylobacter colitis

Campylobacter spp. are Gram-negative spiral bacilli, which were previously (until 1964) classified as *Vibrio* spp. [47]. *Campylobacter* spp. may well be the most frequent cause of bacterial diarrhoea worldwide [48] and also in the UK [49]. *C. jejuni* is far more common a cause than *C. coli*. However, the closely related *Arcobacter* spp. are also increasingly recognised as a cause of acute infectious colitis [50]. In the UK, almost 1/1000 of the population have *Campylobacter* spp. cultured annually from stool, so the true prevalence is probably 5–10 times higher, suggesting that at least 1/200 of the population may get symptomatic *Campylobacter* spp. annually. Similar figures have been obtained from the USA. More infections occur in warm months.

Numerous animal and avian species harbour the organism, including household pets and poultry, in which it is a normal inhabitant of the intestines (as *Salmonella* spp. frequently are) and produces no symptoms. Removal of intestines provides ample opportunity for contamination of the carcass and virtually 100% of chickens harbour the organism [50]. In a case–control study in the UK, the risk for illness associated with recent chicken consumption was much lower for those regularly eating chicken than in those who did not, suggesting a degree of immunological protection. Chicken-related risk factors accounted for 41% of cases, acid-suppressing medication 10% and recent acquisition of a pet dog 1% [49]. Infection may also occur from person to person but is more usually acquired from food, water or domestic pets [51].

Clinically both a small bowel secretory component and an invasive colonic phase seem likely. Initial isolations from humans suggested primary disease in the small intestine (hence *jejuni*) [52,53] but the bacterium is also clearly associated with a procto-colitis and the typical changes of an acute infectious colitis can be seen on colorectal biopsies

[54,55]. Although the mechanism for campylobacter pathogenesis has been unclear, it is apparent that experimentally it is both invasive and toxin-producing [56].

Abdominal pain is a prominent clinical symptom that may result in admission to a surgical ward and subsequent unwarranted surgery [54]. Indeed the organism can induce an appendicitis [53]. Ileo-caecal disease, focal Crohn's disease-like colonic involvement ('focal active colitis') and diffuse disease have all been described at colonoscopy [54]. Rarely, toxic megacolon may develop, requiring surgical resection, but it is usually one of the more 'gentle' infective colitides, at least colonoscopically.

Enteroinvasive *Escherichia coli* diarrhoea

This group of *E. coli* is closely related to *Shigella* spp. Dysentery is produced by destruction of the epithelium in the colon with ulceration and blood, mucus and pus in the stools. Mucosal attachment and plasmids are involved in the pathogenesis [57,58]. Other *E. coli* causing small intestinal disease are considered elsewhere (see Chapter 20).

Enteropathogenic *E. coli*

Haemorrhagic colitis usually results from verotoxin-producing *E. coli* (VTEC), known as Shiga toxin-producing *E. coli* [59–63]. There are two common and distinct cytotoxins: Shiga-like toxin T and Shiga-like toxin II. Enterohaemorrhagic E. coli adhere to the luminal surface, as they do in animals when they elaborate a toxin before absorption of the toxin. The absorption of the toxin, as in shigellosis, interferes with protein synthesis and results in epithelial and endothelial damage [63,64]. The cellular insult is not limited to the bowel. The endothelium of the kidneys is also damaged to produce haemolytic–uraemic syndrome (HUS) and thrombotic thrombocytopaenic purpura (TTP), resulting from the failure of secretion of anticoagulant substances from the damaged vascular endothelial cells, leading to thrombosis in small blood vessels. Unsurprisingly, given the pathogenic mechanisms at play, the bowel may show a close histopathological resemblance to ischaemic colitis.

The incidence of *E. coli* infection is highest in the summer. *E. coli* O157 (EO157) can survive in water and may consequently be associated with water-borne outbreaks. It is also recognised to occur in hamburgers and other processed beef. *E. coli* in such processed meat is more sensitive to heat than other bacteria, but may survive for long periods in extreme cold conditions, even in the domestic freezer [65]. For this reason, there have been many epidemics associated with commercial hamburger outlets, so that thorough cooking of hamburgers is exceptionally important because a minced beef product may carry E. coli in the centre of the product, where it will be less likely to be destroyed during cooking. However, contamination of unchlorinated drinking water can occur and is especially dangerous because rehydration is attempted with contaminated water, perpetuating the disease, and also resulting in an increase in post-infectious irritable bowel syndrome [66].

The incubation period of the colitis is 3–4 days, whereas the infective diarrhoea usually lasts for 2–9 days. Asymptomatic infections may occur, as may a milder form of the disease. Immunocompromised, very young and very elderly individuals are more susceptible to HUS [63] and TTP after EO157 infection. The progression of the syndrome to HUS and TTP does not seem to be influenced by antibiotic therapy.

The clinical differential diagnosis includes ischaemic colitis, pseudo-membranous colitis, chronic inflammatory bowel disease and occasionally acute appendicitis, if the disease is predominantly a right-sided colitis or an ileocolitis. Colonoscopy may reveal a normal-looking mucosa with oozing of blood or pseudo-membrane formation, thereby mimicking pseudo-membranous or ischaemic colitis. Patchy erosions and ulceration may be seen in the right side of the colon. In children, more commonly the entire colon is involved.

The histopathological appearances are fundamentally those of an infective colitis (see below) but mucosal haemorrhage and intravascular platelet thrombi are sometimes conspicuous and may mimic mucosal ischaemia [25,65]. Pseudo-membranes, when present, tend to be small and more of a microscopic, rather than a gross, finding. As the changes are distinctly patchy, multiple biopsies are helpful in achieving the diagnosis, but the severity of the histological changes may relate poorly to the severity of the illness. The focal nature of the change is a useful distinguishing feature in the differential diagnosis between EO157 infection and acute ulcerative colitis. Unexpected pseudo-membranes in biopsies should always raise the possibility of VTEC.

Clostridial infections

Clostridial species are especially implicated in inflammatory and necrotising disease in the small (see Chapter 20) and large intestine. *Clostridium difficile* causes pseudo-membranous colitis and antibiotic-associated colitis as well as sporadic diarrhoea (see 'Pseudo-membranous colitis and antibiotic-associated diarrhoea and colitis' later in this chapter). The enterotoxigenic varieties of *Clostridium perfringens* are implicated in pig-bel and may cause infective colitis [67–69]. Pig-bel is a form of necrotising small bowel infection (enteritis necroticans) usually seen after gorging on undercooked pork along with sweet potato which has been reported from Papua New Guinea [67]. Similar disease had been reported during the Second World War in individuals who consumed abundant pork after a period of starvation. Rare cases have been reported from other parts of the world. Pig-bel has been reported to affect the colon as well as the small bowel and may even be seen in vegetarians [70]. *C. septicum* is one of the putative pathogens in neutropaenic colitis (see below).

The biopsy diagnosis of acute infectious (acute self-limited or infectious-type) colitis

As few patients come to surgery for this condition, the histopathologist is usually asked to make the diagnosis of infective procto-colitis on biopsy material. Perhaps the most critical factor in this assessment is the timing of the biopsy, because the typical changes of infective colitis are usually seen only early in the course of the infection [71,72]. In most cases, the changes begin to resolve or assume a more chronic picture after about 7–10 days. Although it can then become harder to distinguish infective colitis from other forms of inflammatory bowel disease [73–76], in practice architectural preservation is maintained, except in severe culturable infections, whereas for basal plasma cells to extend to the muscularis mucosae needs a good antibody response, which takes at least 2 weeks. This is important to realise because very few patients undergo biopsies in the early phase of an inflammatory disease of the large intestine. Biopsies are often performed when the clinical presentation is unusual, when the symptoms last longer than expected or after partial treatment with antibiotics, and occasionally entirely fortuitously.

In the typical biopsy, the initial impression at low magnification is of architectural preservation but a mucosa widened by oedema and an inflammatory infiltrate, the latter appearing like sprinkled salt grains across the lamina propria with a hint of superficial condensation [73,77–81] (Figures 35.2–35.4). The architecture is distorted only in severe disease, usually when crypts are regenerative, but infection is severe and culturable, such as in severe shigellosis [79]. In addition the crypt bases are often pointed rather than rounded and mucin depletion is readily apparent. There is mucin depletion and the individual crypt

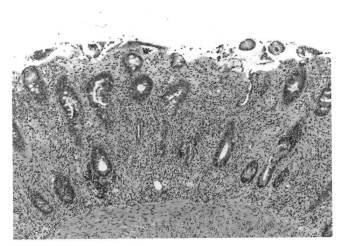

Figure 35.3 Infective colitis: large numbers of neutrophils are caught up between the crypt epithelial cells (incipient crypt abscesses) and the lamina propria, a characteristic feature of infective colitis.

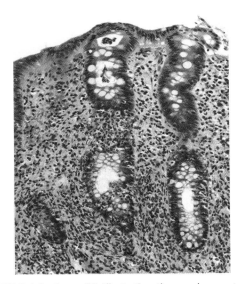

Figure 35.2 Infective colitis illustrating the regular crypt alignment, but the typical acute inflammatory cell infiltrate within the crypts is well seen in the central crypt. Such beaded intracryptal neutrophil polymorph infiltrate has been called the string of pearls sign.

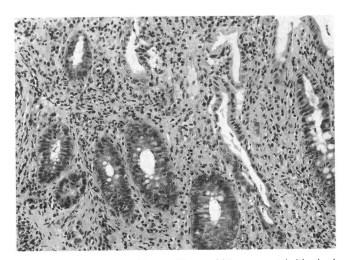

Figure 35.4 Infective colitis: in this rectal biopsy crypt 'withering' with an infiltrate predominantly of neutrophils is seen. The lamina propria contains mostly neutrophils and no significant increase in chronic inflammatory cells.

epithelial cells appear attenuated. This is reflected in dilatation of the superficial half of many of the crypts. In some, this area may degenerate completely (Figure 35.4).

The surface epithelium is reduced in height and mucin and surface neutrophils are common. Luminal pus is frequent and margination of neutrophils prominent within congested capillaries. Focal clusters of neutrophils are also present throughout the biopsy, often adjacent to dilated capillaries or alongside crypts, and are distinctly patchy across the biopsy. Characteristically they are found within the crypt epithelium but not commonly within the crypt lumen. This appearance, the incipient crypt abscess or 'cryptitis' (see Figure 35.3), is in contrast to the true crypt abscess, which does occur in infective colitis but is much more prevalent in active chronic ulcerative colitis and Crohn's disease [73,80,81]. The epithelium associated with these intra-epithelial neutrophils may be degenerate or gathered into small projecting tufts between individual crypts. When present, crypt abscesses tend to be present in the superficial half or two-thirds of the mucosa, and are relatively uncommon at the crypt bases. Peri-cryptal haemorrhage may be striking at low power [80].

The absolute number of plasma cells and lymphocytes within the lamina propria may well be increased but this is partially masked by the oedema. It is the dominance of the polymorphonuclear neutrophils over the chronic inflammatory cell infiltrate, especially plasma cells, that is of key diagnostic importance when making the distinction between infection and other causes of procto-colitis. Epithelial bridges may be present across the crypt lumina, giving an additional feature known as the 'string of pearls' sign [38].

This descriptive account of infective colitis represents the characteristic pattern and as mentioned earlier is common only early in the disease [38]. Inter-observer variability between histopathologists is considerable in the reporting of biopsies showing acute self-limiting colitis [80]. There have been attempts to identify simple, objective criteria for the histological diagnosis of acute colitis, 1–10 weeks after onset [80]. However, such methods, involving cell counting, are difficult to incorporate into routine diagnostic practice. One study of biopsies taken 1–10 weeks after the onset of diarrhoea identified that those without significant inflammation, with irritable bowel syndrome, had a concentration of lamina propria cells in the upper third of the lamina propria, whereas increased lamina propria acute inflammatory cell numbers in the upper and middle third correlated well with infective colitis. In chronic inflammatory bowel disease, there was increased lamina propria cellularity in the lower third of the lamina propria, usually known as a basal plasmacytosis [73].

Not all biopsies in infective colitis, even if taken early in the disease and with positive cultures, show typical features [78]. Indeed there is a range of changes from a virtu-

ally normal appearance, some with oedema, lamina propria haemorrhage and occasional neutrophils (focal active colitis).

The main value of a biopsy in infective disease is in those patients who are culture negative [78]. Here, in the presence of characteristic histology, a confident diagnosis can be made but the terms 'acute self-limited colitis' and 'acute infectious-type colitis' are preferred. It is also important that such patients are not misdiagnosed as having ulcerative colitis or Crohn's disease. Where there is doubt about the diagnosis, a follow-up biopsy, between 6 and 8 weeks later, is often helpful. In the vast majority of cases of infection, the histological appearances will have reverted to normal. This should not be the case in ulcerative colitis. In some series a small number of biopsies from patients with clinical infective disease may have biopsies interpreted as more like Crohn's disease or ulcerative colitis [55,80–85]. However, care needs to be taken in children because some have an appearance indistinguishable from acute infectious colitis, except that the history will indicate that symptoms have been present for months. These children invariably evolve into one or other form of chronic inflammatory bowel disease.

Complications of infective colitis

These can be systemic and include myocarditis, splenitis, liver abscess and effusions into the joints, but they are found only in severe infections, usually with *Shigella* sp., which produces a powerful exotoxin [25,64]. Locally, infection can be followed by a chronic state in which organisms remain in the bowel and ulceration of the intestine persists. Alternatively, the initial inflammation may have been so severe that, despite healing, permanent structural changes are found. These include the appearances known as colitis cystica profunda in which mucus retention cysts are found in the submucosa [86], presumably derived from epithelium misplaced during the acute stage of the disease. This must be distinguished from colitis cystica superficialis, which is an entirely different condition seen occasionally in children dying from debilitating diseases such as leukaemia, pellagra and tropical sprue [87], but can occur with severe infections such as with *Shigella* sp.

'Post-dysenteric colitis' is a term introduced to describe persistent inflammation and irritability of the bowel following attacks of both bacillary and amoebic dysentery, more commonly the latter [42–44,88,89]. The original infecting organism is often no longer present. There are three forms:
1. Non-ulcerative, which is really a problem of abnormal intestinal motility; this is now called post-infectious irritable bowel syndrome [66]
2. Ulcerative, which responds to anti-bacterial or anti-amoebic treatment (persistent infection)
3. Ulcerative, which fails to respond to therapy and may be related to ulcerative colitis or Crohn's disease.

However, severe disease can also destroy the muscularis propria, resulting in fibrosis and the formation of strictures [45].

There has been much controversy in the past over the relationship between acute infectious colitis ('bacillary dysentery') and ulcerative colitis. Anecdotally many patients relate the onset of their chronic inflammatory bowel disease (CIBD) to an acute infection that partially resolved, then reappeared as CIBD. Indeed, in one series, up to a quarter of patients experienced the first attack of CIBD after tropical exposure and a clinical illness indistinguishable from infective enterocolitis [84]. The problem of distinguishing the pathology of acute infectious colitis from ulcerative colitis in surgical specimens does not usually arise, although it may be an important issue in rectal biopsies. However, fulminant colitis can occasionally arise during the course of an infection and lead to a colectomy [88,89]. This is increasingly seen in severe *C. difficile* infection, (invariably the NAP1 strain), although the pseudo-membranes usually make the diagnosis obvious. If these are absent, the diagnosis then depends on recognising any mucosal features of infection against the background of the changes of fulminant disease (see 'Pseudo-membranous colitis and antibiotic-associated diarrhoea and colitis' below). To add to the diagnostic difficulties, the infection can also complicate pre-existing CIBD.

Tuberculosis

Tuberculosis (TB) of the gastrointestinal tract, whether primary or secondary, usually involves the terminal ileum, caecum and appendix [90–93]. Oesophageal involvement, with ulcers or strictures, and gastric involvement, leading to outlet obstruction, have also been reported. Most cases now, with widespread pasteurisation of milk, are due to *Mycobacterium tuberculosis*. *M. bovis* accounts for less than 1.5% of all cases [94,95]. Involvement of the colon and rectum is less common, even in countries where intestinal TB is frequent [90], although there are reports from India [91,93], Israel [90], Iraq [96] and South Africa [97, 98]. It is rare in the UK [99] and the USA [100–102], and is almost always secondary. We have seen few acceptable examples of primary TB of the distal large bowel, although it is documented [103–108], especially in immigrant populations.

The clinical and therapeutic implications of a diagnosis of intestinal TB are so important to the patient that great care must be taken to make a clear distinction from other conditions that give a similar histological picture. In the western world, the differential diagnosis from Crohn's disease is the most important [106]. The most common macroscopic appearance is of sharply defined ulceration with an excavated base covered by slough. The ulcers may be multiple but are usually few in number, and the mucosa between tends to appear normal. The other gross appearance is of stricture formation. In some, ulceration and stricturing occur together. In contrast to Crohn's disease, the ulcers in intestinal TB appear to be transverse or circumferential, and the strictures are shorter. The surrounding bowel is thickened and indurated. Fat wrapping is not usually seen in TB and may therefore be a helpful distinguishing feature from Crohn's disease [107]. Miliary tubercles may be seen on the mucosal and serosal surfaces. Such an appearance is unusual in Crohn's disease, which involves a large length of bowel with more superficial ulceration and/or a cobblestone pattern.

The microscopic distinction between Crohn's disease and TB is discussed below and in Chapter 20. Colonoscopic examination and biopsy ARE proving more and more useful for making the diagnosis [107–109]. In such biopsy work, the diagnostic yield is increased by taking large numbers of biopsies [107]. Special stains for organisms should be performed whenever TB is seriously considered because acid-fast bacilli may be seen when histiocytic foci are present even in the absence of well-formed granulomas [107].

Generally speaking, the diagnosis of intestinal TB should not be accepted without demonstration of the characteristic caseating tubercles or the presence of tuberculous bacilli in histological sections, along with culture. It should also be recognised that the acid-fast stains can be negative (54–85%) in a significant number of cases, which varies markedly between studies [110,111]. Polyclonal and species-specific antibodies against mycobacteria are available for immunohistochemical staining. In one study the organisms were detected in 169 (97.1%) of 174 cases of TB by immunohistochemical staining compared with only 75 (44.3%) cases that were positive with acid-fast stains [112]. PCR-based assays are also now available: these are quite sensitive and specific, and can increase the diagnostic accuracy in equivocal cases. However, one needs to be careful because they can occasionally give false-positive results, especially in Crohn's disease [113].

Although intestinal TB was, until recently, an unusual diagnosis in western Europe, there is evidence of a modest resurgence of the disease, matching the large increase in cases of pulmonary TB seen in these countries in the last 10 years. Nevertheless, the disease remains unusual in patients born and resident in the UK and then it is likely to be secondary to open pulmonary TB. Even now, most cases seen in the British Isles are found in immigrants, from Asian countries in particular.

Yersinia enterocolitica colitis

Besides causing an ileo-colitis (see 'Yersinia', Chapter 20), *Yersinia enterocolitica* can be a frequent cause of colitis. Perversely, up to 25% of stool culture-positive individuals may be asymptomatic [114]. Canada, Scandinavia, Belgium and Germany all have a high incidence of the disease and it is increasing in the UK [115–117]. It may be found in bulk tank milk [118]. It is generally a self-limiting disease or one easily amenable to antibiotics. There are case reports of gut perforation, pancreatitis and a presentation with diverticulitis [119–123]. In patients with haemochromatosis, the medications can increase the potency of pathogens so that innocuous infections become severe [124]. The organism also seems to like the iron-rich environment found in patients with haemochromatosis. *Y. enterocolitica* infection can also be associated with a wide range of autoimmune problems and systemic illnesses which include myocarditis, arthritis and erythema nodosum [123].

There have been several colonoscopic accounts of the colitis of *Y. enterocolitica* [121,122]. In general there is widespread patchy disease which, in half the cases, may spare the lower sigmoid and rectum, making rectal biopsy unreliable [122]. Punched-out or aphthous ulcers are characteristic [123]. Some of the cases may be similar to those seen in the small intestine or appendix, with granulomas consisting of palisaded histiocytes and surrounded by hyperplastic lymphoid tissue. In one series, despite positive stool culture and abdominal symptoms, 50% had a normal colonoscopic examination and biopsy [121]. Microscopy is usually that of a focal inflammation, which disappears with clinical recovery [122]. Granulomas are not usually a feature of *Y. enterocolitica* colitis. When colonoscopy is undertaken, there is usually an enterocolitis with acute infection affecting both the terminal ileum and the large bowel. Yersinia DNA has been found in surgical resections of a significant proportion of patients with Crohn's disease, raising the question that *Yersinia* sp. may be one of a number of infectious triggers of Crohn's disease.

Sexually transmitted infections in the large intestine

The increasing freedom of sexual expression in the last few decades has presented the gastroenterologist with a large array of sexually transmitted infections [125–127]. Although this was initially mainly seen in the homosexual population, anal sex and oral–anal practices are increasingly prevalent among heterosexuals. Apart from the well-established sexually transmitted infections such as gonorrhoea, chlamydia infection and syphilis, it is now appreciated that several gastrointestinal pathogens can be transmitted in this manner, including *Salmonella* and *Campylobacter* spp. At one time these were collectively grouped as the 'gay bowel syndrome' [126] but many of the common pathogens seen in the large intestine of non-immunosuppressed patients also occur in immunosuppressed patients, and many of them will have much more severe consequences in these patients.

Gonorrhoea

Rectal gonorrhoea is virtually always acquired by homosexual contact in males but, in females, it is said that up to 30% of cases are the result of spread from the vagina [128]. Although older papers describe severe histological abnormality, rectal gonorrhoea often presents with normal sigmoidoscopic and histological examinations [129–131]. Indeed a third or more of cases are asymptomatic. In a large series, 84% of cases of rectal gonorrhoea had a normal proctoscopic appearance and 68% a normal rectal biopsy [130]. In the majority with an abnormal biopsy, there was a mild-to-moderate increase in lymphocytes and plasma cells within the lamina propria. Crypt architecture remained normal. Only 5% of cases showed acute inflammatory cells in the lamina propria, with migration into the crypt and surface epithelium in a manner resembling the pattern associated with more common bacterial enteropathogens. Detection of *Neisseria gonorrhoeae* is best carried out by direct culture on specialised media or via a smear preparation from the mucosal surface, from which PCR can also be carried out. A rectal biopsy is simply an aid and does not provide a diagnostic appearance unless culture or PCR is used.

Syphilis

The primary lesion of syphilis occurs at the site of infection. Most large intestinal cases are in homosexual or bisexual males, and seen as chancres at the anal margin or in the anal canal. However, lesions may occur in the rectum and these can mimic a carcinoma, solitary ulcer syndrome, polyp or fistula [132–134]. Biopsy of a syphilitic lesion typically shows large numbers of plasma cells and proliferating capillaries lined by prominent endothelial cells. However, as in the stomach, the morphology can be hugely variable and the liberal use of Warthin–Starry stains, immunohistochemistry and/or PCR is required, as organisms may vary from few to many and be strikingly focal in distribution [135].

In secondary syphilis, a proctitis may be present. In some cases the histological appearance can resemble that of a typical bacterial infection [136] and small granulomas have also been documented. The inflammatory abnormalities in the biopsies of patients with syphilis can be more florid than those in patients with gonorrhoeal infection [136]. Again a high index of suspicion is required. However, most pathologists have probably never ordered any of these stains/tests on rectal biopsies, so the prevalence of rectal syphilis is almost certainly under-estimated.

Chlamydia infection/lymphogranuloma venereum

The L1, L2 and L3 immunotypes of *Chlamydia trachomatis*, an obligate intracellular bacterium, cause lymphogranuloma venereum. Synonyms include lymphogranuloma inguinale, lymphopathia venereum, climatic bubo and

Nicolas–Favre disease. It is important to distinguish inguinal lesions from granuloma inguinale, caused by *Klebsiella granulomatis* (formerly *Calymmatobacterium granulomatis*), and Crohn's disease. In the past, the disease was considered one of tropical and subtropical countries [137], being rare in western Europe. However, with better methods of diagnosis available, it is now realised that anorectal infection is not uncommon in the homosexual population in western countries. The diagnosis of lymphogranuloma venereum can be made by a direct demonstration of the organisms on tissue sections using monoclonal antibodies [138] or by serological detection of changing antibody levels to particular immunotypes.

The primary infection is transmitted by sexual contact. Males tend to develop a lesion on the genitalia, followed by a suppurative inflammatory reaction in the inguinal gland (buboes), which does not usually result in rectal involvement, whereas females usually develop rectal and colonic lesions, presumably as the result of lymphatic spread from the vagina. When lymphogranuloma venereum of the rectum occurs in males, it is invariably the result of homosexual practices and it is possible that, in females, rectal coitus may sometimes cause it. Accidental non-venereal infection has been reported in juveniles.

Lymphogranuloma venereum of the rectum and colon presents in two phases [139]: an initial distal procto-colitis, followed by a chronic stage with the formation of a stricture, usually in the rectum. Similar to other sexually transmitted infections, the acute phase seldom causes severe problems. It can be asymptomatic or present as mild or chronic diarrhoea due to a distal proctitis. Rectal biopsy shows an acute proctitis with neutrophils, plasma cells and lymphocytes infiltrating the mucosa. Crypt abscesses and occasional granulomas may be present, the latter related to damaged crypts. The picture may be confused with Crohn's disease or other causes of acute infectious procto-colitis. The distinction, however, seldom poses a clinical problem, unless the pathologist is misled by a lack of clinical information.

The pathology of the chronic phase of procto-colitis has been documented by sigmoidoscopic and radiological methods [137,140]. The rectal mucosa is granular, nodular and oedematous with rigidity of the underlying tissues. Mild abnormality may extend up as far as the transverse colon and a pancolitis has been documented [141]. The most constant and severe changes are in the rectum. There is therefore a definite right-to-left gradient and severe macroscopic disease in the right colon is very unlikely to be due to lymphogranuloma venereum [141]. Distally there may be associated perirectal abscesses and fistulae.

Strictures of the rectum [127,142] are usually tubular with an abrupt line of demarcation from the non-involved bowel above. The wall of the rectum is thickened and rigid with a severely ulcerated mucosa, and any surviving mucosa appears polypoid and haemorrhagic. There is severe stenosis of the lumen, which may be contracted down to a diameter as small as 10mm. The perirectal tissues may also show fibrosis and there is much scarring of the anus, often with a characteristic bridging of the perianal skin. So-called burnt-out strictures are not uncommon. In these, the rectum is stenosed but the mucosa is smooth and intact.

Microscopically, there is an inflammatory reaction with infiltration by lymphocytes and plasma cells together with much fibrosis. The intensity of scarring, which is often transmural, is greater than in Crohn's disease and neuronal hyperplasia is common. The formation of epithelioid cell granulomas is rare in the chronic form of the disease, although it is well recognised in inguinal lymph nodes in the acute stage. Inflammation diminishes proximal to the sigmoid colon and when present is limited to the mucosa [137].

The pathologist's diagnostic problem is to distinguish the appearances of lymphogranuloma venereum from Crohn's disease (Figure 35.5). The gradient of disease from left to right side is opposite to that in most cases of Crohn's disease, although in some cases with pancolitis the terminal ileum may be involved [141]. On microscopy, transmural fibrosis favours lymphogranuloma venereum and the lymphocytic infiltrate is seldom as packeted as that in Crohn's colitis [142]. Although some have shown that antibodies to a lymphogranuloma venereum strain are present in 69% of patients with Crohn's disease [143], subsequent studies have failed to substantiate this relationship [144].

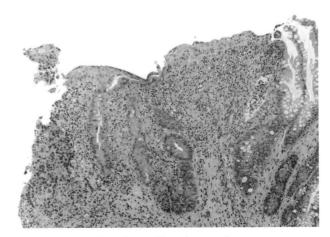

Figure 35.5 Typical histology of lymphogranuloma venereum proctitis: there is patchy active inflammation with chronic features such as crypt architectural distortion, immediately at the anorectal junction (there is anal-type squamous mucosa also present). There is strong mimicry of Crohn's disease.

The incidence of carcinoma in lymphogranulomatous strictures of the rectum is not high [145]: both adenocarcinoma and squamous cell carcinoma are described. The original senior author of this text described three patients with squamous cell carcinoma arising in long-standing strictures of the rectum due to lymphogranuloma venereum. In all cases there was extensive involvement of the rectum and anal canal [146]. The biopsy diagnosis can be difficult because the squamous mucosa of the anal canal tends to grow up over the ulcerated rectum, giving rise to appearances that may be mistaken for malignancy.

Chlamydia trachomatis proctitis

The non-lymphogranuloma venereum immunotypes of *C. trachomatis* are mainly confined to infections of the genito-urinary system but can cause mild proctitis on occasion [147]. Focal collections of neutrophils occur in the lamina propria. Occasionally one can observe granulomas, with or without giant cells, and/or lymphoid follicular hyperplasia (follicular proctitis) [147]. The typical intranuclear inclusions are rarely seen and the diagnosis on biopsy material is aided by immunohistochemical stains or PCR-based assays. The diagnosis should be sought in the correct clinical setting [148,149].

Infections due to other specific bacteria

Intestinal spirochaetosis

Rectal, colonic and occasionally appendiceal mucosa can be colonised by rows of spiral organisms embedded in the epithelial cell border [150,151]. These organisms appear as a violaceous hue on the luminal aspect of the cell when stained routinely with H&E (Figure 35.6), but the periodic

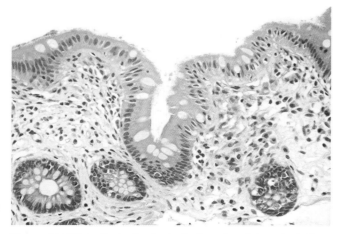

Figure 35.6 Intestinal spirochaetosis: there is patchy colonisation of the luminal surface of the epithelial cells by a haematoxyphilic layer of spirochaetes.

acid–Schiff (PAS) reagent or Warthin–Starry method emphasises the bacterial colonisation of the mucosal surface. In the older literature, it was said that organisms could be found in about 5% of colorectal biopsies from patients attending gastroenterology clinics [150,152] and in up to 36% of biopsies in the homosexual population [153]. However, we see only a few biopsies with this annually, suggesting that the prevalence of this is much lower.

The taxonomy of the organism has been disputed but *Brachyspira aalborgi* and *Brachyspira pilosicoli* are now generally accepted terms for two of the most common species causing intestinal disease [154]. Other groups of spirochaetes similar to those found in the pig intestine have also been isolated from human stool [155].

These epithelial spirochaetes are not normally associated with any morphological abnormalities, although some cases may show a mild or focal increase in inflammatory cells with some cryptitis. If inflammation is prominent, one should look for other causes carefully. However, there are a few reports of spirochaetes within epithelial cells [156], and subepithelial macrophages and the number of IgE-containing plasma cells within the lamina propria may be raised [157]. Degranulation of mast cells has also been demonstrated.

The pathogenic role of these spirochaetes remains contentious, with most opinion favouring the view that they are not of pathological significance [152]. However, some patients with diarrhoea in whom spirochaetosis was the only abnormal finding have been cured by a course of antibiotics, notably metronidazole, which eliminated the organisms [157,158]. Our suspicion is that this organism is a little like *Helicobacter pylori* with symptoms following initial infection and the subsequent ability for the organism to persist in an asymptomatic state. The key to making this diagnosis is to routinely look for organisms, rather than hoping that they will jump up and bite you. There is no substitute for methodological examination of biopsies, so that cryptosporidia and spirochaetosis are always looked for on the surface epithelium of all large bowel biopsies.

Occasionally, other entero-adherent bacteria attach to the glycocalyx and will stain with Warthin–Starry or other silver stains. There is little or no literature on this but anti-escherichia antibodies, PCR or electron microscopy on biopsies could help, although one is always cognisant of the fact that a variety of normal organisms may be sampled, so that it may need laser capture to specifically obtain such organisms and allow their identification.

The electron microscopic appearances of spirochaetosis are characteristic but this is not necessary for the diagnosis. High power examination shows the morphology of the spirochaetes, whereas silver stains often reveal individual organisms in the surface mucus. On occasion, the infestation can be confused with a slightly thick glycocalyx, especially when the haematoxylin stain is especially heavy or uses certain haematoxylin types (e.g. Harris's haematoxylin) that will stain mucus. The infection can be extensive but sometimes found only in one or two of a series of biopsies, often the most proximal, but its limitation to the mouths of the crypts contrasts with that of the mucin staining, which is distinctly patchy. The other main differential diagnosis is other organisms, possibly coliforms, embedded in the surface mucosa. Silver stains will also demonstrate these.

Actinomycosis

The appendix (see 'Actinomycosis', Chapter 29) and the ileo-caecal region (see 'Other bacterial causes of enteritis', Chapter 20) are the most common sites of actinomycosis in the gastrointestinal tract [159]. Caused by the Gram-positive filamentous bacterium, *Actinomyces israelii*, the disease is rare in the colon [160–165] but rather more common in the rectum [162] where it is usually associated with anal fistulae. We have seen one example of actinomycosis in the rectum without associated fistulae [162]. This presented as an induration of the rectum without mucosal ulceration and the diagnosis was made by rectal biopsy in which colonies of *Actinomyces* spp. were found. There are two varieties of rectal involvement: one in which the disease is primary in the rectum, and the other due to spread from the ileo-caecal region. Actinomycosis should be considered in the differential diagnosis of smooth submucosal strictures of the rectum.

It is likely that actinomycosis is invasive only when the intestinal wall has been breached by some other condition such as diverticulitis or trauma [164]. We have seen colonies of *Actinomyces* spp. in the pericolic abscesses of diverticular disease but it is extremely rare for these to provoke much inflammatory reaction. Granulomas forming at the suture line after anterior resection of the sigmoid colon and rectum may contain actinomyces [166] but it is unusual for this to lead to pericolic abscess formation, fibrosis or stenosis of the anastomosis. Intra-abdominal actinomycosis is also associated with use of the intrauterine contraceptive device [167], and the organisms may form tumours that compress the large bowel, resulting in obstruction [168,169].

Aeromonas infection

Aeromonas hydrophila, a Gram-negative bacillus, may cause a procto-colitis in HIV-infected patients. It is also a cause of colorectal infection in both adults and children without HIV. Culture from the tissues will reveal the organism. The pathological changes are similar to any other infectious-type colitis but can be associated with ischaemic-type lesions and right-sided or segmental colitis [170–172]. There can be considerable necrosis in the base of large ulcers and sometimes there is crypt distortion that may mimic CIBD.

Inflammation due to fungi

As with lesions in the more proximal gastrointestinal tract, fungi can secondarily infect primary ulcerating lesions of rectum and colon. There are case reports of primary infection with mucormycosis [173], cryptococcosis [174] and histoplasmosis. *Histoplasma* sp. is the organism most likely to involve the gut and can mimic Crohn's disease [175] or cause perforation [176]. Most cases are seen post mortem in patients dying of haematological diseases, especially those with neutropaenia. Histoplasmosis may also involve the intestines as a complication of AIDS. Most cases of fungal infection of the bowel are unsuspected and the diagnosis relies on identifying the fungus in the histological section. The majority of cases occur as part of disseminated disease or in immunologically suppressed individuals [177]. In the colon fungal infection may mimic ulcerative colitis or present as a mass.

Disseminated histoplasmosis predominantly affects immunocompromised patients but is fairly infrequent in AIDS patients outside endemic areas for histoplasmosis, such as the valleys of the Mississippi and Ohio rivers of the USA, and in Central and South America. Macrophages containing the fungus are usually present in large numbers in mesenteric lymph nodes, liver, spleen and bone marrow. There are occasional reports of histoplasmosis confined to the colon [176]. Such colorectal histoplasmosis may mimic or complicate CIBD.

Protozoal infection

Amoebiasis

Amoebiasis is a primary infection of the large intestine caused by the protozoon *Entamoeba histolytica*. The organism's normal habitat is in the crypts of the caecum and ascending colon [45,178]. It is worldwide in its distribution, although more prevalent in the tropics than in temperate climates. Acute vegetative forms, the trophozoites, are present in the large bowel in people who the disease: these are passed in the stools, encyst into a more resistant form, and may survive in food and fluid vehicles to be reingested. The cysts survive the gastric acid pH and the capsule of the cyst is digested in the small intestine, with the release of four trophozoites which then colonise the right colon. Here their lysosomal enzymes damage the mucosa releasing red blood cells (RBCs), which they ingest. The spread of amoebiasis is by faecal–oral contamination, usually of uncooked foods, such as salads and contaminated water supplies. It is a disease associated with poor hygiene and therefore more common in developing countries. In western countries, patients usually give a history of foreign travel but this is not invariable [179]. In such cases there may readily be confusion with other inflammatory conditions such as diverticulitis [180] and ulcerative colitis [181,182].

Infection is also now accepted as one of the sexually transmitted infections [178,183] but not all forms of *E. histolytica* are pathogenic. Virulence correlates with the position of a phosphoglucomutase band on starched gel electrophoresis of cultured *E. histolytica*. Some 22 different patterns, zymodene types, are recognised and only 9 have been associated with tissue invasiveness [184,185]. It cannot be automatically assumed, therefore, that, as cysts are identified in the stool of a patient, amoebiasis is the cause of disease. Furthermore, asymptomatic carriage of virulent zymodene types is recognised. Such patients usually have positive amoebic serology, in contrast to those carrying the non-virulent forms [186]. Identifying trophozoites with ingested RBCs is indicative of tissue invasion and pathogenicity. In the homosexual population there is dispute as to whether the identification of amoebic cysts, in the presence of proctitis, always signifies infection that requires treatment [186,187]. In a study from India, cyst carriage eradication was noted to occur spontaneously [187]. In addition, homosexuals (and others) can harbour other species of non-pathogenic amoebae such as *E. hartmanni* and *E. coli*.

Macroscopic appearances

The earliest lesions of amoebic colitis are small, yellow elevations of the mucosal surface containing semi-fluid necrotic material infected with the parasite. When these lesions rupture into the lumen, the amoebae continue to proliferate, undermining the adjacent intact mucosa to leave a discrete oval ulcer with overhanging edges (Figure 35.7a) and extending into the submucosa.

Amoebic ulcers are most frequent in the caecum, ascending colon and rectum, but may be scattered throughout the large intestine and are especially numerous in the region of the flexures. Diffuse amoebic colitis involving the entire large bowel is the most dangerous form of the disease (Figure 35.7a). In surgical specimens, the ulcers are oval in shape and tend to lie with their long axis transversely across the bowel. They are flat, without induration of the underlying bowel wall, and have a characteristic hyperaemic edge. Amoebic colitis is one of the causes of 'flask-shaped ulcers', with overhanging mucosa at the edges and deep ulceration of the submucosa. Ragged, yellowish-white membranes cover the floor of the ulcer, especially in severe cases. In severe cases, the ulceration becomes confluent, leaving isolated patches of intact, hyperaemic mucosa among extensive areas of necrosis. Extensive inflammatory polyposis has been demonstrated as a complication of amoebic colitis and this may be a source of confusion with CIBD [188]. We have seen examples of amoebic infection isolated in the appendix presenting clinically as acute appendicitis.

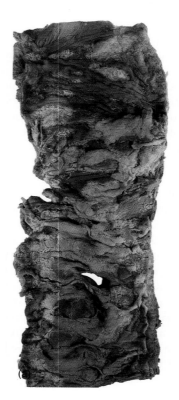

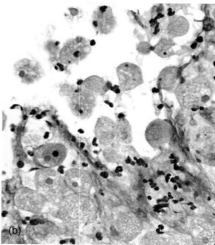

Figure 35.7 Amoebiasis: (a) a segment of colon excised because of perforation due to amoebic colitis. The sloughing ulceration is a typical feature of severe amoebic colitis and a full-thickness defect, the perforation, is readily apparent. (b) A mucosal biopsy of colonic amoebiasis. Multiple amoebae are seen on the surface: they have prominent nuclear karyosomes and contain engulfed erythrocytes.

Microscopic appearances

The accurate diagnosis of amoebic colitis always centres on demonstrating the organisms. What is less well recognised is that the mucosa may show features typical of CIBD, because there has been longstanding inflammation and ulceration. Inflammation can be diffuse or focal. Wherever pus or exudate is seen in colorectal biopsies, the possibility of amoebae must always be considered.

The inflammatory reaction of amoebic colitis is found around the ulcers and, in severe cases, passes right through the bowel wall. There is oedema, vascular congestion and infiltration with leukocytes, especially eosinophils. Amoebae are found on or just beneath the surface of the ulcers (Figure 35.7b), particularly beneath the overhanging margin, but in severe cases they accompany the inflammatory reaction into the bowel wall and may also be seen within blood vessels. They are readily recognised in H&E preparations by their round contour and large size relative to other cells. The PAS reaction can be a useful method for demonstrating them more vividly in histological preparations, especially when formalin fixation has been delayed. Counterstaining with Martius yellow effectively delineates the ingested red cells [189]. Some prefer trichrome stains and CD68 immunohistochemistry can be used to confirm that the organisms are present within histiocytes. The real key to the diagnosis is to always closely examine pus, in which trophozoites are invariably found, as a routine.

The diagnosis of amoebic colitis may be made by finding cysts or active forms of *E. histolytica* in the stools, scrapings from the surface of rectal ulcers or rectal biopsies. With the appreciation of the existence of the numerous non-pathogenic zymodene forms, it is important to identify trophozoites with ingested RBCs. The stools must be unformed in order to achieve this, because only cysts can be found in formed stools [186]. Colorectal biopsies should be taken from the edge of an ulcer, because the amoebae are usually to be found there, lying within a pool of mucus protected by the overhanging edge. If no biopsy material is obtained, it is worth blocking out aspirated mucus [186]. Despite extensive sectioning, amoebae may be identified only in up to 50% of biopsy material [188]. Amoebae are easily recognised as large round cells with small, dark nuclei. The proportion of cytoplasm to nucleus is greater than in other cells, and this will often contain ingested red blood corpuscles, which differentiates *E. histolytica* from *Escherichia coli* and other non-pathogenic intestinal amoebae.

Several stages in the development of the classic flask-shaped ulcer have been described [190–192]. Initially, in a biopsy, there is inflammation with small groups of neutrophil neutrophils near the surface, oedema and congestion, a picture similar to that early in many bacterial infections. Subsequently, focal areas of the mucosa become thinned and depressed followed by surface ulceration. The ulcers are covered by basophilic debris in which the organisms can be seen. Neutrophils are prominent in the mucosa but not crypt abscesses. In the most severe cases, there is marked tissue necrosis and the mucosa is replaced by a thick amorphous grey–blue exudate. Organisms may be seen within this but not inflammatory cells. These are confined to the mucosa on either side. At all stages, only the demonstration of amoebae allows the diagnosis to be made, but a thick acellular basophilic slough with adjacent mucosal changes similar to those seen in bacterial infections should raise suspicions for the diagnosis.

Complications

These are local, the result of migration of amoebae through the bowel wall or adjacent structures, and systemic, after amoebic invasion of blood vessels. Local complications are partly caused by secondary bacterial infection. However, the progress of mucosal disease through transmural invasion to colonic infarction and perforation can be clinically insignificant, with patients often presenting late and in extremis [193]. Toxic megacolon may occur [88] and there can be invasion of the perianal skin with the formation of extensive granulomatous lesions [194]. Likewise, amoebic ulceration of the abdominal wall may occur around colostomies and after the drainage of pericolic and appendiceal abscesses. In cutaneous amoebiasis, the causative organisms can be recovered from the surface of the lesion. Other complications include polyarthritis [195], post-dysenteric colitis [42–44] and haemorrhage [45].

A mass-like lesion, the so-called amoeboma, is a recognised late complication of amoebic colitis [196]. This can develop months or many years after the original infection. It is a chronic form of the disease in which localised secondary infection and fibrosis lead to the formation of a tumour-like mass, which may be mistaken for carcinoma or diverticulitis. Amoebomas are usually single and involve a short segment of colon. They are most common in the right colon and rectum [196,197], and are rarely seen in the transverse colon [188]. Internal fistulae between loops of affected bowel seem to be very rare [191]. In surgical specimens there is pronounced stenosis of the lumen, the result of intra-mural and extra-mural inflammation with fibrosis and abscess formation. Both cysts and active forms of *E. histolytica* can usually be found in the affected tissues, although, in very chronic cases, these may be absent.

The most serious complication of amoebic colitis is invasion of blood vessels within the bowel wall, subsequent spread of amoebae to the liver in the portal bloodstream and the development of amoebic hepatitis or amoebic liver abscess. In amoebic hepatitis, there is an inflammatory reaction in the portal tracts without necrosis or abscess formation. Amoebae are not found. In amoebic liver abscesses, small zones of necrosis of the parenchyma enlarge and coalesce to form cavities filled with sterile pus. A zone of hyperaemia surrounds the lesions, which are often in the right lobe. Bleeding occurs into the abscess, the contents of which become a dark reddish-brown colour and have been likened to anchovy sauce. Microscopically the abscess is characterised by areas of necrosis of liver parenchyma in which amoebae may be found, although in very chronic cases they may be absent. Such an abscess may progress to a chronic state, become encapsulated with fibrous tissue and undergo calcification. It can rupture into the peritoneal cavity or through the diaphragm and into the pleural cavity causing amoebic empyema. Spread to the brain and kidneys may result from invasion of the bloodstream.

Cryptosporidiosis

The protozoon *Cryptosporidium* spp., and the related *Isospora belli*, are recognised causes of diarrhoea in immunocompromised individuals. Cryptosporidiosis is the most common infective cause of diarrhoea in British patients with AIDS [198–201]. However, as well as in immunocompromised patients [201], it is also documented in previously healthy individuals [202], both children and adults, and is a recognised cause of travellers' diarrhoea [202]. *Cryptosporidium parvum* is the only species of the genus known to infect humans. The primary site of infection is the upper small bowel and the interested reader is referred elsewhere for a fuller account of the infection (see 'Cryptosporidiosis', Chapter 20). Notwithstanding its primary site of infection, the disease is most often diagnosed microbiologically in stool samples and colorectal biopsies may demonstrate the protozoa adherent to the surface of colorectal epithelium, on the surface of the mucosa and within crypts. Here they appear as uniform haematoxyphilic dots. Their uniformity helps to distinguish them from mimics, especially small blobs of mucin. Electron microscopy reveals the characteristic forms of the organism's life cycle.

AIDS patients are unable to clear the organism, clearance being the usual defence mechanism in immunocompetent individuals, and infection in AIDS patients will persist for the rest of the patient's life, unless eradicated by appropriate treatment. Such infection is usually seen in patients with CD4 counts of <100. Cryptosporidiosis is often seen in association with other pathogens in the gut, particularly *Giardia* sp., microsporidia and CMV.

Microsporidiosis

Microsporidia are spore-forming intracellular protozoa which may cause encephalitis as well as enterocolitis. They are found as pathogens in birds, fish and some mammals. They are found more commonly in HIV-infected patients. Subtyping requires expertise and electron microscopy. Although these organisms may be seen as intracellular parasites of the colorectal epithelium in AIDS patients [153,203–206], they are primarily an enteric infection, so a more detailed account may be found elsewhere (see 'Microsporidiosis', Chapter 20). At the time of colonoscopy, few

if any abnormalities have been ascribed to the infection, although, if the terminal ileum is entered, some villous abnormalities may be seen.

Balantidiasis

Balantidium coli is a large, ciliated protozoon, which causes changes in the colon and rectum similar to those seen in amoebic colitis [207,208]. Tissue diagnosis depends on recognising the organisms within histological sections. Their numbers associated with severe necrosis and their huge nuclei make recognition easy.

Chagas' disease (intestinal trypanosomiasis)

The colopathy resulting from chronic infection with South American trypanosomiasis, caused by *Trypanosoma cruzi*, results in neuromuscular pathology of the colon and rectum, including colomegaly, neuropathy, loss of myenteric ganglia and muscle hypertrophy. It is dealt with elsewhere (see 'Neurological disorders', Chapter 34).

Helminthic infection

Helminthic infection most commonly occurs in the small intestine and, apart from schistosomiasis, primary infection of the colorectum is not often observed by the practising histopathologist: it is much more common in the small intestine (see 'Helminthic infection', Chapter 20). Occasional cases of hyper-infestation with strongyloidiasis are seen in the large bowel, especially in immunocompromised hosts.

Schistosomiasis

Infestation of the large intestine is most commonly caused by *Schistosoma mansoni* [209] and S. japonicum [210]. S. haematobium is found in the bladder and only rarely involves the intestine [211]. *S. mansoni* is endemic in African and central South American countries, including the Caribbean islands. *S. japonicum* is found in Japan, China and the Philippine Islands, and the countries of south-east Asia. *S. haematobium* is found in Africa, particularly Egypt, and in countries of the near Middle East.

Infection occurs in humans while wading or bathing in water contaminated with the larval stage of the worm, the cercaria. This penetrates the skin and enters venules, from whence it is carried through the heart and systemic circulation to the liver where the cercariae mature to form adult worms. These migrate to the mesenteric veins, and particularly the submucosal vessels of the gut, where they lay their ova. The latter pass through the intestine into the faeces. The cycle is completed in water contaminated with faeces containing eggs. The latter hatch out, liberating larvae that are ingested by the intermediate host, the snail, within which the second larval stage of cercariae develop and eventually emerge in a free-swimming form.

The pathological changes in schistosomiasis are essentially the result of an inflammatory reaction to the eggs in the tissues of the intestinal wall. The severity depends on host immunity and the infecting dose. Lesions are most common in the rectum and left colon, and are then nearly always due to *S. mansoni*. On the right side of the colon and the appendix, *S. japonicum* is more common and *S. haematobium* is only rarely responsible for disease [212].

In the early stages, there is an acute proctitis and colitis, accompanied by oedema, haemorrhage and discharge of eggs into the bowel lumen. There then follows a state of chronic infection, which leads to a great variety of morphological appearances. Localised or diffuse ulceration, strictures due to extensive granulomatous inflammation, pericolic masses and polyposis are the main types. Schistosomal localised or diffuse polyposis, due to the chronic inflammation of the infestation, may be confused with other types, including the inflammatory polyposis caused by ulcerative colitis and familial adenomatous polyposis.

The microscopic appearances of schistosomiasis are characteristic (Figure 35.8). The eggs are surrounded by epithelioid cell histiocytes and giant cells. Outside these, there is infiltration by leukocytes, mainly eosinophils, and proliferation of fibroblasts. In chronic cases, a characteristic concentric fibrosis develops around the granuloma and sometimes the parasitic eggs become completely calcified. Not infrequently, eggs may be embedded in tissue without any surrounding inflammatory reaction. The eggs of *S. mansoni* are oval and possess a lateral spine. In *S. haema-tobium* the egg has a terminal spine but is much the same size and shape. The lateral spine of *S. japonicum* is smaller than that of *S. mansoni* and the egg is more spherical.

The diagnosis of schistosomiasis is made by finding the schistosomal granulomas in rectal biopsies [210,212]. As old or effete ova may invoke no inflammatory response, it is worthwhile examining multiple levels of any biopsy from a patient in whom schistosomiasis is suspected. A Ziehl–Neelsen stain is useful because the chitinous coats of the ova of *S. mansoni* stain red. There is an increased incidence of carcinoma of the large bowel in patients with chronic schistosomal infection [213,214]. Dysplasia probably precedes the development of carcinoma in a fashion similar to ulcerative colitis.

Inflammatory bowel diseases

This is a group of chronic relapsing diseases characterised by chronic diarrhoea that can be bloody or watery. When there are overt endoscopic changes, one is usually dealing with ulcerative colitis or Crohn's disease, or sometimes inflammatory bowel disease of undetermined aetiology (now best termed 'IBDU') [215]. If the endoscopic changes are sparse, one may be dealing with one of the variants of microscopic colitis. However these are well-defined diseases and terms such as 'non-specific inflammatory bowel disease' are discouraged. Indeed the term 'non-specific', whether used as a clinical, endoscopic or histological prefix, is invariably a hedge for ignorance and the omission of this 'prefix' never changes the meaning of the sentence or diagnosis. If the histological changes are those of CIBD but cannot be further categorised, then the diligent pathologist is advised to say so, rather than hiding behind a diagnosis of 'non-specific chronic active colitis', when one really means chronic inflammatory bowel disease of uncertain type.

Ulcerative colitis

Ulcerative colitis is a CIBD of the large intestine, which, with the possible exception of rare patients with diverticular colitis, always begins in the rectum. In some, the disease remains limited to the rectum (ulcerative proctitis), whereas in others it may extend proximally to involve a variable length of the large intestine and sometimes the entire large bowel (pancolitis or extensive colitis) in a continuous or diffuse fashion, although the changes are almost always more severe in the distal large intestine. It is a disease characterised by periods of exacerbation and remission. Less commonly there is continuous low grade activity or an initial single attack which years later causes questions as to whether this was really an infection (hence the need for initial biopsy documentation) or presentation with severe disease, sometimes with dilatation (toxic

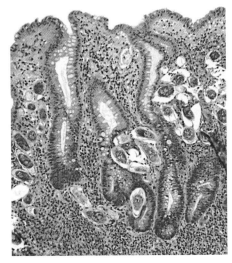

Figure 35.8 Rectal biopsy with multiple schistosome eggs within the lamina propria.

megacolon). Involvement of the terminal ileum can occur in patients with pancolitis, in continuity with disease in the colon, but this has little significance from the treatment viewpoint.

Of importance in the differentiation from Crohn's disease, ulcerative colitis is primarily an inflammatory condition of the mucosa although, in cases of severe disease, deeper layers of the bowel wall can be involved. The appearance of the bowel depends much on the severity and length of history of disease. Although Crohn's disease may also be initially mucosal, the inflammation has a much greater aptitude to involve deeper layers of the bowel.

Surgical resection is usually performed for chronic extensive ulcerative colitis resistant to medical therapy or dependent on unacceptable levels of therapy, for severe disease, and in patients with other complications including dysplasia and/or carcinoma. The study of surgical specimens therefore shows only a limited spectrum of the disease. In biopsies, the great majority of patients have milder and less extensive disease and it is emphasised that ulcerative proctitis is the most common manifestation of the disease.

Ulcerative colitis is classically diffuse in its distribution. However, not all the diseased bowel need be in a similar state of activity and this can create a false impression of segmental involvement, especially after systemic or local treatment. Activity is usually maximal in the rectum unless the patient is receiving local therapy, and tends to decrease proximally but a caecal [216] or peri-appendiceal [217–222] patch may be surprisingly active and discontinuous from more distal disease. This apparent 'skip lesion' is therefore easily interpreted as Crohn's disease and not a proximal patch associated with distal ulcerative colitis. By definition peri-appendiceal or caecal patches should not occur in patients with pancolitis, then being part of the background disease. The reported incidence of appendiceal involvement [21–86%) and caecal patch lesions (10–75%) is highly variable and sometimes similar skip lesions in the ascending colon have also been described in a small subset (4%). One study found that peri-appendiceal disease had a male predominance. None had had a prior appendicectomy but, although there was proximal extension in half, this was no more than in historical controls [223]. Focality of inflammatory activity can also be occasioned by treatment, especially local steroid therapy, by enema, in the rectum.

It is important for pathologists to recognise that, in some patients, there can be reversal of both endoscopic and histological changes, to the point that the biopsies appear absolutely normal [224]. This is seen especially in patients with longstanding disease in surveillance biopsies. The implication of this is that, although we can review biopsies and report 'no evidence of CIBD', we can never say that the patient does not have CIBD. Return to normality after treatment of classic ulcerative colitis may result in so-called 'rectal sparing' which has occasionally been reported [225–227]. Interestingly, in resected specimens, the thickened duplicated muscularis mucosae may be the only recognisable tombstone of previous involvement.

Aetiology and pathogenesis

The aetiology of ulcerative colitis remains unknown, despite extensive research into likely causes, such as infection, diet and environmental factors, primary immunological defects, abnormalities of mucin, genetic defects and psychomotor disorders. Abnormalities have been detected in several of these. The pathogenesis of the disease is ultimately likely to encompass one or more genetic factors in association with the action of external agents (antigens, organisms) and altered host immunology, possibly a failure to down-regulate a normal immune reaction. The other factor essential for developing CIBD is the presence of microbes in the gut, because, in all experimental models of CIBD, the disease cannot be reproduced in a germ-free environment. Although so far no single pathogen has been consistently shown to be associated with CIBD, it seems clear that the interplay between micro-organisms and the immune system plays a central role in the aetiopathogenesis of CIBD. Further, a proportion of patients (25% in one series) developing either ulcerative colitis or Crohn's disease relate their onset to an episode of infection [84].

An intriguing feature of ulcerative colitis is the possibility that prior appendicectomy may protect against the development of ulcerative colitis. The weight of data suggests that appendicectomy does indeed protect against the development of ulcerative colitis [228] and may also delay disease onset, as well as producing a milder CIBD phenotype [229], although the extent of disease may well be greater [230]. The mechanism of this activity is unclear. However, the appendix may act as a reservoir or safe house for maintaining large bowel flora, serving as a reservoir for normal flora when an acute infection is present in the large bowel. Its removal might therefore disturb normal large bowel flora or, if the response is immune mediated, there may be immune mimicry between appendiceal and rectal mucosa, so that inflammation at one site induces inflammation at the other. Most of the time, the activity at one site is similar to the other in ulcerative colitis, suggesting that they behave as a single unit.

Another major factor involved in the aetiology of ulcerative colitis is smoking, because it is clear that, in contrast to Crohn's disease, smoking is preventive and some patients have their first attack when they stop smoking and some patients, including this small subset, are best controlled by unobtrusively smoking a few cigarettes a day. Interestingly nicotine, in other forms, seems not to have the same effect. This could be linked to the finding that the colonic mucosa of smokers demonstrates increased glycoprotein synthesis, compared with that of non-smokers, which would help maintain the protective colonic mucosal barrier [231–233].

Depletion of goblet cell mucin is a characteristic feature of ulcerative colitis and mucus has an important role in preserving the integrity of the colonic mucosa against trauma and bacterial attack. Primary abnormalities of colonic mucus have been demonstrated: several components of colonic mucin have been identified and a reduction in one type found in ulcerative colitis, even in cases in remission [234]. Changes in mucin pattern are not related to alteration in bacterial faecal degradation enzymes or to any differential susceptibility of mucus in ulcerative colitis to desialation or desulphation.

Epidemiological factors

The peak age incidence of initial presentation with ulcerative colitis, for either sex, is in the third decade. However, the disease can present in very young children or elderly people [235–237], in whom the anatomical distribution of the disease may be different [238]. The disease is common in most communities of Anglo-Saxon origin in north-western Europe, North America and New Zealand, with incidence ranging between 58 and 105 per 100 000 of the population. Prevalence figures for Scandinavia and much of North America reach over 100 per 100 000 of the population [239,240]. The disease shares many epidemiological similarities with Crohn's disease and, although it is said to be uncommon in eastern Europe, southern Europe and developing countries, much of this is due to a failure to diagnose the disease, to attribute it to recurrent infections or to require specific histological features for the diagnosis. In Japan and India both major forms of CIBD are well recognised, and large series are starting to appear in the literature from these countries and other developing countries.

Generally the incidence is reported to be stable or gradually rising [239,241], although there are isolated marked rises in some stable well-documented communities [240, 242]. There is a higher incidence of ulcerative colitis in towns and urban communities compared with rural societies [243]. The incidence of Crohn's disease is rising in children, probably for similar reasons, although other factors have been proposed, including infection by *Mycobacterium paratuberculosis* and *Yersinia* spp. [244,245]. At one time MMR (measles, mumps, rubella) immunisation was implicated in the development of Crohn's disease. However, the evidence has since been refuted [246]: this is described more fully elsewhere (see 'Crohn's disease', Chapter 20).

In most studies the incidence rates for ulcerative colitis are higher than for Crohn's disease and an increasing incidence of ulcerative colitis in a population generally precedes an increase in Crohn's disease by a time lag of approximately 15–20 years. In almost all studies, the Jewish population has a greater incidence of ulcerative colitis than in other groupings [247–249], although incidence studies in Israel are not very different from those of other high incidence areas such as the UK and Scandinavia. There is no gender predilection for ulcerative colitis, although, for Crohn's disease, there is a slight female predominance.

Genetics

A genetic factor for CIBD was first thought likely because siblings and first-degree relatives of patients with ulcerative colitis carry an increased risk of developing not only ulcerative colitis but also Crohn's disease. Twin studies show phenotypic concordance of 50% for Crohn's disease versus only 18% for ulcerative colitis. When identical twins with Crohn's disease both have CIBD, they are remarkably similar, although, surprisingly, only about 15% of monozygotic twins both have CIBD [250,251]. Relatives of patients with Crohn's disease have an increased risk of developing ulcerative colitis, calculated to be about eightfold [252]. Patients with HLA-1327 and -BW35 phenotypes also carry an increased risk [253].

A positive family history of CIBD seems to be the single most important factor determining an individual's risk of developing IBD, although both family studies and twin studies indicate a stronger genetic effect for Crohn's disease than for ulcerative colitis. Of 522 patients with Crohn's disease, 187 (35.2%) were found to have an affected family member, of which 87 (16.7%) were first-degree relatives [249]. The equivalent frequency in the group with ulcerative colitis was 20 out of a total of 171 patients (11.7%) [249]. Satsangi found that 41 of 317 (13%) patients with Crohn's disease had a positive family history of CIBD [252]. The greatest risk was in those with a monozygotic twin with Crohn's disease or those who have two affected parents. The risk of getting CIBD if two parents are affected is in the region of 30–40% [253]. Kirsner reported that, of 103 families with more than 1 case of CIBD, 31 families contained both Crohn's disease and ulcerative colitis patients [254]. Two British studies have demonstrated similar findings [249,255].

There are now innumerable 'CIBD' genes. To date, over 60 published CIBD susceptibility loci have been confirmed, of which about a third are associated with both ulcerative colitis and Crohn's disease, about a third specific to ulcerative colitis and about a third to Crohn's disease. New loci for ulcerative colitis include genes implicated in mucosal barrier function (*ECM1*, *CDH1*, *HNF4α* and *laminin B1*). Furthermore, E-cadherin studies are the first to show a genetic correlation between ulcerative colitis and colorectal cancer. Impaired interleukin 10 (IL-10) signalling also seems to be a key pathway in intestinal inflammation [256]. One of these, mutations in the *NOD1/CARD4* gene, codes for a protein that is a cytoplasmic receptor or a tri-peptide moiety of peptidoglycan, found predominantly in Gram-negative bacteria. This receptor leads to activation of NF-κb. Furthermore, patients with ulcerative colitis with the HLA class 2 allele (HLA-DRBI* 0103) are very likely to have severe disease that often requires colectomy.

NOD2 was the first susceptibility gene described in Crohn's disease and is located on chromosome 16. It predisposes to terminal ileal Crohn's disease [257–259]. These data support the notion that Crohn's disease represents an abnormal immune response to enteric bacteria in genetically susceptible individuals. Numerous polymorphisms of the NOD gene have been identified [259] but it is uncertain how many of these are associated with Crohn's disease susceptibility.

A number of other genetic polymorphisms have been reported to play a role in CIBD pathogenesis. Polymorphisms causing a lower expression of the human multidrug resistance 1 gene product, P-glycoprotein, have also been associated with the risk of developing ulcerative colitis or CIBD in general. Toll-like receptors (TLRs) are receptors of the innate immune system that are involved in recognition of bacterial products. The TLR4 Asp299Gly polymorphism has also been associated with CIBD in various studies. Increased intestinal epithelial expression of TLR4 has been noted in CIBD. Thus far, it appears that there are multiple susceptibility genes, some common to both diseases and some linked separately to one disease or the other [256].

Microbiological agents and other environmental factors

The relationship between infections and CIBD is complex. Besides a possible aetiological role, infections play a part in disease exacerbations and its complications. The search for a microbial cause for ulcerative colitis has been inconclusive but has produced fewer false trails than similar work on Crohn's disease [260,261]. Attempts to identify infective agents in the stool and mucosa, or to demonstrate raised antibody titres to particular organisms in patients' sera, are problematic. The difficulty is trying to establish whether an abnormality, when present, is the primary defect or simply a secondary phenomenon. Patients with ulcerative colitis have raised antibody titres to numerous organisms including a lipopolysaccharide extract of *Escherichia coli* O14, an antibody common to most enterobacteria [262,263]. This antibody cross-reacts with goblet cell antigen in colonic epithelium [194]. Similar antibodies are found in first-degree female relatives who have undamaged mucosa [264,265]. The sharing of antigens between the large intestinal epithelium and intestinal bacteria has also proved the basis of methods for inducing experimental colitis in animals [194,266]. As well as *E. coli*, raised antibody titres have been demonstrated to certain *Bacteroides* spp., and eubacterial, peptococcal and *Mycobacterium kansasii* antigens [267,268], suggesting a leaky mucosa

to bacteria and secondary antibody generation. Anti-*Saccharomyces cerevisiae* antibody (ASCA), anti-*neutrophil cytoplasmic* antibody (ANCA) and similar antibodies may occur on the same basis.

None of the common enteropathogens is consistently associated with ulcerative colitis but many of these infections may herald the onset of disease or precipitate a relapse. In one study almost a quarter of patients with an attack of 'colitis' after a recent visit to a tropical environment were shown to have developed ulcerative colitis [83]. The onset of the disease was presumably initiated by an infection or a significant change in colonic flora, e.g. the presence of *Clostridium difficile* may have a role in the relapse of colitis, especially in patients receiving antibiotics [269].

Helicobacters have been isolated from human faeces and, in animal models, they can cause CIBD-like disease, but on the evidence available, *Helicobacter pylori* does not seem to have a role in the cause of CIBD. Viruses studied include measles. In a review of the maternity records of 25 000 babies, 4 mothers had had measles during pregnancy, and 3 of the 4 children had developed severe Crohn's disease [270]. The three cases showed the presence of the measles virus antigen by immunogold electron microscopy. The authors concluded that exposure to measles virus *in utero* or in the perinatal period inferred an increased risk of Crohn's disease. A further study based on the population of the UK suggested that the risk might also apply to children immunised against measles [271]. Immunohistochemical evidence has indicated that the measles protein apparently demonstrated in the human tissues is of human, and not viral, origin; the current conclusion is that there is no specificity to the association between measles exposure and subsequent Crohn's disease [272,273].

Granulomatous Crohn's disease resembles intestinal tuberculosis, both clinically and in its mucosal pathology, whereas *M. paratuberculosis* causes an enterocolitis in cattle, known as Johne's disease, although this has little histological similarity to human intestinal tuberculosis or Crohn's disease. Isolating mycobacteria from CIBD tissue has been very difficult, perhaps because these fastidious organisms are extremely difficult to culture, and the leakiness of the gut in CIBD casts doubt on the significance of any organisms found. *M. paratuberculosis* has been demonstrated in Crohn's disease tissue and less so in ulcerative colitis tissue [274]. However, no consistent results have yet been found to support the notion that this bacterium is specifically involved in the pathogenesis of either form of CIBD, particularly Crohn's disease. The clinical data that immunosuppressive treatment of CIBD is usually beneficial, even in those with profound immunosuppression [275], would suggest that mycobacterial infection is unlikely to cause CIBD.

It is also very likely that there is no single microbe or specific group of pathogens responsible for the development of CIBD, but the alteration in normal gut flora may be involved. The alteration in the resident intestinal microflora may be responsible for the initiation and amplification of the increased intestinal inflammation. The normal colonic flora may also play a role in initiation of the disease and the progression to chronicity. Experimentally, in rats, it has been shown that certain broad-spectrum antibiotics prevent chronicity after colitis induced by trinitrobenzenesulphonic acid. Bacteria or bacterial products seem to be critical to the induction of mucosal ulcerations in the small bowel by indometacin, because germ-fee rats develop minimal lesions. Because of molecular analogy between some bacterial proteins and human heat shock proteins (HSPs), an autoimmune reaction could be induced. Bacterial products (peptidoglycans) can be responsible for an immune reaction and bacterial cell wall fragments can provoke a granulomatous response.

Immunology

To explain the aetiology of ulcerative colitis and the basis for its pathogenesis by an immunological defect is an attractive thesis and this has resulted in a plethora of complex and contentious findings [276]. However, the gut epithelium in CIBD is leaky so that numerous organisms can be found within the wall of the bowel, especially in Crohn's disease, as a secondary effect. Establishing that the observation is of primary and not of secondary importance is difficult.

All limbs of the immune system have been investigated in ulcerative colitis and no consistent antecedent abnormalities in humoral or cell-mediated immunity have been demonstrated. There is increased B-cell activity in the mucosa in ulcerative colitis with alteration in the ratios of IgA and IgG immunoglobulins and in IgG-containing cells [277]. However, nothing is specific to this pattern of immune response.

There have been many attempts to produce experimental colitis in animals. These have used a variety of chemical models and genetic manipulation with knock-out models of numerous genes. Virtually all require the presence of luminal bacteria [278]. These have thrown considerable light mechanistically, although understanding the parallels between murine and other animal models, on the one hand, and human disease, on the other, has proved difficult. The theories behind the immunological aspects of the role of appendicectomy in protecting against ulcerative colitis have already been described (see above).

Macroscopic appearances in surgical specimens

On external examination, the length of the colon and rectum may be shortened in chronic ulcerative colitis, sometimes markedly so with obliteration of the sigmoid loop. This shortening appears to be due to muscular contraction of both muscle layers and is most obvious in the distal colon and rectum. Fibrosis is often present in the submucosa, which may be completely obliterated. Clinically, shortening of the colon is sometimes reversible if remission is maintained [279]. The contraction is accompanied by a reduction in the transverse calibre, which is also particularly marked in the distal large bowel. In the rectum it accounts for the increase in the sacrorectal distance, which is an important sign in the radiographic diagnosis of ulcerative colitis. The serosa is intact and retains its normal shiny surface, although there is considerable congestion and dilatation of blood vessels. The exception is severe disease that has become transmural, including toxic dilatation, either of which can perforate. The regional lymph nodes are sometimes enlarged.

Involvement of the terminal ileum in ulcerative colitis (so-called backwash ileitis) is rarely seen on external examination. Severe involvement is rare but can be associated with a tendency to dilatation, rigidity and muscular thickening of the bowel wall. When these changes are present, the possibility of Crohn's disease should always be considered.

On opening a fresh surgical specimen of ulcerative colitis, the first notable feature in active disease is the amount of dark fluid and blood present within the lumen, justifying the French terminology of *rectocolite hémorrhagique*. The mucosa has a granular or velvety surface appearance and is extremely friable (Figures 35.9 and 35.10). When ulcers are present, the deep (circular) muscle coat may be visible (Figure 35.11). The earliest form of macroscopically recognisable mucosal damage is redness with a prominent vascular pattern and erosion with purulent foci. Full-thickness ulceration of the mucosa is usually patchy but any intact intervening mucosa is always diseased. In severe disease the ulceration may have a linear distribution, especially in the colon where it is related to the line of attachment of the taeniae coli (Figure 35.9). Conversely, in resections for steroid resistance or dysplasia, the disease may be completely quiescent.

Inflammatory changes in ulcerative colitis are continuous with three notable exceptions. The first two are the appendiceal 'skip lesion' [217–222] and the caecal patch lesion [225] (Figure 35.12). However, severely affected areas may sometimes be separated by patches of less obviously involved mucosa, because not all regions of the bowel show equal activity. The other is diverticular-associated colitis, described subsequently, which is usually limited to the sigmoid colon.

The mucosal changes of ulcerative colitis usually involve the rectum initially and may remain localised or spread proximally in continuity until a larger part of, or the entire, large bowel may be involved. In many patients, the disease

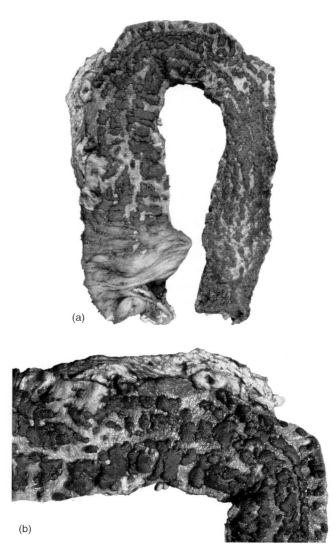

(a)

(b)

Figure 35.9 Severe ulcerative colitis: (a) active disease involves most of the large bowel in a diffuse, continuous fashion from the rectum to the mid-ascending colon. (b) There is widespread ulceration that tends to be linear, interspersed with residual islands of dark, granular, haemorrhagic mucosa.

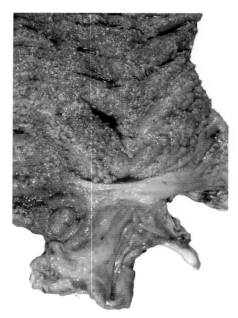

Figure 35.10 Active ulcerative colitis affecting the right side of the colon: the mucosa of the caecum and ascending colon is diffusely inflamed with a uniform, granular, velvety appearance. This extends up to the ileo-caecal valve; the mucosa of the terminal ileum is unaffected.

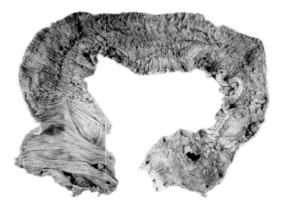

Figure 35.11 Fulminant ulcerative colitis with toxic dilatation: the transverse colon is particularly dilated and shows deep ulceration with residual mucosal islands. Many inflammatory polyps are seen in the left side of the colon.

is extensive at first presentation, so there is nothing to suggest that the disease was ever anything other than extensive. The extent determines whether the diagnosis is that of ulcerative proctitis, ulcerative proctosigmoiditis or distal colitis, left-sided ulcerative colitis (distal to the splenic flexure), substantial colitis (distal to the hepatic flexure) or extensive. Genetic determinants may be important in deciding the extent of disease. Anatomical variations in arterial supply to the colon are, we believe, a less likely explanation [280].

Rectal sparing

Ulcerative colitis with a sigmoidoscopically and histologically normal rectum is very unusual, in our experience, and some believe that it never occurs. In most patients, crypt architectural distortion is present, but, as discussed previously, this can completely resolve, which is different to never being present. Occasionally the rectal mucosa may look endoscopically normal and have no architectural dis-

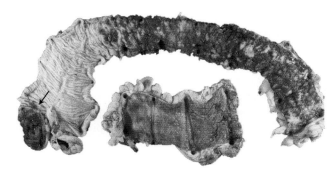

Figure 35.12 Active ulcerative colitis: this specimen shows the colon (above) and the separated rectum (below). There is severe diffuse left-sided disease with a sharp cut-off in the mid-transverse colon. Within the caecum there is a round disc-like area of discontinuous active disease (arrow), a so-called caecal patch lesion.

tortion but thickening and duplication of the muscularis mucosae and a degree of submucosal fibrosis are invariably present. However, such features may not be seen in biopsies and may require resection specimens to demonstrate them [281].

Rectal sparing can be an illusion because the features can be produced by healing in response to local steroid enemas, leading to endoscopic, but not histological, healing. This is best termed 'relative rectal sparing' rather than true rectal sparing. On occasion, relative rectal sparing may occur in some patients with ulcerative colitis in the absence of rectal instillation of anti-inflammatory drugs. However, in two controlled studies in ulcerative colitis associated with primary sclerosing cholangitis, although one study showed a distinct right-sided tendency compared with control individuals [282], the other showed no difference [283]. In both groups there were patients with apparently normal rectal mucosa. There is no way of knowing whether the rectum was never involved in these patients or whether there was active involvement with return to normal because there was no architectural abnormality [284].

In general, the severity of the mucosal changes in surgical specimens is usually greatest in the distal large bowel and tends to diminish proximally. Even in total colitis, the disease is usually more severe in the left colon and rectum (see Figure 35.11). This pattern is very useful when seen in sequential biopsies. Macroscopically, the proximal limit of the disease most frequently shows an abrupt transition from disease to normal mucosa, but a gradual change is more usually seen histologically. Clearly the mucosal appearances will depend on the stage of activity at the time of resection and, in very severe disease, focal ulcers can be present and there may even be transition zones in the form of ulcers both proximally and distally.

One of the significant features of ulcerative colitis is the relative lack of fibrosis in the lamina propria or muscularis propria, although duplication of the muscularis mucosae is often accompanied by a degree of adjacent submucosal fibrosis, identifying sites of prior ulceration. There may be an increase in the amount of collagen in the superficial submucosa, particularly in the rectum, but this is quantitatively relatively small even when there is a long history of severe disease. Rarely strictures occur on the basis of hyperplasia of the muscularis mucosae with submucosal fibrosis [285]. If true fibrous strictures are present in a colon with diffuse inflammation, the diagnosis of Crohn's disease, rather than ulcerative colitis, should be considered. Alternatively stricture formation can be the result of coexistent diverticular disease or malignant change.

Polyps in ulcerative colitis

Polyps are common in ulcerative colitis, being present in about 12–20% of cases and are more commonly associated with bouts of previous severe disease [286,287]. These comprise both mucosal excrescences and re-epithelialised granulation tissue. These inflammatory polyps or mucosal tags may be present in large numbers and adopt bizarre shapes. The term 'pseudo-polyp' is commonly used to describe these post-inflammatory polyps but this is a poor term. How can you have a lesion that looks like something that is raised above an epithelial surface? In our view, 'inflammatory polyp' is a much better designation because it indicates the mechanism of development of the polyps. However these have to be distinguished from mucosal islands, which, ironically, may be genuine 'pseudo-polyps'. They are the result of localised ulceration of the mucosa and usually submucosa, with undermining of adjacent intact mucosa, resembling amoebic ulcers. The remaining mucosa appears raised, but only relative to the adjacent ulcerated mucosa, so that it appears to form a polyp (see Figure 35.11). The polyp is therefore formed by the adjacent ulcers, and the term 'mucosal islands' is actually preferable to 'pseudo-polyp', removing the ambiguity inherent in that term.

Inflammatory polyps can become adherent to form mucosal bridges across the lumen. If healing takes place, forests of polyps may remain as evidence of past disease, so-called colitis polyposa, giant inflammatory polyposis or villiform polyposis (Figure 35.13). This polyposis of ulcerative colitis is more prominent in the colon than the rectum, especially in the descending colon and sigmoid colon, and may be seen proximal to the area of active disease. The polyposis may be so severe as to cause large bowel obstruction. Benign inflammatory polyps rarely become dysplastic.

Adenomas can occur in ulcerative colitis patients, as in the rest of the population, as do adenoma-like masses, and dysplasia-associated lesions or masses (DALMs). However, unless the lesion occurs in non-dysplastic mucosa, when it

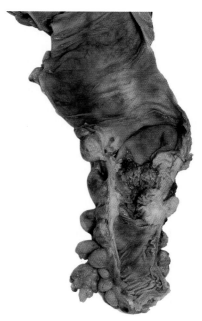

Figure 35.13 Inactive ulcerative colitis: re-epithelialisation after previous ulceration in the descending colon has given rise to a villiform inflammatory polyposis (centrally) with only modest abnormalities (mucosal flattening mainly) in the adjacent mucosa.

has no relationship to the colitic process, the management of all dysplastic lesions in colitic mucosa is identical, so this division is of historical interest only. Both are now treated by polypectomy and biopsy of the surrounding mucosa to ensure that local excision is complete. If excision is proved to be complete, then no further therapy is required for that lesion. If excision is incomplete, the lesion cannot be removed endoscopically or lesions are multiple, then colectomy is required. Adenomas can be straightforward to diagnose in ulcerative colitis if they occur in the adenoma age group, in non-colitic mucosa, especially on the right side of the colon, and are pedunculated. These issues are discussed in more detail subsequently.

Ileal involvement in ulcerative colitis

When the terminal ileum is involved, the mucosal changes are similar to those seen in the colon and are always in continuity with disease in the large bowel, being associated with an open dilated and incompetent ileo-caecal valve. Although the expression 'backwash ileitis' is not necessarily accurate, because there is, as yet, no evidence that ileal disease is the result of such a mechanism, it is in common usage. Ileitis is found in about 10% of colectomy specimens for ulcerative colitis, the extent of involvement varying from 50 mm to 250 mm. Only very rarely is the involved segment considerably longer than this.

Pre-stomal ileitis is a condition usually seen as a complication of ileostomy formation in patients with ulcerative colitis [288]. In this rare disease, ulcers are scattered throughout the ileum and jejunum. The intervening mucosa is normal or oedematous. The ulcers can perforate, resulting in peritonitis and faecal fistulae.

Inflammation of the ileum occurs in pelvic ileal reservoirs with an adaptive colonic phenotypic change of the mucosa to produce a picture similar to the original colitis, and is also seen in the ileum proximal to the pouch (pre-pouch ileitis). For a full account of the small intestinal manifestations of chronic ulcerative colitis, the interested reader is referred to 'Ileal reservoirs and pouchitis', Chapter 20).

Fulminant colitis and toxic megacolon

Between 5% and 12% of patients with ulcerative colitis have a fulminating episode [289,290], either as a first attack or in an acute relapse. In a proportion the colon may be resected as an emergency measure (see Figure 35.11). There is severe diffuse disease and there may also be a segment, most commonly the transverse colon, that becomes acutely dilated. In this so-called toxic megacolon, the bowel wall is markedly thinned. The intestine may have the consistency of wet paper tearing readily, with subsequent perforation and peritonitis. There is extensive mucosal ulceration with surviving islands of mucosa showing intense congestion. Single or multiple perforations of the thinned bowel, either spontaneous or produced at the time of surgery, were at one time common but this is much less commonly seen now.

Fulminant colitis is severe disease usually necessitating resection and can complicate any form of colitis. There is frequently a fibrinous or fibrino-purulent exudate on the peritoneal surface. The caecum and ascending colon are not invariably involved [291]. Furthermore, the lower sigmoid and rectum may be macroscopically spared and so mislead the examining sigmoidoscopist [281,292]. In fulminant ulcerative colitis, there is inflammation beyond the mucosa, often into, and sometimes through, the muscularis propria, unlike that usually seen in ulcerative colitis. However, the pattern of this inflammation is important. In fulminant ulcerative colitis, the active inflammation extends into the muscularis propria as a polymorphous infiltrate. This is quite different from the focal lymphoid hyperplasia with lymphoid aggregates and follicles, which are seen in a transmural distribution in Crohn's disease. The myenteric plexus may be incidentally involved but the colonic dilatation might be due to a primary toxic atrophy of muscle cells [290,293]. Prominent telangiectasia of all blood vessels, including capillaries and myocytolysis, is the hallmark of a fulminant episode of disease.

Fissuring ulcers are part of severe or fulminant disease, irrespective of the underlying aetiology, and do not themselves imply a diagnosis of Crohn's disease. These fissures may extend into, and sometimes through, the muscularis propria but perforation is rare. Again the inflammation may be transmural but it is polymorphous with numerous plasma cells. Granulomas are rare but care has to be taken with mucosal granulomas that are much more frequently secondary to ruptured crypts or foreign material.

The fulminant stage of CIBD in resection specimens is one in which a diagnosis of indeterminate colitis may be appropriate if the histological features do not allow a positive distinction between ulcerative colitis and Crohn's disease [294]. It should also be appreciated that fulminant colitis can occur during the course of the many different types of inflammatory pathology of the colorectum and the intensity and distribution of ulceration may be similar in all, often making it difficult to make a macroscopic diagnosis of the underlying disease in this phase of the disease [295]. In those cases of fulminant colitis where the histological features do not allow the original cause of the colitis to be determined, all clinical, radiological, endoscopic and histological features should be reviewed. It is important to obtain pre-treatment, as well as post-treatment, biopsies, because post-treatment changes may be misleadingly patchy. The length of history may be helpful. If of considerable duration, the disease is unlikely to be due to infection. Stool culture may also be helpful. If there has been a colectomy, with the rectum left *in situ* and an ileostomy formed, the ensuing histological changes in the diverted rectum are helpful only until the features of diversion disease supervene, usually ≥2 months, after which the features of diversion disease dominate the picture and do not allow insight into the underlying disease. The crypt architecture is likely to be normal in most cases of infective procto-colitis but is often abnormal in ulcerative colitis.

In this situation, one helpful feature is the difference in response to diversion shown by Crohn's disease and ulcerative colitis patients. Diversion of the faecal stream in ulcerative colitis will result in severe changes of diversion superimposed on those of ulcerative colitis, whereas in diverted Crohn's disease procto-colitis, there is usually remission of the inflammatory changes [296,297]. Diversion-related changes are usually well established within 3 months [298].

Appendiceal involvement

The appendix is involved in about 75% of total colectomy specimens performed for ulcerative colitis. This may be continuous with extensive colitis or may represent a 'skip lesion' of ulcerative colitis [219–222]. Such a 'skip lesion', although apparently suggestive of Crohn's disease, should not be regarded as a contraindication to pouch surgery. This mucosal appendicitis may extend into the contiguous large bowel as a peri-appendiceal patch lesion. It does not lead on to an acute suppurative appendicitis because the inflammation remains confined to the mucosa, with a histological appearance identical to that seen in ulcerative colitis in the colon and rectum [217].

Ulcerative proctitis

Inflammation localised to the rectal mucosa can be caused by a great variety of pathological entities such as mucosal prolapse, trauma, suppositories, radiation, antibiotic therapy, piles, persistent diarrhoea, Crohn's disease, ulcerative colitis and, in more recent years, increasing numbers of infectious agents, the latter having particular importance in the homosexual population, as well as in women engaging in anal sex. The old viewpoint was that, when these causes have been excluded, one is left with an idiopathic pattern of distal disease [299], for which there were many synonyms, including proctosigmoiditis, idiopathic proctitis, non-specific proctitis, lymphoid follicular proctitis (see below) and ulcerative proctitis. This implies that 'non-specific ulcerative proctitis' is a disease of exclusion. Up to a point this has some validity, if only clinical features are assessed and infections are excluded. However, in biopsies, the changes of ulcerative colitis are relatively specific and, similar to its more proximal counterpart ulcerative proctocolitis, the changes are usually readily discernible on biopsy. The 'non-specific' part of this eponym is therefore a historical title borne of ignorance when all biopsies were called 'non-specific chronic active colitis/proctitis', regrettably a designation still all too common. There was no appreciation that the chronic infections of this region whether sexually transmitted, tuberculous or even amoebic could be diagnosed and treated, and that the architectural distortion and deep plasma cells are the features of CIBD. If the disease is diffuse and there are crypt abscesses in their active phase, then these findings are virtually diagnostic of ulcerative colitis. The other main form of CIBD, Crohn's disease, rarely produces just these features in such a distribution.

The precise extent of the disease can be determined by flexible sigmoidoscopy and biopsy, because it is found that endoscopically normal mucosa may be histologically inflamed [300]. Biopsies above the proximal limit of disease may reveal that the disease is actually much more extensive than the active disease visualised at endoscopy. This is important to document because this finding may identify a patient for surveillance colonoscopies in the future.

In addition, approximately 10% of these patients with distal disease will develop more extensive ulcerative colitis [295], whereas 15% will have recurrent bouts of active disease and 75% will enter permanent remission. Extension of disease usually occurs within 2 years and seldom after 5 years [299]. There is some evidence that distal disease may predominate in an elderly population [238]. The symptoms from severe proctitis may be disabling as a result of defecatory frequency and urgency, with blood but little or no diarrhoea. In addition, chronic ulcerative proctitis may sometimes be remarkably resistant to medical therapy, including 5-aminosalicylic acid, local and even systemic steroids, and/or immunosuppressive agents. Some patients, with only rectal involvement, benefit greatly from restorative proctocolectomy [301]. Morphologically the disease has the features of ulcerative colitis, although the chronic inflammatory component may be more severe than its more extensive disease equivalents, even in remission [302].

Microscopic appearances

The chronic and intermittent nature of ulcerative colitis, with periods of exacerbation and remission, makes it convenient to divide the appearances into active disease, resolving disease and disease in remission.

Active ulcerative colitis

In active ulcerative colitis, the most striking features are:

• Architectural distortion, especially distally and proximally if a caecal patch is present.

• A diffuse chronic inflammatory cell infiltrate extending to the muscularis mucosae, the most reliable feature being the presence of plasma cells extending to the muscularis mucosae. However, in the caecal mucosa, this feature may be present normally in adults.

• Active disease reflected by neutrophils that seem to migrate directly from capillaries into the crypt epithelium (cryptitis) and often form crypt abscesses (neutrophils in the lumen). The latter can progress to focal loss of epithelium with neutrophils extending back into the adjacent lamina propria, erosions (breaks in the surface epithelium) and, less frequently, ulcers.

• Congestion and dilatation of the capillary blood vessels: the vascular changes and mucosal friability account for much of the bleeding tendency experienced during endoscopy.

The mucosa appears thickened and the surface epithelium may take on an undulating or low villiform appearance (Figure 35.14). The inflammation may extend into the superficial submucosa but the muscularis propria and serosa remain free of inflammation, except in severe or fulminant colitis.

An early feature of the histopathology of active ulcerative colitis is the formation of crypt abscesses in the mucosa. It must be emphasised that these reflect active disease and are not specific to ulcerative colitis, because they occur in a great variety of other intestinal inflammatory conditions, including Crohn's disease, infections and acute appendicitis. They are, however, particularly conspicuous in active ulcerative colitis (Figure 35.15). The small micro-abscess created expands and either bursts into the lumen of the

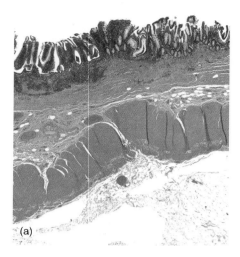

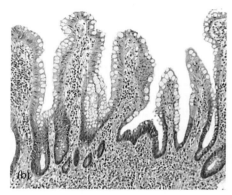

Figure 35.14 (a) Active ulcerative colitis emphasising the mucosal nature of the disease, all the damage and inflammation being limited to this layer of the bowel wall. (b) After prolonged active disease the mucosa can adopt a villiform pattern.

bowel, elaborating pus into the faeces, or spreads into the lamina propria, or, if inflammation is severe, into the submucosa.

It is significant that neutrophils are predominant within the lumen of the crypts in ulcerative colitis whereas, unlike in infective colitis, comparatively small numbers are seen migrating between the epithelial cells. In acute infections, they tend to be more superficial but are invariably plentiful in the lamina propria. This can be a helpful feature in the differentiation of ulcerative colitis from infective proctocolitis. Indeed, although neutrophils can be found in the lamina propria without crypt infiltration in ulcerative colitis, it is sufficiently uncommon that other causes, such as Crohn's disease or an infectious colitis superimposed on ulcerative colitis, should be considered.

Crypt abscesses play an important role in the mechanism of mucosal ulceration and in the formation of inflammatory polyps in ulcerative colitis. In severe disease, they burst

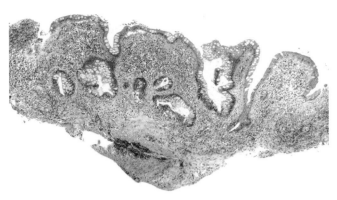

Figure 35.17 Resolving ulcerative colitis: the fading inflammatory infiltrate is becoming somewhat patchy and only focal acute inflammation remains. The goblet cell population is recovering. Regenerative epithelial hyperplasia is seen in the bases of crypts, which themselves show marked distortion.

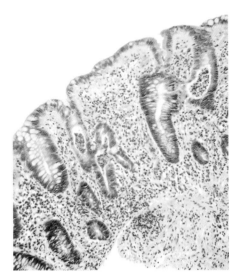

Figure 35.15 Active ulcerative colitis: there is crypt architectural distortion with variation in intercrypt spacing and a diffuse increase in acute and chronic inflammatory cells. Neutrophil neutrophils infiltrate the crypt epithelium to form crypt abscesses.

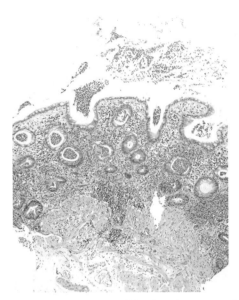

Figure 35.16 Active ulcerative colitis: there is severe active chronic inflammation with crypt abscesses, early crypt rupture, pus on the luminal surface and incipient erosion. The architecture is distorted and the crypt epithelium is attenuated with goblet cell depletion.

into the loose submucosal tissues and there is a tendency to spread longitudinally beneath the mucosal membrane, which sloughs off leaving an ulcer (Figures 35.16 and 35.17). The mucosal margins of these ulcerated areas are further undermined and relatively raised up to form poly-poid tags of mucosa projecting into the lumen. These mucosal tags or inflammatory polyps can be short or extremely long and filiform [303].

The inflammatory damage to the crypts produces a variety of degenerative and regenerative changes in the crypt epithelium. There is loss of mucin from goblet cells (see Figure 35.16), often with enlargement and hyperchromatism of nuclei of the absorptive cells. Such changes must not be mistaken for dysplasia (see below). In the presence of attenuated or restituting epithelium anywhere in the superficial epithelium, the changes in the crypts are almost certainly reactive.

Paneth cells are, with the exception of the right colon, absent from the colon and rectum normally. In chronic ulcerative colitis, they appear in the crypt epithelium [304], and are most common in long-established disease. They produce lysozyme and defensins, regulate the gut flora [305,306] and can be numerous in those patients with long-standing colitis who develop malignant change [307]. Increased numbers of endocrine cells may also be seen in the base of the crypts. Although the absolute numbers of these cells is probably not increased [308], in some patients crypts are completely surrounded by their bright orange subnuclear granules and these cells appear hyperplastic.

The damage to the crypts in chronic ulcerative colitis (see Figure 35.17) produces crypt architectural distortion with branching and sometimes shortening. The distortion may result from re-epithelialisation of irregular crypt abscesses. It may also arise after erosions or ulcers when epithelium grows in from the edge of the erosion. New crypts are formed when the surface mucosa dips irregularly into the ulcer to form new crypts, but in a much more irregular manner than usual. This then develops a lamina propria and new muscularis mucosae, superficial to the original, so it appears duplicated. Physiological crypt division is from the crypt bases up, so they remain straight. Persistent mucosal architectural abnormalities are therefore characteristic of chronic ulcerative colitis but transient irregularities may be observed in regenerating mucosa from many causes, even previous biopsy sites.

Mucin granulomas

A particular problem, in the differential diagnosis of CIBD, is the significance of giant cell reaction and poorly formed granulomas in relation to crypt damage and liberated mucin. These granulomas usually contain mucin and/or neutrophils, histiocytes and occasionally giant cells. However the 'granuloma' may also be very well formed and sarcoid like. The mucin is not always readily visible and often the best clue is that their location is precisely in the location in which a crypt should be, even given the irregularity that can occur in ulcerative colitis. Care needs to be taken to note the location so that this feature is not misinterpreted as representing Crohn's disease. An important clue is that crypt remnants may be visible, although the demonstration may require many levels, a mucin stain or an epithelial immunostain.

So-called cryptolytic granulomas may be seen in Crohn's disease [309] but are also seen in other forms of colitis [310], including ulcerative colitis and the colitis associated with diverticular disease [311], as well as in ileal pouches. These need careful assessment, because genuine basally oriented sarcoid-type granulomas appear not to occur in ulcerative colitis. On the other hand, cryptolytic granulomas should not be used as evidence 'consistent with Crohn's disease', because, once that diagnosis is suggested, it has a habit of sticking and the patient is labelled as having 'histologically proven Crohn's disease'. This may deprive the patient of the advantages of a pelvic ileal pouch in the future. In diverted ulcerative colitis, several types of granuloma have been described in the bowel wall and in draining lymph nodes and, once again, this should not be taken as evidence, as such, of Crohn's disease [312].

In active colitis, accompanying the changes in the crypts and surface epithelium, there is a heavy diffuse infiltrate of inflammatory cells in the lamina propria. These include neutrophils, lymphocytes, plasma cells, eosinophils and mast cells. The presence of deep plasma cells is characteristic of longstanding CIBD. Studies of immunoglobulin-containing plasma cells in ulcerative colitis demonstrate an increase in the major forms of IgA, IgG and IgM [313]. The increase correlates with disease activity and the rise of IgG- and IgM-containing cells is proportionally more than for IgA-containing cells [314].

In some biopsies from ulcerative colitis, large numbers of eosinophils may be seen in the lamina propria and may completely dominate the lamina propria. This infiltrate has been the subject of much study in attempts to correlate it with clinical outcome but there have been few consistent results [314]. It probably reflects the extreme end of the T-cell helper 2 (Th2) response that is said to characterise ulcerative colitis. Furthermore, in developed countries, quiescent ulcerative colitis is by far the most common cause of 'eosinophilic colitis' (see below). The same conclusions have to be made about mast cell numbers [314–316], although difficulties in techniques for demonstrating degranulated mast cells complicate the issue if histochemistry rather than immunohistochemistry is used. In long-standing disease, hyperplasia of mucosal basal lymphoid follicles becomes a prominent feature, particularly in the rectum [317] but in resections transmural inflammation in the form of lymphoid aggregates, characteristic of Crohn's disease, is never seen in ulcerative colitis, although it is a feature of the diverted rectum in ulcerative colitis [312].

Vasculitic lesions of the polyarteritis type, in submucosal vessels, can be seen in ulcerative colitis but are rare [318]. Nevertheless we have seen patients with overt systemic vasculopathy with normal vessels in biopsies. Inflammation within blood vessels may be seen close to ulcerated areas but this is usually a secondary feature. Granulomatous vasculitis, generally the preserve of Crohn's disease [319], has been described in ulcerative colitis only in association with diversion [320].

The assessment of disease activity in CIBD, in routine practice, is usually by clinical and endoscopic criteria. The only exception is the contribution to management, by pathology, in pouchitis. The importance of routine, repeated biopsy examination in CIBD is to reconfirm the diagnosis, to suggest that the biopsy findings are not typical for ulcerative colitis and raise the question of other forms of CIBD, to exclude concurrent infection (if possible), especially those in which organisms may be visible, and to assess for the presence of dysplasia.

Histological scoring of disease activity in ulcerative colitis and Crohn's disease is usually confined to therapeutic trials of new drugs. Several informal scoring systems have been devised for this purpose. Most are not evidence based or tested for their reproducibility, and are based on the presence and site of neutrophils and the amount of crypt and epithelial destruction caused by them. Although Truelove, in Oxford, devised the first recorded method relating to the amount of neutrophil infiltrate and epithelial damage, the Riley system, which is similarly based, is somewhat less exact but has demonstrated that a mild activity score (occasional small groups of neutrophils in the lamina propria) does correlate with early relapse after cessation of treatment [321]. So, activity is worth documenting in biopsy reports, although its quantitation is of dubious value outside clinical trials. However, if a scoring system is to be used, the Geboes system is easy to use and has been tested for its reproducibility [322]. This represents a great advance in standardisation and comparison of results of therapeutic trials.

Active ulcerative colitis – fulminant phase

Ulcerative colitis is primarily a disease of the mucosa and inflammation does not extend beyond the submucosa, except in severe or acute fulminating disease. In acute fulminating disease, inflammation can be focal or diffuse, the mucosa can be either diffusely hemorrhagic or there may be linear ulcers; there may be proximal or distal sparing or both. All variants may show deep fissuring ulcers with myocytolysis and transmural inflammation (Figure 35.18), although this is polymorphous and not in the form of the transmural lymphoid follicles as seen in Crohn's disease.

Extensive loss of mucosa can occur and any surviving mucosa shows intense vascular congestion and oedema, although sometimes with a relatively mild inflammatory cell response. In areas of mucosal ulceration, the submucosal tissues largely disappear laying bare the deep muscle coats, which may be covered by only a thin layer of vascular granulation tissue and also be visible grossly. The fibres of the muscularis propria are separated by oedematous exudate and become stretched and thinned. This may proceed to incipient or complete perforation. Such an appearance must therefore be carefully evaluated in the context of other changes.

Residual mucosa is worthy of careful evaluation. Although there is an excess of chronic inflammation with deep plasma cells to indicate the underlying chronic colitis, there may also be overt architectural changes indicative of prior ulcerative colitis. These can be signed out as severe active ulcerative colitis. However, a second group of patients have virtually no architectural abnormality and most of these present with a first attack of severe disease that is unresponsive to most therapies and may be held in check briefly with tumour necrosis factor (TNF) antagonists, but ultimately come to colectomy. The lack of architectural changes may cause the diagnosis of ulcerative

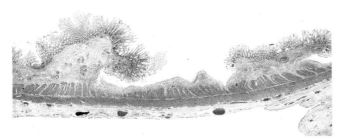

Figure 35.18 Histology of fulminant colitis with toxic dilatation: there is extensive, deep ulceration into the muscularis propria and the surviving mucosa is undermined giving a polypoid appearance.

colitis to (reasonably) be questioned. The key features are that, although polymorphous transmural inflammation and fissuring ulcers may be present, there are no other features to indicate Crohn's disease, whether transmural lymphoid hyperplasia or granulomas, not attributable to mucin or foreign material, and ideally away from fissures or ulceration and along the subserosa. Whether one decides that this is severe ulcerative colitis or CIBD of uncertain aetiology matters little. The important message is that there are no features to indicate that the underlying disease is Crohn's disease and therefore there is nothing to preclude an ileal pouch–anal anastomosis, although the patient may well be at risk for pouchitis.

Resolving ulcerative colitis

The relapses and remissions of ulcerative colitis imply that inflammation may resolve spontaneously. Evidence that this is the case comes from placebo-based studies, when up to about a third of patients in any placebo group go into remission spontaneously. Active drugs therefore need a correspondingly higher response rate to be deemed active. Furthermore, resolution can occur at different rates in different anatomical areas of the colon. This can give a false impression of segmental disease, not only macroscopically but also microscopically [224,226,323]. With resolution of disease, the numbers of inflammatory cells of all types begin to diminish and their distribution becomes uneven. The goblet cell population returns towards normal and, depending on the severity of the attack, the crypt architecture will show evidence of damage. Some crypts may appear short and others branched, the changes invariably being more marked distally.

Quiescent ulcerative colitis

Varying degrees of crypt atrophy and distortion are the hallmarks of quiescent disease. Shortfall of the crypt with regard to the muscularis mucosae and crypt loss is a convenient way of assessing this atrophy, when present, and the lamina propria may show an unusual 'empty' appearance (Figure 35.19). On the other hand, there may be lymphoid follicular hyperplasia in the rectum (Figure 35.20). Crypts are normally present in the large bowel mucosa at a frequency of 6/mm in a biopsy that includes muscularis mucosae. In a biopsy without muscularis mucosae, the mucosa may be stretched out and appear atrophic when it is not. Oedema may also cause mimicry of crypt atrophy: this may follow administration of bowel preparation fluids, especially older hyperosmolar solutions [324].

Although most ulcerative colitis patients have some residual changes of previous damage (crypt distortion, atrophy, Paneth cell metaplasia), it has become increasingly recognised that a group of ulcerative colitis patients may show complete resolution with no evidence of previous disease [224–226]. This must always raise the question of

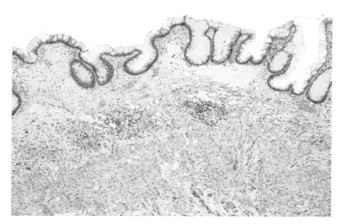

Figure 35.19 Ulcerative colitis in remission (quiescent ulcerative colitis): the crypts are atrophic, branched, and shortened such that they do not reach the thickened muscularis mucosae. Mononuclear cells are sparse in the lamina propria, giving it an 'empty' appearance.

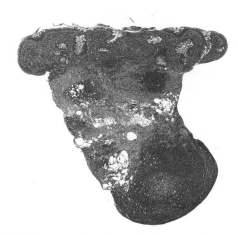

Figure 35.20 Inactive ulcerative colitis in a rectal biopsy: there is lymphoid follicular hyperplasia whereas the mucosa shows chronic inflammation and crypt distortion. This appearance is sometimes termed 'lymphoid follicular proctitis'.

whether the original diagnosis was really ulcerative colitis or an infective colitis and a careful review of all clinical data and histological material is warranted. After such review, there remains a patient group with genuine ulcerative colitis, with collateral evidence for such a diagnosis, including coexistent primary sclerosing cholangitis, who undoubtedly show evidence of complete mucosal recovery, although the colitis of primary sclerosing cholangitis may be more right sided than is usually seen in ulcerative colitis [282].

The patient group with histological evidence of ulcerative colitis, who have crypt architectural distortion, but

normal radiology and colonoscopy, has been termed 'minimal change colitis' [325]. We do not advise widespread use of this term: quiescent ulcerative colitis is much less ambiguous. It should not be confused with microscopic colitis, because there is crypt architectural distortion, not a feature of microscopic colitis. 'Minimal change colitis' may be seen after treatment or at presentation, and indeed may never develop endoscopically recognisable changes, although some authors claim that minor vascular abnormalities may be seen at colonoscopy. It is not clear why some patients will show quite florid atrophy, yet, in others, the mucosa returns to a state of relative normality.

Inflammatory polyps can occur in quiescent disease, although they reflect more a phase of healing after a bout of severe disease rather than being, of necessity, a sign of chronicity. Occasionally thickening of the muscularis mucosae is seen but a characteristic finding in ulcerative colitis, especially in rectal biopsies, is the double muscularis mucosae [326]. The upper layer is thought to be a new layer of smooth muscle, possibly derived from pericryptal fibroblasts. When there has been ulceration and the epithelium regenerates, it does so with new muscularis mucosae, as also seen in Barrett's oesophagus. This may lead to diagnostic confusion on examination of a mucosal biopsy, because inflammatory changes may be misinterpreted as extending beneath the muscularis mucosae if only the superficial neo-muscularis mucosae is included. Mucosal inflammation will then be erroneously thought to be within the submucosa, potentially leading to a misdiagnosis of Crohn's disease. There is often no convenient way to resolve the presence of a double muscularis mucosae in biopsies, but deep inflammation in biopsies should not be used as a definitive criterion to distinguish ulcerative colitis from Crohn's disease.

The rectum in ulcerative procto-colitis after ileo-rectal anastomosis

Ileo-rectal anastomosis is not a widely promulgated technique in ulcerative colitis because the rectum is the main seat of disease and could possibly become neoplastic in the future. Nevertheless, the operation is still very occasionally undertaken in ulcerative colitis and there are many patients who, historically, have had this operation. The macroscopic and histological changes in the rectum after ileo-rectal anastomosis are no different from those in the rectum in continuity with an inflamed colon. Biopsies from just above the anastomosis may be misinterpreted as small bowel metaplasia. It is crucial that the pathologist is made aware of the previous operation, when presented with a biopsy from this area. The dysplasia and carcinoma risk in this circumstance relates to the original disease extent: in total or extensive colitis it would be as high as if the whole colon were still present. The pathological changes of inflammation are quite different from those in the diverted rectum in ulcerative colitis.

The effects of drugs on the macroscopic and microscopic appearances of ulcerative colitis

It is possible that many of the difficulties concerning the classification of CIBD, on mucosal biopsies, arise because of the effects of drug therapy. Furthermore, the difficulties are compounded by variations in the distribution of disease when modified by drug therapy, underpinning the importance of assessing multiple colonoscopic biopsies, from multiple sites, in the accurate diagnosis of CIBD [226,227].

Immunosuppressive agents, such as ciclosporin, have been used as an effective drug in severe ulcerative colitis otherwise unresponsive to conventional medical therapy [327,328]. It has been recognised to have important consequences for the histopathologist and may lead to the misdiagnosis of dysplasia [329]. The changes induced by ciclosporin, usually seen only when given intravenously, are villiform mucosal regeneration and epithelial regenerative changes, which are severe with marked nuclear enlargement, sometimes extending to the mucosal surface, but usually with plentiful eosinophilic cytoplasm. Perhaps the most helpful feature is that the 'pseudo-dysplasia' induced by ciclosporin is strikingly diffuse, with many, and sometimes all, crypts showing similar changes, in a way not usually associated with ulcerative colitis-associated dysplasia. Despite this, it is very important that the clinician alert the pathologist to the fact that the patient has been on ciclosporin and that the pathologist is cautious not to over-diagnose dysplasia in this circumstance.

Increasingly, TNF antagonists may be the drug of choice in steroid-resistant severe ulcerative colitis. These can have a dramatic effect on the amount of inflammation present so that, when resection takes place, the disease often appears relatively quiescent, often with a striking diminution in lamina propria inflammatory cells, although linear ulcers may still be present.

Dysplasia and malignancy in ulcerative colitis

Carcinoma of the large intestine is a well-recognised complication of ulcerative colitis and, in the vast majority of patients, is preceded by morphologically recognisable dysplastic lesions. Cancer in colitis accounts for less than 1% of deaths from large bowel malignancies and, within the ulcerative colitis population, approximately 3–5% of all ulcerative colitis patients will eventually develop a carcinoma [330]. There is geographical variation in the occurrence of cancer in colitis because the incidence of this complication is lower in Israel and central Europe than in Western European countries [331,332].

The risk factors for dysplasia and carcinoma are well known. At maximum risk are those with total or extensive colitis, including those with documented total colitis in the form of backwash ileitis, those with a history of at least 8 years and those with an early age of onset [333,334]. Active disease, primary sclerosing cholangitis and a family history of colorectal carcinoma all increase the risk. Nevertheless, several facts regarding dysplasia in ulcerative colitis are clear:
- Dysplasia, when definitely present, should be graded only low grade and high grade.
- There is no such thing as 'moderate dysplasia'. This is a clinically useless term because there are no management algorithms that use this terminology in patient care. The use of this term and other outmoded classifications should be abandoned.
- There is good inter-observer agreement for neoplastic change at either end of the spectrum (i.e. none and high grade dysplasia), but for 'indefinite for dysplasia' and low grade dysplasia the inter-observer agreement is less.
- Biopsies of endoscopic lesions can be extremely problematic in that some carcinomas show very subtle cytological changes. It may only be the architectural disarray that gives the clue to the fact that the lesion is a carcinoma and needs resection. Some tubulo-glandular carcinomas, or even regular carcinomas with or without a colloid component, can have very little cytological abnormality, in either the mucosa or the underlying invasive component. In some, the diagnosis is almost impossible and it is the clinical suspicion, lack of the ability to carry out mucosal resection (failure of the lesion to rise after submucosal injections to achieve this) or use of endoscopic ultrasonography that determines that there is a deep component.
- The need for a second opinion, when resection is at stake, depends on the expertise of the pathologist and the confidence of the clinician in that pathologist's diagnosis. An expert is not merely someone who sees a lot, speaks a lot or writes a lot, but someone who gets it right a lot.
- Many dysplasias are very easy to diagnose and others more difficult. In a study from the Netherlands most diagnoses of low grade dysplasia were downgraded, potentially saving the patient a resection [335].
- The objectives of surveillance are to prevent the patient dying of carcinoma but, if a carcinoma is present, there is no way to accurately and reproducibly predict its stage. Resection is therefore ideally carried out for patients with high grade dysplasia but its timing is also important.
- Resections are usually advised for high grade dysplasia, suspicious for invasive carcinoma. Visible dysplastic lesions need to be completely removed endoscopically. This can now be achieved with techniques such as EMR (endoscopic mucosal resection) and ESD (endoscopic submucosal dissection). The correct treatment for flat low grade dysplasia remains controversial. Some argue that, as

long as it is stable, it can be followed but the data suggest that following it is fraught with hazard because patients do develop and die from cancer when subjected only to surveillance.

The risk of cancer and its prevention

Assessing the risk of cancer in ulcerative colitis is complex and problematic. Historical data may not be appropriate, because active disease tends to predominate and it has been shown that successful treatment of the disease, much more likely now with so many useful pharmacological agents, is protective against neoplasia. A variety of data, for cancer risk in ulcerative colitis, are available but their validity is dependent on how patient cohorts have been assembled. In some historical series, the risk of cancer reaches 5% at 10 years, >20% at 20 years and >40% at 25 years [337–339]. However, in carefully defined cohorts, patients with extensive colitis had a 19-fold increase in risk compared with the general population, whereas those with left-sided disease had a fourfold increase. Cumulative risks were 7.2% at 20 years and 16.5% at 30 years. Individuals may be at greatest risk of developing cancer at around the age of 50 years. Some patients with extensive colitis may have a genetic predisposition to colorectal cancer [340].

Patients who are dysplasia free, well controlled and undergoing regular surveillance with full colonoscopy after appropriate biopsy protocols rarely die of carcinoma, and the challenge is in deciding when, or if, colectomy should be carried out in patients with dysplasia. Furthermore, there is nothing specific about the 8-year history that is often quoted [341,342] because cancer is well documented in people with colitis but only limited left-sided disease [343], even in those in whom the history is <5 years [344]. In a recent study from the Netherlands, 20% of ulcerative colitis cancers occurred before 8 years, suggesting that 5 years is a better starting time to consider surveillance.

Having defined the type of patient with ulcerative colitis most susceptible to malignant change, the management of the individual patient remains a formidable problem. Prophylactic proctocolectomy after 10 years of disease was, at one time, a valid recommendation but surveillance has now became the standard of care. The notion of detecting dysplasia or early (asymptomatic) carcinoma and, in the absence of other indications for colectomy, limiting colectomy to this group has become the norm. However, this remains imperfect, because both dysplasia and carcinoma can be very difficult to recognise endoscopically. Numerous endoscopic techniques have improved our ability to detect neoplastic lesions and to remove them. Guidelines for management have emerged but are still based on surprisingly few data. Despite surveillance, some patients still develop and die from carcinoma. It is surprisingly easy to find reasons why this happened (patient missed a visit, poor preparation, lesion behind a fold, patient does not want an operation: there is a morbidity and mortality, fear of an ileostomy, complications of pouchitis, etc.) which deflect blaming the managing physician.

The prognosis of cancer in colitis is probably no worse than in the general population, provided that similar stages are compared [339,345,346]. With the appreciation of the significance of dysplasia in colonoscopic and rectal biopsy material [347], a more rational approach to the problem of cancer and colitis is possible [339,345–350].

Terminology of dysplastic lesions and their management

The terminology for dysplastic lesions and their management has been undergoing a quiet revolution in the last decade or so.

Adenomas

These occur in both colitic and non-affected mucosa in ulcerative colitis patients. They can be treated like any other adenoma by complete local excision. However, some lesions that appear to be adenomatous endoscopically extend on to the adjacent mucosa and, without special endoscopic techniques, their margins may be indiscernible. Until they are excised it is unclear whether such lesions are just adenomas or part of a more widespread area of dysplasia (Figures 35.21 and 35.22). Such lesions have been called *adenoma-like masses* (ALMs) but the implication is the same. They need to be demonstrably removed and the mucosa in the stalk or biopsies around the base must demonstrate completeness of excision.

The demise of 'DALM'

The concern with all dysplastic endoscopically discernible lesions is that they may have an underlying invasive carcinoma. This is the rationale behind the introduction of the term 'DALM' and the implication that this was usually a definitive indication for colectomy [351]. This concept was useful, implying that endoscopic dysplastic lesions or masses, including some that looked like adenomas but occurred in colitic mucosa, could well have an underlying invasive component and the presence of this could not be determined until the lesion was resected. With the availability of endoscopic polypectomy and EMR, the DALM concept is now outdated because most lesions that are non-invasive can be removed using these techniques. Those that cannot be removed endoscopically need to be resected anyway and, although theoretically the term DALM can be applied to these lesions, the same applies to similar lesions in the non-colitic population.

Management of endoscopic polyps and dysplastic lesions

Polypectomy can remove many of the polypoid lesions occurring in ulcerative colitis. It is important to emphasise that, in ulcerative colitis patients, biopsies need to be taken around the base of the polypoid lesion to ensure that local excision is really complete and that the lesion is not part of a larger area of dysplasia that is less obvious endoscopically (see Figure 35.21). If biopsies around the base are positive for dysplasia (see Figure 35.22), then EMR, or ESD,

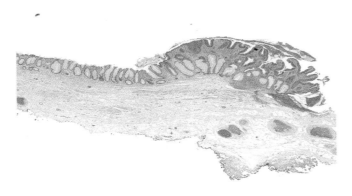

Figure 35.21 Endoscopic resections of a polypoid mass in the sigmoid colon in which the dysplasia is limited to the nodule and the adjacent mucosa (left) is non-dysplastic. Were this amenable to endoscopic resection, biopsies from around the base of the lesion would have been non-dysplastic, confirming that local excision was adequate.

can be used to remove most larger lesions. If this cannot be carried out, resection has to be seriously considered. Where possible, ESD is a better technique, because it removes the entire lesion in one piece rather than the multiple pieces obtained from EMR, so it is easier to assess all margins. However, it takes considerably more time and much of the experience in this technique has been in Japan. As EMR usually results in multiple fragments, it can be impossible to piece these together to determine if margins are free of dysplasia. Some proponents tattoo the area before endoscopic resection to ensure that the entire lesion has been removed. Other options are to return to the site and biopsy around the scar or to take the biopsies when one can see the rim at the time of resection. The latter gives the quickest answer and the edges are very easy to see at that time. If these are dysplasia free, and if there is no dysplasia elsewhere in regular surveillance biopsies, then no further therapy is required for that lesion or until the next surveillance colonoscopy which raises other issues.

Macroscopic features of dysplasia in ulcerative colitis

The gross features of dysplasia are well documented and run the entire gamut of changes. The lesion may be polypoid and resemble an adenoma or be slightly raised and plaque like, resembling flat adenomas [351,352]. It may be villous and/or have a velvety/chamois leather-like mucosal appearance (Figure 35.23). Importantly it can

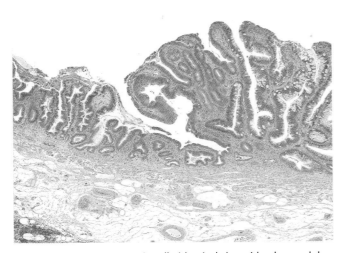

Figure 35.22 Here, in a virtually identical sigmoid colon nodule in another patient, the dysplasia extends into the adjacent mucosa (and to the margin of the resection). The nodule was therefore part of a wider area of dysplasia. Were this nodule amenable to local resection, biopsies around its base would still have been dysplastic showing that the lesion had not been removed in its entirety. Treatment would have to be by colectomy, unless the lesion could be visualised by chromo-endoscopy and/or magnification endoscopy and excised endoscopically.

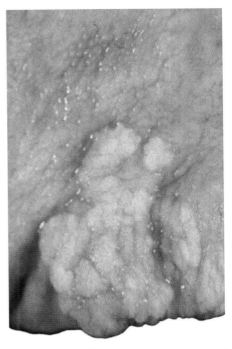

Figure 35.23 The plaque-like appearance of an area of raised dysplasia (formerly termed 'DALM') in chronic ulcerative colitis.

occur in flat and otherwise unremarkable mucosa [353]. Even in dysplastic flat mucosa, the endoscopic pit pattern may be abnormal [354], such changes being visible using chromo-endoscopy with magnification. Surveillance is also demonstrably better using these techniques, which doubles the number of dysplastic lesions identified, compared with taking random biopsies [355]. Indeed, given a 1000-mm length of large bowel 100mm in diameter, it takes 320 regularly spaced biopsies to guarantee finding a 20-mm patch of flat dysplasia. The futility of repeating the colonoscopy to 'confirm the diagnosis', when dysplasia is detected in macroscopically unremarkable mucosa, is apparent. Specialist techniques such as these, narrow-band imaging or confocal endomicroscopy, which allows visualisation of nuclei in crypts, may all have roles to play in the routine surveillance of ulcerative colitis in the near future [356].

Without these tools, the ill-defined nature of the dysplastic lesion makes it difficult for the colonoscopist to select areas for targeted biopsy and greater reliance is placed on regular surveillance biopsies. It has been calculated that the likelihood of a cancer arising without a visible lesion is 2%, whereas 28% of non-cancer-associated dysplasia is undetected macroscopically [357].

Features of neoplasia in surgical specimens
Apart from the background colitis, ulcerative colitis carcinomas are similar to their non-colitic counterparts. However, some features are seen more frequently in colitic cancers:
- Tumours may be multiple, although this tends to apply only to patients presenting with symptoms, which therefore tend to be advanced and develop on a background of widespread or multi-focal dysplasia. It is rare in patients from surveillance programmes undergoing colectomy.
- Cancers in colitis are often flat and infiltrating with an ill-defined edge and can sometimes be felt more easily than seen. Thus they tend to resemble the macroscopic pathology of gastric carcinoma rather than ordinary carcinoma of the colon.
- There is a higher incidence of high grade and mucinous carcinomas than in ordinary colorectal cancer. In non-colitic cancers, it is now known that right-sided mucinous tumours have a better prognosis than left-sided ones. Whether this distinction holds in ulcerative colitis is not yet known.

Cancers in ulcerative colitis are more common on the left side and in the rectum [358,359], so there is little difference in the distribution of cancer between ulcerative colitis patients and patients who are non-colitic [352,360]. It is essential that many sections, from all parts of a colectomy specimen, are examined in the search for small cancers and dysplasia in flat mucosa, which may not be seen with the naked eye, although carcinoma, in contrast to dysplasia, is rare in completely flat mucosa [351,353]. In practice, when examining resected specimens, any mucosa looking different from background mucosa should be sliced through and

the cut surface examined. Usually the mucosal/submucosal junction is linear and readily seen. Carcinomas are visible as yellowish tongues or mucin pools extending into the submucosa or beyond. Adjacent slices are made as close as possible to the first on both sides to determine the maximum depth of tumour grossly and the deepest of these, together with all regional nodes or deposits, also taken for examination. Such flat cancers may also be seen in a retained rectum in ulcerative colitis, because unexpected carcinomas may be found within the proctectomy specimen, not identified on endoscopic or histological examination of mucosal biopsies.

Microscopic features of dysplasia in ulcerative colitis
Histologically, dysplasia in ulcerative colitis reflects all of the macroscopic types of dysplasia, so that it includes raised dysplasia (Figures 35.24 and 35.25), flat dysplasia (Figure 35.26), polypoid and villous dysplasia. Lesions with underlying carcinoma can adopt any of these patterns, including a low villous pattern (Figure 35.24). There are both cytological and architectural criteria for dysplasia in colitis, and these are similar to those applied to other glandular epithelia.

Architectural changes
Architectural changes are important in the diagnosis of dysplasia but it is important to emphasise that quiescent ulcerative colitis can also demonstrate pronounced architectural changes. At one end of the spectrum, dysplasia simply mimics the pre-existing architecture of the crypts so that there is no discernible specific architectural change. However, often there is a degree of crypt budding, as seen in many adenomas [357], so that crypts become more

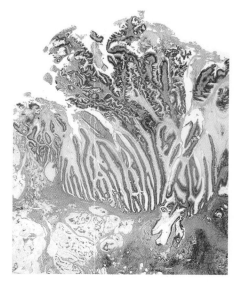

Figure 35.24 Villiform high grade dysplasia in ulcerative colitis with an underlying invasive mucinous adenocarcinoma in the submucosa.

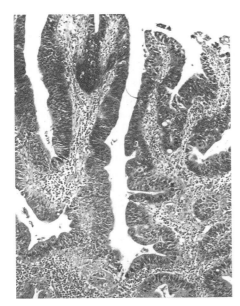

Figure 35.25 High grade dysplasia in ulcerative colitis: the mucosa is both polypoid and villiform and shows very substantial cytological abnormalities.

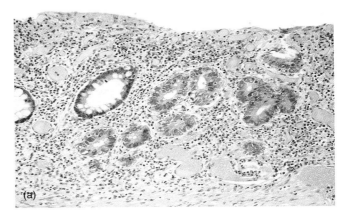

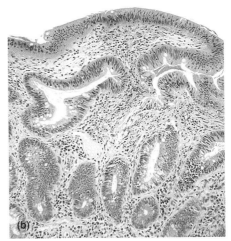

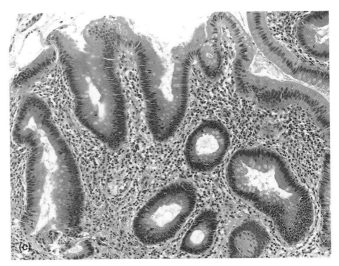

Figure 35.26 Dysplasia in flat mucosa: (a) high grade dysplasia affecting all parts of the crypt uniformly (right). (b) Low grade dysplasia with multilayering of enlarged nuclei extending on to the surface. (c) Indefinite for dysplasia. There is only minor nuclear stratification and crowding with little nuclear pleomorphism and some surface maturation.

tightly packed, in contrast to the decreased or normal number of crypts present in non-dysplastic ulcerative colitis. When this becomes extreme, the point at which budding into the lamina propria becomes invasion into the lamina propria is subjective and not reproducible [361]. As such 'intramucosal carcinoma' has no metastasising potential in the large bowel; it is best regarded as similar to high grade dysplasia for management purposes, although it does have a specific categorisation within the Vienna classification [362]. The most extreme form of architectural distortion is the presence of random crypts with no clear order which invariably represents subtle invasive carcinoma. Unfortunately ulcerative colitis carcinomas often develop without the classic desmoplastic reaction seen in non-ulcerative colitis colorectal carcinoma. There are two notable variants of architectural change that occur.

Villous dysplasia A villiform architecture can be seen in active colitis but is always of concern because the crypt bases often have a degree of hyperchromasia, so that the line between reactive hyperplasia and low grade dysplasia is very subjective. Worse, although the changes of dysplasia are best identified in the surface epithelium, in villous dysplasia the changes are maximal in the crypt bases with a form of maturation toward the surface (so-called 'bottom-up' dysplasia).

This creates an obvious problem because maturation is the prerequisite of reactive epithelium and the usual teaching is that, if it matures, it is wise not to call it dysplasia. There are therefore two options: one is to designate this as 'mucosa indefinite for dysplasia'; and the other is to accept that this variant of dysplasia occurs and call it low/high grade dysplasia with maturation. This type of dysplasia can also be seen especially in villous adenomas, usually in the rectum, where there is apparent surface maturation, and yet there is an invasive component, at the base of the lesion [363]. We do accept the existence of 'bottom-up' dysplasia but diagnose it only when we are sure that the crypt bases are truly dysplastic and there is no alternative explanation for the changes present. The more marked variants of this pattern also have considerable branching at the crypt bases. These are one of the forms of dysplasia often best sent to an 'expert'. However, usually such lesions are visible endoscopically so that this is one situation where correlation with the endoscopic features is paramount. If it is well demarcated, it is likely to be removed endoscopically anyway. If no lesion is visible, then the alternative designation of 'mucosa indefinite for dysplasia' will ensure appropriate close follow-up.

Serrated changes Our preoccupation with serrated pathology of the colorectum has made us very aware of the frequency with which serrated changes are found in both non-dysplastic and dysplastic mucosa in ulcerative colitis. They are usually readily visible at scanning power. Some patients appear to have them fairly diffusely throughout much of the large bowel in the absence of dysplasia, although others have it patchily and still others have serrations only in dysplastic lesions [364,365]. One word of caution is that ulcerated inflammatory polyps invariably have serrations immediately beneath the surface erosion, and so should be regarded as non-significant.

Cytological changes

Cytological changes in the crypt epithelium are a prerequisite for the diagnosis of dysplasia. The *loss of basal–luminal differentiation axis* should be regarded as the most useful criterion for the establishment of the presence of dysplasia in ulcerative colitis (Figure 35.26 and see Figure 35.25). Cytologically there is variation of epithelial nuclear position causing the appearance of stratification of cells within the crypts, which can be marked at one extreme but minimal at the other. Nuclear chromatin varies from dense and hyperchromatic to more open with small nucleoli. Mitoses are variably increased and finding them in the upper third of the crypt is a warning sign to search for other features of dysplasia. Mucin secretion may be marked and occupy most of the cell; alternatively mucin may be limited to the cell apices or completely absent. A highly characteristic feature of dysplasia is the presence of the mucin on the basal side of the nucleus when the nuclei have lost their polarity, so-called dystrophic/inverted goblet cells.

Unfortunately, none of the cytological or architectural features is unique to dysplasia and each can be seen in isolation in inflamed or regenerating epithelium. Extreme caution is necessary before a diagnosis of dysplasia is made in active disease or in the presence of florid regeneration [357], especially after ciclosporin therapy [329]. Some changes more specific to dysplasia in flat mucosa have been described. These include proliferation of enlarged darkly staining cells arranged in a line along the whole length of the crypts and accompanied by eosinophilic cytoplasm, with absent goblet cells. This type of dysplasia often gives rise to a very poorly differentiated type of carcinoma in ulcerative colitis. Sometimes the dysplastic cells become vacuolated, stain poorly with a mucin stain and resemble the clear cell type of carcinoma of the stomach and colorectum. Finally, a variety known as pancellular dysplasia has large hyperchromatic nuclei with loss of polarity and affects all cell lines including Paneth cells, argentaffin and goblet cells.

The distinction from reactive changes

In, or after, active ulcerative colitis, the presence of an acute inflammatory infiltrate of neutrophils, whether in the lamina propria or, especially, within epithelium, is a warning sign to interpret epithelial changes with caution. The resolving and regenerating phase of active disease, when inflammation is less obvious, causes the greatest interpretative problems. The presence of cuboidal (restituting) epithelium anywhere, and maturation at the surface with hyperchromatic nuclei at the base, both tend to suggest that the changes are reactive. Reactive nuclei are enlarged, often vesicular with prominent nucleoli, and, importantly, are separated from each other, with little or no overlap.

A further problem posed in chronic ulcerative colitis is the distinction between regenerative hyperplasia and dysplasia within inflammatory polyps complicating ulcerative colitis (see 'Polyps in ulcerative colitis' above). Fortunately, dysplasia in inflammatory polyps is distinctly uncommon [303]. An important concept for the colonoscopist is that no polypoid lesion in ulcerative colitis should be biopsied or removed in isolation. It must always be accompanied by biopsies from adjacent flat mucosa: these might aid the pathologist in making the distinction between regenerative hyperplasia and dysplasia.

Role of immunohistochemistry

In our practices, we find immunohistochemistry to be of some use but overall we use it to support our impression based on our review of routine preparations. Once overt dysplasia is present, immunohistochemistry is of little additional value. When using wnt signalling pathway antibodies (*p53* and, less well documented, nuclear β-catenin), about 80–85% of ulcerative colitis carcinomas are thought be associated with abnormalities of this pathway and the same applies to the preceding dysplasia. Patients with CIBD have been found to harbour mutations in the *p53* gene before the development of dysplasia [366–369]. However, where one really needs help (indefinite for dysplasia), there is often increased immunoreactivity, limited to the basal halves of the crypts corresponding to the proliferative zone with *bcl-2* negativity. In contrast, sporadic adenoma usually shows *p53* negativity and *bcl-2* positivity [370–372]. However, in our view, these results are neither sufficiently sensitive nor specific to be used diagnostically. Racemase (α-methylacyl-CoA racemase – AMACR) initially showed promise, being increased in 96% of cases with low grade dysplasia, 80% of cases with high grade dysplasia and 71% of cases with carcinoma, but no expression in mucosa negative for dysplasia [373,374]. However, weak or moderate racemase expression has also been shown in patients with CIBD but no neoplasia [375], and that has also been our experience. Certainly overt dysplasia often exhibits immunoreactivity to these antigens, but immunostains do not change the H&E diagnosis or significantly impact on any management algorithm.

The classification and grading of dysplasia

The need to classify dysplasia is based on the belief that increasing degrees of dysplasia have increasing malignant potential [357]. However, this concept is far from absolute and both low grade dysplasia, and some lesions that are hard to classify as having usual dysplasia, may have an associated underlying invasive carcinoma [351]. Nevertheless, the classification of low or high grade dysplasia forms the basis of the clinical management and surveillance programmes.

Grading dysplasia

Grading dysplasia is, inevitably, highly subjective, and only two definitive grades are recommended for use, low grade and high grade, with the term 'indefinite' used for equivocal appearances [357]. It cannot be over-emphasised that the old classification of mild, moderate and severe dysplasia should no longer be used, either singly or in combination with the low and high grade system, in any circumstances, because this may erroneously influence management and there are no current management guidelines for this outmoded classification. However, the Vienna system [362] is an acceptable alternative which uses the term 'non-invasive neoplasia' (NIN) instead of the term 'dysplasia'. It does have an intramucosal carcinoma designation, but this, in the context of ulcerative colitis, is part of high grade dysplasia from a management perspective.

Limiting the number of definitive categories to two, rather than three, aids management of individual patients and makes classification less subject to the vagaries of pathological diagnosis and inter-observer variation [357]. In high grade dysplasia, there is usually architectural abnormality and the cytological changes are marked, the defining factor being the extension of nuclei at least two-thirds of the way to the surface and/or overt loss of nuclear polarity. There are no criteria for how much of the biopsy should be involved, although most like to see more than one crypt. When there is cribriform crypt branching with back-to-back crowding of glands, the diagnosis of high grade dysplasia is usually easy. The most severely dysplastic area determines the final grade. Low grade dysplasia should not have nuclei more than two-thirds of the way to the surface.

The necessity for an *indefinite for dysplasia* category (see Figure 35.26c) emphasises the limitations of light microscopy and routine staining in the diagnosis of dysplasia. The use of the term does not infer that the pathologist is being indefinite but rather that there are changes present in colorectal biopsy or biopsies that could represent dysplasia and accompanying features (most usually inflammation or features of repair or restitution) serve to make the distinction between these changes and dysplasia impossible.

We believe that it is reasonable to make a diagnosis of *indefinite for dysplasia* in five circumstances:

1. When there are cytological changes in the presence of severe active inflammation. This is the most common indication for the use of the term 'indefinite for dysplasia' in many gastrointestinal pathologists' practices. Treatment for active ulcerative colitis may induce remission of the disease, with diminution of the cytological changes associated with active inflammation. Thus, further colonoscopy and multiple biopsies, after this treatment, may allow a clear distinction between regenerative and dysplastic changes to be made.

2. When there are very small foci of possible dysplasia (just a few crypts) [357]. Such microscopic foci demand further assessment by colonoscopy and extensive biopsies, including from the site where the biopsy in question was from.

3. When there is poor orientation of the tissue. The most important diagnostic criterion for dysplasia is failure of maturation of the abnormal cytological changes towards the surface. If the biopsy is tangentially oriented, then full and accurate assessment may not be possible, even after reorientation of the biopsy in the wax block: *indefinite for dysplasia* would be an appropriate diagnosis in this situation with a recommendation for early further colonoscopy and multiple biopsies.

4. When there is low grade 'bottom-up' dysplasia limited to the crypt bases with maturation as the surface is approached (see above).

5. When there are artefactual changes (such as crush artefact of a biopsy) that do not allow the distinction between regeneration and true dysplasia.

Reproducibility Problems of intra- and inter-observer variation mostly arise with the low grade and indefinite categories [357,376–378]. Some biopsies are quite predictably problematic, but others have a morphology identical to adenomas with low grade dysplasia, so the diagnosis of low grade dysplasia is not in doubt. However, the classification has been demonstrated to be reliable [378] among general histopathologists. Not surprisingly, a back-to-back appearance, glandular crowding, villous architecture, nuclear hyperchromasia and nuclear stratification are the features most readily appreciated. It is unusual for high grade dysplasia not to be recognised [378] and the conditional probability for a diagnosis of dysplasia versus no dysplasia has been shown to be 0.759. This means that the chance of one histopathologist, randomly chosen, agreeing with a first pathologist who has diagnosed dysplasia is 75% [379]. Nevertheless there remains a subjective element to this that cannot be ignored.

The implications of dysplasia in ulcerative colitis

The management of non-flat lesions has been discussed previously. The management of flat dysplasia is more difficult, because there are few reliable data in the literature.

Low grade dysplasia in flat mucosa has been shown to be associated with a 59% 5-year risk of progression to high grade dysplasia or colorectal carcinoma [336,380]. Yet although the data regarding flat dysplasia suggest that there is a degree of futility in not treating it, the institutions publishing those data seem not to have heeded their own advice, possibly because, similar to adenomas, some patients really can be followed and seem not to develop carcinoma. However, those who do seem to have quite advanced lesions when resected, which is not the purpose of surveillance [336]. There is less disagreement about multi-focal low grade dysplasia: most would advocate colectomy in this situation. High grade dysplasia is less of an issue, because the data suggest that there is a 40–65% risk of synchronous invasive carcinoma. As more sensitive endoscopic techniques become available, these figures may well reduce but they still probably reflect most current practices and have now become established in new endoscopic techniques in the UK and the USA [381–383].

Currently, finding and treating dysplasia is the best method to prevent carcinoma. Finding lesions that are detectable endoscopically, and potentially the precursor lesions of carcinoma, is increasingly valid. When there is high grade dysplasia, especially in concert with an endoscopic mass or lesion, radical surgery should be considered [347,384,385]. When an endoscopic lesion is present, up to 65% of patients will already have a carcinoma (see Figure 35.24) [347]. However, this is very dependent on the technique used. It is increasingly apparent that chromo-endoscopy with high-resolution (zoom) endoscopy or confocal endomicroscopy all markedly increase the likelihood of detecting dysplastic lesions, to the point that regular surveillance biopsies can be effectively dispensed with [386–388] Yet these techniques are very slow to catch on, in part because of the learning curve but also because

the high resolution or confocal endoscopes may not be readily available.

In flat mucosa showing dysplasia with no endoscopic lesion visible, the likelihood of carcinoma is much less [351,389–391]. Furthermore, probably about 2% of cancers develop in the absence of conventional dysplasia and not every patient with high grade dysplasia necessarily progresses to cancer. The chances of detecting dysplasia in a colonoscopic surveillance programme depend on its extent and the extent of mucosal sampling. A review of the many series has shown that the maximum diagnostic yield of cancer based on finding high grade dysplasia is 62% [353] but advanced endoscopic techniques are more likely to detect both areas of dysplasia and small carcinomas. Data about the utility of rectal biopsy are obsolete and biased, because that was the only means of detecting dysplasia at that time [353].

Patients with long-standing extensive ulcerative colitis are usually part of a cancer surveillance programme and subject to annual colonoscopy. The diagnosis of high grade dysplasia, in flat mucosa, with its concomitant risk of cancer, calls for the immediate consideration of a procto-colectomy. This decision is a clinico-pathological one and the pathologist should attempt to confirm the diagnosis in one of the following ways:
• Documentation of high grade dysplasia in other biopsies from the same examination
• Documentation of high grade dysplasia in the same area at a repeat examination
• Confirmation of the diagnosis by another interested pathologist or, perhaps, an expert gastrointestinal pathologist.

Clinical management after a diagnosis of low grade dysplasia is less certain. Essentially the pathologist should follow the same safeguards. In flat mucosa, low grade dysplasia can be observed by colonoscopic surveillance with extensive biopsies of the entire colon within close time frames. Certainly initially, colonoscopy should be repeated at 3–6 months. Should such close surveillance fail to reveal any further dysplasia, the time between colonoscopic surveillance can be extended. However, some data suggest that procto-colectomy should still be considered because there is a real risk of finding a lethal carcinoma on follow-up. As discussed previously, in the presence of a macroscopic lesion that cannot be removed endoscopically, even if only low grade dysplasia is detected, procto-colectomy should be considered because a cancer is likely to be already present within that lesion [336,351,392,393].

Management of neoplasia complicating ulcerative colitis

Procto-colectomy is the correct treatment for cancer complicating colitis, whatever the site of the primary tumour. This is essential because the entire mucosa of the colon and rectum is cancer prone. The only exception is when distant metastases have already occurred, in which case a more limited or palliative operation such as total colectomy and/or ileo-rectal anastomosis can be justified. Total colectomy and ileo-rectal anastomosis do not remove the disease in the rectum, of course, and this remains at risk from the development of carcinoma. So, patients who have had this operation should be considered for continuing surveillance because of the risk of neoplasia in the remaining rectum.

Despite the presence of high grade dysplasia, between 30% and 50% of patients will not have a cancer on resection [391,394]. Rather than errors of judgement, such cases are the foundation of cancer prevention and should be regarded as a success in any surveillance programme. They provide some evidence that dysplasia does not necessarily progress to cancer. Until improved markers of malignant potential are developed, a small number of patients will continue to undergo potentially unnecessary major surgery. However, these are designed to prolong life, which is the objective.

Whether restorative procto-colectomy (ileal pouch surgery) is appropriate depends on the site of the carcinoma. If the tumour is in the lower third of the rectum, this may not be an appropriate option but, for cancers in the middle third of the rectum and higher, most surgeons would consider ileal pouch surgery. Patients with carcinoma or high grade dysplasia in their colectomy specimen are at risk of developing high grade dysplasia or adenocarcinoma within the columnar cuff of the anal canal [395]. The pouch–anal anastomosis is therefore often performed using a hand-sewn technique with mucosectomy to remove all diseased rectal mucosa [396]. An alternative is to perform the more usual stapled anastomosis, survey the columnar cuff [397] and perform a mucosectomy at a later time if dysplasia develops [395]. The advantages of a stapled anastomosis are the ease of surgery and reduced risk of incontinence in the future.

Other complications of chronic ulcerative colitis

Liver pathology
The liver is often affected in ulcerative colitis and liver function tests are frequently abnormal, with the most common being a raised alkaline phosphatase. The incidence of liver disease depends on the severity and extent of the colitis but significant liver problems occur in between 5 and 8% of patients [398,399]. Involvement of the liver may either be coincidental or have a more direct relationship with ulcerative colitis. Fatty change and viral hepatitis are examples of the former. The chronic nature of ulcerative colitis, and the exposure of the patient to injections, infusions and a hospital environment, all increase the susceptibility of the patient to viral infection. Nutritional and absorptive problems contribute to fatty infiltration. Sclerosing cholangitis,

pericholangitis, cirrhosis, cholangio-carcinoma and chronic active hepatitis are the major complications related more directly to ulcerative colitis. Occasionally granulomas and amyloidosis may be found [399–401].

Pericholangitis and primary sclerosing cholangitis are both diseases of the biliary tract seen most commonly in association with extensive/total ulcerative colitis [402–404]. Indeed 70% of patients with sclerosing cholangitis are found to have ulcerative colitis. Pericholangitis affects small ducts and sclerosing cholangitis larger ducts but both conditions are now considered part of the same disease process and progression from small to large duct involvement has been demonstrated [405]. The basic pathology includes varying degrees of peri-ductular fibrosis and cholangitis, along with portal tract enlargement, leading on to piecemeal necrosis and eventually biliary cirrhosis [406]. Increased copper can be demonstrated in periportal positions. Ductular disease may present before the ulcerative colitis and colectomy does not protect the patient from its progression. The disease can also occur in the absence of ulcerative colitis, suggesting that the two conditions might share a common cause or factor.

Cholangio-carcinoma (adenocarcinoma of the bile duct epithelium) is the most serious hepatic complication associated with ulcerative colitis. The incidence is low (0.4–1.4%) [407] and it may develop years after panprocto-colectomy [408]. The tumour may be relatively slow growing and, if jaundice can be relieved, survival is surprisingly long. Cirrhosis occurs in up to 5% of patients, usually in those with severe and total ulcerative colitis; it may also arise on a basis of long-term autoimmune-type chronic hepatitis [409,410].

Other extra-intestinal manifestations of chronic ulcerative colitis
There are a large number of extra-intestinal manifestations of ulcerative colitis [410,411]. These include arthritis, ankylosing spondylitis, pyoderma gangrenosum, erythema nodosum, pericarditis, uveitis and episcleritis [410]. Amyloidosis is a rare complication [400,401], because many original reports are believed to have actually represented cases of Crohn's disease [401]. Complications may also be the result of therapy. Of the commonly used drugs, both steroids and sulphasalazine have well-documented side effects.

Crohn's disease of the large intestine

The pathology of Crohn's disease and its aetiology, pathogenesis, complications and management have been fully described in Chapter 20. The pathological features of colorectal Crohn's disease are fundamentally the same as those in the small intestine and are therefore described more briefly here.

The original senior author of this text, and his surgical colleague, Lockhart-Mummery, were the first to describe Crohn's disease of the colorectum, back in 1960, when they distinguished its macroscopic and histological features from ulcerative colitis [412,413]. Crohn's colitis usually presents with diarrhoea, rectal bleeding or perianal disease; recurrent abdominal pain and intestinal obstruction are much less conspicuous than in small bowel disease. Anal and perianal disease, including oedematous skin tags, cavitating ulcers, fissures, fistulae, abscesses and anal canal strictures (see Chapter 42) may occur in 75% of patients with colonic Crohn's disease at some time during the course of their illness. Such manifestations are more common during severe attacks when the colon is extensively involved. They are also associated with other extra-intestinal manifestations [411].

Large bowel Crohn's disease may coexist with small intestinal disease, when it is most commonly manifested as involvement of the terminal ileum and the right side of the colon [413], or it may be limited to the colon, a situation found in some 15–30% of patients. Unlike Crohn's disease in the small bowel, when there is often a clear demarcation between diseased and non-diseased intestine, the transition between affected and unaffected areas in the colon is often less clear. Colonic Crohn's disease has three major patterns of distribution: a diffuse colitis that may be difficult to distinguish from ulcerative colitis macroscopically, stricturing disease and Crohn's proctitis. These patterns may coexist or change from one to another during the course of a patient's illness. It is important to remember that the rectum is macroscopically normal in 50% of cases of Crohn's colitis.

Macroscopic appearances

The serosa of the bowel is often hyperaemic and erythematous, with a slightly dusky blue appearance due to vascular congestion and there may be a covering of inflammatory exudate. There may be dense fibrous adhesions to other loops of bowel or other intra-abdominal organs. Fat wrapping may be difficult to assess within the colon but is usually present, and of course this will not be assessable in the lower part of the rectum as it is normally entirely invested by fat.

The pathological hallmark of Crohn's disease in the large bowel, as in the small intestine, is discontinuous, patchy or focal disease and this is seen most obviously from the mucosal aspect. Accordingly, ulceration may vary within a single specimen from deep serpiginous fissuring ulcers (Figure 35.27) to tiny aphthous ulcers surrounded by normal or mildly oedematous bowel (Figure 35.28). Such aphthous ulcers are thought to represent the earliest manifestations of Crohn's disease and appear to start as erosions of mucosa overlying lymphoid follicles. Larger ulcers are

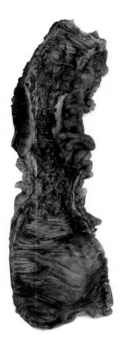

Figure 35.27 Crohn's disease of the colon: the terminal ileum is visible at bottom right. In the ascending colon, there is the typical focal pathology with ulceration and cobblestone appearance that characterises colonic Crohn's disease.

usually discrete with oedematous, overhanging, slightly violaceous edges and they are often stellate in outline [412–416]. Other examples have a more linear 'tramline' appearance with two or more roughly parallel lines of discrete ulceration running along the length of the colon, often, but not always, related to the point of mesocolic vascular entry into the bowel wall. After ulcer healing tramline indentations of the mucosal surface frequently remain. Cobblestoning of the mucosal surface of the colon, resulting from areas of marked oedema of the mucosa and submucosa separated by crevices which represent narrow fissuring ulcers (see Figure 35.27), is rarely as conspicuous as in the small bowel and is not unique to Crohn's disease, being sometimes seen in ischaemic colitis.

Fistulae are found in up to 60% of patients, whereas overt perforation of active colonic Crohn's disease is uncommon. This probably reflects the fact that the inflammatory process penetrates the tissue planes slowly and causes loops of inflamed bowel to adhere to each other, effectively walling off any perforation or abscess that may have formed. Fistulae, perforations and abscesses form from the base of the fissuring ulcers, where there is extension of the inflammatory process into the serosa and adjacent structures. It can be difficult to find fistulae. The exit point may be detectable and may have been oversewn at the time of surgery, but fistulae may also be present between adherent loops of

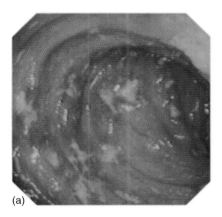

(a)

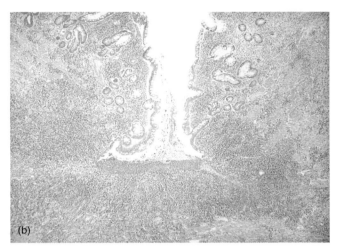

(b)

Figure 35.28 (a) Endoscopic appearance of multiple aphthous ulcers in Crohn's disease. (b) Histology of an aphthoid ulcer with ulcer slough overlying a lymphoid follicle surrounded by mucosa with focal crypt architectural distortion and patchy chronic inflammation.

bowel when they are more difficult to detect. They may be found by gentle probing, especially if recesses in the mucosa are probed and inflammatory polyps gently pushed aside because the opening may be immediately adjacent to them (so-called sentinel polyps). As a last resort, strictures can be bread sliced as thinly as possible (block thickness), when they will usually be revealed. Indeed it is quite good practice to do this routinely to find unexpected fistulae and even the occasional carcinoma.

Colonic strictures in Crohn's disease, similar to those in the small bowel, usually result from transmural inflammation, fibrosis and fibromuscular proliferation. They have no particular macroscopic distinguishing features from those due to ischaemia, chronic infective disorders and drug-induced strictures (see below) but they may serve in the distinction from ulcerative colitis, in which they are very uncommon. On the other hand, diffuse colonic involvement with Crohn's disease, although uncommon, can be

difficult to distinguish macroscopically from ulcerative colitis. Useful pointers towards Crohn's disease include rectal sparing and the presence of anal or perianal inflammation. Mucosal inflammatory polyps (also known misguidedly as pseudo-polyps) may be seen in Crohn's disease, sometimes adopting giant proportions up to 50 mm in maximum dimension [417,418]. Tall, narrow filiform polyps may also be seen. So-called giant inflammatory polyposis or filiform polyposis may be seen in colonic Crohn's disease but is less common than in ulcerative colitis. A particular feature of some cases of Crohn's disease is the presence of a 'sentinel' inflammatory polyp on the proximal side of an ulcerated stricture.

Microscopic appearances

The diagnosis of Crohn's disease is usually made by a combination of clinical, endoscopic, radiological, operative and pathological findings. It is an important, lifelong diagnosis for the patient and should not be made lightly. The pathological diagnosis is usually easier on the resected specimen than in a mucosal biopsy [415,416]; both are considered briefly here.

Mucosal biopsy appearances of Crohn's disease

The most typical histological feature of Crohn's disease in mucosal biopsies is patchy active chronic inflammation. The mucosa contains an infiltrate of lymphocytes, plasma cells and macrophages that varies from place to place, even within a small biopsy, both vertically and longitudinally in the mucosa, but it is especially noticeable when multiple biopsies are examined from the same patient, either synchronously or metachronously [302,419–421]. In deep biopsies it may be seen to extend into the submucosa, where its density may be proportionately greater than in the mucosa. Sometimes the infiltrate contains eosinophils or mast cells but the most useful diagnostic finding is the presence of aggregates of epithelioid macrophages (microgranulomas) (Figure 35.29) or more classic non-caseating epithelioid cell granulomas.

Active disease is manifested by the presence of neutrophils and typically these are also seen to have a patchy or focal distribution, such that apparently single crypts, or even segments of crypts, may be acutely inflamed whereas their neighbours are apparently unaffected [74] (Figure 35.30). This so-called focal active colitis on a background of patchy chronic inflammation is highly characteristic of Crohn's disease but it must be distinguished from 'isolated' focal active colitis (when there is no background chronic inflammation), which can be found in a number of other conditions (see above and 'Focal active colitis' later in this chapter) [422,423].

Migration of neutrophils into crypt lumina may result in crypt abscess formation and rupture of inflamed crypts

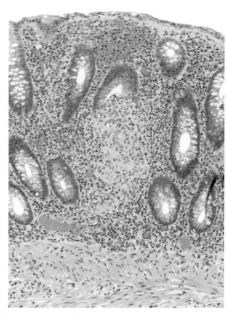

Figure 35.29 Crohn's disease with a cryptolytic granuloma: there is a circumscribed granulomatous reaction to a crypt, which appears half destroyed. However similar lesions can be seen in many forms of inflammatory pathology in the colon, including ulcerative colitis.

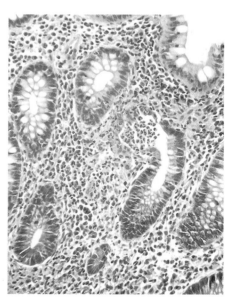

Figure 35.30 Crohn's disease: focal acute and chronic inflammation destroying part of a single crypt while leaving the remainder of that crypt and the adjacent crypts unaffected.

releases mucus into the surrounding lamina propria. As described above in ulcerative colitis, this can sometimes result in pericryptal aggregates of macrophages, so-called cryptolytic granulomas, and it is important to recognise these for what they are and not attribute to them the same diagnostic relevance as 'proper' granulomas and microgranulomas [424–426]. In some biopsies of Crohn's colitis, the acute inflammation is more diffuse, especially when the disease is highly active with ulceration and, in these cases, the pattern can be indistinguishable from ulcerative colitis. Nevertheless, the inflammation often fails to induce marked mucus (goblet cell) depletion and the crypt architecture is often surprisingly preserved. In long-standing cases the epithelium may show metaplasia, with the appearance of either Paneth cells or pseudo-pyloric metaplasia (ulcer-associated cell lineage) [427], although the latter is less common in colonic Crohn's disease than in the small bowel [428].

Resection specimens

In most resection specimens, the most striking histological feature is ulceration that characteristically takes the form of deep, knife-like fissures which are lined by ulcer slough and surrounded by inflammatory granulation tissue. These extend into and often through the colonic wall to form fistulae, to terminate in an extramural abscess or communicate with other fissuring ulcers, extending laterally to produce a complex network of sinuses and fistulae. In other cases there may be more widespread mucosal ulceration with large, deep, but still discrete, mucosal defects with overhanging oedematous edges. Despite the severity of the ulceration, it is often remarkable that, in Crohn's disease, the mucosa within a few millimetres may be virtually normal. On the other hand, the very earliest lesions, the so-called aphthous ulcers, result from superficial erosion over reactive mucosal lymphoid follicles. Ulcer healing in Crohn's disease may result in entrapment or misplacement of epithelium from the mucosa into the deeper layers of the bowel wall, usually with some accompanying lamina propria. This may give rise to intramural mucus-filled cysts (colitis cystica profunda) and confusion with carcinoma should be resisted.

The patchiness of the inflammation that is the histological hallmark of Crohn's disease, described above in mucosal biopsies, extends throughout the full thickness of the bowel wall (see Figure 35.28), where it is manifested as round or ovoid lymphoid aggregates which may measure up to a few millimetres in diameter. These may be found in all layers of the bowel wall but they are most obvious in the submucosa and when they line up along the outer aspect of the muscularis propria to form a 'Crohn's rosary' [225] in the subserosal tissues. Associated with the transmural inflammation is gross bowel wall thickening, involving all the layers, with oedema and fibrosis being especially prominent in the sub-

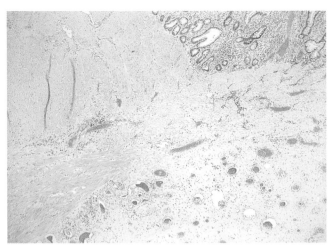

Figure 35.31 Connective tissue changes throughout all layers of the bowel in Crohn's disease. There is muscularisation of the submucosa and neuromuscular hyperplasia in the muscularis propria. Perineural chronic inflammation is also noted in the myenteric plexus.

mucosa. Lymphangiectasia is also a common feature and is best appreciated in the submucosa and subserosa. Intramural epithelioid cell granulomas are seen in 50% of cases of Crohn's colitis. They too may be present in all layers of the bowel wall and in the regional lymph nodes, although they are generally inconspicuous in the lymph nodes unless numerous within the bowel wall. They are commonly found alongside blood vessels and, especially, adjacent to lymphatics. Sometimes there may be a full-blown granulomatous lymphangitis, phlebitis or even arteritis.

Connective tissue changes of Crohn's disease (Figure 35.31) affecting all layers of the bowel wall [416,429,430] include thickening and disruption of the muscularis mucosae, fibrosis and focal muscularisation of the submucosa, fibrous scarring of the muscularis propria and marked neuronal hyperplasia of the intra- and extra-mural nerve fibres [429,430]. Perineural chronic inflammation may be seen in the submucosal (Meissner's) plexus, as well as in the myenteric (Auerbach's) plexus. The presence of the latter at resected margins may be associated with an increased risk of recurrence [431,432]. Cases have been described in which the histological features of Crohn's disease are limited to the mucosa and submucosa [433]. These have been termed 'superficial Crohn's disease' but are very rare in our experience.

The differential diagnosis of Crohn's disease and ulcerative colitis

In this section we are mainly concerned with the important differentiation between colorectal Crohn's disease and chronic ulcerative colitis, the two main forms of CIBD. This account therefore concentrates on the means at the disposal of the diagnostic pathologist for differentiating these conditions, because such a distinction has important management implications for the patient. First, it should be stated clearly that it is occasionally impossible, on pathological evidence alone, to make an accurate and confident distinction between these two disorders. Even in long-term disease that has been subject to innumerable colonoscopic biopsies the distinction may still not be possible.

Macroscopic differences from ulcerative colitis in resection specimens

The distinction between ulcerative colitis and large intestinal Crohn's disease can, in many cases, be made solely on the macroscopic pathology. Indeed the importance of taking into account the macroscopic features of the disease process cannot be over-emphasised. Too often we see pathologists trying to make the distinction on the basis of microscopic features alone and taking no account of important macroscopic features of resection specimens. The ease with which this can be achieved does depend on the way the surgical specimen has been prepared. It is important that the fresh colectomy specimen is promptly fixed in formalin solution in a way that preserves the pathological anatomy, and in particular allows close inspection of the mucosal surface.

In Table 35.1 the main differences in the macroscopic pathology of these two diseases are demonstrated. It must be emphasised that these differences are not definitive and, in some cases, there is considerable overlap. The comparative macroscopic pathology of ulcerative colitis and large intestinal Crohn's disease can be summarised as follows:
1. Ulcerative colitis is an inflammatory disease primarily of the mucosa of the colon and rectum. It spreads from the rectum in continuity to involve part or the whole of the large intestine. In contrast, Crohn's disease is nearly always a discontinuous process. Commonly, there are diseased areas widely separated by normal tissue. Even with extensive involvement, there are usually small patches of uninvolved bowel. A segmental colitis with histologically normal bowel on either side is most unlikely to represent ulcerative colitis [414,433,434], although after treatment macroscopic patchiness may be apparent.
2. The rectum is always involved in ulcerative colitis. It must be emphasised that sigmoidoscopy alone is not enough to determine this, because occasionally a diseased mucosa may be found histologically when the sigmoidoscopic appearances reveal no abnormality. The rectum may also be involved in Crohn's disease but the presence of CIBD affecting only the colon, with a normal rectum, is highly suggestive of Crohn's disease. In a minority of cases of ulcerative colitis, the mucosal changes in the rectum can be minimal and easily overlooked.

Table 35.1 Macroscopic differences in the pathology of ulcerative colitis and Crohn's disease in the large intestine

Ulcerative colitis	Crohn's disease
Disease in continuity	Disease usually discontinuous
Rectum almost always involved	Rectum normal in 50%
Terminal ileum involved in 10%	Terminal ileum involved in 30%
Granular and ulcerated mucosa (no fissuring)	Discretely ulcerated mucosa; cobblestone appearance; fissuring
Often intensely vascular	Vascularity seldom intense
Normal serosa (except in acute fulminating colitis)	Serositis common
Muscular shortening of colon; fibrous strictures very rare	Shortening due to fibrosis; fibrous strictures common
Never internal spontaneous fistulae	Enterocutaneous or intestinal fistulae in 10%
Inflammatory polyposis common and extensive	Inflammatory polyposis less prominent and less extensive
Dysplasia and malignant change well recognised	Malignant change possibly less common
Anal lesions in less than 25%; acute fissures, excoriation and oedematous anal tags less common	Anal lesions in 75%; anal fistulae (often multiple); anal ulceration

3. The terminal ileum is involved in only 10% of colectomy specimens for ulcerative colitis. Often this involvement is for a very short distance but uncommonly it may affect as much as 250 mm of the most distal ileum. Involvement is much more common in Crohn's disease. However, ileal involvement in ulcerative colitis is always in continuity with disease in the proximal colon, across the ileo-caecal valve, usually with a patulous ileo-caecal valve. The activity cannot be more severe in the terminal ileum than in the mucosa distal to the ileo-caecal valve.

4. In ulcerative colitis there is a granular haemorrhagic appearance of the mucosa, sometimes with patchy superficial ulceration but without fissuring. The appearance is in marked contrast with Crohn's disease, which shows a thickened wall, stenosis of the lumen and serpiginous mucosal ulceration, often with a cobblestone appearance and the presence of fissures (see Figure 35.27). Discontinuous disease may be present, a feature that is not usually seen in ulcerative colitis, the exception being a caecal or peri-appendiceal patch, which may have normal intervening mucosa between the right- and left-sided disease. This feature is quite acceptable for ulcerative colitis and does not indicate a skip lesion of Crohn's disease. An impression of discontinuous disease in ulcerative colitis may be given if one area of the mucosa is less active than others or in specific situations such as the caecal patch lesion (see above).

5. Fresh operative specimens of ulcerative colitis are often intensely vascular and congested, especially in very active disease. Vascularity is not a prominent feature of Crohn's disease, in which oedema is a better index of activity.

6. Inspection of the serosal surface of a colectomy specimen with ulcerative colitis will show normal shiny peritoneum, except in fulminating disease with toxic megacolon. Serositis, with or without granuloma formation, is a regular feature of Crohn's disease. Fat wrapping may also be seen in Crohn's disease of the colon but it may be more difficult to evaluate in the colon compared with the small intestine.

7. In ulcerative colitis, there is a striking shortening of the large intestine. This is never due to fibrosis but is the result of a muscle abnormality, which is sometimes reversible and also accounts for the loss of the haustral pattern, such a valuable sign in the radiographic diagnosis. If a true stricture is present in chronic ulcerative colitis, then it is malignant until proven otherwise, but may alternatively be due to coexistent diverticular disease. Crohn's disease characteristically produces fibrous strictures.

8. Spontaneous internal or enterocutaneous fistulae are a feature of Crohn's disease and effectively never occur in ulcerative colitis, unless there has been previous surgery. They are caused by a fissure penetrating right through the bowel wall and causing a serosal reaction, which then leads to adherence to neighbouring bowel or adjacent structures such as bladder or the anterior abdominal wall. For the same reason, chronic pericolic abscess formation occurs only in Crohn's disease.

9. Extensive inflammatory polyposis in the form of mucosal tags is common in colectomy specimens of ulcerative colitis and involves the colon more than the rectum. In Crohn's disease polyposis is a less prominent [430] and extensive

Table 35.2 Microscopic differences in the pathology of ulcerative colitis and Crohn's disease of the large intestine

Ulcerative colitis	Crohn's disease
Mucosal and submucosal inflammation (except in acute fulminating colitis)	Patchy transmural inflammation
Width of submucosa normal or reduced	Width of submucosa normal or increased
Often intense vascularity; little oedema	Vascularity seldom prominent; oedema marked
Focal lymphoid hyperplasia restricted to the mucosa and superficial submucosa	Focal lymphoid hyperplasia (lymphoid aggregates) in mucosa, submucosa, subserosa and pericolic tissues
'Crypt abscesses' very common	'Crypt abscesses' fewer in number
Mucus secretion grossly impaired	Mucus secretion slightly impaired
Paneth cell metaplasia common	Paneth cell metaplasia rare
Formed epithelioid cell granulomas absent from bowel and lymph nodes	Formed epithelioid cell granulomas in 60–70% of patients in bowel and local lymph nodes
'Fissuring' absent	'Fissuring' very common
Pre-cancerous epithelial change more common	Pre-cancerous epithelial change uncommon
Anal pathology rare: usually non-specific inflammation	Anal pathology: epithelioid cell granulomas often present

feature, although cobblestoning in Crohn's disease can mimic the presence of multiple polyps.

10. Malignant change is a well-established feature of ulcerative colitis. There is an increased risk of malignancy throughout the gastrointestinal tract in Crohn's disease [435] but cancer surveillance for the detection of dysplasia is usually recommended for extensive large bowel disease.

11. Anal lesions are much more common in Crohn's disease than in ulcerative colitis. In the latter there may be acute superficial ulceration of the anal canal and excoriation of the skin around the anus, but chronic lesions such as fistulae, ulceration and oedematous anal tags are characteristic of Crohn's disease. In operative specimens, extensive perianal and perirectal chronic inflammation is seen in Crohn's disease but in ulcerative colitis the inflammation is more superficial. Nevertheless an occasional fistula *in ano* can be seen in ulcerative colitis as in the non-CIBD population.

Microscopic differences from ulcerative colitis

When analysing a resection specimen of the colon and/or rectum removed for CIBD, sections should be taken from all parts of the colectomy specimen, especially from those areas that may be most productive of the important microscopic signs of fissuring ulceration and transmural inflammation. Lymph nodes should be extensively sampled, especially those draining areas of active disease, for microscopic examination in order to detect epithelioid cell granu-

lomas. The principal microscopic differences between these two diseases are given in Table 35.2 and are summarised as follows:

1. Ulcerative colitis is essentially a superficial inflammation of the mucosa of the rectum and colon, with involvement of the submucosal layer only in the presence of full-thickness mucosal ulceration. Even in very chronic long-standing cases, the muscularis propria and serosa remain free of inflammatory infiltration. The exception is in fulminant colitis and toxic megacolon, when the intense inflammatory reaction causes separation and splitting of the muscle fibres of the muscularis propria with eventual perforation through the greatly thinned bowel wall. In contrast, Crohn's disease is a transmural inflammation spreading throughout the bowel wall.

2. In ulcerative colitis the width of the submucosal layer is normal or reduced whereas it is characteristically widened in Crohn's disease to a variable extent by oedema, fibrosis and inflammatory cell infiltration. There are other submucosal signs such as lymphangiectasia, neuronal hyperplasia, muscularisation and vascular changes, all of which are features of Crohn's disease and are not seen in ulcerative colitis.

3. Intense congestion and dilatation of the blood supply to the bowel wall (particularly capillaries and veins) are more prominent in the submucosa in severe ulcerative colitis, particularly with very active disease; they are not conspicuous in Crohn's disease.

4. Focal hyperplasia of lymphoid tissue is restricted to the base of the mucosa and the superficial submucosa in ulcerative colitis, and is most common in the rectum. In Crohn's disease such focal collections of lymphocytic cells are characteristically distributed across the bowel wall, particularly in the submucosa and just outside the muscularis propria where they present as a 'Crohn's rosary'. There may be a third row in the myenteric plexus. They may be found quite some way out in the pericolic fat. This *transmural inflammation in the form of lymphoid aggregates* (transmural lymphoid hyperplasia) is one of the most distinctive and specific features of Crohn's disease in both the large and small intestine.

5. Crypt abscesses are not specific for ulcerative colitis: they can be found in a wide variety of inflammations of gut, including acute appendicitis, in infective colitis, adjacent to inflamed tumours and in Crohn's disease. They indicate activity. However, they are a particularly common feature of ulcerative colitis because of the great extent of mucosal inflammation.

6. In ulcerative colitis there is much epithelial destruction with goblet cell depletion and a corresponding impairment in the amount of mucin secretion. In Crohn's disease, areas of involved gut will often retain what is an almost normal population of goblet cells despite considerable adjacent inflammation. It is a useful histological sign that can be detected in routine sections as well as with special stains.

7. The cycles of epithelial destruction and repair in ulcerative colitis may lead to Paneth cell metaplasia, especially in very long-standing disease. Paneth cell metaplasia is less conspicuous in Crohn's disease.

8. Granulomas are variably found in Crohn's colitis resections and seem to be getting less common. They consist of collections of epithelioid cells and giant cells of Langhans' type without central caseation. They may be found anywhere in the affected bowel wall as well as in the regional lymphatic glands. Their numbers vary greatly from specimens in which they are very sparse indeed to others in which they are abundant. In about 30–40% of cases of Crohn's disease, no granulomas can be found. They are not usually found in the regional lymph glands without also being present in the bowel wall. Classic, basally oriented, well-formed, epithelioid cell granulomas are not a feature of chronic ulcerative colitis. However, giant cells and histiocytes, in aggregation, may be seen in association with damaged crypts in ulcerative colitis and a careful evaluation of such appearances is necessary. Some patients develop granulomas in response to crypt rupture. Granulomas at the site of crypts need to be treated with extreme caution. They are not synonymous with Crohn's disease but those at the base of the mucosa or deeper are much more likely to represent Crohn's disease than those at the site of a crypt rupture.

9. Fissuring ulceration is the most important sign of Crohn's disease and can be found in most cases if looked for carefully. Fissures appear as knife-like linear ulcers, which are lined by a layer of necrotic inflammatory cells surrounded by granulation tissue. They may also appear in histological sections as intramural or submucosal abscesses, but their shape depends on the way that the section has been cut. They are not a feature, as such, of chronic ulcerative colitis but are a feature of all severe acute colitides, irrespective of cause.

10. Dysplasia is much more common in ulcerative colitis. It is well described, but is rare, in colonic Crohn's disease. The main impact of ulcerative colitis is on the mucosa of the large bowel, leading to repeated cycles of diffuse epithelial destruction and repair, which may at least partly explain the proneness to malignant change. In contrast, the intestinal epithelium is relatively unaffected by this process in Crohn's disease.

11. Epithelioid cell granulomas can also be found in the anal lesions of Crohn's disease, sometimes widely involving the tissues of the perianal region. They are never found in the perianal region in ulcerative colitis.

12. After anti-TNF-α therapy, many of the changes of Crohn's disease may disappear. Inflammation may be minimal, the transmural lymphoid hyperplasia may be very restricted and areas of ulceration, beneath which one might expect to find abundant inflammation, may have a dearth of inflammation. However, these therapies tend to increase the amount of fibrosis and structuring, which may also be devoid of inflammation. This is in contrast with other forms of therapy that may cause symptomatic improvement but rarely affect the amount of inflammation present.

Crohn's disease in biopsies

The diagnosis can usually be made if the gastroenterologist has provided information on the extent, distribution and focality of disease present. Ideally the biopsy series should start in the terminal ileum and biopsies taken from each major named segment, finishing in the rectum. Rectal biopsies should always be included, because rectal sparing can be a major distinguishing feature. In a study of features distinguishing CIBD from non-CIBD (crypt atrophy, architectural distortion, basal cell plasmacytosis and Paneth cell metaplasia distal to the hepatic flexure were the distinguishing features), and also ulcerative colitis from Crohn's disease, the features that indicated Crohn's disease to be the underlying disease were segmental distribution (focality) of crypt atrophy and distortion, segmental distribution (focal) of loss of mucin, mucin preservation at an ulcer edge (as opposed to ulcerative colitis where erosions or ulcers are on a background of diffuse mucin depletion) and focal mononuclear infiltration (the greater the number of biopsies the better) [436].

Indeterminate colitis and IBDU

Examination of multiple biopsies allows a correct diagnosis of the type of CIBD to be made in 66–75% of newly diagnosed patients. The addition of endoscopic and clinical data increases this figure to >90% [437]. Terminology for patients without a definite diagnosis is not uniform and terms such as 'unclassified' and 'uncertain' colitis have been proposed as well as 'indeterminate colitis'. The last term has become widely used but with a variety of definitions [438]. The common feature of all definitions is that the aetiology and type of colitis cannot be identified properly.

The term 'indeterminate colitis' has been used in many ways and this has undoubtedly resulted in a diminution in its diagnostic utility and much confusion. Thus, the term has been used for patients with endoscopic and histological inflammation in the colorectum but uncertainty as to whether or not the patient has CIBD, and also for patients with CIBD but of uncertain type, in both biopsy material and resections. Unless pathologists are aware of this they will assume that a clinical diagnosis of indeterminate colitis means that the patient has CIBD which may not be the case [438]. For this reason the Montreal classification has suggested that the term 'indeterminate colitis' be reserved only for those cases where colectomy has been performed and pathologists are unable to make a definitive diagnosis of either Crohn's disease or ulcerative colitis after full examination. This is a recommendation with which we strongly concur. Where patients have CIBD but do not clearly fall into with either ulcerative colitis or Crohn's disease, they also propose the term 'inflammatory bowel disease, type unclassified' (IBDU). This is suggested for patients in whom there is evidence on clinical and endoscopic grounds for CIBD affecting the colon, without small bowel involvement, and no definitive histological or other evidence to favour either Crohn's disease or ulcerative colitis. In these patients, infection has been ruled out before the term IBDU is applied [215,439].

In practice, this distinction is of major importance only where an ileal pouch anal anastomosis are being considered. As it makes no difference whether the large bowel resection is called 'ulcerative colitis' or 'indeterminate colitis', the only issue is in ensuring that features of Crohn's disease are not present. In resected specimens this means either the typical transmural inflammation in the form of lymphoid aggregates (but not polymorphous transmural inflammation), in the submucosa and, especially, in the subserosa, or granulomas that are not crypt (mucin) or foreign material related. Using these criteria, the patient's history and prior biopsies, resections fall fairly easily into the following categories: ulcerative colitis, Crohn's colitis and severe (fulminant) colitis without features of ulcerative colitis or Crohn's disease (or uncertain aetiology). If the term 'indeterminate colitis' is to be used, it is this last group to which it is applied. There is a residual group that looks similar to ulcerative colitis but has rare subserosal lymphoid aggregates, usually close to the distal margin of resection. It is difficult to call this outright Crohn's disease and deny the patient a pouch, but neither is one comfortable using any of the alternative categories. An approach is to call these 'severe colitis with some features of Crohn's disease' (which is invariably the case), together with a comment that the final construction of the pouch should be delayed for a few months, but can go ahead provided that the disease is limited to the large bowel (no ileal or anal disease) and there is no evidence of Crohn's elsewhere (after upper gastrointestinal endoscopy, ileoscopy through the ileostomy and some form of examination of the residual small bowel ideally by capsule or enteroscopy). Some advocate the use of this philosophy and thus no longer use the admittedly ambiguous term 'indeterminate colitis'. At the end of the day, the key is to ensure that the clinician, and anybody else involved in the patient's care, know clearly and unambiguously what the pathologist is seeing, how it is being interpreted and its implications.

When all of the distinguishing features between ulcerative colitis and Crohn's disease have been considered, there will still be approximately 10% of specimens of CIBD in which the diagnosis remains in doubt [294,437]. It has been stated that these difficulties in differential diagnosis are due either to the overlapping histological features of the two diseases or to the fact that ulcerative colitis and Crohn's disease represent ends of the spectrum of one disease [433,434,440–442].

The term 'indeterminate colitis' was coined to describe those operative specimens, representing about 10% of the total, that do not conform to the standard macroscopic and microscopic features of ulcerative colitis and Crohn's disease [294,442] (Figures 35.32 and 35.33). However, they do conform to a recognisable clinical and pathological pattern. Mostly, the difficult cases are examples of extensive acute and severe colitis, often with some degree of dilatation of the colon. In this state, the maximal overlap of the pathology of Crohn's disease and ulcerative colitis is present and discriminating attributes are few or unreliable, e.g. relative rectal sparing is an accepted feature in many cases of Crohn's disease of the large bowel, yet this can be seen in fulminant ulcerative colitis, mainly because the predominant impact of the disease is seen in the more proximal, especially the transverse, colon. This accentuates relative sparing of the lower left colon and rectum. The healing effect of steroid enemas is another factor responsible for such appearances. Another misleading appearance

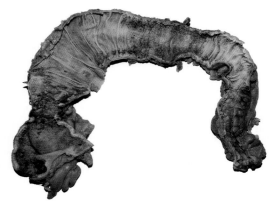

Figure 35.32 Indeterminate colitis: there is extensive ulceration on the right side of the colon with discontinuous disease, and ulceration, in the transverse colon and left colon. The histological features were equivocal for ulcerative colitis and Crohn's disease and hence the designation 'indeterminate colitis'.

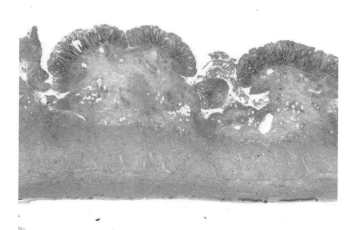

Figure 35.33 The histology of indeterminate colitis: at low power, there is deep, somewhat fissuring, ulceration with the surviving mucosal islands showing only modest evidence of active chronic inflammatory bowel disease.

is the discontinuous ulceration caused by the unusually variable intensity of the inflammation in fulminant colitis, of any cause, including ulcerative colitis. The minor histological changes in intact mucosa between ulcerated areas suggest previous inflammation that has resolved and may be the only clue that genuine skip lesions are not present.

Fissuring ulceration is an accepted parameter of Crohn's disease but is seen in severe colitis of any cause including acute ulcerative colitis. However, the quality of the fissuring is different. Typically the fissures in acute colitis are clefts, sparsely lined by inflammatory cells, whereas in Crohn's disease they tend to be serpiginous and covered by granulation tissue, although these features cannot

be used to make an unequivocal distinction. Transmural inflammation with myocytolysis of the muscularis propria can occur in both types of CIBD and is also common to toxic megacolon of any cause.

Examination of the surgical specimen alone may not reveal sufficient discriminating criteria for a diagnosis of ulcerative colitis or Crohn's disease, and thus the microscopic features are the key to the diagnosis. Clues to the correct diagnosis may be also found in the study of preoperative or postoperative rectal and colonic biopsies and, of course, in the subsequent progress of the disease, which may in later surgical material reveal diagnostic criteria. The importance of establishing a sequential record of rectal and colonic biopsy appearances in all cases of CIBD cannot be over-emphasised. The terminology indeterminate colitis is essentially a temporary classification until such a time that further clinical and pathological criteria become available to establish a diagnosis of either Crohn's disease or ulcerative colitis. Careful follow-up eventually provides this evidence in most cases. In particular, follow-up of the diverted rectum may be helpful. Crohn's disease tends to recover with diversion [443–446], whereas ulcerative colitis tends to develop more marked inflammation [445].

It has become particularly important to differentiate between colonic Crohn's disease and ulcerative colitis since the advent of restorative procto-colectomy (pelvic ileal reservoir surgery) [447–449]. The long-term results of pelvic ileal reservoir construction in patient groups with indeterminate colitis show that those who subsequently develop Crohn's disease usually have a poor outcome, whereas the majority, probably in excess of 80% of patients with a diagnosis of indeterminate colitis, have an outcome similar to that of pouch patients with ulcerative colitis [448], although one study has suggested a 19% failure rate for pouches in indeterminate colitis as opposed to 8% failure in the ulcerative colitis group [448]. A further study from Canada has reported a 95% success rate for pouches in ulcerative colitis and an 81% success rate for pouches in cases of indeterminate colitis [450]. In comparing ulcerative colitis patients with those with a diagnosis of indeterminate colitis, at the time of total colectomy, there appear to be clear-cut differences in rates of pelvic sepsis and perineal complications and patients and surgeons need to be warned of this potential problem in the indeterminate colitis patient group [451].

Synchronous and metachronous Crohn's disease and ulcerative colitis

There are rare reports, some not entirely convincing, that Crohn's disease and ulcerative colitis can occur in the same patient simultaneously [452,453]. Although we are aware of the very occasional case where the colorectum has shown the classic pathology of ulcerative colitis, with the small bowel showing unequivocal features of Crohn's disease, we believe that extreme caution is appropriate before concluding that Crohn's disease and ulcerative colitis are synchronous in the same patient. Most of these cases will represent only Crohn's disease. We, and others, have certainly seen extremely unusual cases of metachronous ulcerative colitis and Crohn's disease, the former usually occurring first, with the patient later developing small intestinal Crohn's disease [454].

The role of upper gastrointestinal biopsies in differentiating Crohn's disease from ulcerative colitis

Focal active gastritis and focal active duodenitis, in the absence of *H. pylori*, can be demonstrated in up to 40% of cases of Crohn's disease where the endoscopic appearances are normal. This may provide additional helpful information in distinguishing Crohn's disease from ulcerative colitis, particularly, it would seem, in children. However, studies have shown evidence of focal active gastritis in ulcerative colitis patients and the duodenum may also show active inflammation in ulcerative colitis. In one study, 12% of ulcerative colitis patients showed a chronic active gastritis [455]. The topic of inflammatory change in the mucosa of the stomach and duodenum in both Crohn's disease and ulcerative colitis is dealt with more extensively in the appropriate section (see Chapters 11 and 20).

Inflammatory polyposis in CIBD

There is a variety of florid (giant) inflammatory polyposis of the colorectum, which occurs in both major types of CIBD, but is much more common in ulcerative colitis [417]. It is also occasionally seen in diverticular disease, usually restricted to the sigmoid colon, and occasionally as a complication of chronic infective colitis, especially schistosomiasis. In such CIBD cases the mucosa is replaced by a thick polypoid mass of mucosal fronds. This type of polyposis has a macroscopic appearance similar to that of seaweed or even spaghetti. Sometimes the polyps are remarkably thin and filiform, and they may have a curious resemblance to worms. The polyposis is often segmental or focal and may completely fill the lumen of the colon, producing obstructive symptoms (Figure 35.34). Ulceration is conspicuous by its absence on macroscopic inspection and adjacent flat mucosa can appear quite normal. The appropriate histological diagnosis should be sought by ignoring the polyposis and examining the background mucosa for the usual discriminating criteria between ulcerative colitis and Crohn's disease. If there is no ulceration or transmural inflammation, and the disease is confined to the polypoid mucosa, then a diagnosis of ulcerative colitis is more likely. Faeces tend to become trapped within the maze of mucosal

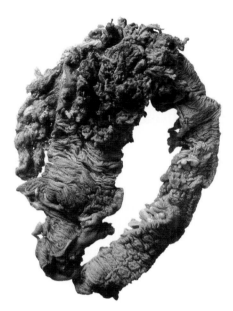

Figure 35.34 'Giant inflammatory polyposis' in ulcerative colitis: there is a huge exophytic mass composed of irregular haemorrhagic mucosal fronds filling the transverse colon. The proximal and distal mucosa is relatively unaffected but showed histological features of inactive ulcerative colitis.

fronds and this can cause local inflammation. The pathogenesis of this inflammatory polyposis reflects previous severe ulceration, islands of preserved inflamed and oedematous mucosa that eventually take the shape of polyps [417,456]. Over time the intervening ulcers heal and become re-epithelialised. When the disease is limited to a single segment, this may prove to be Crohn's disease but caution is appropriate (see below). The main problems with these lesions are that they may cause obstructive symptoms and it is also virtually impossible to carry out surveillance, so their presence leads to serious consideration of colectomy.

In ulcerative colitis, such (giant) inflammatory polyposis of the colorectum has especial features for which there have been few sensible explanations. First, the disease is often very sharply localised, especially in the descending colon and sigmoid colon, whereas the rest of the colorectum shows characteristic features of ulcerative colitis but without very much inflammatory polyposis. This may provide that unusual indication in the management of ulcerative colitis – for a segmental colectomy (often because of obstructive symptoms). Second, it is a characteristic feature that, although the flat mucosa shows the distinctive changes of ulcerative colitis, especially in the form of crypt architectural distortion, the mucosa lining the filiform polyps often appears relatively normal having few, if any, features of chronic ulcerative colitis. The importance of examining the mucosa away from the polyposis areas for evidence of ulcerative colitis cannot be over-emphasised in this situation. A third feature is that (giant) inflammatory polyposis of the colorectum complicating ulcerative colitis is especially prone to submucosal epithelial misplacement (colitis cystica profunda), and this may show profound mimicry of, admittedly very well differentiated, adenocarcinoma.

Diverticular disease and CIBD of the large intestine

Diverticular disease of the sigmoid colon is common in developed countries and it is not surprising that sometimes it occurs in patients with either Crohn's disease or ulcerative colitis [457,458]. However, in some cases the inflammatory bowel disease-like changes in the colon are limited to the segment involved by diverticulosis and have been termed 'diverticular colitis', 'diverticular disease associated chronic colitis' or 'segmental colitis associated with diverticulosis' (SCAD) [459–462]. The inflammatory changes are then seen in the luminal mucosa of the colon. The histology ranges from a mild increase in chronic inflammation, which may extend to the muscularis mucosae, or may strongly mimic CIBD, with granulomas, to being indistinguishable from ulcerative colitis, except for its distribution.

The key to the diagnosis is that changes are limited to the regional mucosa, so that normal biopsies from proximal to the diverticular disease and also from the rectum will indicate inflammation localised to the segment afflicted by diverticular disease (Figure 35.35). Potential for confusion with Crohn's disease is also apparent, given the focal nature of the changes. It is also one occasion where a disease that looks identical to ulcerative colitis has rectal sparing.

Crohn's disease-like pathology can be superimposed upon that of diverticular disease of the sigmoid colon, especially when there has been abscess formation and a degree of resolution. Worse, because one of the complications of complex diverticular disease is fistula formation, the presence of fistulae can further confuse the picture. The changes of complex diverticular disease can therefore be seen occasionally in colectomy specimens removed for diffuse ulcerative colitis and Crohn's disease. Transmural

lymphoid hyperplasia mimicking the changes of Crohn's disease can be found under these circumstances and granulomatous inflammation, sometimes even with granulomatous vasculitis and other characteristic pathological and radiological features of Crohn's disease, have also been described [463–465]. However, unless the patient is known to have Crohn's disease or has a separate focus of disease, this is just a mimic and there are no data to support this evolving into typical Crohn's disease. Sometimes the character of the transmural inflammation, such a distinctive feature of Crohn's disease, is subtly different in complicated diverticular disease compared with that seen in Crohn's disease. In complicated diverticular disease, the lymphoid aggregates radiate away from an inflamed diverticulum and do not have the rosary-like distinction that is so characteristic of colonic Crohn's disease. This distinction can be quite subtle and not always easy to detect.

When the pathologist is examining surgical specimens of diverticular disease, he or she should be alert for the presence of any macroscopic or microscopic criteria for either type of CIBD. In some cases of diverticulosis, the mucosa between the diverticula may be normal. There are reports of a limited segmental sigmoid colitis where inflammation of the luminal mucosa between diverticula is present, apparently unassociated with concomitant Crohn's disease or ulcerative colitis [460,461,466]. Mechanical damage to the redundant mucosa, a feature of diverticular disease, may account for this.

In one recent endoscopic and biopsy study, 'diverticular colitis' showed three endoscopic patterns: 'crescentic fold disease' (about half), an 'ulcerative colitis-like' pattern (about a third), and a 'Crohn's colitis-like' pattern (11%). Most patients with the first and second patterns showed histological alterations resembling moderate ulcerative colitis, whereas those in the Crohn's-disease like group showed most variation [467].

We would recommend that this CIBD-like pathology in the sigmoid colon, especially when seen in biopsy material and correlating with signs of endoscopic luminal mucosal inflammation, now be termed 'diverticular colitis' (which

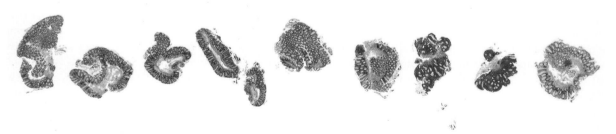

Figure 35.35 A case of 'diverticular colitis': these are colonoscopic biopsies taken from the caecum (at left) right through to the rectum (at right). Only two biopsies (towards the right-hand end) show chronic inflammatory changes with crypt architectural distortion and these derive from the sigmoid colon. This demonstration serves to emphasise the importance of distribution of inflammatory changes in the diagnosis of chronic inflammatory bowel disease and its 'mimics'.

seems to us the most simple and applicable appellation) or diverticulosis-associated colitis. The term 'diverticular-associated colitis' has been widely used but is quite simply etymologically unacceptable, because association with an adjective is not appropriate.

This is yet another example of inflammatory pathology in the intestines where the differentiation from both types of CIBD requires sound clinico-pathological correlation. The key to excluding ulcerative colitis is to take biopsies from the rectum, because these will be normal. However, an important caveat here is that a small number of cases of diverticular colitis, without evidence of rectal involvement, will ultimately evolve into classic ulcerative colitis [460,466,468]. This is one of the few examples when ulcerative colitis does not start in the rectum.

Diverticular colitis represents an unusual spectrum of pathology in the sigmoid colon afflicted by diverticulosis. In many cases, it appears to represent a unique entity related to diverticulosis whereas long-term follow-up studies suggest that some patients do evolve into classic CIBD, especially ulcerative colitis, often years later [459, 460,462,468,470]. The treatment response reflects the clinical and histological ambiguities, some cases responding to acute diverticulitis-like treatment and some requiring CIBD-type therapy [469]. Some may even require surgical resection of the involved segment. On the one hand, pathologists, examining biopsy material from the sigmoid colon afflicted by diverticulosis, should heed all clinical and endoscopic evidence while, on the other, during examination of the surgical specimens of diverticulosis, they should carefully evaluate the presence of any macroscopic or microscopic inflammatory changes occurring in the luminal mucosa and recognise potential CIBD mimicry, especially Crohn's disease [459–461].

Other granulomatous pathology in the large intestine

Reports of sarcoidosis [471] of the colorectum should be treated with caution, if isolated to the intestine, because these are more likely to be examples of segmental Crohn's disease or intestinal tuberculosis. A similar histological appearance can also be seen as a local reaction to malignant disease [472]. Involvement of the large bowel in sarcoidosis is extremely rare and is usually clinically silent [473,474].

Active chronic inflammation of the large intestinal mucosa with granulomas has recently been described in the cord colitis syndrome [475], a novel form of intestinal inflammation occurring in recipients of stem cell transplants with umbilical cord blood (but not with other allogeneic haematopoietic tissues). The condition appears to be different from graft-versus-host disease and usually responds to antibiotics, despite an inability to demonstrate any infective agent (see Chapter 40).

Biopsy in the differential diagnosis of CIBD and infective procto-colitis

In a biopsy with inflamed colorectal mucosa, the most common differential diagnoses to consider are CIBD, both ulcerative colitis and Crohn's disease, and infective colitis. However, there are many other conditions that may mimic these entities: appreciation of the clinical context, including age and previous treatment, be it medical or surgical, cannot be over-emphasised because many such iatrogenic pathological entities, and numerous other conditions, can closely mimic CIBD. Ischaemia, for example, is a consideration in elderly people but is very unlikely in a teenager. Recent antibiotics or recent travel may also direct attention to the relevant clinical diagnosis. The correct classification of CIBD clearly has important long-term implications for the patient. Classification is bedevilled by the problem that there is no single histological feature that is invariably present in any one condition and invariably absent from the others. Thus even a granuloma, although it may help to exclude chronic ulcerative colitis, does not necessarily imply a diagnosis of Crohn's disease, because it may indicate an infective granulomatous pathology.

The diagnostic problems in biopsy work usually centre on the active phases of the various forms of CIBD and the resolving phase of ulcerative colitis. In remission, the architectural distortion so typical of chronic ulcerative colitis seldom causes diagnostic confusion. Crypt architectural distortion, a villiform surface, goblet cell depletion, prominent crypt abscesses and a diffuse, predominantly plasma cell infiltrate of the lamina propria, point strongly to a diagnosis of ulcerative colitis. By contrast, in infective procto-colitis, the crypts remain aligned but some degree of crypt degeneration is seen (Figure 35.36). Neutrophils are the most conspicuous inflammatory cell, migrating in a characteristic way between the crypt epithelial cells to produce a cryptitis, and also seen clustered in the lamina propria. There is frequently obvious mucosal oedema and the plasma cell infiltrate is light to moderate. In general the diagnosis of infective procto-colitis is suggested by appreciating that there is an absence of the features that characterise Crohn's disease and ulcerative colitis [38], most notably by assessment of the acute:chronic inflammatory cell ratio.

Although granulomas are undeniably useful in the diagnosis of Crohn's disease, their identification is neither specific nor sensitive for that diagnosis. They are present only in 25–28% of biopsy material in Crohn's disease. Granulomas may occur in campylobacter colitis, chlamydia proctitis, yersiniosis and of course tuberculosis [91,104]. There has to be careful interpretation of mucosal giant cells associated with an ill-defined clustering of inflammatory cells and histiocytes formed secondarily and adjacent to damaged crypts, so-called cryptolytic granulomas or mucin

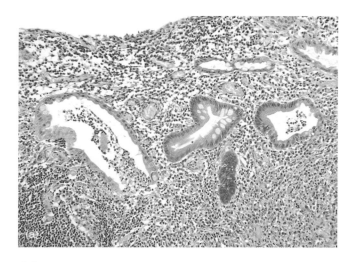

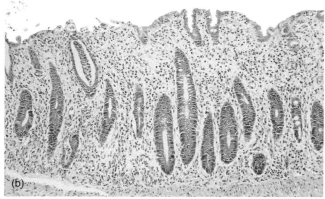

Figure 35.36 (a) Active chronic ulcerative colitis (UC) and (b) acute infective colitis. Important differences are in the crypt architecture (distorted in UC, preserved in infective colitis) and in the content of the lamina propria (oedema and predominantly acute inflammation in infective colitis, heavy diffuse acute and chronic inflammation in UC). Note the 'pointed crypts' that tends to be characteristic of infection.

granulomas (Figure 35.37). These can be seen in ulcerative colitis and Crohn's disease, besides other inflammatory conditions, so are not specific for any.

In Crohn's disease, in the face of a moderate inflammatory cell infiltrate, the crypts remain aligned with little mucin depletion. This infiltrate is often patchy and basal lymphoid aggregates are a useful sign. Neutrophils may form crypt abscesses but their numbers seldom match those seen in ulcerative colitis or infection, although at times they can be more intense and also exquisitely focal. Micro-granulomas [476,477], focal collections of inflammatory cells including histiocytes but not crypt related, are a useful pointer to Crohn's disease. In the absence of granulomas, patchy chronic inflammation on a background of regular crypt architecture favours Crohn's disease, as does observing inflammatory cells in the submucosa. A pitfall is the biopsy appearance of a patient with resolving ulcerative colitis. Here the goblet cell population is recovering,

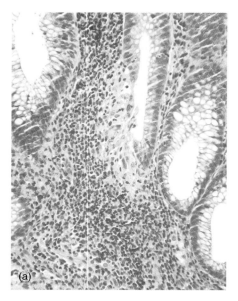

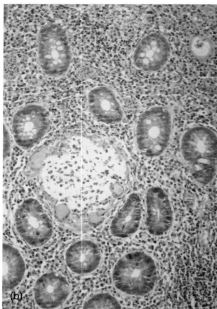

Figure 35.37 (a) A cryptolytic granuloma that appears to be destroying part of a crypt in a segmental manner in Crohn's disease. (b) Foreign body-type giant cells surround mucus at the site of a ruptured crypt in a patient with ulcerative colitis.

the acute inflammatory infiltrate diminished, and the distribution of plasma cells and lymphocytes often patchy. Considerable reliance must be placed on crypt distortion with the caveat that this can be irregular in areas of healing ulceration of whatever aetiology. The presence of crypt irregularity has been shown to be reliable in several studies militating against a diagnosis of infection [72,73,478–481]. In severe shigella dysentery, however, extensive crypt distortion is well described [26,28]. This may indicate that *Shigella* sp. can be an exception or that in severe inflammation the value of architectural damage as a distinguishing attribute is less valid.

Both ulcerative colitis and Crohn's disease may present in a similar way to infective colitis or be precipitated by it [39]. Also, patients with CIBD are susceptible to acute infections. A problem facing the pathologist is to know how often a biopsy of these two conditions may mimic infection or vice versa. Reports suggest that between 7 and 30% of biopsies from patients who are culture positive or carry a confident clinical diagnosis of infective colitis can have a biopsy more in keeping with ulcerative colitis or Crohn's disease [481,482]. Children are notorious in this regard and what looks like 'classic' acute infectious colitis may be accompanied by a history of months of diarrhoea, ultimately evolving into one or other major form of CIBD. Figures for the converse, patients with Crohn's disease or ulcerative colitis but with biopsies resembling infection, are around 5–7%. However, as the mucosal appearances in infective colitis and ulcerative colitis vary with the time from the onset of disease, such figures must be viewed with caution. Emphasis is laid on the value of the study of sequential biopsies to solve these diagnostic dilemmas: ultimately these diseases usually declare themselves.

Special stains are of little value in this important differential diagnosis. A change in goblet cell mucin pattern from predominant sulpho-mucin to sialo-mucin is common to both ulcerative colitis and Crohn's disease, and simply reflects disease activity [234,483,484] but is useless diagnostically. In an individual biopsy the distribution of immunoglobulin-containing plasma cells is of little value [485], although there is a suggestion that the plasma cell IgG:IgM ratio is permanently raised in Crohn's disease [485,486] and the plasma cell IgG:IgM and IgG:IgA ratios remain low in infection [485].

The widespread use of colonoscopic examination allows the assessment of the distribution and focality of pathology in the colon and rectum [487], and reduces the sampling error inherent in a single biopsy. Indeed, although it is usually possible to separate ulcerative colitis from infection on one or two appropriately involved rectal biopsies, it is usually foolhardy to do the same in distinguishing ulcerative colitis from Crohn's disease. The distinguishing histological attributes of the patterns of CIBD are no different in a colonoscopic biopsy from those in a rectal biopsy. A series of diffusely inflamed colonoscopic biopsies throughout the left colon and a normal right colon favour the diagnosis of ulcerative colitis even though the rectal biopsy might have been equivocal. On the other hand, variation in the intensity of inflammation between biopsy sites and within individual biopsies suggests Crohn's disease, even if there are no specific microscopic features seen. Indeed it is this focal and patchy active inflammation that is, in biopsies, one of the most useful pathological findings in colonoscopic biopsies. Patients with the common causes of infective procto-colitis seldom require colonoscopy but the biopsies

are usually uniformly inflamed, with the characteristics described earlier [482].

Colonoscopic patterns of inflammation will be altered by treatment, because not all areas of the colon may respond equally. The rectum, after local steroid enemas, may appear relatively spared, perhaps suggesting Crohn's disease. Of considerable diagnostic importance is the colonoscopist's account of the macroscopic pathology. This can be diagnostic even when the biopsies may be considered non-specific. An accuracy of 89% has been claimed for colonoscopic examination in distinguishing Crohn's disease from ulcerative colitis, with most difficulty occurring in cases of severe inflammatory activity, as one might expect [487]. By contrast it must be remembered that biopsies may be abnormal when colonoscopy appears normal. Published interobserver variation studies in the diagnostic utility of multiple colonoscopic biopsies in CIBD are rare. A recent study shows poor agreement but does suggest that some of the features used by experts may be taught to non-experts [488].

Sequential biopsy is an aid to diagnosis, differentiating the varied natural histories of the main forms of CIBD. In infective procto-colitis, most cases return to normal within 2–3 weeks and are virtually always normal within 3 months [478,481,482]. In ulcerative colitis, besides the waxing and waning of the inflammatory infiltrate, permanent crypt architectural damage develops usually over many months, but may also slowly return to normal in the face of quiescent disease. In Crohn's disease, a pattern of exacerbation and remission is not microscopically evident and the crypt alignment tends to remain intact, except where there have been ulcers, hence the usefulness of focal architectural distortion in making a diagnosis of Crohn's disease (see above). Therefore, in the clinical context of any individual patient, in whom there is difficulty in interpreting the rectal biopsy, a colonoscopic series and subsequent follow-up biopsies are invaluable, and usually result in a definitive diagnosis. An adequate colonoscopic series of biopsies (from the terminal ileum, caecum, ascending colon, transverse colon, descending colon, sigmoid colon and rectum, in separate containers) will usually supply important diagnostic information on the distribution and focality of active inflammation.

Drug-induced procto-colitis

Drugs are important causes of colorectal inflammation. Apart from the antibiotic-associated colitides described below, a wide range of other drugs may directly cause inflammation in pre-existing normal large bowel mucosa or activate CIBD that has previously been in remission. When drugs produce colitides in their own right, the pattern of inflammation is variable. Occasionally the microscopic appearances are sufficiently characteristic to allow the histopathologist to suggest the probable aetiology but more often they are less specific, encompassing those of acute self-limiting colitis, microscopic colitis (see below), focal active colitis (see below) or idiopathic CIBD.

Non-steroidal anti-inflammatory drugs and procto-colitis

It is now well established that the consumption of non-steroidal anti-inflammatory drugs (NSAIDs) may result in the reactivation of CIBD, especially ulcerative colitis [489]. However, in some patients, this group of drugs has also been implicated in initiating ulcerative colitis, in that there is sometimes a clear association between therapy and the onset of disease. In both of these scenarios the histological appearances of colorectal biopsies are usually indistinguishable from those in ulcerative colitis patients where there is no drug history, although occasionally some of the features described below, more particularly linked with NSAIDs, may also be found.

The most useful histological feature in distinguishing NSAID-related colitis from other forms of inflammation is an increase in apoptotic bodies in the crypt epithelium where, in normal circumstances, they are hardly ever seen [490]. Sometimes they may also be prominent in the lymphocytes and mononuclear cells of the superficial lamina propria. This increased apoptotic activity may result in the accumulation of a lipofuscin pigment, producing a modest melanosis coli [491]. There is often a generalised increase in chronic inflammatory cells in the lamina propria and there may also be a striking eosinophil leukocyte infiltrate, increased intra-epithelial T lymphocytes or thickening of the subepithelial collagen plate, resulting in a picture resembling eosinophilic colitis, lymphocytic colitis and collagenous colitis, respectively (see below). Accordingly, in all cases of colitis that do not easily fit a typical histological pattern, the pathologist should consider the possibility of an NSAID-induced colitis, especially in cases of microscopic colitis with unusual histological features, including a triumvirate of mucosal eosinophilia, epithelial cell apoptosis and surface intra-epithelial lymphocytosis [492].

NSAIDs may also cause isolated ulcers in the right side of the colon, which may mimic Crohn's disease or give rise to bowel strictures or diaphragms [493,494]. The latter are fully recognised in the colon, especially in the right colon, but are much less common than their small intestinal equivalents (see 'Diaphragm disease', Chapter 20). Colonic diaphragms provide a close radiological mimic to the 'apple core' strictures of cancer on barium studies.

When used as suppositories, NSAIDs may give rise to a localised proctitis, ulceration of the rectum resembling the solitary rectal ulcer syndrome and rectal strictures [495,496]. In a review of causes of 'colitis', one study found that 3% of the overall 'colitis' group were drug-related. The ultimate drug-related diagnoses included microscopic colitis (50%), eosinophil-rich infiltrate of the left colon (34%), ischaemic-type colitis (11%), pseudo-membranous colitis (3%) and apoptotic colopathy (2%). The drugs most frequently associated with these colitides were the NSAIDs [497]. In another study by the same group, a left-sided eosinophilic colitis was usually associated with medications and the drugs implicated were NSAIDs (70%), anti-platelet agents (19%) and oestro-progestogenic agents (11%) [498].

Colitis related to heavy metal therapy

The colitides associated with heavy metal therapy are uncommon. It is, however, important to be aware of them because they may have severe consequences. Gold, mercury, silver and arsenic therapy may all cause colitis [499,500]. Gold is the most common of these in clinical practice because it is used for the treatment of intractable rheumatoid arthritis and, although gold-induced colitis is uncommon, it was sufficiently severe to result in death in 42% of cases in one series. Macroscopically (or endoscopically) the picture is of multiple petechial haemorrhages [501], focal ulceration or an appearance resembling pseudo-membranous colitis [502]. Toxic megacolon may develop. Histologically there is diffuse chronic mucosal inflammation rich in eosinophils [501], usually with relative preservation of crypt architecture, apart from occasional crypt drop-out. The mechanism of gold-induced colitis is not clear but it may be either a direct toxic effect or a hypersensitivity reaction [501].

Colitis related to chemotherapeutic agents

Chemotherapy is designed to have an effect on cells in mitosis in order to be useful in tumour treatment. The agents used also affect other mitotically active cells including colonocytes. The pattern of colitis is characteristic and readily recognisable, the clue being the random admixture of crypts in various sages of regeneration, some being relatively normal, although often mucin depleted, and then a whole range of crypts in varying stages of restitution, some being almost endothelial thin, others more cuboidal, low columnar, etc., but all totally random without the geographical pattern of the withering crypts that characterise ischaemic colitis. Early on, there is a marked increase in apoptosis [490], the crypt epithelium becomes degenerate with markedly atypical pyknotic and karyorrhectic nuclei, and there may be superficial mucosal necrosis (Figure 35.38). Epithelial restitution and ulcer healing may result in enlarged nuclei with bizarre morphology and hyperplastic, disorganised and cystically dilated crypts [503,504].

It is important to recognise this variant of 'colopathy' (inflammatory cells being virtually absent), because the cause is often readily identifiable. In our experience it is often the result of a miscalculation of chemotherapy dose.

The most common drug responsible is 5-fluorouracil, which is used as part of the chemotherapy for colorectal cancer. Rarely similar changes can follow herbal enemas, which may contain agents such as vinca alkaloids (vincristine/vinblastine) if the Madagascan periwinkle (*Catharanthus roseus*) is used in patients with diarrhoeal diseases. This is known to result in constipation and is a known constituent of Chinese herbal medicines, grown worldwide. Mucosal effects may be seen at about 4 days after the start of treatment. Colchicine and taxanes can cause a diagnostic histopathological picture with crypt epi-

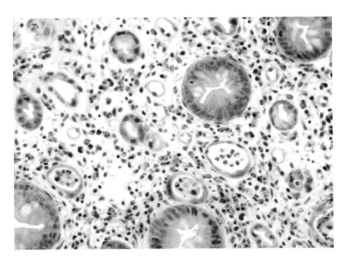

Figure 35.38 Apoptotic colopathy typical of the changes found after chemotherapy. There is no architectural distortion but the crypts are in various stages of repair from tall columnar to thin attenuated epithelium, and all stages in between. In this example eosinophils are prominent but this is not always the case.

thelium showing numerous 'ring mitoses', because these agents halt mitotic activity at the metaphase stage (so-called metaphase arrest) [505].

Drug-induced ischaemic colitis

Ischaemic colitis may be a consequence of therapy with ergotamine for migraine and interleukin-2 and interferon-α therapy [506]. It may also be seen with oral contraceptive therapy with oestrogens and progesterones [507] when it can mimic CIBD clinically [508]. Cocaine body packers involved in drug smuggling may also develop ischaemic colitis if the contents of one of their ingested packages is released into the intestine [509] and cocaine is probably the single most common cause of intestinal ischaemia in young people. However, a variety of other medications that promote vasoconstriction can cause ischaemic entero-colitis if ingested in sufficient quantities. These include sumatriptan or ergot used for migraine, alosetron (irritable bowel syndrome) and even anti-congestives, if used in large enough amounts [510].

Kayexalate colitis

Kayexalate sorbitol (sodium polystyrene sulphonate), which is given orally or as an enema for the treatment of hyperkalaemia, primarily in post-operative, dialysis and/or transplantation patients, has been reported to induce ischaemia and intestinal necrosis in uraemic patients [511] (Figure 35.39). The mechanism of the mucosal damage is unclear although local reduction of blood flow has been suggested as playing a role. Mucosal necrosis is observed in the stomach, small intestine or colon. Experimental evidence suggests that the sorbitol component of the drug,

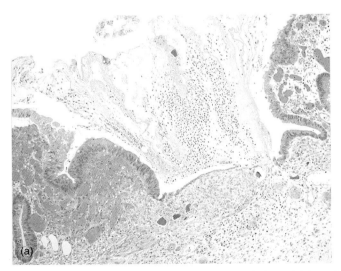
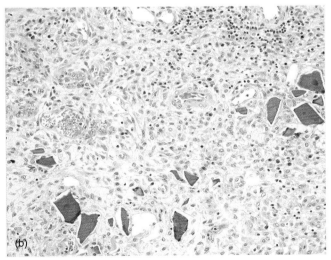

Figure 35.39 Kayexalate-associated ischaemic pathology: (a) large bowel with an ulcer that has a pseudo-membrane and is being re-epithelialised. Kayexalate crystals have been incorporated into the ulcer base. (b) Detail of Kayexalate crystals.

rather than Kayexalate itself, is involved in the pathogenesis of the necrosis. However, there is a suggestion that a related compound (Kalimate), which has morphologically identical Kayexalate crystals and does not contain sorbitol, has been demonstrated to cause similar ischaemic colitis [512]. The disease has been reported at all ages from infants to elderly people [513,514]. It is associated with a considerable mortality, especially given the associated underlying diseases [513].

The lesions induced by Kayexalate can be recognised due to the presence of the characteristic Kayexalate crystals in the bed of the ulcers. The crystals, on H&E staining, are polygonal, opaque and slightly basophilic to amphophilic. They are not birefringent. Other resins besides Kayexalate, e.g. cholestyramine (Questran), which is administered orally, has a similar crystalline morphology but is not associated with ischaemic colitis. Crystals within the lamina propria or in a pseudo-membrane are therefore almost guaranteed to be Kayexalate. Compared with Kayexalate, Questran crystals tend to be more opaque and more pinkish. With the use of acid-fast stains, Kayexalate crystals are more maroon whereas Questran crystals are more pink.

Other drugs that occasionally cause colitis

Methyldopa and penicillamine may cause occasional cases of diffuse 'colitis'. Isotretinoin and aciclovir can produce an allergic colitis [515,516]. Isotretinoin may also activate idiopathic CIBD [515].

Colitis related to immunomodulatory drugs

Mycophenolate mofetil, an immunosuppressive agent, is used after bone marrow and solid organ transplantation, and has been known to cause variety of gastrointestinal side effects, of which diarrhoea is most common. Colonic biopsies show a variety of changes and the histological features have been reported to mimic 'self-limited colitis', graft-versus-host disease and CIBD: they thus pose diagnostic and management difficulties [517,518]. In one study of 40 patients with solid organ transplantation on mycophenolate mofetil, the histological changes were categorised as normal/near normal (31%), CIBD like (28%), graft-versus-host disease like (19%), ischaemia like (3%) and self-limited colitis like (16%) [518]. Similar changes have also been described in children [519]. Withdrawal of the drug or reduction in the dosage resulted in resolution of the symptoms.

Colitis due to the anti-CTLA4 antibody, ipilimumab, which has been used for the treatment of melanoma, has been recently reported [520,521]. The histological features either are non-specific or resemble an infectious-type colitis pattern. It is the most frequent serious toxicity of the drug and, if untreated, may lead to intestinal perforation. The colitis seems to respond to steroids and is believed to be immune-mediated. Some even refer it to as autoimmune enteropathy like. Rare cases with inflammatory enteric neuropathy leading to constipation have also been reported [522].

Fibrosing colonopathy in cystic fibrosis

Fibrosing colonopathy is an uncommon condition that affects children and young adults with cystic fibrosis who take high-dose, enteric-coated, pancreatic enzyme supplements [523]. Patients present with watery diarrhoea, abdominal distension and anorexia [523]. Since the advent of low-dose pancreatic enzyme supplements, cases are much less common. The condition may affect the whole colon or part of it, usually the more proximal part. Macroscopically there is stricturing with superimposed ulceration and the affected bowel may be cobblestoned in appearance. The main histological abnormality is marked submucosal fibrosis with dense mature collagen bands, sometimes with associated haemorrhage. There may also be thickening of the muscularis propria, whereas the overlying mucosal changes are of non-specific chronic and acute inflammation.

Pseudo-membranous colitis and antibiotic-associated diarrhoea and colitis

Terminology

Clostridium difficile toxins are the main cause of pseudo-membranous colitis but there is a spectrum of clinical and pathological findings and patterns of inflammatory pathology of the colorectum. Pseudo-membranous colitis provides a pathognomonic, colonoscopic, macroscopic and histological picture. Antibiotic-associated colitis refers to patients with diarrhoea after a recent course of antibiotics with histological evidence of 'colitis' that is not pseudo-membranous. Antibiotic-associated diarrhoea defines patients with diarrhoea related to a recent course of antibiotics but with no microscopic evidence of mucosal disease [524,525]. Within these definitions, *C. difficile* and its toxin are seen in 6% of patients with antibiotic-associated diarrhoea, 38% with antibiotic-associated colitis and 97% with pseudo-membranous colitis [526,527].

Pseudo-membranous colitis

Pseudo-membranous colitis is regarded as an iatrogenic disease associated with antibiotics and caused by the bacterium *C. difficile* and its associated toxins [528–531]. However, it was described before antibiotics were discovered [532], and in the pre-antibiotic period seems to have been mostly a complication of intestinal surgery, involving any site in the gastrointestinal tract. Until the discovery of its bacterial aetiology, the pathogenesis of the disease was believed to be ischaemic. In these early reports it is not always possible to separate ischaemic necrosis from the confluent mucosal damage seen in severe cases of pseudo-membranous colitis [533]. Unlike the pre-antibiotic era cases, antibiotic-associated pseudo-membranous colitis is largely limited to the colon and rectum, although occasionally involvement of the terminal ileum is seen (see Chapter 20) and the disease has also been described in ileal conduits [534].

Macroscopic appearances

In the established case of pseudo-membranous colitis, there are discrete raised indurated creamy-yellow plaques usually from about 15 mm in diameter, which are firmly attached to the underlying mucosa and separated from each other by congested but otherwise normal areas of mucosa (Figure 35.40). The firm attachment of the plaques means that a very characteristic endoscopic feature of the disease is that the raw mucosa bleeds when the plaques are removed at the time of colonoscopic/sigmoidoscopic examination. With more extensive involvement, the plaques may coalesce and the necrotic membrane formed may then be indistinguishable from those seen in some cases of ischaemic enterocolitis with superficial infarction. The disease is primarily mucosal and, at laparotomy, surgeons may fail to detect any peritoneal abnormality. However, there can be slight dilatation of the bowel and serosal hyperaemia. Toxic megacolon is a rare occurrence [535] as is perforation [536].

The rectum is frequently but not invariably involved, so that in most patients the plaques can be seen and biopsied at proctoscopy and/or sigmoidoscopy [537]. The factors controlling the distribution and growth of the lesions are not known but, in patients coming to surgery, it is customary to find the major length of the large bowel involved. The examining clinicians must, however, be aware that the rectum and sigmoid colon can be spared [538].

Microscopic appearances

The histological picture corresponding to the discrete plaque is characteristic [539,540]. Each plaque represents a small focus of disrupted crypts (Figure 35.41a). The base of each crypt often survives, whereas the superficial two-thirds is dilated and filled with degenerative absorptive cells and goblet cells, liberated mucus, fibrin and acute inflammatory cells. These coalesce to form the yellow plaque visible on the mucosal surface. Although the cellular components of the crypts are lost, their ghost outlines

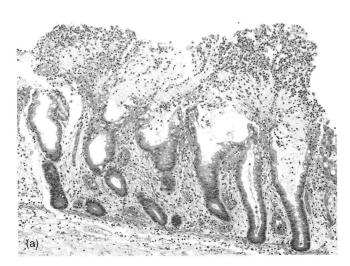

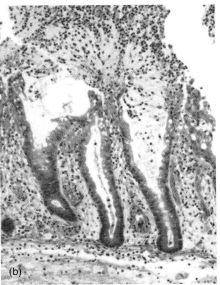

Figure 35.41 The typical histological features of pseudo-membranous colitis: (a) at the low power, the classic features of summit/volcano lesions are seen. (b) At high power, an early lesion with a wisp of inflammatory cells exuding from the mucosal surface between two crypts is evident, along with modest inflammatory changes and oedema in the lamina propria.

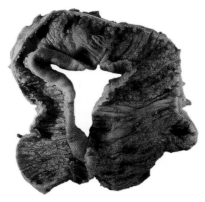

Figure 35.40 A total colectomy specimen showing pseudo-membranous colitis with discrete, raised and indurated mucosal plaques.

remain. Initially the mucosa between such foci can be normal or slightly oedematous or show small clusters of neutrophils involving individual crypts and surface epithelium. As the lesions enlarge the crypt destruction becomes more complete, so that a stage is reached when a layer of inflammatory slough rests on the muscularis mucosae. At this point of full-thickness mucosal necrosis, the features are no longer diagnostic and merge with other diseases capable of producing complete mucosal necrosis, such as arterial ischaemia.

In the early stages of development of the typical lesion, and before recognisable macroscopic lesions, one may find tiny superficial intercryptal erosions (Figure 35.41b). Between two crypts the surface epithelium is destroyed and replaced by a wisp of fibrin and acute inflammatory cells. This *summit lesion* [540] represents the earliest stage at which a confident morphological diagnosis can be made. However, it is important to examine the adjacent mucosa, because superficial erosions of the mucosa are a feature of many different types of mucosal pathology, caused by many different aetiological factors. Moreover they are usually accompanied by changes appropriate to the conditions in question, e.g. in the solitary ulcer (mucosal prolapse) syndrome in the rectum and in acute appendicitis. Failure to appreciate this may account for lesions of pseudo-membranous colitis being described in an unusual clinical setting [541].

The three patterns described, the summit lesion, focal crypt lesion and state of confluent mucosal necrosis, represent three stages in the evolution of the pathology, types I, II and III, respectively [539]. In cases coming to colectomy, although all stages can be seen, obviously more extensive necrosis is more common. Capillary micro-thrombi are a variable accompaniment and these were, at one time, felt to be of prime aetiological importance. It cannot be ruled out that toxins of *C. difficile* may mediate mucosal damage via a vascular mechanism, thereby implicating ischaemia in, at least, part of the pathogenesis. In line with the notion that vascular factors are important in the pathogenesis of pseudo-membranous colitis, it is notable that identical histological changes may be seen in multi-focal mucosal ischaemia from other causes, especially the small vessel disease produced by 'shower' cholesterol emboli from an atheromatous aortic aneurysm, usually seen after aortic aneurysm surgery.

The role of *C. difficile*

Clostridium difficile and/or its toxin can be detected in all but a few isolated reports of pseudo-membranous colitis [542,543]. Indeed it should be emphasised that there is a significant false-negativity rate in the microbiological identification of toxin in the stools and, often, multiple samples may be required. In most cases there is a strong association with antibiotics but this is not invariable [544–546]. In many cases the disease develops after the course of antibiotic therapy has been completed. The relationship between *C. difficile* and the disease is complex, and this complexity is exemplified by the observation that toxigenic organisms are carried by up to 64% of healthy neonates [542] and by a small percentage of adults without any diarrhoea [529,530,547]. It is clear that, after antibiotics, some individuals can harbour the organism and its toxin without developing diarrhoea and that, in others with diarrhoea, the organism, but no toxin, can be found. In general, the higher the faecal toxin titres, the more likely a membrane is to be found [526,529,548]. It is not clear why some patients, after exposure to antibiotics and colonisation by *C. difficile*, will develop pseudo-membranous colitis, yet others will develop only antibiotic-associated diarrhoea. This could be explained by variations in pathogenicity among strains of *C. difficile* [527,547].

The organism produces four toxins, the main ones being toxin A, a potent enterotoxin, and toxin B, a cytotoxin [530,547–549]. Both are believed necessary to produce disease and may act synergistically. Toxin B acts systemically on sites initially damaged by local production of toxin A. Both can be present in the absence of disease [542]. Variation in ratios between the toxins and the inhibitory action of other gut flora may account for the wide spectrum of patterns of *C. difficile*-associated colonic disease [525,550]. Indeed in the hamster model, exposure to antibiotics and *C. difficile* is insufficient to cause disease if the animals are caged in sterile conditions. Clearly expression of the disease requires not only the organism but also additional susceptibility factors within the bowel lumen or in the colonic mucosa [551]. The organism and its toxins may also induce relapses of CIBD, both ulcerative colitis and Crohn's disease [548], and it has a minor role in cases of sporadic diarrhoea in the community [541].

The epidemic NAP1 strain of *C. difficile*

The emergence of the NAP1 isolates of *C. difficile* (officially known as PCR ribotype 027 but also sometimes referred to as BI/NAP1/027) appears to coincide with the increasing incidence of *C. difficile* infections throughout the developed world, particularly in the USA, Canada and Europe, and has resulted in massive outbreaks both in hospitals and in the community [552,553]. Furthermore, it is more likely to be resistant to the usual antibiotics used in its treatment. NAP1 strains produce about 20 times more toxin A and B, and this is thought to be the result of a frameshift mutation within a gene (TcdC) that normally down-regulates the amount of toxin produced. The resulting infection is more often associated with severe disease and with higher rates of colectomy for severe unresponsive disease and of mortality. In addition, infections are more frequently spontaneous, occurring in the community. They are also more frequent in children and more likely to complicate CIBD.

The NAP1 isolates produce a third toxin that disrupts the actin cytoskeleton of its target cells. Controversy persists about which of the toxins are responsible for disease, and it is increasingly apparent that this is dependent on the model used, as well as its age and how the toxins are administered [552,553]. The diagnosis of *C. difficile* including its NAP1 strain is now far quicker using multiplex PCR techniques.

Antibiotic-associated colitis

In antibiotic-associated colitis, by definition no membrane is present and the three patterns of pseudo-membranous colitis are conspicuous by their absence. The disease is specifically a biopsy diagnosis, as such patients do not warrant surgery. However, the mucosa often shows mild changes, akin to those seen in infectious procto-colitis [525,541]. Mild focal inflammation of the mucosa is present with clusters of neutrophils and only a minimal increase in plasma cells. The neutrophils are usually superficial and infiltrate the upper halves of the crypts. Tiny micro-abscesses can be seen in the surface epithelium [525] and the surface epithelial cells can take on a crenated appearance. These might be forerunners to the summit lesions [525].

This picture cannot be considered diagnostic but may form the basis of a helpful clinical suggestion when reporting such a biopsy. It occurs only in a minority of patients with antibiotic-associated colitis, the remainder having minor mucosal inflammatory changes but without any distinctive patterns. A transient right-sided, haemorrhagic, antibiotic-associated colitis has been described with ampicillin and penicillin [525,554], but no pathological details are documented. This may be related to the haemorrhagic colitis in connection with toxin-producing *E. coli* O157:H17.

Antibiotic-associated diarrhoea

In antibiotic-associated diarrhoea, there is no demonstrable mucosal abnormality, despite a history of recent antibiotics. Few such patients are subject to colonoscopic examination, which is the only sure way to exclude evidence of colonic disease. In only 10–20% of such cases can *C. difficile* be demonstrated. This serves to emphasise that, for most cases of diarrhoea associated with antibiotics, the cause is unknown [528].

Biopsy in the differential diagnosis of *C. difficile*-related pathology

The recognition of the typical type I and II lesions of pseudo-membranous colitis is seldom a problem in the differential diagnosis of inflammatory disorders of the colon and rectum. Care is needed in the interpretation of the type I summit lesion, because similar intercryptal erosions can be seen in the solitary ulcer syndrome and even on the surface of polyps when they have been subject to intraluminal trauma. Looking for the ghost outlines of crypts beneath the inflammatory membrane in the type II pattern of pseudo-membranous colitis may help distinguish it from ischaemic mucosal necrosis. In the latter, the adjacent mucosa, if any is present, may often be haemorrhagic or show other ischaemic features. Mucosa adjacent to lesions in pseudo-membranous colitis is only mildly abnormal, showing oedema and focal inflammatory cells. A heavy plasma cell infiltrate and crypt irregularity are generally features against a diagnosis of pseudo-membranous colitis at any stage.

The biopsy in antibiotic-associated colitis cannot be confidently distinguished from mild changes seen in other forms of infective procto-colitis, although there may be a few morphological clues [525]. In such cases, stool culture and a toxin test are indicated. Deeper levels through the paraffin block may reveal summit lesions and the patient should be carefully questioned about recent antibiotics.

Brainerd diarrhoea

An outbreak of chronic diarrhoea of sudden onset occurred in 122 residents of Brainerd, Minnesota between December 1983 and July 1984 [555]. The disease had a characteristic sudden onset and marked urgency, with a secretory diarrhoea, lack of systemic symptoms and no response to antibiotics. It has been associated with consumption of raw milk and, in another outbreak, with water on a ship [556].

Histologically, there is a surface intra-epithelial lymphocytosis (but not in the crypt epithelium) with no thickening of the subepithelial collagen plate or crypt distortion [557]. There is no excess of lamina propria cells. This superficial intra-epithelial lymphocytosis was demonstrated in 20 of 22 cases. Three cases had a focal active colitis and two were completely normal. All cases had normal duodenal mucosal biopsies [557]. Although the disease is self-limiting and is likely to be of viral aetiology [556], its importance to pathologists is that its histological features are not those usually associated with acute self-limiting colitis and are more like those of lymphocytic colitis. However, making a histological diagnosis requires care because one is effectively attributing symptoms to a surface intra-epithelial lymphocytosis and suggesting that the disease is largely untreatable but will resolve in anything from weeks to 18 months.

Focal active colitis

Focal active colitis is a relatively recently recognised histological diagnosis in colorectal biopsies which describes focal crypt infiltration by neutrophils in the absence of any other significant microscopic abnormality [422,423]. It is not an uncommon finding in biopsy practice and, although it can be observed in some biopsies from patients who have Crohn's disease, it is certainly not specific for that condition and may be found in several other colitides, including ischaemic colitis, infective colitis and partially treated or newly presenting ulcerative colitis. The real problem is that focal active colitis really needs to be distinguished from focal chronic active CIBD.

The first study of the disease was a group of 42 patients with no past history of idiopathic CIBD and no other diagnostic biopsy features [422]. It found that 19 patients had had an acute self-limiting colitis, 4 had an antibiotic-associated colitis, 2 had ischaemic colitis, 6 had irritable bowel syndrome and 11 had isolated focal active colitis in the absence of any endoscopic abnormality or any symptoms. No patient developed CIBD on follow-up. It was noted that 20 patients were immunosuppressed and 19 were taking NSAIDs. Another study of 31 cases [423] produced broadly similar findings, with 15 being related to infection and 3 to ischaemia. Nine were incidental findings in patients being screened for colorectal neoplasia but four patients were found to have Crohn's disease. It would appear, therefore, that many cases of focal active colitis are infective in origin and others may be related to NSAIDs or ischaemia. In a more recent study, campylobacter DNA was found in the faeces of about 10% of patients with focal active colitis [558].

Although the demonstration of the lesion of focal active colitis should always lead to consideration of the possibility of Crohn's disease, in the absence of any other findings it should not be used to label a patient with this diagnosis. Focal active colitis in children is much more likely to be a harbinger of CIBD than it is in adults, particularly in teenagers [559]. Second, in a very recent study from the UK, focal active colitis was associated with an ultimate diagnosis of CIBD, predominantly Crohn's disease but also ulcerative colitis in two cases, in about 15% of cases [560]. However, we would emphasise that the features seen in focal active colitis are much more likely to be an indicator of a diagnosis of Crohn's disease in the presence of other, especially chronic, features, such as chronic inflammation, crypt architectural changes and granulomas [559,560].

Radiation procto-colitis

Patients who have received radiation therapy to the pelvis and/or abdomen may be subject to bowel injury with subsequent complications, which may occur immediately or at variable times after treatment, even as long as 20–30 years later. The late changes have an ischaemic aetiology, consequent on the vascular damage, which is one of the hallmarks of radiation injury [561–563]. The radiotherapy is usually for cervical or bladder cancer, and the distal colon and rectum, or the ileo-caecal area, are the common sites of damage, these being fixed sites and, in the case of the rectosigmoid area, in close proximity to the target organ. Between 1 and 12% of patients may develop complications [561,564]. The complications include proctitis, radionecrotic ulceration with stenosis, intestinal obstruction, internal fistulae, perforation, haemorrhage into the lumen and mucosal inflammation [561,564,565].

The precision of modern radiotherapy means that it is now rare to see the early acute changes in patients treated for cancer elsewhere [566]. However, with the recent advent of short- and long-course preoperative radiotherapy for rectal cancer, the diagnostic histopathologist is now exposed to such acute radiation pathology in sections of rectal mucosa. Occasionally this can have a disturbing appearance due to the cytological atypia of the crypt epithelium (Figure 35.42). The changes are diffuse with cytological abnormalities, reduced mitotic activity and the rare but highly characteristic eosinophil crypt abscess [566]. These changes may also be seen in the small percentage of patients presenting with proctitis in the first month after radiotherapy of other cancers [566]. Fortunately they are rarely biopsied. However, short-course radiation therapy for rectal cancer (usually a full course of radiation in five divided doses over 5 consecutive days the week before the operation) results in inevitable changes in the adjacent mucosa of rectal cancer resections (see Figure 35.41c,d).

More common are patients with chronic radiation proctocolitis who present within 3 months to 2 years and the remainder over a much longer period. The macroscopic picture reveals a granular and haemorrhagic mucosa. There may be multiple ulcers covered by yellowish-white slough. Stenosis of the colon is common with serosal fibrosis and adhesions. Perforation is also a common presentation [562].

On microscopic examination, the pathology is evident in connective tissue and blood vessels, the brunt being borne by the submucosa. The connective tissue is first oedematous and myxoid before becoming homogeneous and eosinophilic [566]. Bizarre/stellate fibroblasts are especially characteristic. The blood vessels, especially arteries and arterioles, show varying degrees of intimal fibrosis accompanied by fibrinoid necrosis in some instances and commonly fibrin thrombi [563]. Endothelial cells are prominent and atypical, often alongside intimal foamy macrophages. These latter cells were thought diagnostic of radiation damage at one time [563] but similar cells are one of the hallmarks of the vascular changes in eclampsia in the placental bed [567].

Mucosal changes are often ischaemic in appearance with a degree of hyalinisation of the lamina propria with dilated capillaries that are often thrombosed. Withering crypts may be present and they are often mucin depleted. Telangiectasia is common and believed to occur because of the developing rigidity in the connective tissue [563]. After healing of areas of ulceration permanent damage to the

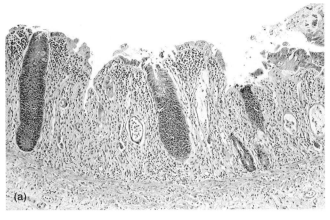

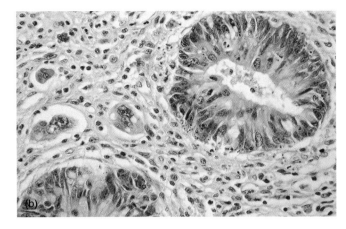

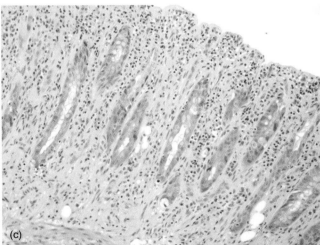

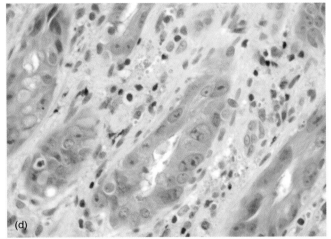

Figure 35.42 Acute radiation proctitis: (a) there is mucosal oedema and acute inflammation, but the most noticeable feature at low power is the 'withering' of crypts with cystic dilatation. Surviving crypts are enlarged and show marked regenerative hyperplasia. (b) High power shows residual crypt fragments in the lamina propria marked by groups of isolated pleomorphic, degenerate epithelial cells. Surviving whole crypts show regenerative changes, but also prominent apoptotic bodies.

(c) Changes seen in short-term radiation therapy given the week preceding proctectomy for rectal carcinoma. Note the lack of architectural distortion but there is mucin depletion and attenuated crypts superficially with resulting stripping of luminal epithelium (d) Detail of crypt bases showing marked nuclear atypia, apparent hyperplasia of Kulchitsky's cells and occasional apoptotic bodies and foci of regeneration. Lamina propria fibrosis is apparent, despite the short time interval between radiation and resection.

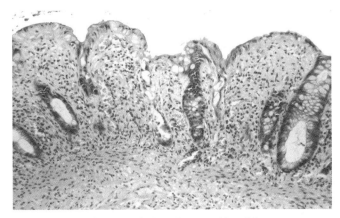

Figure 35.43 Chronic radiation change with mild crypt architectural distortion, lamina propria fibrosis, vascular ectasia and focal crypt 'withering'.

mucosa is manifest by crypt atrophy together with the features above. This can be appreciated in mucosal biopsies (Figure 35.43). The vascular changes also occur adjacent to obviously involved bowel. This is important for the surgeon to appreciate when carrying out a resection and also for the pathologist when examining what may appear a normal biopsy.

The long delay in presentation in many cases of radiation procto-colitis reflects the slow development of the vascular changes, but presentation is accelerated in patients with diabetes mellitus and/or hypertension in whom there will be superimposed atherosclerotic vascular disease. Radiation proctitis has occasionally been treated by local instillation of formalin enemas [568,569]. Biopsies after this treatment are usually haemorrhagic and not well preserved; it is difficult to identify consistent changes.

Diversion procto-colitis

Pathological changes peculiar to defunctioning of the whole or part of the large intestine, by ileostomy or colostomy, to divert the faecal stream, were first described in an earlier edition of this very textbook. However, the term 'diversion colitis' was coined by Glotzer and colleagues [570]. The inflammation may mimic that of CIBD [571] but crypt distortion is usually absent [572]. The pathological changes may resolve after restoration of the faecal stream [572,573]. Amelioration of the pathological changes has also been shown after butyrate enemas, suggesting that this condition is a result of a diminution or absence of butyrate, a fatty acid critical for colonic epithelial cell proliferation, due to a lack of intraluminal bacteria [573]. However, the only controlled trial of butyrate therapy for diversion procto-colitis did not show a consistent response [574] and increased numbers of nitrate-producing bacteria have been suggested as a cause for the inflammation in diversion procto-colitis [575].

Before the development of colectomy and ileostomy, usually for CIBD, it was customary to perform caecostomy alone and such patients were sometimes left with a defunctioned bowel for many years. Such patients have allowed the comprehensive study of diversion procto-colitis. With increasing time, the bowel contracts down until its lumen is as small as 10 mm in diameter [576]. The mucosa is granular in appearance due to the distinctive lymphoid follicular hyperplasia and aphthous ulceration that occurs in diversion procto-colitis (Figure 35.44) [577–579]. There is also diffuse chronic inflammation in the lamina propria. Some authors have referred to this as 'diversion reaction' [580], restricting the use of the term 'diversion procto-colitis' for those cases with ulceration and acute inflammation together with lymphoid follicular hyperplasia and diffuse mucosal chronic inflammation. The important feature of diversion procto-colitis is the relative lack of crypt architectural distortion. This allows its distinction, often, from CIBD [572]. In diversion disease, the submucosa and serosa contain an excess of adipose tissue and the muscularis propria is thickened, accounting for the luminal restriction of chronic diversion.

The pre-diversion condition of the large intestine is important in determining the outcome after diversion. Diversion of the faecal stream from pre-existing normal large bowel mucosa, as in diverticular disease, carcinoma or Hirschsprung's disease, results in the endoscopic and histological changes of diversion procto-colitis as described above. However, if the bowel has been previously involved by Crohn's disease, the inflammation is characteristically ameliorated by diversion of the faecal stream [296,444,581,582]. Conversely, in ulcerative colitis patients, in whom the rectum is diverted as part of the three-stage ileal pouch procedure, the superimposition of

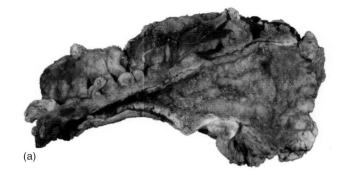

(a)

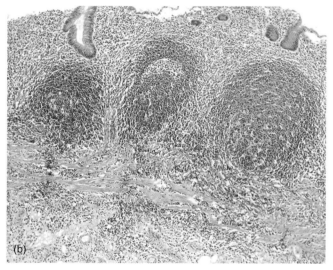

(b)

Figure 35.44 Diverted rectum from a patient with ulcerative colitis: (a) macroscopically the mucosa shows focal ulceration and a diffuse granular or nodular appearance due to lymphoid follicular hyperplasia, confirmed histologically as seen in (b). (b) The crypt architecture is distorted due to the coexisting ulcerative colitis; it is not a feature of 'pure' diversion colitis.

diversion changes upon those of ulcerative proctitis tends to exacerbate the inflammatory changes [572,581]. Furthermore, in such a diverted rectum, the combination of ulcerative colitis and diversion-induced pathology, possibly with additional ischaemic changes induced by surgery, incites additional pathological changes, including transmural inflammation (often in the form of lymphoid aggregates), fissuring ulceration and micro-granulomas (including within draining lymph nodes), such that the pathology closely mimics Crohn's disease [312]. It could be the ischaemic component of the pathology that also produces an appearance similar to that of pseudo-membranous procto-colitis [312].

It should be emphasised that the effects of surgery, particularly diversion, may produce perplexing histological appearances. We strongly advocate that a diagnosis of ulcerative colitis or indeterminate colitis must never be changed to Crohn's disease based solely on the pathological assessment of the diverted rectum [312,572]. All pathological material, particularly that of the original colectomy, should be reviewed, along with all available clinical, radiological and endoscopic information [312,572].

Although diversion in the rectum of ulcerative colitis shows these dramatic pathological appearances, the histological appearances of diverted Crohn's disease typically show 'burnt-out disease' with fibrosis and a lack of active inflammation. Granulomas become effete and hyalinised. Probably a reflection of the age and relative inactivity of the granulomatous pathology is the distinctive presence of Schaumann's bodies (which are an unusual feature in Crohn's colitis) within these granulomas [572]. Microcarcinoids have also been reported in the diverted rectum in ulcerative colitis [583].

In summary, diversion procto-colitis can provide perplexing histological appearances that closely mimic CIBD of both types, in specific situations. It is clearly important not to make an unwarranted diagnosis of Crohn's disease or ulcerative colitis in previously diverted large intestine. Indeed, once diversion disease is established, there are no good criteria for distinguishing it from Crohn's disease, so clinicians should not take biopsies with this question, pathologists should not attempt to answer it and, most importantly, pathologists should not indicate that 'the changes are consistent with Crohn's disease'. It is clear that any inflammation associated with diversion subsides when bowel continuity is restored [571,572] or in some cases with the instillation of butyrate enemas [573,574].

Necrotising colitis

A gangrenous process involving patches of colon has been described and attributed to infection with *Clostridium perfringens* [584–586]. However, it is difficult to know whether this is simply acute ischaemia with tissue necrosis followed by secondary invasion by *C. perfringens* from the faeces. The literature contains a confusing host of conditions encompassing terms such as necrotising enterocolitis [584], haemorrhagic enterocolitis [587] and phlegmonous enterocolitis, in which it is difficult to separate primary, usually clostridial, infections from secondary infection subsequent to ischaemia. The picture is seen in both small and large bowel. The term 'acute intestinal failure' has also been coined for this group.

Neonatal necrotising enterocolitis and the necrotising enteritis of pig-bel, which may also have specific clostridial associations, are described elsewhere (see Chapter 20). There remain a number of cases in which the term 'necrotising colitis' has to be used. There is a variable length of large bowel, which is deeply discoloured black or purple. The mucosa ranges from being frankly gangrenous and covered by a yellow–green membrane (hence the original inclusion of pseudo-membranous colitis) to, in mild cases, being simply congested and oedematous. On microscopy, the mucosa has undergone varying degrees of necrosis and haemorrhage. There is submucosal oedema and, depending on severity, the muscle coat shows signs of myocytolysis. Clostridial organisms in the tissue should be sought but, as mentioned, it is difficult to eliminate a primary ischaemic insult, especially as most patients will be elderly, post-operative or have a chronic debilitating medical disease.

Neutropaenic colitis

This is a segmental necrotising and ulcerating inflammatory condition primarily affecting the terminal ileum, caecum and ascending colon, although it can be more extensive in some cases [588–594]. Clinically it resembles acute appendicitis with abdominal pain and fever. It occurs in patients with neutropaenia [593] from a wide variety of causes [591–595]. Most cases are believed to be due to invasion by *Clostridium septicum* and the organisms can be demonstrated invading the mucosa and submucosa [586,594,596]. It is interesting that, although this organism is not a normal inhabitant of the colon, it is found in the normal appendix. Mucosal damage may be the result of leukaemic infiltration, cytotoxic therapy or haemorrhage in the patient group with thrombocytopaenia. Occasionally other clostridia may be implicated [585]. In patients at risk, it is important to be alert for the condition and institute specific therapy. Until more recently the condition usually went undiagnosed and was uniformly fatal [597].

The affected bowel shows ulceration and necrosis, haemorrhage and pronounced oedema, these features overlapping with ischaemia and the type III pattern of pseudomembranous colitis. In some cases ulceration is minimal with submucosal oedema and patchy necrosis of the muscularis being predominant [590]. In preserved areas of mucosa, crypt degeneration reminiscent of infection may be seen but with no acute inflammatory cell accompaniment.

Neonatal necrotising enterocolitis

Neonatal necrotising enterocolitis is a disease of premature infants, occurring during neonatal intensive care in over 90% of cases [598–600]. It happens most often in the first 2 weeks of life and after enteric feeding has commenced. The most consistent risk factor identified is prematurity. Other risk factors may roughly be grouped into three categories: transient ischaemia of the intestine, local/ systemic inflammation predisposing the bowel to injury and therapeutic interventions [599]. Genetic polymorphisms in pro-inflammatory cytokines such as the IL-4 receptor α chain and IL-18, involved in prematurity, have been implicated in necrotising enterocolitis [599].

The hallmark of the diagnosis is the radiological demonstration of pneumatosis intestinalis [595]. The terminal ileum and ascending colon are the most common sites but the entire gastrointestinal tract may be involved [595,596, 600]. The bowel is congested and thickened due to oedema and the presence of gas-filled cysts. With time it becomes necrotic, covered by fibrinous exudate. There is often perforation. The mucosa may be intact and have a cobblestone appearance due to the gas cysts, but usually it is necrotic and covered by a membrane.

Microscopy shows submucosal gas-filled cysts, vascular congestion, oedema, and a variable inflammatory infiltrate in the mucosa and submucosa. The inflammatory component may appear relatively minor in the face of such extensive mucosal necrosis [595]. Small vessel thrombosis can be seen and giant cells may line the gas-filled cysts [595]. Gas-filled cysts are not always apparent [598] and, in their absence, the pathology simply merges into the group of conditions collectively known as the necrotising enterocolopathies. Whether such cases have a different aetiology is not currently known. The role for bacteria has, for many years, been proposed as at least one component of the disease but, as with other varieties of necrotising bowel disease, whether this role is primary or secondary remains a conundrum. Indeed, one bacterium may initiate damage only later to be overgrown by opportunistic flora. A wide range of organisms, including viruses, has been implicated in causing neonatal necrotising enterocolitis but clostridia have usually been implicated, in particular *C. butyricum* [601], *C. perfringens* and *C. difficile*. This is because of the similarities of the disease to other clostridial enterotoxaemias in animals and adult humans, namely pig-bel, neutropaenic enterocolitis and pseudo-membranous colitis.

Microscopic colitis

This term refers to a group of patients with a triumvirate of clinico-pathological features, namely long-standing chronic diarrhoea that is often watery, normal or near-normal colonoscopy and microscopic chronic inflammation [602–605]. There may be rectal sparing in up to 30% of cases [492]. The term is used to encompass specific histological conditions, most notably collagenous colitis and lymphocytic colitis, and their variants. The term can also be used for a group of idiosyncratic reactive colopathies, especially drug reactions, in which there may be non-specific histological features or changes more specific to drug reactions such as a prominent eosinophilic infiltrate in the lamina propria, pronounced apoptotic activity and modest melanosis coli.

In the patient group originally described as having 'microscopic colitis', colonoscopic biopsies show a modest increase in plasma cells and lymphocytes throughout the colon with or without some neutrophils [604]. Cryptitis or crypt abscesses are few and when prominent a component of infection should be considered in the differential diagnosis. Usually there is no crypt distortion; however, mild crypt distortion and/or Paneth cell metaplasia can be seen [605]. The terminal ileum may also be involved in a minority of cases of either collagenous colitis or lymphocytic colitis [606].

In most cases, there are none of the typical features of ulcerative colitis, Crohn's disease or infection. There is no or little crypt distortion. However, occasionally, morphological or clinical overlaps do occur, either sequentially (infections followed by microscopic colitis, microscopic colitis followed by CIBD or patients with CIBD developing features of microscopic colitis, the last especially as a result of treatment of the CIBD). Sometimes the overlap is morphological with features of one form of microscopic colitis but also features of CIBD.

Patho-physiological studies [607] have shown a depressed colonic absorption of water and altered sodium, chloride and bicarbonate exchange. There remains considerable dispute as to whether this condition of 'microscopic colitis' is a definite entity or simply part of the spectrum of collagenous colitis and lymphocytic colitis. These conditions should not be confused with so-called minimal change colitis, which is a pattern of mild CIBD seen within the spectrum of Crohn's disease and ulcerative colitis.

'Non-specific' chronic colitis

We would strongly recommend that the use of this term be avoided, unless very specifically qualified, e.g. all inflammation is non-specific unless it has diagnostic features usually when causative organisms (such as those causing amoebiasis or spirochaetosis) or specific viral cytopathic effect is demonstrable. Alternatively, descriptive terms, such as pseudo-membranous, lymphocytic or collagenous colitis, are used when a specific feature dominates the morphological picture but this is still a description, the cause of which still needs to be determined. Furthermore, the term 'colitis' infers that there is an unequivocal increase in inflammatory cells over that normally expected in the large bowel. This is hugely subjective and, as there is so little documentation of normal, relies on experience. This is actually site and age dependent. Children have very little inflammation throughout the large bowel whereas, in later life, there is more 'inflammation' around the ileo-caecal valve where deep 'inflammation' including plasma cells is normal. In the same patient in the distal large bowel, or in children, both of these are abnormal and the same may also be geography dependent akin to changes seen in the small bowel in developing countries. The variation with time throughout the large bowel and with age is obviously hugely subjective or may not be appreciated at all.

We also believe that the use of the term 'non-specific colitis' may be a hedge for ignorance, if used unqualified, or worse for economy of effort. Whenever a diagnosis of 'non-specific colitis' or 'mild non-specific chronic inflammation' is rendered, if there is no endoscopic abnormality, one has effectively just made a diagnosis of microscopic colitis (inflammation without an endoscopic abnormality). Ultimately the term 'non-specific colitis' could, and we believe should, be completely eradicated from our lexicon without any ill effect. In contradistinction, its abandonment could save many patients from being unnecessarily labelled with microscopic colitis or CIBD, when they actually have no good evidence for these diseases. The message we would wish to convey is that, if a biopsy is within normal physiological limits, then it should be called 'normal' or 'without significant abnormality'. If there is unequivocal inflammation, then that should be described and the further features assessed, along with clinical and endoscopic correlation, to determine whether a designation of microscopic colitis, CIBD or any other form of inflammatory pathology of the large intestine is appropriate.

Lymphocytic colitis

The characteristic presentation of lymphocytic colitis is with chronic watery diarrhoea that may be continuous or intermittent. It may have a sudden explosive onset and may persist for many years. The watery diarrhoea is thought to result from decreased water absorption in some patients [608,609] whereas in others it may be related to bile acid malabsorption [610,611]. Crampy abdominal pain and weight loss can occasionally occur but they are not typical. Some patients also show features of malabsorption and the condition may be associated with a lymphocytic enteritis that may or may not respond to gluten withdrawal [610–617] or with tropical sprue [618,619]. Conversely, about 40% of coeliac disease patients have increased intra-epithelial lymphocytes (IELS) in the large bowel mucosa, although this is generally much less marked than in lymphocytic colitis. Lymphocytic colitis is also associated with collagenous colitis (see below) and with lymphocytic gastritis [613].

It affects individuals of a wide age range, including children, and occurs equally in men and women [608,615, 620,621]. A sero-negative non-destructive arthritis is seen in some, raising the possibility that the condition may be related to a systemic immunological disturbance or to therapeutic agents such as NSAIDs, proton pump inhibitors, H_2-receptor antagonists, anti-platelet medications, Cyclo 3 Fort (in France) and food allergies.

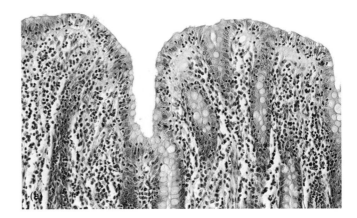
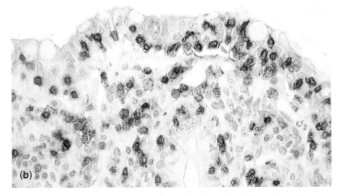

Figure 35.45 Lymphocytic colitis: (a) there is diffuse chronic mucosal inflammation and a normal crypt architecture. (b) Intra-epithelial lymphocytes are markedly increased and are shown to be T cells by CD3 immunostaining.

The diagnostic hallmark of lymphocytic colitis is a diffuse increase in IELs (T cells) in excess of 20 per 100 epithelial cells [609] (Figure 35.45). There is also diffuse lamina propria chronic inflammation, with increased lymphocytes and plasma cells and sometimes prominent eosinophils and/or mast cells. Neutrophils may be seen in the lamina propria, usually in small numbers, but they rarely invade the crypt epithelium. The surface epithelium is usually degenerate and sometimes becomes detached from the underlying lamina propria, a feature more usually and more prominently seen in collagenous colitis. Unlike collagenous colitis, there is no thickening of the subepithelial collagen plate and the disease is usually relatively diffusely distributed throughout the colonic mucosa. Paneth cell metaplasia may be seen and does not imply a diagnosis of CIBD. It is important to realise that the intra-epithelial lymphocytosis of lymphocytic colitis is diffuse and not focal. Focal intra-epithelial lymphocytosis may be seen in Crohn's disease, some mucosal polyps and diverticular disease [492].

One large series found that, in most patients, lymphocytic colitis is an isolated condition with a clinical course that is benign and self-limiting. After a mean period of 38 months, the watery diarrhoea had resolved in 25 of 27 cases, the histological changes had returned to normal in all but 3 of these and none progressed to collagenous colitis [621]. Whether any form of medical therapy influences the outcome is uncertain. The condition has been associated with a variety of medications, so a careful medication history including over-the-counter medications is initially indicated, because stopping the causative agent may be all that is required where that is possible. Anti-diarrhoeals, cholestyramine and budesonide are the most common therapies, the last often being regarded as the treatment of choice.

Brainerd diarrhoea has already been described (see above) in which an intra-epithelial lymphocytosis occurs, usually only in the superficial epithelium, and probably represents a viral infection. We also recognise that certain bacterial infections, especially salmonellosis, may be associated with an intra-epithelial lymphocytosis. Lymphocytic colitis has been associated with additional pathological features that may cause pathological consternation [622]. It is now well recognised that there is both a giant cell variant [623,624] and a granulomatous variant [625,626] of lymphocytic colitis. The latter, in particular, can provide histological mimicry of Crohn's disease and yet has been especially ascribed to the effects of drugs, notably allopurinol [626].

More recently described is a variant associated with a notably reduced amount of inflammation, so-called 'pauci-cellular lymphocytic colitis' [627,628]. In one study this was more common than either lymphocytic or collagenous colitis and was characterised by a dearth of FoxP3/CD25 regulatory T cells, which were present in about two-thirds of both the other subtypes. There was no relationship with coeliac disease or NSAIDs. Criteria used for the diagnosis of pauci-cellular lymphocytic colitis were: a diffuse or a patchy pattern of involvement, with the presence of an increased number of IELs (>7% but <20%) and a chronic inflammatory infiltrate (plasma cells and lymphocytes) in the lamina propria; the absence of a thickened subepithelial collagen layer and flattening of epithelial cells; epithelial loss and detachment or an IEL count >20%, but with a patchy distribution of epithelial lymphocytosis (in more than one biopsy sample but not in all); a chronic inflammatory infiltrate in the lamina propria; and an absence of both a thickened subepithelial collagen layer and epithelial abnormalities [627,628]. There is clearly more to come in our understanding of lymphocytic colitis and its variants.

Collagenous colitis

The diagnosis of collagenous colitis is also an entirely microscopic one and can be made only from histological analysis of colonoscopic biopsies, because other investigations are usually unhelpful. In most patients the presentation is similar to that of lymphocytic colitis but the disease may run a notably different course, e.g. rarely the disease is so severe and unresponsive to therapy that colectomy may be considered. Patients whom we have seen with major clinical problems from the disease are those who have multi-organ involvement including the stomach or small intestine or both (so-called collagenous gastro-enterocolitis). The combination of collagenous colitis and enteritis is associated with a high morbidity and appreciable mortality [629]. Rarely patients come to colectomy because of perforation. However, in some cases failing to respond to medical treatment, diversion of the faecal stream has been successful.

Clinical features

The patients are predominantly women, with a sex ratio of at least 4:1. Persistent chronic watery, bloodless diarrhoea, often severe enough to present with incontinence, is an invariable symptom. The length of history is variable, from weeks up to 20 years in some cases [492,603]. Laboratory investigations and barium studies are usually unhelpful. Occasionally the white count and blood viscosity are raised. Sigmoidoscopy and colonoscopy are normal [492] or, at most, show minor abnormalities such as alteration of the vascular pattern or slight mucosal friability, although the thickened collagen band can be visualised using confocal endo-microscopy.

There may be an association with rheumatoid arthritis and thyroid disease such that a link with autoimmunity has been suggested [620]. Despite the often long history and the frequency of bowel action, with up to 20 stools per day being recorded [620], patients have few complications, provided that there is adequate fluid balance during the exacerbations of diarrhoea. One well-recognised endoscopic abnormality in collagenous colitis, belying the endoscopic normality that is said to characterise the condition, is bleeding linear 'ulcers' occurring primarily in the right colon, often under direct visualisation during endoscopy ('fractured colon', 'mucosal cracking' and 'cat scratch' are terms that have been used to describe them); surgery, in the form of a right hemicolectomy, may have to be undertaken [630,631]. Further, there is one special and relatively rare form of the disease, called pseudo-membranous collagenous colitis, that, unsurprisingly given its name, is also often associated with endoscopic abnormalities [632]. This condition shows the combination of the pathological features of pseudo-membranous colitis (often with classic summit lesions) and the thickened collagen band of collagenous colitis. It appears to represent a more severe form of collagenous colitis, with the pseudo-membranous changes perhaps a reflection of mucosal ischaemia, in that only very rarely do the clinical features of *C. difficile*-related pathology manifest and only rarely are *C. difficile* toxins detectable [632].

Pathology

Most patients with collagenous colitis have rectal involvement but this is not invariable [492,620] because up to 30% have rectal sparing, with histologically normal rectal biopsies. It is therefore unwise to rely on rectal biopsies to make the diagnosis, although additional biopsies from the left colon usually suffice. However, occasionally the collagen band is found only in the right colon and would therefore require full colonoscopy for its diagnosis. Colonoscopic biopsies are necessary for complete investigation, because the transverse colon and proximal colon are most likely to show the changes of the disease, and are also the areas most likely to be maximally involved. The diagnosis depends on demonstrating a thickened collagen band immediately beneath the surface epithelium [633–635] (Figure 35.46). This is often accompanied by stripping of the surface epithelium, so that, whenever surface epithelium has been stripped in mucosal biopsies, it is worth analysing the biopsy at high power to ensure there is no underlying

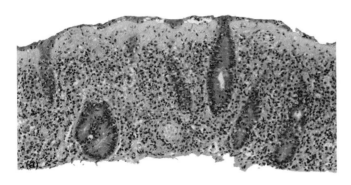

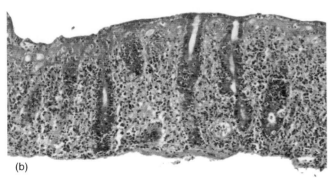

Figure 35.46 Collagenous colitis: (a) there is diffuse chronic inflammation and eosinophilic thickening of the subepithelial collagen plate, (b) confirmed by van Gieson's staining for collagen. Focal separation of the surface epithelium from the underlying connective tissue is a common feature in this condition.

thickened collagen band. Subtle increases in the thickness of the collagen band are also easy to miss.

The accompanying changes are variable but are usually those of a chronic inflammatory pathology, the mucosa being infiltrated by variable numbers of chronic inflammatory cells and occasionally giant cells [624]. There may be an infiltrate of IELs without crypt damage and, in our experience, as well as that of others, this can predate the appearance of a thickened collagen band. Indeed, in some patients, there seems to be an admixture of both lymphocytic and collagenous colitis, although, under these circumstances, the diagnosis of collagenous colitis seems to trump that of lymphocytic colitis. Nevertheless it has long been recognised that some patients progress from one of the major types of 'microscopic colitis' to the other, usually lymphocytic colitis to collagenous colitis [492,636].

Beneath the surface epithelium in the normal colorectal mucosa is a basal lamina that includes a thin band of collagen. Before making the diagnosis of collagenous colitis, the thickness of the normal collagen band must be appreciated and any increase in thickness assessed only on a well-oriented specimen. The normal subepithelial collagen plate is 3–7 μm thick [637] and varies according to site, increasing slightly from right to left colon [633]. It has been shown to be 3 μm thick when measured in a postmortem population of otherwise healthy people involved in fatal road traffic accidents [612]. In 4% of this series of 457 patients, it was >10 μm but only in those with a thickness of >15 μm were there clinical features such as diarrhoea. In the literature there is a wide range of collagen band thickness associated with collagenous colitis, from a minimum of 10 μm up to 70 μm [636]. As the collagen band thickness has been found to vary both in the time course of the disease [634] and by biopsy site, it is important to take the average of several measurements along any one biopsy and to study several biopsies. Only by these procedures can a confident diagnosis be made. There are documented examples of an abnormal band developing over several years [613], which means that sequential biopsies are also an important part of the diagnostic procedures in prolonged, unexplained, intermittent diarrhoea. It is also important to appreciate that the abnormal band may be present at times when diarrhoea is absent.

The abnormal collagen band does not normally extend downwards alongside the crypts. That it is collagen should always be confirmed by any of the standard collagen stains, because superficial oedema of the lamina propria and amyloidosis may give rise to similar appearances. The band is birefringent under polarised light and stains pale pink using the PAS reagent. The mucosal inflammatory infiltrate that accompanies the abnormal band does not have any characteristic features but, whatever the aetiology of the thickened band, there is a background element of chronic inflammation. In occasional cases this inflammatory cell infiltrate may be particularly florid and associated with a marked neutrophil polymorph infiltrate. This form of severe collagenous colitis is usually associated with surface epithelial degeneration and superficial erosions. It is usually these severe forms of collagenous colitis that are associated with the modest colonoscopic abnormalities that have been described in the disease, especially in the more proximal colon.

The collagenous nature of this subepithelial band when studied with the electron microscope has been confirmed [637]. Collagen typing has been carried out and the band has been shown to be mostly type III with some type I collagen [637]. This is a pattern indicating a derivation from myofibroblasts, and supports the concept that the abnormality originates in the pericryptal myofibroblasts.

Pathogenesis

It was initially postulated that the thickened collagen band interfered with water absorption. However, in one case the diarrhoea was shown to be secretory in nature with a net secretion of fluid and electrolytes into the lumen [607]. It was suggested the anionic secretion could be prostaglandin mediated. This in turn could have been activated by mucosal hypoxia from the collagenous diffusional barrier. The pericryptal fibroblast is considered the source of the increased collagen and is recognised to be responsible for normal subepithelial collagen production: it may be demonstrated by a specific monoclonal antibody [638].

Abnormal amounts of subepithelial collagen have been found in hyperplastic/serrated polyps [492,638–640], and such polyps are believed to result from decreased apoptosis, rather than qualitative changes in maturation. Thus these polyps may be hypermature and such a state might equally apply to the pericryptal fibroblast sheath in collagenous colitis. The other main theory for the pathogenesis of collagenous colitis is an inflammatory one. Bile has also been implicated in the pathogenesis of collagenous colitis and bile is known to be fibrogenic although it tends to promote cell turnover. There are documented cases of an established intramucosal chronic inflammatory cell infiltrate colitis preceding the development of the abnormal collagen band by 1–2 years, suggesting a primary inflammatory pathology as the initial event. This is supported by the inter-relationship between lymphocytic colitis and collagenous colitis, with cases of the former evolving into the latter. Some patients have both 'collagenous sprue' and collagenous colitis, and clearly have a worse prognosis, sometimes needing immunosuppressive therapy with a distinct mortality [629]. Abnormal collagen plates can be found in patients with adenocarcinoma [640], megacolon, polyps and diverticular disease. There are also cases of microscopic colitis, including both collagenous and lymphocytic colitis, that are unequivocally directly related to drug therapy, especially NSAID therapy [641].

At present the aetiology of collagenous colitis is unknown and its specificity has even been questioned [642]. We are developing some understanding of the mechanisms of collagen band thickening but often the clinical course of the condition is unpredictable, certainly more so than in lymphocytic colitis. Some cases are clearly drug-related [492,621,641,643] whereas others seem to follow an episode of infection.

Mastocytic enterocolitis

Mast cells are key regulators of intestinal secretory and motor function, and have been known to increase in number in a wide range of inflammatory disorders involving the colon, including primary mast cell disorders. Although a mild increase in mast cells is one of numerous minor abnormalities that can be found in some patients with irritable bowel syndrome [644], an increase in mast cells has also be seen in the colonic biopsies of a group of patients with apparent intractable diarrhoea who do not have any underlying systemic mast cell disease or cutaneous mastocytosis but present with watery diarrhoea and a normal colonoscopic examination, similar to microscopic colitis [645–647]. Biopsies from colon or duodenum either appear normal or show a minimal increase in lamina propria mixed inflammatory cells. However, an increase in mast cell numbers can be demonstrated by using immunohistochemical markers such as mast cell tryptase or CD117 as, often, histochemical stains such as toluidine blue for mast cells are unreliable. In one of these studies, a level of >20 mast cells per high power field was used to diagnose 'mastocytic enterocolitis' [645]. Despite this study being published in 2006, there has to date been no further evidence base to test the notion of whether or not this is a specific condition. No cause for the diarrhoea is usually found in these patients, although in some symptomatic relief is achieved with anti-histamine medications, either mast cell stabilisers or H_2-receptor antagonists.

So, data supporting the use of routine mast cells stains in patients with diarrhoea are currently lacking. Until we have more comprehensive data to demonstrate whether or not this condition actually does exist, we cannot recommend the routine use of these stains and, currently, the role of mast cells in the genesis of inflammatory disorders of the bowel remains controversial and uncertain.

Phlegmonous colitis

This rare form of inflammatory disease of the intestines is manifest mainly as a cellulitis of the submucosa which can affect any region of the gastrointestinal tract. It is more common in the stomach than at other sites and most commonly seen in patients with cirrhosis and portal hypertension [597,648,649]. The serosal aspect of the colon is congested and the affected length slightly thickened. The mucosa is usually intact with thickened mucosal folds and there is obvious submucosal oedema and sometimes ulceration. As many patients have portal hypertension, changes of portal colopathy, such as venous ectasia, are usually present [649]. There may be extensive thrombophlebitis and obliteration of vessels. Histology reveals an intense diffuse infiltrate of neutrophils in the oedematous submucosa throughout the involved segment. There is variable spillover of the inflammation into the muscle coat and mucosa. The latter is usually intact but may show focal ulceration or haemorrhage. A Gram stain may demonstrate organisms in the submucosa. Cases have shown Gram-negative rods, Gram-positive rods and rarely Gram-positive cocci. The involved segment is of variable length but the whole small and large intestine is occasionally affected. Although a variety of organisms, including pneumococci, group B-haemolytic streptococci and *Escherichia coli*, have been grown from the blood, a focus of infection is often not found and the route by which the organism comes to preferentially involve the submucosa is also unknown. The outcome is generally poor and most cases are diagnosed post mortem.

Transient colitis and acute self-limiting (acute infectious type) colitis

The term 'transient colitis' was coined to delineate a group of patients who have a single attack of relatively mild colitis of short duration, clinically believed to be infective in causation but with negative stool cultures. This is not unexpected because, in about half of patients clearly having an acute infectious colitis, no pathogen is found. The biopsy diagnosis of a single attack of proctitis or procto-colitis, in the absence of positive bacteriology or specific histological features to suggest CIBD, is a frequent problem in pathological practice. The microscopic picture in a biopsy is similar to that of culture-positive infective colitis, but may include some with a picture more in favour of Crohn's disease or ulcerative colitis. It also includes biopsies from patients with unexplained spontaneously resolving diarrhoea in whom the biopsy appearances, although clearly inflamed, cannot be categorised further. Only a prolonged follow-up period can confidently exclude Crohn's disease or ulcerative colitis. Even so, there remains a group of patients who have had single attacks of documented ulcerative colitis, usually only affecting the rectum.

The term 'acute self-limiting colitis' or 'infectious-type colitis' is a term favoured in American studies and describes a patient with signs and symptoms of infectious diarrhoea with a corresponding biopsy picture [80]. Both culture-positive and culture-negative cases are included. It is therefore a broader term than transient colitis. Rectal biopsies taken from healthy volunteers in countries with a high background incidence of infective diarrhoea may show

increased inflammatory cells in the lamina propria and structural abnormalities at electron microscopy. This tropical colopathy has been compared with similar findings in the small intestine in such areas [184].

Obstructive colitis

The term 'obstructive colitis' denotes the occurrence of a segment of colonic inflammation and ulceration proximal to a complete or partial obstruction, due to an obstructing tumour, diverticular disease, Crohn's disease, radiation colitis, chronic ischaemic colitis, volvulus or food impaction [650–652]. The affected segment may measure up to 250 mm in length and typically is separated from the site of obstruction by a length of normal, or only slightly dilated, colon of ≥350 mm [653]. Indeed, this normal segment may even involve virtually the whole length of the colon because the caecum is a relatively common place for the pathology to occur irrespective of how distal the obstruction is (Figure 35.47).

The condition may closely mimic CIBD, with the diffuse nature of the involvement and predominant mucosal pathology perhaps suggesting ulcerative colitis, whereas the segmental nature of the disease, with a length of normal mucosa beyond it is reminiscent of Crohn's disease [652]. A similar change may be seen in colonic pseudo-obstruction due to Hirschsprung's disease or in Ogilvie's syndrome (Figure 35.47), a complication of pregnancy, orthopaedic and other surgery, and major states of debilitation, in which the colon becomes grossly dilated, especially the caecum and/or ascending colon, often leading to perforation. Obstructive colitis is more common in elderly people, particularly those with a history of hypertension, diabetes or

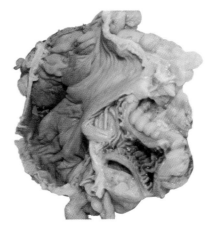

Figure 35.47 Obstructive colitis in a right hemicolectomy specimen: there is an area of inflammation, ulceration and perforation in the lateral wall of the caecum. The cause in this case was acute colonic pseudo-obstruction (Ogilvie's syndrome) in a post-puerperal woman.

other chronic illness, who may also have a background of generalised atherosclerosis and cardiac insufficiency. Rarely obstructive pathology, with similar macroscopic and microscopic pathology, is seen in the small intestine [654] (see Chapter 20).

The pathology is likely largely caused by ischaemia, especially of the mucosa, and mechanical causes may be partly at play, with stretching of the mucosa as a result of dilatation leading to relative mucosal ischaemia with haemorrhage and oedema. Nevertheless, in its early phases especially, the disease may show a primary inflammatory pathology of the mucosa and many have been deluded into thinking that a combination of a distal stricture with a proximal 'skip lesion' and inflammatory pathology in the mucosa may represent Crohn's disease. As the lesion progresses there is ischaemic-type ulceration, sometimes with fissures and fibrosis, which may progress to transmural necrosis and perforation. In the large bowel one can also see 'stercoral' ulcers secondary to faecal impaction (see Chapter 40), primarily in bedridden individuals in whom a degree of pseudo-obstruction may be present. Thus there may a distinct overlap between the 'obstructive colitis' of pseudo-obstruction and stercoral pathology.

Behçet's disease

Large intestinal involvement with Behçet's disease is uncommon and the macroscopic and microscopic appearances mirror those seen in the small intestine (see Chapter 20). Caecal lesions frequently accompany ileal disease, particularly in cases from the Far East [655], and typically there are multiple, discrete, deeply penetrating punched-out ulcers of varying sizes that may perforate (Figure 35.48)

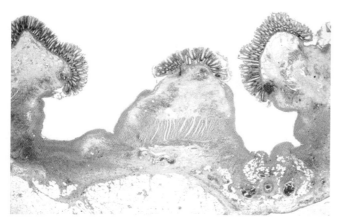

Figure 35.48 Colonic ulceration in Behçet's disease: the ulcers are 'punched out' and can be deep and perforating. There is a characteristic lack of inflammatory or other reaction in the tissue adjacent. This is a section of colon removed from a patient known to have Behçet's disease who presented with an acute abdomen. The colon had perforated.

[656]. The intervening mucosa is often remarkably normal. Rare cases, particularly from western countries, involve the colon and rectum more extensively [657,658], giving a gross appearance that may mimic Crohn's disease, or even ulcerative colitis. Histological features include deep, crater-like ulcers that penetrate the serosa, typically without fissures, lymphoid aggregates or granulomas, which helps in the distinction from Crohn's disease [656]. The presence of a lymphocytic vasculitis, which may be active or healing and located in the vicinity of the ulceration or at some distance from it [658], in the appropriate clinical context of orogenital and ocular inflammation usually allows the diagnosis to be made.

References

1. Denno DM, Stapp JR, Boster DR, et al. Etiology of diarrhea in pediatric outpatient settings. *Pediatr Infect Dis J* 2005;**24**:142.
2. Fowler CJ, Dunlap J, Troyer D, Stenzel P, Epner E, Maziarz RT. Life-threatening adenovirus infections in the setting of the immunocompromised allogeneic stem cell transplant patients. *Adv Hematol* 2010;601548.
3. Nicolas JC, Ingrand D, Fortier B, Bricout F. A one-year virological survey of acute intussusception in childhood. *J Med Virol* 1982;**9**:267.
4. Lamps LW. Appendicitis and infections of the appendix. *Semin Diagn Pathol* 2004;**21**:86.
5. Francis N. Light and electron microscopic appearances of pathological changes in HIV gut infection. *Baillière's Clin Gastroenterol* 1990;**4**:495.
6. Blanshard C, Francis N, Gazzard BG. Investigation of chronic diarrhoea in acquired immunodeficiency syndrome. A prospective study of 155 patients [see comment]. *Gut* 1996;**39**:824.
7. Surawicz CM, Myerson D. Self-limited cytomegalovirus colitis in immunocompetent individuals. *Gastroenterology* 1988;**94**:194.
8. Rabinowitz M, Bassan I, Robinson MJ. Sexually transmitted cytomegalovirus proctitis in a woman. *Am J Gastroenterol* 1988;**83**:885.
9. Rompalo AM. Diagnosis and treatment of sexually acquired proctitis and proctocolitis: an update. *Clin Infect Dis* 1999;**28**(suppl 1):S84.
10. Mate del Tio M, Pena Sanchez de Rivera JM, Larrauri Martinez J, Garces Jimenez MC, Barbado Hernandez FJ. [Association of cytomegalovirus colitis and the 1st episode of ulcerative colitis in an immunocompetent patient]. *Gastroenterol Hepatol* 1996;**19**:206.
11. Rasmussen E, Gronbaek K, Linnemann D. [Cytomegalovirus colitis in immunocompetent young male.] *Ugeskr Laeger* 2009;**171**:1298.
12. Goodman ZD, Boitnott JK, Yardley JH. Perforation of the colon associated with cytomegalovirus infection. *Dig Dis Sci* 1979;**24**:376.
13. Meiselman MS, Cello JP, Margaretten W. Cytomegalovirus colitis. Report of the clinical, endoscopic, and pathologic findings in two patients with the acquired immune deficiency syndrome. *Gastroenterology* 1985;**88**:171.
14. Frager DH, Frager JD, Wolf EL, et al. Cytomegalovirus colitis in acquired immune deficiency syndrome: radiologic spectrum. *Gastrointest Radiol* 1986;**11**:241.
15. Cooper HS, Raffensperger EC, Jonas L, Fitts WT Jr. Cytomegalovirus inclusions in patients with ulcerative colitis and toxic

dilation requiring colonic resection. *Gastroenterology* 1977;**72**: 1253.

16. Hunt NAC, Jewell D, Mortensen N, Warren B. Cytomegalovirus infection complicating ulcerative colitis. *CPD Bull Cell Pathol* 1999;**1**:72.

17. Daley AJ, Craven P, Holland AJ, Jones CA, Badawi N, Isaacs D. Herpes simplex virus colitis in a neonate. *Pediatr Infect Dis J* 2002;**21**:887.

18. Goodell SE, Quinn TC, Mkrtichian E, Schuffler MD, Holmes KK, Corey L. Herpes simplex virus proctitis in homosexual men. Clinical, sigmoidoscopic, and histopathological features. *N Engl J Med* 1983;**308**:868.

19. Kotter DP, Gaetz HP, Lange M, Klein EB, Holt PR. Enteropathy associated with acquired immunodeficiency syndrome. *Ann Intern Med* 1984;**101**:421.

20. Nelson JA, Wiley CA, Reynolds-Kohler C, Reese CE, Margaretten W, Levy JA. Human immunodeficiency virus detected in bowel epithelium from patients with gastrointestinal symptoms. *Lancet* 1988;**i**:259.

21. Kotler DP, Weaver SC, Terzakis JA. Ultrastructural features of epithelial cell degeneration in rectal crypts of patients with AIDS. *Am J Surg Pathol* 1986;**10**:531.

22. Francis N. Infectious complications of HIV disease: a selective review. *Curr Diagn Path* 1994;**1**:142.

23. Donohue-Rolfe A, Keusch GT, Edson C, Thorley-Lawson D, Jacewicz M. Pathogenesis of Shigella diarrhea. IX. Simplified high yield purification of Shigella toxin and characterization of subunit composition and function by the use of subunit-specific monoclonal and polyclonal antibodies. *J Exp Med* 1984;**160**:1767.

24. Speelman P, Kabir I, Islam M. Distribution and spread of colonic lesions in shigellosis: a colonoscopic study. *J Infect Dis* 1984;**150**:899.

25. Tesh VL, O'Brien AD. The pathogenic mechanisms of Shiga toxin and the Shiga-like toxins. *Mol Microbiol* 1991;**5**:1817.

26. McElfatrick RA, Wurtzebach LR. Collar-button ulcers of the colon in a case of shigellosis. *Gastroenterology* 1973;**65**:303.

27. Takeuchi A, Sprinz H, LaBrec EH, Formal SB. Experimental bacillary dysentery. An electron microscopic study of the response of the intestinal mucosa to bacterial invasion. *Am J Pathol* 1965;**47**:1011.

28. Gonzalez-Licea A, Yardley JH. A comparative ultrastructural study of the mucosa in idiopathic ulcerative colitis, shingellosis and other human colonic diseases. *Bull Johns Hopkins Hosp* 1966;**118**:444.

29. Rout WR, Formal SB, Giannella RA, Dammin GJ. Pathophysiology of *Shigella* diarrhea in the rhesus monkey: intestinal transport, morphological, and bacteriological studies. *Gastroenterology* 1975;**68**:270.

30. Christie AB. Salmonellosis. *Br J Hosp Med* 1971;**5**:331.

31. Mandal BK, Mani V. Colonic involvement in salmonellosis. *Lancet* 1976; **i**:887.

32. McGovern VJ, Slavutin LJ. Pathology of salmonella colitis. *Am J Surg Pathol* 1979;**3**:483.

33. Boyd JF. Pathology of the alimentary tract in *Salmonella typhimurium* food poisoning. *Gut* 1985;**26**:935.

34. Appelbaum PC. Colonic involvement in salmonellosis. *Lancet* 1976;**ii**:102.

35. Boyd JF. *Salmonella typhimurium*, colitis and pancreatitis. *Lancet* 1969;**ii**:901.

36. Axon AT, Poole D. Salmonellosis presenting with cholera-like diarrhoea. *Lancet* 1973;**i**:745.

37. Radsel-Medvescek A, Zargi R, Acko M, Zajc-Satler J. Colonic involvement in salmonellosis. *Lancet* 1977;**i**:601.

38. Day DW, Mandal BK, Morson BC. The rectal biopsy appearances in *Salmonella* colitis. *Histopathology* 1978;**2**:117.

39. Dronfield MW, Fletcher J, Langman MJ. Coincident salmonella infections and ulcerative colitis: problems of recognition and management. *BMJ* 1974;**i**:99.

40. Mandal B. Letter: Ulcerative colitis and acute salmonella infection. *BMJ* 1974;**i**:326.

41. Black PH, Kunz LJ, Swartz MN. Salmonellosis – a review of some unusual aspects. *N Engl J Med* 1960;**262**:921 concl.

42. Fung WP, Monteiro EH, Ang HB, Kho KM, Lee SK. Ulcerative postdysenteric colitis. *Am J Gastroenterol* 1972;**57**:341.

43. Stewart GT. Post-dysenteric colitis. *BMJ* 1950;**i**:405.

44. Powell SJ, Wilmot AJ. Ulcerative post-dysenteric colitis. *Gut* 1966;**7**:438.

45. Patterson M, Schoppe LE. The presentation of amoebiasis. *Med Clinics North Am* 1982;**66**:689.

46. Harries J. Amoebiasis: a review. *J R Soc Med* 1982;**75**:190.

47. Lambert ME, Schofield PF, Ironside AG, Mandal BK. Campylobacter colitis. *BMJ* 1979;**i**:857.

48. Mead PS, Slutsker L, Griffin PM, Tauxe RV. Food-related illness and death in the united states reply to dr. hedberg. *Emerg Infect Dis* 1999;**5**:841.

49. Tam CC, Higgins CD, Neal KR, Rodrigues LC, Millership SE, O'Brien SJ. Chicken consumption and use of acid-suppressing medications as risk factors for *Campylobacter* enteritis, England. *Emerg Infect Dis* 2009;**15**:1402.

50. Son I, Englen MD, Berrang ME, Fedorka-Cray PJ, Harrison MA. Prevalence of *Arcobacter* and *Campylobacter* on broiler carcasses during processing. *Int J Food Microbiol* 2007;**113**:16.

51. Gubina M, Zajc-Satler J, Dragas AZ, Zeleznilc Z, Mehle J. Enterotoxin activity of campylobacter species. In: *Campylobacter: Epidemiology, pathogenesis and biochemistry.* Lancaster: MTP Press Ltd, 1982.

52. Blaser MJ, LaForce FM, Wilson NA, Wang WL. Reservoirs for human campylobacteriosis. *J Infect Dis* 1980;**141**:665.

53. Megraud F, Tachoire C, Latrille J, Bondonny JM. Appendicitis due to *Campylobacter jejuni. BMJ (Clin Res Ed)* 1982;**285**:1165.

54. Loss RW Jr, Mangla JC, Pereira M. Campylobacter colitis presentin as inflammatory bowel disease with segmental colonic ulcerations. *Gastroenterology* 1980;**79**:138.

55. Blaser MJ, Parsons RB, Wang WL. Acute colitis caused by *Campylobacter fetus* ss. *jejuni. Gastroenterology* 1980;**78**:448.

56. Malagon I, Garcia S, Heredia N. Adherence, invasion, toxigenic, and chemotactic properties of Mexican campylobacter strains. *J Food Prot* 2010;**73**:2093.

57. Candy DC, McNeish AS. Human *Escherichia coli* diarrhoea. *Arch Dis Child* 1984;**59**:395.

58. Riley LW, Remis RS, Helgerson SD, et al. Hemorrhagic colitis associated with a rare *Escherichia coli* serotype. *N Engl J Med* 1983;**308**:681.

59. Pai CH, Gordon R, Sims HV, Bryan LE. Sporadic cases of hemorrhagic colitis associated with *Escherichia coli* O157:H7. Clinical, epidemiologic, and bacteriologic features. *Ann Intern Med* 1984;**101**:738.

60. Smith HR, Rowe B, Gross RJ, Fry NK, Scotland SM. Haemorrhagic colitis and vero-cytotoxin-producing Escherichia coli in England and Wales. *Lancet* 1987;**i**:1062.

61. Morrison DM, Tyrrell DL, Jewell LD. Colonic biopsy in verotoxin-induced hemorrhagic colitis and thrombotic thrombocytopenic purpura (TTP). *Am J Clin Pathol* 1986;**86**:108.

62. Kelly JK, Pai CH, Jadusingh IH, Macinnis ML, Shaffer EA, Hershfield NB. The histopathology of rectosigmoid biopsies from adults with bloody diarrhea due to verotoxin-producing *Escherichia coli. Am J Clin Pathol* 1987;**88**:78.

63. Richardson SE, Karmali MA, Becker LE, Smith CR. The histopathology of the hemolytic uremic syndrome associated with verocytotoxin-producing Escherichia coli infections. *Human Pathol* 1988;**19**:1102.

64. Van Heyningen WE, Gladstone GP. The neurotoxin of *Shigella shigae*. IV. A semi-micro method for the flocculation assay of the toxin. *Br J Exp Pathol* 1953;**34**:230.

65. Doyle MP, Schoeni JL. Survival and growth characteristics of *Escherichia coli* associated with hemorrhagic colitis. *Appl Environ Microbiol* 1984;**48**:855.

66. Thabane M, Simunovic M, Akhtar-Danesh N, et al. An outbreak of acute bacterial gastroenteritis is associated with an increased incidence of irritable bowel syndrome in children. *Am J Gastroenterol* 2010;**105**:933.

67. Murrell TG, Walker PD. The pigbel story of Papua New Guinea. *Trans R Soc Trop Med Hyg* 1991;**85**:119.

68. Borriello SP, Larson HE, Welch AR, Barclay F, Stringer MF, Bartholomew BA. Enterotoxigenic Clostridium perfringens: a possible cause of antibiotic-associated diarrhoea. *Lancet* 1984; i:305.

69. Borriello SP. Newly described clostridial diseases of the gastrointestinal tract: *Clostridium perfringens* enterotoxin-associated diarrhea and neutropenic enterocolitis due to *Clostridium septicum*. In: Borriello SP (ed.), *Clostridia in Gastrointestinal Disease*. Boca Raton, FL: CRC Press Inc., 1985.

70. Farrant JM, Traill Z, Conlon C, et al. Pigbel-like syndrome in a vegetarian in Oxford [see comment]. *Gut* 1996;**39**:336.

71. Kumar NB, Nostrant TT, Appelman HD. The histopathologic spectrum of acute self-limited colitis (acute infectious-type colitis). *Am J Surg Pathol* 1982;**6**:523.

72. Talbot I, Price A. Infective colitis. In: *Biopsy Pathology of Colorectal Disease*. London: Chapman & Hall, 1987.

73. Surawicz CM. The role of rectal biopsy in infectious colitis. *Am J Surg Pathol* 1988;**12**(suppl 1):82.

74. Tanaka M, Riddell RH, Saito H, Soma Y, Hidaka H, Kudo H. Morphological criteria applicable to biopsy specimens for effective distinction of inflammatory bowel disease from other forms of colitis and of Crohn's disease from ulcerative colitis. *Scand J Gastroenterol* 1999;**34**:55.

75. Lessells AM, Beck JS, Burnett RA, et al. Observer variability in the histopathological reporting of abnormal rectal biopsy specimens. *J Clin Pathol* 1994;**47**:48.

76. Jenkins D, Goodall A, Scott BB. Simple objective criteria for diagnosis of causes of acute diarrhoea on rectal biopsy. *J Clin Pathol* 1997;**50**:580.

77. Choudari CP, Mathan M, Rajan DP, Raghavan R, Mathan VI. A correlative study of etiology, clinical features and rectal mucosal pathology in adults with acute infectious diarrhea in southern India. *Pathology* 1985;**17**:443.

78. Allison MC, Hamilton-Dutoit SJ, Dhillon AP, Pounder RE. The value of rectal biopsy in distinguishing self-limited colitis from early inflammatory bowel disease. *Q J Med* 1987;**65**:985.

79. Anand BS, Malhotra V, Bhattacharya SK, et al. Rectal histology in acute bacillary dysentery. *Gastroenterology* 1986;**90**:654.

80. Surawicz CM, Belic L. Rectal biopsy helps to distinguish acute self-limited colitis from idiopathic inflammatory bowel disease. *Gastroenterology* 1984;**86**:104.

81. Dickinson RJ, Gilmour HM, McClelland DB. Rectal biopsy in patients presenting to an infectious disease unit with diarrhoeal disease. *Gut* 1979;**20**:141.

82. Koplan JP, Fineberg HV, Ferraro MJ, et al. Value of stool cultures. *Lancet* 1980;**ii**:413.

83. Harries AD, Myers B, Cook GC. Inflammatory bowel disease: a common cause of bloody diarrhoea in visitors to the tropics. *BMJ (Clin Res Ed)* 1985;**291**:1686.

84. Mandal BK, Schofield PF, Morson BC. A clinicopathological study of acute colitis: the dilemma of transient colitis syndrome. *Scand J Gastroenterol* 1982;**17**:865.

85. Willoughby CP, Piris J, Truelove SC. Campylobacter colitis. *J Clin Pathol* 1979;**32**:986.

86. Goodall HB, Sinclair ISR. Colitis cystica profunda. *J Pathol Bacteriol* 1957;**73**:33.

87. Denton J. The pathology of pellagra. *Am J Trop Med* 1925; **5**:173.

88. Luvuno FM, Mtshali Z, Baker LW. Toxic dilatation complicating fulminant amoebic colitis. *Br J Surg* 1982;**69**:56.

89. Anderson JB, Tanner AH, Brodribb AJ. Toxic megacolon due to Campylobacter colitis. *Int J Colorectal Dis* 1986;**1**:58.

90. Gefel A, Pruzanski W, Altman R. The clinical picture and rare variants of primary gastro-intestinal tuberculosis. *Gastroenterologia* 1963;**99**:359.

91. Ukil AC. Early diagnosis and treatment of intestinal tuberculosis. *Indian Med Gaz* 1942;**77**:613.

92. Anscombe AR, Keddie NC, Schofield PF. Caecal tuberculosis. *Gut* 1967;**8**:337.

93. Tandon HD, Prakash A, Rao VB, Prakash O, Nair SK. Ulceroconstrictive disorders of the intestine in northern India: a pathologic study. *Indian J Med Res* 1966;**54**:129.

94. de la Rua-Domenech R. Human *Mycobacterium bovis* infection in the United Kingdom: Incidence, risks, control measures and review of the zoonotic aspects of bovine tuberculosis. *Tuberculosis (Edinb)* 2006;**86**:77.

95. de Kantor IN, LoBue PA, Thoen CO. Human tuberculosis caused by *Mycobacterium bovis* in the United States, Latin America and the Caribbean. *Int J Tuberc Lung Dis* 2010; **14**:1369.

96. Hamandi WJ, Thamer MA. Tuberculosis of the bowel in Iraq: A study of 86 cases. *Dis Colon Rectum* 1965;**8**:158.

97. Dinner M. Tuberculosis of the gastrointestinal tract in the non-white population of the Transvaal. *S Afr Med J* 1965;**39**:97.

98. Schuurmans-Stekhoven JH. Tuberculous enterocolitis. A study of 19 cases seen at Edendale Hospital, Pietermaritzburg, Natal, 1959–1964. *S Afr Med J Suid-Afrikaanse Tydskrif Vir Geneeskunde* 1965;**39**:1199.

99. Hawley PR, Wolfe HR, Fullerton JM. Hypertrophic tuberculosis of the rectum. *Gut* 1968;**9**:461.

100. Davis JW. Hyperplastic tuberculosis of the rectum. *Am J Surg* 1957;**93**:490.

101. Rhoades ER, Klein LJ, Welsh JD. A case of probable tuberculosis of the distal colon. *Gastroenterology* 1960;**38**:654.

102. Need RL, Behnke RH. Tuberculous ulcers of the distal colon. *Am Rev Respir Dis* 1963;**88**:69.

103. Chaudhary A, Gupta NM. Colorectal tuberculosis. *Dis Colon & Rectum* 1986;**29**:738.

104. Klimach OE, Ormerod LP. Gastrointestinal tuberculosis: a retrospective review of 109 cases in a district general hospital. *Q J Med* 1985;**56**:569.

105. Kwiniemi H, Ristkari S, Ramo J. Tuberculosis of the large bowel. *Acta Chir Scand* 1984;**150**:345.

106. Ehsannulah M, Isaacs A, Filipe MI, Gazzard BG. Tuberculosis presenting as inflammatory bowel disease. Report of two cases. *Dis Colon & Rectum* 1984;**27**:134.

107. Franklin GO, Mohapatra M, Perrillo RP. Colonic tuberculosis diagnosed by colonoscopic biopsy. *Gastroenterology* 1979; **76**:362.

108. Koo J, Ho J, Ong GB. The value of colonoscopy in the diagnosis of Ileo-caecal tuberculosis. *Endoscopy* 1982;**14**:48.

109. Radhakrishnan S, Al Nakib B, Shaikh H, Menon NK. The value of colonoscopy in schistosomal, tuberculous, and amebic colitis. Two-year experience. *Dis Colon Rectum* 1986;**29**:891.

110. Dasgupta A, Singh N, Bhatia A. Abdominal tuberculosis: a histopathological study with special reference to intestinal perforation and mesenteric vasculopathy. *Indian J Pathol Microbiol* 2010;**53**:418.

111. Yonal O, Hamzaoglu HO. What is the most accurate method for the diagnosis of intestinal tuberculosis? *Turk J Gastroenterol* 2010;**21**:91.

112. Goel MM, Budhwar P. Species-specific immunocytochemical localization of Mycobacterium tuberculosis complex in fine needle aspirates of tuberculous lymphadenitis using antibody to 38 kDa immunodominant protein antigen. *Acta Cytol* 2008; **52**:424.

113. Marchetti G, Gori A, Catozzi L, Vago L, et al. Evaluation of PCR in detection of Mycobacterium tuberculosis from formalin-fixed, paraffin-embedded tissues: comparison of four amplification assays. *J Clin Microbiol* 1998;**36**:1512.

114. Snyder JD, Christenson E, Feldman RA. Human *Yersinia enterocolitica* infections in Wisconsin. Clinical, laboratory and epidemiologic features. *Am J Med* 1982;**72**:768.

115. Weir WRC. *Yersinia* infection. *Curr Opin Gastroenterol* 1985; **1**:135.

116. Editorial. Yersiniosis today. *Lancet* 1984;**i**:84.

117. Vantrappen G, Ponette E, Geboes K, Bertrand P. Yersinia enteritis and enterocolitis: gastroenterological aspects. *Gastroenterology* 1977;**72**:220.

118. Cover TL, Aber RC. Yersinia enterocolitica. *N Engl J Med* 1989; **321**:16.

119. Leino R, Granfors K, Havia T, Heinonen R, Lampinen M, Toivanen A. Yersiniosis as a gastrointestinal disease. *Scand J Infect Dis* 1987;**19**:63.

120. Rabinovitz M, Stremple JF, Wells KE, Stone BG. *Yersinia enterocolitica* infection complicated by intestinal perforation. *Arch Intern Med* 1987;**147**:1662.

121. Simmonds SD, Noble MA, Freeman HJ. Gastrointestinal features of culture-positive *Yersinia enterocolitica* infection. *Gastroenterology* 1987;**92**:112.

122. Rutgeerts P, Geboes K, Ponette E, Coremans G, Vantrappen G. Acute infective colitis caused by endemic pathogens in western Europe: endoscopic features. *Endoscopy* 1982;**14**:212.

123. O'Loughlin EV, Humphreys G, Dunn I, et al. Clinical, morphological, and biochemical alterations in acute intestinal yersiniosis. *Pediatr Res* 1986;**20**:602.

124. Mazzoleni G, deSa D, Gately J, Riddell RH. *Yersinia enterocolitica* infection with ileal perforation associated with iron overload and deferoxamine therapy. *Dig Dis Sci* 1991;**36**:1154.

125. Hawe P. Fibrous stricture of the rectum due to lymphogranuloma venereum. *Proc R Soc Med* 1951;**44**:426.

126. Kazal HL, Sohn N, Carrasco JI, Robilotti JG, Delaney WE. The gay bowel syndrome: clinico-pathologic correlation in 260 cases. *Ann Clin Lab Sci* 1976;**6**:184.

127. Weller IV. The gay bowel. *Gut* 1985;**26**:869.

128. Nicol CS. Some aspects of gonorrhea in the female with special reference to infection of the rectum. *Br J Vener Dis* 1948; **24**:26.

129. Kilpatrick ZM. Gonorrhoeal proctitis. *N Engl J Med* 1972; **287**:967.

130. McMillan A, Gilmour HM, Slatford K, McNeillage GJ. Proctitis in homosexual men. A diagnostic problem. *Br J Vener Dis* 1983; **59**:260.

131. Klein EJ, Fisher LS, Chow AW, et al. Anorectal gonococcal infection. *Ann Intern Med* 1977;**86**:340.

132. Wells BT, Kierland RR, Jackman RJ. Rectal chancre. Report of a case. *Am Med Assoc Arch Dermatol* 1959;**79**:179.

133. Marino AW Jr. Proctological lesions observed in male homosexuals. *Dis Colon Rectum* 1964;**7**:121.

134. Smith D. Infectious syphilis of the rectum. Report of a case. *Dis Colon Rectum* 1965;**8**:57.

135. Quinn TC, Lukehart SA, Goodell S, Mkrtichian E, Schuffler MD, Holmes KK. Rectal mass caused by *Treponema pallidum*: confirmation by immunofluorescent staining. *Gastroenterology* 1982;**82**:135.

136. McMillan A, Lee FD. Sigmoidoscopic and microscopic appearance of the rectal mucosa in homosexual men. *Gut* 1981; **22**:1035.

137. Saad EA, Filho PD, Dacorso Filho P, Teixeira D, Pereira AA, Erthal A. Ano-rectal-colonic lymphogranuloma venereum. *Gastroenterogy (Basel)* 1962;**97**:89.

138. Klotz SA, Drutz DJ, Tam MR, et al. Hemorrhagic proctitis due to lymphogranuloma venereum serogroup L2. Diagnosis by fluorescent monoclonal antibody. *N Engl J Med* 1983;**308**:1563.

139. Annamunthodo H. Rectal lymphogranuloma venereum in Jamaica. *Ann R Coll Surg of Engl* 1961;**29**:141.

140. Annamunthodo H, Marryatt J. Barium studies in intestinal lymphogranuloma venereum. *Br J Radiol* 1961;**34**:53.

141. de la Monte S, Hutchins GM. Follicular proctocolitis and neuromatous hyperplasia with lymphogranuloma venereum. *Hum Pathol* 1985;**16**:1025.

142. Miles RP. Rectal lymphogranuloma venereum. *Br J Surg* 1957; **45**:180.

143. Schuller JL, Piket-van Ulsen J, Veeken IV, Michel MF, Stolz E. Antibodies against *Chlamydia* of lymphogranuloma-venereum type in Crohn's disease. *Lancet* 1979;**1**:19.

144. Swarbrick ET, Kingham JG, Price HL, et al. *Chlamydia*, cytomegalovirus, and *Yersinia* in inflammatory bowel disease. *Lancet* 1979;**ii**:11.

145. Levin I, Romano S, Steinberg M, Welsh RA. Lymphogranuloma venereum: Rectal stricture and carcinoma. *Dis Colon Rectum* 1964;**7**:129.

146. Morson BC. Anorectal venereal disease. *Proc R Soc Med* 1964; **57**:179.

147. Quinn TC, Goodell SE, Mkrtichian E, et al. *Chlamydia trachomatis* proctitis. *N Engl J Med* 1981;**305**:195.

148. Munday PE, Dawson SG, Johnson AP, et al. A microbiological study of non-gonococcal proctitis in passive male homosexuals. *Postgrad Med J* 1981;**57**:705.

149. McMillan A, Kell P, Ward H. Diagnosing chlamydia and managing proctitis in men who have sex with men: current UK practice. *Sex Transm Infect* 2008;**84**:97.

150. Nielsen RH, Orholm M, Pedersen JO, Hovind-Hougen K, Teglbjaerg PS, Thaysen EH. Colorectal spirochetosis: clinical significance of the infestation. *Gastroenterology* 1983;**85**:62.

151. Henrik-Nielsen R, Lundbeck FA, Teglbjaerg PS, Ginnerup P, Hovind-Hougen K. Intestinal spirochetosis of the vermiform appendix. *Gastroenterology* 1985;**88**:971.

152. Lee FD, Kraszewski A, Gordon J, Howie JG, McSeveney D, Harland WA. Intestinal spirochaetosis. *Gut* 1971;**12**:126.

153. Cone LA, Woodard DR, Potts BE, Byrd RG, Alexander RM, Last MD. An update on the acquired immunodeficiency syndrome (AIDS). Associated disorders of the alimentary tract. *Dis Rectum Colon* 1986;**29**:60.

154. Hovind-Hougen K, Birch-Andersen A, Henrik-Nielsen R, et al. Intestinal spirochetosis: morphological characterization and cultivation of the spirochete *Brachyspira aalborgi* gen. *nov.*, sp. *nov. J Clin Microbiol* 1982;**16**:1127.

155. Tompkins DS, Foulkes SJ, Godwin PG, West AP. Isolation and characterisation of intestinal spirochaetes. *J Clin Pathol* 1986; **39**:535.

156. Antonakopoulos G, Newman J, Wilkinson M. Intestinal spirochaetosis: an electron microscopic study of an unusual case. *Histopathology* 1982;**6**:477.

157. Gebbers JO, Ferguson DJ, Mason C, Kelly P, Jewell DP. Spirochaetosis of the human rectum associated with an intraepithelial mast cell and IgE plasma cell response. *Gut* 1987;**28**:588.

158. Douglas JG, Crucioli V. Spirochaetosis: a remediable cause of diarrhoea and rectal bleeding? *BMJ (Clin Res Ed)* 1981;**283**:1362.

159. Mahant TS, Kohli PK, Mathur JM, Bhushurmath SR, Wig JD, Kaushik SP. Actinomycosis caecum. A case report. *Digestion* 1983;**27**:53.

160. James AW, Phelps AH. Actinomycosis of the colon. *Can J Surg* 1977;**20**:150.

161. Machaffie RA, Zaayer RL, Saichek H, Sciortino AL. An unusual case of actinomycosis manifested as an abdominal wall abscess. *Gastroenterology* 1957;**33**:830.

162. Morson BC. Primary actinomycosis of the rectum. *Proc R Soc Med* 1961;**54**:723.

163. Miller AG. Actinomycosis of the colon: Case report. *Dis Colon Rectum* 1964;**7**:207.

164. Klaaborg KE, Kronborg O, Olsen H. Enterocutaneous fistulization due to Actinomyces odontolyticus. Report of a case. *Dis Colon Rectum* 1985;**28**:526.

165. Saha S, Mukherjee AJ, Agarwal N, Chumber S, Karak AK. Colonic actinomycosis masquerading as perforated colonic carcinoma. *Trop Gastroenterol* 2007;**28**:74.

166. Whitaker BL. Actinomycetes in biopsy material obtained from suture-line granulomata following restorative resection of the rectum. *Br J Surg* 1964;**51**:445.

167. Asuncion CM, Cinti DC, Hawkins HB. Abdominal manifestations of actinomycosis in IUD users. *J Clin Gastroenterol* 1984;**6**:343.

168. Lee YK, Bae JM, Park YJ, Park SY, Jung SY. Pelvic actinomycosis with hydronephrosis and colon stricture simulating an advanced ovarian cancer. *J Gynecol Oncol* 2008;**19**:154.

169. Muezzinoglu B, Kus E. Intrauterine device associated actinomycosis mimicking sigmoid colon tumor. *Indian J Pathol Microbiol* 2010;**53**:848.

170. Lin YC. Segmental ascending colitis associated with *Aeromonas veronii* biovar *sobria*. *Pediatr Int* 2006;**48**:334.

171. Alperi A, Figueras MJ. Human isolates of *Aeromonas* possess Shiga toxin genes (stx1 and stx2) highly similar to the most virulent gene variants of *Escherichia coli*. *Clin Microbiol Infect* 2010;**16**:1563.

172. Holthouse DJ, Chen F, Leong RW, Chleboun J, Hallam L. *Aeromonas hydrophilia* colitis mimicking ischaemic colitis in an elderly woman. *J Gastroenterol Hepatol* 2007;**22**:1554.

173. De Feo E. Mucormycosis of the colon. *Am J Roentgenol Radium Ther Nucl Med* 1961;**86**:86.

174. Unat EK, Pars B, Kosyak JP. A case of cryptococcosis of the colon. *BMJ* 1960;**2**:1501.

175. Alberti-Flor JJ, Granda A. Ileocecal histoplasmosis mimicking Crohn's disease in a patient with Job's syndrome. *Digestion* 1986;**33**:176.

176. Lee SH, Barnes WG, Hodges GR, Dixon A. Perforated granulomatous colitis caused by Histoplasma capsulatum. *Dis Colon Rectum* 1985;**28**:171.

177. Cappell MS, Mandell W, Grimes MM, Neu HC. Gastrointestinal histoplasmosis. *Dig Dis Sci* 1988;**33**:353.

178. Goldmeier D, Sargeaunt PG, Price AB, et al. Is *Entamoeba histolytica* in homosexual men a pathogen? *Lancet* 1986;**i**:641.

179. Morton TC, Neal RA, Sage M. Indigenous amoebiasis in Britain. *Lancet* 1951;**i**:766.

180. McAllister TA. Diagnosis of amoebic colitis on routine biopsies from rectum and sigmoid colon. *BMJ* 1962;**1**:362.

181. Tucker PC, Webster PD, Kilpatrick ZM. Amebic colitis mistaken for inflammatory bowel disease. *Arch Intern Med* 1975;**135**:681.

182. Berkowitz D, Bernstein LH. Colonic pseudopolyps in association with amebic colitis. *Gastroenterology* 1975;**68**(4 Part 1):786.

183. McMillan A, Gilmour HM, McNeillage G, Scott GR. Amoebiasis in homosexual men. *Gut* 1984;**25**:356.

184. Mathan MM, Mathan VI. Rectal mucosal morphologic abnormalities in normal subjects in southern India: a tropical colonopathy? *Gut* 1985;**26**:710.

185. Sargeaunt PG, Williams JE, Grene JD. The differentiation of invasive and non-invasive Entamoeba histolytica by isoenzyme electrophoresis. *Trans R Soc Trop Med Hyg* 1978;**72**:519.

186. Alvarez-Fuertes G, Pelaez M, Gomez Velasco A. Paraffin inclusion of rectal mucus for diagnosis of amebiasis: preliminary results. *Dis Colon Rectum* 1963;**6**:172.

187. Nanda R, Baveja U, Anand BS. *Entamoeba histolytica* cyst passers: clinical features and outcome in untreated subjects. *Lancet* 1984;**2**:301.

188. Prathap K, Gilman R. The histopathology of acute intestinal amebiasis. A rectal biopsy study. *Am J Pathol* 1970;**60**:229.

189. Hulman G, Taylor LA. *Entamoeba histolytica*: demonstration by PAS/Martius yellow technique. *Med Lab Sci* 1987;**44**:396.

190. Hadley GP, Mickel RE. Fulminating amoebic colitis in infants and children. *J R Coll Surg Edinb* 1984;**29**:370.

191. Adams EB, MacLeod IN. Invasive amebiasis. II. Amebic liver abscess and its complications. *Medicine (Baltimore)* 1977;**56**:325.

192. Pittman FE, Hennigar GR. Sigmoidoscopic and colonic mucosal biopsy findings in amebic colitis. *Arch Pathol* 1974;**97**:155.

193. Cade D, Webster GD. Amoebic perforation of the intestine in children. *Br J Surg* 1974;**61**:159.

194. Perlmann P, Hammarstrom S, Lagercrantz R, Campbell D. Autoantibodies to colon in rats and human ulcerative colitis: cross reactivity with Escherichia coli O:14 antigen. *Proc Soc Exp Biol Med* 1967;**125**:975.

195. Rappaport EM, Rossien AX, Rosenblum LA. Arthritis due to intestinal amebiasis. *Ann Intern Med* 1951;**34**:1224.

196. Rominger JM, Shah AN. Ameboma of the rectum. *Gastrointest Endosc* 1979;**25**:71.

197. Gabriel WB. A case of amoebic ulceration of the rectum and anus. *Proc R Soc Med* 1939;**32**:b902.

198. Casemore DP, Sands RL, Curry A. *Cryptosporidium* species a 'new' human pathogen. *J Clin Pathol* 1985;**38**:1321.

199. Current WL, Reese NC, Ernst JV, Bailey WS, Heyman MB, Weinstein WM. Human cryptosporidiosis in immunocompetent and immunodeficient persons. Studies of an outbreak and experimental transmission. *N Engl J Med* 1983;**308**:1252.

200. Soave R, Danner RL, Honig CL, et al. Cryptosporidiosis in homosexual men. *Ann Intern Med* 1984;**100**:504.

201. Fletcher A, Sims TA, Talbot IC. Cryptosporidial enteritis without general or selective immune deficiency. *BMJ (Clin Res Ed)* 1982;**285**:22.

202. Jokipii L, Pohjola S, Jokipii AM. *Cryptosporidium*: a frequent finding in patients with gastrointestinal symptoms. *Lancet* 1983;**ii**:358.

203. Cook GC. Opportunistic parasitic infections associated with the acquired immune deficiency syndrome (AIDS): parasitology, clinical presentation, diagnosis and management. *Q J Med* 1987;**65**:967.

204. Dworkin B, Wormser GP, Rosenthal WS, et al. Gastrointestinal manifestations of the acquired immunodeficiency syndrome: a review of 22 cases. *Am J Gastroenterol* 1985;**80**:774.

205. Modigliani R, Bories C, Le Charpentier Y, et al. Diarrhoea and malabsorption in acquired immune deficiency syndrome: a

study of four cases with special emphasis on opportunistic protozoan infestations. *Gut* 1985;**26**:179.

206. DeHovitz JA, Pape JW, Boncy M, Johnson WD Jr. Clinical manifestations and therapy of Isospora belli infection in patients with the acquired immunodeficiency syndrome. *N Engl J Med* 1986;**315**:87.

207. Mc CA. Balantidiasis in South Persia. *BMJ* 1952;**i**:629.

208. Baskerville L, Ahmed Y, Ramchand S. Balantidium colitis. Report of a case. *Am J Dig Dis* 1970;**15**:727.

209. Prata A. Schistosomiasis mansoni. *Clin Gastroenterol* 1978;**7**:49.

210. Warren KS. Schistosomiasis japonica. *Clin Gastroenterol* 1978;**7**:77.

211. Azar JE, Schraibman IG, Pitchford RJ. Some observations on *Schistosoma haematobium* in the human rectum and sigmoid. *Trans R Soc Trop Med Hyg* 1958;**52**:562.

212. Kruatrachue M, Bhaibulaya M, Harinasuta C. Evaluation of rectal biopsy as a diagnostic method in *Schistosoma japonicum* infection in man in Thailand. *Ann Trop Med Parasitol* 1964;**58**:276.

213. Ch'en MC, Hu JC, Chang PY, et al. Pathogenesis of carcinoma of the colon and rectum in schistosomiasis japonica: a study on 90 cases. *Chin Med J* 1965;**84**:513.

214. Chen MC, Chang PY, Chuang CY, et al. Colorectal cancer and schistosomiasis. *Lancet* 1981;**i**:971.

215. Satsangi J, Silverberg MS, Vermeire S, Colombel JF. The Montreal classification of inflammatory bowel disease: controversies, consensus, and implications. *Gut* 2006;**55**:749.

216. D'Haens G, Geboes K, Peeters M, Baert F, Ectors N, Rutgeerts P. Patchy cecal inflammation associated with distal ulcerative colitis: a prospective endoscopic study. *Am J Gastroenterol* 1997;**92**:1275.

217. Davison AM, Dixon MF. The appendix as a 'skip lesion' in ulcerative colitis. *Histopathology* 1990;**16**:93.

218. Hewavisenthi SJ, Deen KI. An appendiceal skip lesion in ulcerative colitis. *Ceylon Med J* 1998;**43**:244.

219. Groisman GM, George J, Harpaz N. Ulcerative appendicitis in universal and nonuniversal ulcerative colitis. *Mod Pathol* 1994;**7**:322.

220. Cohen T, Pfeffer RB, Valensi Q. 'Ulcerative appendicitis' occurring as a skip lesion in chronic ulcerative colitis; report of a case. *Am J Gastroenterol* 1974;**62**:151.

221. Channer JL, Smith JH. 'Skip lesions' in ulcerative colitis. *Histopathology* 1990;**17**:286.

222. Yang SK, Jung HY, Kang GH, et al. Appendiceal orifice inflammation as a skip lesion in ulcerative colitis: an analysis in relation to medical therapy and disease extent. *Gastrointest Endosc* 1999;**49**:743.

223. Rubin DT, Rothe JA. The peri-appendiceal red patch in ulcerative colitis: review of the University of Chicago experience. *Dig Dis Sci* 2010;**55**:3495.

224. Levine TS, Tzardi M, Mitchell S, Sowter C, Price AB. Diagnostic difficulty arising from rectal recovery in ulcerative colitis. *J Clin Pathol* 1996;**49**:319.

225. Tanaka M, Riddell RH. The pathological diagnosis and differential diagnosis of Crohn's disease. *Hepatogastroenterology* 1990;**37**:18.

226. Kleer CG, Appelman HD. Ulcerative colitis: patterns of involvement in colorectal biopsies and changes with time. *Am J Surg Pathol* 1998;**22**:983.

227. Kim B, Barnett JL, Kleer CG, Appelman HD. Endoscopic and histological patchiness in treated ulcerative colitis. *Am J Gastroenterol* 1999;**94**:3258.

228. Rutgeerts P, D'Haens G, Hiele M, Geboes K, Vantrappen G. Appendicectomy protects against ulcerative colitis. *Gastroenterology* 1994;**106**:1251.

229. Radford-Smith GL, Edwards JE, et al. Protective role of appendicectomy on onset and severity of ulcerative colitis and Crohn's disease. *Gut* 2002;**51**:808.

230. Radford-Smith GL. What is the importance of appendicectomy in the natural history of IBD? *Inflamm Bowel Dis* 2008;**14** (suppl 2):S72.

231. Logan RF, Edmond M, Somerville KW, Langman MJ. Smoking and ulcerative colitis. *BMJ (Clin Res Ed)* 1984;**288**:751.

232. Vessey M, Jewell D, Smith A, Yeates D, McPherson K. Chronic inflammatory bowel disease, cigarette smoking, and use of oral contraceptives: findings in a large cohort study of women of childbearing age. *BMJ (Clin Res Ed)* 1986;**292**:1101.

233. Cope GF, Heatley RV, Kelleher JK. Smoking and colonic mucus in ulcerative colitis. *BMJ (Clin Res Ed)* 1986;**293**:481.

234. Podolsky DK, Isselbacher KJ. Glycoprotein composition of colonic mucosa. Specific alterations in ulcerative colitis. *Gastroenterology* 1984;**87**:991.

235. Coll I, Stevenson DL. Case of infantile ulcerative colitis. *BMJ* 1958;**2**:952.

236. Mir-Madjlessi SH, Michener WM, Farmer RG. Course and prognosis of idiopathic ulcerative proctosigmoiditis in young patients. *J Pediatr Gastroenterol Nutr* 1986;**5**:571.

237. Brocklehurst JC. Colonic disease in the elderly. *Clin Gastroenterol* 1985;**14**:725.

238. Zimmerman J, Gavish D, Rachmilewitz D. Early and late onset ulcerative colitis: distinct clinical features. *J Clin Gastroenterol* 1985;**7**:492.

239. Mayberry JF. Some aspects of the epidemiology of ulcerative colitis. *Gut* 1985;**26**:968.

240. Binder V, Both H, Hansen PK, Hendriksen C, Kreiner S, Torp-Pedersen K. Incidence and prevalence of ulcerative colitis and Crohn's disease in the County of Copenhagen, 1962 to 1978. *Gastroenterology* 1982;**83**:563.

241. Calkins BM, Lilienfeld AM, Garland CF, Mendeloff AI. Trends in incidence rates of ulcerative colitis and Crohn's disease. *Dig Dis Sci* 1984;**29**:913.

242. Kirsner JB, Shorter RG. Recent developments in nonspecific inflammatory bowel disease (second of two parts). *N Engl J Med* 1982;**306**:837.

243. Monk M, Mendeloff AI, Siegel CI, Lilienfeld A. An epidemiological study of ulcerative colitis and regional enteritis among adults in Baltimore. II. Social and demographic factors. *Gastroenterology* 1969;**56**:847.

244. Hermon-Taylor J. Protagonist. *Mycobacterium avium* subspecies *paratuberculosis* is a cause of Crohn's disease. *Gut* 2001;**49**:755.

245. White SA, Nassau E, Burnham R, Stanford JL, Lennard-Jones JE. Further evidence for a mycobacterial aetiology of Crohn's disease. *Gut* 1978;**19**:A443.

246. Montgomery SM, Morris DL, Pounder RE, Wakefield AJ. Measles vaccination and inflammatory bowel disease. *Lancet* 1997;**350**:1774.

247. Mayberry JF, Rhodes J, Newcombe RG. Familial prevalence of inflammatory bowel disease in relatives of patients with Crohn's disease. *BMJ* 1980;**280**:84.

248. McConnell RB. Genetic factors. In: Brooke BN, Wilkinson AW (eds), *Inflammatory Disease of the Bowel*. London: Pitman Medical, 1980: 8.

249. Lewkonia RM, McConnell RB. Progress report. Familial inflammatory bowel disease – heredity or environment? *Gut* 1976;**17**:235.

250. Halfvarson J. Genetics in twins with Crohn's disease: less pronounced than previously believed? *Inflamm Bowel Dis* 2011;**17**:6.

251. Halfvarson J, Bodin L, Tysk C, Lindberg E, Jarnerot G. Inflammatory bowel disease in a Swedish twin cohort: a long-term

follow-up of concordance and clinical characteristics. *Gastroenterology* 2003;**124**:1767.

252. Satsangi J, Rosenberg WM, Jewell DPJ. The prevalence of inflammatory bowel disease in relatives of patients with Crohn's disease. *Eur J Gastroenterol Hepatol* 1994;**6**:413.

253. Parkes M, Satsangi J. Genetic factors. In: Jewell DP, Mortensen NJ, Warren BF (eds), *Challenges in Inflammatory Bowel*. Oxford: Blackwell Science, 2001.

254. Kirsner JB. Genetic aspects of inflammatory bowel disease. *Clin Gastroenterol* 1973;**2**:555.

255. Probert CS, Jayanthi V, Hughes AO, Thompson JR, Wicks AC, Mayberry JF. Prevalence and family risk of ulcerative colitis and Crohn's disease: an epidemiological study among Europeans and south Asians in Leicestershire. *Gut* 1993;**34**:1547.

256. Thompson AI, Lees CW. Genetics of ulcerative colitis. *Inflamm Bowel Dis* 2011;**17**:831.

257. Hugot JP, Chamaillard M, Zouali H, et al. Association of NOD2 leucine-rich repeat variants with susceptibility to Crohn's disease. *Nature* 2001;**411**:599.

258. Ogura Y, Bonen D, Inohara N, et al. A frameshift mutation in NOD2 associated with susceptibility to Crohn's disease. *Nature* 2001;**411**:603.

259. McGovern DP, van Heel DA, Ahmad T, Jewell DP. NOD2 (CARD15), the first susceptibility gene for Crohn's disease. *Gut* 2001;**49**:752.

260. Beeken WL. Transmissible agents in inflammatory bowel disease: 1980. *Med Clinics North Am* 1980;**64**:1021.

261. Cave D, Kirsner JB, McClaren L. Infectious agents in inflammatory bowel disease (IBD), a status report. *Gastroenterogy* 1980;**78**:440.

262. Thayer WR, Brown M, Sangree MH, Katz J, Hersh T. *Escherichia coli* O:14 and colon hemagglutinating antibodies in inflammatory bowel disease. *Gastroenterology* 1969;**57**:311.

263. Carlsson HE, Lagercrantz R, Perlmann P. Immunological studies in ulcerative colitis. VIII. Antibodies to colon antigen in patients with ulcerative colitis, Crohn's disease, and other diseases. *Scand J Gastroenterol* 1977;**12**:707.

264. Hodgson HJ, Potter BJ, Jewell DP. Immune complexes in ulcerative colitis and Crohn's disease. *Clin Exp Immunol* 1977;**29**:187.

265. Potter BJ, Brown DJ, Watson A, Jewell DP. Complement inhibitors and immunoconglutinins in ulcerative colitis and Crohn's disease. *Gut* 1980;**21**:1030.

266. Lagercrantz R, Perlmann P, Hammarstrom S. Immunological studies in ulcerative colitis. V. Family studies. *Gastroenterology* 1971;**60**:381.

267. Perlmann P, Hammarstrom S, Lagercrantz R. Immunological features of idiopathic ulcerative colitis and Crohn's disease. *Gastroenterology* 1973;**5**:17.

268. Asherson GL, Holborow EJ. Autoantibody production in rabbits. VII. Autoantibodies to gut produced by the injection of bacteria. *Immunology* 1966;**10**:161.

269. Greenfield C, Aguilar Ramirez JR, et al. *Clostridium difficile* and inflammatory bowel disease. *Gut* 1983;**24**:713.

270. Ekbom A, Daszak P, Kraaz W, Wakefield AJ. Crohn's disease after in-utero measles virus exposure. *Lancet* 1996;**348**:515.

271. Thompson NP, Montgomery SM, Pounder RE, Wakefield AJ. Is measles vaccination a risk factor for inflammatory bowel disease? *Lancet* 1995;**345**:1071.

272. Metcalf J. Is measles infection associated with Crohn's disease? *BMJ* 1998;**316**:166.

273. Iizuka M, Chiba M, Yukawa M, et al. Immunohistochemical analysis of the distribution of measles related antigen in the intestinal mucosa in inflammatory bowel disease. *Gut* 2000; **46**:163.

274. Sanderson JD, Moss MT, Tizard ML, Hermon-Taylor J. *Mycobacterium paratuberculosis* DNA in Crohn's disease tissue. *Gut* 1992;**33**:890.

275. James SP. Remission of Crohn's disease after human immunodeficiency virus infection. *Gastroenterology* 1988;**95**:1667.

276. Jewell DP, Rhodes JM. Immunology of ulcerative colitis. In: Allen RN, Keighley MR, Alexander-Williams J, Hawkins C (eds), *Inflammatory Bowel Disease*. Edinburgh: Churchhill Livingstone, 1983: 155.

277. Van Spreeuwal JP, Meyer CJ, Rosekrans PC, Lindeman J. Immunoglobulin-containing cells in gastrointestinal pathology – diagnostic applications. In: Sommers SC, Rosen RP, Fechner RE, (eds), *Pathology Annual*. Connecticut: Appleton-Century Crofts, 1986: 295.

278. Mizoguchi A, Mizoguchi E, Chiba C, Bhan AK. Role of appendix in the development of inflammatory bowel disease in TCR-alpha mutant mice. *J Exp Med* 1996;**184**:707.

279. Kirsner JB, Palmer WL, Klotz A. Reversibility in ulcerative colitis; clinical and roentgenologic observations. *Radiology* 1951;**57**:1.

280. Hamilton MI, Dick R, Crawford L, Thompson NP, Pounder RE, Wakefield AJ. Is proximal demarcation of ulcerative colitis determined by the territory of the inferior mesenteric artery? [see comment] [erratum appears in *Lancet* 1995;**345**:1584] *Lancet* 1995;**345**:688.

281. Spiliadis CA, Lennard-Jones JE. Ulcerative colitis with relative sparing of the rectum. Clinical features, histology, and prognosis. *Dis Colon Rectum* 1987;**30**:334.

282. Ye BD, Yang SK, Boo SJ, et al. Clinical characteristics of ulcerative colitis associated with primary sclerosing cholangitis in Korea. *Inflamm Bowel Dis* 2011;**17**:1901.

283. Joo M, Abreu-e-Lima P, Farraye F, et al. Pathologic features of ulcerative colitis in patients with primary sclerosing cholangitis: a case-control study. *Am J Surg Pathol* 2009;**33**:854.

284. Odze R, Antonioli D, Peppercorn M, Goldman H. Effect of topical 5-aminosalicylic acid (5-ASA) therapy on rectal mucosal biopsy morphology in chronic ulcerative colitis. *Am J Surg Pathol* 1993;**17**:869.

285. Goulston SJ, McGovern VJ. The nature of benign strictures in ulcerative colitis. *N Engl J Med* 1969;**281**:290.

286. Jalan KN, Walker RJ, Sircus W, McManus JP, Prescott RJ, Card WI. Pseudopolyposis in ulcerative colitis. *Lancet* 1969;**ii**:555.

287. Kelly JK, Gabos S. The pathogenesis of inflammatory polyps. *Dis Colon Rectum* 1987;**30**:251.

288. Knill-Jones RP, Morson B, Williams R. Prestomal ileitis: clinical and pathological findings in five cases. *Q J Med* 1970;**39**:287.

289. Fazio VW. Toxic megacolon in ulcerative colitis and Crohn's colitis. *Clinic Gastroenterol* 1980;**9**:389.

290. Lumb G, Protheroe RH, Ramsay GS. Ulcerative colitis with dilatation of the colon. *Br J Surg* 1955;**43**:182.

291. Lumb G, Protheroe RH. Ulcerative colitis; a pathologic study of 152 surgical specimens. *Gastroenterology* 1958;**34**:381.

292. Burnham WR, Ansell ID, Langman MJ. Normal sigmoidoscopic findings in severe ulcerative colitis, an important and common occurrence. *Gut* 1980;**21**:A460.

293. Sampson PA, Walker FC. Dilatation of the colon in ulcerative colitis. *BMJ* 1961;**ii**:1119.

294. Price AB. Overlap in the spectrum of non-specific inflammatory bowel disease – 'colitis indeterminate'. *J Clin Pathol* 1978;**31**:567.

295. Ritchie JK, Powell-Tuck J, Lennard-Jones JE. Clinical outcome of the first ten years of ulcerative colitis and proctitis. *Lancet* 1978;**i**:1140.

296. Edwards CM, George B, Warren BF. Diversion colitis: new light through old windows. *Histopathology* 1999;**35**:86.

297. Edwards CM, George BD, Jewell DP, Warren BF, Mortensen NJ, Kettlewell MG. Role of a defunctioning stoma in the management of large bowel Crohn's disease. *Br J Surg* 2000;**87**:1063.

298. Roe AM, Warren BF, Brodribb AJ, Brown C. Diversion colitis and involution of the defunctioned anorectum. *Gut* 1993;**34**:382.

299. Farmer RG. Nonspecific ulcerative proctitis. *Gastroenterol Clinics North Am* 1987;**16**:157.

300. Das KM, Morecki R, Nair P, Berkowitz JM. Idiopathic proctitis. I. The morphology of proximal colonic mucosa and its clinical significance. *Am J Dig Dis* 1977;**22**:524.

301. Samarasekera DN, Stebbing JF, Kettlewell MG, Jewell DP, Mortensen NJ. Outcome of restorative proctocolectomy with ileal reservoir for ulcerative colitis: comparison of distal colitis with more proximal disease. *Gut* 1996;**38**:574.

302. Jenkins D, Balsitis M, Gallivan S, Dixon MF, Gilmour HM, Shepherd NA, et al. Guidelines for the initial biopsy diagnosis of suspected chronic idiopathic inflammatory bowel disease. The British Society of Gastroenterology Initiative. *J Clin Pathol* 1997;**50**:93.

303. Kelly JK, Langevin JM, Price LM, Hershfield NB, Share S, Blustein P. Giant and symptomatic inflammatory polyps of the colon in idiopathic inflammatory bowel disease. *Am J Surg Pathol* 1986;**10**:420.

304. Watson AJ, Roy AD. Paneth cells in the large intestine in ulcerative colitis. *J Pathol Bacteriol* 1960;**80**:309.

305. Elmes ME, Stanton MR, Howells CH, Lowe GH. Relation between the mucosal flora and Paneth cell population of human jejunum and ileum. *J Clin Pathol* 1984;**37**:1268.

306. Wehkamp J, Stange EF. Paneth disease. *J Crohns Colitis* 2010;**4**:523.

307. Morson BC, Pang LS. Rectal biopsy as an aid to cancer control in ulcerative colitis. *Gut* 1967;**8**:423.

308. Gledhill A, Enticott ME, Howe S. Variation in the argyrophil cell population of the rectum in ulcerative colitis and adenocarcinoma. *J Pathol* 1986;**149**:287.

309. Lee FD, Maguire C, Obeidat W, Russell RI. Importance of cryptolytic lesions and pericryptal granulomas in inflammatory bowel disease. *J Clin Pathol* 1997;**50**:148.

310. Warren BF, Shepherd NA, Price AB, Williams GT. Importance of cryptolytic lesions and pericryptal granulomas in inflammatory bowel disease. *J Clin Pathol* 1997;**50**:880.

311. Burroughs SH, Bowrey DJ, Morris-Stiff GJ, Williams GT. Granulomatous inflammation in sigmoid diverticulitis: two diseases or one? *Histopathology* 1998;**33**:349.

312. Warren BF, Shepherd NA, Bartolo DC, Bradfield JW. Pathology of the defunctioned rectum in ulcerative colitis. *Gut* 1993;**34**:514.

313. Wilders MM, Drexhage HA, Kokje M, Verspaget HW, Meuwissen SG. Veiled cells in chronic idiopathic inflammatory bowel disease. *Clin Exp Immunol* 1984;**55**:377.

314. Sarin SK, Malhotra V, Sen Gupta S, Karol A, Gaur SK, Anand BS. Significance of eosinophil and mast cell counts in rectal mucosa in ulcerative colitis. A prospective controlled study. *Dig Dis Sci* 1987;**32**:363.

315. Rosekrans PC, Meijer CJ, van der Wal AM, Cornelisse CJ, Lindeman J. Immunoglobulin containing cells in inflammatory bowel disease of the colon: a morphometric and immunohistochemical study. *Gut* 1980;**21**:941.

316. Heatley RV, James PD. Eosinophils in the rectal mucosa. A simple method of predicting the outcome of ulcerative proctocolitis? *Gut* 1979;**20**:787.

317. Flejou JF, Potet F, Bogomoletz WV, et al. Lymphoid follicular proctitis. A condition different from ulcerative proctitis? *Dig Dis Sci* 1988;**33**:314.

318. Warren S, Sommers SC. Pathogenesis of ulcerative colitis. *Am J Pathol* 1949;**25**:657.

319. Wakefield AJ, Sankey EA, Dhillon AP, et al. Granulomatous vasculitis in Crohn's disease. [Erratum appears in *Gastroenterology* 1991;**101**:595] *Gastroenterology* 1991;**100**(5 Part 1):1279.

320. Rice AJ, Abbott CR, Mapstone NM. Granulomatous vasculitis in diversion procto-colitis.[see comment]. *Histopathology* 1999;**34**:276.

321. Riley SA, Mani V, Goodman MJ, Dutt S, Herd ME. Microscopic activity in ulcerative colitis: what does it mean? *Gut* 1991;**32**:174.

322. Geboes K, Riddell R, Ost A, Jensfelt B, Persson T, Lofberg R. A reproducible grading scale for histological assessment of inflammation in ulcerative colitis. *Gut* 2000;**47**:404.

323. Bernstein CN, Shanahan F, Anton PA, Weinstein WM. Patchiness of mucosal inflammation in treated ulcerative colitis: a prospective study. *Gastrointest Endosc* 1995;**42**:232.

324. Teague RH, Manning AP. Preparation of the large bowel for endoscopy. *J Intern Med Res* 1977;**5**:374.

325. Elliott PR, Williams CB, Lennard-Jones JE, et al. Colonoscopic diagnosis of minimal change colitis in patients with a normal sigmoidoscopy and normal air-contrast barium enema. *Lancet* 1982;**i**:650.

326. Soundy VC, Davies SE, Warren BF. The double muscularis mucosae in ulcerative colitis: is it all new? *Histopathology* 1998;**32**:484.

327. Lichtiger S, Present DH, Kornbluth A, et al. Cyclosporine in severe ulcerative colitis refractory to steroid therapy. *N Engl J Med* 1994;**330**:1841.

328. Hyde GM, Thillainayagam AV, Jewell DP. Intravenous cyclosporin as rescue therapy in severe ulcerative colitis: time for a reappraisal? *Eur J Gastroenterol Hepatol* 1998;**10**:411.

329. Hyde GM, Jewell DP, Warren BF. Histological changes associated with the use of intravenous cyclosporin in the treatment of severe ulcerative colitis may mimic dysplasia. *Colorectal Dis* 2002;**4**:455.

330. Mottet NK. Histopathologic spectrum of regional enteritis and ulcerative colitis. In: Bennington JL (ed.), *Major Problems in Pathology*. Philadelphia, PA: WB Saunders, 1971: 220.

331. Gilat T, Fireman Z, Grossman A, et al. Colorectal cancer in patients with ulcerative colitis. A population study in central Israel. *Gastroenterology* 1988;**94**:870.

332. Maratka Z, Nedbal J, Kocianova J, Havelka J, Kudrmann J, Hendl J. Incidence of colorectal cancer in proctocolitis: a retrospective study of 959 cases over 40 years. *Gut* 1985;**26**:43.

333. Baker WN, Glass RE, Ritchie JK, Aylett SO. Cancer of the rectum following colectomy and ileorectal anastomosis for ulcerative colitis. *Br J Surg* 1978;**65**:862.

334. Lennard-Jones JE, Morson BC, Ritchie JK, Williams CB. Cancer surveillance in ulcerative colitis. Experience over 15 years. *Lancet* 1983;**2**:149.

335. van Schaik FD, Ten Kate FJ, Offerhaus GJ, et al. Misclassification of dysplasia in patients with inflammatory bowel disease: Consequences for progression rates to advanced neoplasia. *Inflamm Bowel Dis* 2011;**17**:1108.

336. Ullman T, Croog V, Harpaz N, Sachar D, Itzkowitz S. Progression of flat low grade dysplasia to advanced neoplasia in patients with ulcerative colitis. *Gastroenterology* 2003;**125**:1311.

337. De Dombal FT, Watts JM, Watkinson G, Goligher JC. Local complications of ulcerative colitis: stricture, pseudopolyposis, and carcinoma of colon and rectum. *BMJ* 1966 Jun;**1**:1442.

338. Devroede GJ, Taylor WF, Sauer WG, Jackman RJ, Stickler GB. Cancer risk and life expectancy of children with ulcerative colitis. *N Engl J Med* 1971;**285**:17.

339. MacDermott RP. Review of clinical aspects of cancer of the colon in patients with ulcerative colitis. *Dig Dis Sci* 1985; **30**(12 suppl):114S.

340. Gyde SN, Prior P, Allan RN, et al. Colorectal cancer in ulcerative colitis: a cohort study of primary referrals from three centres. *Gut* 1988;**29**:206.

341. van Schaik FD, Offerhaus GJ, Schipper ME, Siersema PD, Vleggaar FP, Oldenburg B. Endoscopic and pathological aspects of colitis-associated dysplasia. *Nat Rev Gastroenterol Hepatol* 2009;**6**:671.

342. Lutgens MW, Vleggaar FP, Schipper ME, et al. High frequency of early colorectal cancer in inflammatory bowel disease. *Gut* 2008;**57**:1246.

343. Greenstein AJ, Sachar DB, Smith H, et al. Cancer in universal and left-sided ulcerative colitis: factors determining risk. *Gastroenterology* 1979;**77**:290.

344. Allen DC, Biggart JD, Pyper PC. Large bowel mucosal dysplasia and carcinoma in ulcerative colitis. *J Clin Pathol* 1985;**38**:30.

345. Jones HW, Grogono J, Hoare AM. Surveillance in ulcerative colitis: burdens and benefit. *Gut* 1988;**29**:325.

346. Hinton JM. Risk of malignant change in ulcerative colitis. *Gut* 1966;**7**:427.

347. Collins RH Jr, Feldman M, Fordtran JS. Colon cancer, dysplasia, and surveillance in patients with ulcerative colitis. A critical review. *N Engl J Med* 1987;**316**:1654.

348. Manning AP, Bulgim OR, Dixon MF, Axon AT. Screening by colonoscopy for colonic epithelial dysplasia in inflammatory bowel disease. *Gut* 1987;**28**:1489.

349. Lennard-Jones JE. Compliance, cost, and common sense limit cancer control in colitis. *Gut* 1986;**27**:1403.

350. Fozard JB, Dixon MF. Colonoscopic surveillance in ulcerative colitis – dysplasia through the looking glass. *Gut* 1989;**30**:285.

351. Blackstone MO, Riddell RH, Rogers BH, Levin B. Dysplasia-associated lesion or mass (DALM) detected by colonoscopy in long-standing ulcerative colitis: an indication for colectomy. *Gastroenterology* 1981;**80**:366.

352. Granqvist S, Gabrielsson N, Sundelin P, Thorgeirsson T. Precancerous lesions in the mucosa in ulcerative colitis. A radiographic, endoscopic, and histopathologic study. *Scand J Gastroenterol* 1980;**15**:289.

353. Lennard-Jones JE, Morson BC, Ritchie JK, Shove DC, Williams CB. Cancer in colitis: assessment of the individual risk by clinical and histological criteria. *Gastroenterology* 1977;**73**:1280.

354. Huang Q, Fukami N, Kashida H, et al. Interobserver and intraobserver consistency in the endoscopic assessment of colonic pit patterns. *Gastrointest Endosc* 2004;**60**:520.

355. Kiesslich R, Fritsch J, Holtmann M, et al. Methylene blue-aided chromoendoscopy for the detection of intra-epithelial neoplasia and colon cancer in ulcerative colitis. *Gastroenterology* 2003; **124**:880.

356. Vucelic B. Inflammatory bowel diseases: controversies in the use of diagnostic procedures. *Dig Dis* 2009;**27**:269.

357. Riddell RH, Goldman H, Ransohoff DF, et al. Dysplasia in inflammatory bowel disease: standardized classification with provisional clinical applications. *Hum Pathol* 1983;**14**:931.

358. Butt JH, Konishi F, Morson BC, Lennard-Jones JE, Ritchie JK. Macroscopic lesions in dysplasia and carcinoma complicating ulcerative colitis. *Dig Dis Sci* 1983;**28**:18.

359. Muto T, Bussey HJ, Morson BC. The evolution of cancer of the colon and rectum. *Cancer* 1975;**36**:2251.

360. Slater G, Greenstein AJ, Gelernt I, Kreel I, Bauer J, Aufses AH Jr. Distribution of colorectal cancer in patients with and without ulcerative colitis. *Am J Surg* 1985;**149**:780.

361. Downs-Kelly E, Mendelin JE, Bennett AE, et al. Poor interobserver agreement in the distinction of high grade dysplasia and adenocarcinoma in pretreatment Barrett's esophagus biopsies. *Am J Gastroenterol* 2008;**103**:2333; quiz 41.

362. Schlemper RJ, Riddell RH, Kato Y, et al. The Vienna classification of gastrointestinal epithelial neoplasia. *Gut* 2000;**47**:251.

363. Levi GS, Harpaz N. Intestinal low grade tubuloglandular adenocarcinoma in inflammatory bowel disease. *Am J Surg Pathol* 2006;**30**:1022.

364. Srivastava A, Redston M, Farraye FA, Yantiss RK, Odze RD. Hyperplastic/serrated polyposis in inflammatory bowel disease: a case series of a previously undescribed entity. *Am J Surg Pathol* 2008;**32**:296–303.

365. Rubio CA. Serrated neoplasias and de novo carcinomas in ulcerative colitis: a histological study in colectomy specimens. *J Gastroenterol Hepatol* 2007;**22**:1024.

366. Ajioka Y, Watanabe H, Matsuda K. Over-expression of p53 protein in neoplastic changes in ulcerative colitis: immunohistochemical study. *J Gastroenterol* 1995;**30**(suppl 8):33.

367. Brentnall TA, Crispin DA, Rabinovitch PS, et al. Mutations in the p53 gene: an early marker of neoplastic progression in ulcerative colitis. *Gastroenterology* 1994;**107**:369.

368. Sato A, MacHinami R. p53 immunohistochemistry of ulcerative colitis-associated with dysplasia and carcinoma. *Pathol Int* 1999;**49**:858.

369. Harpaz N, Peck AL, Yin J, et al. p53 protein expression in ulcerative colitis-associated colorectal dysplasia and carcinoma. *Hum Pathol* 1994;**25**:1069.

370. Noffsinger AE, Belli JM, Miller MA, Fenoglio-Preiser CM. A unique basal pattern of p53 expression in ulcerative colitis is associated with mutation in the p53 gene. *Histopathology* 2001;**39**:482.

371. Hao XP, Ilyas M, Talbot IC. Expression of *Bcl-2* and *p53* in the colorectal adenoma-carcinoma sequence. *Pathobiology* 1997; **65**:140.

372. Schneider A, Stolte M. Differential diagnosis of adenomas and dysplastic lesions in patients with ulcerative colitis. *Z Gastroenterol* 1993;**31**:653.

373. Dorer R, Odze RD. AMACR immunostaining is useful in detecting dysplastic epithelium in Barrett's esophagus, ulcerative colitis, and Crohn's disease. *Am J Surg Pathol* 2006; **30**:871.

374. Strater J, Wiesmuller C, Perner S, Kuefer R, Moller P. Alpha-methylacyl-CoA racemase (AMACR) immunohistochemistry in Barrett's and colorectal mucosa: only significant overexpression favours a diagnosis of intra-epithelial neoplasia. *Histopathology* 2008;**52**:399.

375. Marx A, Simon P, Simon R, et al. AMACR expression in colorectal cancer is associated with left-sided tumor localization. *Virchows Arch* 2008;**453**:243.

376. Ransohoff DF, Riddell RH, Levin B. Ulcerative colitis and colonic cancer. Problems in assessing the diagnostic usefulness of mucosal dysplasia. *Dis Colon Rectum* 1985;**28**:383.

377. Dixon MF, Brown LJ, Gilmour HM, et al. Observer variation in the assessment of dysplasia in ulcerative colitis. *Histopathology* 1988;**13**:385.

378. Eaden J, Abrams K, McKay H, Denley H, Mayberry J. Inter-observer variation between general and specialist gastrointestinal pathologists when grading dysplasia in ulcerative colitis. *J Pathol* 2001;**194**:152.

379. Biasco G, Migholi M, Di Febo G, et al. Cancer and dysplasia in ulcerative colitis: preliminary report of a prospective study. *Ital J Gastroenterol* 1984;**16**:212.

380. Connell WR, Lennard-Jones JE, Williams CB, Talbot IC, Price AB, Wilkinson KH. Factors affecting the outcome of endoscopic surveillance for cancer in ulcerative colitis. *Gastroenterology* 1994;**107**:934.

381. Cairns SR, Scholefield JH, Steele RJ, et al. Guidelines for colorectal cancer screening and surveillance in moderate and high risk groups (update from 2002). *Gut* 2010;**59**:666.

382. Farraye FA, Odze RD, Eaden J, Itzkowitz SH. AGA technical review on the diagnosis and management of colorectal neoplasia in inflammatory bowel disease. *Gastroenterology* 2010;**138**:746, 74 e1; quiz e12.

383. Farraye FA, Odze RD, Eaden J, Itzkowitz SH, McCabe RP, Dassopoulos T, et al. AGA medical position statement on the diagnosis and management of colorectal neoplasia in inflammatory bowel disease. *Gastroenterology* 2010;**138**:738.

384. Kewenter J, Hulten L, Ahren C. The occurrence of severe epithelial dysplasia and its bearing on treatment of longstanding ulcerative colitis. *Ann Surg* 1982;**195**:209.

385. de Dombal FT, Softley A. Cancer and inflammatory bowel disease – changing perspectives. In: de Dombal FT, Myran J, Bouchier IA, Watkinson G (eds), *Inflammatory Bowel Disease, Some International Data and Reflections.* Oxford: Oxford University Press, 1985: 247.

386. Hurlstone DP, Kiesslich R, Thomson M, Atkinson R, Cross SS. Confocal chromoscopic endomicroscopy is superior to chromoscopy alone for the detection and characterisation of intraepithelial neoplasia in chronic ulcerative colitis. *Gut* 2008;**57**:196.

387. Hurlstone DP, Sanders DS, Lobo AJ, McAlindon ME, Cross SS. Indigo carmine-assisted high-magnification chromoscopic colonoscopy for the detection and characterisation of intraepithelial neoplasia in ulcerative colitis: a prospective evaluation. *Endoscopy* 2005;**37**:1186.

388. Kiesslich R, Goetz M, Lammersdorf K, et al. Chromoscopy-guided endomicroscopy increases the diagnostic yield of intraepithelial neoplasia in ulcerative colitis. *Gastroenterology* 2007;**132**:874.

389. Talbot IC, Price AB. Dysplasia in inflammatory bowel disease. In: *Biopsy Pathology in Colorectal Disease.* London: Chapman & Hall, 1987: 149.

390. Brostrom O, Lofberg R, Ost A, Reichard H. Cancer surveillance of patients with longstanding ulcerative colitis: a clinical, endoscopical, and histological study. *Gut* 1986;**27**:1408.

391. Butt JH, Price AB, Williams CB. Dysplasia and cancer in ulcerative colitis. In: Allen RN, Keighley MR, Alexander-Williams J, Hawkins C (eds), *Inflammatory Bowel Disease.* Edinburgh: Churchill Livingstone, 1983: 140.

392. Dobbins WO 3rd. Current status of the precancer lesion in ulcerative colitis. *Gastroenterology* 1977;**73**:1431.

393. Yardley JH, Bayless TM, Diamond MP. Cancer in ulcerative colitis. *Gastroenterology* 1979;**76**:221.

394. Rosenstock E, Farmer RG, Petras R, Sivak MV Jr, Rankin GB, Sullivan BH. Surveillance for colonic carcinoma in ulcerative colitis. *Gastroenterology* 1985;**89**:1342.

395. Ziv Y, Fazio VW, Sirimarco MT, Lavery IC, Goldblum JR, Petras RE. Incidence, risk factors, and treatment of dysplasia in the anal transitional zone after ileal pouch-anal anastomosis. *Dis Colon Rectum* 1994;**37**:1281.

396. Parks AG, Nicholls RJ. Proctocolectomy without ileostomy for ulcerative colitis. *BMJ* 1978;**2**:85.

397. Thompson-Fawcett MW, Rust NA, Warren BF, Mortensen NJ. Aneuploidy and columnar cuff surveillance after stapled ileal pouch-anal anastomosis in ulcerative colitis. *Dis Colon Rectum* 2000;**43**:408.

398. Dew MJ, Thompson H, Allan RN. The spectrum of hepatic dysfunction in inflammatory bowel disease. *Q J Med* 1979;**48**:113.

399. Perrett AD, Higgins G, Johnston HH, Massarella GR, Truelove SC, Wright R. The liver in ulcerative colitis. *Q J Med* 1971; **40**:211.

400. Rand JA, Brandt LJ, Becker NH, Lynch J. Ulcerative colitis complicated by amyloidosis. *Am J Gastroenterol* 1980;**74**:185.

401. Shorvon PJ. Amyloidosis and inflammatory bowel disease. *Am J Dig Dis* 1977;**22**:209.

402. Chapman RW, Arborgh BA, Rhodes JM, et al. Primary sclerosing cholangitis: a review of its clinical features, cholangiography, and hepatic histology. *Gut* 1980;**21**:870.

403. Meuwissen SG, Feltkamp-Vroom TM, De La Riviere AB, Von Dem Borne AE, Tytgat GN. Analysis of the lympho-plasmacytic infiltrate in Crohn's disease with special reference to identification of lymphocyte-subpopulations. *Gut* 1976;**17**:770.

404. Ludwig J, Laruso N, Wiesner R. Primary sclerosing cholangitis of small bile ducts. In: Peters R, Craig J (eds), *Liver Pathology.* Edinburgh: Churchill Livingstone, 1986: 193.

405. Wee A, Ludwig J. Pericholangitis in chronic ulcerative colitis: primary sclerosing cholangitis of the small bile ducts? *Ann Intern Med* 1985;**102**:581.

406. Barbatis C, Grases P, Shepherd HA, et al. Histological features of sclerosing cholangitis in patients with chronic ulcerative colitis. *J Clin Pathol* 1985;**38**:778.

407. Mir-Madjlessi SH, Farmer RG, Sivak MV Jr. Bile duct carcinoma in patients with ulcerative colitis. Relationship to sclerosing cholangitis: report of six cases and review of the literature. *Dig Dis Sci* 1987;**32**:145.

408. Ritchie JK, Allan RN, Macartney J, Thompson H, Hawley PR, Cooke WT. Biliary tract carcinoma associated with ulcerative colitis. *Q J Med* 1974;**43**:263.

409. Olsson R, Hulten L. Concurrence of ulcerative colitis and chronic acitve hepatitis, Clinical courses and results of colectomy. *Scand J Gastroenterol* 1975;**10**:331.

410. Mayer L, Janowitz HD. Extra-intestinal manisfestations of ulcerative colitis including reference to Crohn's disease. In: Allan RN, Keighley MR, Alexander-Williams J, Hawkins C (eds), *Inflammatory Bowel Disease.* Edinburgh: Churchill Livingstone, 1983: 121.

411. Greenstein AJ, Janowitz HD, Sachar DB. The extra-intestinal complications of Crohn's disease and ulcerative colitis: a study of 700 patients. *Medicine (Baltimore)* 1976;**55**:401.

412. Lockhart-Mummery HE, Morson BC. Crohn's disease (regional enteritis) of the large intestine and its distinction from ulcerative colitis. *Gut* 1960;**1**:87.

413. Cornes JS, Stecher M. Primary Crohn's disease of the colon and rectum. *Gut* 1961;**2**:189.

414. Kent TH, Ammon RK, DenBesten L. Differentiation of ulcerative colitis and regional enteritis of colon. *Arch Pathol* 1970;**89**:20.

415. Morson BS. Histopathology of Crohn's disease. *Proc R Soc Med* 1968;**61**:79.

416. Lockhart-Mummery HE, Morson BC. Crohn's disease of the large intestine. *Gut* 1964;**5**:493.

417. Joffe N. Localised giant pseudopolyposis secondary to ulcerative or granulomatous colitis. *Clin Radiol* 1977;**28**:609.

418. Buchanan WM, Fyfe AH. Giant pseudopolyposis in granulomatous colitis. *J Pathol* 1979;**127**:51.

419. Bentley E, Jenkins D, Campbell F, Warren B. How could pathologists improve the initial diagnosis of colitis? Evidence from an international workshop. *J Clin Pathol* 2002;**55**:955.

420. Riddell RH. Pathology of idiopathic inflammatory bowel disease. In: Kirsner JB, Shorter RG (eds), *Inflammatory Bowel Disease.* Philadelphia: Lea & Febiger, 1988: 325.

421. Haggitt RC. The differential diagnosis of idiopathic inflammatory bowel disease. In: Norris HT (ed.), *Pathology of the Colon, Small Intestine and Anus.* New York: Churchill Livingstone, 1983: 21.

422. Greenson JK, Stern RA, Carpenter SL, Barnett JL. The clinical significance of focal active colitis. *Hum Pathol* 1997;**28**:729.

423. Volk EE, Shapiro BD, Easley KA, Goldblum JR. The clinical significance of a biopsy-based diagnosis of focal active colitis: a clinicopathologic study of 31 cases. *Mod Pathol* 1998;**11**:789.

424. Rotterdam H, Korelitz BI, Sommers SC. Microgranulomas in grossly normal rectal mucosa in Crohn's disease. *Am J Clin Pathol* 1977;**67**:550.

425. Cook MG, Dixon MF. An analysis of the reliability of detection and diagnostic value of various pathological features in Crohn's disease and ulcerative colitis. *Gut* 1973;**14**:255.

426. Schmitz-Moormann P, Pittner PM, Sangmeister M. Probability of detecting a granuloma in a colorectal biopsy of Crohn's disease. *Pathol Res Pract* 1984;**178**:227.

427. Hanby AM, Wright NA. The ulcer-associated cell lineage: the gastrointestinal repair kit? *J Pathol* 1993;**171**:3.

428. Longman RJ, Warren BF. Is the colonic reparative cell lineage yet to be discovered? *Gut* 2000;**47**:307.

429. Borley NR, Mortensen NJ, Kettlewell MG, George BD, Jewell DP, Warren BF. Connective tissue changes in ileal Crohn's disease: relationship to disease phenotype and ulcer-associated cell lineage. *Dis Colon Rectum* 2001;**44**:388.

430. Borley NR, Mortensen NJ, Jewell DP, Warren BF. The relationship between inflammatory and serosal connective tissue changes in ileal Crohn's disease: evidence for a possible causative link. *J Pathol* 2000;**190**:196.

431. Sokol H, Polin V, Lavergne-Slove A, et al. Plexitis as a predictive factor of early postoperative clinical recurrence in Crohn's disease. *Gut* 2009;**58**:1218.

432. Ferrante M, de Hertogh G, Hlavaty T, et al. The value of myenteric plexitis to predict early postoperative Crohn's disease recurrence. *Gastroenterology* 2006;**130**:1595.

433. Lewin K, Swales J. Granulomatous colitis and atypical ulcerative colitis. *Gastroenterology* 1966;**50**:211.

434. Margulis AR, Goldberg HI, Lawson TL, et al. The overlapping spectrum of ulcerative and granulomatous colitis: a roentgenographic-pathologic study. *Am J Roentgenol Radium Ther Nucl Med* 1971;**113**:325.

435. Gyde SN, Prior P, Macartney JC, Thompson H, Waterhouse JA, Allan RN. Malignancy in Crohn's disease. *Gut* 1980;**21**:1024.

436. Tanaka M, Saito H, Fukuda S, Sasaki Y, Munakata A, Kudo H. Simple mucosal biopsy criteria differentiating among Crohn disease, ulcerative colitis, and other forms of colitis: measurement of validity. *Scand J Gastroenterol* 2000;**35**:281.

437. Geboes K, Van Eyken P. Inflammatory bowel disease unclassified and indeterminate colitis: the role of the pathologist. *J Clin Pathol* 2009;**62**:201.

438. Geboes K, Colombel JF, Greenstein A, et al. Indeterminate colitis: a review of the concept – what's in a name? *Inflamm Bowel Dis* 2008;**14**:850.

439. Silverberg MS, Satsangi J, Ahmad T, et al. Toward an integrated clinical, molecular and serological classification of inflammatory bowel disease: Report of a Working Party of the 2005 Montreal World Congress of Gastroenterology. *Can J Gastroenterol* 2005;**19**(suppl A):5.

440. Kleer CG, Appelman HD. Ulcerative colitis: patterns of involvement in colorectal biopsies and changes with time. *Am J Surg Pathol* 1998;**22**:983.

441. Kent TH, Ammon RK, DenBesten L. Differentiation of ulcerative colitis and regional enteritis of colon. *Arch Pathol Lab Med* 1970;**89**:20.

442. Lee KS, Medline A, Shockey S. Indeterminate colitis in the spectrum of inflammatory bowel disease. *Arch Pathol Lab Med* 1979;**103**:173.

443. Harper PH, Truelove SC, Lee EC, Kettlewell MG, Jewell DP. Split ileostomy and ileocolostomy for Crohn's disease of the colon and ulcerative colitis: a 20 year survey. *Gut* 1983;**24**:106.

444. Winslet MC, Andrews H, Allan RN, Keighley MR. Fecal diversion in the management of Crohn's disease of the colon. *Dis Colon Rectum* 1993;**36**:757.

445. Edwards CM, George B, Warren B. Diversion colitis – new light through old windows. *Histopathology* 1999;**34**:1.

446. Warren BF, Shepherd NA. The role of pathology in pelvic ileal reservoir surgery. *Int J Colorectal Dis* 1992;**7**:68.

447. Geboes K. Crohn's disease, ulcerative colitis or indeterminate colitis – how important is it to differentiate? *Acta Gastroenterol Belgica* 2001;**64**:197.

448. Yu CS, Pemberton JH, Larson D. Ileal pouch-anal anastomosis in patients with indeterminate colitis: long-term results. *Dis Colon Rectum* 2000;**43**:1487.

449. McIntyre PB, Pemberton JH, Wolff BG, Dozois RR, Beart RW Jr. Indeterminate colitis. Long-term outcome in patients after ileal pouch-anal anastomosis. *Dis Colon Rectum* 1995;**38**:51.

450. Atkinson KG, Owen DA, Wankling G. Restorative proctocolectomy and indeterminate colitis. *Am J Surg* 1994;**167**:516.

451. Koltun WA, Schoetz DJ Jr, Roberts PL, Murray JJ, Coller JA, Veidenheimer MC. Indeterminate colitis predisposes to perineal complications after ileal pouch-anal anastomosis. *Dis Colon Rectum* 1991;**34**:857.

452. White CL, III, Hamilton SR, Diamond MP, Cameron JL. Crohn's disease and ulcerative colitis in the same patient. *Gut* 1983;**24**:857.

453. Eyer S, Spadaccini C, Walker P, Ansel H, Schwartz M, Sumner HW. Simultaneous ulcerative colitis and Crohn's disease. Report of a case. *Am J Gastroenterol* 1980;**73**:345.

454. Dwarakanath AD, Nash J, Rhodes JM. 'Conversion' from ulcerative colitis to Crohn's disease associated with corticosteroid treatment. *Gut* 1994;**35**:1141.

455. Parente F, Cucino C, Bollani S, et al. Focal gastric inflammatory infiltrates in inflammatory bowel diseases: prevalence, immunohistochemical characteristics, and diagnostic role. *Am J Gastroenterol* 2000;**95**:705.

456. Kelly JK, Langevin JM, Price LM, Hershfield NB, Share S, Blustein P. Giant and symptomatic inflammatory polyps of the colon in idiopathic inflammatory bowel disease. *Am J Surg Pathol* 1986;**10**:420.

457. Schmidt GT, Lennard-Jones JE, Morson BC, Young AC. Crohn's disease of the colon and its distinction from diverticulitis. *Gut* 1968;**9**:7.

458. Sladen GE, Filipe MI. Is segmental colitis a complication of diverticular disease? *Dis Colon Rectum* 1984;**27**:513.

459. Makapugay LM, Dean PJ. Diverticular disease-associated chronic colitis. *Am J Surg Pathol* 1996;**20**:94.

460. Gore S, Shepherd NA, Wilkinson SP. Endoscopic crescentic fold disease of the sigmoid colon: the clinical and histopathological spectrum of a distinctive endoscopic appearance. *Int J Colorectal Dis* 1992;**7**:76.

461. Van Rosendaal GM, Andersen MA. Segmental colitis complicating diverticular disease. *Can J Gastroenterol* 1996;**10**:361.

462. Goldstein NS, Leon-Armin C, Mani A. Crohn's colitis-like changes in sigmoid diverticulitis specimens is usually an idiosyncratic inflammatory response to the diverticulosis rather than Crohn's colitis. *Am J Surg Pathol* 2000;**24**:668.

463. Gledhill A, Dixon MF. Crohn's-like reaction in diverticular disease. *Gut* 1998;**42**:392.

464. Shepherd NA. Diverticular disease and chronic idiopathic inflammatory bowel disease: associations and masquerades. *Gut* 1996;**38**:801.

465. Meyers MA, Alonso DR, Morson BC, Bartram C. Pathogenesis of diverticulitis complicating granulomatous colitis. *Gastroenterology* 1978;**74**:24.

466. Makapugay LM, Dean PJ. Diverticular disease-associated chronic colitis. *Am J Surg Pathol* 1996;**20**:94.

467. Tursi A, Elisei W, Brandimarte G, et al. The endoscopic spectrum of segmental colitis associated with diverticulosis. *Colorectal Dis* 2010;**12**:464.

468. Pereira MC. Diverticular disease-associated colitis: progression to severe chronic ulcerative colitis after sigmoid surgery [see comment]. *Gastrointest Endosc* 1998;**48**:520.

469. Tursi A. Segmental colitis associated with diverticulosis: complication of diverticular disease or autonomous entity? *Dig Dis Sci* 2011;**56**:27.

470. Lamps LW, Knapple WL. Diverticular disease-associated segmental colitis. *Clin Gastroenterol Hepatol* 2007;**5**:27.

471. Gourevitch A, Cunningham IJ. Sarcoidosis of the sigmoid colon. *Postgrad Med J* 1959;**35**:689.

472. Gregorie HB Jr, Othersen HB Jr, Moore MP Jr. The significance of sarcoid-like lesions in association with malignant neoplasms. *Am J Surg* 1962;**104**:577.

473. Tobi M, Kobrin I, Ariel I. Rectal involvement in sarcoidosis. *Dis Colon Rectum* 1982;**25**:491.

474. Gould SR, Handley AJ, Barnardo DE. Rectal and gastric involvement in a case of sarcoidosis. *Gut* 1973;**14**:971.

475. Herrera AF, Soriano G, Bellizzi AM, et al. Cord colitis syndrome in cord-blood stem-cell transplantation. *N Engl J Med* 2011;**365**;815.

476. Petri M, Poulsen SS, Christensen K, Jarnum S. The incidence of granulomas in serial sections of rectal biopsies from patients with Crohn's disease. *Acta Pathol Microbiol Immunol Scand A* 1982;**90**:145.

477. Rotterdam H, Korelitz BI, Sommers SC. Microgranulomas in grossly normal rectal mucosa in Crohn's disease. *Am J Clin Pathol* 1977;**67**:550.

478. Nostrant TT, Kumar NB, Appelman HD. Histopathology differentiates acute self-limited colitis from ulcerative colitis. *Gastroenterology* 1987;**92**:318.

479. Green FH, Fox H. The distribution of mucosal antibodies in the bowel of patients with Crohn's disease. *Gut* 1975;**16**:125.

480. Anonymous. Which type of colitis? *Lancet* 1988;**i**:336.

481. Surawicz CM, Belic L. Rectal biopsy helps to distinguish acute self-limited colitis from idiopathic inflammatory bowel disease. *Gastroenterology* 1984;**86**:104.

482. Surawicz CM. Diagnosing colitis. Biopsy is best. *Gastroenterology* 1987;**92**:538.

483. Rhodes JM, Black RR, Gallimore R, Savage A. Histochemical demonstration of desialation and desulphation of normal and inflammatory bowel disease rectal mucus by faecal extracts. *Gut* 1985;**26**:1312.

484. Sheng YH, Hasnain SZ, Florin TH, McGuckin MA. Mucins in inflammatory bowel disease and colorectal cancer. *J Gastroenterol Hepatol* 2012;**27**:28.

485. van Spreeuwel JP, Lindeman J, Meijer CJ. A quantitative study of immunoglobulin containing cells in the differential diagnosis of acute colitis. *J Clin Pathol* 1985;**38**:774.

486. Skinner JM, Whitehead R. The plasma cells in inflammatory disease of the colon: a quantitative study. *J Clin Pathol* 1974;**27**:643.

487. Pera A, Bellando P, Caldera D, et al. Colonoscopy in inflammatory bowel disease. Diagnostic accuracy and proposal of an endoscopic score. *Gastroenterology* 1987;**92**:181.

488. Bentley E, Jenkins D, Campbell F, Warren B. How could pathologists improve the initial diagnosis of colitis? Evidence from an international workshop [see comment]. *J Clin Pathol* 2002;**55**:955.

489. Kaufmann HJ, Taubin HL. Nonsteroidal anti-inflammatory drugs activate quiescent inflammatory bowel disease. *Ann Intern Med* 1987;**107**:513.

490. Lee FD. Importance of apoptosis in the histopathology of drug related lesions in the large intestine. *J Clin Pathol* 1993;**46**:118.

491. Byers RJ, Marsh P, Parkinson D, Haboubi NY. Melanosis coli is associated with an increase in colonic epithelial apoptosis and not with laxative use. *Histopathology* 1997;**30**:160.

492. Warren BF, Edwards CM, Travis SP. 'Microscopic colitis': classification and terminology. *Histopathology* 2002 Apr;**40**:374.

493. Robinson MH, Wheatley T, Leach IH. Nonsteroidal antiinflammatory drug-induced colonic stricture. An unusual cause of large bowel obstruction and perforation. *Dig Dis Sci* 1995;**40**:315.

494. Fellows IW, Clarke JM, Roberts PF. Non-steroidal anti-inflammatory drug-induced jejunal and colonic diaphragm disease: a report of two cases. *Gut* 1992;**33**:1424.

495. Gizzi G, Villani V, Brandi G, Paganelli GM, Di Febo G, Biasco G. Ano-rectal lesions in patients taking suppositories containing non-steroidal anti-inflammatory drugs (NSAID). *Endoscopy* 1990;**22**:146.

496. Levy N, Gaspar E. Letter: Rectal bleeding and indomethacin suppositories. *Lancet* 1975;**i**:577.

497. Villanacci V, Casella G, Bassotti G. The spectrum of drug-related colitides: Important entities, though frequently overlooked. *Dig Liver Dis* 2011;**43**:523.

498. Casella G, Villanacci V, Fisogni S, et al. Colonic left-side increase of eosinophils: a clue to drug-related colitis in adults. *Aliment Pharmacol Ther* 2009;**29**:535.

499. Fam AG, Paton TW, Shamess CJ, Lewis AJ. Fulminant colitis complicating gold therapy. *J Rheumatol* 1980;**7**:479.

500. Szpak MW, Johnson RC, Brady CE. Gold induced enterocolitis. *Gastroenterology* 1979;**76**:1257.

501. Jackson CW, Haboubi NY, Whorwell PJ, Schofield PF. Gold induced enterocolitis. *Gut* 1986;**27**:452.

502. Reinhart WH, Kappeler M, Halter F. Severe pseudomembranous and ulcerative colitis during gold therapy. *Endoscopy* 1983;**15**:70.

503. Floch MH, Hellman L. The effect of five-fluorouracil on rectal mucosa. *Gastroenterology* 1965;**48**:430.

504. Miller SS, Muggia AL, Spiro HM. Colonic histological changes induced by 5 fluorouracil. *Gastroenterology* 1962;**43**:391.

505. Daniels JA, Gibson MK, Xu L, et al. Gastrointestinal tract epithelial changes associated with taxanes: marker of drug toxicity versus effect. *Am J Surg Pathol* 2008;**32**:473.

506. Sparano JA, Dutcher JP, Kaleya R, et al. Colonic ischemia complicating immunotherapy with interleukin-2 and interferon-alpha. *Cancer* 1991;**68**:1538.

507. Deana DG, Dean PJ. Reversible ischemic colitis in young women. Association with oral contraceptive use. *Am J Surg Pathol* 1995;**19**:454.

508. Tedesco FJ, Volpicelli NA, Moore FS. Estrogen- and progesterone-associated colitis: a disorder with clinical and endoscopic features mimicking Crohn's colitis. *Gastrointest Endosc* 1982;**28**:247.

509. Nalbandian H, Sheth N, Dietrich R, Georgiou J. Intestinal ischemia caused by cocaine ingestion: report of two cases. *Surgery* 1985;**97**:374.

510. Montgomery E, Riddell RH. Ischemic colitis in a young patient. *Pathol Case Rev* 2004;**9**:93.

511. Rashid A, Hamilton SR. Necrosis of the gastrointestinal tract in uremic patients as a result of sodium polystyrene sulfonate (Kayexalate) in sorbitol: an underrecognized condition. *Am J Surg Pathol* 1997;**21**:60.

512. Joo M, Bae WK, Kim NH, Han SR. Colonic mucosal necrosis following administration of calcium polystyrene sulfonate (Kalimate) in a uremic patient. *J Korean Med Sci* 2009;**24**:1207.

513. McGowan CE, Saha S, Chu G, Resnick MB, Moss SF. Intestinal necrosis due to sodium polystyrene sulfonate (Kayexalate) in sorbitol. *South Med J* 2009;**102**:493.

514. Rugolotto S, Gruber M, Solano PD, Chini L, Gobbo S, Pecori S. Necrotizing enterocolitis in a 850 gram infant receiving sorbitol-free sodium polystyrene sulfonate (Kayexalate): clinical and histopathologic findings. *J Perinatol* 2007;**27**:247.

515. Martin P, Manley PN, Depew WT, Blakeman JM. Isotretinoin-associated proctosigmoiditis. *Gastroenterology* 1987;**93**:606.

516. Moshkowitz M, Konikoff FM, Arber N, Baratz M, Gilat T. Acyclovir-associated colitis. *Am J Gastroenterol* 1993;**88**:2110.

517. Behling KC, Foster DM, Edmonston TB, Witkiewicz AK. Graft-versus-host disease-like pattern in mycophenolate mofetil related colon mucosal injury: Role of FISH in establishing the diagnosis. *Case Rep Gastroenterol* 2009;**3**:418.

518. Selbst MK, Ahrens WA, Robert ME, Friedman A, Proctor DD, Jain D. Spectrum of histologic changes in colonic biopsies in patients treated with mycophenolate mofetil. *Mod Pathol* 2009;**22**:737.

519. Phatak UP, Seo-Mayer P, Jain D, Selbst M, Husain S, Pashankar DS. Mycophenolate mofetil-induced colitis in children. *J Clin Gastroenterol* 2009;**43**:967.

520. Lord JD, Hackman RC, Moklebust A, et al. Refractory colitis following anti-CTLA4 antibody therapy: analysis of mucosal FOXP3+ T cells. *Dig Dis Sci* 2010;**55**:1396.

521. Minor DR, Chin K, Kashani-Sabet M. Infliximab in the treatment of anti-CTLA4 antibody (ipilimumab) induced immune-related colitis. *Cancer Biother Radiopharm* 2009;**24**:321.

522. Bhatia S, Huber BR, Upton MP, Thompson JA. Inflammatory enteric neuropathy with severe constipation after ipilimumab treatment for melanoma: a case report. *J Immunother* 2009;**32**:203.

523. Ramsden WH, Moya EF, Littlewood JM. Colonic wall thickness, pancreatic enzyme dose and type of preparation in cystic fibrosis. *Arch Dis Child* 1998;**79**:339.

524. Welkon CJ, Long SS, Thompson CM Jr, Gilligan PH. *Clostridium difficile* in patients with cystic fibrosis. *Am J Dis Child* 1985;**139**:805.

525. Lishman AH, Al-Jumaili IJ, Record CO. Spectrum of antibiotic-associated diarrhoea. *Gut* 1981;**22**:34.

526. Burdon DW, George RH, Mogg GA, et al. Faecal toxin and severity of antibiotic-associated pseudomembranous colitis. *J Clin Pathol* 1981;**34**:548.

527. Borriello SP, Ketley JM, Mitchell TJ, et al. *Clostridium difficile* – a spectrum of virulence and analysis of putative virulence determinants in the hamster model of antibiotic-associated colitis. *J Med Microbiol* 1987;**24**:53.

528. Bartlett JG, Chang TW, Gurwith M, Gorbach SL, Onderdonk AB. Antibiotic-associated pseudomembranous colitis due to toxin-producing clostridia. *N Engl J Med* 1978;**298**:531.

529. Gerding DN, Olson MM, Peterson LR, et al. *Clostridium difficile*-associated diarrhea and colitis in adults. A prospective case-controlled epidemiologic study. *Arch Intern Med* 1986;**146**:95.

530. Taylor NS, Thorne GM, Bartlett JG. Comparison of two toxins produced by *Clostridium difficile*. *Infect Immun* 1981;**34**:1036.

531. Larson HE, Price AB. Pseudomembranous colitis: Presence of clostridial toxin. *Lancet* 1977;**ii**:1312.

532. Penner A, Bernheim AI. Acute post-operative enterocolitis. *Arch Pathol* 1939;**27**:966.

533. Whitehead R. Ischaemic enterocolitis: an expression of the intravascular coagulation syndrome. *Gut* 1971;**12**:912.

534. Shortland JR, Spencer RC, Williams JL. Pseudomembranous colitis associated with changes in an ileal conduit. *J Clin Pathol* 1983;**36**:1184.

535. Cone JB, Wetzel W. Toxic megacolon secondary to pseudomembranous colitis. *Dis Colon Rectum* 1982;**25**:478.

536. Snooks SJ, Hughes A, Horsburgh AG. Perforated colon complicating pseudomembranous colitis. *Br J Surg* 1984;**71**:291.

537. Seppala K, Hjelt L, Sipponen P. Colonoscopy in the diagnosis of antibiotic-associated colitis. A prospective study. *Scand J Gastroenterol* 1981;**16**:465.

538. Tedesco FJ, Corless JK, Brownstein RE. Rectal sparing in antibiotic-associated pseudomembranous colitis: a prospective study. *Gastroenterology* 1982;**83**:1259.

539. Price AB, Davies DR. Pseudomembranous colitis. *J Clin Pathol* 1977;**30**:1.

540. Price AB. Histopathology of clostridial gut disease in man. In: Borriello SP (ed.), *Clostridia in Gastrointestinal Disease*. Boca Raton, FL: CRC Press, 1985: 177.

541. Price AB, Day DW. Pseudomembraneous and infective colitis. In: Anthony PP, MacSween RNM (eds), *Recent Advances in Histopathology*. Edinburgh: Churchill Livingstone, 1981. p. 99.

542. Holst E, Helin I, Mardh PA. Recovery of *Clostridium difficile* from children. *Scand J Infect Dis* 1981;**13**:41.

543. Dickinson RJ, Rampling A, Wight DG. Spontaneous pseudomembranous colitis not associated with *Clostridium difficile*. *J Infect* 1985;**10**:252.

544. Cundy T, Trafford JA, Thom BT, Somerville PG. *Clostridium difficile* and non-antibiotic-associated colitis. *Lancet* 1980;**ii**:595.

545. Rocca JM, Pieterse AS, Rowland R, Hecker R, Rich GE. *Clostridium difficile* colitis. *Austr N Z J Med* 1984;**14**:606.

546. Wald A, Mendelow H, Bartlett JG. Non-antibiotic-associated pseudomembranous colitis due to toxin-producing Clostridia. *Ann Intern Med* 1980;**92**:798.

547. Wren B, Heard SR, Tabaqchali S. Association between production of toxins A and B and types of Clostridium difficile. *J Clin Pathol* 1987;**40**:1397.

548. Meyers S, Mayer L, Bottone E, Desmond E, Janowitz HD. Occurrence of *Clostridium difficile* toxin during the course of inflammatory bowel disease. *Gastroenterology* 1981;**80**:697.

549. Sullivan NM, Pellett S, Wilkins TD. Purification and characterization of toxins A and B of Clostridium difficile. *Infect Immun* 1982;**35**:1032.

550. Larson HE, Price AB, Borriello SP. Epidemiology of experimental enterocecitis due to Clostridium difficile. *J Infect Dis* 1980;**142**:408.

551. Keighley MR, Burdon DW, Alexander-Williams J, et al. Diarrhoea and pseudomembranous colitis after gastrointestinal operations. A prospective study. *Lancet* 1978;**ii**:1165.

552. Carter GP, Rood JI, Lyras D. The role of toxin A and toxin B in *Clostridium difficile*-associated disease: Past and present perspectives. *Gut Microbes* 2010;**1**:58.

553. Freeman J, Bauer MP, Baines SD, et al. The changing epidemiology of *Clostridium difficile* infections. *Clin Microbiol Rev* 2010;**23**:529.

554. Duerr RH, Targan SR, Landers CJ, Sutherland LR, Shanahan F. Anti-neutrophil cytoplasmic antibodies in ulcerative colitis. Comparison with other colitides/diarrheal illnesses.[see comment]. *Gastroenterology* 1991;**100**:1590.

555. Osterholm MT, MacDonald KL, White KE, et al. An outbreak of a newly recognized chronic diarrhea syndrome associated with raw milk consumption. *JAMA* 1986;**256**:484.

556. Mintz ED, Weber JT, Guris D, et al. An outbreak of Brainerd diarrhea among travelers to the Galapagos Islands. *J Infect Dis* 1998;**177**:1041.

557. Bryant DA, Mintz ED, Puhr ND, Griffin PM, Petras RE. Colonic epithelial lymphocytosis associated with an epidemic of chronic diarrhea. *Am J Surg Pathol* 1996;**20**:1102.

558. Schneider EN, Havens JM, Scott MA, Goldblum JR, Greenson JK, Shaffer RA, et al. Molecular diagnosis of Campylobacter jejuni infection in cases of focal active colitis. *Am J Surg Pathol* 2006;**30**:782.

559. Xin W, Brown PI, Greenson JK. The clinical significance of focal active colitis in paediatric patients. *Am J Surg Pathol* 2003;**27**:1134.

560. Shetty S, Anjarwalla SM, Gupta J, et al. Focal active colitis: a prospective study of clinico-pathological correlations in 90 patients. *Histopathology* in press.

561. Schofield PF, Holden D, Carr ND. Bowel disease after radiotherapy. *J R Soc Med* 1983;**76**:463.

562. Perkins DE, Spjut HJ. Intestinal stenosis following radiation therapy. *Am J Roentgenol Radium Ther Nucl Med* 1962;**88**:953.

563. Hasleton PS, Carr N, Schofield PF. Vascular changes in radiation bowel disease. *Histopathology* 1985;**9**:517.

564. Berthrong M, Fajardo LF. Radiation injury in surgical pathology. Part II. Alimentary tract. *Am J Surg Pathol* 1981;**5**:153.

565. DeCosse JJ, Rhodes RS, Wentz WB, Reagan JW, Dworken HJ, Holden WD. The natural history and management of radiation induced injury of the gastrointestinal tract. *Ann Surg* 1969;**170**:369.

566. Gelfand MD, Tepper M, Katz LA, Binder HJ, Yesner R, Floch MH. Acute irradiation proctitis in man: development of eosinophilic crypt abscesses. *Gastroenterology* 1968;**54**:401.

567. McFadyen IR, Price AB, Geirsson RT. The relation of birthweight to histological appearances in vessels of the placental bed. *Br J Obstet Gynaecol* 1986;**93**:476.

568. Counter SF, Froese DP, Hart MJ. Prospective evaluation of formalin therapy for radiation proctitis. *Am J Surg* 1999;**177**:396.

569. Pikarsky AJ, Belin B, Efron J, Weiss EG, Nogueras JJ, Wexner SD. Complications following formalin installation in the treatment of radiation induced proctitis. *Int J Colorectal Dis* 2000;**15**:96.

570. Glotzer DJ, Glick ME, Goldman H. Proctitis and colitis following diversion of the fecal stream. *Gastroenterology* 1981;**80**:438.

571. Geraghty JM, Talbot IC. Diversion colitis: histological features in the colon and rectum after defunctioning colostomy. *Gut* 1991;**32**:1020.

572. Warren BF, Shepherd NA. Diversion proctocolitis. *Histopathology* 1992;**21**:91.

573. Harig JM, Soergel KH, Komorowski RA, Wood CM. Treatment of diversion colitis with short-chain-fatty acid irrigation. *N Engl J Med* 1989;**320**:23.

574. Guillemot F, Colombel JF, Neut C, et al. Treatment of diversion colitis by short-chain fatty acids. Prospective and double-blind study. *Dis Colon Rectum* 1991;**34**:861.

575. Neut C, Guillemot F, Colombel JF. Nitrate-reducing bacteria in diversion colitis: a clue to inflammation? *Dig Dis Sci* 1997;**42**:2577.

576. Roe AM, Warren BF, Brodribb AJ, Brown C. Diversion colitis and involution of the defunctioned anorectum. *Gut* 1993;**34**:382.

577. Yeong ML, Bethwaite PB, Prasad J, Isbister WH. Lymphoid follicular hyperplasia – a distinctive feature of diversion colitis. *Histopathology* 1991;**19**:55.

578. Lusk LB, Reichen J, Levine JS. Aphthous ulceration in diversion colitis. Clinical implications. *Gastroenterology* 1984;**87**:1171.

579. Murray FE, O'Brien MJ, Birkett DH, Kennedy SM, LaMont JT. Diversion colitis. Pathologic findings in a resected sigmoid colon and rectum. *Gastroenterology* 1987;**93**:1404.

580. Haque S, Eisen RN, West AB. The morphologic features of diversion colitis: studies of a pediatric population with no other disease of the intestinal mucosa. *Hum Pathol* 1993;**24**:211.

581. Harper PH, Lee EC, Kettlewell MG, Bennett MK, Jewell DP. Role of the faecal stream in the maintenance of Crohn's colitis. *Gut* 1985;**26**:279.

582. Korelitz BI, Cheskin LJ, Sohn N, Sommers SC. The fate of the rectal segment after diversion of the fecal stream in Crohn's disease: its implications for surgical management. *J Clin Gastroenterol* 1985;**7**:37.

583. Griffiths AP, Dixon MF. Microcarcinoids and diversion colitis in a colon defunctioned for 18 years. Report of a case. *Dis Colon Rectum* 1992;**35**:685.

584. Killingback MJ, Williams KL. Necrotizing colitis. *Br J Surg* 1961;**49**:175.

585. Wade DS, Nava HR, Douglass HO Jr. Neutropenic enterocolitis. Clinical diagnosis and treatment. *Cancer* 1992;**69**:17.

586. Newbold KM, Lord MG, Baglin TP. Role of clostridial organisms in neutropenic enterocolitis. *J Clin Pathol* 1987;**40**:471.

587. Kay AW, Richards RL, Watson AJ. Acute necrotizing (pseudomembranous) enterocolitis. *Br J Surg* 1958;**46**:45.

588. Taylor AJ, Dodds WJ, Gonyo JE, Komorowski RA. Typhlitis in adults. *Gastrointest Radiol* 1985;**10**:363.

589. Alt B, Glass NR, Sollinger H. Neutropenic enterocolitis in adults. Review of the literature and assessment of surgical intervention. *Am J Surg* 1985;**149**:405.

590. Kies MS, Luedke DW, Boyd JF, McCue MJ. Neutropenic enterocolitis: two case reports of long-term survival following surgery. *Cancer* 1979;**43**:730.

591. Moir DH, Bale PM. Necropsy findings in childhood leukaemia, emphasizing neutropenic enterocolitis and cerebral calcification. *Pathology* 1976;**8**:247.

592. Mulholland MW, Delaney JP. Neutropenic colitis and aplastic anemia: a new association. *Ann Surg* 1983;**197**:84.

593. King A, Rampling A, Wight DG, Warren RE. Neutropenic enterocolitis due to *Clostridium septicum* infection. *J Clin Pathol* 1984;**37**:335.

594. Rifkin GD. Neutropenic enterocolitis and *Clostridium septicum* infection in patients with agranulocytosis. *Arch Intern Med* 1980;**140**:834.

595. Santulli TV, Schullinger JN, Heird WC, et al. Acute necrotizing enterocolitis in infancy: a review of 64 cases. *Pediatrics* 1975;**55**:376.

596. Kliegman RM, Fanaroff AA. Neonatal necrotizing enterocolitis: a nine-year experience. *Am J Dis Child* 1981;**135**:603.

597. Rosen Y, Won OK. Phlegmonous enterocolitis. *Am J Dig Dis* 1978;**23**:248.

598. Kliegman RM, Fanaroff AA. Neonatal necrotizing enterocolitis in the absence of pneumatosis intestinalis. *Am J Dis Child* 1982;**136**:618.

599. Treszl A, Tulassay T, Vasarhelyi B. Genetic basis for necrotizing enterocolitis – risk factors and their relations to genetic polymorphisms. *Front Biosci* 2006;**11**:570.

600. Kliegman RM, Fanaroff AA. Neonatal necrotizing enterocolitis: a nine-year experience. II. Outcome assessment. *Am J Dis Child* 1981;**135**:608.

601. Howard FM, Flynn DM, Bradley JM, Noone P, Szawatkowski M. Outbreak of necrotising enterocolitis caused by Clostridium butyricum. *Lancet* 1977;**ii**:1099.

602. Lindstrom CG. 'Collagenous colitis' with watery diarrhoea – a new entity? *Pathol Eur* 1976;**11**:87.

603. Bogomoletz WV. Collagenous colitis: a clinicopathological review. *Surv Dig Dis* 1983;**1**:19.

604. Kingham JG, Levison DA, Ball JA, Dawson AM. Microscopic colitis-a cause of chronic watery diarrhoea. *BMJ (Clin Res Ed)* 1982;**285**:1601.

605. Ayata G, Ithamukkala S, Sapp H, et al. Prevalence and significance of inflammatory bowel disease-like morphologic features in collagenous and lymphocytic colitis. *Am J Surg Pathol* 2002;**26**:1414.

606. Sapp H, Ithamukkala S, Brien TP, et al. The terminal ileum is affected in patients with lymphocytic or collagenous colitis. *Am J Surg Pathol* 2002;**26**:1484.

607. Rask-Madsen J, Grove O, Hansen MG, Bukhave K, Scient C, Henrik-Nielsen R. Colonic transport of water and electrolytes in a patient with secretory diarrhea due to collagenous colitis. *Dig Dis Sci* 1983;**28**:1141.

608. Mullhaupt B, Guller U, Anabitarte M, Guller R, Fried M. Lymphocytic colitis: clinical presentation and long term course. *Gut* 1998;**43**:629.

609. Lazenby AJ, Yardley JH, Giardiello FM, Jessurun J, Bayless TM. Lymphocytic ('microscopic') colitis: a comparative histopathologic study with particular reference to collagenous colitis. *HumPathol* 1989;**20**:18.

610. Bossart R, Henry K, Booth CC, Doe WF. Subepithelial collagen in intestinal malabsorption. *Gut* 1975;**16**:18.

611. Rampton DS, Baithun SI. Is microscopic colitis due to bile-salt malabsorption? *Dis Colon Rectum* 1987;**30**:950.

612. Gledhill A, Cole FM. Significance of basement membrane thickening in the human colon. *Gut* 1984;**25**:1085.

613. Christ AD, Meier R, Bauerfeind P, Wegmann W, Gyr K. [Simultaneous occurrence of lymphocytic gastritis and lymphocytic colitis with transition to collagenous colitis.] *Schweiz Med Wochenschr* 1993;**123**:1487.

614. Saul SH. The watery diarrhea-colitis syndrome. A review of collagenous and microscopic/lymphocytic colitis. *Int J Surg Pathol* 1993;**1**:65.

615. Bo-Linn GW, Vendrell DD, Lee E, Fordtran JS. An evaluation of the significance of microscopic colitis in patients with chronic diarrhea. *J Clin Invest* 1985;**75**:1559.

616. Hamilton I, Sanders S, Hopwood D, Bouchier IA. Collagenous colitis associated with small intestinal villous atrophy. *Gut* 1986;**27**:1394.

617. Bogomoletz WV. Collagenous, microscopic and lymphocytic colitis. An evolving concept. *Virchows Arch* 1994;**424**:573.

618. Fine KD, Lee EL, Meyer RL. Colonic histopathology in untreated celiac sprue or refractory sprue: is it lymphocytic colitis or colonic lymphocytosis? *Hum Pathol* 1998;**29**:1433.

619. DuBois RN, Lazenby AJ, Yardley JH, Hendrix TR, Bayless TM, Giardiello FM. Lymphocytic enterocolitis in patients with 'refractory sprue'. *JAMA* 1989;**262**:935.

620. Bohr J, Tysk C, Jarnerot G. Microscopic colitis. *Medicine* 1998;**26**:93.

621. Fraser AG, Warren BF, Chandrapala R, Jewell DP. Microscopic colitis: a clinical and pathological review. *Scand J Gastroenterol* 2002;**37**:1241.

622. Chang F, Deere H, Vu C. Atypical forms of microscopic colitis: morphological features and review of the literature. *Adv Anat Pathol* 2005;**12**:203.

623. Brown IS, Lambie DL. Microscopic colitis with giant cells: a clinico-pathological review of 11 cases and comparison with microscopic colitis without giant cells. *Pathology* 2008;**40**:671.

624. Libbrecht L, Croes R, Ectors N, Staels F, Geboes K. Microscopic colitis with giant cells. *Histopathology* 2002;**40**:335.

625. Iwai H, Hisamatsu T, Iizuka H, et al. Microscopic colitis with granuloma which responded to steroid therapy. *Intern Med* 2007;**46**:1551.

626. Saurine TJ, Brewer JM, Eckstein RP. Microscopic colitis with granulomatous inflammation. *Histopathology* 2004;**45**:82.

627. Fernandez-Banares F, Casalots J, Salas A, et al. Paucicellular lymphocytic colitis: is it a minor form of lymphocytic colitis? A clinical pathological and immunological study. *Am J Gastroenterol* 2009;**104**:1189.

628. Goldstein NS, Bhanot P. Paucicellular and asymptomatic lymphocytic colitis: expanding the clinicopathologic spectrum of lymphocytic colitis. *Am J Clin Pathol* 2004;**122**:405.

629. Maguire AA, Greenson JK, Lauwers GY, et al. Collagenous sprue: a clinicopathologic study of 12 cases. *Am J Surg Pathol* 2009;**33**:1440.

630. Allende DS, Taylor SL, Bronner MP. Colonic perforation as a complication of collagenous colitis in a series of 12 patients. *Am J Gastroenterol* 2008;**103**:2598.

631. Sherman A, Ackert JJ, Rajapaksa R, West AB, Oweity T. Fractured colon: an endoscopically distinctive lesion associated with colonic perforation following colonoscopy in patients with collagenous colitis. *J Clin Gastroenterol* 2004;**38**:341.

632. Yuan S, Reyes V, Bronner MP. Pseudomembranous collagenous colitis. *Am J Surg Pathol* 2003;**10**:1375.

633. Jessurun J, Yardley JH, Giardiello FM, Hamilton SR, Bayless TM. Chronic colitis with thickening of the subepithelial collagen layer (collagenous colitis): histopathologic findings in 15 patients. *Hum Pathol* 1987;**18**:839.

634. Teglbjaerg PS, Thaysen EH, Jensen HH. Development of collagenous colitis in sequential biopsy specimens. *Gastroenterology* 1984;**87**:703.

635. Hwang WS, Kelly JK, Shaffer EA, Hershfield NB. Collagenous colitis: a disease of pericryptal fibroblast sheath? *J Pathol* 1986;**149**:33.

636. Chetty R, Govender D. Lymphocytic and collagenous colitis: an overview of so-called microscopic colitis. *Nat Rev Gastroenterol Hepatol* 2012;**21**:209.

637. Fausa O, Foerster A, Hovig T. Collagenous colitis. A clinical, histological, and ultrastructural study. *Scand J Gastroenterol Suppl* 1985;**107**:8.

638. Richman PI, Tilly R, Jass JR, Bodmer WF. Colonic pericrypt sheath cells: characterisation of cell type with new monoclonal antibody. *J Clin Pathol* 1987;**40**:593.

639. Pascal RR, Kaye GI, Lane N. Colonic pericryptal fibroblast sheath: replication, migration, and cytodifferentiation of a mesenchymal cell system in adult tissue. I. Autoradiographic studies of normal rabbit colon. *Gastroenterology* 1968;**54**:835.

640. Kaye GI, Fenoglio CM, Pascal RR, Lane N. Comparative electron microscopic features of normal, hyperplastic, and adenomatous human colonic epithelium. Variations in cellular structure relative to the process of epithelial differentiation. *Gastroenterology* 1973;**64**:926.

641. Riddell RH, Tanaka M, Mazzoleni G. Non-steroidal anti-inflammatory drugs as a possible cause of collagenous colitis: a case-control study. *Gut* 1992;**33**:683.

642. Williams GT, Rhodes J. Collagenous colitis: disease or diversion? *BMJ (Clin Res Ed)* 1987;**294**:855.

643. Kakar S, Pardi DS, Burgart LJ. Colonic ulcers accompanying collagenous colitis: implication of nonsteroidal anti-inflammatory drugs. *Am J Gastroenterol* 2003;**98**:1834.

644. Kirsch R, Riddell RH. Histopathological alterations in irritable bowel syndrome. *Mod Pathol* 2006;**19**:1638.

645. Jakate S, Demeo M, John R, Tobin M, Keshavarzian A. Mastocytic enterocolitis: increased mucosal mast cells in chronic intractable diarrhea. *Arch Pathol Lab Med* 2006;**130**:362.

646. Ogilvie-McDaniel C, Blaiss M, Osborn FD, Carpenter J. Mastocytic enterocolitis: a newly described mast cell entity. *Ann Allergy Asthma Immunol* 2008;**101**:645.

647. Ramsay DB, Stephen S, Borum M, Voltaggio L, Doman DB. Mast cells in gastrointestinal disease. *Gastroenterol Hepatol (NY)* 2010;**6**:772.

648. Blei ED, Abrahams C. Diffuse phlegmonous gastroenterocolitis in a patient with an infected peritoneo-jugular venous shunt. *Gastroenterology* 1983;**84**:636.

649. Holzer T, Gervaz P, Spahr L, McKee T, Bucher P, Morel P. Phlegmonous colitis: another source of sepsis in cirrhotic patients? *BMC Gastroenterol* 2009;**9**:94.

650. Toner M, Condell D, O'Briain DS. Obstructive colitis. Ulceratoinflammatory lesions occurring proximal to colonic obstruction. *Am J Surg Pathol* 1990;**14**:719.

651. Moriwaki Y, Sugiyama M, Toyoda H, et al. Lethal obstructive colitis: how and when patients with colonic obstruction should be prevented from falling into a lethal condition. *Hepatogastroenterology* 2009;**56**:659.

652. Gratama S, Smedts F, Whitehead R. Obstructive colitis: an analysis of 50 cases and a review of the literature. *Pathology* 1995;**27**:324.

653. Rettig PJ. Campylobacter infections in human beings. *J Pediatr* 1979;**94**:855.

654. Levine TS, Price AB. Obstructive enterocolitis: a clinicopathological discussion. *Histopathology* 1994;**25**:57.

655. Leonard N, Palazzo J, Jameson J, Denman AM, Talbot IC, Price AB. Behçet's colitis has distinctive pathological features. *Int J Surg Pathol* 1998;**6**:1.

656. Kasahara Y, Tanaka S, Nishino M, Umemura H, Shiraha S, Kuyama T. Intestinal involvement in Behcet's disease: review of 136 surgical cases in the Japanese literature. *Dis Colon Rectum* 1981;**24**:103.

657. Smith GE, Kime LR, Pitcher JL. The diagnosis of Behcet's disease: a separate entity? Colonoscopic findings and literature review. *Am J Dig Dis* 1973;**18**:987.

658. Lee RG. The colitis of Behcet's syndrome. *Am J Surg Pathol* 1986;**10**:888.

CHAPTER 36

Vascular disorders of the large intestine

Cian Muldoon

St James's Hospital, Dublin, Ireland

Anatomy

The colon is supplied by both the superior mesenteric and the inferior mesenteric arteries. The latter artery becomes the superior rectal artery when it crosses the pelvic brim. It supplies most of the rectum, bifurcating into left and right branches, which pass downwards on either side of the mesorectum. The middle and inferior rectal arteries, derived from the internal iliac and pudendal arteries, respectively, contribute to the blood supply of the lower rectum. Two important anastomotic links exist between the inferior and superior mesenteric arteries which, after occlusion of one of the major vessels, have a role in maintaining the viability of the bowel. The marginal artery is an arterial arcade situated along the mesocolic surface of the entire colon, connecting the main branches of the inferior and superior mesenteric vessels. The second anastomotic link is the 'arc of Riolan' between the left colic artery and the middle colic artery. The splenic flexure is potentially a vulnerable region, being at the junction of the main distribution zones of the superior and inferior mesenteric vessels. However, injection studies suggest that there is not consistently a 'watershed' at this point and an analysis of cases reveals more lower left-sided ischaemic colitis than disease at the splenic flexure [1,2]. Venous return is to the portal system. The internal rectal plexus outside the rectal wall communicates via the superior and inferior rectal veins with the portal and systemic venous systems, respectively. Portosystemic anastomoses are present around the lower rectum and anus.

Nomenclature

The terminology used in the setting of ischaemic colitis is varied and potentially confusing. Terms such as 'gangrene', 'haemorrhagic necrosis' and 'haemorrhagic necrotising colitis' have been variably employed to describe severe acute ischaemic colitis. This confusion is only added to by the apparent overlap with disorders such as necrotising enterocolitis. These terms are better avoided and use of the terms 'ischaemic colitis' and, where appropriate, 'infarction' is recommended. The former can be qualified by terms reflecting severity and duration of the ischaemic episode.

Causes of ischaemic colitis

The causes of large intestinal ischaemia are numerous and, although a single cause may be identified in a minority of cases, the pathogenesis is often multifactorial. Ischaemic injury to the large bowel can be the result of arterial impairment, venous impairment or any cause of a low flow state. The aetiology and pathogenesis are very similar to those affecting the small bowel (see Chapter 22) and the same factors of gradual arterial occlusion, more acute blockage and hypotension are equally applicable in the large intestine.

Both inferior and superior mesenteric arteries are liable to atheromatous narrowing, especially at their origins from the aorta. Of the two, the superior mesenteric artery is more prone to occlusion by thrombosis or embolism because of its larger calibre and less acute angle of take-off from the aorta. Other causes of arterial impairment include aortic dissection and systemic vasculitis. Possible causes of intestinal venous impairment include mesenteric vein thrombosis, vasculitis, enterocolic lymphocytic phlebitis and idiopathic myointimal hyperplasia of mesenteric veins. Vascular compression due, for instance, to volvulus, intussusception, tumour or prolapse may have similar consequences. Likewise, microangiopathic disorders such as those seen in diabetes, hypertension and some hypercoagulable states may result in ischaemic colitis.

As with small intestinal ischaemia, in up to 30% of cases no vascular lesion is evident. Ischaemic colitis can occur purely as a result of any cause of a low flow state such as cardiogenic shock, sepsis or haemorrhage [3]. It has also been described in long distance runners [4] and in pregnancy [5].

In those cases in which no cause is immediately apparent, it is important to remember that drugs can be responsible for ischaemic colitis. Most frequent causes among these are non-steroidal anti-inflammatory drugs, which tend to affect the right side of the colon more than the left and, in addition to flat ulcers, can cause diaphragm-like strictures [6]. Other drugs shown to cause ischaemic colitis are cocaine [7], pseudoephedrine [8], widely used in patent cough medicines, and 5-hydroxytryptamine (5HT) agonists used in the treatment of migraine such as sumatriptan [9]. Oral contraceptive agents and hormone replacement therapy are also associated with increased risk [10,11].

Ischaemic lesions

Ischaemic lesions in the large bowel, whether full thickness with necrosis or less extensive with predominantly mucosal damage and subsequent stricture formation, bear a striking similarity to those seen in the small bowel. The reaction of the colon to ischaemia can be divided into three phases [2]:

(1) acute, with haemorrhage and necrosis

(2) reparative, with granulation tissue formation and fibrosis

(3) residual pathology, with ischaemic stricture and chronic complications.

The location and extent of ischaemic lesions in the colon are a reflection of the anatomy and physiology of the blood supply. Compared with the small bowel, the blood supply of the colon is relatively poor and this is particularly true of the supply to the left side. The importance of the anastomotic vessels between the superior and inferior mesenteric vessels has already been mentioned. In a review of over 1000 cases of ischaemic colitis, the distribution was: right colon 8%, transverse colon 15%, splenic flexure 23%, descending colon 27%, sigmoid colon 23% and rectum 4% [12]. Rectal involvement is being recognised with increas-

ing frequency [12,13], can result in gross appearances resembling carcinoma [14] and can occur after aortic surgery [15]. There are a few case reports of caecal ischaemia [16], although right-sided disease was reported in 25% of one series of ischaemic colitis [17]. It must be remembered that combined involvement of small and large intestine is not infrequent [18]. The susceptibility of the colon to ischaemia can be demonstrated post mortem when careful microscopic examination often reveals early mucosal lesions, many of which are agonal in nature.

Macroscopic appearance

The appearances of colonic ischaemia vary with the severity and duration of the ischaemic insult and with the interval between that insult and the time of examination, the latter determining the degree of regeneration present. The hallmark of ischaemic lesions is, however, their sharp demarcation from the adjacent unaffected bowel.

In the earliest stages the bowel is pale and oedematous with patchy mucosal granularity and erythema. With time this is replaced by a more darkly and diffusely congested and oedematous mucosa with a cobblestone-type appearance (Figure 36.1). Mucosal necrosis leads to greenish–grey ulceration, which is typically superficial and linear in distribution but is less often deeper. Occasionally the ulceration is confluent and extensive. The lumen is filled with altered blood. Inflammatory polyposis due to undermining ulceration of mucosa with the formation of mucosal tags can occasionally arise. Submucosal oedema is usually extremely marked. In cases of greater severity there may be an inflammatory peritoneal reaction, sometimes with frank perforation. The overall appearance can mimic that seen in fulminating ulcerative colitis with toxic megacolon.

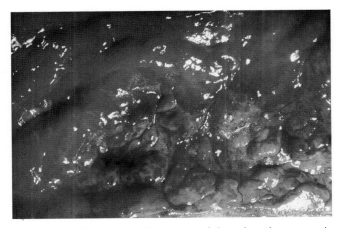

Figure 36.1 Acute ischaemic necrosis of the colon: the mucosa is deeply congested and coarsely cobblestoned due to submucosal oedema and haemorrhage.

When infarction of the colon involves only part of the thickness of the wall, mucosal necrosis may give rise to a shaggy white or grey membrane, loosely adherent to the luminal surface. This can lead to confusion with pseudo-membranous colitis, particularly in cases where the ischaemic changes are multifocal rather than segmental. This distinction can at times also be difficult to make at microscopy (see below). Transmural necrosis, on the other hand, may cause initial pallor, followed by a black or a more congested and haemorrhagic red/purple discoloration. Perforation may then ensue.

In patients who survive an episode of ischaemia for some days or longer, signs of resolution will appear. The bowel wall becomes thicker, contracted and indurated; the very dark appearance gradually diminishes; and the changes fade slowly into the stage of stricture formation with pallor, contraction and thickening of the bowel wall. With the formation of a stricture and the disappearance of any acute changes, the macroscopic picture may be less specifically ischaemic and may resemble a Crohn's disease stricture.

The vascular supply to the bowel wall should always be examined for evidence of aneurysm, atherosclerosis, thrombosis or embolism. Likewise at post mortem examination the abdominal aorta and origins of the main mesenteric vessels should be inspected for evidence of vascular abnormalities.

Microscopic appearance

Acute ischaemia

The microscopic features of ischaemic colitis are relatively distinctive and can usually be readily distinguished from acute ulcerative colitis and other inflammatory bowel diseases. There is haemorrhage into the mucosa and sometimes the submucosa, with oedema and necrosis. In more severe cases only a shadowy outline of the normal histology remains, with so-called 'ghost outlines' of crypts and vessels evident within the necrotic mucosal compartment (Figure 36.2). In less severe cases the mucosal crypts often show loss of their more superficial epithelial components with preservation of their deeper elements. There may be deposition of fibrin and necrotic tissue on the denuded luminal surface (Figure 36.3). Occasionally this material takes the form of mushroom-like collections that appear to originate from dilated crypt remnants. Therein lies the potential confusion at a microscopic level with *Clostridium difficile*-related pseudo-membranous colitis.

There is only a sparse neutrophilic infiltrate during the early stages. This helps to distinguish ischaemia from acute colitis due to infection or inflammatory bowel disease, although cryptitis and crypt abscesses may occasionally be seen in acute ischaemic colitis. Later the inflammatory infiltrate usually becomes more intense and is accompanied by mucosal ulceration and sloughing. Fibrin thrombi within

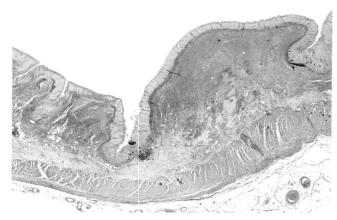

Figure 36.2 Acute colonic ischaemia, with mucosal necrosis (pale zone), prominent submucosal oedema and haemorrhage.

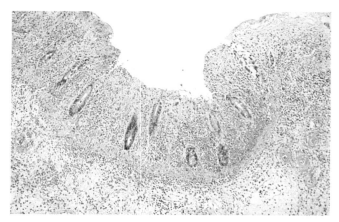

Figure 36.3 Acute colonic ischaemia, showing dissolution of the upper parts of the crypts. There is haemorrhage, oedema and a mild acute inflammatory infiltrate.

mucosal and submucosal capillaries are often found and are non-specific [19]. Frequently, after ischaemic ulceration, there is an acute endophlebitis of veins draining the ulcerated areas, within the submucosa and bowel wall. This may even extend along the veins to involve the extramural mesenteric veins, in the manner of a pyelophlebitis. It has been suggested that such a picture can arise anew, and be the cause rather than the effect of ischaemic ulceration, but this is very difficult to confirm in an individual case.

In many examples of acute ischaemic disease of the colon the histological changes are confined to the mucosa and submucosa. This is, at a microscopic level, usually patchy with intact normal intervening mucosa that is raised up by submucosal oedema or haemorrhage. This gives a 'cobblestone' appearance that accounts for the characteristic 'thumbprinting' radiological sign. It would appear that the muscularis propria is relatively resistant to the effects of acute deprivation of blood. However, as in early small intestinal ischaemia, the muscle fibres may show impaired staining and loss of nuclei. With greater severity and duration of ischaemia there is necrosis of the muscularis propria and often of the subserosa with associated perforation and peritoneal inflammation.

Distinction of ischaemic colitis from *Clostridium*-induced pseudo-membranous colitis can, as mentioned above, be difficult both macroscopically and histologically. This is in part explained by the probable role of exotoxin-induced ischaemia in the latter disorder. Differentiation of these diseases on biopsy histology can be particularly difficult. The presence of lamina propria fibrosis and haemorrhage, full-thickness mucosal necrosis or small atrophic residual crypts is said to favour ischaemic colitis. The presence of fibrosis is particularly useful and can be confirmed, if necessary, using a trichrome stain [20]. Correlation with clinical, endoscopic and microbiological features is imperative in this setting.

Reparative phase

The effects of acute ischaemia are followed by subacute and chronic inflammation, with the formation of granulation tissue and a mixed population of acute and chronic inflammatory cells. Capillary proliferation, macrophage activity and fibroblast production complete the picture until the mucosal epithelium begins to regenerate. Microscopic fissures may lead down to or into the muscularis propria at points of deeper anoxic damage (Figure 36.4). Entrapped particles of foreign material may provoke a giant cell reaction. The granulation tissue reaction is generally exuberant and, together with the residual islands of inflamed and sometimes hyperplastic mucosal glands, presents a pattern mimicking Crohn's disease or active fulminant ulcerative colitis. Eosinophils and iron pigment-laden histiocytes are a variable element. The presence of iron-positive granules

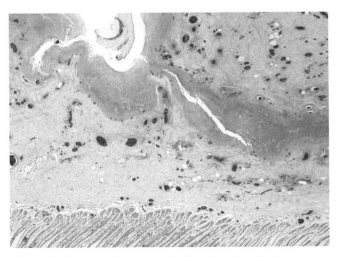

Figure 36.4 Mucosal necrosis with fissuring ulceration in ischaemic colitis.

in histiocytes reflects previous haemorrhage in the submucosa and mucosa, and can be useful in differentiating ischaemia from inflammatory bowel disease. Epithelial cell regeneration is visible at the margin of the mucosal ulcers in the form of a thin layer of cells extending across a bed of inflamed granulation tissue or mingling with the fibrin, leukocyte exudate, and lymphocytes and histiocytes on the gut luminal surface. Bacteria can sometimes be demonstrated at the mucosal surface but rarely penetrate deep tissues. The regenerating epithelium can show considerable cellular atypia such that confusion with dysplasia is possible [21]. Regenerated glands may also show irregularity of outline that can be mistaken for the architectural distortion of chronic inflammatory bowel disease.

Ischaemic strictures

Most cases of severe and extensive infarction of the colon never reach the stage of stricture because the small intestine is also involved and the patient dies of shock. Thus, most ischaemic strictures treated by surgical excision are relatively short. They are uncommon in the right colon and rare in the rectum. They occur relatively frequently in the left colon, at the 'watershed' of the blood supply between the territories of the superior and inferior mesenteric arteries although, as mentioned above [1,12], they may not be as specifically located at the splenic flexure as has been alleged. Ischaemic colitis in general, as mentioned earlier, predominates in the descending and sigmoid colon. The strictures may be tubular or fusiform and in some there is striking sacculation of the gut wall. In all cases there is obvious fibrosis that may extend deeply into the pericolic tissue. The submucosa is characteristically widened and filled with white granulation tissue (Figure 36.5). Mucosal ulceration tends to be patchy. The differential diagnosis from segmental Crohn's disease of the colon may be difficult before microscopic examination.

The principal histological features of ischaemic stricture are seen in all layers of the bowel wall (Figure 36.6). The mucosa shows patchy atrophy and irregularity of crypts, typical of healed ulceration. There may be persisting ulceration, lined by granulation tissue packed with dilated capillaries. There is splaying of the fibres and fibrosis of the muscularis mucosae. The submucosal layer is initially widened and filled with oedematous granulation tissue, with conspicuous fibroblasts and a sprinkling of chronic inflammatory cells, including lymphocytes, eosinophils and plasma cells.

As the healing progresses, the submucosa becomes less cellular, denser and thinner. Fibrous tissue extends downwards between the fascicles of the inner muscularis propria, which become attenuated and separated (Figure 36.6c,d). At the edge of ulcerated areas epithelial regeneration is present with columnar epithelium beginning to grow over

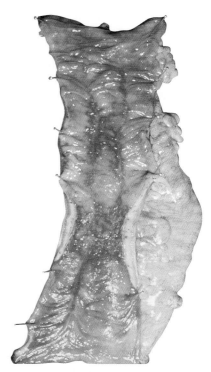

Figure 36.5 Fusiform ischaemic stricture of descending colon: the submucosa at the site of the stricture is thickened by white fibrous tissue. There is longitudinal linear ulceration of the mucosa above and below the stricture, together with cobblestoning due to submucosal oedema.

the surface (Figure 36.6a). Neighbouring intact mucosa is not always normal but shows patchy atrophy and irregularity of crypts, suggestive of healing with incomplete restitution. Macrophages containing haemosiderin pigment are sometimes a prominent feature of the cellular infiltrate and, when present, are of considerable diagnostic use. The submucosal arterioles tend to be thick walled and tortuous. There may be fibrinoid necrosis of the walls of submucosal vessels near the surface of the ulcerated bowel, but this is likely to be due to proximity to the reparative inflammatory process rather than a primary vasculitis. The muscularis propria in ischaemic stricture is relatively spared but may show patchy fibrosis, with replacement and separation of its fibres by granulation tissue (Figure 36.6b), contiguous with that seen in the submucosal layer. The inflammatory process may also involve the serosa and pericolic tissues in a patchy fashion.

Thus, the histological picture at this stage of ischaemic colitis is quite distinct from the microscopic pathology of Crohn's disease. Crypt abscesses are only occasionally seen. Transmural hyperplasia of lymphoid tissue with lymphoid aggregates is not prominent, fissuring ulceration

is unusual and epithelioid granulomas are conspicuously absent.

Transient ischaemic colitis

Apart from full-thickness infarction of the colon or superficial necrosis with healing and later stricture formation, there is also a transient form of ischaemia, sometimes referred to as reversible or evanescent colitis [22–25]. In a typical case there is a short illness characterised by cramping abdominal pain and diarrhoea with minimal-to-moderate rectal bleeding and radiological features of ischaemia, which quickly revert to normal. Although the diagnosis is often made clinically, the pathologist may obtain biopsy material. Sequential biopsies show features of acute haemorrhagic necrosis of the mucosa with a subsequent return to normal or to a regenerative mucosal pattern (Figure 36.7) [23]. Transient or prodromal episodes may be a part of chronic ischaemia in the patients described by Marston who have major vessel stenosis [26]. Transient ischaemic disease may also occur in younger adults and be part of the pathological picture produced by the contraceptive pill [10].

Obstructive colitis

This entity is mentioned here because of its strikingly ischaemic morphology on histology, although it is more fully discussed in Chapter 35. It is a segmental inflammatory and ulcerating condition that occurs proximal to an obstructing colorectal lesion, typically separated from it by a length of normal-appearing colon measuring up to 350 mm or more [27,28].

Endoscopic features and biopsy

In ischaemic colitis endoscopy typically reveals a relatively well delineated segmental abnormality, most commonly on the left side. The exact endoscopic features depend on the severity and stage of ischaemia. Cases of acute ischaemia show petechial haemorrhages, oedema, mucosal fragility and erythema with scattered erosions or linear ulceration. There is contact bleeding [29,30]. More chronic cases tend to show stricturing, often with loss of mucosal folds and more diffuse ulceration with or without evidence of re-epithelialisation.

Biopsy is seldom carried out or warranted in acute gangrenous ischaemia, being more usual in non-resolving disease and in transient colitis [23]. Characteristic of such less severe disease is the damage to the superficial half of the mucosa (Figures 36.8 and 36.9) [18]. The epithelial cells appear flattened or degenerate and there can be complete loss of occasional crypts, so-called 'crypt dropout' (Figure 36.9). The more severe the ischaemia, the greater the crypt loss. The lamina propria takes on a dense eosinophilic

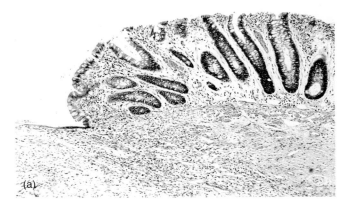

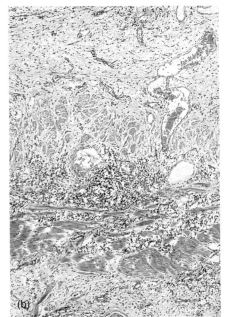

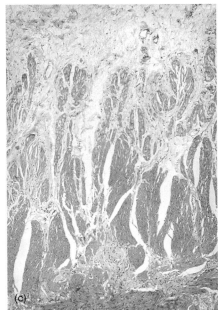

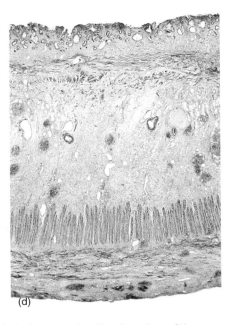

Figure 36.6 (a) Histology of ischaemic colitis: regenerating epithelium is growing over the edge of ulcerated mucosa. The submucosa is filled with granulation tissue. (b) Ischaemic colitis: the bundles of the muscularis propria are separated by young fibrous tissue. Note the chronic inflammatory cell infiltrate, most prominent in the region of the myenteric plexus, more loosely arranged than in Crohn's disease and unlike ulcerative colitis. (c) Healing phase of ischaemic colitis: there is maturation of the fibrous tissue that separates the fascicles of the muscularis propria. (d) Ischaemic colonic stricture: trichrome stain showing marked widening of the submucosa and striking transmural fibrosis.

quality due to deposition of fibrin and subsequent fibrosis. Inflammatory cells are present in small numbers compared with ulcerative colitis and Crohn's disease, although any submucosa present can appear oedematous.

Biopsy during the recovering phases of ischaemia will show regenerative hyperplasia of the crypts. They can be distorted and, depending on the initial severity, present a variable picture of crypt atrophy. Fibrosis of the lamina propria is to be expected with healing. There is little inflammation but iron-laden macrophages are a characteristic feature (Figure 36.10). Both iron and trichrome stains can be usefully employed in this setting.

Relatively uncommon is the discovery in a biopsy of evidence a primary vascular lesion. This may be a focus of vasculitis, thrombus or embolism. Cholesterol athero-emboli are occasionally observed in patients with aortic aneurysm and/or recent aortic surgery (Figure 36.11) [15]. Caution must, as described above, be applied in interpreting vessel wall changes in proximity to an area of ulceration.

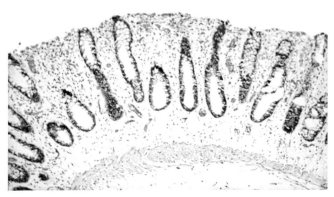

Figure 36.7 A colonoscopic biopsy from a patient with a self-limiting episode of ischaemic colitis, showing oedema and some haemorrhage but with little inflammation. The crypt epithelium is regenerating.

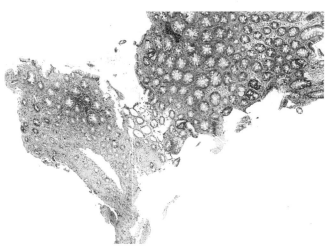

Figure 36.9 Ischaemic colitis with lamina propria fibrosis, attenuation of epithelium of the superficial components of the crypts and 'crypt dropout' in the left half of this field. Note the relative paucity of inflammatory cells present.

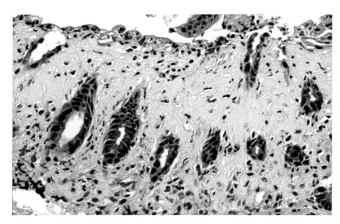

Figure 36.8 Ischaemic colitis: biopsy from an area of linear ulceration at the splenic flexure showing degenerative damage to the epithelium of the surface with 'withering' of the crypts. The luminal half of the lamina propria is eosinophilic due partly to collagen but partly to fibrin. This should not be confused with the discrete collagen band seen in collagenous colitis.

The differential diagnosis of the acute ischaemic biopsy is from pseudo-membranous colitis, other infective colitides and collagenous colitis. If there is severe mucosal necrosis a distinction from the type III lesion of pseudo-membranous colitis may not be possible. Although there is damage to the superficial half of the crypts in both the early lesions of pseudo-membranous colitis and ischaemia, in the latter they look thinned and degenerate rather than distended by mucinous debris as in the former. The glandular attenuation in the upper half of the crypts in ischaemia can also resemble the crypt 'withering' characteristic of infective colitis. However, the accompanying inflammatory infiltrate in infection is usually considerably more intense than is typical with ischaemia.

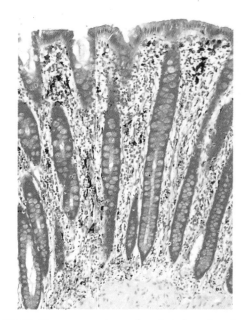

Figure 36.10 Mucosa covering a chronic ischaemic colonic stricture, stained by Perls' method. Haemosiderin-laden macrophages in the lamina propria are the only clue to the underlying diagnosis.

Occasionally the fibrosis of the lamina propria may cause confusion with collagenous colitis. A trichrome stain will help delineate the extent of collagen deposition. This is likely to extend considerably deeper on a broader front in healing ischaemic colitis than in collagenous colitis, in which it is typically denser, better defined and more super-

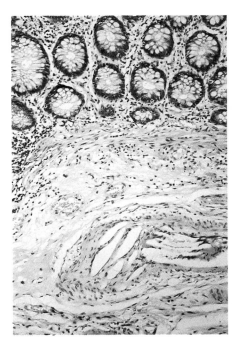

Figure 36.11 Cholesterol atheroembolus in a colonic submucosal artery: the patient had recently undergone surgery for an aortic aneurysm.

ficial, with more elongate tendril-like processes. There is usually a moderate inflammatory infiltrate, sometimes with intra-epithelial lymphocytosis, in collagenous colitis. Perls' stain for haemosiderin, which should be negative in collagenous colitis, and procurement of an accurate clinical history will distinguish the vast majority of cases in this differential scenario.

In biopsies of chronic ischaemia the crypt irregularity of healed ulceration may suggest a more quiescent phase ulcerative colitis or perhaps even Crohn's disease. Again the presence of haemosiderin and prominent mucosal fibrosis favour ischaemia, whereas the presence of more than occasional foci of cryptitis or crypt abscess formation or of epithelioid granulomas strongly favours chronic inflammatory bowel disease. Many of the characteristic features of chronic ischaemic damage in the mucosa are to be seen in the mucosal prolapse syndrome and mucosal ischaemia undoubtedly occurs when mucosa prolapses, due to mechanical stress on small blood vessels (see Chapter 34). Clinico-pathological correlation is crucial in making this distinction.

Angiodysplasia

Angiodysplasia is an ectasia of pre-existing colonic submucosal veins with or without ectasia of the overlying mucosal capillaries. This vascular malformation is claimed by some authors to be the most common cause of bleeding in elderly people [31], although post mortem studies have reported a wide range in incidence from 2% to 50% [32]. Angiodysplasias are considered degenerative lesions [31]. They are believed to result from chronic low grade obstruction of the submucosal veins where they traverse the muscularis propria. This occurs over a timescale of many years until the submucosal veins become dilated and tortuous. The resulting back pressure causes further dilatation of the mucosal vessels draining into these veins. The lesions are often multiple and are most common in the right colon [33–35]. This predilection of angiodysplasias for the right side is due to the intramural tension on the right side being greater than in other segments: according to Laplace's principle, the tension in the wall for a given intraluminal pressure is highest in the segment with the greatest diameter, i.e. the right colon.

Most patients with angiodysplasia are aged >60 but there are some well documented cases in younger patients [35,36]. There is no associated clinical syndrome as there is with some telangiectasias. Aortic stenosis may be associated with angiodysplasia [31] but is unlikely to be causally related. It seems more probable that patients with angiodysplasia are more likely to bleed when aortic stenosis is present.

The diagnosis is most often made radiologically with selective mesenteric angiography. More recently radionuclide scanning and helical CT angiography have also been employed. At endoscopy the contour of the mucosa is seldom altered but the endoscopist may see prominent vessels radiating from a raised cherry-red central point, or a localized 7- to 10-mm blush of dilated superficial vessels [37]. They are friable to touch and bleed easily.

Histopathological diagnosis is difficult in both biopsies and surgical resections. Macroscopically, under a dissecting microscope, the normal mucosal honeycomb vascular pattern is replaced by clusters of tortuous vessels resembling a coral reef [32,38]. These ectatic mucosal capillaries communicate with enlarged submucosal veins and venules. It is the latter that are believed to be the primary and constant abnormality. However, because of the wide range in size and tortuosity of submucosal vessels [32], it is unwise to make the diagnosis of angiodysplasia in the absence of mucosal abnormalities [32,38]. The mucosa can present a spectrum of change from just one or two ectatic capillaries to crypts pushed apart by large numbers (Figure 36.12) [32,39].

In biopsy work the abnormal submucosal veins may not be sampled and the number of ectatic mucosal capillaries is variable. They also are frequently disrupted in the biopsy process. Consequently, biopsy fails to substantiate the diagnosis in up to 50% of cases [32,40].

In the surgical specimen the lesions are tiny and fixation causes additional shrinkage. The cases are often surgical emergencies done at night and the bowel is well fixed by

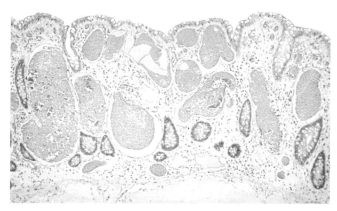

Figure 36.12 Angiodysplasia of the colon, with markedly ectatic mucosal vessels: this is a section of a colon following arterial perfusion of an aqueous suspension of barium sulphate before fixation.

the time the pathologist inspects it the next day. For a reasonable chance of identifying any angiodysplasia the bowel needs to be received fresh and unopened. The major vessels can then be sought and injected with contrast media such as barium sulphate, with or without warm gelatin solution [38]. Still unopened, the bowel should be rinsed out, then distended with formalin and fixed for 48 hours. At this stage a radiograph can be taken. Only then is it opened and the mucosa inspected for lesions. Another radiograph is often helpful at this stage. If difficulty is still present the specimen can be rendered transparent using dehydration procedures [41] and examined under the dissecting microscope. An alternative method, using transillumination to examine mucosa stripped away from the deeper layers of the fixed bowel wall [42], has been claimed to avoid the need to perform vascular perfusion, but we have found it to be of only limited value.

Portal (hypertensive) colopathy

It is well recognised that patients with portal hypertension develop a variety of vascular abnormalities in the upper gastrointestinal tract. It is, however, less well recognised that these patients may also develop mucosal vascular ectasias and even varices in the large bowel. One series demonstrated such abnormalities at endoscopy in as many as 66% of patients with cirrhosis. It also indicated that, as the severity of portal hypertension increases, the prevalence of portal hypertensive colopathy also increases [43–45].

Vasculitides

The large intestine is occasionally affected by vasculitic processes although rarely it is the sole site of involvement.

When the colon is involved the pathology is similar to that seen in the small intestine (see Chapter 22). Colonic involvement in particular vasculitic disorders is, however, outlined here.

Polyarteritis nodosa

Segmental involvement of the colon in polyarteritis nodosa is rare but may occur as a manifestation of generalised disease or as an isolated lesion apparently confined to the bowel. We have had experience of one case of sigmoid involvement in which a rectal biopsy revealed the characteristic histology in the arterioles of the submucosal layer. A subsequent resection of the sigmoid colon was performed and the specimen showed patchy mucosal ulceration and gangrene with a curious peach-like colour of the intervening intact mucosa. The pericolic fatty tissue was indurated and microscopic examination revealed extensive fat necrosis. In other aspects, the histology was typical. Polyarteritis nodosa presenting with perforation of the colon has been reported [46–48].

Systemic lupus erythematosus

Although systemic lupus erythematosus (SLE) is quite often accompanied by gastrointestinal symptoms, colonic lesions are rare, occurring in as few as 0.2% of cases [49,50]. Pathological changes associated with gastrointestinal vasculitis occur in the small vessels of the intestinal wall rather than in medium-sized mesenteric arteries [50]. In addition to occasionally causing ischaemic colitis, SLE has been linked with a severe ischaemic proctitis [49].

ANCA-associated vasculitides, including Wegener's granulomatosis

In a review of six patients with Wegener's granulomatosis who developed ischaemic colitis, specific vasculitic features were seen in mucosal biopsies of three. Four perforations occurred and surgical intervention was required six times [51]. Other anti-neutrophil cytoplasmic antigen (ANCA)-associated vasculitides [52] such as Churg–Strauss syndrome have been reported to cause perforating colonic as well as enteric ulceration [53].

Idiopathic enterocolic lymphocytic phlebitis

There have been several reports of patients with ischaemic colitis as well as ischaemic enteritis in whom the mesenteric veins show a florid mural inflammatory infiltrate, mainly lymphocytic, with or without associated thrombosis [54–56]. Despite careful documentation, it is uncertain whether this is a primary phlebitis or a secondary phenomenon following idiopathic ischaemic colitis, akin to a pyelophlebitis, such as may occur as a complication of appendicitis. In some cases the endophlebitis is granulomatous in nature [57].

Idiopathic myointimal hyperplasia of mesenteric veins

This rare condition predominantly affects young, previously healthy, males. It presents as a procto-sigmoiditis and thus may be misdiagnosed clinically as chronic inflammatory bowel disease [58–60]. Biopsies, however, show ischaemic changes and may show hyalinised vessels in the lamina propria [58]. Segmental resection is curative and examination of the mesenteric veins shows focal myointimal hyperplasia. Some authors believe that the condition may represent a late reparative stage of enterocolic lymphocytic phlebitis [55], whereas others suggest that it may be related to previous trauma [60].

References

1. Binns JC, Isaacson P. Age-related changes in the colonic blood supply: their relevance to ischaemic colitis. *Gut* 1978;**19**:384.
2. Alschibaya T, Morson BC. Ischaemic bowel disease. *J Clin Pathol* 1977;**30**(suppl 11):68.
3. Zeitz M. Shock-associated nonocclusive ischemic colitis: a very rare event in young patients after trauma. *Int J Colorectal Dis* 2001;**16**:58.
4. Lucas W, Schroy PC III. Reversible ischemic colitis in a high endurance athlete. *Am J Gastroenterol* 1998;**93**:2231.
5. Okamoto Y, Fujii M, Shinpei T, et al. A case of ischemic colitis during pregnancy. *J Gastroenterol* 2003;**38**:1195.
6. Puspok A, Kiener HP, Oberhuber G. Clinical, endoscopic, and histologic spectrum of nonsteroidal anti-inflammatory drug-induced lesions in the colon. *Dis Colon Rectum* 2000;**43**:685.
7. Linder JD, Monkemuller KE, Raijman I, Johnson L, Lazenby AJ, Wilcox CM. Cocaine-associated ischemic colitis. *South Med J* 2000;**93**:909.
8. Dowd J, Bailey D, Moussa K, Nair S, Doyle R, Culpepper-Morgan JA. Ischemic colitis associated with pseudoephedrine: four cases. *Am J Gastroenterol* 1999;**94**:2430.
9. Knudsen JF, Friedman B, Chen M, Goldwasser JE. Ischemic colitis and sumatriptan use. *Arch Intern Med* 1998;**158**:1946.
10. Deana DG, Dean PJ. Reversible ischemic colitis in young women. Association with oral contraceptive use. *Am J Surg Pathol* 1995;**19**:454.
11. Zervoudis S, Grammatopoulos T, Iatrakis G, et al. Ischemic colitis in postmenopausal women taking hormone replacement therapy. *Gynecol Endocrinol* 2008;**24**:257.
12. Reeders JWAJ, Tytgat GNJ, Rosenbusch G, Gratama S. *Ischaemic Colitis*. The Hague: Martinus-Nijhoff, 1984.
13. Bharucha AE, Tremaine WJ, Johnson CD, Batts KP. Ischemic proctosigmoiditis. *Am J Gastroenterol* 1996;**91**:2305.
14. Jeck T, Sulser H, Heer M. Local ischemia causes carcinoma-like changes of the rectum. *Dis Colon Rectum* 1996;**39**:1026.
15. Jaeger HJ, Mathias KD, Gissler HM, Neumann G, Walther LD. Rectum and sigmoid colon necrosis due to cholesterol embolization after implantation of an aortic stent-graft. *J Vasc Interv Radiol* 1999;**10**:751.
16. Schuler JG, Hudlin MM. Cecal necrosis: infrequent variant of ischemic colitis. Report of five cases. *Dis Colon Rectum* 2000;**43**:708.
17. Arnott ID, Ghosh S, Ferguson A. The spectrum of ischaemic colitis. *Eur J Gastroenterol Hepatol* 1999;**11**:295.
18. Whitehead R. The pathology of intestinal ischaemia. *Clin Gastroenterol* 1972;**1**:613.
19. Brandt LJ, Gomery P, Mitsudo SM, Chandler P, Boley SJ. Disseminated intravascular coagulation in nonocclusive mesenteric ischemia: the lack of specificity of fibrin thrombi in intestinal infarction. *Gastroenterology* 1976;**71**:954.
20. Dignan CR, Greenson JK. Can ischemic colitis be differentiated from *C. difficile* colitis in biopsy specimens? *Am J Surg Pathol* 1997;**21**:706.
21. Zhang S, Ashraf M, Schinella R. Ischemic colitis with atypical reactive changes that mimic dysplasia (pseudodysplasia). *Arch Pathol Lab Med* 2001;**125**:224.
22. Heron HC, Khubchandani IT, Trimpi HD, Sheets JA, Stasik JJ. Evanescent colitis. *Dis Colon Rectum* 1981;**24**:555.
23. Dawson MA, Schaefer JW. The clinical course of reversible ischemic colitis. Observations on the progression of sigmoidoscopic and histological changes. *Gastroenterology* 1971;**60**:577.
24. Boley SJ, Schwartz S, Lash J, Sternhill V. Reversible vascular occlusion of the colon. *Surg Gynecol Obstet* 1963;**116**:53.
25. Marston A, Pheils MT, Thomas ML, Morson BC. Ischaemic colitis. *Gut* 1966;**7**:1.
26. Marston A, Clarke JM, Garcia Garcia J, Miller AL. Intestinal function and intestinal blood supply: a 20 year surgical study. *Gut* 1985;**26**:656.
27. Toner M, Condell D, O'Briain DS. Obstructive colitis. Ulceratoinflammatory lesions occurring proximal to colonic obstruction. *Am J Surg Pathol* 1990;**14**:719.
28. Levine TS, Price AB. Obstructive enterocolitis: a clinicopathological discussion. *Histopathology* 1994;**25**:57.
29. Scowcroft CW, Sanowski RA, Kozarek RA. Colonoscopy in ischemic colitis. *Gastrointest Endosc* 1981;**27**:156.
30. Zou X, Cao J, Yao Y, Liu W, Chen L. Endoscopic findings and clinicopathologic characteristics of ischemic colitis: a report of 85 cases. *Dig Dis Sci* 2009;**54**:2009.
31. Boley SJ, Sammartano R, Adams A, DiBiase A, Kleinhaus S, Sprayregen S. On the nature and etiology of vascular ectasias of the colon. Degenerative lesions of aging. *Gastroenterology* 1977;**72** (4 Part 1):650.
32. Price AB. Angiodysplasia of the colon. *Int J Colorectal Dis* 1986;**1**:121.
33. Meyer CT, Troncale FJ, Galloway S, Sheahan DG. Arteriovenous malformations of the bowel: an analysis of 22 cases and a review of the literature. *Medicine (Baltimore)* 1981;**60**:36.
34. Richter JM, Hedberg SE, Athanasoulis CA, Schapiro RH. Angiodysplasia. Clinical presentation and colonoscopic diagnosis. *Dig Dis Sci* 1984;**29**:481.
35. Hochter W, Weingart J, Kuhner W, Frimberger E, Ottenjann R. Angiodysplasia in the colon and rectum. Endoscopic morphology, localisation and frequency. *Endoscopy* 1985;**17**:182.
36. Allison DJ, Hemingway AP. Angiodysplasia: does old age begin at nineteen? *Lancet* 1981;**ii**:979.
37. Danesh BJ, Spiliadis C, Williams CB, Zambartas CM. Angiodysplasia – an uncommon cause of colonic bleeding: colonoscopic evaluation of 1050 patients with rectal bleeding and anaemia. *Int J Colorectal Dis* 1987;**2**:218.
38. Pounder DJ, Rowland R, Pieterse AS, Freeman R, Hunter R. Angiodysplasias of the colon. *J Clin Pathol* 1982;**35**:824.
39. Mitsudo SM, Boley SJ, Brandt LJ, Montefusco CM, Sammartano RJ. Vascular ectasias of the right colon in the elderly: a distinct pathologic entity. *Hum Pathol* 1979;**10**:585.
40. Stamm B, Heer M, Buhler H, Ammann R. Mucosal biopsy of vascular ectasia (angiodysplasia) of the large bowel detected

during routine colonoscopic examination. *Histopathology* 1985; **9**:639.

41. Reynolds DG. Injection techniques in the study of intestinal vasculature under normal conditions and in ulcerative colitis. In: Boley SJ, Schwartz SS, Williams LF (eds), *Vascular Disorders of the Intestine*. New York: Appleton-Century Crofts, 1971: 383.

42. Thelmo WL, Vetrano JA, Wibowo A, DiMaio TM, Cruz-Vetrano WP, Kim DS. Angiodysplasia of colon revisited: pathologic demonstration without the use of intravascular injection technique. *Hum Pathol* 1992;**23**:37.

43. Ito K, Shiraki K, Sakai T, Yoshimura H, Nakano T. Portal hypertensive colopathy in patients with liver cirrhosis. *World J Gastroenterol* 2005;**11**:3127.

44. Diaz-Sanchez A, Nuñez-Martinez O, Gonzalez-Asanza C, et al. Portal hypertensive colopathy is associated with portal hypertension severity in cirrhotic patients. *World J Gastroenterol* 2009; **15**:4781.

45. Goenka MK, Kochhar R, Nagi B, Mehta SK. Rectosigmoid varices and other mucosal changes in patients with portal hypertension. *Am J Gastroenterol* 1991;**86**:1185.

46. Burke AP, Sobin LH, Virmani R. Localized vasculitis of the gastrointestinal tract. *Am J Surg Pathol* 1995;**19**:338.

47. Tanakaya K, Konaga E, Takeuchi H, et al. Penetrating colon ulcer of polyarteritis nodosa. *Dis Colon Rectum* 2001;**44**:1037.

48. Okada M, Konishi F, Sakuma K, Kanazawa K, Koiwai H, Kaizaki Y. Perforation of the sigmoid colon with ischemic change due to polyarteritis nodosa. *J Gastroenterol* 1999;**34**:400.

49. Reissman P, Weiss EG, Teoh TA, Lucas FV, Wexner SD. Gangrenous ischemic colitis of the rectum: a rare complication of systemic lupus erythematosus. *Am J Gastroenterol* 1994;**89**:2234.

50. Lee JR, Paik CN, Kim JD, Chung WC, Lee KM, Yang JM. Ischemic colitis associated with intestinal vasculitis: histological proof in systemic lupus erythematosus. *World J Gastroenterol* 2008;**14**:3591.

51. Storesund B, Gran JT, Koldingsnes W. Severe intestinal involvement in Wegener's granulomatosis: report of two cases and review of the literature [see comments]. *Br J Rheumatol* 1998; **37**:387.

52. Gross WL. Systemic necrotizing vasculitis. *Baillière's Clin Rheumatol* 1997;**11**:259.

53. Kurita M, Niwa Y, Hamada E, et al. Churg–Strauss syndrome (allergic granulomatous angiitis) with multiple perforating ulcers of the small intestine, multiple ulcers of the colon, and mononeuritis multiplex. *J Gastroenterol* 1994;**29**:208.

54. Flaherty MJ, Lie JT, Haggitt RC. Mesenteric inflammatory veno-occlusive disease. A seldom recognized cause of intestinal ischemia. *Am J Surg Pathol* 1994;**18**:779.

55. Saraga E, Bouzourenne H. Enterocolic (lymphocytic) phlebitis: a rare cause of intestinal ischemic necrosis: a series of six patients and review of the literature. *Am J Surg Pathol* 2000;**24**:824.

56. Tuppy H, Haidenthaler A, Schandalik R, Oberhuber G. Idiopathic enterocolic lymphocytic phlebitis: a rare cause of ischemic colitis. *Mod Pathol* 2000;**13**:897.

57. Martinet O, Reis ED, Joseph JM, Saraga E, Gillet TM. Isolated granulomatous phlebitis: rare cause of ischemic necrosis of the colon: report of a case. *Dis Colon Rectum* 2000;**43**:1601.

58. Abu-Alfa AK, Ayer U, West AB. Mucosal biopsy findings and venous abnormalities in idiopathic myointimal hyperplasia of the mesenteric veins. *Am J Surg Pathol* 1996;**20**:1271.

59. Savoie LM, Abrams AV. Refractory proctosigmoiditis caused by myointimal hyperplasia of mesenteric veins: report of a case. *Dis Colon Rectum* 1999;**42**:1093.

60. Sherman J, Kao PC, West AB, Blaszyk H. Focal myointimal hyperplasia of mesenteric veins is associated with previous trauma in surgical specimens. *Pathol Res Pract* 2006;**202**:517.

CHAPTER 37

Polyps and tumour-like lesions of the large intestine

Andrew D. Clouston and Neal I. Walker

University of Queensland; Envoi Specialist Pathologists, Brisbane, QLD, Australia

When broadly defined as projections from the colonic mucosal surface, polyps of the large intestine are readily detected and encompass a wide range of lesions. The great majority of these are adenomas and hyperplastic polyps, but other lesions of the mucosa and submucosa may be observed at the time of colonoscopy or radiological imaging as mucosal elevations. A classification of these is shown in Table 37.1, and includes benign and malignant epithelial tumours, inflammatory and reactive polyps, stromal tumours, endocrine neoplasms and other less common lesions.

Conventional adenoma

Conventional adenomas, well characterised and commonly seen in gastrointestinal pathology practice, are the precursor lesions for most colorectal adenocarcinomas. They are defined by the presence of dysplasia [1] which, in turn, is defined as unequivocal intra-epithelial neoplastic change [2]. The 'conventional' adenomas – tubular, tubulo-villous and villous adenomas – are the best characterised of the colorectal adenomas, but more recently it has been recognised that other forms such as sessile serrated, traditional serrated and flat adenomas play an incompletely defined role in colonic carcinogenesis. These lesions are discussed in subsequent sections.

Epidemiology

The prevalence of conventional adenomas varies throughout the world. The highest frequency is seen in North America, western Europe and Australia, where they are found in up to 50% or more of older individuals [3,4], or at lower rates of around 20% in colonoscopic screening programmes [5]. Although they may be seen in younger adults, the presence of adenomas increases sharply after 50 years of age [6] and this is taken into account in screening programmes. In addition to advancing age, other factors associated with adenoma formation include smoking, obesity, increased alcohol intake and dietary factors such as high fat-containing diets, low folate and reduced amounts of fresh fruit and vegetables [7–9]. However, interventions to alter dietary habits have not had a major effect on reducing adenomas unless rigorously followed [10]. Similarly, chemopreventive strategies with non-steroidal anti-inflammatory drugs, selenium or calcium have shown only modest effects [9].

Macroscopic features

Macroscopically, several features of adenomas relate to their behaviour. The size of the adenoma is important for several reasons. It is related to the likelihood of malignant transformation [11–13], and also to the risk of synchronous and metachronous adenomas [14]. Diminutive polyps <5 mm only rarely (<2%) have advanced features, i.e. villous architecture or high grade dysplasia, and are not associated with carcinoma [15]. Small lesions 5–10 mm diameter have been shown to have advanced features in 10% and carcinoma in almost 1%, so they have a low but definite malignancy risk. The majority of adenomas removed, over 80–90%, are tubular adenomas <10 mm [16,17]. Adenomas

Morson and Dawson's Gastrointestinal Pathology, Fifth Edition. Edited by Neil A. Shepherd, Bryan F. Warren, Geraint T. Williams, Joel K. Greenson, Gregory Y. Lauwers and Marco R. Novelli.
© 2013 Blackwell Publishing Ltd. Published 2013 by Blackwell Publishing Ltd.

Table 37.1 Classification of colorectal polyps

Epithelial
Conventional adenoma
   Tubular
   Tubulovillous
   Villous
   Flat adenoma
Serrated polyp
   Hyperplastic (microvesicular, goblet cell, mucin poor)
   Sessile serrated adenoma
   Mixed polyp
   Traditional serrated adenoma
Polypoid adenocarcinoma

Inflammatory
Mucosal prolapse-associated polyp (includes polypoid
   prolapsing mucosal fold, inflammatory cloacogenic polyp,
   inflammatory myoglandular polyp, inflammatory cap polyp)
Inflammatory pseudo-polyp
Polypoid granulation tissue
Infection-associated polyp (cytomegalovirus, schistosomiasis)

Hamartomatous
Peutz–Jeghers polyp
Juvenile polyp
Cowden syndrome and Bannayan–Riley–Ruvalcaba syndrome
Cronkite–Canada syndrome

Stromal
Inflammatory fibroid polyp
Fibroblastic polyp/peri-neurioma
Schwann cell hamartoma
Neurilemmoma and nerve sheath tumour variants
Ganglio-neuroma
Leiomyoma of muscularis mucosae
Lipoma
Lipohyperplasia of ileo-caecal valve
Gastrointestinal stromal tumour
Neurofibroma
Granular cell tumour

Lymphoid
Prominent lymphoid follicle/rectal tonsil
Lymphomatous polyposis

Endocrine
Well differentiated endocrine (carcinoid) tumour

Other
Prominent mucosal fold
Everted appendiceal stump or caecal diverticulum
Elastotic (elastofibromatous) polyp
Endometriosis
Mucosal xanthoma
Melanoma/clear cell sarcoma
Metastasis

Table 37.2 The Paris endoscopic classification of superficial gastrointestinal neoplastic lesions

Endoscopic appearance		Features
Polypoid type	0–Ip	Pedunculated lesion
	0–Is	Sessile lesion
	0–Isp	Semi-pedunculated lesion
Non-polypoid type	0–IIa	Slightly elevated lesion
	0–IIb	Flat lesion
	0–IIc	Slightly depressed lesion without ulcer

Reproduced from Participants in the Paris Workshop. The Paris endoscopic classification of superficial neoplastic lesions: esophagus, stomach, and colon: November 30 to December 1, 2002. Gastrointestinal Endoscopy, 2003; 58: S3.

>10 mm are regarded as advanced adenomas, but even so most do not progress to invasive adenocarcinoma. In a follow-up study of barium enema-detected polyps >10 mm found before the routine use of colonoscopy, 37% of the polyps increased in size and 10% of patients developed carcinoma at the site of the polyp over a mean period of 108 months [18]. Importantly these polyps had not been biopsied and so the precise identification of the initial lesion is not known. In that study, actuarial analysis suggested an 8% carcinoma risk at 10 years and 25% at 20 years. In addition, 5% of patients developed a colorectal adenocarcinoma remote from the original polyp.

Macroscopically, adenomas have traditionally been described as pedunculated or sessile. More recently, this has been refined to include flat and depressed lesions. The Paris classification (Table 37.2) [19], used particularly by endoscopists and modified from earlier Japanese classifications, recognises several macroscopic patterns of which some carry an increased risk of malignancy. Protruded polypoid lesions are readily observed projecting from the mucosal surface and may be pedunculated (Figure 37.1), sub-pedunculated with an inconspicuous pedicle drawn up into the polyp head (Figure 37.2) or sessile (Figure 37.3). In these lesions, foci of irregular ulceration should raise the possibility of carcinoma arising in the adenoma.

A second group of lesions is non-polypoid (flat adenomas). Although initially more commonly described in Japan, it is now clear that flat adenomas are also present in appreciable numbers in western populations, making up more than a quarter of resected adenomas [20]. Most of these lesions are subtly elevated from the surrounding mucosa (Paris type IIa). Standardised definitions are lacking [21] but the elevation is generally less than the height of closed biopsy forceps (2.5 mm), or histologically less than twice the height of the adjacent mucosa [19,22].

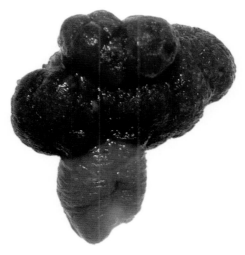

Figure 37.1 Pedunculated adenoma: the stalk is covered by paler non-dysplastic mucosa.

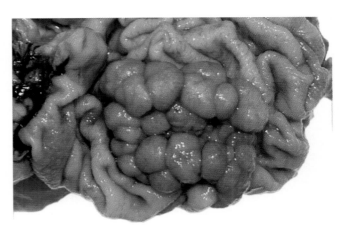

Figure 37.3 Sessile adenoma with a lobulated appearance.

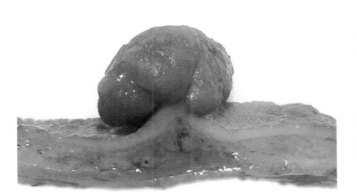

Figure 37.2 Semi-pedunculated adenoma with an inconspicuous pedicle drawn up into the lesion.

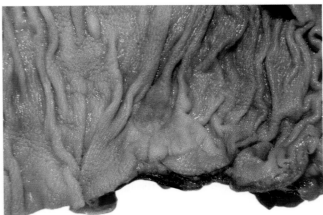

Figure 37.4 Flat adenoma, with no elevation above the surrounding mucosa. A colour difference compared with the surrounding mucosa may be the only macroscopic change.

These adenomas can spread laterally, becoming large and carpet like; others probably evolve into polypoid adenomas [23]. Another group of non-polypoid adenoma is rare, difficult to detect and truly flat compared with the surrounding colonic surface (Paris type IIb) (Figure 37.4). The least common variant has a slightly depressed central area without ulceration (Paris type IIc) and the greatest correlation with malignancy. When central depression is combined with a raised edge, the malignant risk is particularly high [24,25]. Truly flat and depressed adenomas are difficult to detect, often showing only slight congestion macroscopically.

Classification of the adenoma type is often not possible during initial handling, but at one end of the spectrum villous tumours often have fine papillary processes that can be recognised (Figure 37.5). Tubulovillous adenomas do not have these fine papillae, but rather a lobulated contour with a finer gyriform or cerebriform pattern that is visible by magnified chromo-endoscopy [26] and is responsible for the areas with a villous appearance histologically. The mouths of crypts from tubular adenomas can also be recognised by chromoendoscopy as rounded openings that are larger than the normal adjacent crypts.

Secondary changes are common. Macroscopic changes that can be recognised include haemorrhage, torsion-associated congestion, ulceration or diathermy change from the polypectomy. Prolapsing pedunculated adenomas may show pseudo-invasion with mucin or mucosal displacement into the stalk, causing thickening in this area as well as mucinous cysts and extravasates on the cut face.

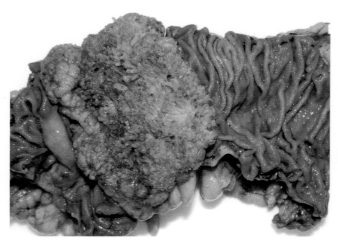

Figure 37.5 Large villous adenoma in the rectum with a shaggy appearance.

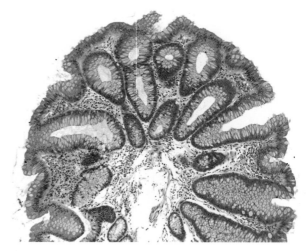

Figure 37.6 Tubular adenoma.

Microscopic appearances

Adenomas arise as single crypts lined by dysplastic epithelium (monocryptal adenomas), probably following mutation or epigenetic gene silencing in colonic stem cells located at the crypt bases [27,28]. With continued proliferation of dysplastic epithelium, adenomas are believed to grow by both crypt fission with vertical branching and growth of the abnormal epithelium into adjacent crypts [28,29]. Aberrant crypt foci can be detected *in situ* by high magnification chromoscopic colonoscopy and are characterised by an altered shape of the luminal opening, thickened epithelium and larger than normal crypts [30]. Increased numbers of these foci have been described in patients who also have adenomas or carcinoma [31].

Microscopically, two key features are used to define and classify conventional adenomas – the architecture and the degree of dysplasia (intraepithelial neoplasia). The architectural pattern assesses the proportion of tubular elements, characterised by epithelial glands surrounded by lamina propria, and villous elements in which the epithelial lining contains the lamina propria. Thus, the tubular and villous elements in an adenoma can be likened to the structure of crypts and villi in the small intestine. Tubular adenoma is composed of tubular crypts (Figure 37.6), usually more closely packed than the adjacent normal mucosa, and by definition has less than 20% of villous elements using the World Health Organization (WHO) criteria [1,32]. Other authors have suggested a cut-off of 25% villous elements [16] but the distinction is somewhat semantic because the assessment is made by estimation. Tubulovillous adenoma has a combination of crypts and villous structures (Figure 37.7), the latter comprising 20–80% of the polyp. In villous adenoma the villous elements predominate, comprising more than 80% of the polyp [1,32] (Figure 37.8). Distinction between the polyp types may not

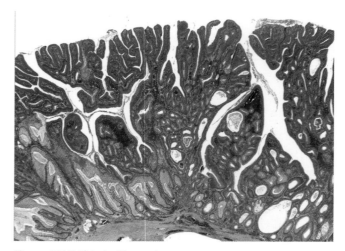

Figure 37.7 Tubulovillous adenoma.

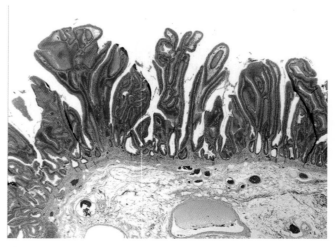

Figure 37.8 Villous adenoma.

always be straightforward because of problems in determining whether structures are villi or open tubules [1], as well as the need to estimate the degree of villosity. It has been noted that the reproducibility of this classification based on the proportion of villous elements is imperfect [33,34] and at best only moderate [35,36], but an attempt is encouraged because of the importance of classification in determining the future neoplastic risk and follow-up screening intervals [37].

Dysplasia (intra-epithelial neoplasia) is characterised by hypercellularity, nuclear enlargement with hyperchromasia and crowding. The nuclei show a variable degree of loss of polarity and stratification, are mitotically active [32] and in most cases have a pencillate shape. More severely dysplastic nuclei may be oval and vesicular with a prominent nucleolus. Some conventional adenomas have intensely eosinophilic cytoplasm. Mucin is variably reduced and atypical or dystrophic goblet cells may occur, often with reversed or 'upside-down' polarity. Previously graded as mild, moderate or severe, dysplasia in adenomas is now graded using a two-tier system of low grade and high grade, following the recommendations initially described for dysplasia in inflammatory bowel disease [2]. In low grade dysplasia the nuclei are relatively uniform and pencillate, and mostly located in the basal half of the cell with cytoplasm on the luminal side (Figure 37.9). Invariably rare nuclei will extend into the apical half, but this is not prominent. Conversely, high grade dysplasia shows more marked stratification with nuclei extending prominently into the apical half of the cells and having greater nuclear pleomorphism (Figure 37.10). Glandular complexity including cribriform glands can occur in some cases. It is common in adenomas to see more than one grade of dysplasia and conventionally the highest grade of dysplasia is the one used [2,32], but only when it affects more than 'one or two crypts' [2].

With regard to the nomenclature of high grade dysplasia, it is recognised that it can show a spectrum of changes that includes lesions with marked cytological and architectural complexity – the hallmarks of adenocarcinoma *in situ*. It is recommended that the latter term be avoided, as it may lead to confusion and over-treatment because of the use of the word 'carcinoma' [17,38]. More problematic are the lesions where there is focal invasive adenocarcinoma with a desmoplastic stromal reaction that is confined to the mucosa, indicating intramucosal adenocarcinoma. With the possible exception of poorly differentiated intramucosal adenocarcinoma (see discussion below in 'Adenocarcinoma arising in an adenoma'), these do not have any metastatic potential and can be treated conservatively if completely excised at polypectomy. For this reason, some have advocated classifying such lesions as adenomas with high grade dysplasia and not using the term 'intramucosal adenocarcinoma', thus avoiding over-treatment [17]. If the term is used, the histological report must clearly state that the lesion does not invade into the submucosa and therefore has no metastatic potential [38].

Flat adenoma is a variant of adenoma with a low profile. Although initially described more often by Japanese workers, increasing awareness of this form of adenoma in the west has led to increasing consensus on its importance [23]. Histologically it has a height that is less than twice the thickness of the adjacent mucosa, but rare cases are not elevated or are even depressed. Most cases are slightly elevated (Paris type IIa) and these have only a low risk of high grade dysplasia [23]. Conversely, those that are completely flat and not elevated above the level of surrounding mucosa, or are slightly depressed, are more likely to show high grade dysplasia or adenocarcinoma on histological examination [19,23,39] (Figure 37.11). Carcinoma is particularly frequent in depressed lesions, although these are the rarest form and represent less than 5% of flat lesions [19,23,39,40].

As well as the usual dysplastic colonocytes and goblet cells, adenomas can contain other elements. These often

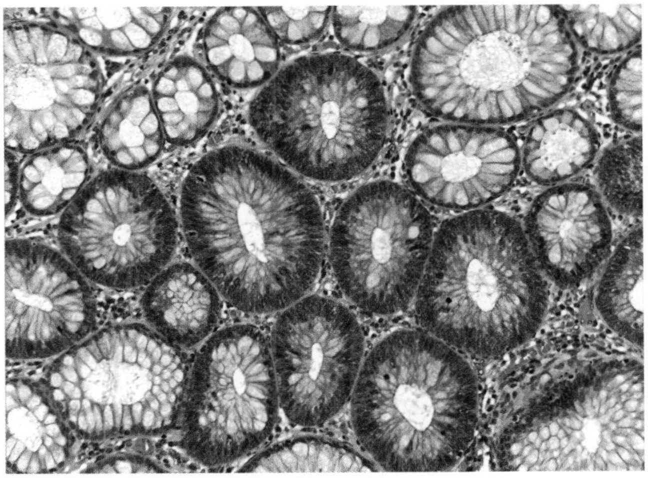

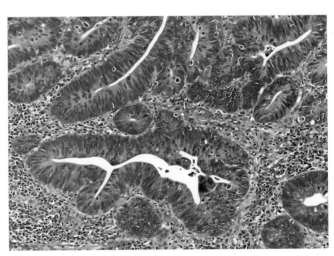

Figure 37.9 Low grade adenomatous dysplasia.

Figure 37.10 High grade adenomatous dysplasia.

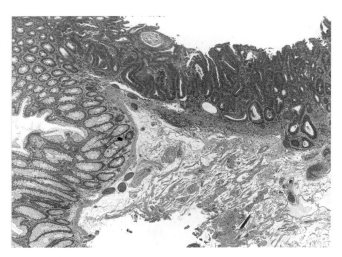

Figure 37.11 Flat adenoma with high grade dysplasia: there is early adenocarcinoma invading the submucosa at 3 o'clock in the picture. This was seen to a greater degree in another area of the polyp.

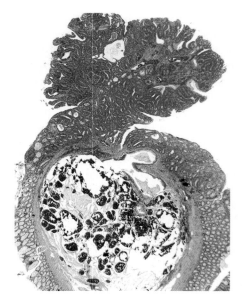

Figure 37.12 Pseudo-invasion of the stalk of a tubulovillous adenoma, with formation of a mucous cyst.

include Paneth cells and endocrine cells [2,41,42], and rarely intraglandular morules that are cytokeratin-20 negative [43,44], foci of squamous metaplasia [41,44,45], clear cell areas with a high proliferative index [46,47], osseous metaplasia [48] and melanocytes [41]. One report of an adenoma from the ileal pouch of a patient with familial adenomatous polyposis described over 90% of the cells as Paneth cells and the name Paneth cell adenoma was applied [49]. Secondary changes are common and include acute, subacute and chronic inflammation, ulceration, fibrosis and haemorrhage. In more extreme examples there can be secondary mucosal prolapse changes, particularly at the anal verge where admixed inflammatory cloacogenic polyp and adenoma has been described [50]. Immunostaining for p53 and Ki67 can be used to highlight the adenomatous glands [50].

Epithelial misplacement (pseudo-invasion)

Pseudo-invasion, or epithelial misplacement, of adenomatous mucosa into the submucosa is commonly seen in larger pedunculated polyps (Figure 37.12), probably occurring secondarily to repeated torsional or traction injury [51]. It has been found in 2–10% of adenomas [51,52]. The misplacement is particularly likely in the sigmoid where most of these lesions are found [51]. Bleeding associated with the traction injury may be detected in bowel cancer screening programmes using faecal occult blood testing, and for this reason it is likely that these problem polyps will be seen with increasing frequency. In many cases the diagnosis is straightforward, but in others the interpretation is difficult and requires the assessment of several histological changes (Table 37.3). Features of pseudo-invasion

include rounded nests of dysplastic epithelium in the submucosa, with the dysplastic glands having a similar cytological appearance to the rest of the adenoma. Usually the dysplastic glands are low grade, but pseudo-invasion with high grade dysplastic glands occurs [53,54]. Focal cystic dilatation of glands is common [51]. Lamina propria may be evident at least focally around the displaced epithelium in the submucosa, but other cases have a more fibrotic stroma (Figure 37.13). Haemorrhage is commonly seen due to the initiating torsional injury; haemosiderin subsequently forms and is evident in routine haematoxylin and eosin (H&E) sections in 80–90% of cases without the need to use Perls' staining [51,52]. Rupture of cystic glands not infrequently leads to mucin extravasation and dissection into the surrounding submucosa, and this feature can be of concern. Benign mucin extravasates are generally rounded and may be acellular or lined by dysplastic epithelium, but free-floating epithelial clusters are not typical in benign lesions [52,55] (Figure 37.14).

The above features are distinct from invasive adenocarcinoma, which shows infiltrative glands with irregular architecture, angulated glands and more marked cytological atypia compared with the overlying adenoma. In making the comparison it is important to be aware of any intramucosal adenocarcinoma, which will have similar features to the submucosal component. Adenocarcinoma induces a desmoplastic reaction, has no or little haemosiderin and does not have a component of lamina propria. Invasive mucinous carcinoma is characterised by irregular dissecting pools containing floating clusters of atypical epithelial cells. In particularly difficult cases it has been shown

Table 37.3 Comparison of features of epithelial misplacement into the submucosa (pseudo-invasion) versus invasive adenocarcinoma

	Epithelial misplacement	**Invasive adenocarcinoma**
Glandular epithelial atypia	Same as adenoma	Usually higher grade
Shape of glandular nests	Rounded	Irregular and infiltrative
Cystic glands	Common	Rare
Lamina propria present	Often	No
Stroma	Loose with muscle fibres; occasionally dense sclerosis	Desmoplastic
Haemosiderin	Common	Uncommon and focal
Mucin pools	Sometimes	Sometimes
Epithelium in mucin pools	Confined to periphery	Floating in mucin

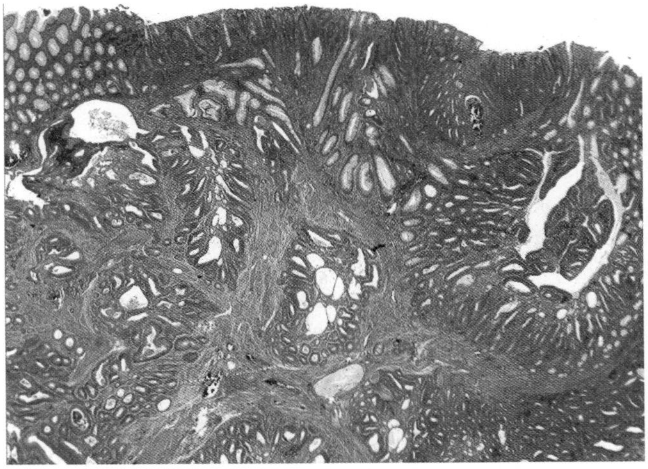

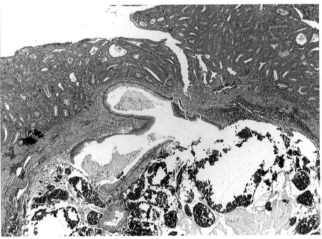

Figure 37.13 Pseudo-invasion of adenoma: the submucosal glands form rounded nests with residual lamina propria and haemosiderin deposition in the surrounding fibrotic stroma.

Figure 37.14 Mucus extravasation into the submucosa of an adenoma, also seen in Figure 37.12. The epithelium is confined to the wall of the extravasate. Lamina propria and haemorrhage are present and support the diagnosis of pseudo-invasion.

that decreased or discontinuous immunohistochemical expression of E-cadherin and collagen IV is seen in 65% and 96% respectively of carcinomas but not in foci of pseudo-invasion [54].

Post-biopsy epithelial misplacement has also been described after adenoma biopsy, generally of sessile rather than pedunculated lesions [56]. The appearances differ somewhat from those described above, with small pools of mucin embedded in granulation tissue and containing small groups of dysplastic epithelium forming small papillary projections [56]. Helpful diagnostic features include a history of recent polyp biopsy, the very small size, lack of frankly malignant cytology, presence of surrounding granulation tissue, evidence of previous haemorrhage and a prominent eosinophilic infiltrate.

Adenocarcinoma arising in an adenoma ('malignant colorectal adenoma')

A malignant adenoma is defined as adenocarcinoma invading into the submucosa of a polypoid adenoma (Figures 37.15 and 37.16). These early lesions, potentially curable by endoscopic polypectomy alone if certain conditions for low-risk lesions are met, have been estimated to account for up to 3–9% of adenomas resected at colonoscopy [57], although in contemporary practice the frequency is lower.

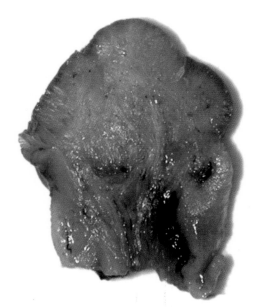

Figure 37.15 Carcinoma arising in an adenomatous polyp: there is a blurred interface between the mucosa and submucosa on the cut surface.

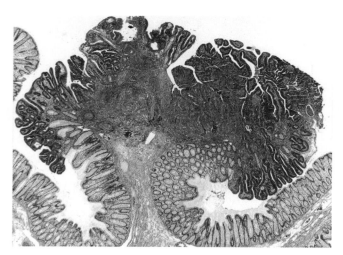

Figure 37.16 Carcinoma arising in an adenomatous polyp, invading the submucosa.

Carcinoma confined to the mucosa generally has been regarded as incapable of metastatic spread and is cured by complete excision (see discussion later in this section), but invasion by the carcinoma beyond the muscularis mucosae into the submucosa gives access to lymphatic and other vessels and the potential risk of nodal or less commonly haematogenous spread [38,57–61]. For this reason, malignant adenomas must be carefully assessed and fully reported to allow an informed decision to be made about the requirement for further surgery. Most cases seen have

focal carcinoma occupying a variable amount of the polyp, but some lesions are purely polypoid carcinoma without an adenomatous component [57,58]. These are regarded as equivalent to malignant adenoma and the same criteria are applied to determine the risk of adverse outcome [62,63].

Careful pathological handling is important to allow malignant adenomas to be fully assessed. In some cases an area of irregular ulceration or surface excavation may look suspicious, and ideally sectioning should be oriented to give the best view of these areas in relation to the resection margin. Pedunculated adenomas should have the diathermied margin identified, and be trimmed to allow the central stalk and resection margin to be blocked and serially sectioned. Peripheral parts of the polyp head often need to be placed in further blocks due to polyp size. Inking of the stalk margin is generally not required because diathermy change is readily identified macroscopically and histologically. Sessile polyps ideally should be sectioned into sequential slices as is currently recommended for other mucosal resections [64]; inking can be useful with the larger sessile polyps now being removed, and also assists in correct orientation during embedding. Large lesions should be pinned out during fixation and blocked completely. If the polyp has been removed piecemeal the margins generally cannot be accurately assessed, although sometimes a definite stalk and final margin can be identified among the fragments.

Conservative management of malignant adenomas is now standard practice if the polyp features suggest that there is a low risk of an adverse outcome such as residual and recurrent adenocarcinoma, lymph nodal or haematogenous metastases, or increased cancer-related mortality on follow-up [38,65]. Lesions are segregated into low-risk and high-risk groups depending on the presence of unfavourable histological features in the carcinomatous component. The best recognised ones are poor differentiation (grade III), positive margins and, in some studies, lymphovascular invasion. Others have suggested that the level of invasion ('Haggitt level') (Table 37.4), dimensions of the submucosal adenocarcinoma and tumour budding impact on the risk, as discussed below. Many studies have clearly shown that it is the high risk group with unfavourable histology that harbours the cases where adenocarcinoma may recur or spread, with a 10–30% risk of an adverse outcome [57,58, 63,65]. This is usually residual adenocarcinoma at the polypectomy site, but it is important to recognise that even in these cases up to 90% of colectomies will not show residual malignancy. Features to include in the histological report are shown in Table 37.5.

Poorly differentiated adenocarcinoma
The carcinomatous component is graded on the worst area as well, moderately or poorly differentiated (grades I–III respectively). Poorly differentiated adenocarcinoma

Table 37.4 Haggitt's levels of invasion of malignant adenomas

Level 0	Carcinoma *in situ* or intramucosal carcinoma
Level 1	Invasion of submucosa of polyp head above junction with stalk (head)
Level 2	Carcinoma invading to junction of adenoma and stalk (neck)
Level 3	Carcinoma invading to any other part of the polyp (stalk)
Level 4	Invasion into submucosa below the stalk of a pedunculated polyp or the submucosa of a sessile polyp

Table 37.5 Features to include in the histological report for malignant adenoma

Site

Maximum diameter

Adenocarcinoma grade

Level of invasion

Lymphovascular invasion

Adjacent adenoma type and grade (if present)

Margin involvement by adenocarcinoma (includes diathermied zone)

Minimum clearance from adenocarcinoma to margin

Optional items

Tumour budding [70]

Dimensions of adenocarcinoma in submucosa

includes signet ring and undifferentiated types [57]. These are not common; overall approximately 7.2% of lesions are poorly differentiated [65] and these tumours carry a significant risk of nodal metastases or cancer-related death, found in up to 30–50% of cases [57,58,61–63,65,66]. Commonly other unfavourable histological features are also present. As has been pointed out [67], early studies of all colorectal adenocarcinomas confined to the submucosa found that less than 5% had nodal metastases and most of these were poorly differentiated [68]. This reinforces that poor differentiation is an important adverse feature.

Positive polypectomy resection margin
A positive margin is predictive of a higher risk of residual carcinoma at the polyp site [65]. Many cases have no further

adenocarcinoma found at the time of colectomy, probably reflecting fulguration at the time of the original procedure. As a result of this some have recommended re-excision of the polypectomy site before making a final decision on definitive colectomy if no other adverse features are present [69], although most centres would progress to colectomy if the margin is reported as positive. Different definitions of an adequate clear resection margin have been used in the literature. Many reports simply required the adenocarcinoma to be unequivocally clear of the margin and the adjacent diathermied area [57,62,70], and this is the minimum needed in clinical practice. Other authors have regarded adequate clearance as 1 mm [58] or 2 mm [61] from the margin, although lesions in the latter study with margins between 0 and 2 mm were associated with other unfavourable histology in the majority (64%) of cases. Netzer and colleagues found that 28% of completely excised polyps with unequivocal clear margins had a clearance of <2 mm from carcinoma, but these cases did not have any adverse events on follow-up [66].

Lymphovascular invasion
This feature is more controversial as an independent adverse histological feature in malignant polyps [65,66] due to its frequent occurrence with other changes such as poorly differentiated tumours, but some studies have found it to be important [57,58,70]. Described in up to 17.6% of malignant polyps, but less common in our experience, definite invasion of lymphatics is associated with an increased risk for nodal metastasis [65]. As it may be difficult to distinguish from retraction artefact, its identification has been shown to have only fair to substantial agreement between pathologists [58]. In cases where the finding is uncertain it should be reported as 'indefinite' and correlated with the presence of other adverse features, as well as the patient's condition and age. Immunohistochemical staining of lymphatic endothelium with the monoclonal antibody D2-40 may be of use, but often small foci cut out quickly, thus limiting its usefulness. In those rare cases where lymphatic invasion is the only adverse feature, it 'would be imprudent to ignore' [67]. Venous invasion is uncommon but is of similar significance.

Level of invasion other features
Haggitt et al. described four levels of invasion of pedunculated polyps (see Table 37.4) from the polyp head to the submucosa of the underlying colonic wall [71]. In Haggitt's study the level of invasion was found to be important in determining the disease course, with only level 4 lesions being associated with an unfavourable outcome, defined by them as death from colorectal carcinoma, patients alive with disease or positive nodes at colectomy. Sessile polyps, because of the absence of a stalk, are all level 4, but these

lesions are also associated with a greater incidence of other adverse features that could affect the prognosis [57,58]. A number of centres have reported that sessile polyps are not all high risk, and can be stratified for risk using the factors described above [58,67,70]. In addition, more recent data suggest that other features may identify the high-risk group. Ueno et al. found that tumour budding (single tumour cells or small tumour cell clusters of more than five cells, with five or more foci in a 200 × [or 0.785 mm²] field) imparted a high risk. They also suggested that the absolute dimensions of adenocarcinoma in the submucosa provide an objective measure of risk. Submucosal carcinoma measuring <4 mm across or <2 mm in depth from the muscularis mucosae had a low frequency of adverse outcome [70]. Another study suggested that nodal metastasis could occur when the carcinomatous component had a submucosal tumour depth (measured from the muscularis mucosae) of ≥1.25 mm, and suggested this as the maximum depth for conservative management [72].

Purely intramucosal poorly differentiated adenocarcinoma

It is widely stated that an adenoma containing a focus of adenocarcinoma that is invasive but confined to the mucosa does not have metastatic potential [17,38,57]. Very rarely, the intramucosal carcinoma is poorly differentiated. As poorly differentiated tumours have the highest risk of adverse outcome [67], there is a theoretical risk that tumour cells could invade lymphatic vessels present in the deepest aspect of the mucosa and muscularis mucosae [73]. These lymphatics can sometimes be readily seen in routine practice if a carcinoma has very extensive lymphatic invasion. In a recent study of 15 patients with adenomas containing purely intramucosal, poorly differentiated adenocarcinoma, no metastatic disease was identified from these lesions [74]. However, subsequent correspondence described two similar cases from the Memorial Sloan Kettering Cancer Centre. One developed distant metastases despite colectomy after the initial polypectomy, and the second showed invasion of lymphatic vessels in the deep mucosa, without any submucosal invasion [75]. This suggests that poorly differentiated adenocarcinoma should prompt consideration of colectomy, even if confined to the mucosa. The frequency of this appears to be increasing [74] and further studies are needed.

Pathogenesis of conventional adenoma

There is a full discussion of colorectal carcinogenesis in Chapter 38 and a brief overview only is given here. In most cases, colorectal carcinoma begins with the initiation and progression of a colonic adenoma through a series of genetic alterations affecting genes that are associated with key intracellular pathways [76,77]. Biallelic loss of APC is

the initiator of adenoma formation in the mucosa of patients with familial adenomatous polyposis, but in sporadic cases it remains unclear whether the earliest mutation is in APC or in other genes encoding different proteins inhibiting Wnt signalling [30,78]. By the time that the adenoma is macroscopically visible, APC mutation is found in two-thirds [79]. Loss of the functional protein, which is a negative regulator of the Wnt signalling pathway, allows the accumulation and nuclear translocation of β-catenin, resulting in the increased expression of genes affecting proliferation, differentiation and cellular migration [80]. The APC protein also has a role in promoting chromosomal stability [81]. Conventional adenomas begin as monocryptal adenomas and recent studies suggest that mutation in the crypt stem cell is necessary to give rise to a growing, dysplastic lesion [27]. Deletion of APC in the putative stem cell in mice caused intestinal microadenoma formation within 8 days and the development of a lethal tumour burden by 36 days. Conversely, deletion of APC in the proliferative transit-amplifying cells but not in the stem cells was associated with only microadenoma formation, the growth of which ceased early. Later, the acquisition of other mutations in genes such as KRAS is associated with adenoma progression [76,78], which may include increased villosity [82]. Recent gene mapping studies have suggested that there is considerable heterogeneity in the actual mutations that occur in individual colorectal tumours [83], but these appear to affect genes encoding proteins in about 10–20 critical intracellular pathways [77,83]. The mutation of TP53, leading to loss of function of this key tumour-suppressor gene, signals the progression to accelerated chromosomal instability and malignant progression [77,81].

Flat adenomas appear to have a different pattern of mutation, which may explain their unusual appearance. These lesions have a lower frequency of APC and KRAS mutation (<10% for both) and apparent frequent early mutation of TP53 (reviewed in Kudo et al. [23]).

Serrated polyps

Serrated polyps (SPs) have a serrated or 'saw-tooth' appearance on histology as a result of crypt epithelial cell accumulation and luminal inbudding secondary to inhibition of apoptosis [84,85]. The latter is caused by KRAS or BRAF mutations [86,87], which are believed to initiate SP formation [87–89]. A serrated neoplasia pathway is well documented that leads to colorectal cancer (CRC) involving sequential BRAF or KRAS mutation, DNA CpG island methylation (CIMP) and microsatellite instability (MSI) [86–88,90,91]. Serrated polyps in this pathway are the hyperplastic polyp (HP), sessile serrated adenoma (SSA), mixed polyp (MP) and traditional serrated adenoma (TSA).

Table 37.6 Clinical and molecular features of serrated polyps

	Frequency (%)		Molecular changes (%)				
	Proportion of removed polyps	Proportion of serrated polyps	*BRAF* mutation	*KRAS* mutation	CIMP high	MSI high	References
Hyperplastic polyp – goblet cell	8.5	24–30	20–23	42–50	14–15		[88,89,93,98, 122,151]
Hyperplastic polyp – microvesicular	15	40–50	29–76	11–13	47		[88,89,93,98, 122,151]
Hyperplastic polyp – mucin poor	1.5	4–5					
Sessile serrated adenoma (lesion, polyp)	9	23	78–90	7–8	75–76		[20,89,98,122]
Mixed polyp	0.7–1.7	1.9–4.2	40–100 (proximal)	43–50 (distal)			[98,112,122,151]
Traditional serrated adenoma	0.6–2.5	2–7	36–77	8–9 (distal)	68 (proximal)	7–51	[98,122,124,127, 144,151]

CIMP, DNA CpG island methylation; MSI, microsatellite instability.

Hyperplastic polyp

Although traditionally HPs have been regarded as inconsequential non-neoplastic lesions [86,92,93], subsequent identification of clonal genetic aberrations, including *KRAS* mutation, chromosome 1p deletions and MSI [92,93], indicated that they are in fact neoplastic. More recently, based on microscopic features, classic or harmless HPs have been distinguished from larger, usually right-sided lesions of similar appearance, designated SSAs, which may progress to CRC [87,93–95].

Classic HPs are common diminutive lesions predominantly located in the distal colon and rectum [93,96]. They represent approximately 25% of endoscopically removed polyps but 70–85% of all serrated polyps (Table 37.6). Endoscopically they are pale, sessile, slightly raised lesions <5 mm across that flatten with air insufflation [97] (Figure 37.17). Histologically serration is limited to the upper third to half of the crypt, varying from lesion to lesion. The deeper crypts appear straight and tubular, similar to adjacent normal crypts, and show symmetrical expansion of the proliferative zone without basal crypt dilation (Figure 37.18). The collagen plate underlying the surface epithelium is usually thickened. Detailed analysis of a series of SPs identified three morphological subtypes of classic HP: microvesicular, goblet cell rich and mucin poor [93]. Although at this time no specific clinical importance is attached to these subtypes, there appears to be a molecular basis for the subclassification [88,98].

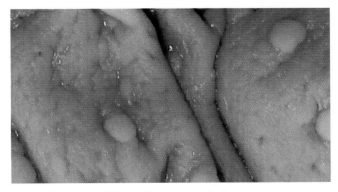

Figure 37.17 Small hyperplastic polyps in the rectum.

Microvesicular HPs, 59% of HPs, represent the typical HP of the distal colon and rectum where almost all are located. They are generally thicker than the adjacent mucosa and comprise vesicular mucin-containing epithelial cells and goblet cells, the latter in decreased numbers compared with normal crypts. Goblet cell abnormalities are common. Ki67 staining shows a symmetrically expanded proliferative compartment occupying the lower half of the crypt [99]. Minimal nuclear atypia is seen in most cases and nuclear stratification, although not prominent, occurs in crypts and at the surface. Endocrine cells with eosinophilic or clear cytoplasm are usually increased in number or enlarged. Thickening of the subepithelial collagen plate is usual, as is thickening of the muscularis mucosae, with extension of muscle fibres into the lamina propria between crypts

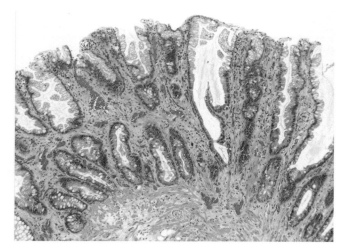

Figure 37.18 Hyperplastic polyp, microvesicular type: the muscularis mucosae is thickened.

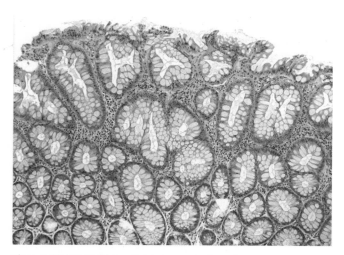

Figure 37.19 Goblet cell-rich hyperplastic polyp.

(Figure 37.18). *BRAF* mutations are commonly found in this HP variant (Table 37.6).

Goblet cell-rich HPs, accounting for 34% of HPs, almost all occur in the left colon and rectum. They show mucosal thickening, elongation of crypts with increased goblet cells (Figure 37.19), goblet cell-type mucin only, and serration limited to the upper third of the crypt or the surface only. There is minimal nuclear atypia or stratification and thickening of the subepithelial collagen plate, and the muscularis mucosae is thickened in most. They resemble hyperplastic colonic mucosa adjacent to mass lesions. *KRAS* mutations are predominant (Table 37.6).

Mucin-poor HPs are rare and occur only in the left colon and rectum. They contain little or no microvesicular mucin. The epithelial cells appear smaller with less cytoplasm, and goblet cells are absent or decreased with an irregular distribution. There are uniform and prominent serrations with

a micropapillary pattern and crypts may appear dilated. Nuclear hyperchromasia and anisocytosis may be prominent and typically there is hyperplasia of clear endocrine cells. The mucin-poor polyp was identified only through statistical analysis of the datasets, and the cytological changes suggest that these lesions may represent regenerative change in an injured microvesicular HP.

Sessile serrated adenoma (sessile serrated lesion, sessile serrated polyp)

In 1996, Torlakovic and Snover reported a study of polyps from six patients with hyperplastic polyposis (HPP), four of whom developed CRC [95]. The polyps differed from classic HPs by way of larger size, architectural distortion, cytologically atypical nuclei, focal nuclear crowding with dispolarity and decreased endocrine cells, but they lacked conventional dysplasia of the type seen in traditional serrated adenomas. In a follow-up study published in 2003 [93] the same atypical polyps, tentatively named sessile serrated adenomas (SSAs), represented 18% of 'hyperplastic' polyps in non-polyposis patients. The same year, Goldstein reported identical polyps preceding sporadic MSI-high CRCs in the same colonic segment [94]. Molecular evidence supports SSAs as precursors of these cancers [87,88,100]. Despite this, the lack of overt dysplasia makes many pathologists reluctant to use the word 'adenoma' for these growths, preferring the terms 'sessile serrated lesion' (SSL) and 'sessile serrated polyp' (SSP).

SSAs are common, and represented 9% of all polyps and 23% of non-dysplastic SPs (HPs and SSAs) identified by magnifying chromoendoscopy in a recent series of consecutive, unselected colonoscopy patients [98]. They tend to be multiple, right sided and larger than conventional HPs, often exceeding 10 mm in diameter and sometimes reaching several centimetres [93,95,98,100]. Endoscopically they are easily missed, malleable, smooth, sessile lesions, pale to yellow in colour and covered with mucus that may be difficult to remove [98,101–103] (Figure 37.20).

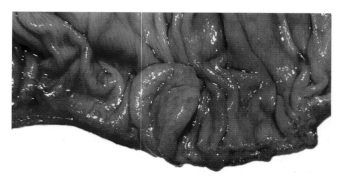

Figure 37.20 Sessile serrated adenoma (lesion): the lesion is slightly elevated.

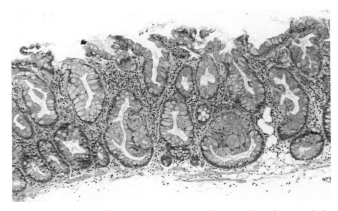

Figure 37.21 Sessile serrated adenoma (lesion): the characteristic dilated and horizontal crypt bases are well seen. Usual adenomatous dysplasia is not seen in most lesions.

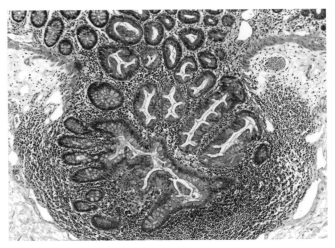

Figure 37.22 Herniation of sessile serrated adenoma (lesion) into the submucosa.

The histological differentiation of SSAs from HPs is predominantly architecture dependent. Characteristic findings are branched crypts, dilated crypt bases, inverted L- and T-shaped crypts with horizontal extension along the muscularis mucosae (Figure 37.21), exaggerated serration that can extend to the crypt base, prominent intraluminal mucin and inverted growth, where crypt bases extend through the muscularis mucosae into the superficial submucosa, often in the region of lymphoid follicles [87,93–95] (Figure 37.22). As many of the diagnostic changes are seen in crypt bases, accurate diagnosis is dependent on well orientated sections and examination of deeper levels may be required to achieve this [87,100].

Other histological findings reflect abnormal cell proliferation and dysmaturation. These include nuclear atypia in the form of irregular contours, open chromatin pattern, small prominent nucleoli and failed surface maturation,

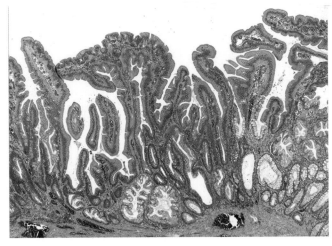

Figure 37.23 Mixed polyp with areas of sessile serrated adenoma seen at the central base of the polyp and traditional serrated adenoma overlying this.

dystrophic goblet cells, goblet cell or gastric foveolar cell phenotype replacing the normal proliferative zone in crypt bases, mitosis in the middle and upper crypts, and Ki67 staining that is irregular along the length of the crypt and often asymmetrical there. Focal surface nuclear stratification and eosinophilic change resembling TSA cytology and a reduction in endocrine cells also occur. Other differentiating features from HPs are lack of basement membrane thickening and focal loss of MLH1 and/or MSH2 positivity [87,93–95,99]. The molecular changes found most commonly are *BRAF* mutations and CIMP-high (Table 37.6). A morphological continuum and overlapping molecular biology support the origin of SSAs in preceding microvesicular HPs [87,88,100,104,105].

Recent studies show that serrated polyps, particularly large SSAs outside the setting of HPP, are strongly associated with synchronous and subsequent serrated polyps and advanced neoplasia, notably right-sided MSI-high colorectal adenocarcinoma [106–110].

Mixed polyps

In 1984, Urbanski et al. reported a CRC arising in a mixed hyperplastic and adenomatous polyp and reviewed previous reports of similar lesions [111]. Also called mixed hyperplastic/adenomatous polyps, sessile serrated polyps with dysplasia or advanced sessile serrated adenomas, mixed polyps have a non-dysplastic serrated component of HP or SSA and a dysplastic component comprising conventional adenoma, TSA or morphologically variable but distinctive non-TSA-type serrated dysplasia [112–114] (Figure 37.23). Mixed polyps are uncommon (see Table 37.6).

The different non-dysplastic serrated and dysplastic elements of a mixed polyp usually show similar molecular

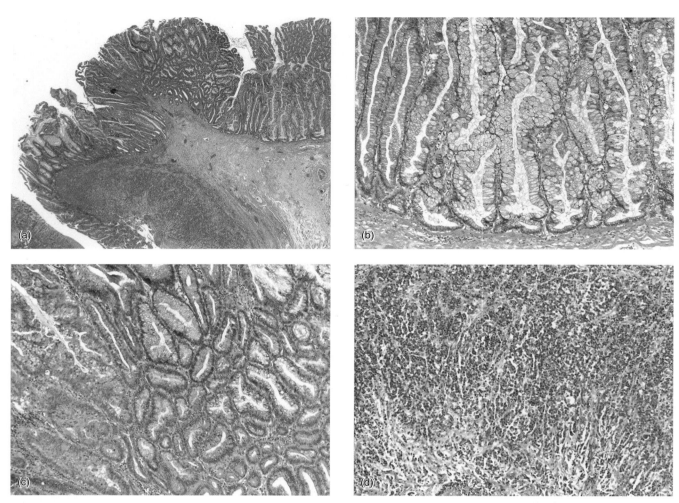

Figure 37.24 Signet-ring adenocarcinoma arising in a mixed polyp: (a) sessile serrated adenoma (SSA; lesion) at the top right of the image shows transition into traditional serrated adenoma and then the carcinoma at the lower left. The traditional serrated adenomatous and carcinomatous components showed loss of MLH1 immunostaining, indicating microsatellite instability. MLH1 staining was preserved in the SSA. (b) At higher power there are typical features of SSA at the edge and within the lesion. (c) Transitional zone with serrated dysplasia at higher power. (d) Signet ring adenocarcinoma at higher power.

profiles [88,115,116], indicating that the dysplasia arises in a pre-existing non-dysplastic SP, typically SSA, and constitutes an intermediate step in the progression to cancer [87,100,117,118]. Nuclear β-catenin expression, seen in 30% of SSAs and all components of most if not all mixed polyps, may precede dysplastic change and indicate SSA at risk of neoplastic progression [113,117]. Loss of MLH1 is often seen in the high grade adenomatous component of a mixed polyp and significantly increases the risk of carcinomatous transformation, but may not be required to initiate dysplastic change [113,119–121]. A significant minority of mixed polyps show loss of *O*-6-methylguanine-DNA methyltransferase (MGMT) or aberrantly express p53 in the dysplastic components [113,117]. *BRAF* mutations are more common in the proximal colonic mixed polyps whereas *KRAS* mutations occur particularly in distal lesions [98,112,122] (see Table 37.6).

Malignant transformation of mixed polyps is frequent even in lesions ≤10 mm in size [113,119,120], consistent with genetic instability promoting rapid neoplastic progression [113] (Figure 37.24). These early carcinomas are most common in the right colon and tend to directly invade the submucosa without lateral spread. They may be well, moderately or poorly differentiated and are often mucinous or serrated in type. Lymph node metastasis is unusual.

Traditional serrated adenoma

First described by Longacre and Fenoglio-Preiser in 1990, serrated adenomas have the saw-toothed configuration

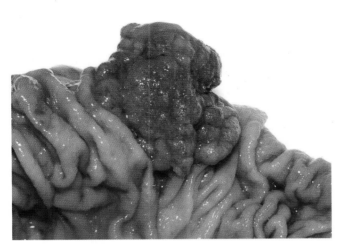

Figure 37.25 Traditional serrated adenoma with polypoid growth.

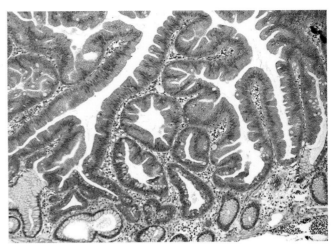

Figure 37.26 Traditional serrated adenoma with characteristic serration of crypts and abundant eosinophilic cytoplasm of the dysplastic epithelium.

of an HP but show dysplasia in the upper crypt and surface epithelium [123,124]. Termed TSAs in 2003 to differentiate them from SSAs [93], serrated adenomas reported in the literature are heterogeneous, probably including SSAs, mixed polyps and some conventional adenomatous polyps [112,125,126]. As a result, TSAs remain poorly characterised.

TSAs are uncommon at colonoscopy and represent 1–3% of adenomas (see Table 37.6). The mean age at diagnosis is 60–65 years and males outnumber females 2:1 [96]. Although TSAs occur throughout the large intestine, up to two-thirds are found in the rectosigmoid region [124,127,128]. This is distinct from SSAs, which are typically right sided.

Two-thirds of TSAs are polypoid and the remainder flat or sessile [127–131]. The polypoid lesions are more common distally, show reddish coloration and a granulo-lobular or lobular appearance with cerebriform or petal-like pit patterns (Figure 37.25). Sessile and flat lesions tend to be larger, more often proximal, white or the colour of adjacent mucosa, and show HP-like, small, round, elongated oval or stellate crypt openings. Lesions vary in size from 1 mm to 2 mm up to ≥70 mm [124,129,132–134], and may be multiple in some patients [124,128,135].

Histologically, sessile and flat TSAs show a tubular architecture and polypoid TSAs a more complex tubulovillous or villous growth pattern with convoluted serrated crypts and dysplastic epithelial cells (Figure 37.26). The latter typically have abundant eosinophilic cytoplasm, which is a useful histological feature (Figure 37.27). The nuclei in most lesions are uniform, mildly stratified and centrally placed. They are somewhat hyperchromatic and elongated, with a pencillate shape and dispersed chromatin, and have small but conspicuous eosinophilic nucleoli and smooth nuclear contours. Surface epithelial tufting or papillation is seen and mitoses are uncommon or absent [124,131,136].

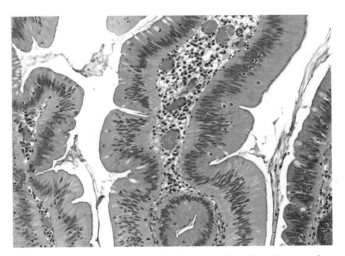

Figure 37.27 Typical cytological features of traditional serrated adenoma.

Nuclei are less stratified and show less atypia than conventional adenomatous polyps. Components of HP, SSA and conventional adenomatous polyp may be found in some TSAs.

High grade dysplasia, seen in more than 10% of TSAs in many series and particularly found in larger polyps [124,131,137–139], is manifested by glandular epithelial cells that have vesicular nuclei with prominent nucleoli and complex glandular budding, branching and back-to-back placement [140] (Figure 37.28). Carcinoma is seen in 1–6.5% of TSAs [124,132,135,138,141] and TSA is found immediately adjacent to 5.8% of CRCs [142]. TSAs are a substantial risk factor for separate synchronous and metachronous CRC and have a higher growth rate, recur more

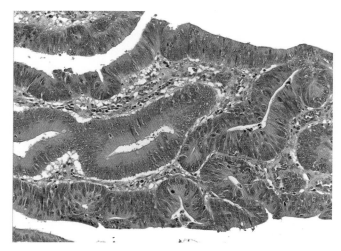

Figure 37.28 High grade dysplasia in a traditional serrated adenoma.

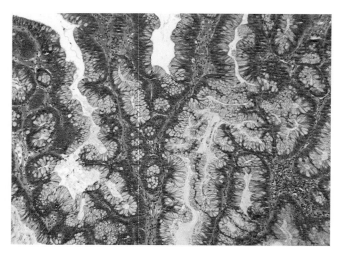

Figure 37.29 Traditional serrated adenoma with more conventionally appearing dysplasia but with conspicuous ectopic crypt foci (see text).

frequently and are more predictive of concurrent SPs and subsequent SAs than conventional adenomatous polyps [127,132,137,143].

Two major histological subtypes of TSA have been recognised [112,126]. The first and best known, with the morphological features described above, usually shows a *BRAF* or less commonly a *KRAS* mutation [144]. Those with a *BRAF* mutation are found throughout the colon and are usually low grade, with elements of precursor HP or SSA, with which they share similar genetic changes. Those with a *KRAS* mutation are predominantly left sided, lack precursor elements and are more likely to be high grade. They are also more likely to harbour conventional adenomatous dysplasia and progress to adenocarcinoma. The second subtype, which has also been called conventional adenoma with serrated architecture, shows serration, villous change and adenomatous dysplasia characterised by cytoplasmic basophilia (rather than eosinophilia) and elongated, hyperchromatic, pseudo-stratified nuclei without prominent nucleoli [112,126] (Figure 37.29). This form of TSA correlates with *KRAS* mutation, MSI low or stable and loss of MGMT that results in mutations causing chromosomal instability and loss of heterozygosity [117]. The relationship of this subtype with 'fusion' characteristics to the serrated and conventional pathways of neoplastic progression remains uncertain [126,145].

TSAs have an overall low proliferative index with Ki67-positive cells distributed irregularly in ectopic crypt foci (ECFs) oriented perpendicular to larger crypts. These are recognised as variably sized, often tiny crypts budding from the sides of larger crypts (Figure 37.29). The ECFs fail to reach the underlying muscularis mucosae as normal crypts do, possibly accounting for the protuberant growth typical of TSAs [99]. Using ECFs to recognise TSAs may standardise their identification and allow improved char-

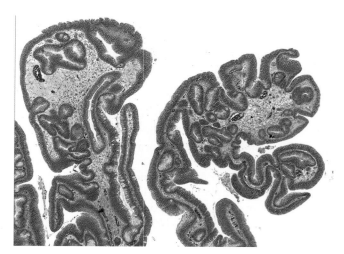

Figure 37.30 Filiform serrated adenoma.

acterisation. Diagnosis of TSAs on this basis reveals frequent and sometimes predominant goblet cell differentiation. Mucinous differentiation has also been reported [140].

A variant of TSA, *filiform serrated adenoma*, is almost exclusively located in the rectosigmoid and has been described in older adults, particularly women [146]. It shows predominant, thin, finger-like, villiform projections with distended bulbous tips, tall columnar epithelial cells with eosinophilic cytoplasm, serrated contours, variable goblet cell component and frequent ulceration, erosion and oedema consistent with traumatic injury (Figure 37.30). Over 50% contain components of HP, SSA and conventional adenomatous polyp; foci of high grade dysplasia and invasive carcinoma are seen in some larger polyps.

Results of molecular studies of TSAs are highly variable, reflecting the heterogeneity of the lesions studied. *BRAF* or

KRAS mutations can be found [88,89,112,116,144,147] with *KRAS* mutations most common in left-sided polyps [116,147]. CIMP-high (two or more markers positive) is commonly seen and increases with advanced histology, proximal location, size >5 mm and *BRAF* mutation [88,89,148, 149]. MSI and loss of MLH1 can occur [115,147,148,150]. Partial or complete loss of MGMT is seen in 13–29% [112, 113,141,151], and methylation of the MLH1 and MGMT promoter sites occurs in 48% and 45% respectively [88]. Overexpression of p53, usually in areas of high grade dysplasia [112,113,139,141,152], nuclear staining for β-catenin [117,153], loss of heterozygosity [141,150,152] and aneuploidy with near diploid DNA [127] occur in some cases.

Serrated polyposis

Serrated (formerly hyperplastic) polyposis (SPP), recognised as an entity by Williams et al. in 1980 [154], encompasses considerable heterogeneity [155–158]. This is reflected in the current WHO diagnostic criteria:
1. At least five histologically diagnosed SPs proximal to the sigmoid colon, of which two are >10 mm in diameter
2. Any number of SPs occurring proximal to the sigmoid colon in an individual who has a first-degree relative with SPP
3. More than 20 HPs of any size, but distributed throughout the colon [159].

Inclusion of advanced SPs and the use of a cumulative total of polyps removed over time are recommended for the purpose of meeting the definition [84]. Although many published reports use these definitions [157,160,161], others have applied less stringent criteria [156,158,162–165].

SPP is most commonly diagnosed in the fifth to seventh decades [166] with an age range of 10–79 years [162,163, 167,168]. Although some series show a male predominance [154,157,169], in most there are relatively equal numbers of males and females [158,160,161,163,168]. Most SPP patients reported are from western countries. A large proportion has been from Australia and New Zealand [155,170], the latter almost entirely of Celtic origin [163]. Although considered rare [154,157,168,171], it is likely that SPP is under-diagnosed [157]. One study using the previous WHO criteria established a prevalence of 1 in 3000 in 55–64 year olds [172].

In 1996, Torlakovic and Snover reported six patients, four of whom developed CRC, with multiple large atypical SPs (later to be called SSAs), and they called this condition 'serrated adenomatous polyposis' [93,95]. In an accompanying editorial Burt suggested that there may be at least two subtypes of SPP, sessile serrated adenomatosis and another characterised by very large numbers of small typical HPs, which he and others had personally seen [100,173]. In 2007 Jass named these type I and type II HPP respectively [155] (Figure 37.31).

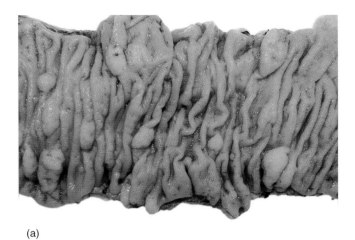

(a)

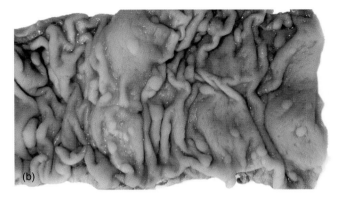

(b)

Figure 37.31 Serrated polyposis (SPP). Two broad groups are recognised: (a) type I SPP has fewer, larger serrated polyps, and (b) type II SPP has numerous small hyperplastic polyps.

Type I HPP is characterised by five or more SPs, at least two >10 mm in diameter, with SSA architecture located proximal to the sigmoid; dysplastic SPs (mixed polyps and TSAs) and coexisting conventional adenomatous polyps are frequent [95,156,157,159–165,168,170,173–176]. *BRAF* mutations and DNA methylation are common [86,121, 174,177,178] whereas *KRAS* mutation is almost never seen [156,161]. There is a high risk of CRC [95,155,173] (see below), with 33% of CRCs MSI high and showing inactivation of *MLH1* through promoter methylation [155]. MSI may also be seen in dysplastic serrated polyps in these patients [161,175,177,178].

Type II SPP generally shows large numbers (≥30) of small and morphologically typical HPs, each 1–10 mm in diameter and in a pancolonic distribution [155,156,159,173]. It is likely that most patients in the series of Williams et al. and Fernandez et al., and the dense polyposis group of Buchanan et al., fit into this category [154,158,169]. These patients tend to be younger males with very large numbers of polyps, often ≥80, and a lower risk of developing or having a family history of CRC. Dysplastic SPs and adenomas tend not to occur in this type of SPP [155]. *KRAS* rather than *BRAF* mutations have been demonstrated [121,156,162]. A separate group may show loss of heterozygosity (LOH) for chromosome 1p [156], with polyps that are less methylated [121]. Some in this category may be forme frustes of type I SPP [155].

SPP patients are at increased risk of CRC in the range 33–69% [155,158,170]. The CRCs tend to occur in younger patients and are more commonly right sided, multiple and present at the time of diagnosis of SPP or shortly after [95,156–158,160,161,163,164,167,168,170,176,178–180]. The cancer risk increases with an increasing number of polyps [158], the size of the SPs [160,178] and the presence of dysplastic serrated polyps [161] or conventional adenomas [158]. Tumours first identified in colectomy specimens and during surveillance may be very small with appearances similar to non-cancerous polyps [161,178]. In a surveillance series, the cumulative risk of CRC was 7% after 5 years [165]. The cancers in SPP may be MSI high, MSI low or MS stable [155,161,170,178,180].

A family history of CRC is seen in 18–59% of SPP patients, usually in those with type I disease [156,158,160–164,168,170,181]. Familial SPP is seen infrequently with both autosomal dominant and recessive inheritance described [156,160,163,181]. One SPP patient with biallelic *MUTYH* (*MYH*) mutations was identified in a recent SPP series [163], and conversely 18% of patients with *MUTYH*-associated polyposis met the criteria for SPP [182] (see below). Extensive DNA methylation in both normal colonic mucosa and the polyps in SPP suggests a hypermethylation phenotype related to specific carcinogen exposure or genetic predisposition [84,175,177,183]. Cigarette smoking is associated with CIMP and *BRAF* mutation [183], and may act as a modifier of SPP phenotype [158,184].

Familial adenomatous polyposis

Familial adenomatous polyposis (FAP) is an inherited autosomal dominant disorder caused by mutations, usually truncating, in the *APC* gene at chromosome 5q21. It is characterised by the development of hundreds to thousands of adenomas throughout the colon, appearing first at adolescence, with the early development of adenocarcinoma by the age of 40. By definition, affected patients have more than 100 adenomas [185], but there are usually many more. There are also specific abnormalities at extra-colonic sites including gastric fundic gland polyps, small intestinal adenomas and adenocarcinomas, congenital hypertrophy of retinal pigmented epithelium (CHRPE) and fibromatosis.

Colonic manifestations

Responsible for <1% of colorectal adenocarcinoma, classic FAP has a high penetrance and an incidence of approxi-

mately 1 in 8000–13 000 [155,186,187]. About 75% of cases have a clear inherited basis but the remaining 25% are the result of new mutations in the *APC* gene [155,186]. Adenoma formation usually begins in adolescence, initially in the rectum and then spreading proximally to affect all areas of the colon. Some cases have rectal sparing [188]. The early adenomas are tiny, forming from monocryptal adenomas or aberrant crypt foci that can be detected by chromoendoscopy. The use of dye spray helps to enumerate the number of adenomas present more accurately [187]. Adenocarcinomas begin to develop 10 years or so after the appearance of the adenomas and most, 70–80%, occur in the left colon [189] although any part of the colon may be involved. Prophylactic colectomy is generally performed by the patients' early 20s when the risk of malignancy begins to increase [190]. Submitted colonic specimens typically are carpeted with adenomas of varying size throughout the colon (Figure 37.32), abruptly ceasing at the ileo-caecal valve. Most lesions are sessile and <10 mm but larger lesions do occur. As all lesions cannot be assessed histologically for practical reasons, all larger lesions, ulcerated areas and polyps with any irregular contours should be sampled and examined. A small group of patients has flat adenomas, which are raised only slightly above the mucosal surface and have a height of less than two times the normal mucosa [191–193]. Although most of these cases have an attenuated phenotype, with fewer than 100 polyps and a right-sided predominance [194], cases with >100 adenomas are described. Flat adenomas can also be seen in the rectal stump after colectomy with ileo-rectal anastomosis [195]. Similarly, flat/depressed adenocarcinoma has been described in a rectal stump [196]. Since the advent and widespread use of pouch surgery in the 1980s, it is clear that adenomas also develop in the adapted ileal pouch and

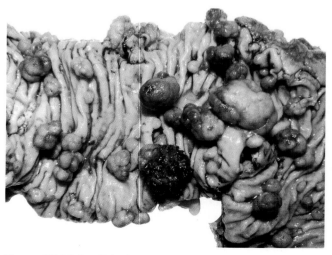

Figure 37.32 Familial adenomatous polyposis.

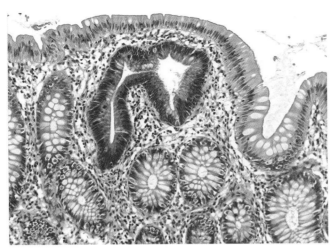

Figure 37.33 Microadenoma in familial adenomatous polyposis.

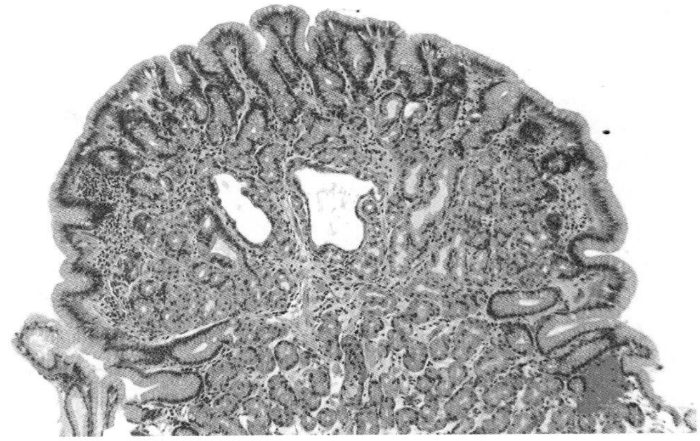

Figure 37.34 Fundic gland polyp in familial adenomatous polyposis with subtle foveolar dysplasia overlying the cystic glands. This is seen in about half the lesions.

can be found in about a third of patients after 10 years and three-quarters after 15 years [197]. However, the development of adenocarcinoma from these is extremely rare [80].

Histologically, most of the lesions in patients with FAP are sessile tubular adenomas, with some larger lesions having a tubulovillous architecture. The adenomas themselves are identical to conventional sporadic ones, but unicryptal and submacroscopic adenomas are often found in the mucosa adjacent to sampled adenomas (Figure 37.33) and may also be seen in the mucosa covering the polyp stalks of any pedunculated lesions. Serrated polyps are not usual; if seen, consideration should be given to *MUTYH*-associated polyposis which, although usually having an attenuated phenotype with <100 polyps, can be associated in some instances with a greater number of adenomas of various types (see below) and be confused with FAP [187,198]. However, the authors have seen some patients with atypical FAP and documented germline *APC* mutation in whom proximal serrated polyps have occurred, so that correlation with the genotype is required.

Clinically, classic FAP is often detected at screening. In others, including those with new mutations, presenting complaints include rectal bleeding and mucous discharge [185].

Extracolonic manifestations

As well as adenomas and colorectal adenocarcinomas, FAP has distinctive extracolonic manifestations [199].

Fundic gland polyps of stomach

These occur in up to 60% of patients and can precede the appearance of adenomas in the colon [80]. They closely resemble sporadic fundic gland polyps that are commonly seen now in the context of proton pump inhibitor therapy used for gastric acid suppression, with cystically dilated glands lined variously by parietal, chief and mucus cells, causing dome-shaped polyps (see Chapter 12). In FAP, however, approximately 50% of the polyps have hyperchromasia and crowding of the surface foveolar epithelium that impart a distinctive appearance [200,201]. This was called 'foveolar hyperproliferation' in the Padova classification of gastric dysplasia [202], but more recently has been recognised as foveolar dysplasia. The cells have rounded, relatively uniform but crowded nuclei, eosinophilic cytoplasm and low grade dysplasia (Figure 37.34). Despite the frequent presence of foveolar dysplasia in these polyps, the development of high grade foveolar dysplasia or malignant transformation does not appear to be a significant problem. Gastric adenomas of usual intestinal type do occur but are rare, and probably account for the rare cases of gastric adenocarcinoma seen in about 1% of patients [203].

Duodenal, ampullary, small intestinal, adenomas

Adenomas in the small intestine occur one to two decades after the colonic polyps in up to 90% of patients [204] and are most numerous in the duodenum and peri-ampullary region. These lesions are an increasing problem in patients who have undergone colectomy and screening programmes now include upper gastrointestinal surveillance [205]. Adenomas can increase in size, number and severity of dysplasia but the risk of malignant progression is much lower than in the colon, with a 5% risk of progression to adenocarcinoma over 10 years [204]. The Spigelman stage assesses number, villosity and degree of dysplasia of the duodenal adenomas to predict if and when surgery may be necessary [206]. This is usually when there are >20 adenomas, with tubulovillous adenomas and high grade dysplasia. However, many patients can be controlled with endoscopic polypectomy [207]. Adenomas more distally in the small intestine are less common but are particularly prone to develop in the ileal pouch [208].

Fibromatosis (desmoid tumour)

Occurring in about 15% of patients [80], fibromatoses are principally seen in the abdominal wall, mesentery and retroperitoneum, with occasional instances at other sites such as the pancreas. Many cases follow surgery or trauma, including colectomy, with lesions growing gradually before presenting on average 2–4 years after the initiating insult [199,209]. They form rounded, infiltrative masses of scar-like collagen with uniform fibroblastic cells, but smaller two-dimensional plaques are also seen [209]. Retroperitoneal tumours may have myxoid areas. The association of FAP and fibromatosis, as well as osteomas and epidermal cysts, has been given the eponymous name Gardner's syndrome [210], but in fact it does not represent a distinct syndrome [80].

Eye, skin, teeth, stromal tissues

In the eyes, CHRPE can be seen in most affected patients as grey–brown patches on the retinal surface, but is variable between families. Dental abnormalities include supernumerary teeth, dentigerous cysts and fused roots [199]. Osteomas, of the skull and mandible in particular, lipomas, epidermal cysts and nasopharyngeal angiofibromas have been described [80,203].

Endocrine tumours

There is an increased risk of papillary carcinoma of the thyroid in young women – around 160 times normal [155]. Women are affected more than men at a rate of 17:1 [199]. The carcinomas may have an unusual cribriform or morular pattern [211]. Adrenal cortical adenoma is increased in frequency [212]. Often small and incidental, some are functional.

Liver and biliary tree

Apart from peri-ampullary adenomas, involvement of the liver and biliary tree is uncommon. Hepatoblastoma has a significantly increased risk particularly in male infants, but nevertheless is still rare in FAP and is seen in less than 1% of patients [155,199,213]. Lesions described in the bile ducts include adenoma [214] and adenocarcinoma [214,215], as well as dysplasia of the gallbladder epithelium [216], but all of these lesions are rare.

CNS

Turcot's syndrome refers to polyposis, colorectal cancer and central nervous system (CNS) tumours. It is heterogeneous and includes patients with both Lynch syndrome (hereditary non-polyposis colorectal cancer or HNPCC)

and FAP. In the cohort with an *APC* mutation, medulloblastoma is the most common tumour, although high grade astrocytoma and ependymoma occur [199].

Genetics and genotype–phenotype correlations

The APC protein is widely expressed and coded from a relatively large gene on the long arm of chromosome 5. It is a negative regulator of the Wnt signalling pathway. With normal function as part of a complex of proteins, it binds β-catenin, downregulating its activity. Mutation usually leads to APC protein truncation and loss of function, resulting in the accumulation of β-catenin; this then binds several transcription factors, causing abnormal expression of proteins involved in regulating proliferation, differentiation, migration and apoptosis of enterocytes and other cells [80,217]. APC protein also binds microtubules at the chromosomal ends, promoting chromosomal stability, so that its loss compounds chromosomal instability when acting in concert with *TP53* mutation and telomere dysfunction [203].

There are hundreds of described mutations in FAP, commonly causing truncation in the middle of the protein [80,155]. Most are found in the central region of the *APC* gene that corresponds to the 5′-coding region of exon 15. This mutation cluster region (MCR) contains 60% of mutations, most commonly at codons 1309 and 1061, which together account for ≥15% of identified mutations [187]. The location of mutation can affect the phenotypic expression of disease in individuals and families. Most strikingly, mutations at the extremes of the *APC* gene, either the 5′-end of the gene or at the 3′-end of exon 15, as well as in the alternatively spliced region of exon 9, are associated with attenuated FAP, characterised by <100 adenomas, later onset of adenocarcinoma and fewer extra-intestinal manifestations (see below). Conversely, mutation between codons 1250 and 1464 can be associated with a marked polyposis [155,218]. Although not precise, other phenotypic correlations with the approximate sites of mutation include the following: fibromatosis (codons 1309–1580), CHRPE (463–1445), osteoma (767–1578) and carcinoma of the thyroid (140–1309) [199]. The *I1307K* mutation found in 7% of Ashkenazi Jews does not cause APC protein truncation but renders the gene more susceptible to further mutation, leading to a 10–20% risk of colorectal cancer [203].

Attenuated FAP

Attenuated FAP is characterised by a familial tendency for increased colorectal adenomas and colorectal carcinoma, but unlike classic FAP is characterised by fewer adenomas and a later onset. Patients with attenuated FAP have fewer than 100 adenomas (Figure 37.35), often located more prox-

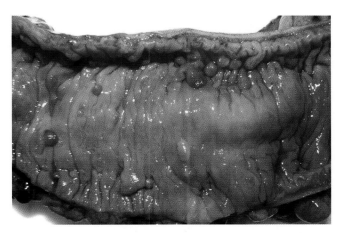

Figure 37.35 Attenuated familial adenomatous polyposis: there were 75 adenomas in this 30-year-old man. He was diagnosed when his father presented with colorectal carcinoma and polyposis at age 68. An *APC* mutation was found in this family. Interestingly, the polyps in the right colon were serrated polyps, not conventional adenomas.

imally in the right colon and a later onset of adenocarcinoma development that trails classic cases by approximately 15 years, with a mean age of 50–55 [80,219–221]. In some instances the adenomas are flat [194]. Upper gastrointestinal manifestations of FAP, particularly fundic gland polyps and duodenal adenomas, can be seen [192], but other extraintestinal manifestations of FAP are uncommon.

It is important to note that the *APC* mutation is only one cause of this pattern of disease. It is now clear that a second, more recently described familial syndrome, *MUTYH-* (or *MYH*)-associated polyposis, can give a similar phenotype (see below). However, *MUTYH*-associated polyposis differs somewhat because it has an autosomal recessive inheritance and therefore shows a horizontal rather than vertical familial clustering and may be associated with both conventional and serrated polyps. Early reports suggested that *APC* and *MUTYH* mutations still accounted for only a minority of cases of attenuated FAP, but recent reports have found that mutations in these two genes probably account for most cases where there is a clear family history, and particularly when there are in excess of 20–30 polyps [222,223].

MUTYH-associated polyposis

MUTYH- (*MYH*)-associated polyposis (MAP) is an autosomal recessive disorder caused by biallelic inherited mutations in the *MUTYH* gene (also called *MYH*) that result in increased colorectal adenomas and colorectal adenocarcinoma [224,225]. In most patients, the adenomatous polyposis has an attenuated phenotype, with two-thirds of patients having between 10 and 100 adenomas [225]. A significant minority, however, have >100 adenomas [198,

225,226], although never the very large number (>1000) seen in germline *APC* mutation [227]. Carcinoma development in these patients is also typically later than in classic FAP and is similar to cases of attenuated FAP, with a mean age at diagnosis of around 48 years [225,227]. Such cancers are microsatellite stable [166]. Whether there is a preferential localisation to the right side remains controversial [227,228], but it is likely that there is phenotypic heterogeneity and each family should be carefully characterised to determine how the disease is likely to express itself, because this may guide the type of surgery offered. Multiple colorectal cancers, either synchronous or metachronous, have been described in a third of patients [225]. In addition, it is noteworthy that a third or more of patients can present with adenocarcinoma in the absence of any polyposis [229].

The *MUTYH* (*MYH*) gene encodes a base-excision repair protein that has an important role in correcting reactive oxygen species-induced DNA damage. When deficient, it leads to a characteristic G:C → T:A transversion mutation, on failure to recognise and correct an oxidised guanine (8-oxo-dG) that mispairs with adenine [166,230]. This mutational profile is particularly likely to induce mutation in *APC*, which has a high number of prone GAA sites [227], but it also leads to frequent mutation of *KRAS* [230,231]. Importantly, the latter is associated with the development of serrated polyps and these are now recognised as part of the spectrum of lesions that can be seen in affected individuals [182]. Some cases even fulfil the criteria for hyperplastic polyposis, although the coexistence of significant numbers of conventional adenomas should alert the correct diagnosis. Thus, MAP should be considered not only if there is a horizontal (recessive) pedigree and a moderate adenomatous polyposis, but also if there is a mixture of adenomas and serrated polyps. In addition, it emphasises the importance of endoscopic sampling of both larger and smaller polyps when an index colonoscopy is being performed [230].

The carrier frequency of *MUTYH* mutations is 0.3–2% [166,232], giving a biallelic mutation frequency estimated between 1 per 10 000 and 1 per 40 000 births [187]. Despite a high penetrance approaching 100%, MAP nevertheless has variable expression. At least a part of this has been linked to genotype–phenotype associations. In European populations approximately 70% of mutations are found at two sites: *Y179C* and *G396D* (previously annotated as *Y165C* and *G382D*). Patients homozygous for *Y179C* have been shown to have a more severe phenotype, including a greater number of adenomas and an earlier onset of adenocarcinoma compared with compound heterozygotes or *G382D* homozygotes [226]. As a result of phenotypic variation, careful assessment of the distribution and frequency of polyps in a particular case is necessary to plan the most appropriate surgical treatment. Despite the frequency of the two major mutations, there are many other mutations described so that gene sequencing is the favoured diagnostic method when available.

Extra-colonic tumours occur in MAP. Duodenal adenomas are the most frequent and have been found in almost 20% of patients; fundic gland polyps are also seen [233]. Sebaceous neoplasms are described but appear to be infrequent [233].

Juvenile polyp

Juvenile polyps are the most common polyp found in children, generally occurring singly or in small numbers in the rectum. Typically presenting with rectal bleeding or less commonly prolapse or torsion-induced autoamputation, the polyps are usually pedunculated and oval or spherical, with a smooth red and ulcerated surface. The stalk is generally fine and less than 10% are sessile. These are hamartomatous lesions and, as such, are characterised by an admixture of tissues native to the colorectal site but showing disorganised architecture. On the cut face small mucus-filled cysts can be seen macroscopically (Figure 37.36). Histologically, juvenile polyps have an expanded and inflamed lamina propria containing cystically dilated crypts that impart a lattice-like appearance on low power (Figure 37.37). The epithelium may have reactive changes but true dysplasia is exceptional in sporadic lesions [234]. Separating the crypts, oedema and a granulation tissue-like stroma are common. Smooth muscle fibres in the lamina propria are not a usual feature, which helps to distinguish them from other reactive polypoid lesions arising secondary to mucosal fold prolapse (see Chapter 34). These include inflammatory myoglandular polyps and prolapsing fold polyps around colonic diverticula, usually seen in older patients. The surface epithelium is often eroded.

Autosomal dominant inherited hamartomatous polyposis syndromes

Forming a smaller component of the inherited polyposis syndromes, there are a number of disorders in which polyps are of hamartomatous type. Most of these syndromes are associated with an increased risk of colorectal malignancy, or with malignancy in other organs. Correct classification of the polyp type, usually obtained at colonoscopic examination, allows the correct correlation with the type of polyposis and helps to guide appropriate genetic testing. In addition, the hamartomatous polyps generally precede the onset of malignancy, allowing the use of appropriate screening.

The major hamartomatous polyposes with colonic manifestations are familial juvenile polyposis, Peutz–Jeghers syndrome, Cowden's syndrome and Bannayan–Riley–Ruvalcaba syndrome. The recently described hereditary mixed polyposis syndrome is currently regarded as a variant of juvenile polyposis [235]. The genes causing these syndromes are now identified and shown in Table 37.7.

Juvenile polyposis

Juvenile polyposis is a hamartomatous polyposis with multiple juvenile polyps and an increased risk of colorectal adenocarcinoma, often inherited as an autosomal dominant trait. It is defined either by the presence of more than five juvenile polyps, or juvenile polyps located throughout the gastrointestinal tract, or any number of juvenile polyps in an individual with a family history of juvenile polyposis [236] (Figure 37.38). Although the most common of the hamartomatous polyposes [235], it is still rare with a frequency of 1 per 100 000. Several clinical forms are described [155,237]: a rare form presenting in infancy with a severe

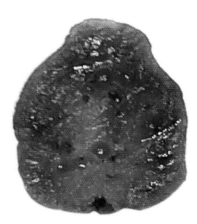

Figure 37.36 Juvenile polyp with cystic crypts on the cut face.

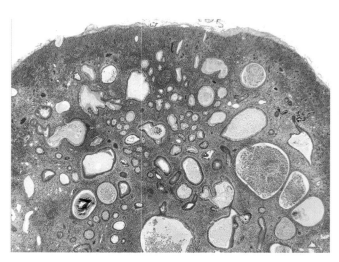

Figure 37.37 Juvenile polyp with surface ulceration and dilated, lattice-like crypts in an inflamed and expanded lamina propria.

Table 37.7 Intestinal polyposes and their related genes

Polyposis	Gene
Familial	
Familial adenomatous polyposis (FAP)	*APC*
Turcot's syndrome	*APC* in two-thirds of patients
Attenuated FAP	*APC* in some
MUTYH-associated polyposis	*MYH* (*MUTYH*)
Serrated polyposis	Unknown
Peutz–Jeghers syndrome	*LKTB1*
Familial juvenile polyposis	*SMAD4, BMPR1A*, possibly *ENG*
Cowden's and Bannayan–Riley–Ruvalcaba syndromes	*PTEN*
Hereditary mixed polyposis syndrome	Unknown
Non-familial	
Cronkhite–Canada syndrome	N/A
Inflammatory cap polyposis	N/A

Modified with permission from Rustgi AK. The genetics of hereditary colon cancer. Genes & Development, 2007; 21: 2525.

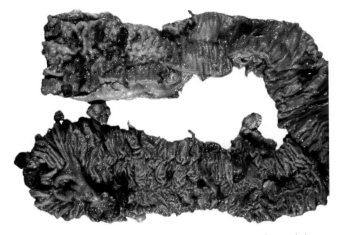

Figure 37.38 Juvenile polyposis: colectomy was performed, but the patient died from small intestinal adenocarcinoma (before the advent of small intestinal screening technology). (Courtesy of Professor Barbara Leggett.)

phenotype and generally with no family history; polyposis confined to the colorectum; and a generalised polyposis throughout the gastrointestinal tract, particularly affecting the stomach.

Macroscopically, almost all patients show colonic involvement with between 5 and 200 polyps distributed uniformly. Most of the polyps are spherical and pedunculated with the typical macroscopic appearance of juvenile polyps, but about 20% may be multi-lobated, sessile or papillary [236], sometimes with bizarre-shaped surface projections. Colorectal carcinoma develops in 30–50% of patients at a mean age of 45 years [238,239].

Histologically, as well as demonstrating the usual appearances of juvenile polyps, some lesions may have atypical features [155] including a relative lack of stromal expansion and epithelial dysplasia. Adenomas and adenocarcinomas may also be seen, the cancers often showing poorly differentiated or mucinous histology [155]. Similarly, gastric cancers are increased in the 20% of patients who have gastric polyposis, and these also show poorly differentiated (diffuse) morphology [239].

Juvenile polyposis commonly presents with rectal bleeding, pain or mucus secretion, and when marked these may lead to rectal prolapse, anaemia, hypokalaemia or protein-losing enteropathy. A minority of patients have extra-intestinal manifestations including cardiac and vascular anomalies and CNS defects. In about 40–50% of patients, mutations can be found in either *SMAD4/DPC4* on chromosome 18q21 or *BMPR1A* at 10q22-23 [240,241]. Those with *SMAD4* mutations are particularly prone to gastric involvement, necessitating upper gastrointestinal screening; some overlap with hereditary haemorrhagic telangiectasia occurs due to common involvement of the *SMAD4* gene in both conditions [242]. The severe infantile form has been linked in some cases to multigenic deletions of chromosome 10q23, which affect both *BMPR1A* and neighbouring *PTEN* [243].

Hereditary mixed polyposis syndrome is a very rare, autosomal dominant polyposis found in occasional Ashkenazi Jewish families [244–248]. Several polyp types are described, including serrated, conventional adenomatous and atypical juvenile polyps. The individual polyps frequently have overlapping features of several polyp types [245,248] and the polyp stroma is often markedly oedematous. There is an increased risk of colonic adenocarcinoma.

Peutz–Jeghers syndrome

The Peutz–Jeghers syndrome is discussed in Chapter 23. In about half of all cases, one or more polyps are found in the colon and rectum [249]. Although rarely of clinical significance, anal extrusion of polyps, rectal bleeding and colonic intussusception may occur [249]. Individuals with this syndrome, more importantly, carry a very high relative and cumulative risk of CRC [250,251]. A hamartoma–adenoma–carcinoma sequence is supported histologically and biochemically [252–255]. Occasionally one or more polyps of Peutz–Jeghers syndrome appearance are found in the colorectum in the absence of polyps in the stomach or small intestine. Grossly these mimic adenoma and histologically

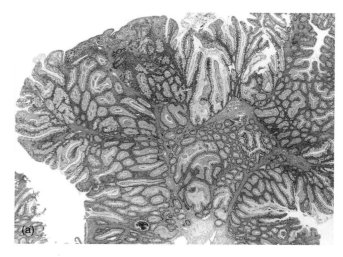

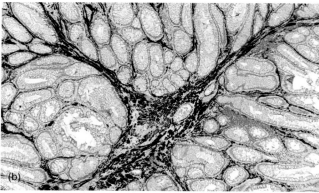

Figure 37.39 (a) Peutz–Jeghers polyp of colon: disorganised colonic crypts are supported by a branching framework of smooth muscle that can be highlighted by (b) desmin immunostaining.

show a tree-like branching of smooth muscle derived from the muscularis mucosae that is covered by normal-appearing colonic mucosa (Figure 37.39). They can be difficult to differentiate from prolapse lesions and, in fact, true sporadic Peutz–Jeghers polyps may be extremely rare [256].

PTEN hamartoma tumour syndromes – Cowden's and Bannayan–Riley–Ruvalcaba syndromes

Several syndromes are caused by germline mutation of *PTEN*, a tumour-suppressor gene at chromosome 10q23, and these are now grouped together as the PTEN hamartoma tumour syndromes (PHTSs) [239,257]. They include the rare clinical entities of Cowden's syndrome, Bannayan–Riley–Ruvalcaba syndrome and proteus syndrome. Only the first two have significant colonic polyposis, but lipomatous involvement of the colon has been described in proteus syndrome. Although most patients can be readily subcate-

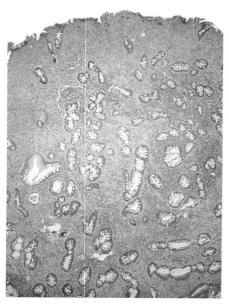

Figure 37.40 Hamartomatous polyp in an individual with Cowden's syndrome.

gorised as either Cowden's or Bannayan–Riley–Ruvalcaba syndrome, overlapping phenotypes are found consistent with the common genetic origin [239].

Cowden's syndrome (multiple hamartoma syndrome) is an autosomal dominant disorder that usually presents in adulthood and is characterised by benign and malignant lesions, with elements derived from all three germ-cell layers [258]. The syndrome is diagnosed using major and minor criteria, which include facial trichilemmomas, acral keratoses, oral mucosal papillomas, mental impairment and a high frequency of carcinomas in the breast, thyroid (principally follicular) and endometrium [258]. It is rare, with 75% of cases having a family history and about 25% being new mutations [235].

In the gastrointestinal tract, polyps occur in approximately 60% of patients [259] and in the colon these are usually distal to the splenic flexure [260]. The polyps are usually small, measuring 2–5 mm, and dome shaped, but some larger lesions can occur [260,261]. The polyp density is variable; many cases with gastrointestinal involvement have 10–15 polyps, with up to 50 developing over a 10-year period [260]. In keeping with the hamartomatous nature, most of the polyps are composed of irregularly arranged crypts in a fibrous stroma, which is arranged concentrically around the crypts [155,260] (Figure 37.40). Crypts are generally not significantly dilated and the stroma is not oedematous or inflamed, which distinguishes them from juvenile polyps [155]. The muscularis mucosae may be splayed and increased [260] but there is no muscular scaffold as seen in Peutz–Jeghers polyps. Ganglion cells [155] or adipose tissue [260] may be present, and discrete lipomas and ganglio-neuromas are described [262]. Descriptions of juvenile and inflammatory polyps in these patients may be incorrect and reflect a misinterpretation of the hamartomatous fibrotic stroma. One patient was found to have an epithelioid 'leiomyoma', but this was described before the recognition of gastrointestinal stromal tumours [260]. Adenomas are also described [263]. The risk of colorectal malignancy is not believed to be increased, despite earlier reports of an association [155,260].

Bannayan–Riley–Ruvalcaba syndrome, initially believed to represent a distinct syndrome, is also a manifestation of *PTEN* mutation and related to Cowden's syndrome [264,265]. It is characterised by macrocephaly, lipomas, haemangiomas and pigmented macules of the glans penis [258]. In contrast to Cowden's syndrome, it is detected in infancy. Gastrointestinal polyps may be more numerous than in Cowden's syndrome [266], with associated intussusception described in the small bowel. Microscopic descriptions of the gastrointestinal polyps have not been extensive and the literature has few illustrations. Two groups have called them juvenile polyps [267,268] but it is conceivable that they are similar to the more fibrotic hamartomatous polyps seen in Cowden's syndrome. Further descriptions are needed.

A small group of patients may have other types of polyps but overlapping phenotypic features of PHTS. A recent study of such patients, including careful genetic analysis and sequencing, found two patients with the *PTEN* mutation who developed multiple hyperplastic polyps and tubular adenomas [171], suggesting that a clear genotype–phenotype correlation may not be present in every case. In addition, the genes mutated in PHTS and some cases of juvenile polyposis syndrome are neighbouring, and gene deletions in some cases of juvenile polyposis syndrome have also been shown to affect *PTEN* [269].

Cronkhite–Canada syndrome

Cronkhite–Canada syndrome is a rare form of gastrointestinal polyposis affecting patients of European and Asian descent, with a mean age of onset of 59 years (range 31–86). There is a male:female ratio of 3:2 [270,271]. Affected individuals present with ectodermal changes including skin pigmentation, alopecia and nail atrophy, as well as diarrhoea, malabsorption, protein-losing enteropathy and severe electrolyte disturbances [270–272]. In some cases the clinical symptoms can mimic inflammatory bowel disease (IBD) [273]. The gastrointestinal manifestations may be difficult to control, and this syndrome is often fatal. The cause is unknown and there is no familial tendency. It should be noted that severe juvenile polyposis presenting in infancy is sometimes (erroneously) described as infantile Cronkhite–Canada syndrome.

The macroscopic and microscopic appearances of the polyps are similar throughout the gastrointestinal tract, although the oesophagus is characteristically spared [270]. In the colon the polyps are numerous and broad based (Figure 37.41), and the latter feature distinguishes them from the typically pedunculated appearance of juvenile polyps [274]. Otherwise, the microscopic features are similar to juvenile polyps, with mucosa that is diffusely thickened and shows cystic dilatation of elongated crypts, with epithelial flattening (Figure 37.42). The lamina propria is typically expanded and oedematous. There is a variable inflammatory cell content and some polyps have relatively little inflammation. Rarely, eosinophils are prominent [275].

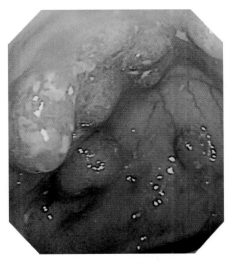

Figure 37.41 Cronkhite–Canada syndrome: there was a diffuse polyposis affecting the gastric body and antrum, small intestine and colon. The last is shown here at endoscopy, with multiple broad-based sessile polyps. (Courtesy of Dr Florian Grimpen.)

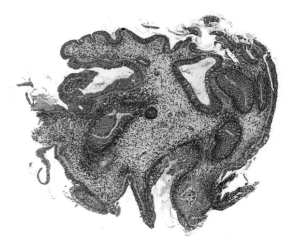

Figure 37.42 Cronkhite–Canada polyp, resembling juvenile polyp but with a broad, sessile base.

Muscle fibres are not conspicuous [274]. The diagnosis can be made by colorectal, gastric or jejunal biopsy. Carcinomas of stomach, colon and rectum, and adenomatous change in the syndromic colonic polyps are described in some patients [271,276].

Inflammatory polyps

A variety of polyps may evolve as a reaction to some form of injury to the mucosa and are characterised by non-dysplastic crypts within an inflamed stroma. The appearance and number of the polyps varies depending on the initiating insult; most cases can be attributed to localised mucosal prolapse, IBD or less commonly a variety of other insults.

Mucosal prolapse-associated polyps

Mucosal prolapse causes reactive polypoid changes in the mucosal crypts and lamina propria (see Chapter 34). These include slight cryptal irregularity, elongation and serration. Secondary erosion of the surface, sometimes with a cap of granulation tissue seen as a pale covering macroscopically, is common and some crypts may become cystic. There is solidification of the lamina propria by fibromuscular proliferation, which displaces the normal inflammatory cell component and imparts an eosinophilic rather than basophilic appearance on low power examination (Figure 37.43). Haemorrhage is seen in some cases and small amounts of stromal haemosiderin may be detected in macrophages using Perls' stain.

Inflammatory polyps occurring secondary to mucosal prolapse have been given a variety of names based on the dominant histological changes, associated conditions and location [277]. They have a predilection for the sigmoid colon, particularly in association with diverticular disease and chronic constipation with straining at stool, as well as the anorectal junction. Polyps with general features of mucosal prolapse have been called *polypoid prolapsing fold* [278], or *inflammatory cloacogenic polyp* when at the anorectal verge. Some very small lesions form *prominent mucosal folds*, only a few millimetres in diameter, showing just subtle stromal fibrosis and slight splitting of the muscularis mucosae. Larger lesions with prominent cystically dilated crypts and inflamed stroma resembling juvenile polyps, but with stromal smooth muscle proliferation, are known as *inflammatory myoglandular polyps* [279]. When surface ulceration is dominant, causing a 'cap' of granulation tissue, the name *inflammatory cap polyp* has been used. These lesions may be multiple, particularly in the sigmoid colon and rectum, a condition that has been variously labelled (*inflammatory*) *cap polyposis* or *eroded polypoid hyperplasia of rectosigmoid* [280–282]. Although mechanical factors are the probable cause of the polyposis, one case without predisposing mucosal prolapse that responded to infliximab therapy has been described, suggesting that this may be a heterogeneous group [283]. Prolapse-related polyps are also common in areas of diverticular disease, arising as a result of the redundant folds that commonly form around diverticular openings [284].

Inflammatory bowel disease-associated inflammatory pseudo-polyps

Inflammatory pseudo-polyps are commonly found in patients with IBD (see Chapter 35). They can be composed of granulation tissue, inflamed mucosa with crypt distortion as seen in typical IBD or uninflamed mucosa with a variable degree of cryptal distortion. The last form can be associated with long, filiform mucosal polyps [285] (filiform polyposis) in both Crohn's disease and ulcerative colitis (Figure 37.44). Marked inflammatory polyposis,

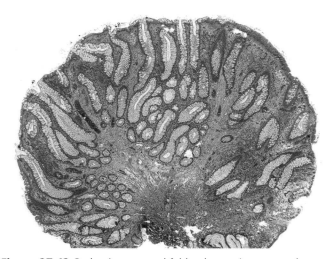

Figure 37.43 Prolapsing mucosal fold polyp: various names have been applied to these lesions depending on the location, degree of stromal muscle or inflammation or surface ulceration.

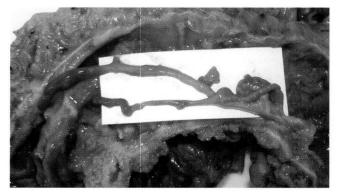

Figure 37.44 Filiform inflammatory pseudo-polyps in Crohn's disease.

including giant pseudo-polyps up to ≥50 mm, can be complicated by pain, obstruction, intussusception, chronic blood loss, misinterpretation as malignancy or difficulty in screening for dysplasia and malignancy [286–289]. Occasional pseudo-polyps have bizarre multinucleated stromal cells or a pseudo-sarcomatous appearance of the stroma [290,291].

Inflammatory polyps from other causes

Polypoid *granulation tissue*, occurring either as a sporadic polyp [292], at surgical anastomoses, or associated with diverticulitis, is common. Diverticular disease is also often associated with intramucosal ganglion cells and these should not be interpreted as ganglio-neuromas [293]. Inflammatory polyps may follow ischaemic colitis [294]. Rare cases of diffuse filiform polyposis occurring in patients without coexistent IBD have been described [295,296] and the cause of this remains unclear. Polypoid reactions may be seen in some infectious diseases, including cytomegalovirus in severely immunosuppressed patients and schistosomal egg-induced polyps [297,298]. Pyogenic granuloma of colon has been described [299].

Other polyps

Inflammatory fibroid polyp

Most inflammatory fibroid polyps occur in the stomach and small intestine, and are only rarely found in the colon and rectum. Here they may be symptomatic or present with abdominal pain, bloody stools, weight loss, diarrhoea, anaemia or intussusception [300–303]. They show a smooth sessile or pedunculated profile, most arising in the right colon. The pathological features are identical to those found in proximal locations of the gastrointestinal tract (see Chapters 12 and 25).

Fibroblastic polyp/peri-neurioma

Originally separately described but with overlapping features, fibroblastic polyps/peri-neuriomas occur as solitary incidental flat/sessile or rounded/pedunculated polyps 2–15 mm in diameter, represent 0.2% of all polyps and arise predominantly in the rectosigmoid [304–307]. The lesions comprise cytologically bland, monomorphic, plump, spindle cells with blunt, oval or tapered nuclei, abundant pale eosinophilic cytoplasm and indistinct cell borders centred on the lamina propria, but sometimes involving submucosa (Figure 37.45). No mitosis or necrosis is seen. The intervening stroma contains collagen, mast cells, rare lymphocytes and sometimes eosinophils. Abundant small calibre blood vessels may be present. The tumours are

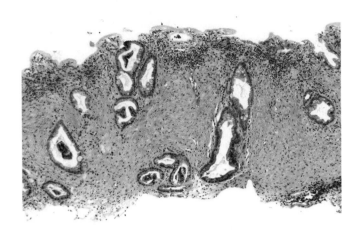

Figure 37.45 Fibroblastic polyp of colon.

unencapsulated with pushing margins, widely separate crypts and are often intimately associated with SPs, particularly HPs. There is separation from overlying intact epithelium by a thin layer of lamina propria and close association with the muscularis mucosae, the fibres of which may be split or extend perpendicularly towards the mucosal surface. Superficially tumour cells form bundles parallel to the mucosal surface but elsewhere are haphazardly arranged with few peri-glandular and peri-vascular concentric arrangements.

Initially shown to be strongly and diffusely positive for vimentin, but negative for most other markers, including epithelial membrane antigen (EMA), with higher antibody concentrations, a prolonged incubation time and extended antigen retrieval the tumour cells were subsequently shown to be positive for EMA as well as other peri-neurioma markers: claudin 1, GLUT-1 and collagen IV [305,308]. Electron microscopy demonstrated peri-neurioma features, including spindle cells with long bipolar cytoplasmic processes and prominent pinocytotic vesicles, surrounded by discontinuous basal lamina. All have behaved as benign tumours with no recurrences or metastases recorded.

Schwann cell hamartoma

These are small, incidental sessile polyps 1–6 mm in diameter, occurring predominantly in the rectosigmoid [309]. Affected individuals have no neural polyps on follow-up and no evidence of neurofibromatosis type 1 or other syndromes. Histologically, the lesions comprise a diffuse lamina propria proliferation of uniform spindle cells with elongated tapering or wavy nuclei, abundant dense eosinophilic cytoplasm and indistinct cell borders that entrap adjacent crypts (Figure 37.46a). The lesions are poorly circumscribed and have an irregular interface with adjacent

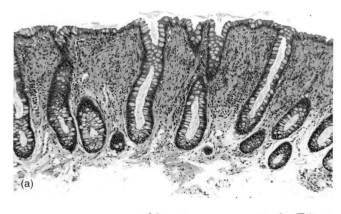

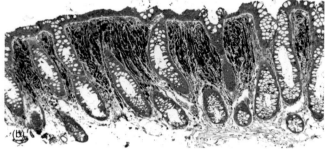

Figure 37.46 Schwann cell hamartoma: (a) Schwann cells slightly expand the lamina propria. (b) There is strong immunoreactivity for S-100.

lamina propria. Component cells stain strongly with S-100 (Figure 37.46b) and rare axons are identified with immunostaining for neurofilament protein. No ganglion cells are seen.

Mucosal benign epithelioid (peripheral) nerve sheath tumours

These are small, incidental polyps up to 10 mm in diameter, occurring mainly in the left colon. Usually unencapsulated with an infiltrative growth pattern, they comprise small spindled to predominantly epithelioid cells with uniform round-to-oval nuclei, frequent nuclear pseudo-inclusions and clear-to-eosinophilic fibrillary cytoplasm arranged as nests and whorls [310]. Although usually centred on the lamina propria, they frequently involve the superficial submucosa. Tumour cells are diffusely positive for S-100; CD34-positive supporting cells may be seen but no neuraxons can be identified. No patient has had neurofibromatosis and the tumours followed a benign course with no recurrences at follow-up.

Other rare nerve sheath tumours that have been reported as single cases only include the microcystic/reticular schwannoma [311], hybrid schwannoma/perineurioma [312] and psammomatous melanotic schwannoma [313].

Ganglioneuroma

This is a mucosal proliferation of ganglion cells and S-100-positive spindle cell elements. It most commonly presents as a small, solitary and sporadic lesion [314,315]. Other clinical presentations include multiple ganglio-neuromatous polyposis or diffuse ganglio-neuromatosis associated with areas of diffuse colonic wall thickening [314]. Sporadic lesions are not associated with other diseases, but multiplicity should raise the possibility of neurofibromatosis type I or multiple neuro-endocrine neoplasia type 2b [314].

Granular cell tumour

This is uncommon in the large intestine. A recent series described predominance in the right colon [316]. In addition to the usual features of nests of cuboidal cells with abundant eosinophilic granular cytoplasm seen in lesions from the proximal gastrointestinal tract, colonic granular cell tumours frequently have nuclear atypia, dystrophic calcification, hyalinisation and prominent lymphoid cuffing [316,317]. Recurrence can be seen after incomplete resection, particularly for lesions with a submucosal component.

Leiomyomas of the muscularis mucosae

These are incidental, typically sessile but occasionally pedunculated polyps 1–22 mm in diameter (median 4 mm) that occur predominantly in the rectosigmoid [318,319]. Macroscopically they form pale circumscribed nodules covered by grossly intact colonic mucosa. Histologically they are circumscribed lesions obliterating and merging with the muscularis mucosae and comprising fasciculated, spindled, smooth muscle cells. The overlying mucosa is mildly attenuated. Eosinophilic cytoplasmic globules, interpreted on electron microscopy as aggregates of desmin and intermingled actin, have been described [318]. Nuclear atypia and mitoses are rare, and such lesions are regarded as 'symplastic' leiomyomas. Tumour cells are strongly positive for smooth muscle actin and desmin and negative for CD34, S-100 and CD117. Described lesions have been uniformly benign, but complete excision and follow-up for lesions with atypia or mitotic activity has been recommended.

Prominent lymphoid follicles

These occur as one or more follicles located in the mucosa or upper submucosa, and can present as a polyp (Figure 37.47). They are most commonly found in the right colon and rectum, and single proximal examples are probably seen increasingly as colonoscopic resolution continues to improve. Rectal lesions may be relatively large due to the aggregation of confluent follicles, termed a 'rectal tonsil'

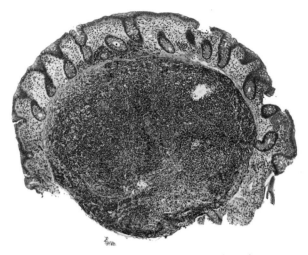

Figure 37.47 Prominent lymphoid follicle in the colon.

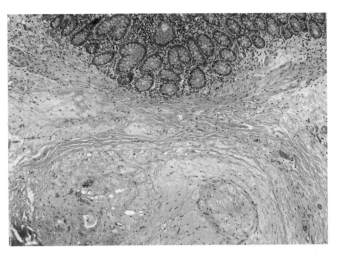

Figure 37.48 Elastofibromatous polyp.

[320,321]. Intra-epithelial lymphocytosis, including infiltration of the crypts, overlying these follicles should not be misdiagnosed as lymphoma.

Lymphomatous polyposis

This is the classic gastrointestinal presentation for mantle cell lymphoma, but other categories of malignant lymphoma can be associated with a polypoid mucosal appearance. These entities are discussed in Chapter 39.

Everted appendiceal stump

Late eversion of the appendiceal stump is a rare lesion that produces a caecal pole polyp with a central dimple [322,323]. Histologically, biopsies show mucosa with prominent lymphoid tissue, as is usually the case in appendiceal mucosa, and can be a clue to the correct diagnosis. In rare cases there may be intussusception of an intact appendix, which at colonoscopy gives a polypoid appearance that has been likened to a foreskin [324–326]. Elsewhere in the caecum, eversion of caecal diverticula has also been described [327], producing polyps with a central dimple.

Elastotic and elasto-fibromatous polyp

A focal increase of elastic fibres in the muscularis mucosae or submucosa of the colon can give rise to a polyp, usually mistaken for an adenoma clinically [328–330]. It is likely that this is an under-recognised cause of polyp formation. The elastic fibres form amphophilic amorphous or fibrillar masses sometimes resembling solar elastosis of the skin, and may be admixed with collagen fibres (elasto-fibromatous change) [328] (Figure 37.48). When present around blood vessels the elastosis can mimic amyloid dep-

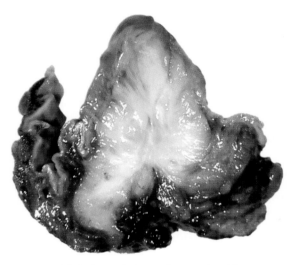

Figure 37.49 Endometriosis causing a polypoid appearance in the colonic mucosa.

osition, but staining for elastic fibres (with negative Congo red staining) correctly identifies the nature of the lesion. The cause remains obscure.

Endometriosis

This can have a number of presentations when affecting the colorectum (see Chapter 40). Occasionally it gives rise to a mucosal polypoid lesion [331], which may be challenging to correctly diagnose in this unusual location (Figure 37.49). The recognition of benign glands with different morphological appearances to the colonic crypts, presence of endometrial stroma and stromal haemosiderin help in making the diagnosis.

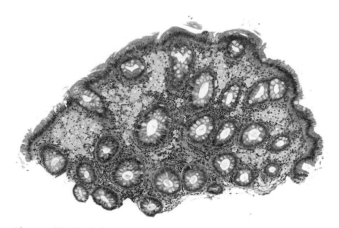

Figure 37.50 Colonic xanthoma.

Xanthoma (xanthelasma)

Xanthoma of colorectal mucosa causes small polyps, generally sessile, which may be yellow or reddish in colour and are located distally [332]. Collections of foamy macrophages are present in the mucosa (Figure 37.50) and the cells are strongly positive by CD68 immunostaining.

References

1. Hamilton SR, Vogelstein B, Kudo S, et al. Carcinoma of the colon and rectum. In: Hamilton SR, Aaltonen LA (eds), *World Health Organization Classification of Tumours: Pathology and genetics of tumours of the digestive system*. Lyon: IARC Press, 2000: 103.
2. Riddell RH, Goldman H, Ransohoff DF, et al. Dysplasia in inflammatory bowel disease: standardized classification with provisional clinical applications. *Hum Pathol* 1983;**14**:931.
3. Lieberman D, Moravec M, Holub J, Michaels L, Eisen G. Polyp size and advanced histology in patients undergoing colonoscopy screening: Implications for CT colonography. *Gastroenterology* 2008;**135**:1100.
4. Neugut AI, Jacobson JS, De Vivo I. Epidemiology of colorectal adenomatous polyps. *Cancer Epidemiol Biomarkers Prev* 1993; **2**:159.
5. Kahi CJ, Rex DK, Imperiale TF. Screening, surveillance, and primary prevention for colorectal cancer: a review of the recent literature. *Gastroenterology* 2008;**135**:380.
6. Pendergrass CJ, Edelstein DL, Hylind LM, et al. Occurrence of colorectal adenomas in younger adults: an epidemiologic necropsy study. *Clin Gastroenterol Hepatol* 2008;**6**:1011.
7. Jacobs ET, Ahnen DJ, Ashbeck EL, et al. Association between body mass index and colorectal neoplasia at follow-up colonoscopy: a pooling study. *Am J Epidemiol* 2009;**169**:657.
8. Giovannucci E. Epidemiologic studies of folate and colorectal neoplasia: a review. *J Nutr* 2002;**132**:2350S.
9. Marshall JR. Prevention of colorectal cancer: diet, chemoprevention, and lifestyle. *Gastroenterol Clin North Am* 2008;**37**:73.
10. Sansbury LB, Wanke K, Albert PS, et al. The effect of strict adherence to a high-fiber, high-fruit and -vegetable, and low-fat eating pattern on adenoma recurrence. *Am J Epidemiol* 2009; **170**:576.
11. Muto T, Bussey HJR, Morson BC. Evolution of cancer of colon and rectum. *Cancer* 1975;**36**:2251.
12. Shinya H, Wolff WI. Morphology, anatomic distribution and cancer potential of colonic polyps – analysis of 7,000 polyps endoscopically removed. *Ann Surg* 1979;**190**:679.
13. O'Brien MJ, Winawer SJ, Zauber AG, et al. The National Polyp Study. Patient and polyp characteristics associated with high-grade dysplasia in colorectal adenomas. *Gastroenterology* 1990; **98**:371.
14. Mattar W, Rex DK. Large sessile adenomas are associated with a high prevalence of synchronous advanced adenomas. *Clin Gastroenterol Hepatol* 2008;**6**:877.
15. Butterly LF, Chase MP, Pohl H, Fiarman GS. Prevalence of clinically important histology in small adenomas. *Clin Gastroenterol Hepatol* 2006;**4**:343.
16. Martinez ME, Baron JA, Lieberman DA, et al. A pooled analysis of advanced colorectal neoplasia diagnoses after colonoscopic polypectomy. *Gastroenterology* 2009;**136**:832.
17. Rex DK, Bond JH, Winawer S, et al. Quality in the technical performance of colonoscopy and the continuous quality improvement process for colonoscopy: Recommendations of the US Multi-Society Task Force on Colorectal Cancer. *Am J Gastroenterol* 2002;**97**:1296.
18. Stryker SJ, Wolff BG, Culp CE, Libbe SD, Ilstrup DM, Maccarty RL. Natural history of untreated colonic polyps. *Gastroenterology* 1987;**93**:1009.
19. Participants in the Paris Workshop. The Paris endoscopic classification of superficial neoplastic lesions: esophagus, stomach, and colon: November 30 to December 1 2002. *Gastrointest Endosc* 2003;**58**:S3.
20. O'Brien M J, Winawer SJ, Zauber AG, et al. Flat adenomas in the National Polyp Study: is there increased risk for high-grade dysplasia initially or during surveillance? *Clin Gastroenterol Hepatol* 2004;**2**:905.
21. Suzuki N, Saunders BP, Brown G. Flat colorectal neoplasms: endoscopic detection, clinical relevance and management. *Tech Coloproctol* 2004;**8**(suppl 2):s261.
22. Tsuda S, Veress B, Toth E, Fork FT. Flat and depressed colorectal tumours in a southern Swedish population: a prospective chromoendoscopic and histopathological study. *Gut* 2002;**51**:550.
23. Kudo SE, Lambert R, Allen JI, et al. Nonpolypoid neoplastic lesions of the colorectal mucosa. *Gastrointest Endosc* 2008;**68**:S3.
24. Hurlstone DP. The detection of flat and depressed colorectal lesions: Which endoscopic imaging approach? *Gastroenterology* 2008;**135**:338.
25. Kudo S, Kashida H, Tamura T, et al. Colonoscopic diagnosis and management of nonpolypoid early colorectal cancer. *World J Surg* 2000;**24**:1081.
26. Kudo S. Endoscopic mucosal resection of flat and depressed types of early colorectal-cancer. *Endoscopy* 1993;**25**:455.
27. Barker N, Ridgway RA, van Es JH, et al. Crypt stem cells as the cells-of-origin of intestinal cancer. *Nature* 2009;**457**:608.
28. Humphries A, Wright NA. Colonic crypt organization and tumorigenesis. *Nat Rev Cancer* 2008;**8**:415.
29. Leedham SJ, Wright NA. Expansion of a mutated clone: from stem cell to tumour. *J Clin Pathol* 2008;**61**:164.
30. Gupta AK, Pretlow TP, Schoen RE. Aberrant crypt foci: What we know and what we need to know. *Clin Gastroenterol Hepatol* 2007;**5**:526.
31. Hurlstone DP, Karajeh M, Sanders DS, Drew K, Cross SS. Rectal aberrant crypt foci identified using high-magnification-chromoscopic colonoscopy: Biomarkers for flat and depressed neoplasia. *Am J Gastroenterol* 2005;**100**:1283.
32. Konishi F, Morson BC. Pathology of colorectal adenomas – a colonoscopic survey. *J Clin Pathol* 1982;**35**:830.

33. Appelman HD. High-grade dysplasia and villous features should not be part of the routine diagnosis of colorectal adenomas. *Am J Gastroenterol* 2008;**103**:1329.

34. Odze R. Pathologist–clinician interaction is essential. *Am J Gastroenterol* 2008;**103**:1331.

35. Costantini M, Sciallero S, Giannini A, et al. Interobserver agreement in the histologic diagnosis of colorectal polyps: the experience of the multicenter adenoma colorectal study (SMAC). *J Clin Epidemiol* 2003;**56**:209.

36. Terry MB, Neugut AI, Bostick RM, Potter JD, Haile RW, Fenoglio-Preiser CM. Reliability in the classification of advanced colorectal adenomas. *Cancer Epidemiol Biomarkers Prevent* 2002;**11**:660.

37. Rex DK, Goldblum JR. Should HGD or degree of villous changes in colon polyps be reported? *Am J Gastroenterol* 2008;**103**:1327.

38. Riddell RH. Hands off cancerous large bowel polyps. *Gastroenterology* 1985;**89**:432.

39. Rembacken BJ, Fujii T, Cairns A, et al. Flat and depressed colonic neoplasms: a prospective study of 1000 colonoscopies in the UK. *Lancet* 2000;**355**:1211.

40. Soetikno RM, Kaltenbach T, Rouse RV, et al. Prevalence of non-polypoid (flat and depressed) colorectal neoplasms in asymptomatic and symptomatic adults. *JAMA* 2008;**299**:1027.

41. Bansal M, Fenoglio CM, Robboy SJ, King DW. Are metaplasias in colorectal adenomas truly metaplasias. *Am J Pathol* 1984;**115**:253.

42. Joo M, Shahsafaei A, Odze RD. Paneth cell differentiation in colonic epithelial neoplasms: evidence for the role of the Apc/beta-catenin/Tcf pathway. *Hum Pathol* 2009;**40**:872.

43. Sarlin JG, Mori K. Morules in epithelial tumors of the colon and rectum. *Am J Surg Pathol* 1984;**8**:281.

44. Ueo T, Kashima K, Daa T, Kondo Y, Sasaki A, Yokoyama S. Immunohistochemical analysis of morules in colonic neoplasms: Morules are morphologically and qualitatively different from squamous metaplasia. *Pathobiology* 2005;**72**:269.

45. Almagro UA, Pintar K, Zellmer RB. Squamous metaplasia in colorectal polyps. *Cancer* 1984;**53**:2679.

46. Domoto H, Terahata S, Senoh A, Sato K, Aida S, Tamai S. Clear cell change in colorectal adenomas: its incidence and histological characteristics. *Histopathology* 1999;**34**:250.

47. Reed RJ, Love GL, Harkin JC. Consultation case. *Am J Surg Pathol* 1983;**7**:597.

48. Groisman GM, Benkov KJ, Adsay V, Dische MR. Osseous metaplasia in benign colorectal polyps. *Arch Pathol Lab Med* 1994;**118**:64.

49. Rubio CA. Paneth cell adenoma of the ileum. *Anticancer Res* 2004;**24**:4187.

50. Parfitt JR, Shepherd NA. Polypoid mucosal prolapse complicating low rectal adenomas: beware the inflammatory cloacogenic polyp! *Histopathology* 2008;**53**:91.

51. Muto T, Bussey HJR, Morson BC. Pseudo-carcinomatous invasion in adenomatous polyps of colon and rectum. *J Clin Pathol* 1973;**26**:25.

52. Qizilbash AH, Meghji M, Castelli M. Pseudocarcinomatous invasion in adenomas of the colon and rectum. *Dis Colon Rectum* 1980;**23**:529.

53. Pascal RR, Hertzler G, Hunter S, Goldschmid S. Pseudoinvasion with high-grade dysplasia in a colonic adenoma – distinction from adenocarcinoma. *Am J Surg Pathol* 1990;**14**:694.

54. Yantiss RK, Bosenberg MW, Antonioli DA, Odze RD. Utility of MMP-1, p53, E-cadherin, and collagen IV immunohistochemical stains in the differential diagnosis of adenomas with misplaced epithelium versus adenomas with invasive adenocarcinoma. *Am J Surg Pathol* 2002;**26**:206.

55. Molavi D, Argani P. Distinguishing benign dissecting mucin (stromal mucin pools) from invasive mucinous carcinoma. *Adv Anat Pathol* 2008;**15**:1.

56. Dirschmid K, Kiesler J, Mathis G, Beller S, Stoss F, Schobel B. Epithelial misplacement after biopsy of colorectal adenomas. *Am J Surg Pathol* 1993;**17**:1262.

57. Coverlizza S, Risio M, Ferrari A, Fenogliopreiser CM, Rossini FP. Colorectal adenomas containing invasive-carcinoma – pathologic assessment of lymph-node metastatic potential. *Cancer* 1989;**64**:1937.

58. Cooper HS, Deppisch LM, Gourley WK, et al. Endoscopically removed malignant colorectal polyps – clinicopathological correlations. *Gastroenterology* 1995;**108**:1657.

59. Fenoglio CM, Pascal RR. Colorectal adenomas and cancer – pathologic relationships. *Cancer* 1982;**50**:2601.

60. Muto T, Kamiya J, Sawada T, et al. Colonoscopic polypectomy in diagnosis and treatment of early carcinoma of the large-intestine. *Dis Colon Rectum* 1980;**23**:68.

61. Volk EE, Goldblum JR, Petras RE, Carey WD, Fazio VW. Management and outcome of patients with invasive-carcinoma arising in colorectal polyps. *Gastroenterology* 1995;**109**:1801.

62. Morson BC, Whiteway JE, Jones EA, Macrae FA, Williams CB. Histopathology and prognosis of malignant colorectal polyps treated by endoscopic polypectomy. *Gut* 1984;**25**:437.

63. Stein BL, Coller JA. Management of malignant colorectal polyps. *Surg Clinics North Am* 1993;**73**:47.

64. Lauwers GY, Forcione DG, Nishioka NS, et al. Novel endoscopic therapeutic modalities for superficial neoplasms arising in Barrett's esophagus: a primer for surgical pathologists. *Mod Pathol* 2009;**22**:489.

65. Hassan C, Zullo A, Risio M, Rossini FP, Morini S. Histologic risk factors and clinical outcome in colorectal malignant polyp: A pooled-data analysis. *Dis Colon Rectum* 2005;**48**:1588.

66. Netzer P, Forster C, Biral R, et al. Risk factor assessment of endoscopically removed malignant colorectal polyps. *Gut* 1998;**43**:669.

67. Jass JR. Malignant colorectal polyps. *Gastroenterology* 1995;**109**:2034.

68. Morson BC. Factors influencing prognosis of early cancer of rectum. *Proc R S Med* 1966;**59**:607.

69. Seitz U, Bohnacker S, Seewald S, et al. Is endoscopic polypectomy an adequate therapy for malignant colorectal adenomas? Presentation of 114 patients and review of the literature. *Dis Colon Rectum* 2004;**47**:1789.

70. Ueno H, Mochizuki H, Hashiguchi Y, et al. Risk factors for an adverse outcome in early invasive colorectal carcinoma. *Gastroenterology* 2004;**127**:385.

71. Haggitt RC, Glotzbach RE, Soffer EE, Wruble LD. Prognostic factors in colorectal carcinomas arising in adenomas – implications for lesions removed by endoscopic polypectomy. *Gastroenterology* 1985;**89**:326.

72. Tamura S, Ohkawauchi K, Yokoyama Y, Onishi S. Indications and techniques for endoscopic mucosal resection in the lesions of a colorectal tumor. *Dig Endosc* 2003;**15**(suppl):S39.

73. Fenoglio CM, Kaye GI, Lane N. Distribution of human colonic lymphatics in normal, hyperplastic, and adenomatous tissue – its relationship to metastasis from small carcinomas in pedunculated adenomas, with 2 case reports. *Gastroenterology* 1973;**64**:51.

74. Lewin MR, Fenton H, Burkart AL, Sheridan T, Abu-Alfa AK, Montgomery EA. Poorly differentiated colorectal carcinoma with invasion restricted to lamina propria (intramucosal carcinoma): A follow-up study of 15 cases. *Am J Surg Pathol* 2007;**31**:1882.

75. Shia J, Klimstra DS. Intramucosal poorly differentiated colorectal carcinoma: Can it be managed conservatively? *Am J Surg Pathol* 2008;**32**:1586.

76. Fearon ER, Vogelstein B. A genetic model for colorectal tumorigenesis. *Cell* 1990;**61**:759.

77. Vogelstein B, Kinzler KW. Cancer genes and the pathways they control. *Nat Med* 2004;**10**:789.

78. Takayama T, Ohi M, Hayashi T, et al. Analysis of K-ras, APC, and beta-catenin in aberrant crypt foci in sporadic adenoma, cancer, and familial adenomatous polyposis. *Gastroenterology* 2001;**121**:599.

79. Powell SM, Zilz N, Beazer-Barclay Y, et al. APC mutations occur early during colorectal tumorigenesis. *Nature* 1992;**359**:235.

80. Galiatsatos P, Foulkes WD. Familial adenomatous polyposis. *Am J Gastroenterol* 2006;**101**:385.

81. Pino MS, Chung DC. The chromosomal instability pathway in colon cancer. *Gastroenterology* 2010;**138**:2059.

82. Jass JR, Baker K, Zlobec I, et al. Advanced colorectal polyps with the molecular and morphological features of serrated polyps and adenomas: concept of a 'fusion' pathway to colorectal cancer. *Histopathology* 2006;**49**:121.

83. Wood LD, Parsons DW, Jones S, et al. The genomic landscapes of human breast and colorectal cancers. *Science* 2007;**318**:1108.

84. Higuchi T, Jass JR. My approach to serrated polyps of the colorectum. *J Clin Pathol* 2004;**57**:682.

85. Tateyama H, Li WX, Takahashi E, Miura Y, Sugiura H, Eimoto T. Apoptosis index and apoptosis-related antigen expression in serrated adenoma of the colorectum – The saw-toothed structure may be related to inhibition of apoptosis. *Am J Surg Pathol* 2002;**26**:249.

86. Kambara T, Simms LA, Whitehall VLJ, et al. BRAF mutation is associated with DNA methylation in serrated polyps and cancers of the colorectum. *Gut* 2004;**53**:1137.

87. Snover DC, Jass JR, Fenoglio-Preiser C, Batts KP. Serrated polyps of the large intestine – A morphologic and molecular review of an evolving concept. *Am J Clin Pathol* 2005;**124**:380.

88. O'Brien MJ, Yang S, Mack C, et al. Comparison of microsatellite instability, CpG island methylation phenotype, BRAF and KRAS status in serrated polyps and traditional adenomas indicates separate pathways to distinct colorectal carcinoma end points. *Am J Surg Pathol* 2006;**30**:1491.

89. Yang S, Farraye FA, Mack C, Posnik O, O'Brien MJ. BRAF and KRAS mutations in hyperplastic polyps and serrated adenomas of the colorectum – Relationship to histology and CpG island methylation status. *Am J Surg Pathol* 2004;**28**:1452.

90. Hawkins NJ, Ward RL. Sporadic colorectal cancers with microsatellite instability and their possible origin in hyperplastic polyps and serrated adenomas. *J Natl Cancer Inst* 2001;**93**:1307.

91. Jass JR. Serrated route to colorectal cancer: back street or super highway? *J Pathol* 2001;**193**:283.

92. Jass JR. Serrated adenoma and colorectal cancer. *J Pathol* 1999;**187**:499.

93. Torlakovic E, Skovlund E, Snover DC, Torlakovic G, Nesland JM. Morphologic reappraisal of serrated colorectal polyps. *Am J Surg Pathol* 2003;**27**:65.

94. Goldstein NS. Hyperplastic-like colon polyps preceding microsatellite-unstable adenocarcinomas – The author's reply. *Am J Clin Pathol* 2003;**120**:634.

95. Torlakovic E, Snover DC. Serrated adenomatous polyposis in humans. *Gastroenterology* 1996;**110**:748.

96. Huang CS, O'Brien MJ, Yang S, Farraye FA. Hyperplastic polyps, serrated adenomas, and the serrated polyp neoplasia pathway. *Am J Gastroenterol* 2004;**99**:2242.

97. Waye JD, Bilotta JJ. Rectal hyperplastic polyps – now you see them, now you don't – a differential point. *Am J Gastroenterol* 1990;**85**:1557.

98. Spring KJ, Zhao ZZ, Karamatic R, et al. High prevalence of sessile serrated adenomas with BRAF mutations: A prospective study of patients undergoing colonoscopy. *Gastroenterology* 2006;**131**:1400.

99. Torlakovic EE, Gomez JD, Driman DK, et al. Sessile serrated adenorna (SSA) vs. Traditional serrated adenoma (TSA). *Am J Surg Pathol* 2008;**32**:21.

100. Batts KP. Serrated colorectal polyps. An update. *Pathol Case Rev* 2004;**9**:173.

101. Anderson JC, Pollack BJ. Predicting of hyperplastic histology by endoscopic features. *Gastrointest Endosc* 2000;**52**:149.

102. Langdon DE. Large hyperplastic polyps of the right colon. *Gastrointest Endosc* 1998;**48**:659.

103. Rex DK, Rahmani EY. New endoscopic finding associated with hyperplastic polyps. *Gastrointest Endosc* 1999;**50**:704.

104. Baker K, Zhang Y, Jin C, Jass JR. Proximal versus distal hyperplastic polyps of the colorectum: different lesions or a biological spectrum? *J Clin Pathol* 2004;**57**:1089.

105. Chung SM, Chen YT, Panczykowski A, Schamberg N, Klimstra DS, Yantiss RK. Serrated polyps with 'Intermediate features' of sessile serrated polyp and microvesicular hyperplastic polyp – A practical approach to the classification of nondysplastic serrated polyps. *Am J Surg Pathol* 2008;**32**:407.

106. Li D, Jin C, McCulloch C, et al. Association of large serrated polyps with synchronous advanced colorectal neoplasia. *Am J Gastroenterol* 2009;**104**:695.

107. Lu FI, van Niekerk de W, Owen D, Tha SP, Turbin DA, Webber DL. Longitudinal outcome study of sessile serrated adenomas of the colorectum: an increased risk for subsequent right-sided colorectal carcinoma. *Am J Surg Pathol* 2010;**34**:927.

108. Pai RK, Hart J, Noffsinger AE. Sessile serrated adenomas strongly predispose to synchronous serrated polyps in non-syndromic patients. *Histopathology* 2010;**56**:581.

109. Schreiner MA, Weiss DG, Lieberman DA. Proximal and large hyperplastic and nondysplastic serrated polyps detected by colonoscopy are associated with neoplasia. *Gastroenterology* 2010;**139**:1497.

110. Hiraoka S, Kato J, Fujiki S, et al. The presence of large serrated polyps increases risk for colorectal cancer. *Gastroenterology* 2010;**139**:1503.

111. Urbanski SJ, Kossakowska AE, Marcon N, Bruce WR. Mixed hyperplastic adenomatous polyps – an underdiagnosed entity. Report of a case of adenocarcinoma arising within a mixed hyperplastic adenomatous polyp. *Am J Surg Pathol* 1984;**8**:551.

112. Jass JR, Baker K, Zlobec I, et al. Advanced colorectal polyps with the molecular and morphological features of serrated polyps and adenomas: concept of a 'fusion' pathway to colorectal cancer. *Histopathology* 2006;**49**:121.

113. Oh K, Redston M, Odze RD. Support for hMLH1 and MGMT silencing as a mechanism of tumorigenesis in the hyperplastic-adenoma-carcinoma (serrated) carcinogenic pathway in the colon. *Hum Pathol* 2005;**36**:101.

114. Ensari A, Bosman FT, Offerhaus GJ. The serrated polyp: getting it right! *J Clin Pathol* 2010;**63**:665.

115. Iino H, Jass JR, Simms LA, et al. DNA microsatellite instability in hyperplastic polyps, serrated adenomas, and mixed polyps: a mild mutator pathway for colorectal cancer? *J Clin Pathol* 1999;**52**:5.

116. Lee EJ, Choi C, Park CK, et al. Tracing origin of serrated adenomas with BRAF and KRAS mutations. *Virchows Arch* 2005;**447**:597.

117. Jass JR. Classification of colorectal cancer based on correlation of clinical, morphological and molecular features. *Histopathology* 2007;**50**:113.

118. Lash RH, Genta RM, Schuler CM. Sessile serrated adenomas: prevalence of dysplasia and carcinoma in 2139 patients. *J Clin Pathol* 2010;**63**:681.

119. Goldstein NS. Small colonic microsatellite unstable adenocarcinomas and high-grade epithelial dysplasias in sessile serrated adenoma polypectomy specimens – A study of eight cases. *Am J Clin Pathol* 2006;**125**:132.

120. Sheridan TB, Fenton H, Lewin MR, et al. Sessile serrated adenomas with low- and high-grade dysplasia and early carcinomas. An immunohistochemical study of serrated lesions 'caught in the act'. *Am J Clin Pathol* 2006;**126**:564.

121. Wynter CVA, Walsh MD, Higuchi T, Leggett BA, Young J, Jass JR. Methylation patterns define two types of hyperplastic polyp associated with colorectal cancer. *Gut* 2004;**53**:573.

122. Carr NJ, Mahajan H, Tan KL, Hawkins NJ, Ward RL. Serrated and non-serrated polyps of the colorectum: their prevalence in an unselected case series and correlation of BRAF mutation analysis with the diagnosis of sessile serrated adenoma. *J Clin Pathol* 2009;**62**:516.

123. Hamilton SR, Aaltonen LA, eds. *World Health Organization Classification of Tumours: Pathology and genetics of tumours of the digestive system.* Lyon: IARC Press, 2000.

124. Longacre TA, Fenogliopreiser CM. Mixed hyperplastic adenomatous polyps serrated adenomas – a distinct form of colorectal neoplasia. *Am J Surg Pathol* 1990;**14**:524.

125. Cunningham KS, Riddell RH. Serrated mucosal lesions of the colorectum. *Curr Opin Gastroenterol* 2006;**22**:48.

126. O'Brien M J, Yang S, Huang CS, Shepherd C, Cerda S, Farraye FA. The serrated polyp pathway to colorectal carcinoma. *Diagn Histopathol* 2008;**14**:78.

127. Iwabuchi M, Sasano H, Hiwatashi N, et al. Serrated adenoma: A clinicopathological, DNA ploidy, and immunohistochemical study. *Anticancer Res* 2000;**20**:1141.

128. Matsumoto T, Mizuno M, Shimizu M, Manabe T, Iida M, Fujishima M. Serrated adenoma of the colorectum: colonoscopic and histologic features. *Gastrointest Endosc* 1999;**49**:736.

129. Jaramillo E, Tamura S, Mitomi H. Endoscopic appearance of serrated adenomas in the colon. *Endoscopy* 2005;**37**:254.

130. Morita T, Tamura S, Miyazaki J, Higashidani Y, Onishi S. Evaluation of endoscopic and histopathological features of serrated adenoma of the colon. *Endoscopy* 2001;**33**:761.

131. Oka S, Tanaka S, Hiyama T, et al. Clinicopathologic and endoscopic features of colorectal serrated adenoma: differences between polypoid and superficial types. *Gastrointest Endosc* 2004;**59**:213.

132. Chandra A, Sheikh AA, Cerar A, Talbot IC. Clinico-pathological aspects of colorectal serrated adenomas. *World J Gastroenterol* 2006;**12**:2770.

133. Jiao YF, Nakamura S, Sugai T, Yamada N, Habano W. Serrated adenoma of the colorectum undergoes a proliferation versus differentiation process: New conceptual interpretation of morphogenesis. *Oncology* 2008;**74**:127.

134. Lee SK, Chang HJ, Kim TI, et al. Clinicopathologic findings of colorectal traditional and sessile serrated adenomas in Korea: A multicenter study. *Digestion* 2008;**77**:178.

135. Jaramillo E, Watanabe M, Rubio C, Slezak P. Small colorectal serrated adenomas: endoscopic findings. *Endoscopy* 1996;**28**:1.

136. Bariol C, Hawkins NJ, Turner JJ, Meagher AP, Williams DB, Ward RL. Histopathological and clinical evaluation of serrated adenomas of the colon and rectum. *Mod Pathol* 2003;**16**:417.

137. Lazarus R, Junttila OE, Karttunen TJ, Makinen MJ. The risk of metachronous neoplasia in patients with serrated adenoma. *Am J Clin Pathol* 2005;**123**:349.

138. Rubio CA, Jaramillo E. Flat serrated adenomas of the colorectal mucosa. *Jpn J Cancer Res* 1996;**87**:305.

139. Yao T, Kouzuki T, Kajiwara M, Matsui N, Oya M, Tsuneyoshi M. 'Serrated' adenoma of the colorectum, with reference to its gastric differentiation and its malignant potential. *J Pathol* 1999;**187**:511.

140. Jass JR. Serrated adenoma of the colorectum. *Curr Diagn Pathol* 2002;**8**:42.

141. Sawyer EJ, Cerar A, Hanby AM, et al. Molecular characteristics of serrated adenomas of the colorectum. *Gut* 2002;**51**:200.

142. Makinen MJ, George SMC, Jernvall P, Makela J, Vihko P, Karttunen TJ. Colorectal carcinoma associated with serrated adenoma – prevalence, histological features, and prognosis. *J Pathol* 2001;**193**:286.

143. Glazer E, Golla V, Forman R, Zhu H, Levi G, Bodenheimer HC. Serrated adenoma is a risk factor for subsequent adenomatous polyps. *Dig Dis Sci* 2008;**53**:2204.

144. Kim KM, Lee EJ, Kim YH, Chang DK, Odze RD. *KRAS* mutations in traditional serrated adenomas from Korea herald an aggressive phenotype. *Am J Surg Pathol* 2010;**34**:667.

145. Leggett B, Whitehall V. Role of the serrated pathway in colorectal cancer pathogenesis. *Gastroenterology* 2010;**138**:2088.

146. Yantiss RK, Oh KY, Chen YT, Redston M, Odze RD. 'Filiform' serrated adenomas – A clinicopathologic and immunophenotypic study of 18 cases. *Am J Surg Pathol* 2007;**31**:1238.

147. Konishi K, Yamochi T, Makino R, et al. Molecular differences between sporadic serrated and conventional colorectal adenomas. *Clin Cancer Res* 2004;**10**:3082.

148. Park SJ, Rashid A, Lee JH, Kim SG, Hamilton SR, Wu TT. Frequent CpG island methylation in serrated adenomas of the colorectum. *Am J Pathol* 2003;**162**:815.

149. Dong SM, Lee EJ, Jeon ES, Park CK, Kim KM. Progressive methylation during the serrated neoplasia pathway of the colorectum. *Mod Pathol* 2005;**18**:170.

150. Yashiro M, Laghi L, Saito K, et al. Serrated adenomas have a pattern of genetic alterations that distinguishes them from other colorectal polyps. *Cancer Epidemiol Biomarkers Prevent* 2005;**14**:2253.

151. Higuchi T, Sugihara K, Jass JR. Demographic and pathological characteristics of serrated polyps of colorectum. *Histopathology* 2005;**47**:32.

152. Kang M, Mitomi H, Sada M, et al. Ki-67, p53, and bcl-2 expression of serrated adenomas of the colon. *Am J Surg Pathol* 1997;**21**:417.

153. Yachida S, Mudali S, Martin SA, Montgomery EA, Iacobuzio-Donahue CA. Beta-catenin nuclear labeling is a common feature of sessile serrated adenomas and correlates with early neoplastic progression after BRAF activation. *Am J Surg Pathol* 2009;**33**:1823.

154. Williams GT, Arthur JF, Bussey HJR, Morson BC. Metaplastic polyps and polyposis of the colorectum. *Histopathology* 1980;**4**:155.

155. Jass JR. Gastrointestinal polyposes: Clinical, pathological and molecular features. *Gastroenterol Clinics North Am* 2007;**36**:927.

156. Rashid A, Houlihan PS, Booker S, Petersen GM, Giardiello FM, Hamilton SR. Phenotypic and molecular characteristics of hyperplastic polyposis. *Gastroenterology* 2000;**119**:323.

157. Rubio CA, Stemme S, Jaramillo E, Lindblom A. Hyperplastic polyposis coli syndrome and colorectal carcinoma. *Endoscopy* 2006;**38**:266.

158. Buchanan DD, Sweet K, Drini M, et al. Phenotypic diversity in patients with multiple serrated polyps: a genetics clinic study. *Int J Colorectal Dis* 2010;**25**:703.

159. Snover DC, Ahnen DJ, Burt RW, Odze RD. Serrated polyps of the colon and rectum and serrated polyposis. In: Bosman FT, Carneiro F, Hruban RH, Theise ND (eds), *World Health Organization Classification of Tumours of the Digestive System*. 4th edition. Lyon: IARC Press, 2010:160.

160. Lage P, Cravo M, Sousa R, et al. Management of Portuguese patients with hyperplastic polyposis and screening of at-risk first-degree relatives: A contribution for future guidelines based on a clinical study. *Am J Gastroenterol* 2004;**99**:1779.

161. Leggett BA, Devereaux B, Biden K, Searle J, Young J, Jass J. Hyperplastic polyposis – Association with colorectal cancer. *Am J Surg Pathol* 2001;**25**:177.

162. Carvajal-Carmona LG, Howarth KM, Lockett M, et al. Molecular classification and genetic pathways in hyperplastic polyposis syndrome. *J Pathol* 2007;**212**:378.

163. Chow E, Lipton L, Lynch E, et al. Hyperplastic polyposis syndrome: Phenotypic presentations and the role of MBD4 and MYH. *Gastroenterology* 2006;**131**:30.

164. Hyman NH, Anderson P, Blasyk H. Hyperplastic polyposis and the risk of colorectal cancer. *Dis Colon Rectum* 2004;**47**:2101.

165. Boparai KS, Mathus-Vliegen EMH, Koornstra JJ, et al. Increased colorectal cancer risk during follow-up in patients with hyperplastic polyposis syndrome: a multicentre cohort study. *Gut* 2010;**59**:1094.

166. Lindor NM. Hereditary colorectal cancer: MYH-associated polyposis and other newly identified disorders. *Best Pract Res Clin Gastroenterol* 2009;**23**:75.

167. Keljo DJ, Weinberg AG, Winick N, Tomlinson G. Rectal cancer in an 11-year-old girl with hyperplastic polyposis. *J Pediatr Gastroenterol Nutr* 1999;**28**:327.

168. Renaut AJ, Douglas PR, Newstead GL. Hyperplastic polyposis of the colon and rectum. *Colorectal Dis* 2002;**4**:213.

169. Ferrandez A, Samowitz W, DiSario JA, Burt RW. Phenotypic characteristics and risk of cancer development in hyperplastic polyposis: Case series and literature review. *Am J Gastroenterol* 2004;**99**:2012.

170. Yeoman A, Young J, Arnold J, Jass J, Parry S. Hyperplastic polyposis in the New Zealand population: a condition associated with increased colorectal cancer risk and European ancestry. *N Z Med J* 2007;**120**:U2827.

171. Sweet K, Willis J, Zhou XP, et al. Molecular classification of patients with unexplained hamartomatous and hyperplastic polyposis. *JAMA* 2005;**294**:2465.

172. Lockett MJ, Atkin WS. Hyperplastic polyposis: Prevalence and cancer risk. *Gut* 2001;**48**:011.

173. Burt RW, Samowitz WS. Serrated adenomatous polyposis: A new syndrome? *Gastroenterology* 1996;**110**:950.

174. McCann BG. A case of metaplastic polyposis of the colon associated with focal adenomatous change and metachronous adenocarcinomas. *Histopathology* 1988;**13**:700.

175. Minoo P, Baker K, Goswami R, et al. Extensive DNA methylation in normal colorectal mucosa in hyperplastic polyposis. *Gut* 2006;**55**.

176. Shepherd NA. Inverted hyperplastic polyposis of the colon. *J Clin Pathol* 1993;**46**:56.

177. Chan AOO, Issa JPJ, Morris JS, Hamilton SR, Rashid A. Concordant CpG island methylation in hyperplastic polyposis. *Am J Pathol* 2002;**160**:529.

178. Jass JR, Iino H, Ruszkiewicz A, et al. Neoplastic progression occurs through mutator pathways in hyperplastic polyposis of the colorectum. *Gut* 2000;**47**:43.

179. Bengoechea O, Martinez-Penuela JM, Larrinaga B, Valerdi J, Borda F. Hyperplastic polyposis of the colorectum and adenocarcinoma in a 24-year-old man. *Am J Surg Pathol* 1987;**11**:323.

180. Hawkins NJ, Gorman P, Tomlinson IPM, Bullpitt P, Ward RL. Colorectal carcinomas arising in the hyperplastic polyposis syndrome progress through the chromosomal instability pathway. *Am J Pathol* 2000;**157**:385.

181. Jeevaratnam P, Cottier DS, Browett PJ, VandeWater NS, Pokos V, Jass JR. Familial giant hyperplastic polyposis predisposing to colorectal cancer: A new hereditary bowel cancer syndrome. *J Pathol* 1996;**179**:20.

182. Boparai KS, Dekker E, van Eeden S, et al. Hyperplastic polyps and sessile serrated adenomas as a phenotypic expression of MYH-associated polyposis. *Gastroenterology* 2008;**135**:2014.

183. Young J, Jenkins M, Parry S, et al. Serrated pathway colorectal cancer in the population: Genetic consideration. *Gut* 2007;**56**:1453.

184. Walker RG, Landmann JK, Hewett DG, et al. Hyperplastic polyposis syndrome is associated with cigarette smoking, which may be a modifiable risk factor. *Am J Gastroenterol* 2010;**105**:1642.

185. Talbot IC, Burt R, Jarvinen H, Thomas G. Familial adenomatous polyposis. In: Hamilton SR, Aaltonen LA (eds), *World Health Organization Classification of Tumours: Pathology and genetics of tumours of the digestive system*. Lyon: IARC Press, 2000: 120.

186. Bisgaard ML, Fenger K, Bulow S, Niebuhr E, Mohr J. Familial adenomatous polyposis (FAP) – frequency, penetrance, and mutation-rate. *Hum Mut* 1994;**3**:121.

187. Half E, Bercovich D, Rozen P. Familial adenomatous polyposis. *Orphanet J Rare Dis* 2009;**4**:22.

188. Perry RE, Christensen MA, Thorson AG, Williams T. Familial polyposis – colon cancer in the absence of rectal polyps. *Br J Surg* 1989;**76**:744.

189. Bjork J, Akerbrant H, Iselius L, Alm T, Hultcrantz R. Epidemiology of familial adenomatous polyposis in Sweden: Changes over time and differences in phenotype between males and females. *Scand J Gastroenterol* 1999;**34**:1230.

190. Jarvinen HJ. Time and type of prophylactic surgery for familial adenomatosis coli. *Ann Surg* 1985;**202**:93.

191. Cohen M, Thomson M, Taylor C, Donatone J, Quijano G, Drut R. Colonic and duodenal flat adenomas in children with classical familial adenomatous polyposis. *Int J Surg Pathol* 2006;**14**:133.

192. Lynch HT, Smyrk TC, Watson P, et al. Hereditary flat adenoma syndrome – a variant of familial adenomatous polyposis. *Dis Colon Rectum* 1992;**35**:411.

193. Masaki T, Sheffield JP, Talbot IC, Williams CB. Non-polypoid adenoma of the large-intestine. *Int J Colorectal Dis* 1994;**9**:180.

194. Lynch HT, Smyrk T, McGinn T, et al. Attenuated familial adenomatous polyposis (AFAP) – a phenotypically and genotypically distinctive variant of FAP. *Cancer* 1995;**76**:2427.

195. Jenner DC, Levitt S. Rectal cancer following colectomy and ileorectal anastomosis for familial adenomatous polyposis. *Austr NZ J Surgery* 1998;**68**:136.

196. Saito Y, Fujii T, Akasu T, et al. Development of an aggressive depressed cancer in a case of familial adenomatous polyposis. *Endoscopy* 2002;**34**:421.

197. Parc YR, Olschwang S, Desaint B, Schmitt G, Parc RG, Tiret E. Familial adenomatous polyposis: Prevalence of adenomas in the ileal pouch after restorative proctocolectomy. *Ann Surg* 2001;**233**:360.

198. Sieber OM, Lipton L, Crabtree M, et al. Multiple colorectal adenomas, classic adenomatous polyposis, and germ-line mutations in MYH. *N Engl J Med* 2003;**348**:791.

199. Groen EJ, Roos A, Muntinghe FL, et al. Extra-intestinal manifestations of familial adenomatous polyposis. *Ann Surg Oncol* 2008;**15**:2439.

200. Abraham SC, Nobukawa B, Giardiello FM, Hamilton SR, Wu TT. Fundic gland polyps in familial adenomatous polyposis – Neoplasms with frequent somatic adenomatous polyposis coli gene alterations. *Am J Pathol* 2000;**157**:747.

201. Wu TT, Kornacki S, Rashid A, Yardley JH, Hamilton SR. Dysplasia and dysregulation of proliferation in foveolar and surface epithelia of fundic gland polyps from patients with familial adenomatous polyposis. *Am J Surg Pathol* 1998;**22**:293.

202. Rugge M, Correa P, Dixon MF, et al. Gastric dysplasia: the Padova international classification. *Am J Surg Pathol* 2000;**24**:167.

203. Rustgi AK. The genetics of hereditary colon cancer. *Genes Develop* 2007;**21**:2525.

204. Groves CJ, Saunders BP, Spigelman AD, Phillips RKS. Duodenal cancer in patients with familial adenomatous polyposis (FAP): results of a 10 year prospective study. *Gut* 2002;**50**:636.

205. Gallagher MC, Phillips RKS, Bulow S. Surveillance and management of upper gastrointestinal disease in Familial Adenomatous Polyposis. *Famil Cancer* 2006;**5**:263.

206. Spigelman AD, Talbot IC, Williams CB, Domizio P, Phillips RKS. Upper gastrointestinal cancer in patients with familial adenomatous polyposis. *Lancet* 1989;**ii**:783.

207. Cordero-Fernandez C, Garzon-Benavides M, Pizarro-Moreno A, et al. Gastroduodenal involvement in patients with familial adenomatous polyposis. Prospective study of the nature and evolution of polyps: evaluation of the treatment and surveillance methods applied. *Eur J Gastroenterol Hepatol* 2009;**21**:1161.

208. Burke CA, Santisi J, Church J, Levinthal G. The utility of capsule endoscopy small bowel surveillance in patients with polyposis. *Am J Gastroenterol* 2005;**100**:1498.

209. Hartley JE, Church JM, Gupta S, McGannon E, Fazio VW. Significance of incidental desmoids identified during surgery for familial adenomatous polyposis. *Dis Colon Rectum* 2004; **47**:334.

210. Gardner EJ. Follow-up study of a family group exhibiting dominant inheritance for a syndrome including intestinal polyps, osteomas, fibromas and epidermal cysts. *Am J Hum Genet* 1962; **14**:376.

211. Harach HR, Williams GT, Williams ED. Familial adenomatous polyposis associated thyroid carcinoma – a distinct type of follicular neoplasia. *Histopathology* 1994;**25**:549.

212. Marchesa P, Fazio VW, Church JM, McGannon E. Adrenal masses in patients with familial adenomatous polyposis. *Dis Colon Rectum* 1997;**40**:1023.

213. Hughes LJ, Michels VV. Risk of hepatoblastoma in familial adenomatous polyposis. *Am J Med Genet* 1992;**43**:1023.

214. Jarvinen HJ, Nyberg M, Peltokallio P. Biliary involvement in familial adenomatosis coli. *Dis Colon Rectum* 1983;**26**:525.

215. Lees CD, Hermann RE. Familial polyposis coli associated with bile-duct cancer. *Am J Surg* 1981;**141**:378.

216. Nugent KP, Spigelman AD, Talbot IC, Phillips RKS. Gallbladder dysplasia in patients with familial adenomatous polyposis. *Br J Surg* 1994;**81**:291.

217. Goss KH, Groden J. Biology of the adenomatous polyposis coli tumor suppressor. *J Clin Oncol* 2000;**18**:1967.

218. Nieuwenhuis MH, Vasen HFA. Correlations between mutation site in APC and phenotype of familial adenomatous polyposis (FAP): A review of the literature. *Crit Rev Oncol Hematol* 2007; **61**:153.

219. Knudsen AL, Bisgaard ML, Bülow S. Attenuated familial adenomatous polyposis (AFAP). A review of the literature. *Familial Cancer* 2003;**2**:43.

220. Spirio L, Olschwang S, Groden J, et al. Alleles of the *APC* gene – an attenuated form of familial polyposis. *Cell* 1993;**75**:951.

221. Knudsen AL, Bulow S, Tomlinson I, Moslein G, Heinimann K, Christensen IJ. Attenuated familial adenomatous polyposis (AFAP). Results from an international collaborative study. *Colorect Dis* 2010;**12**:e243.

222. Filipe B, Baltazar C, Albuquerque C, et al. *APC* or *MUTYH* mutations account for the majority of clinically well-characterized families with FAP and AFAP phenotype and patients with more than 30 adenomas. *Clin Genet* 2009;**76**:242.

223. Nielsen M, Hes FJ, Nagengast FM, et al. Germline mutations in *APC* and *MUTYH* are responsible for the majority of families with attenuated familial adenomatous polyposis. *Clin Genet* 2007;**71**:427.

224. Al-Tassan N, Chmiel NH, Maynard J, et al. Inherited variants of MYH associated with somatic G:C → T:A mutations in colorectal tumors. *Nat Genet* 2002;**30**:227.

225. Sampson JR, Jones N. MUTYH-associated polyposis. *Best Pract Res Clin Gastroenterol* 2009;**23**:209.

226. Nielsen M, Joerink-Van de Beld MC, Jones N, et al. Analysis of *MUTYH* Genotypes and Colorectal Phenotypes in Patients with *MUTYH*-associated polyposis. *Gastroenterology* 2009;**136**:471.

227. Poulsen MLM, Bisgaard ML. MUTYH associated polyposis (MAP). *Curr Genom* 2008;**9**:420.

228. Lubbe SJ, Di Bernardo MC, Chandler IP, Houlston RS. Clinical implications of the colorectal cancer risk associated with MUTYH mutation. *J Clin Oncol* 2009;**27**:3975.

229. Terdiman JP. MYH-associated disease: attenuated adenomatous polyposis of the colon is only part of the story. *Gastroenterology* 2009;**137**:1883.

230. Jass JR. What's new in hereditary colorectal cancer? *Arch Pathol Lab Med* 2005;**129**:1380.

231. Lipton L, Halford SE, Johnson V, et al. Carcinogenesis in MYH-associated polyposis follows a distinct genetic pathway. *Cancer Res* 2003;**63**:7595.

232. Wang L, Baudhuin LM, Boardman LA, et al. *MYH* mutations in patients with attenuated and classic polyposis and with young-onset colorectal cancer without polyps. *Gastroenterology* 2004;**127**:9.

233. Vogt S, Jones N, Christian D, et al. Expanded extracolonic tumor spectrum in MUTYH-associated polyposis. *Gastroenterology* 2009;**137**:1976.

234. Aaltonen LA, Jass JR, Howe JR. Juvenile polyposis. In: Hamilton SR, Aaltonen LA, eds. *World Health Organization Classification of Tumours: Pathology and genetics of tumours of the digestive system*. Lyon: IARC Press, 2000:130.

235. Schreibman IR, Baker M, Amos C, McGarrity TJ. The hamartomatous polyposis syndromes: A clinical and molecular review. *Am J Gastroenterol* 2005;**100**:476.

236. Jass JR, Williams CB, Bussey HJR, Morson BC. Juvenile polyposis – a precancerous condition. *Histopathology* 1988;**13**:619.

237. Sachatello CR, Griffen WO. Hereditary polypoid diseases of gastrointestinal-tract working classification. *Am J Surg* 1975; **129**:198.

238. Brosens LAA, van Hattem A, Hylind LM, et al. Risk of colorectal cancer in juvenile polyposis. *Gut* 2007;**56**:965.

239. Calva D, Howe JR. Hamartomatous polyposis syndromes. *Surg Clinics North Am* 2008;**88**:779.

240. Calva-Cerqueira D, Chinnathambi S, Pechman B, Bair J, Larsen-Haidle J, Howe JR. The rate of germline mutations and large deletions of SMAD4 and BMPR1A in juvenile polyposis. *Clin Genet* 2009;**75**:79.

241. Howe JR, Sayed MG, Ahmed AF, et al. The prevalence of *MADH4* and *BMPR1A* mutations in juvenile polyposis and

absence of *BMPR2, BMPR1B,* and *ACVR1* mutations. *J Med Genet* 2004;**41**:484.

242. Gallione CJ, Repetto GM, Legius E, et al. A combined syndrome of juvenile polyposis and hereditary haemorrhagic telangiectasia associated with mutations in *MADH4* (*SMAD4*). *Lancet* 2004;**363**:852.

243. Delnatte C, Sanlaville D, Mougenot JF, et al. Contiguous gene deletion within chromosome arm 10q is associated with juvenile polyposis of infancy, reflecting cooperation between the *BMPR1A* and *PTEN* tumor-suppressor genes. *Am J Hum Genet* 2006;**78**:1066.

244. Jaeger EEM, Woodford-Richens KL, Lockett M, et al. An ancestral Ashkenazi haplotype at the HMPS/CRAC1 locus on 15q13-q14 is associated with hereditary mixed polyposis syndrome. *Am J Hum Genet* 2003;**72**:1261.

245. Cheah PY, Wong YH, Chau YP, et al. Germline bone morphogenesis protein receptor 1a mutation causes colorectal tumorigenesis in hereditary mixed polyposis syndrome. *Am J Gastroenterol* 2009;**104**:3027.

246. Jaeger E, Webb E, Howarth K, et al. Common genetic variants at the CRAC1 (HMPS) locus on chromosome 15q13.3 influence colorectal cancer risk. *Nat Genet* 2008;**40**:26.

247. Whitelaw SC, Murday VA, Tomlinson IPM, et al. Clinical and molecular features of the hereditary mixed polyposis syndrome. *Gastroenterology* 1997;**112**:327.

248. Jass JR. Colorectal polyposes: from phenotype to diagnosis. *Pathol Res Pract* 2008;**204**:431.

249. Utsunomiya J, Gocho H, Miyanaga T, Hamaguchi E, Kashimure A. Peutz–Jeghers syndrome: its natural course and management. *Johns Hopkins Med J* 1975;**136**:71.

250. Giardiello FM, Brensinger JD, Tersmette AC, et al. Very high risk of cancer in familial Peutz–Jeghers syndrome. *Gastroenterology* 2000;**119**:1447.

251. van Lier MG, Wagner A, Mathus-Vliegen EM, Kuipers EJ, Steyerberg EW, van Leerdam ME. High cancer risk in Peutz–Jeghers syndrome: a systematic review and surveillance recommendations. *Am J Gastroenterol* 2010;**105**:1258.

252. Gruber SB, Entius MM, Petersen GM, et al. Pathogenesis of adenocarcinoma in Peutz–Jeghers syndrome. *Cancer Res* 1998;**58**:5267.

253. Hizawa K, Iida M, Matsumoto T, Kohrogi N, Yao T, Fujishima M. Neoplastic transformation arising in Peutz–Jeghers polyposis. *Dis Colon Rectum* 1993;**36**:953.

254. Miyaki M, Iijima T, Hosono K, et al. Somatic mutations of LKB1 and beta-catenin genes in gastrointestinal polyps from patients with Peutz–Jeghers syndrome. *Cancer Res* 2000;**60**:6311.

255. Narita T, Eto T, Ito T. Peutz–Jeghers syndrome with adenomas and adenocarcinomas in colonic polyps. *Am J Surg Pathol* 1987;**11**:76.

256. Burkart AL, Sheridan T, Lewin M, Fenton H, Ali NJ, Montgomery E. Do sporadic Peutz–Jeghers polyps exist? Experience of a large teaching hospital. *Am J Surg Pathol* 2007;**31**:1209.

257. Liaw D, Marsh DJ, Li J, et al. Germline mutations of the PTEN gene in Cowden disease, an inherited breast and thyroid cancer syndrome. *Nat Genet* 1997;**16**:64.

258. Pilarski R, Eng C. Will the real Cowden syndrome please stand up (gain)? Expanding mutational and clinical spectra of the PTEN hamartoma tumour syndrome. *J Med Genet* 2004;**41**:323.

259. Starink TM, Vanderveen JPW, Arwert F, et al. The Cowden syndrome – a clinical and genetic-study in 21 patients. *Clin Genet* 1986;**29**:222.

260. Carlson GJ, Nivatvongs S, Snover DC. Colorectal polyps in Cowden's disease (multiple hamartoma syndrome). *Am J Surg Pathol* 1984;**8**:763.

261. Eng C, Talbot IC, Burt R. Cowden syndrome. In: Hamilton SR, Aaltonen LA (eds), *World Health Organization Classification of Tumours: Pathology and genetics of tumours of the digestive system.* Lyon: IARC Press; 2000:132.

262. Lashner BA, Riddell RH, Winans CS. Ganglioneuromatosis of the colon and extensive glycogenic acanthosis in Cowdens disease. *Dig Dis Sci* 1986;**31**:213.

263. Hizawa K, Iida M, Matsumoto T, et al. Gastrointestinal manifestations of Cowden's disease – report of 4 cases. *J Clin Gastroenterol* 1994;**18**:13.

264. Arch EM, Goodman BK, VanWesep RA, et al. Deletion of *PTEN* in a patient with Bannayan–Riley–Ruvalcaba syndrome suggests allelism with Cowden disease. *Am J Med Genet* 1997;**71**:489.

265. Marsh DJ, Dahia PLM, Zheng ZM, et al. Germline mutations in *PTEN* are present in Bannayan–Zonana syndrome. *Nat Genet* 1997;**16**:333.

266. Hendriks YMC, Verhallen JTCM, van der Smagt JJ, et al. Bannayan–Riley–Ruvalcaba syndrome: further delineation of the phenotype and management of *PTEN* mutation-positive cases *Familial Cancer* 2003;**2**:79.

267. Haggitt RC, Reid BJ. Hereditary gastrointestinal polyposis syndromes. *Am J Surg Pathol* 1986;**10**:871.

268. Lowichik A, White FV, Timmons CF, et al. Bannayan–Riley–Ruvalcaba syndrome: Spectrum of intestinal pathology including juvenile polyps. *Pediatr Develop Pathol* 2000;**3**:155.

269. Van Hattem WA, Brosens LAA, de Leng WWJ, et al. Large genomic deletions of SMAD4, BMPR1A and PTEN in juvenile polyposis. *Gut* 2008;**57**:623.

270. Daniel ES, Ludwig SL, Lewin KJ, Ruprecht RM, Rajacich GM, Schwabe AD. The Cronkhite–Canada syndrome. An analysis of clinical and pathologic features and therapy in 55 patients. *Medicine (Baltimore)* 1982;**61**:293.

271. Ward EM, Wolfsen HC. Review article: the non-inherited gastrointestinal polyposis syndromes. *Aliment Pharmacol Ther* 2002;**16**:333.

272. Cronkhite LW Jr, Canada WJ. Generalized gastrointestinal polyposis: an unusual syndrome of polyposis, pigmentation, alopecia and onychotrophia. *N Engl J Med* 1955;**252**:1011.

273. Ryall RJ. Polypoid hypertrophy of the gastrointestinal mucosa presenting as ulcerative colitis. *Proc R Soc Med* 1966;**59**:614.

274. Burke AP, Sobin LH. The pathology of Cronkhite–Canada polyps. A comparison to juvenile polyposis. *Am J Surg Pathol* 1989;**13**:940.

275. Anderson RD, Patel R, Hamilton JK, Boland CR. Cronkhite–Canada syndrome presenting as eosinophilic gastroenteritis. *Proc (Bayl Univ Med Cent)* 2006;**19**:209.

276. Katayama Y, Kimura M, Konn M. Cronkhite–Canada syndrome associated with a rectal cancer and adenomatous changes in colonic polyps. *Am J Surg Pathol* 1985;**9**:65.

277. Chetty R, Bhathal PS, Slavin JL. Prolapse-induced inflammatory polyps of the colorectum and anal transitional zone. *Histopathology* 1993;**23**:63.

278. Tendler DA, Aboudola S, Zacks JF, O'Brien MJ, Kelly CP. Prolapsing mucosal polyps: An underrecognized form of colonic polyp – A clinicopathological study of 15 cases. *Am J Gastroenterol* 2002;**97**:370.

279. Nakamura SI, Kino I, Akagi T. Inflammatory myoglandular polyps of the colon and rectum – a clinicopathological study of 32 pedunculated polyps, distinct from other types of polyps. *Am J Surg Pathol* 1992;**16**:772.

280. Burke AP, Sobin LH. Eroded polypoid hyperplasia of the rectosigmoid. *Am J Gastroenterol* 1990;**85**:975.

281. Ng KH, Mathur P, Kumarasinghe AP, Eu KW, Seow-Choen F. Cap polyposis: Further experience and review. *Dis Colon Rectum* 2004;**47**:1208.

282. Campbell AP, Cobb CA, Chapman RWG, et al. Cap polyposis – an unusual cause of diarrhea. *Gut* 1993;**34**:562.

283. Bookman ID, Redston MS, Greenberg GR. Successful treatment of cap polyposis with infliximab. *Gastroenterology* 2004; **126**:1868.

284. Kelly JK. Polypoid prolapsing mucosal folds in diverticular-disease. *Am J Surg Pathol* 1991;**15**:871.

285. Brozna JP, Fisher RL, Barwick KW. Filiform polyposis – an unusual complication of inflammatory bowel-disease. *J Clin Gastroenterol* 1985;**7**:451.

286. Balazs M. Giant inflammatory polyps associated with idiopathic inflammatory bowel-disease – an ultrastructural-study of 5 cases. *Dis Colon Rectum* 1990;**33**:773.

287. Sheikholeslami MR, Schaefer RF, Mukunyadzi P. Diffuse giant inflammatory polyposis – A challenging clinicopathologic diagnosis. *Arch Pathol Lab Med* 2004;**128**:1286.

288. Maldonado TS, Firoozi B, Stone D, Hiotis K. Colocolonic intussusception of a giant pseudopolyp in a patient with ulcerative colitis. *Inflamm Bowel Dis* 2004;**10**:41.

289. Yada S, Matsumoto T, Kudo T, et al. Colonic obstruction due to giant inflammatory polyposis in a patient with ulcerative colitis. *J Gastroenterol* 2005;**40**:536.

290. Jessurun J, Paplanus SH, Nagle RB, Hamilton SR, Yardley JH, Tripp M. Pseudosarcomatous changes in inflammatory pseudopolyps of the colon. *Arch Pathol Lab Med* 1986;**110**:833.

291. Pitt MA, Knox WF, Haboubi NY. Multinucleated stromal giant-cells of the colonic lamina propria in ulcerative-colitis. *J Clin Pathol* 1993;**46**:874.

292. Hizawa K, Nakamori M, Taniguchi M, Matsumoto T, Iida M. Gastrointestinal: Inflammatory granulation polyp of the colon. *J Gastroenterol Hepatol* 2008;**23**:1307.

293. Oh HE, Chetty R. Intramucosal ganglion cells are common in diverticular disease. *Pathology* 2008;**40**:470.

294. Levine DS, Surawicz CM, Spencer GD, Rohrmann CA, Silverstein FE. Inflammatory polyposis 2 years after ischemic colon injury. *Dig Dis Sci* 1986;**31**:1159.

295. Oakley GJ, Schraut WH, Peel R, Krasinskas A. Diffuse filiform polyposis with unique histology mimicking familial adenomatous polyposis in a patient without inflammatory bowel disease. *Arch Pathol Lab Med* 2007;**131**:1821.

296. Vainer B, Jess T, Andersen PS. Rapid tumour-like growth of giant filiform polyposis in a patient without a history of chronic bowel inflammation. *APMIS* 2007;**115**:1306.

297. Mohamed ARE, Alkarawi MA, Yasawy MI. Schistosomal colonic disease. *Gut* 1990;**31**:439.

298. Yu XR, Chen PH, Xu JY, Xiao S, Shan ZJ, Zhu SJ. Histological classification of schistosomal egg induced polyps of colon and their clinical significance. An analysis of 272 cases. *Chin Med J (Engl)* 1991;**104**:64.

299. González-Vela MC, Val-Bernal JF, Garijo MF, García-Suárez C. Pyogenic granuloma of the sigmoid colon *Ann Diagn Pathol* 2005;**9**:106.

300. de la Plaza R, Picardo AL, Cuberes R, et al. Inflammatory fibroid polyps of the large intestine. *Dig Dis Sci* 1999;**44**:1810.

301. Park YB, Cheung DY, Kim JI, et al. A large inflammatory fibroid polyp in the sigmoid colon treated by endoscopic resection. *Intern Med* 2007;**46**:1647.

302. Shalom A, Wasserman I, Segal M, Orda R. Inflammatory fibroid polyp and Helicobacter pylori. Aetiology or coincidence? *Eur J Surg* 2000;**166**:54.

303. Wysocki AP, Taylor G, Windsor JA. Inflammatory fibroid polyps of the duodenum: a review of the literature. *Dig Surg* 2007;**24**:162.

304. Eslami-Varzaneh F, Washington K, Robert ME, Kashgarian M, Goldblum JR, Jain D. Benign fibroblastic polyps of the colon: a histologic, immunohistochemical, and ultrastructural study. *Am J Surg Pathol* 2004;**28**:374.

305. Groisman GM, Polak-Charcon S. Fibroblastic polyp of the colon and colonic perineurioma:2 names for a single entity? *Am J Surg Pathol* 2008;**32**:1088.

306. Groisman GM, Polak-Charcon S, Appelman HD. Fibroblastic polyp of the colon: clinicopathological analysis of 10 cases with emphasis on its common association with serrated crypts. *Histopathology* 2006;**48**:431.

307. Zamecnik M, Chlumska A. Fibroblastic polyp of the colon shares features with Vanek tumor. *Am J Surg Pathol* 2004; **28**:1397.

308. Hornick JL, Fletcher CD. Intestinal perineuriomas: clinicopathologic definition of a new anatomic subset in a series of 10 cases. *Am J Surg Pathol* 2005;**29**:859.

309. Gibson JA, Hornick JL. Mucosal Schwann cell 'hamartoma': clinicopathologic study of 26 neural colorectal polyps distinct from neurofibromas and mucosal neuromas. *Am J Surg Pathol* 2009;**33**:781.

310. Lewin MR, Dilworth HP, Abu Alfa AK, Epstein JI, Montgomery E. Mucosal benign epithelioid nerve sheath tumors. *Am J Surg Pathol* 2005;**29**:1310.

311. Lee SM, Goldblum J, Kim KM. Microcystic/reticular schwannoma in the colon. *Pathology* 2009;**41**:595.

312. Hornick JL, Bundock EA, Fletcher CD. Hybrid schwannoma/perineurioma: clinicopathologic analysis of 42 distinctive benign nerve sheath tumors. *Am J Surg Pathol* 2009;**33**:1554.

313. Chetty R, Vajpeyi R, Penwick JL. Psammomatous melanotic schwannoma presenting as colonic polyps. *Virchows Arch* 2007; **451**:717.

314. Shekitka KM, Sobin LH. Ganglioneuromas of the gastrointestinal tract. Relation to Von Recklinghausen disease and other multiple tumor syndromes. *Am J Surg Pathol* 1994;**18**:250.

315. Srinivasan R, Mayle JE. Polypoid ganglioneuroma of colon. *Dig Dis Sci* 1998;**43**:908.

316. Singhi AD, Montgomery EA. Colorectal granular cell tumor: a clinicopathologic study of 26 cases. *Am J Surg Pathol* 2010;**34**: 1186.

317. Hong R, Lim SC. Granular cell tumor of the cecum with extensive hyalinization and calcification: a case report. *World J Gastroenterol* 2009;**15**:3315.

318. Matsukuma S, Takeo H, Ohara I, Sakai Y. Endoscopically resected colorectal leiomyomas often containing eosinophilic globules. *Histopathology* 2004;**45**:302.

319. Miettinen M, Sarlomo-Rikala M, Sobin LH. Mesenchymal tumors of muscularis mucosae of colon and rectum are benign leiomyomas that should be separated from gastrointestinal stromal tumors–a clinicopathologic and immunohistochemical study of eighty-eight cases. *Mod Pathol* 2001;**14**:950.

320. Kojima M, Itoh H, Motegi A, Sakata N, Masawa N. Localized lymphoid hyperplasia of the rectum resembling polypoid mucosa-associated lymphoid tissue lymphoma: a report of three cases. *Pathol Res Pract* 2005;**201**:757.

321. Farris AB, Lauwers GY, Ferry JA, Zukerberg LR. The rectal tonsil: a reactive lymphoid proliferation that may mimic lymphoma. *Am J Surg Pathol* 2008;**32**:1075.

322. Koff JM, Choi JR, Hwang I. Inverted appendiceal orifice masquerading as a cecal polyp on virtual colonoscopy. *Gastrointest Endosc* 2005;**62**:308; discussion 308.

323. Taban S, Dema A, Lazar D, Sporea I, Lazar E, Cornianu M. An unusual 'tumor' of the cecum: the inverted appendiceal stump. *Rom J Morphol Embryol* 2006;**47**:193.

324. Fazio RA, Wickremesinghe PC, Arsura EL, Rando J. Endoscopic removal of an intussuscepted appendix mimicking a polyp – an endoscopic hazard. *Am J Gastroenterol* 1982;**77**:556.

325. Chijiiwa Y, Kabemura T, Toyota T, Tanaka A, Misawa T. Endoscopic appearance of the intussuscepted appendix and accurate preoperative diagnosis. *Am J Gastroenterol* 1988;**83**:1301.

326. Ryu BY, Kim TH, Jeon JY, Kim HK, Choi YH, Baik GH. Colonoscopic diagnosis of appendiceal intussusception: a case report. *J Korean Med Sci* 2005;**20**:680.

327. Posner R, Solomon A. Dilemma of an inverted cecal diverticulum simulating a pedunculated polyp: CT appearance. *Abdom Imaging* 1995;**20**:440.

328. Hobbs CM, Burch DM, Sobin LH. Elastosis and elastofibromatous change in the gastrointestinal tract: a clinicopathologic study of 13 cases and a review of the literature. *Am J Clin Pathol* 2004;**122**:232.

329. Vesoulis Z, Ravichandran P, Agamanolis D, Roe D. Elastofibromatous polyp of the sigmoid colon–a case report and review of gastrointestinal elastofibromas. *Can J Gastroenterol* 2003;**17**:275.

330. Goldblum JR, Beals T, Weiss SW. Elastofibromatous change of the rectum. A lesion mimicking amyloidosis. *Am J Surg Pathol* 1992;**16**:793.

331. Bozdech JM. Endoscopic diagnosis of colonic endometriosis. *Gastrointest Endosc* 1992;**38**:568.

332. Nakasono M, Hirokawa M, Muguruma N, et al. Colorectal xanthomas with polypoid lesion: report of 25 cases. *APMIS* 2004;**112**:3.

CHAPTER 38

Malignant epithelial neoplasms of the large bowel

Shaun V. Walsh and Frank A. Carey
Ninewells Hospital and Medical School, Dundee, UK

Introduction

In the last chapter we have already seen that benign epithelial neoplasms of the large bowel are extremely common. The evidence for an adenoma–carcinoma sequence in the development of colorectal carcinoma now seems beyond doubt. It is therefore not surprising that epithelial cancers of the large bowel (the overwhelming majority of which will be adenocarcinomas) are among the most common human malignancies. In affluent developed societies colorectal cancer is the third most common cancer in terms of incidence (if non-melanoma skin cancer is excluded) and also the third most common cause of cancer death [1]. There are often regional variations in incidence within countries so that in the UK, for example, the incidence is higher in Scotland (and particularly the north of Scotland) than in England [1].

In this chapter we consider the epidemiology and pathogenesis of large bowel cancer. There is clearly overlap with adenomas in these areas. However, not all adenoma-bearing individuals will progress to cancer and understanding the factors important to this progression is crucial. Molecular biology has made a major contribution to the understanding of tumorigenesis in the colon and rectum. We will see that the application of molecular techniques in determining prognosis and, perhaps more importantly, in predicting response to specific therapy is a major developing field.

The aim of this chapter is not to teach pathologists how to diagnose colorectal cancer. This can be done only through practical exposure to diagnostic material. Rather we hope to review aspects of epidemiology, biology and modern therapy that will provide a richer understanding of the context in which a particular specimen is interpreted. Thus, we consider advances in the surgical approach to treatment (many of which were pioneered with the active involvement of pathologists) and the increasingly complex reporting standards required to maintain a high-quality service to patients. Not so long ago, the surgical pathologist's contribution to prognostication did not extend further than producing a Dukes' staging. Histological examination can now produce a far more powerful dataset, which is used in practice and in clinical trials to stratify patient treatment. It is increasingly recognised that good pathology is the 'gold standard' in this regard [2]. Ensuring completeness of clinical reporting is a major effort and a number of national and international guidelines have been developed to aid pathologists in this [3].

Epidemiology

Age and gender

Colorectal cancer is, in general, a disease of older people with a peak incidence in the early 70s. Cancers have been described at all ages including in children. Large bowel malignancy in younger people will always raise a suspicion of an inherited cancer syndrome (disorders such as polyposis can occur new as a mutation). Many clinical guidelines recommend genetic screening in any patient presenting before the age of 50. We see that the pathologist has an important role in this context, particularly in raising

Morson and Dawson's Gastrointestinal Pathology, Fifth Edition. Edited by Neil A. Shepherd, Bryan F. Warren, Geraint T. Williams, Joel K. Greenson, Gregory Y. Lauwers and Marco R. Novelli.
© 2013 Blackwell Publishing Ltd. Published 2013 by Blackwell Publishing Ltd.

a suspicion of Lynch syndrome (hereditary non-polyposis colorectal cancer, HNPCC).

Adenocarcinoma of the colorectum is common in both males and females. In the following section we see that there are differences in the site distribution between the sexes. The precise cause of this difference is not known but it has been suggested that sex hormones may have a direct role. The contribution of gender is somewhat confounded by behavioural differences between the sexes in terms of diet, smoking, alcohol consumption and physical exercise [4].

Topographical distribution

In gathering clinical and population data, cancers of all parts of the large bowel are often considered as the same disease. The epithelium of the proximal colon is, however, subtly different in cellular composition and mucin histochemistry from that lining the distal colon and rectum. The right colon is also usually exposed to a different luminal environment when compared with the distal bowel (rapid transit of fluid contents versus relatively stationary solid bulky stool respectively).

Proximal colonic cancers in general have a different biological profile. They tend to be chromosomally diploid and to have a relatively higher incidence of microsatellite instability (MSI). Right-sided cancers also become more common with advancing age and are relatively more frequent in women [5].

In recent years there has been a suggestion that right-sided large bowel cancers have been increasing in incidence compared with more distal tumours. This area of study is complicated by differences in case ascertainment. Some populations, for example, have better access to colonoscopy services. Development of colorectal cancer screening has also complicated this issue. Large-scale population-based studies extending over several decades have tended to show, however, that there is no fundamental anatomical shift that cannot be explained by age and gender differences [6].

Aetiology

The aetiology of colorectal cancer encompasses both environmental and endogenous influences. Colorectal carcinoma may begin with the inheritance of a mutated tumour-suppressor gene as with familial polyposis coli and Lynch syndrome (HNPCC). Alternatively, carcinogenesis may be acquired by the mutagenic action of the environment on specific genes. Accumulating genetic damage then drives an evolutionary process forward, leading to the development of increasingly dysplastic adenomas and then carcinoma [7]. This is described in more detail in the section 'Pathogenesis of colorectal neoplasia'. The precise

weighting of endogenous and environmental influence on the development of colorectal carcinoma is likely to vary greatly between different individuals. Importantly, the boundaries of distinction between what is constitutional predisposition and what is environmental effect are being redefined as studies reveal evidence of hitherto unknown genetic variants that are strongly associated with a high risk of developing colorectal carcinoma [8,9].

Exogenous factors: environmental effects

The colorectal epithelium acts as a functional barrier between the luminal colonic environment and the internal milieu. As such it is heavily exposed to the effects of the environment as transmitted by diet and other swallowed substances. The importance of this epithelial environmental interaction is underlined by the known geographical variation in the incidence of colorectal cancer and by studies of migrant populations who acquire the risk of colorectal carcinoma appropriate to their adopted country [10–12]. This dominant environmental effect appears to occur despite differences in underlying genetic predisposition [13]. Dietary materials are critical components of the colonic epithelial environment, and they have been extensively studied with respect to risk of colorectal carcinoma development. The main focus of interest has been on the deleterious effects of a diet rich in meat, animal fat and carbohydrate [14–16]. Other studies have highlighted the importance of fibre, fruit and vegetables and trace elements [17–20]. It is apparent that many dietary components will be coincident with each other and with other so-called lifestyle risk factors such as smoking, obesity and lack of exercise. The effect of repeated colonic mucosal injury and repair, as occurs in chronic idiopathic inflammatory bowel disease (IBD), undoubtedly provides an environment conducive to the development of colorectal carcinoma. This is discussed in detail in Chapter 35.

Bile acids

Early in vitro and animal studies suggested that bile acids and their metabolites derived from bacterial action could act as potential carcinogens [21–24]. This mutagenic effect was augmented in animals by a diet rich in fat [25]. In humans, epidemiological studies were the first to reveal evidence for bile acids as carcinogens [26]. Later studies identified a mutagenic lipid compound (fecapentaene) that is produced in the human colon by anaerobic bacteria. Synthesis of this lipid is stimulated by high concentrations of faecal bile acids [27] and fecapentaene may then cause DNA damage directly by oxidation [28]. Recent molecular genetic studies have demonstrated that bile acids can produce DNA damage through oxidative stress and particular targets may include the *KRAS* gene [29]. Nicotine derived from smoking may act synergistically with bile acids to cause oxidative stress [30].

High meat and fat diets

There is much experimental and epidemiological evidence linking excess of red meat, processed meat and animal fat with colorectal carcinoma [14,15,21,31–36]. A high fat and high beef diet significantly increases levels of faecal bile acids, which could then provide a mechanism for carcinogenesis [26]. However, the strength of the association with red meat has been debated and the level of fat content and cooking method may also be important. A recent review of prospective epidemiological studies could not support an overall independent positive association between red meat and colonic carcinoma, although it noted a weak positive association in men alone [37]. This study also emphasised the difficulty of conducting these analyses due to difficulty in separating out red meat effects from other tightly associated dietary and lifestyle habits such as low fibre, low fruit, low vegetables, high sugar, high alcohol, smoking, obesity and lack of exercise. The risk of colorectal carcinoma carried by a diet rich in meat fat may not be entirely separable from constitutional influences, because genetic studies have identified polymorphisms in fatty acid metabolism-related genes that are also associated with increased colorectal cancer risk [38].

Fibre

Epidemiological studies of populations with diets rich in fibre have produced strong evidence for a protective effect of fibre against colorectal carcinoma [36,39]. Many potential mechanisms have been considered and have included decreased transit time, effects on luminal bacteria, fermentation, butyrate production, dilution of carcinogens and adsorption of bile acids [17,19,40–42]. Stimulated by these data, fibre supplementation has been used as a dietary intervention to try to prevent development of new tumours in patients with a history of colorectal adenomas. Although randomised controlled trials showed no influence over the development of new adenomas [43–45], these studies may have been limited by the use of adenoma recurrence as an outcome, because this would seem to be a poor surrogate marker for demonstrating adenoma prevention. Further analysis of one trial suggested that patients with very strict adherence to a diet low in fat, high in fibre, high in vegetables and fruit did in fact have a reduced risk of adenoma recurrence [46]. Larger dietary-based studies, which aim to reassess these questions, are ongoing [47].

Obesity

Of great interest is the association of obesity, a high fat diet and reduced physical exercise with colon cancer [48–52]. The link between obesity and colon cancer risk is clearer for men than women and the association is strongest with adult weight gain rather than body mass index (BMI) before the age of 18 years [53]. Abdominal obesity itself (waist size) has been associated with increased risk of colorectal carcinoma in men but not women [54]. In contrast, abdominal obesity has been associated with increased risk of adenoma development in women, especially in the distal colon [55]. Other hormonal effects may be critical because one study has revealed an increased risk of colorectal carcinoma in women with increased BMI after the menopause [56]. The subtype of carcinoma may vary according to obesity status, because one study has shown that obese patients are more likely to develop microsatellite-stable (MSS) tumours rather than microsatellite-unstable (MSI) ones [57]. Although the mechanism of how obesity increases colorectal cancer risk is unknown, attention has centred on the effect of accompanying type 2 diabetes mellitus and the possible trophic effects of insulin and insulin-like growth factors (IGFs). Type 2 diabetes is positively associated with adenoma and colorectal cancer development [58,59]. The effects of diabetes on colonic epithelium could be direct, through hyperinsulinaemia stimulating cell proliferation, or indirect, by providing an enhanced environment for tumour growth that is rich in glucose and fat [60]. Despite the obvious attractions of these theories, a large multicentre European study found only a modest association between IGF-1 levels and the risk of colorectal cancer [61]. Future studies will no doubt attempt to further unravel mechanisms associating nutrition and colorectal carcinoma as part of cancer prevention strategies [62].

Smoking and alcohol

The association of colorectal cancer with alcohol consumption, particularly beer, is well founded [12]. It appears that the risk of colorectal cancer increases in a linear fashion as alcohol intake increases [63]. Smoking is implicated particularly in the aetiology of adenomas [64–68] and smoking at least 20 pack-years has been associated with increased numbers of serrated aberrant crypt foci in the sigmoid colon and rectum [69]. Several studies have also found smoking to be associated with an increased risk of colorectal carcinoma, but with no clear agreement on whether distal or proximal tumours are more liable to occur [70–72]. In contrast to the effect of obesity, smoking has been associated with increased risk of MSI-high colorectal carcinoma in most studies, although not in all [73–78].

Vitamins, calcium and selenium

There have been numerous studies into the effects of vitamin deficiency on the risk of colorectal cancer. Vitamins B_2, B_6, B_{12}, C and D may all be mildly protective [79–84]. There is some evidence for a protective effect for calcium supplementation, possibly through an action on bile acids, but this is still uncertain [85–88]. The role of folate in colorectal carcinogenesis is controversial, with disagreement between studies that have examined the effects of folate supplementation on recurrent adenoma development [89–91]. Of greater concern are recent reports of an increased risk of colorectal adenoma and carcinoma in patients with high plasma folate levels [92,93]. In contrast to these studies, others have concluded that levels of folate in colorectal mucosa may have a mild protective effect for proximal adenomas [94]. There appears to be no link between dietary folate supplementation to prevent congenital neural tube defects and colorectal carcinoma [95].

Selenium reduces the development of intestinal cancers in experimental animals and, in mice, selenium-enriched dairy proteins can suppress the development of aberrant crypt foci and *KRAS* mutations [96–98]. Selenium may help prevent oxidative damage to DNA via interactions with glutathione peroxidase [99]. In initial epidemiological studies selenium deficiency had been linked to right-sided colonic cancer but a subsequent prospective study did not find an overall increased risk of colorectal cancer in patients with low selenium levels [100,101]. However, a recent multi-ethnic study of patients with distal colorectal carcinoma did find a relationship between selenium levels and a lowered risk in African–Americans [102].

Others

It has been proposed that colorectal carcinoma is associated with a high carbohydrate diet [103–105]. Cruciferous vegetables such as broccoli may exert a protective influence and this has been extensively investigated in vitro and in animal models [18,106–108]. However, conclusive epidemiological evidence of an effect on colonic carcinoma development in human populations is still awaited [109].

Aspirin and colorectal carcinoma

In the human colon there is an undoubted association between chronic mucosal injury due to chronic inflammatory bowel disease and the development of colorectal carcinoma. Experimental data also suggest that artificial induction of an inflammatory environment within the colon can augment adenoma development [110]. There is growing evidence in support of a protective role for aspirin in preventing carcinoma [68,111–113] in the colon and other organs [114,115]. The preventive effect of aspirin may be greatest in the proximal colon and is likely to be mediated through inhibition of the cyclo-oxygenase 2 (COX-2) enzyme, which is upregulated in colorectal adenomas and carcinoma [114,116].

Endogenous factors

Endocrine effects

Although adenomas are more common in males than in females, adenomas in females are likely to be larger [117–119]. It has been suggested that female sex hormones, or

the expression of hormone receptors, might be important in adenoma progression and that adenomas in females are more likely to become malignant [120–122]. In contrast, recent studies find a mild inverse relationship between oral contraceptive use and risk of colorectal carcinoma [123–125]. A similar protective effect has been noted for hormone replacement therapy with regard to distal carcinoma [126]. Further studies are needed to clarify the differential effects of exogenous and endogenous female hormones but it may be that hormone replacement therapy confers a protective effect in the distal colon [127]. Individuals with acromegaly are at increased risk of developing colorectal adenomas and carcinomas [128,129]. Experimental studies have strongly supported a role for gastrin in colorectal carcinoma angiogenesis and cell proliferation, [130–132] but clinical studies have been inconclusive [133,134].

Genetic factors

Classic inherited colorectal cancer syndromes

Colorectal cancer is overwhelmingly a sporadic disease with comparatively few cases being clearly attributable to inherited gene mutations. Nevertheless, mutation in genes such as *APC*, which are most commonly somatic [135], may occur in the germline and studies of such inherited cancer syndromes have provided major insights into the molecular pathogenesis of the disease. The *APC* gene is the tumour-suppressor gene implicated in the autosomal dominant disorder familial adenomatous polyposis (FAP) [136]. A second example is the inheritance of a mutated DNA-mismatch repair (MMR) gene responsible for the autosomal dominant disorder HNPCC or Lynch syndrome [137]. Polyposis syndromes other than FAP and Lynch syndrome are associated with an increased risk of colorectal cancer. These include juvenile polyposis that is associated with inherited *SMAD4* mutations [138], Cowden's syndrome with *PTEN* mutations [139] and serrated polyposis (previously termed hyperplastic polyposis) for which the genetic defect is unknown [140]. *MUTYH*-associated polyposis (MAP) is an autosomal recessive disorder characterised by multiple colorectal adenomas and increased risk of colorectal carcinoma [141]. Although resembling FAP, MAP is distinguished by the later development of 10–100 colorectal adenomas, later onset of colorectal carcinoma, duodenal adenomas and cancers and increased risk of ovarian, bladder and skin cancers [141,142]. This syndrome is not caused by mutations in the *APC* gene but by biallelic mutations in the base excision-repair gene *MUTYH*. Turcot's syndrome, the familial association of colorectal carcinoma and malignant central nervous system (CNS) tumours, may not be a distinct entity as most affected families turn out to have either FAP or HNPCC [143]. Similarly, the Muir–Torre syndrome (combining colorectal cancer and other malignancies, notably multiple cutaneous neoplasms of sebaceous type) appears to be synonymous with HNPCC [144]. The epidemiology, inheritance patterns and pathology of the classic inherited pathways to colorectal carcinoma are discussed in Chapter 37. The complex pathogenic mechanisms underlying these syndromes and their sporadic counterparts are discussed in detail in 'Pathogenesis of colorectal neoplasia' below.

Non-classic inherited pathways

The *APC* I1307K mutation occurring in Ashkenazi Jews does not of itself cause classical FAP but creates a short hypermutable mononucleotide repeat in *APC* that is susceptible to further frameshift mutations that may inactivate APC function. The resulting phenotype is an increased frequency of adenomas and a roughly twofold increased risk of carcinoma in affected families [145,146]. Other rare variants in the *APC* gene that may theoretically affect its function have also been reported [147].

Recently, kindreds that develop Lynch syndrome but without an overt germline mutation in any MMR gene have been identified. Constitutional epimutation of the *MLH1* gene by allele-specific promoter methylation is responsible, due to an inherited predisposition to soma-wide methylation of *MLH1* [148–150]. Carcinomas in these families are MSI high and DNA CpG island methylation positive (see below) without MMR gene mutation and can be easily mistaken for sporadic tumours unless a family history is sought. These complex cases illustrate the need for the close collaboration of histopathologists, molecular geneticists, clinical geneticists and clinicians to identify covert examples of inherited colorectal neoplasia, with their implications for family counselling and surveillance.

Inherited contribution to sporadic colorectal carcinoma

When all the well-characterised inherited syndromes are excluded there still appears to be evidence of an inherited basis to colorectal cancer in 15–25% of cases [151,152]. Numerous families have been described with increased numbers of adenomas and carcinomas but without detectable inherited mutations [153–157]. Recent studies of rare variants in different genes such as *AXIN1* and *CTNNB1* have been suggested that they may account for such families [158]. Genome-wide association studies have discovered several single nucleotide polymorphisms at susceptibility loci including 6q26, 7q31, 8q23, 8q24, 10p24, 11q23, 11q24 and 15q13 that are associated with increased risk of colorectal carcinoma and differ significantly in different ethnic populations [8,9,159–164].

An inherited predisposition to pathogenic metabolism of environmental mutagens may also contribute to colorectal cancer risk. Interest has focused on acetylation and in particular on allelic variants of the *N*-acetyl transferase genes (*NAT1, NAT2*) [165–169]. A recent study highlighted a link between heterocyclic amine production derived from tobacco smoke and NAT2 function, which together influence colorectal cancer risk [170]. This study provides an example of synergy between environmental mutagens and genetically governed metabolic predisposition towards the development of colorectal carcinoma. A second metabolic enzyme with important effects on carcinogen detoxification is glutathione *S*-transferase (GST). The GST-null genotype has been associated with an increased risk of colorectal cancer, although this is disputed [171–173], but a recent meta-analysis of epidemiological studies revealed *GSTM1* polymorphism to be associated with increased cancer risk in white people but not in other ethnic groups [174]. A third focus of enquiry has centred on polymorphisms of methylenetetrahydrofolate reductase *(MTHFR)* that influence enzyme activity. Individuals with the less active form were at lower risk of colorectal cancer in two studies [175,176]. Data from a meta-analysis of 25 populations revealed that individuals who are homozygous for the *MTHFR C677T* polymorphism are at reduced risk of colorectal carcinoma, and suggested that other variants of this gene could also contribute to cancer susceptibility [177]. Apolipoprotein E (ApoE) regulates cholesterol metabolism. Individuals with the ε4 allele absorb a greater percentage of dietary cholesterol, and this allele may be less common in individuals with proximal colorectal cancers [178]. However, the effect of ApoE may be even more subtle because ApoE isoforms appear to alter the risk of MSI-H and MSS/L colorectal cancers among high red meat consumers, which in turn suggests another possible interaction with bile acids [179].

The cytochromes P450 (CYP1A1 and CYP2D6) are implicated in the conversion of polycyclic aromatic hydrocarbons to their DNA-binding carcinogenic forms [168]. Homozygosity for the *MspI* mutant genotype of *CYP1A1* has been associated with colorectal cancer [180] and polymorphic variation in *CYP1A2* and *CYP1B1* may also play a role in colorectal cancer susceptibility [181]. There is also evidence that that expression of *CYP1B1*, but not *CYP1A1*, is downregulated by promoter methylation in colorectal cancer [182].

Summary

Attempting to unravel the complex interactions between genes and the environment in the aetiology of colorectal cancer is a difficult task. Several specific interactions have been proposed (Table 38.1). New studies must be designed on the basis that colorectal cancer is a heterogeneous disease, and stratification of study groups by genetic background will be needed to accurately assess the impact of any proposed dietary or environmental mutagen. The clear goal of these studies must be to present populations with lifestyle advice, given each individual's genetic risk, in order to prevent the development of colorectal carcinoma.

Table 38.1 Proposed environment–gene interactions

1. Bile acids–*KRAS*
2. Selenium–*KRAS*
3. Aspirin–cyclo-oxygenase 2 *(COX2)*
4. Smoking–*NAT2*
5. Folate–*MTHFR*

Table 38.2 Pathways to colorectal carcinoma

1. **Inherited pathways**
   a. Familial adenomatous polyposis
   b. Lynch syndrome (HNPCC)
   c. *MYH*-associated polyposis
   d. Serrated polyposis
   e. Juvenile polyposis
2. **Sporadic pathways**
   a. Conventional
   b. Serrated
3. **Inflammatory bowel disease-associated pathway**

Pathogenesis of colorectal neoplasia

In the past it had been suggested that the molecular pathogenesis of colorectal carcinoma was possibly the most understood of all the common cancers. Certainly it has been extensively studied. However, recent research has unearthed greater complexity than previously imagined, and new molecular pathways from normal colonic epithelium to adenoma and then carcinoma have been accepted. Simultaneously, advances in the treatment of colorectal carcinoma, predicated on the molecular genetic nature of an individual's colorectal cancer, have become available and present the pathologist with a new diagnostic challenge. This book is primarily written for practising diagnostic histopathologists and emphasis has been deliberately placed on broader pathogenic mechanisms rather than on complex and evolving molecular data. However, it is now impossible to ignore key genetic mutations and processes relevant to modern pharmacogenomics and these are discussed in some detail.

Pathways to colorectal adenocarcinoma development

Several broad clinicopathological pathways that lead to the development of colorectal carcinoma are now recognised (Table 38.2). FAP and HNPCC exemplify inherited pathways, whereas longstanding IBD is considered a separate pathway arising from repeated mucosal injury. The remaining bulk of colorectal carcinoma, most often termed 'sporadic' to distinguish it from the other pathways, was at first considered a homogenous entity. Progression of adenoma to carcinoma, central to tumour development in FAP patients, was identified by Morson as the most likely pathway for the pathogenesis of sporadic tumours too: the adenoma–carcinoma sequence [181]. The initiation of tumorigenesis through *APC* gene mutation, followed by progressive accumulation of genetic and chromosomal damage, was related by Vogelstein and colleagues to progression from early adenoma to adenoma with high grade dysplasia and then to adenocarcinoma [7]. However, more recent clinicopathological and molecular genetic studies have identified sporadic tumours that do not fit this classic model and are instead thought to arise along a novel pathway often termed the 'serrated pathway' [183–185].

Such tumours lack an initiating *APC* gene mutation, exhibit high levels of DNA methylation and MSI and demonstrate a serrated architecture on histopathological examination. Even as new, apparently distinct, pathways are identified their boundaries soon become blurred with overlap between different routes to carcinoma development. Despite this complexity, individual pathways to colorectal carcinoma will be considered separately here. Concepts arising from the main inherited pathways are discussed first, allowing the introduction of specific molecular genetic data where appropriate. The so-called sporadic pathways are then discussed, emphasising the place of critical gene mutations. Finally we examine new attempts at molecular classification of colorectal carcinoma as a whole.

Inherited pathways to colorectal carcinoma: models of colorectal cancer pathogenesis

The spectrum of hereditary conditions that predispose to colorectal carcinoma is ever expanding. The classic condition FAP and Lynch syndrome (HNPCC) have been joined by *MUTYH*-associated polyposis, serrated polyposis and juvenile polyposis [186]. The recognition of these rare conditions, accounting for less than 10% of all colorectal carcinomas, has contributed massively to our understanding of the molecular pathogenesis of the more common sporadic carcinomas. The clinical and pathological features of these conditions are discussed in Chapter 37.

Concepts from familial adenomatous polyposis: the *APC* gene, normal-appearing mucosa, ACFs, stem cells and microadenomas, genetic instability, chromosome instability

Familial polyposis coli and the APC gene This autosomal dominant condition leads to the development of thousands of adenomas within an affected patient and without intervention the inevitable advent of adenocarcinoma. Studies on this condition first led to the conclusion that colorectal adenocarcinomas are derived from adenomas [187], and all subsequent work in this field owes a great deal to this seminal observation. FAP is caused by inherited mutations in *APC*, a large gene of 15 exons located on the long arm of chromosome 5 [136,188–190]. Patients usually inherit one mutated allele and acquire a second hit or somatic mutation in the other allele early in life. However, approximately a quarter of FAP cases are due to new germline mutations [191]. Ninety per cent of germline *APC* mutations result in a truncated protein and these patients develop classic FAP [192]. Mutational hotspots at codons 1061 and 1309 are associated with approximately a third of cases. However, new mutations, effects of mosaicism and possible pathogenic variants that may vary in different geographical populations are continually being described [147,158,193–195]. The specific germline mutation type has been shown to associate with disease severity, including the development of attenuated forms of FAP, allowing correlation of genotype with phenotype [191,196]. Interestingly, location in the large bowel also appears to influence the *APC* gene mutations observed in FAP adenomas [197].

The initial germline mutation may also influence the nature of the second somatic hit on the other *APC* allele, suggesting that this must be 'just right' to allow for growth advantage without risking catastrophic cell dysfunction and apoptosis [198–200]. Unusual allelic variants have already been discussed above. There is evidence that inactivation of the wild-type *APC* allele initiates the development of adenomas in FAP [201] and inactivation of both alleles has been observed in small adenomas in FAP patients [202], underlining its importance in the early development of adenomas.

APC protein function: canonical Wnt signalling Extensive studies of FAP patients and murine models such as the APCmin model have yielded a wealth of data on APC function and the central role of the *APC* gene as a multifunctional tumour suppressor is now universally accepted [203,204] (Figure 38.1). APC protein has been shown to exert control over intestinal cell proliferation and differentiation through its inhibition of β-catenin/T-cell factor (TCF)-dependent transcription in the so-called canonical Wnt signalling pathway [205]. Evidence from many studies suggests that the APC protein binds and phosphorylates β-catenin and targets it for destruction via the ubiquitin–proteosomal pathway [206,207]. Mutated APC protein cannot complex with β-catenin, allowing it to accumulate in the cytoplasm, form complexes with DNA-binding proteins of the TCF/LEF (lymphoid enhancer family) group, translocate to the nucleus and co-transactivate several *Wnt* target genes [204,208–210] (Figure 38.2). Wnt target genes may include cell cycle regulators such as *c-Myc* and *cyclin D1* and others important in epithelial interaction with stroma such as matrix metalloprotease 7/Matrilysin and *CD44* [211–213]. Several other important components of the

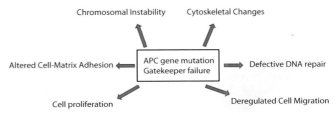

Figure 38.1 *APC* gene mutation and consequent gatekeeper failure initiate multiple deleterious cytogenetic events that produce a defective stem cell phenotype.

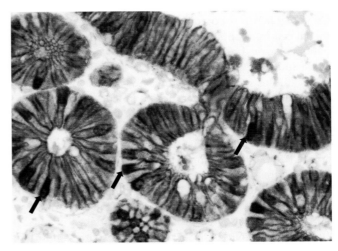

Figure 38.2 Conventional tubular adenoma with β-catenin expression in nuclei (arrows) as well as cytoplasmic and membranous cellular compartments.

Wnt signalling pathway are known, including *axin* and *GSKIII*, as well as several negative-feedback regulators. Other signalling proteins may also influence β-catenin levels including KRAS [214]. The complete Wnt signalling pathway has been excellently reviewed elsewhere [215].

In addition to Wnt-dependent functions, experimental data suggests that APC protein is also important in cell adhesion [216–218], interacts with the cytoskeleton [219], affects directed cell migration [220], interacts with RNAs in cell protrusions, affects mitotic spindle formation and may play a role in chromosomal instability, DNA repair and DNA replication [221–227].

Not all the data gleaned from FAP patient adenomas, in vitro studies and APCmin mice concur, e.g. there is ongoing debate about whether biallelic *APC* mutation is sufficient to produce nuclear translocation of β-catenin in very early adenomas or whether another genetic event such as *KRAS* mutation is also required [214,228–234]. Studies in APC1322T mice, linking low nuclear β-catenin levels and Wnt signalling with increased crypt stem cells and a severe polyposis phenotype, provide an attractive alternative mechanism for low levels of nuclear β-catenin/Wnt signalling driving tumorigenesis, and concur with the 'just right' hypothesis [235].

The mechanics of how *APC* mutation-driven disruption of these processes yields the development of morphologically identifiable adenomas in FAP patients is the subject of extensive ongoing research. Research into the morphological correlates of early neoplasia has focused on three areas: changes in histologically normal crypts, aberrant crypt foci, and effects on stem cells and the formation of microadenomas.

CHANGES IN HISTOLOGICALLY NORMAL CRYPTS Every epithelial cell from apparently normal colonic mucosa in FAP patients carries a germline mutation in at least one *APC* allele and the effects of this 'one hit' have been measured. Early studies of normal colonic mucosa in FAP patients detected expanded proliferation in patches of crypts [236] but its extent was disputed [237,238]. Later studies using monoclonal antibodies provided convincing evidence of a shift in the proliferative compartment into the upper crypts [239]. Other changes described in morphologically normal-appearing FAP mucosa include increased crypt fission, somatic gene mutation and alterations in apoptosis in response to a COX-2 inhibitor [240–242]. The advent of proteomics has provided the clearest evidence of one-hit effects with changes in the expression of proteins important in cell adhesion, apoptosis, motility, cytoskeleton structure, oxidative stress, mitosis and others [243]. Information derived from such proteomics data may well be used to assess the effectiveness of interventions aimed at preventing neoplasia in FAP patients in the future.

ABERRANT CRYPT FOCI Aberrant crypt foci are thought by some to be the earliest morphologically recognisable lesion in the development of colorectal neoplasia but their role is still controversial [244]. These lesions were first described in experimental animals exposed to carcinogens [245] and shortly afterwards in human colonic mucosa, including increased numbers in a case of Gardner's syndrome [246]. Subsequently they have been studied in normal colons and in those from patients with FAP and sporadic colorectal cancer by low-power en face stereomicroscopy after methylene blue staining [247]. By this method ACFs appear as distinct foci of darkly staining crypts, which are slightly larger than usual and often have slit-like openings [247]. They have also been recognised in the Min mouse model of FAP [248] and recently in patients with ulcerative colitis [249]. They are identifiable in vivo using magnification chromoscopic endoscopy [231].

Histologically, ACFs consist of variably sized clusters of crypts with a variety of appearances. Some appear similar to microadenomas with dysplasia [247,250] whereas others are more like small hyperplastic polyps with enlarged crypts that have a serrated appearance and abnormal-appearing goblet cells extending slightly above the mucosal surface. Colonic mucosa from FAP patients has more ACFs per cm^2 with a greater degree of dysplasia than mucosa from sporadic carcinoma patients [247,251]. One study found somatic *APC* gene mutations in all lesions [231]. The spectrum of histopathological appearances associated with ACFs has led some to classify them into dysplastic or hyperplastic types, and to further subclassify hyperplastic ACFs into serrated or non-serrated forms [251,252]. Molecular genetic studies have provided some support for this approach, with different rates of *KRAS* and *BRAF* mutations between the subtypes [231,251–253].

Many authors have recently expressed doubt about the validity of ACFs as biomarkers for colorectal carcinoma in research studies [244,254,255]. Previously identified ACFs could be identified only at follow-up endoscopy in less than half the cases in one study [256], and no endoscopic criteria predicted histological confirmation of ACFs in another [254]. It seems unlikely that histopathologists will be required to recognise ACFs in routine practice in the near future.

STEM CELLS AND MICROADENOMAS The presence within crypts of stem cells that can reconstitute the different epithelial cell types of the colonic mucosa by cell division is central to new theories of adenoma development [257–259]. Colonic crypts have been estimated to have between four and six stem cells per crypt [260,261], forming a 'niche' at the crypt base. These estimates have been made despite the fact that stemness-specific markers, such as the Wnt–β-catenin target *Lgr-5*, are just beginning to emerge [262]. The regulation of stem cell populations is highly complex, involving interactions between epithelium and stromal cells within the stem cell niche. Regulatory pathways are numerous and are known to include *Wnt*, *Hedgehog*, *Notch*, *PI3Kinase* and *BMP* pathways. These pathways and their role in stem cell regulation and early tumour development are thoroughly reviewed elsewhere [263,264]. Established experimental evidence from FAP patients and animal models suggests that stem cells may experience enhanced survival ability, proliferate in an unregulated fashion and overpopulate crypts after *APC* gene mutation [257,265]. The acquisition of progenitor or stem cell phenotype by the APC-deficient mutant cells is characterised by a failure to migrate up the crypt with continuing uncontrolled proliferation [266,267]. These mutated basal crypt cells have a selective advantage and gradually replace the progeny of other stem cells, a process described as niche succession, leading to clonal expansion of neoplastic cells that grow from the bottom up [259,268–270].

This process best explains how, in FAP patients, unicryptal microadenomas populated by severely abnormal and proliferating cells become recognisable to the histopathologist as a clearly dysplastic crypt and are the earliest morphologically detectable abnormality. Unicryptal adenomas then expand, most probably by crypt fission, to produce multi-cryptal adenomas [269,271]. Early adenomas such as these may appear initially flat or depressed but subsequently become polypoid as they enlarge [272,273]. The discovery that larger FAP adenomas may be polyclonal in nature raises the possibility of multiple unicryptal adenomas contributing progeny to these later lesions [274]. Polyclonality has also been detected in some sporadic adenomas [275].

Genetic instability: chromosomal instability After initiation of neoplasia, progressive replacement of older adenoma cells by more aggressive and biologically advantaged subclones has been deemed to be the mechanism by which adenomas progress. How adenomas, with progressively advancing genetic damage, continue to survive, proliferate and avoid triggering apoptosis requires a further mechanism. This is provided by the concept of genetic instability [276]. Genetic instability provides a cellular environment that ensures that progressive mutational events are more likely. There are two forms of genetic instability that have generally been thought to be mutually exclusive, although this has been recently challenged [277,278]. The first is termed chromosomal instability (CIN) affecting parts of or whole chromosomes. The second is MSI, affecting the DNA sequence, which is discussed later.

Chromosome instability Chromosomal instability in tumours may be characterised by aneuploidy, defined as having a number of chromosomes that is not an exact multiple of the haploid number, and/or structural abnormalities in chromosomes such as insertions, deletions or translocations. Failure to faithfully replicate chromosome copy number and integrity during mitosis leads to either gains or losses of chromosomes and encourages genetic diversity among daughter cells (Figure 38.3). This chromosomal instability may be caused by defects in the mitotic machinery [279,280]. Aneuploidy induced by chromosomal instability is distinct from DNA aneuploidy as measured by flow cytometry (see below). The precise causes of CIN are unclear and probably complex. *APC* mutation has been suggested as a possible driver of CIN [227] but other genes controlling chromosomal segregation, such as *Mad, Bub, Nup, Rae, Chfr* and *CENPE*, are also under investigation [281].

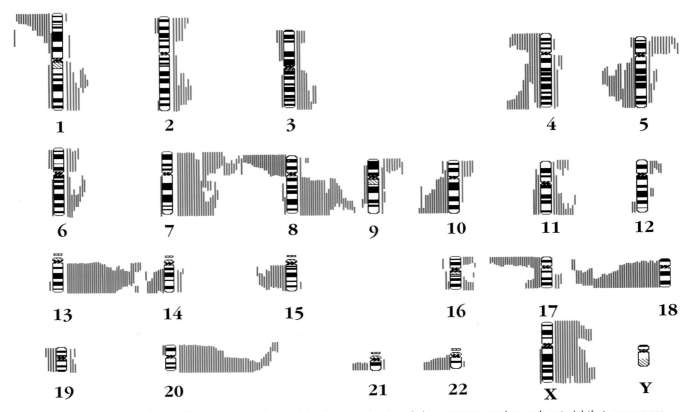

Figure 38.3 Chromosomal instability produces widely variable losses and gains of chromosome number and material that encourages genetic diversity. Summary of data from 50 colorectal carcinomas detected by comparative genomic hybridisation. Green represents areas of gain and red represents areas of loss. (Image courtesy of Dr Norman Pratt, Ninewells Hospital, Dundee.)

CIN is associated with both gains and losses of chromosomal material in colorectal carcinoma [282], but it is the losses of 8p, 17p and 18q that have been most closely studied because they are associated with loss of heterozygosity (LOH) for critical tumour-suppressor genes. Depending on the series being reviewed, CIN is thought to be critical in the development of 60–85% of colorectal carcinomas. It is characteristic of those sporadic carcinomas that are thought to arise via the conventional adenoma–carcinoma sequence. However, it also characterises a subset of carcinomas that are associated with *KRAS* mutation and part of the serrated pathway. CIN is generally viewed as being an engine, driving later steps in the adenoma–carcinoma sequence, in both FAP and conventional-type sporadic carcinomas [283]. Recent studies have suggested that CIN+ colorectal carcinomas have a poorer prognosis [277].

Concepts from Lynch syndrome (HNPCC): DNA-mismatch repair, genetic instability, MSI

Studies of the autosomal dominant condition Lynch syndrome or HNPCC have greatly enhanced our understanding of an entirely different pathway to colorectal cancer. Lynch syndrome is caused by inherited mutations in genes responsible for MMR, and colorectal carcinomas arising in patients with this condition exhibit MSI as a biomarker of defective MMR function. Subsequent studies of MSI in sporadic colorectal carcinomas have confirmed a further important role for this type of genetic instability in a subset of sporadic carcinomas as well (see 'Serrated adenoma–carcinoma sequence' below).

Lynch syndrome and mismatch repair Lynch syndrome or HNPCC is caused by a germline mutation affecting one of a family of MMR genes (*hMLH1, hMSH2, hMSH6, hPMS1, hPMS2*) [137,284–289] with *hMLH1* and *hMSH2* being implicated in the great majority of affected families (30% and 60%, respectively). Loss of DNA repair proficiency follows somatic inactivation of the second or wild-type allele [290]. The MMR proteins encoded by these genes recognise and repair mismatched DNA basepair errors and insertion deletion loops, which can occur during replication [291]. At least seven key genes in the MMR system are known: *hMLH1, hMLH3, hMSH2, hMSH3, hMSH6, hPMS1* and *hPMS2*; these genes are highly conserved from bacteria to humans [292]. The MMR proteins function together as an integrated complex in which all of the component parts are necessary. MSH2 and MSH6 function as a heterodimeric mutation recognition complex whereas MLH1 and PMS2 function as a heterodimeric repair complex. Loss of a single component protein, such as MSH2, will lead to ineffective overall complex formation and further reduce function by failing to provide a binding partner for MSH6, which will then be rapidly degraded [291,293,294]. Similarly, MLH1 must bind with PMS2 for effective repair complex formation [295,296].

Failure to repair mismatched basepairs leads to the development of numerous DNA replication errors (RERs), described also as the mutator phenotype, for which MSI serves as a biomarker. Oncogenesis results from the mutational inactivation of many additional genes implicated in the regulation of growth and differentiation, providing a suitable environment for further neoplastic progression. In HNPCC this is characterised by the development of multiple adenomas that although derived from a different molecular pathway most often appear identical to conventional adenomas. Finally, it appears that MMR protein alterations may not be restricted to the adenomatous phase of colorectal cancer development because loss of MSH6 expression has recently been noted in colorectal carcinomas after neoadjuvant therapy [297].

DNA microsatellite instability Microsatellites are non-encoding regions within the genome comprising repetitive tracts of DNA. These may be either mononucleotide (e.g. AAAAAA) or dinucleotide (e.g. CACACA) runs. These tracts are prone to mismatch errors during DNA replication that are normally repaired by MMR proteins. Impaired function of this caretaker system can lead to 'slippage' in DNA replication and the production of a different number of sequence repeats within a microsatellite in daughter DNA. These errors are not corrected and the number of repeats can vary with each replication cycle, producing MSI (Figure 38.4). This is easily demonstrated by bandshifts in tumour DNA on gel electrophoresis. The presence of MSI in tumour-derived DNA (in contrast to germline DNA) serves as a biomarker for DNA instability and occurs in almost all HNPCC neoplasms (although variably with *MSH6* mutations) and in up to 30% of sporadic colorectal cancers. The list of genes susceptible to MSI-driven mutation is long and includes many genes with critical roles in oncogenesis and tumour suppression such as *TGFBII, Caspase 5, MSH3, MSH6, APC, β-catenin, Axin, Bax, IGF2* and many others [298–305]. It is interesting to note that genes central to the conventional pathway, including *APC* and *β-catenin*, may be mutated in this fashion, providing a potential link between conventional and serrated pathways of colorectal carcinogenesis (see below).

Testing for MSI and MSI-L When assessing a tumour for MSI, usually five DNA microsatellite regions (two mononucleotide and three dinucleotide) from the 'Bethesda panel' of markers are tested [306]. These include BAT25, BAT26, D5S346, D2S123 and D17S250. When MSI can be demonstrated in at least 40% of a panel of microsatellite markers, a tumour is classified as MSI-high (MSI-H). Lower frequencies of instability identify MSI-low (MSI-L) tumours (one marker positive) and those with no demonstrable

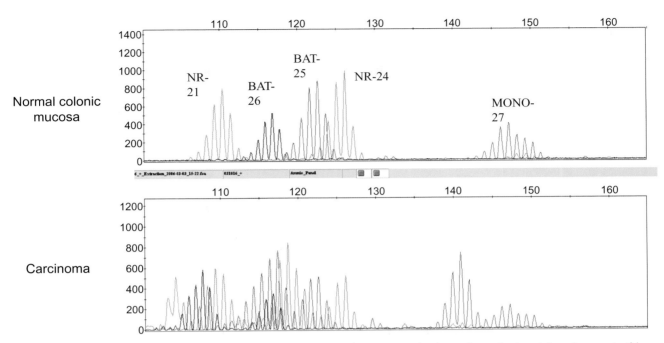

Figure 38.4 Microsatellite instability (MSI) provides a mechanism of tumour progression in a subset of colorectal carcinomas. In this example, tumour instability is observed at several loci (MSI-high) and is easily distinguished from normal signature. (Image courtesy of Nicola Andrews, Ninewells Hospital, Dundee.)

defect are said to be MSS. The significance of MSI-L is uncertain [307] and many cancers may have a minor degree of instability depending on the number of markers tested [308]. The type of marker used is also critical, with mononucleotide markers such as BAT26 and BAT40 being more sensitive for MSI-H than MSI-L. Unlike MSI-H tumours, MSI-L tumours have been shown to demonstrate considerable overlap with conventional or MSS tumours in terms of clinicopathological features [309]. However, there is good evidence that MSI-L colorectal cancers represent an important subgroup with a distinct biological basis. The evidence has been reviewed by Jass [183] and includes an association between MSI-L and the activity of the RAS-induced senescence1 gene (*RIS1*), effects on outcome and effects on DNA methylation when associated with *KRAS* mutation [310–313]. Possible mechanisms to explain MSI-L include partial methylation of *hMLH1* and loss of the DNA-repair protein *O-6*-methylguanine DNA methyltransferase (MGMT) [183], which repairs G:C to A:T transversions [314]. This pathway may be important in a subset of sporadic serrated carcinomas.

MSI in sporadic carcinomas MSI-H cancers show a significantly reduced frequency of *APC*, *KRAS* and *TP53* mutations; LOH or allelic imbalance at 5q, 17p and 18q is very uncommon [315–319]. As these genetic alterations are implicated in the initiation and progression of adenomas, a different spectrum of mutations must occur in the precur-

sors of MSI-H cancers. Earlier studies of MSI in adenomas rarely found MSI-H (other than those occurring in HNPCC) [320,321], and this led to the conclusion that MSI-H must always be a late event in sporadic adenomas. Subsequently, MSI-H and loss of expression of the MMR gene *hMLH1* (Figure 38.5) has been found to occur relatively frequently in the dysplastic components of mixed hyperplastic polyps/adenomas and in serrated adenomas [322,323]. Serrated polyps are now thought to be the precursors of a defined subset of sporadic colorectal cancers, particularly those showing DNA MSI. The mechanism by which sporadic tumours develop MSI is most commonly thought to be by epigenetic silencing of the *hMLH1* gene through promoter methylation [324], rather than mutation, and characterises a large number of tumours that arise via the serrated pathway (see below).

Utility of MSI: screening for Lynch syndrome and prognosis The knowledge that sporadic cancers and Lynch syndrome-derived cancers may both show MSI means that MSI alone cannot be used as a biomarker for Lynch syndrome. Moreover, it must be borne in mind that MSI-L has been associated with *MSH6* mutation. The choice and methodology of the microsatellite analysis may be critical here, because MSH6 deficiency does not affect dinucleotide repeats [325]. The judicious use of immunohistochemistry for MMR proteins can be beneficial as a complementary test [291]. Methylation assays are not routinely used. MSI

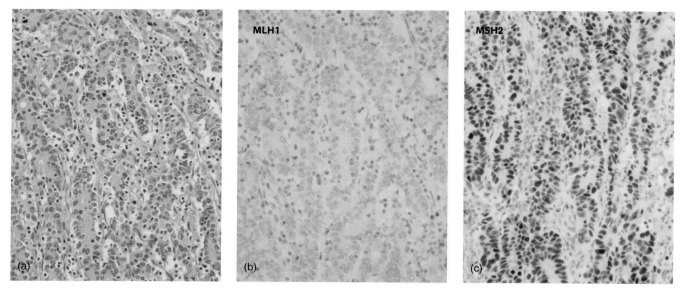

Figure 38.5 Sporadic microsatellite instability (MSI) adenocarcinoma with abundant tumour infiltrating lymphocytes (a). Methylation of the *hMLH1* promoter silences MLH1 expression in tumour cells (b) whereas expression of MSH2 is retained (c).

status may be predictable using pathological features of tumours [326], but there is continuing controversy over the influence of MSI status on prognosis and response to chemotherapy [327–330]. This is discussed further below.

Epigenetics: methylation and genomic silencing
Both hypo- and hypermethylation of DNA have been linked to colorectal carcinogenesis.

Methylation Methylation of DNA commonly occurs at CpG islands [331]. The promoter regions of certain genes are CpG island rich and methylation will lead to transcriptional silencing of those genes [332]. Colorectal cancers with evidence of CpG island methylation are termed 'CIMP positive'. However, methylation in colorectal cancer is not limited to CpG islands or promoters but occurs also in more distant regions of DNA termed 'CpG island shores' [333]. The mechanisms by which CIMP occurs are also uncertain. Constitutional epimutation of *hMLH1* has been reported to account for rare cases of Lynch syndrome [148,150] and some workers have suggested a possible genetic predisposition to methylation, but this is not universally accepted [334–336]. Environmental factors have also been implicated in CIMP including smoking [337,338].

Definition of CIMP CIMP-positive colorectal cancers are commonly defined by using a panel of CpG island methylation markers. Unfortunately, unlike MSI, no consensus yet exists on which panel to use, which technique to use or how to grade the results [339]. This uncertainty creates difficulty in comparing studies of colorectal cancer with CIMP,

and the assessment of CIMP is not yet in routine use in most laboratories. The most commonly used system of CIMP grading divides tumours into CIMP high (CIMP1) and CIMP low (CIMP2). CIMP1 tumours are associated with *BRAF* mutations and show methylation of many markers [340,341]. In contrast, CIMP2 tumours have a high frequency of *KRAS* mutations and a less generalised pattern of methylation [340,341].

Other genes subject to methylation In addition to *hMLH1*, other genes inactivated by methylation in colorectal cancer include *p16* [331], *p14^{ARF}* [342], *COX-2* [343], oestrogen receptor (*ER*) [344], the DNA-repair gene *MGMT* [345], *RASSF1, RASSF2, NORE1* and *MST1*. The *APC* gene promoter can also be subject to methylation but this is uncommon [346].

Hypomethylation When compared with normal cells, adenoma and colorectal cancer cells show a reduction in total methylation [347,348]. Defective methylation might interfere with the genomic imprinting of important regulatory genes such as insulin-like growth factor 2 (*IGF2*). One copy of this allele (usually paternally derived) is silenced by methylation, and defective methylation could lead to loss of imprinting. Loss of imprinting of *IGF2* has been associated with MSI-H colorectal cancer [349].

Non-inherited pathways to colorectal carcinoma: sporadic colorectal carcinoma
Although inherited pathways to colorectal carcinoma have greatly enhanced our understanding of basic mechanisms

in colorectal cancer development, they remain clinically rare. The great bulk of colorectal carcinomas encountered in the developed world have no apparent familial tendency or linkage and such carcinomas are termed 'sporadic'. Instead of germline mutations being responsible as initiating events, interactions between environmental carcinogens and the colonocyte genome are presumed to be the underlying cause. The separation between hereditary and sporadic may well be artificial, as non-classic genetic variations that contribute to the loading of risk without producing a predictable pattern of inheritance are identified (see above). Likewise, a single stepwise sequence of genetic events governing the development of sporadic colorectal carcinoma is no longer thought to explain sufficiently the clinical and pathological varieties of colorectal tumour that are observed in practice.

The conventional model of Vogelstein and Fearon, in which morphologically conventional adenomas give rise via the suppressor pathway to MSS carcinomas, accounts for approximately 60–85% of colorectal cancers [339,350], with most of the remainder arising via the serrated pathway, with sessile serrated adenomas giving rise to CpG island methylated carcinomas that may be MSI-H or stable [184,185]. Although treated separately here, there is probably considerable overlap between pathways. The molecular classification of colorectal carcinoma is a pressing issue and has been extensively reviewed [183,215]. This interest is in large part driven by the need to identify targeted therapies for colorectal cancer patients that are focused on the underlying molecular genetic drivers.

The conventional adenoma–carcinoma sequence (the suppressor, canonical and CIN pathways): *APC, KRAS, DCC, TP53*

This well-known model developed by Fearon and Vogelstein [351] integrates molecular insights (loss or mutation of the tumour-suppressor genes *APC, TP53* and *DCC*, and mutation of *KRAS*) with the evolution of normal epithelium to adenoma and transition to carcinoma. In this pathway adenoma development is thought to pursue a series of steps, with *APC* inactivation as a common initiating event followed by further genetic changes, including *KRAS* mutation and *TP53* inactivation, leading to the development of aggressive subclones of adenoma and ultimately carcinoma [7,351] (Figure 38.6). This model also incorporates chromosomal instability, marked by aneuploidy, with notable loss of critical chromosomal material including 5q (*APC*), 17p (*TP53*) and 18q (*DCC, SMAD4*) [352]. In this model early adenomas are small and most commonly show a tubular architecture. A small number of these progress to become larger adenomas, acquire a villous architecture and, with increasing size, develop high grade dysplasia and ultimately progress to carcinoma. Adenomas arising by this pathway show a smooth non-serrated epi-

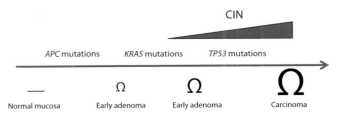

Figure 38.6 The conventional adenoma–carcinoma sequence considered responsible for the development of most colorectal carcinomas. Adenomas accumulate genetic damage in a stepwise fashion beginning with loss of the gatekeeper APC. Chromosomal instability (CIN) is a later event associated with the development of carcinoma.

thelial lining and are termed conventional to distinguish them from serrated adenomas. The morphology of conventional adenomas is discussed in Chapter 37.

Genetic changes in early conventional adenomas

APC APC gene mutations occur in 60–80% of sporadic colorectal neoplasms [215,353]. The initiating role of the gatekeeper *APC* gene has already been discussed in detail above. This gene appears to play a role in many different tumour-suppressive mechanisms and appears very centrally placed in cellular homeostasis [204]. Disruption of its function is an early and critical event in the sporadic pathway, because mutations are found in early adenomas as well as carcinomas [351,353]. In sporadic tumours both alleles are inactivated by somatic mutation or by a combination of LOS and somatic mutation [354–357]. Mutations most frequently occur in a cluster region important for β-catenin binding and regulation [358]. Mutations at codons 1309 and 1450 are the most common and produce an inactive truncated protein [358], leading to increased Wnt signalling and downstream effects. Most adenomas do not progress to carcinoma [359]. Therefore although *APC* mutation may be sufficient to produce early adenoma, progression to carcinoma is not obligatory and further genetic damage is required.

Genetic changes in intermediate (progressed) adenomas

KRAS This proto-oncogene encodes a 21-kDa GTP-binding protein that is important in adenoma progression, the role of which is not limited to the conventional pathway. RAS proteins are a family of intracellular signal transducers, which help transmit extracellular signalling from bound transmembrane growth factor receptors and cytokine receptors [360]. Cellular processes partly governed by RAS signalling include proliferation, cell–cell adhesion, cell–matrix interactions, cytoskeletal structure and cell motility [360]. *KRAS* mutation, most commonly in codon 12 but sometimes in codon 13 or rarely in codon 61, causes loss of protein GTPase activity. This leads to constitutive activation of the mitogen-activated protein kinase (MAPK) and the PI3-K/Akt pathways [360]. Constitutional activation of the MAPK pathway effectively bypasses growth factor receptor-mediated cellular regulation. Interestingly, *KRAS* mutation has been associated with the mutagenic effects of bile acids [29].

The presence of *KRAS* mutations in conventional adenomas is closely related to adenoma size and the degree of dysplasia [7]. *KRAS* mutations are infrequent in conventional adenomas <10 mm in size but occur in almost half of adenomas >10 mm. They have therefore been associated with an intermediate phase of adenoma progression. They are also associated with increasing villous architecture [361], even in adenomas with small amounts of villosity [362]. *KRAS* mutations are generally thought to occur before the development of chromosomal instability and aneuploidy, providing further evidence of their place as an intermediate step in adenoma progression [363]. They may be found in approximately 40% of colorectal carcinomas and are thought to influence tumour progression and spread [364–366]. The type of *KRAS* mutation from adenoma to carcinoma to metastasis remains remarkably stable, with clear implications for therapy, as discussed below [367,368].

Changes in advanced conventional adenomas

DCC and SMAD family The deleted in colorectal carcinoma (*DCC*) gene is located on chromosome 18q21.1; 60–70% of colonic carcinomas show LOH at this site [7,369], whereas approximately 50% of larger adenomas and less than 10% of smaller adenomas show this change [351]. *DCC* encodes a transmembrane receptor that is important in apoptosis, cell cycle control and cell migration, through interactions with Cdc42 and Rac1 [370,371]. Although originally thought to be very important in the adenoma–carcinoma sequence, later studies have cast doubt on this [372].

More recently, the role of the DCC ligand netrin-1 has come to prominence. Important in central nervous system development, netrin-1 is also a transcriptional target of NF-κB, an important pro-inflammatory signal. Netrin-1 has been detected in IBD-associated carcinomas and it has been suggested that its receptor, DCC, may be a link in the development of inflammation-associated colorectal cancers [373].

Other genes situated at the same locus (18q21.1) and also affected by allelic loss include *SMAD 2* and *SMAD4* [374]. These genes produce components of the transforming growth factor β (TGF-β) pathway that is important in the regulation of apoptosis and cell proliferation, among other functions. *SMAD4* mutations increase in frequency with advancing stages of the adenoma–carcinoma sequence

[375,376]. Inherited mutations in *SMAD4* are thought to be responsible for juvenile polyposis syndrome [377].

TP53 The *TP53* gene, located on 17p13, is a tumour suppressor mutated in many human cancers [378]. Colorectal cancers often show loss of heterozygosity at 17p [7] and the remaining *TP53* allele is commonly mutated, most often a missense mutation. Frameshift, nonsense mutations and deletions also rarely occur [379,380]. Most *TP53* mutations fall within its DNA-binding region [381] and mutant p53 protein can exert a dominant negative effect by binding to wild-type p53 and impeding its interaction with DNA [382–384]. Mutant p53 protein may accumulate in the nucleus and become detectable by immunohistochemistry.

The p53 protein is a key regulator of genes with activity at cell cycle checkpoints. In response to a variety of cellular stresses it can induce cell cycle arrest, allowing time for DNA repair during replication [378]. Alternatively, if the extent of genetic damage is too extreme, it can trigger apoptotic pathways that lead to the destruction of the damaged cell [385–387]. The complex regulation of p53 by proteins such as mouse double minute 2 (*MDM2*) and downstream effector pathways of p53 are fully reviewed elsewhere [388–390]. In addition to key roles in cell cycle control and apoptosis, there is evidence to suggest roles in autophagy and micro-RNA processing [391–393]. Mutation of *TP53* leads to rapidly accumulating genetic damage and uncontrolled cell proliferation [387,394,395].

TP53 inactivation is generally considered to be a late event in the conventional colorectal cancer pathway, with LOH for *TP53* found in about 10% of adenomas [7,379]. In one study *TP53* mutations were found in 4–26% of adenomas, 50% of adenomas with invasive cancer and 50–75% of colorectal carcinomas [396]. In another series, large adenoma size (≥10 mm), high grade dysplasia and villous histology were all independently associated with p53 overexpression [397]. Therefore *TP53* inactivation appears to be an important pathway contributing to neoplastic progression.

CHROMOSOMAL INSTABILITY (CIN) CIN provides a mechanism for ongoing neoplastic progression by generating clonal diversity and contributes through LOH to inactivation of important tumour-suppressor genes, such as *SMAD4* and *TP53*. It is generally considered a late event in the conventional adenoma–carcinoma sequence [351,376]. A more detailed discussion is given above.

Pathogenic events in progression of adenoma to carcinoma The final converting step of adenoma to adenocarcinoma must be a rate-limiting step because adenomas are relatively numerous in comparison to carcinomas. Furthermore, this step is accompanied by a multiplicity of phenotypic changes implicating enzymes in metabolic pathways [398], increased telomerase activity [399], growth factors promoting stromal proliferation and angiogenesis [400–402], proteolytic enzymes facilitating local invasion [403–405], numerous changes to secretory and membrane-associated glycoproteins [406], alterations in cell adhesion molecules [407] and the development of aneuploidy [408]. Finally, although most attention has been correctly directed at epithelial events in the adenoma–carcinoma sequence, the response of the lamina propria may also be important in these events [409].

The serrated adenoma–carcinoma sequence (the mutator pathway, the non-canonical, MSI and CIMP pathways)

The discovery of this pathway of adenoma development and progression extended from the investigation of tumours that did not neatly fit into the conventional pathway, and also from studies of serrated polyposis [334,410–412]. Tumours arising by this pathway are commonly associated with activating mutations in the *BRAF* oncogene. They do not show CIN but instead, similar to Lynch syndrome tumours, show MSI or the mutator phenotype. This is not due to germline mutations in the MMR genes but instead results from widespread DNA methylation at CpG islands. This feature gives rise to the name CIMP. In this pathway the methylation of the *hMLH1* promoter, and consequent epigenetic silencing of the gene, forms the basis for the MSI observed. Thus both epigenetic silencing of key genes and MSI-driven mutations in other genes provide the necessary genetic engine for neoplastic progression. However, many questions remain as yet unanswered, e.g. although *BRAF* mutation is strongly associated with CIMP+ it is unclear whether the mutation is causal for CIMP. In addition not all *BRAF*-mutated, CIMP+ carcinomas show MSI. A second arm of this pathway is characterised by tumours with *KRAS* mutations, MSS, low level CIMP and CIN with LOH for *TP53*. These tumours are thus more similar to those derived from the conventional adenoma–carcinoma sequence.

In addition to these distinct molecular genetic profiles, lesions developing by this route show distinct histopathological features, most notably serration. Such lesions include different types of hyperplastic polyps and serrated adenomas [184,185,413]. It has been proposed, if not universally accepted, that the *BRAF*-associated pathway is morphologically characterised by a stepwise progression from ACFs to microvesicular hyperplastic polyps (MVHPs). Some of these hyperplastic polyps may then progress to sessile serrated adenomas, to sessile serrated adenomas with dysplasia or mixed polyps, to traditional serrated adenomas or direct to serrated carcinomas [184,185,414,415] (Figure 38.7). The origins and key steps of the *KRAS* branch of the serrated pathway are less certain but it has also been

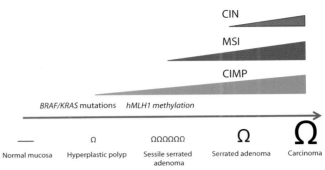

Figure 38.7 The serrated adenoma–carcinoma sequence considered responsible for the development of a subset of colorectal carcinomas. *BRAF* or *KRAS* mutations are likely initiating lesions, followed by CpG island methylation (CIMP) and later by the appearance of microsatellite instability (MSI) and chromosomal instability (CIN).

proposed to follow a stepwise progression from serrated adenoma to serrated adenoma with tubulovillous phenotype (conventional type), and then to carcinoma. The most important genes and molecular processes are discussed in terms of their morphological correlates below. These associations must be tempered by the fact that there is no universal agreement on terminology and different studies have assigned very different names to very similar lesions. A more complete description of the histopathological features is given in Chapter 37. General concepts in MSI and methylation have already been discussed above.

Aberrant crypt foci and microvesicular hyperplastic polyps The *BRAFV600E* mutation has been discovered in ACFs and MVHPs and is thought to be among the earliest changes in this pathway [361,416,417]. In particular, *BRAF* mutations are strongly associated with serrated-type hyperplastic ACFs when compared with non-serrated ACFs [252]. *BRAF* encodes a kinase that is a downstream effector of *RAS* and exerts its effects through MAPK signalling. This pathway is implicated in the control of numerous cellular processes that are relevant to oncogenesis, including cell proliferation and apoptosis. Of particular interest is the association of *BRAF* mutations with cellular senescence [418,419]. A similar effect is seen in dermal naevi, and it is a possible mechanism for the hypermature or senescent features of the upper crypt cells of MVHPs, as seen by electron microscopy [420,421]. Inhibition of apoptosis probably plays a role in the development of serrated epithelial morphology [422]. The process thought most likely to drive progression of MVHPs is CIMP. CIMP, through epigenetic silencing of important growth control genes, leads to a suitably unstable genetic field for further mutations to occur, which could inactivate MVHP senescence. Interestingly CIMP has been demonstrated in MVHPs [423,424] and is more evident in those MVHP derived from the proximal colon. This could explain the predominantly right-sided location of the more advanced sessile serrated adenoma. The specific genetic targets for CIMP are under investigation and differential methylation of important genes such as *CDX2* and *hMLH1* may be important in progression [425].

Goblet cell serrated polyps Goblet cell serrated polyps (GCSPs) are most commonly small hyperplastic polyps typically found in the rectum [413]. They frequently show *KRAS* mutations that might serve as an initiating event. In contrast to MVHPs, they do not show *BRAF* mutations and are much less likely to show evidence of CIMP [416,424]. Whether these GCSP lesions play a role in carcinogenesis is still a matter of debate.

Sessile serrated adenomas Sessile serrated adenomas (SSAs; also termed 'sessile serrated polyps' or 'sessile serrated lesions' because of the frequent absence of overt classic changes of dysplasia) are most commonly, but not exclusively, located on the right side of the colon and may account for almost 10% of adenomas detected at colonoscopy [426]. Their histopathological features are reviewed in Chapter 37. They are typically sessile lesions that are characterised by serration that extends deep into the crypts, irregularly shaped crypts (notably inverted T or L shapes) and usually without conventional dysplasia, although variable features of dysmaturation are seen. On a molecular genetic level, they appear closely related to MVHPs with many studies finding *BRAFV600E* mutations in a high percentage of cases, but rarely *KRAS* mutations [416,417, 424,426]. They show higher levels of CIMP than MVHPs [416,425] and may show loss of MMR proteins MLH1 and MSH2 on immunohistochemistry [413,427,428]. The location, morphology and genetic data all suggest that MVHPs are the precursors of SSAs. Recent follow-up studies have shown that patients with SSAs are predisposed to synchronous serrated polyps and are at increased risk for right-sided colorectal carcinoma of the MSI-H phenotype [429,430].

Sessile serrated adenoma with dysplasia (mixed polyps) These rare lesions show features of SSAs but have areas of frank dysplasia resembling conventional adenomas. They may represent a transient lesion in the process of acquiring further genetic damage and dysplastic features, because the morphological features are intermediate between SSAs and conventional adenomas. Proximal lesions tend to harbour *BRAF* mutations and distal lesions have *KRAS* mutations, suggesting that there could be two different origins for these lesions. *BRAF* mutations have been found in all histological components of mixed polyps, implying that this is an early event. Further immunohistochemical studies have revealed nuclear expression of β-catenin in all components, loss of MLH1, loss of MGMT and aberrant expression of p53 in the dysplastic components, which

suggest that these proteins are involved in progression [417,431,432]. Overall, the molecular evidence also supports the theory that mixed polyps might exhibit fusion characteristics between serrated and conventional pathways [361,433,434].

Traditional serrated adenomas (dysplastic serrated adenomas) Traditional serrated adenomas (TSAs) combine the serrated features of a hyperplastic polyp but also show dysplasia in the upper third of crypts [413,435]. As with SSAs and mixed polyps, difficulties with diagnostic inclusion criteria, nomenclature and classification make the underlying pathogenesis of these lesions difficult to dissect out. Approximately two-thirds are located in the rectosigmoid region and two-thirds are polypoid in shape [436,437]. TSAs may, in addition to areas of serrated dysplasia, show areas of SSA, conventional adenoma, high grade dysplasia and rarely carcinoma. These findings underline the probable relationship of TSAs to precursors described above and their ability to progress. This is supported by immunohistochemical evidence of increased Ki67 labelling in admixed tubular adenoma-like areas and in so-called ectopic crypts (see Chapter 37) [438]. TSAs may exhibit *BRAF* or *KRAS* mutations or neither [361,416,423,426,439, 440]. *BRAF*-mutated TSAs are more commonly right sided and are likely to show CIMP [423,441,442]. CIMP-high serrated adenomas have been associated with the development of high grade dysplasia [443]. The development of MSI is also thought to occur later in the development in these lesions and to be associated with high grade dysplasia and carcinoma [416,443].

KRAS-mutated TSAs are more frequently left sided and not associated with a known precursor lesion. Whether they are histologically distinguishable from *BRAF*-driven lesions is debatable [185]. As these lesions progress they are more likely to show histological features seen in conventional adenomas, including the development of villous architecture. They are mostly CIMP low and MSI-L or MSS but, in tandem with the development of conventional morphology and high grade dysplasia, they exhibit CIN and LOH. A possible mechanism for the genetic instability required to drive these changes in *KRAS*-mutated TSAs is the loss of the *MGMT* gene and consequent defective DNA repair [361]. The overlap with the conventional *APC* pathway again suggests a possible fusion of pathways.

It is now accepted that serrated adenomas are premalignant lesions but the exact level of cancer risk for patients with serrated polyps is unclear [414]. The balance of the early evidence suggested that serrated adenomas had an increased risk of malignant progression compared with conventional adenomas [444,445] and subsequent studies appear to confirm this [446].

Serrated carcinomas It has been estimated that 7.5% of all colorectal carcinomas may be derived from the serrated pathway with the majority arising proximally [414]. Their histopathological features are discussed in detail later but cardinally include epithelial serration, clear or eosinophilic cytoplasm, vesicular nuclei, mucin production and absence of necrosis [447]. The molecular genetic evidence from these serrated carcinomas reflects that found in putative precursor serrated lesions. The rate at which these progress to carcinoma is unknown but some have speculated that the rate of such transformation may be faster than for the conventional pathway. Lastly, proximal MSI-H serrated carcinomas appear to have a better prognosis than distal MSS/MSI-L serrated carcinomas [448].

The molecular classification of colorectal carcinoma

Many lines of evidence from histopathological and genetic research suggest that colorectal carcinoma is most probably a group of related carcinomas that differ in their pathogenesis but share many common features. Based on the growing understanding of the different pathogenic subtypes of colorectal carcinoma, attempts have been made to classify colorectal carcinoma on a molecular genetic basis. These efforts have in part been driven by the clinical need to separate out patients with particular types of colorectal carcinoma in order to deliver the most appropriate therapy [368]. Currently, two or three molecular genetic tests that can personalise therapy have entered routine practice. These are *RAS/RAF* testing and MSI status. It is likely that there will be many more.

Identifying this clinical need for stratification, a molecular genetic classification system for colorectal carcinoma has been proposed by Jass and has received much attention [183]. It divides colorectal carcinoma into five groups (Figure 38.8 and Table 38.3). It is envisioned that groups 1 and 2 arise from serrated adenomas, whereas groups 4 and 5 arise from conventional adenomas. Group 3 colorectal cancers with *KRAS* mutations could theoretically arise from either serrated or conventional adenomas. Although this separation fits well with the evidence, it does not exclude overlaps and these have recently been emphasised by others [184]. There are tumours with mixed morphological features and several genes such as *TGFβ* and *KRAS* are components of conventional and serrated pathways. It is therefore likely that the Jass groups are representative of the main avenues to colorectal carcinoma, but that less common and possibly mixed routes must also exist. Indeed wider mutational analysis of large numbers of oncogenes and tumour-suppressor genes has revealed that every colorectal carcinoma is, to a large degree, genetically unique. Finally, while attempts at molecular genetic classification are ongoing, it should not be forgotten that the development of every colorectal carcinoma will also depend on the interaction between molecular lesions and the individual patient's unique environment.

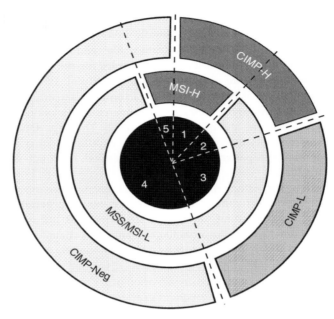

Figure 38.8 Molecular pathogenic classification of colorectal carcinoma, according to Jass [183]. The characteristics of the five groups are given in Table 38.3 below. (Reproduced from Jass JR. Classification of colorectal cancer based on correlation of clinical, morphological and molecular features. Histopathology 2007; 50:113–30.)

Table 38.3 Molecular genetic classification of colorectal carcinoma

Group 1	*BRAF* mutation, CIMP-high, MSI-H, CIN– (serrated)
Group 2	*BRAF* mutation, CIMP-high, MSI-L/MSS, CIN– (serrated)
Group 3	*KRAS* mutation, CIMP-low, MSI-L/MSS, CIN+ (serrated/conventional)
Group 4	*APC* mutation, CIMP negative, MSS, CIN+ (conventional, FAP)
Group 5	MMR gene mutation, CIMP negative, MSI-H, CIN– (conventional, Lynch syndrome/HNPCC)

CIMP, CpG island methylation; CIN, chromosomal instability; H, high; HNPCC, hereditary non-polyposis colorectal carcinoma; L, low; MMR, mismatch repair; MSI, micro-satellite instability; MSS, macro-satellite stability.

The clinical pathology of colorectal adenocarcinoma

Macroscopic pathology

Carcinomas of the large bowel present in a range of macroscopic appearances. These vary somewhat with the anatomical site of origin within the colorectum. The varying features are described in this section.

In clinical pathology practice gross pathology is concerned with the visual identification/confirmation of disease-related abnormality (rather like endoscopy and radiology) and with selection of samples for microscopic examination. More recently, and particularly in colorectal cancer, there has been a subtle shift in emphasis to evaluating the entire surgical resection specimen in terms of oncological outcome and quality standards [2]. The importance of high-quality macroscopic pathology handling in obtaining the best patient outcome is described in detail in Chapter 32.

Conventionally a number of distinct macroscopic forms of large bowel cancer have been recognised: polypoid, exophytic/fungating, ulcerating, stenosing and diffusely infiltrating. These morphological subtypes have been defined largely by pathologists who were looking at fully opened specimens. As current gross dissection protocols more commonly call for preservation of the intact tumour during fixation and subsequent examination in transverse sections, the macroscopic features seen by the pathologist are modified from the 'classic' features.

Most colorectal cancers start as polyps and early carcinomas can be macroscopically indistinguishable from adenomas. These specimens are usually removed at endoscopy. The important features and distinction of early cancer from epithelial misplacement are described in Chapter 37. The earliest grossly visible changes include formation of depressed areas on the polyp surface. Eventually the carcinoma overwhelms the adenoma, leaving an ulcer with raised rolled edges. Sometimes the polypoid nature of the tumour is evident even in quite large lesions (Figure 38.9). Superficial ulceration and excavation in larger polyps will lead to an exophytic or fungating appearance. All of these bulkier macroscopic types are more frequently seen in the caecum and ascending colon, perhaps reflecting the fact that there is relatively more luminal space for growth in these parts of the large bowel.

As a tumour enlarges there is a tendency towards circumferential involvement of the bowel. Cancers arising in sessile or flat adenomas progress more rapidly to ulcerative, deeply invasive lesions. The classic ulcerated tumour plaque with raised rolled edges is most commonly seen in the rectum (Figure 38.10). In the transverse colon, descending colon and sigmoid cancers often present as tightly stenosing lesions. On cross-section the normal bowel wall has 'disappeared' and been replaced by an infiltrative, scarred, tumour that can be surprisingly lacking in bulk (Figure 38.11). A few cancers (normally of signet-ring microscopic type) present as a diffuse thickening of the bowel wall, in a manner reminiscent of the 'linitis plastica' variant seen in gastric carcinoma [449].

Gross identification of mucinous areas in a colorectal cancer is common, reflecting the origin from a mucin-producing glandular epithelium. In some instances, par-

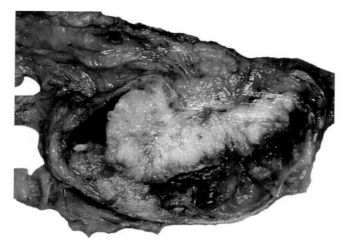

Figure 38.9 Caecal carcinoma seen in transverse section as a macroscopically polypoid mass lesion filling much of the lumen. The tumour was invasive into the stalk but not beyond the submucosa.

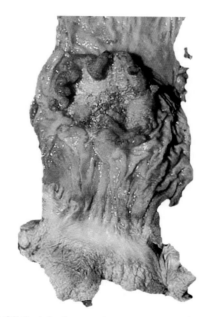

Figure 38.10 Rectal adenocarcinoma seen as a classic centrally ulcerated lesion with raised rolled edges.

ticularly in the right colon, the cancer may have a striking shiny cut surface with obvious accumulation of large pools of mucin throughout the tumour (Figure 38.12). Similar changes may be seen in lymph nodes reflecting the presence of metastatic deposits.

The extent of invasion of a cancer can often be relatively easily defined grossly both within the bowel wall (Figure 38.13) and in terms of invading peritoneum and/or adjacent organs (see Chapter 32).

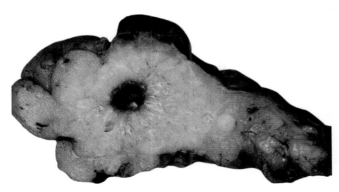

Figure 38.11 Stenosing cancer of the sigmoid colon with marked circumferential encroachment on the lumen. The wall of the bowel has been completely obliterated. The tumour has an irregular stellate cross-section. It infiltrates widely into pericolic fat and encroaches close to the peritoneal surface (arrow) and a mesenteric lymph node.

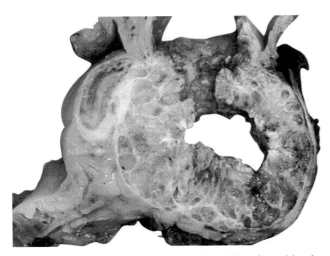

Figure 38.12 Mucinous carcinoma of the right colon arising in the vicinity of the ileo-caecal valve. The cut surface of the gross specimen shows abundant glistening mucus.

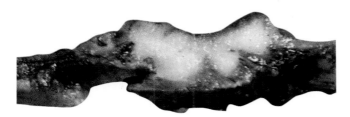

Figure 38.13 Transanal endoscopic microsurgical (TEMS) excision of rectal tumour. Section through the lesion shows obvious tumour invasion into the wall of rectum. Note the proximity to the inked deep margin.

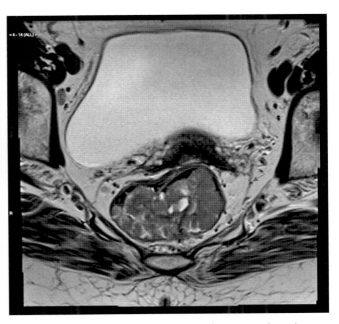

Figure 38.14 MRI of the pelvis in a rectal cancer patient. A polypoid tumour is clearly seen in the lumen of the bowel. The mesorectal fascia is also clearly visible (red arrow).

In practice, interpretation of gross pathological findings may usefully be compared with preoperative clinical imaging by computed tomography and, particularly for rectal cancers, magnetic resonance imaging (Figure 38.14).

Microscopic pathology

When compared with many other visceral carcinomas, colorectal cancers are remarkably homogeneous on microscopic examination with the great majority being moderately differentiated adenocarcinomas. As with other epithelial cancers differentiation is used as a pathological descriptor of variation from the norm in terms of glandular morphology (Figure 38.15).

Well differentiated cancers tend to show an 'adenoma-like' morphology with recognisable tubular structures lined by columnar cells. Moderately differentiated cancers show a lesser resemblance to adenomatous epithelium and often show accumulation of necrotic debris and acute inflammatory cells within the neoplastic glandular lumina. Poorly differentiated cancers are perhaps best defined by a tendency to lose glandular architecture, with the tumour being made up of sheets or discohesive clumps of neoplastic cells, often showing higher grade cytological atypia.

There are some morphological differences between right- and left-sided cancers, mainly reflecting the higher proportion of right-sided tumours arising via the serrated and/or MMR pathway. Carcinomas arising via this route are more often poorly differentiated, more likely to have a Crohn's

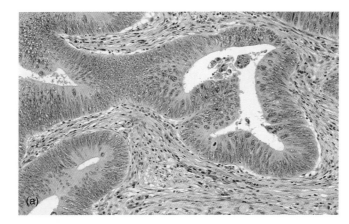

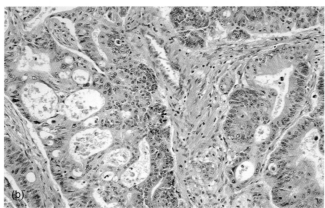

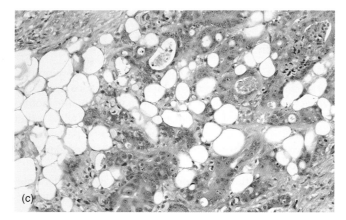

Figure 38.15 Well differentiated (a), moderately differentiated (b) and poorly differentiated (c) adenocarcinoma of large bowel showing a progressive variance from normal epithelial morphology.

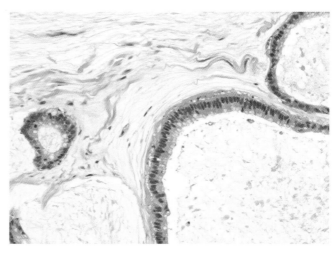

Figure 38.16 Microscopic section of a grossly obvious mucinous carcinoma (Figure 38.12) showing that the mucin is produced by a well differentiated carcinoma with an obviously mucinous epithelium.

cinoma' is reserved for cases where substantial extracellular deposits of mucus are seen in over 50% of the cut surface of the tumour. This can often be appreciated on gross inspection of the tumour cut surface (Figure 38.16 and see Figure 38.12). These cancers show a range of differentiation. The most poorly differentiated examples are often of the signet ring type. It has been considered in the past that mucinous cancer has a worse prognosis. This may be true for mucinous cancers of the sigmoid colon and rectum [450] but does not hold for right-sided mucinous cancers that are often associated with serrated histology, MSI and a relatively better prognosis. Mucinous histology is not therefore considered to be a clinically important independent prognostic indicator.

Inflammatory and lymphoid cell infiltration of the tumour is another prominent feature of many colorectal cancers and one that is again associated with MSI and the mutator phenotype. The inflammatory reaction can be very striking. In some cases lymphoid aggregates are seen at the advancing edge of the tumour and in the pericolic fat, a pattern often referred to as a Crohn's disease-like lymphoid reaction (Figure 38.17). Although not all studies confirm the effect, there appears to be a positive prognostic benefit in patients whose tumours have a high number of intra-epithelial lymphocytes (i.e. within the sheets of malignant cells) [451]. Prominent macrophages and eosinophils are also seen at the advancing front of some neoplasms, again with some positive prognostic association [452,453] (Figure 38.18).

Invasion in a colorectal carcinoma is usually associated with development of a desmoplastic stromal fibrous response. Although an important feature in diagnosing cancer in biopsies and in lesions excised as adenomas,

disease-like inflammatory reaction and increased numbers of intra-epithelial lymphocytes, and to show mucinous differentiation.

Mucinous tumours account for approximately 10% of colorectal cancers. Focal mucin production is a very common feature in carcinoma and the term 'mucinous car-

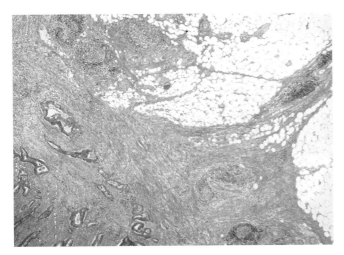

Figure 38.17 Crohn's disease-like inflammatory response manifest as lymphoid aggregates at the advancing tumour edge seen within the bowel wall and in the immediately adjacent pericolic fat.

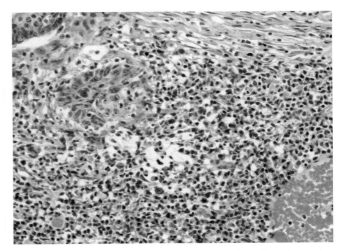

Figure 38.18 Inflammatory infiltrate at the edge of a colorectal cancer. Numerous eosinophil polymorphs are identified.

desmoplasia is not a universal feature of carcinoma and is sometimes absent, particularly in well differentiated carcinomas with a papillary architecture. The definition of invasion in colorectal cancer is tumour penetration through the muscularis mucosae into the submucosa. This feature may not always be clear in small endoscopic biopsies, and definitive diagnosis of cancer should be made in conjunction with endoscopic and radiological features. In many instances the decision is somewhat academic once neoplasia is confirmed because therapy will be surgical in any event. In the rectum a definitive diagnosis of malignancy is more important because patients will often be treated by chemotherapy and/or radiotherapy before surgical excision. It is always important to confirm at the very least that

a suspicious lesion is an epithelial neoplasm. Benign conditions such as mucosal prolapse can look remarkably like cancers (see Chapter 34). Similarly, other rarer forms of malignancy such as lymphoma (which may be best treated by chemotherapy) need to be ruled out.

Carcinomas invading the bowel wall may be said to have either an expanding or an infiltrative pattern at the advancing margin on low power examination (Figure 38.19), and the former tend to be less aggressive. Closer inspection of the invasive front of many colorectal cancers will reveal isolated clusters of tumour cells (no more than four or five in any one group) within the stroma. This phenomenon has been termed 'tumour budding' (Figure 38.20). It is more often seen in flatter non-polypoid tumours and in those with an infiltrative margin and may also correlate with the presence of venous invasion [454].

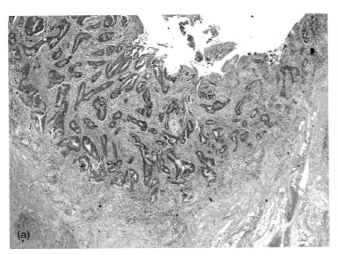

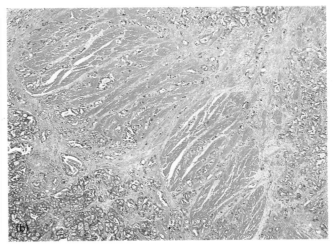

Figure 38.19 Classification of tumour margin: tumour (a) shows a well-defined 'pushing' or 'expanding' margin. In (b) the malignant epithelium shows a ragged 'infiltrative' margin as it dissects through the muscle of the bowel wall.

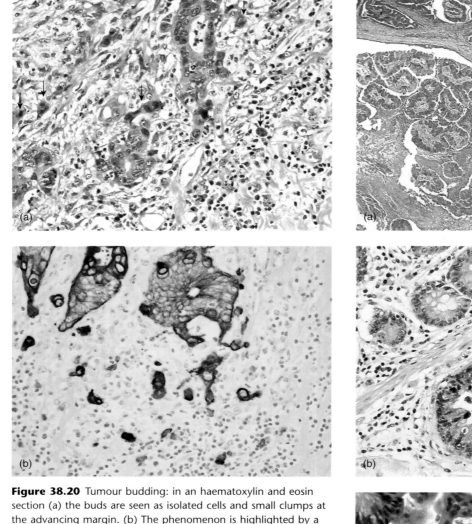

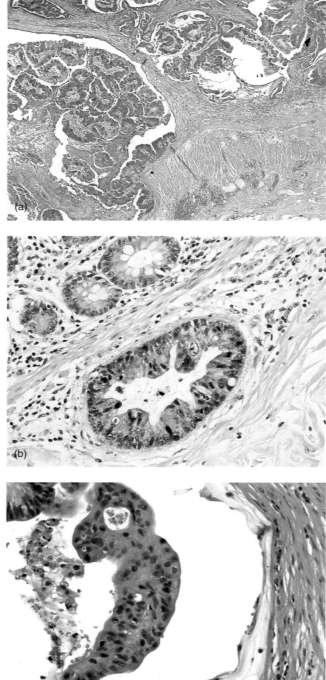

Figure 38.20 Tumour budding: in an haematoxylin and eosin section (a) the buds are seen as isolated cells and small clumps at the advancing margin. (b) The phenomenon is highlighted by a cytokeratin immunostain.

Serrated carcinoma

The concept of the serrated polyp (hyperplastic polyp, serrated adenoma and sessile serrated lesion/adenoma) is discussed in Chapter 37, and the biology put in context earlier in this chapter. It is now clear that these are truly neoplastic lesions that may lead to carcinoma, particularly in the right colon. Carcinomas arising in this way tend to be rather flat grossly and often have a mucoid cut surface. Biologically the cancers arising through this pathway are characterised by *BRAF* mutation. There is gene-promoter hypermethylation with the pattern of methylation varying. Thus the cancers may be MSI-H (in association with *MLH1* methylation) or MSI-L and characterised by MGMT methylation [414]. There is an associated morphological phenotype that maintains epithelial serration, often with eosinophilic cytoplasm (Figure 38.21). However, the clinical robustness of

Figure 38.21 Serrated adenocarcinoma of the colon. (a) The serrated nature of the epithelium is just visible at low power. The tumour does not show obvious necrosis and there is a Crohn's-like lymphoid response. (b) A malignant serrated gland in the submucosa showing a characteristic 'saw-tooth' epithelial architecture. (c) There is striking epithelial eosinophilia and formation of papillary projections into mucinous lakes.

this classification is yet to be established, with one study showing no more than reasonable inter-observer reproducibility in making the diagnosis [455]. In most published series serrated adenocarcinoma makes up no more than 10% of all large bowel cancers [455].

Flat colorectal cancer

We have already seen that flat adenomas are well-described precursor lesions of cancer, recognised particularly in Japan (see Chapter 37). These lesions have some distinct biological features and may have a worse prognosis [456]. Although *TP53* mutation is common, *KRAS* mutation is relatively rarer than in polypoid neoplasms [457]. Flat adenomas tend to give rise to depressed cancers that readily infiltrate the deep submucosa (Figure 38.22). There is some evidence that the cancers arising in this way may show increased expression of CD10 by immunohistochemistry and have an increased tendency to early haematogenous spread to the liver [458]. Recognition of early flat neoplasms, including cancers, may be problematic on routine colonoscopy. They may therefore be missed in population screening programmes.

Grading and cellular heterogeneity

Microscopic grading of colorectal cancer has long been part of routine pathology practice. Grading is based on assessing the degree of deviation from normal, mainly in architecture but also in cytology. By convention grading is done on the predominant pattern of the tumour. Glandular architecture is obvious in most colorectal cancers and is characteristic of well differentiated and moderately differentiated neoplasms. Poorly differentiated tumours, on the other hand, do not show acinar differentiation as a predominant pattern and tend to grow as sheets of solid undifferentiated cells. Poorly differentiated mucinous carcinomas often have a signet-ring cell morphology (Figure 38.23). Despite the foregoing there are no agreed standardised criteria for tumour grading and there is marked inter-observer variation when this is studied systematically [459].

Any of the cell types of the normal intestinal crypt may be seen in colorectal adenomas and carcinomas (colonocyte, goblet cell, endocrine cell, Paneth cell). This is not surprising because the stem cell that gives rise to the cancer has the potential to differentiate along any of these lines. Endocrine cells are particularly common, being seen in up to 50% of cancers, particularly if immunohistochemistry is used to aid in their identification.

Assessment of response to therapy

Preoperative (neoadjuvant) chemotherapy and radiotherapy are increasingly used in downstaging rectal cancer. The

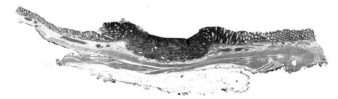

Figure 38.22 Flat carcinoma of the rectum: the tumour is is not raised significantly above the contour of the normal background mucosa. Residual precursor adenomatous epithelium remains at the edges of the central invasive element. The carcinoma infiltrates into the deepest third of the submucosa (sm3 in the Kikuchi classification). The specimen was excised by transanal endoscopic microsurgery (TEMS). Note that both muscle coats of the rectum are present. The deep margin has been inked to aid assessment of completeness of excision.

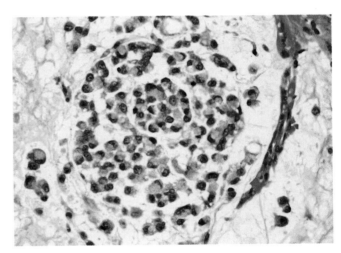

Figure 38.23 Biopsy specimen showing poorly differentiated adenocarcinoma with clumps of malignant epithelial cells, including signet-ring types, floating in mucin lakes.

aim is to decrease the incidence of local recurrence after surgery and ultimately to improve patient prognosis. When the patient does come to surgery the pathologist should be made aware that such therapy has been given. Macroscopically there may be no evident therapy-associated change. In other instances the primary lesion may not be identifiable even after careful examination and selection of many blocks (designated as ypT0 in the TNM staging). More often there are intermediate features with evidence of mucosal healing and necrosis of tumour in the wall (Figure 38.24). Microscopically the pathologist will be expected to comment on regression. Specific grading systems have been used in this context. The Mandard system has five regression grades ranging from 1 (complete response) to 5 (no identifiable response) [460]. Although this system was originally described in oesophageal carcinoma it has been

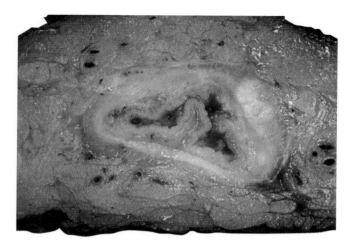

Figure 38.24 Effect of neoadjuvant chemotherapy plus radiotherapy on a rectal cancer. The mucosal surface has regenerated and appears grossly intact. The only visible abnormality is a yellowish necrotic focus in the muscle. This contained occasional foci of viable tumour.

applied to rectal cancer and shown to be of benefit [461]. Other similar classifications have been derived specifically for rectal carcinomas [462]. Some guidelines, recognising that the evidence for any one regression grading system is not yet established, recommend that a simpler three-tier approach be taken (no response, partial response, complete response) [3].

Sometimes mucin lakes devoid of neoplastic cells are seen, either in the wall of the rectum or in lymph nodes, after oncological treatment. It is prudent to carefully sample these and to examine several levels microscopically. If no neoplastic cells are found these areas are not classed as tumorous [462].

Synchronous colorectal cancers

In patients presenting with colorectal carcinoma a second (synchronous) carcinoma is identified in 1–5% of cases [463]. This is more commonly seen in those with predisposing conditions such as familial cancer syndromes and IBD. In many individuals the presence of synchronous malignancy reflects a tendency to adenoma formation. A different phenomenon is evident in IBD where the presence of multiple neoplasms may be a reflection of 'field cancerisation', a carcinogenic pathway more often seen in squamous epithelia of the head and neck and in Barrett's oesophagus. In this instance mutational and ploidy changes can be demonstrated in flat epithelium extending over wide areas of mucosa around and between cancers [464].

Individuals presenting with synchronous large bowel neoplasms have a worse clinical prognosis. In terms of

tumour biology *BRAF* mutations are more frequent and the cancers tend to be both CIMP high and MSI-H [465].

Colorectal carcinoma in patients with IBD

We have already seen (in Chapter 35) that large bowel carcinoma is increased in incidence in patients with long-standing IBD. The risk applies to both ulcerative colitis and Crohn's disease. The cancers are often of a mucinous phenotype, *TP53* mutation is common and they have a high prevalence of DNA aneuploidy [466].

Spread of colorectal cancer

As with any carcinoma colorectal cancer can spread by direct local invasion, through lymphatics and blood vessels, and along nerve trunks.

Local invasion may involve adjacent viscera (other parts of intestine, urogenital tract), the anterior abdominal wall or the retroperitoneum. Direct involvement of the peritoneal (serosal) covering of the bowel is an important route of tumour spread. Once the serosa is penetrated malignant cells can readily cross the peritoneal cavity. Spread in this way quite commonly causes presentation as a large ovarian tumour mass and distinction from primary ovarian mucinous adenocarcinoma may prove difficult. The clinical relevance of identifying peritoneal breach has been demonstrated in well-characterised series of both colonic and rectal cancers [467,468]. It is important that the serosal surface of a cancer be carefully examined macroscopically and that this surface is well sampled for microscopic examination. It has been shown that peritoneal penetration is most often seen in the areas where the serosa reflects off the bowel at an acute angle. It has recently been pointed out that these areas are relatively deficient in elastic tissue, and there may well be value in performing elastic stains to better define and classify this phenomenon [469]. This approach has already been adopted in the staging of lung cancer [470]. Several grades of tumour involvement of peritoneum have been described. At present (and for staging purposes) this parameter is defined by complete ulceration of the peritoneal surface (i.e. an irregular surface with no mesothelial cells lying between the neoplastic cells and the serosal cavity) (Figure 38.25). Quality standards such as those published by the Royal College of Pathologists specify that serosal involvement should be reported in at least 20% of colonic cancers and 10% of rectal cancer resections [3]. Systematic sampling would push these figures up to approximately 55% (colon) and 25% (rectum) [468].

Lymphatic spread has long been recognised as a major prognostic parameter. It is very common to see clumps of tumour cells in thin-walled vessels in the wall of the colon (a feature that is, of itself, of clinical relevance only in localised resections for cancer). Detection of metastases in

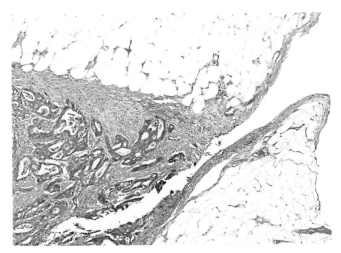

Figure 38.25 Microscopic evidence of peritoneal ulceration by tumour.

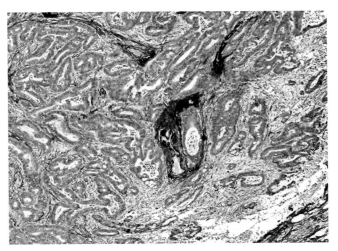

Figure 38.26 Elastic–van Gieson's stain showing carcinoma lying within a muscular vein. This focus was not readily visible on routine haematoxylin and eosin staining.

lymph nodes forms a major component of all prognostic systems. By the TNM/UICC convention this is defined as a nodal deposit seen on routine haematoxylin and eosin examination and measuring ≥0.2 mm in diameter [471]. Smaller deposits are classified as either micro-metastases or isolated tumour cells, depending on whether or not they are aggregated into tumour cell clumps [472]. Current UK practice is for any deposit seen without the use of immunohistochemistry to be counted for staging purposes. By using immunohistochemistry (usually for cytokeratins but sometimes for other epithelial antigens) at least 25% of otherwise node-negative cancers harbour some evidence of possible tumour spread to lymph nodes. This proportion is doubled if molecular techniques are used [473]. Use of these adjuvant techniques is not currently advocated because it is not clear that there is added value over high-quality routine histopathology. It is also well noted that the variety of techniques used makes comparison and standardisation of results difficult [474]. The concept of detecting 'early' node metastasis is also highlighted in studies in which the 'sentinel' node for a tumour is identified at the time of first treatment and therapy planned on whether or not this node is involved. This concept is well established in melanoma and breast cancer but its role in the colorectum has yet to be established [475].

Spread of tumour through veins draining ultimately to the portal vein and liver is the primary route through which metastases in liver, lungs and ultimately other distant body sites may develop. Detection of venous invasion in the primary tumour is a marker of propensity to spread in this fashion. Systematic studies have looked at the clinical implication of both intramural (within the wall of the bowel) and extramural venous invasion [476]. In the past terms such as 'lymphovascular invasion' were used in

describing spread of colorectal cancer. In surgical resection specimens this term should not be used (it is entirely appropriate in describing tumour invasion of thin-walled vascular structures in the submucosa of localised resections). Prognostic studies have clearly shown that it is the presence of malignant cells in *muscular veins* that is of major clinical significance. This can be seen on routine haematoxylin and eosin preparations (and can be suspected macroscopically – Figure 38.26), but detection is markedly improved by using high-quality elastic staining [477]. It has also been suggested that taking at least one block tangential to the cut surface of the tumour can increase the yield of venous invasion [3]. As a quality measure in the reporting of colorectal cancer specimens the Royal College of Pathologists recommends that extramural venous invasion should be detectable in at least 25% of cases [3].

Perineural invasion by tumour is not uncommon, particularly in rectal cancers. There is evidence that this feature is an indicator of high risk of local recurrence and poor outcome (Figure 38.27) [478].

Measurement of the maximum distance of spread of tumour beyond the outer limit of the muscularis propria is useful for correlating with preoperative imaging, and has also been shown to be of prognostic use [479].

Immunohistochemical markers of colorectal carcinoma

Colorectal carcinoma cells generally show strong staining with broad-spectrum cytokeratins, but this has little diagnostic utility apart from distinguishing an anaplastic carcinoma from, for example, lymphoma or melanoma. Cytokeratin (CK) 20 is an acidic cytokeratin that is generally expressed in the colorectal mucosa and its epithelial

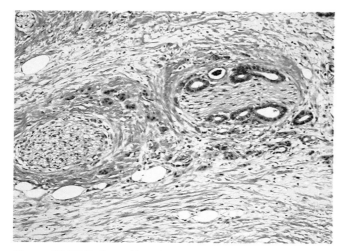

Figure 38.27 Perineural invasion by carcinoma in a surgically resected rectal cancer.

neoplasms (the exception being some tumours of endocrine type). Testing of an adenocarcinoma of unknown primary site with both CK20 and CK7 (a basic cytokeratin) is a common strategy. Colorectal cancers show CK20 expression in the great majority of cases. CK7 is usually negative apart from some cancers from the anorectal region that express both cytokeratins. CK7 expression in the absence of CK20 is unusual in a large bowel primary and should raise the possibility of a tumour originating elsewhere such as the lung, breast, pancreato-biliary tree or ovary (serous or endometrioid carcinomas; CK profiling is of less use in differentiating colorectal cancer from primary ovarian mucinous carcinoma).

Carcinoembryonic antigen (CEA) is frequently used as a clinical serum marker for follow-up of patients with bowel cancer. Immunohistochemically, CEA is expressed in the great majority of colorectal adenocarcinomas but it is also seen in high proportions of pulmonary adenocarcinomas and cancers arising elsewhere in the gastrointestinal tract and pancreas.

The homeobox protein CDX2 is a nuclear transcription factor that is part of a family of genes that is essential for gut organogenesis. It is widely expressed in fetal tissues but shows a much more restricted expression in adults, being largely confined to the pancreas and intestines (it is expressed in the stomach only as part of the phenotype of intestinal metaplasia). As would be expected for a transcription factor, CDX2 is expressed as a positive nuclear signal in the normal gut and in almost all colorectal adenocarcinomas. It is almost always absent from adenocarcinomas of the lung, breast and prostate and is increasingly used together with CK20 as a positive marker of a large bowel primary origin. Unfortunately, from a diagnostic point of view, CDX2 is relatively frequently seen in carci-

nomas of stomach, oesophagus (adenocarcinoma) and biliary tree (perhaps reflecting the high proportion of these cancers that have developed an intestinal differentiation) [480]. There is some evidence that CDX2 may act as a tumour suppressor in a small number of cancers where loss of expression is associated with MSI and a poorly differentiated morphology [481].

Villin is a brush border-associated marker of intestinal differentiation. Although commonly expressed in colorectal cancer it is a less sensitive marker than CDX2. The two antigens show a similar spread of expression across a range of neoplasms [482].

Mucin immunohistochemistry

At least 19 distinct epithelial mucins are recognised. Mucin overproduction and change in mucin phenotype is common in adenocarcinomas arising at a number of sites. Mucin and lectin histochemistry of classical type are not routinely used in the diagnosis and prognostic evaluation of colorectal cancers. Instead, most relevant mucin gene products can now be identified by standard immunohistochemical procedures. MUC1 is not usually expressed in large intestinal epithelium but its acquired expression has been associated with an adverse prognosis in colorectal adenocarcinoma [483]. MUC2 is the most characteristic intestinal epithelial mucin. Its expression has been suggested as an intestinal cancer marker though it appears to offer no advantage over CDX2. Gastric type mucins such as MUC5AC and MUC6 are aberrantly expressed in some colorectal hyperplastic polyps, adenomas and cancers [484]. This phenomenon is of interest in studying tumour histogenesis but currently has no clinical application.

Pathological staging of colorectal cancer

As with most visceral malignancies, the prognosis for a patient with colorectal carcinoma is heavily dependent on tumour stage. Dukes' staging (originally described in rectal cancer in 1932) was the first attempt to combine some measure of local tumour invasion with spread to lymph nodes [485]. Dukes' C tumours, defined by the presence of nodal metastasis, have a worse prognosis than Dukes' A tumours that are confined to the bowel wall or Dukes' B tumours that have penetrated the muscle coat of the colorectum (Table 38.4). The main problem with this classification is that most resected cancers are Dukes' B and better selection is needed to identify those in this group that are at most risk of progressive disease.

Modifications and developments of Dukes' approach, including those of Astler and Coller, have addressed some of the issues in the older classification [486]. The Astler–Coller system (Table 38.4) has advantages in that it defines a larger number of prognostically distinct groups but, as with many cancers, international opinion has now largely

Table 38.4 Staging of colorectal cancer

	TNM	Dukes	Astler–Coller
Direct spread			
Mucosa	Tis (TIE and TIM)[a]	–	A
Submucosa	T1	A	B1
Muscle coat	T2	A	B1
Beyond muscle	T3	B	B2
Transperitoneal (free surface)	T4A	B	B2
Involving adjacent organs	T4B	B	B2
Lymph node spread			
None	N0	(A/B)	(A/B1/B2)
1–3	N1	C1	C1/C2[b]
>3	N2	C1	C1/C2[b]
Apical node	N1/N2	C2	C1/C2[b]
Residual local tumour (transection of tumour)	R1[c]	[d]	[d]
Distant spread	M1[e]	[d]	[d]

[a]TIE, intra-epithelial; TIM, intramucosal.
[b]C1, direct spread confined to wall; C2, spread beyond muscle coat.
[c]R0, no residual tumour; R1, microscopic residual disease; R2, macroscopic residual disease.
[d]Absent, curative; present, palliative.
[e]M0, no distant spread; M1, distant spread.

come to accept the TNM (tumour, node, metastasis) approach, which has the same advantages but avoids the confusing overlap in the 'ABC' nomenclature. The TNM classification (Table 38.4) is now in its seventh edition [471]. Its main benefits in terms of prognosis are in separating T3 from T4 tumours and in separating N0 from N1. Patients with metastatic (M1) disease have the worst outcomes. There has been notable international disagreement concerning changes to the definition of node-positive disease between the fifth (TNM5) and the sixth and seventh editions of the TNM system. The main issue arises in the interpretation of tumour deposits identified in mesorectal or mesocolic fat (Figure 38.28). When these are distinct from the primary tumour mass they may, on the one hand, reflect growth from malignant cells that have spread along vessels or nerves. On the other hand, they may represent lymph node metastases that have overrun and replaced the original nodal structure. Different interpretation could mean that a tumour is staged as pN0 or pN1. Until TNM5, an arbitrary definition was used whereby a deposit of ≥3 mm was defined as an involved lymph node [487]. Recognising that this is almost certainly not always the case, the more recent TNM publications have attempted to differentiate vascular-based 'discontinuous' local spread from nodal deposits on morphological criteria. The main objection to this approach is that it is not evidence based and has not been shown to be reproducible. The issue is further complicated in TNM7 by placing all such mesorectal/

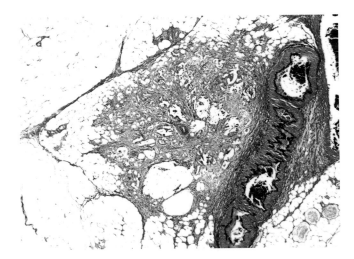

Figure 38.28 A 'tumour deposit' in pericolic fat. This elastic–van Gieson-stained section shows an irregular carcinomatous deposit measuring 3.5 mm lying close to a vessel. Several sections were cut, all showing no evidence of tumour in the wall of the vessel. There is no residual node tissue. In TNM5 this would be classed as a nodal deposit. Classification in subsequent TNM editions would depend on the pathologist's subjective judgement as to whether or not the deposit had the contour of a node.

mesocolic tumour deposits in a new category, N1c, imply-ing that they are nodal deposits; this inevitably shifts more tumours into a 'node positive' stage, with potential thera-peutic implications. For these reasons some clinical com-munities, particularly in the UK and the Netherlands, have elected to retain the TNM5 classification in their national reporting guidelines [488]. Clearly, it is important for pathologists to indicate which version of the TNM staging classification they have used in their reports.

The concept of intramucosal carcinoma in the colorectum

In some parts of the gastrointestinal tract lymphatics are readily identified in the mucosal lamina propria and inva-sive neoplasms confined to the mucosa have a small but definite probability of developing metastases. This is the case in the stomach and the columnar-lined (Barrett's) oesophagus. In these instances it is worth differentiating between the highest grades of dysplasia (that have no metastatic potential) and 'intramucosal carcinoma' (that does). Lymphatics are scantier in the large bowel mucosa and there are no convincing clinical series showing metas-tases from epithelial neoplasms confined to this tissue compartment [489]. Although apparently invasive neo-plasms of this type can be seen in the colorectum (and carcinoma *in situ* is included as Tis in the TNM classifica-tion), many authorities would avoid using the term 'intra-mucosal carcinoma' and use high grade dysplasia in its stead (Figure 38.29) [3]. The term 'early colorectal cancer' is also sometimes used. It tends to have different mean-

ings in different parts of the world. In Japan the term would include lesions considered elsewhere to be adeno-mas (or dysplasia in IBD). In Europe and North America early colorectal cancer would more usually be defined as a T1 primary lesion. Probably the term is best avoided in formal descriptions.

Prognostic indicators in colorectal cancer

In this section the pathological factors of use in determin-ing survival are highlighted. An important distinction is between those (such as staging) that are purely prognostic and others (such as *KRAS* mutation) that are predictive of response to therapy [490]. The latter category is only just emerging in colorectal cancer but is a major drive in research and is likely to become an increasing part of the pathologist's workload in the not too distant future. It is important to recognise that pathological predictors are only part of a bigger picture and that clinical, biochemical and radiological factors will all have to be considered for the individual patient.

Tumour staging, as discussed in the last section, remains the mainstay of prognostic prediction after surgical resec-tion, and detailed guidance on specimen handling and block taking in order to optimise staging is given in Chapter 32. Lymph node metastasis, and the absolute number of nodes involved, both have independent prognostic signifi-cance. Accordingly all lymph nodes in a resection specimen should be harvested for histological examination. It is widely accepted that at least 12 are needed for reliable nodal staging and this is now used as a quality standard in pathology reporting [3]. However, recent studies have sug-gested that the lymph node ratio (the number of tumour-containing nodes expressed as a fraction of total node yield) may be an even more powerful prognostic tool, and this is currently being evaluated in prospective trials [491]. Detection of micrometastases is still largely in the research sphere, at least until an agreed consensus panel of antibod-ies and/or molecular approaches has been defined [474].

Tumour grading has been a routine part of histopatho-logical reporting since the days of Dukes [485]. In a single centre study of over 2000 patients approximately 20% were classified as well differentiated, 60% moderately differenti-ated and 20% poorly differentiated. The respective cor-rected 5-year survival rates for these groups were 77%, 61% and 30%. Grading has, however, proven to be very prone to inter-observer variation. In a review of specimens from 22 different centres entered into a clinical trial, the propor-tion of cancers classified as well differentiated ranged from 3% to 93% [492]. In many reporting guidelines, such as those produced by the Royal College of Pathologists, tumours are classified by the *predominant* pattern of dif-ferentiation [3]. Some studies have, however, shown that it is the *worst* grade of differentiation present that best

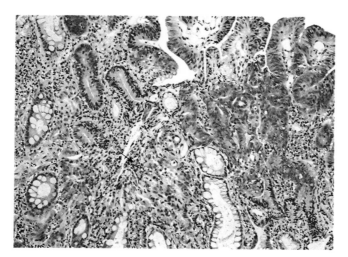

Figure 38.29 A case reported as intramucosal carcinoma. The architecture is complex and there are areas where there appears to be infiltration of the lamina propria (arrow). There is no metastatic potential and the case is best considered as 'high grade dysplasia'.

predicts an adverse outcome [493]. The biggest problem remaining is that grading remains essentially subjective.

Jass described an attempt to systematically pull together probable prognostic indicators into a combined staging and grading system [451]. In this, the degree of local invasion is combined with node involvement and two microscopic grading elements. These are peri-tumoral lymphocytic infiltrate and assessment of the advancing margin (low power) as either pushing or infiltrative. Although this system has been shown to be prognostically useful in several studies it has not achieved widespread acceptance.

Tumour spread by the portal and systemic vasculature has long been recognised as the main route of development of hepatic, pulmonary and more distant metastases. These metastases may be present at the time of clinical presentation, but more commonly appear months to years after treatment of the primary lesion by surgical resection. It is assumed that, unless the original surgical excision was incomplete, clinically evident metastases grow from microscopic deposits that were undetectable at the time of primary staging and treatment. Demonstration of venous invasion predicts the future appearance of distant metastasis, and Shepherd and colleagues have combined this with three other parameters (peritoneal involvement, surgical margin positivity and tumour perforation) to provide a powerful prognostic score in Dukes' B colon cancer [476]. Uncertainty over the prognostic significance of venous invasion in early studies may well have been largely due to methodological differences in terms of the number and orientation of blocks selected and the use of elastic stains. More recently Foulis and colleagues have shown it to be among the most powerful of prognostic indicators. Using systematic elastin staining, fully 58% of cancers were shown to have evidence of vascular invasion. These had a significantly worse survival, irrespective of whether the invasion was intra- or extramural and venous invasion predicted the vast majority of patients who were to progress to systemic disease. It is therefore advocated that elastic staining should become part of routine pathological assessment [477,494].

The effect of tumour genetic abnormalities on prognosis

The complex molecular events underlying the pathogenesis of colorectal cancer have thrown up a bewildering array of candidate markers of potential prognostic utility. The range of potential biomarkers has included those identified by immunohistochemistry and proteomics, mutations in key oncogenes and tumour-suppressor genes, LOH at tumour-suppressor gene loci and chromosomal changes detected by comparative genomic hybridisation but their clinical application has been somewhat confounded by the heterogeneity of techniques used. Studies of the tumour-suppressor TP53 provide a good example. This gene is

frequently mutated in colorectal cancer and both LOH and loss of chromosome 17p (the genetic locus for the TP53 gene) have also been demonstrated. A number of different antibodies to p53 have also been developed, with subtly differing staining patterns and variable relation to gene mutation. A comprehensive review has therefore, not surprisingly, concluded that there is no clear pattern of clinical relevance in the many published studies [495].

In molecular pathology it is likely that issues of technical methodology and sample selection will be crucial in ensuring that laboratories achieve comparable results. Involving pathologists is also crucial in ensuring that the samples analysed contain a suitable proportion of tumour cells, and estimation of this parameter should be included in molecular pathology reports. Where neoplastic cells constitute only a small proportion of the cellular population of a sample to be analysed, there may be a need for microdissection [496].

KRAS is a good model of how the future is likely to look for molecular pathology testing in cancer. It is now clear, from both multicentre studies and smaller series, that those cancers with mutation of this gene have a worse clinical outcome than those with wild-type KRAS [497]. This appears to be particularly the case for mutations in codon 12 of the gene. The effect is, however, small when compared with staging and other conventional pathological parameters, and KRAS mutational analysis has not been adopted as a clinical prognostic marker. More recently, the importance of the gene as a predictive marker has become clear, with a significant impact on diagnostic pathology services. Clinical trials of the monoclonal antibody cetuximab, an epidermal growth factor receptor (EGFR) antagonist, in patients with metastatic colorectal cancer initially showed little or no efficacy. When the results were re-analysed in the context of KRAS mutation as a biomarker, it became clear that while mutant tumours did not respond, there was clear therapeutic benefit in patients with wild-type cancers [498]. Cetuximab is now licensed both in Europe and the USA, with a requirement that KRAS mutational testing is carried out on tumour samples to identify likely responders. The effect of KRAS mutation is easily explained because the mutant gene is constitutively active and acts on the same downstream pathway as EGFR, so that receptor inhibition is futile. There is some evidence that BRAF mutation (that is mutually exclusive with KRAS mutation in colorectal cancer) may have a similar effect but analysis of this gene has not yet been consolidated in clinical practice.

More global markers of genetic abnormality also have potential advantages as prognostic indicators in colorectal cancer. Thus tumours with MSI have a better clinical outcome than MSS cancers [329] and there is disputed evidence that they might also be less sensitive to 5-fluorouracil-based chemotherapy regimens. Measurement of the degree

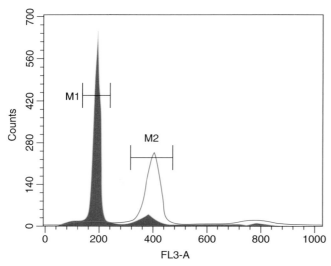

Figure 38.30 DNA flow cytometry: a nuclear preparation from a tumour sample is stained with propidium iodide. Tumour cells are separately identified by cytokeratin staining (green) and show an abnormal near tetraploid DNA content when compared with the stromal cells (red peak) that are used as an internal control. (Courtesy of Dr Jasbani Dayal.)

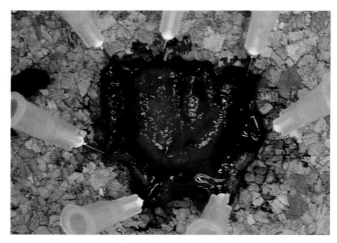

Figure 38.31 Transanal endoscopic microsurgical resection of a small rectal cancer: the fresh specimen has been pinned on cork by the surgeon. It is fixed by floating in formalin and subsequently inked on the underside before cutting. (See Figure 38.22 for a histological preparation.)

to which overall tumour cell DNA deviates from normal can be useful as a rough global surrogate of chromosomal instability. This is achieved by use of dyes that bind to DNA in a stoichiometric fashion. In static image analysis techniques, Feulgen staining is used whereas in DNA flow cytometry fluorescent DNA-binding dyes such as propidium iodide are used [499]. With these techniques tumours containing cell populations with abnormal DNA content are described as DNA aneuploid (Figure 38.30) and there have been numerous publications over the years suggesting that they have an adverse prognosis [500,501]. Not surprisingly DNA aneuploidy is associated more with distal cancers and with the MSS phenotype.

Pathological considerations in localised resections for colorectal cancer

Advances in endoscopic and surgical technique have made it possible to locally resect colorectal neoplasms that would previously have required formal surgical excision. These lesions often do not have a preoperative malignant diagnosis and are resected as large high-risk adenomas. Occasionally there will be a local resection of a known cancer either through patient choice or because the individual is not fit for full surgical excision. Currently there is also interest in combining local resection with sentinel node mapping to better aid staging and selection for adjuvant therapy [475] but this approach has not yet been validated.

The most common scenario is the detection of focal invasive cancer in a simple polypectomy and this is discussed in detail in Chapter 37. More complex resections include endoscopic mucosal resection (EMR) and transanal endoscopic microsurgery (TEMS). EMR is a specialised procedure that can potentially excise sessile lesions in any part of the gastrointestinal tract [502]. TEMS is a more complex procedure using a specialised operating microscope [503] and is applicable only to rectal lesions. These procedures generate flat irregular specimens, the pathological assessment of which can be challenging and close clinical correlation is essential to ensure an optimum report. The specimen should be pinned to a flat corkboard immediately on removal, before dispatch to the laboratory (Figure 38.31) and floated intact in fixative. Once fixed, block selection must ensure thorough sampling of all margins (edge and deep) that will have been painted beforehand. Often, the entire lesion will be submitted for microscopy. It is important to note that the full thickness of the bowel wall, including both muscular layers, will be usual in TEMS specimens (see Figure 38.22).

Microscopic examination of cancers excised in this way is directed towards ensuring that complete excision has been achieved (usually with a microscopic clearance of at least 1 mm) and that other pathological indicators of adverse outcome are identified. One of these is the depth of submucosal invasion. In polypectomy specimens this is often assessed using Haggitt's criteria (see Chapter 37), but for sessile lesions the classification of Kikuchi and colleagues [504] is preferred. Invasion is classified as sm1, sm2 or sm3, depending on whether the invasion reaches the superficial, middle or deepest third of the submucosa (see

Figure 38.22). Ueno and colleagues have also shown that incomplete excision, poor tumour differentiation, the presence of significant tumour budding, vascular invasion and extensive submucosal invasion are the key parameters in predicting an adverse outcome in these patients [505]. With the exception (for now) of budding, these parameters have been included in reporting guidelines for early colorectal cancers, including those identified in screening programmes [506,507].

Endocrine tumours

Endocrine cell neoplasms of the large intestine, previously known as carcinoid tumours, are uncommon, accounting for less than 1% of all colorectal neoplasms, but about 30% of all endocrine cell tumours of the gastrointestinal tract [508]. In England approximately 8% of all gastrointestinal endocrine tumours arise in the rectum, whereas 13% are located in the right colon and caecum [509]. The aetiology of these tumours is uncertain, but a Swedish study has found an increased relative risk in individuals with parental carcinoid tumours, implying that genetic factors could play a role [510]. No sex difference in incidence has been noted [509] but there may be a slight increase in incidence among black and Asian populations. Endocrine cell tumours are reported to occur in patients with ulcerative colitis but there is no evidence that their incidence is increased compared with non-colitic patients [511]. Small colorectal endocrine cell tumours are discovered at endoscopy and their incidence is likely to increase with increasing endoscopy, especially for cancer screening. However, many colorectal carcinoids are incidentally discovered in resection specimens for carcinoma [512]. The most common colorectal endocrine cell tumours arise in the appendix and are considered in Chapter 30. All gastrointestinal endocrine tumours are now classified according to the World Health Organization (WHO) criteria and graded according to mitotic rate and Ki67 labelling index. However, published recommendations including proformas for reporting colorectal endocrine tumours are site specific, because tumours arising at different sites differ in their biology and outcomes. Colorectal endocrine tumours are staged according to the TNM classification system for mid- and hindgut [513].

Right-sided tumours

Right-sided endocrine cell tumours usually present as bulky polypoid or ulcerating masses that are macroscopically indistinguishable from carcinomas; many will have already metastasised to regional lymph nodes and distant sites [514]. The great majority are enterochromaffin (EC) cell neoplasms similar to those arising in the ileum and appendix (see Chapters 24 and 30) and are composed of solid clumps or islands of uniform cells with eosinophilic granular cytoplasm that is argentaffin and argyrophil and stains for 5-hydroxytryptamine (5HT). The larger, overtly malignant varieties show mitotic activity and necrosis. However, an associated carcinoid syndrome is uncommon, even in the presence of liver metastases. Right hemicolectomy is warranted for all but small superficial lesions that can be completely excised endoscopically; an overall 5-year survival rate of only 23% has been reported [508].

Left-sided and rectal tumours

Left-sided and rectal endocrine tumours are mostly L-cell tumours that are argyrophil but not argentaffin. These lesions are most commonly asymptomatic and discovered incidentally. They may occasionally be multiple but are almost always non-functioning clinically [515]. Rectal endocrine tumours present in two macroscopic forms [516]. The usual finding is that of a small nodule or plaque <10 mm in diameter and discovered fortuitously. The cut surface is pink or tan. These superficial tumours are often mobile and can be safely treated by local excision, provided that removal is complete. Less commonly, the tumour presents as a large growth with ulceration that can mimic a rectal carcinoma, often with metastasis at presentation.

Three histological patterns are encountered, of which the ribbon type is the most common. The ribbons comprise two or more layers of cells arranged along a delicate core of vascular connective tissue. The ribbons may be straight, convoluted or interlacing. The next most common pattern is an acinar or tubular type, with the tubular component often being the more conspicuous. This pattern may be accompanied by an 'Indian file' appearance of infiltrating cords of cells, the third and least common pattern to be found in its pure form. Distal colorectal endocrine tumours show variable immunostaining for chromogranin A but more consistent staining for chromogranin B and synaptophysin. Many are positive for prostatic acid phosphatase but not prostate-specific antigen (PSA) [517]. The acinar and infiltrative growth patterns, when lacking chromogranin A expression, may lead the pathologist to consider the diagnosis of metastatic adenocarcinoma, in particular from the prostate. Synaptophysin expression and absence of PSA are helpful guides here. Although there may be a little diastase-periodic acid–Schiff (DPAS)- and Alcian blue-positive material in the lumina of the acinar subtype, intracellular mucin is absent, a feature that distinguishes these neoplasms from goblet cell carcinoids [517]. Although not diagnostically useful, L-cell neoplasms are known to coexpress a range of enteroglucagons or glicentin-related peptides, including glucagon-29, glucagon-37, glicentin, proglucagon cryptic fragments, peptide YY (PYY), pancreatic polypeptide (PP) and pro-PP icosapeptide, and regularly contain minor populations of serotonin (5HT), substance P, somatostatin, insulin, enkephalin, β-endorphin, neurotensin, α-human chorionic gonadotrophin (α-hCG) and motilin-containing cells [518].

Features of colorectal endocrine tumours that indicate malignancy include size >20 mm, vascular invasion, spread into and beyond the muscularis propria, nuclear pleomorphism, high mitotic activity and necrosis. Lymph node metastases are recorded in 60–80% of such cases [515,519]. On the other hand, well differentiated tumours measuring <10 mm that are confined to the mucosa or submucosa and show none of these 'atypical' histological features virtually never metastasise and can be safely treated by local excision [520–522].

Goblet cell carcinoid

It is not always a simple matter to distinguish malignant endocrine tumours from adenocarcinomas that have either adopted a 'carcinoid-like' growth pattern or contain a conspicuous population of endocrine cells. An example of the latter is the so-called goblet cell carcinoid, which has been described in the colon as well as the appendix (see Chapter 30). These are rare but aggressive lesions in the colon and rectum that are frequently metastatic and carry a poor prognosis [523]. Consideration must always be given to the possibility of metastasis from the appendix, which was reported in 25% of cases in one study [523]. In this multi-institutional series, colorectal goblet cell carcinoids were frequently misdiagnosed as signet-ring cell carcinomas [523].

That such difficulties of classification should arise is not surprising, in light of the fact that endocrine cells and other epithelial cells arise from a common stem cell. It is of interest that an association exists between colorectal endocrine neoplasia and both synchronous (including contiguous) and metachronous epithelial neoplasia [516]. Endocrine cell hyperplasia and neoplasia has been recorded in patients with longstanding ulcerative colitis, with [524] and without [525] synchronous dysplasia and cancer. These observations indicate the possible sharing of aetiological factors in the processes of endocrine and non-endocrine epithelial neoplasia.

Small cell carcinoma

Small cell undifferentiated carcinoma (SCUC, 'oat cell') may be placed at the most malignant end of the spectrum of colorectal endocrine neoplasms. It may arise in association with conventional colorectal adenocarcinoma and occasionally within an adenoma. Several case reports exist of small cell carcinoma arising in patients with ulcerative colitis [526], but overall small cell carcinomas are rare,

comprising <1% of colon and rectal cancers [527]. Their pathogenesis is unknown but one recent study suggested CIN as a possible pathogenic mechanism, as they almost always express MMR proteins [528]. SCUCs occur throughout the colon and rectum and are roughly equally distributed between the right and left side. They are often metastatic at the time of diagnosis and carry a poor prognosis [527]. They usually display hallmark features of small cell carcinoma, with smudged nuclear chromatin, nuclear moulding, smearing artefact, frequent apoptotic bodies and necrosis. SCUCs are variably positive for endocrine markers such as chromogranin and synaptophysin [527,528]. In common with many extrapulmonary small cell carcinomas, they may express thyroid transcription factor-1 (TTF-1) [529]. Therefore, histopathologically and immunophenotypically they may appear identical to metastatic bronchogenic small cell carcinoma. A prudent review of clinical and radiological findings may be required to exclude this rare possibility.

Rare forms of colorectal cancer

Squamous cell carcinoma

Primary squamous cell carcinoma of the colon and rectum does occur but is extremely rare [530–534]. Before such a condition can be accepted as genuine, care must be taken to exclude metastatic tumour presenting as a primary growth. This is most likely to come from the uterine cervix or the anus. There may be great difficulty in deciding whether such a tumour is primarily arising from rectal mucosa or whether it is really an upward extension of a carcinoma of the anal canal. Additional care must be taken in the case of anorectal fistulae in which squamous carcinomas can arise. Some cases may arise from squamous differentiation within colorectal adenomas and the frequency distribution of squamous carcinoma around the colorectum mirrors that of adenocarcinoma [535]. It is generally a disease of adults and more common in women than in men [532].

Squamous carcinoma of the rectum complicating chronic ulcerative colitis has been reported on a number of occasions [536] and has rarely been associated with adjacent and pre-existent squamous metaplasia [537]. Indeed, although it would appear to account for only 1–2% of all cancers complicating ulcerative colitis, this represents a relative incidence 50–100 times greater than in the general population. It is also exceedingly rarely described as a complication of Crohn's disease.

The role of human papillomavirus (HPV) is controversial. Frizelle et al., in a large series, did not find any evidence of HPV in rectal squamous cell carcinomas by *in situ* hybridisation [534]. This finding has been supported by Nahas et al. and Audeau et al. in separate series [538,539].

However, three other smaller recent studies have found evidence of HPV infection [540–542]. Differences in the molecular techniques employed between the studies makes drawing firm conclusions difficult. In one case squamous cell carcinoma of the rectum has also been reported in association with HPV in an HIV-positive patient [541].

Squamous cell carcinoma of the large intestine presents with similar symptoms to colorectal adenocarcinoma and the prognosis depends largely on stage. One series found the overall 5-year survival rate to be 33% for squamous cell carcinomas of the rectum [532]. The primary treatment in the past has been surgical, but more recently encouraging results with chemoradiotherapy have been reported and this has been suggested as an alternative first-line therapy [411,543].

Adenosquamous carcinoma

This is a very rare tumour in the colorectum, in which both adenocarcinoma and squamous carcinoma elements are present. Either carcinoma subtype may predominate. Adenosquamous carcinoma can be found in all parts of the large bowel, although some claim that it is seen mostly in the right colon and rectum. These tumours may behave in an aggressive manner and the squamous component may have the greater metastatic potential [544].

Carcinosarcoma

There are now over 20 reports of carcinosarcoma of the colon in the published literature worldwide, particularly in the Asian population, but in practice this tumour remains exceedingly rare [545,546]. It occurs in adults with no sex predilection and in any part of the colon and rectum [546]. Although the diagnosis requires the simultaneous demonstration of divergent epithelial and mesenchymal differentiation within the same tumour, it may be that some cases could be reclassified as sarcomatoid colorectal carcinoma, depending on the stringency of morphological and immunohistochemical diagnostic criteria applied. Osteosarcomatous and chondrosarcomatous components have been reported [547]. In females an origin from the gynaecological tract should be excluded before ascribing a primary origin to the colorectum. The prognosis is usually dismal and is related to stage.

Secondary carcinoma

The stomach is probably the most common source of both solitary and multiple secondary carcinomatous deposits in the colon and rectum. These may present as single or multiple strictures mimicking primary colorectal cancer and even Crohn's disease or ulcerative colitis. The last is simulated when there is widespread and diffuse mural spread of malignant cells, giving rise to a shortened, tubular colon on radiological examination. Symptoms may be referable to the colon only, and the primary disease in the stomach may be difficult to demonstrate, even at laparotomy. Colorectal metastases from carcinoma of the breast, especially lobular carcinoma, can produce a similar picture [548,549]. Accurate clinical information is paramount in resolving these cases and morphological appearances on haematoxylin and eosin (H&E) staining that are not typical of colorectal carcinoma should always arouse the suspicions of the pathologist. In most cases the distinction is easily made between primary and metastatic carcinoma; however, in difficult cases, in particular when signet-ring cell carcinoma of the colon is being considered, immunohistochemistry may be prudent. Expression of CK20 and CDX2 with absence of CK7 may be helpful in confirming a colorectal phenotype.

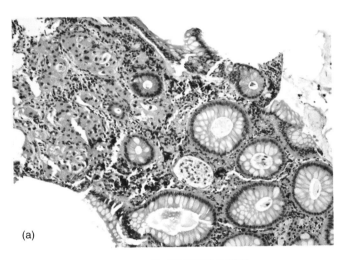

(a)

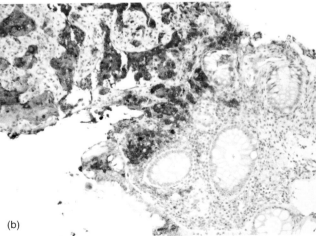

(b)

Figure 38.32 Metastatic prostate carcinoma in rectal mucosa (a). The tumour shows strong immunoreactivity for prostate-specific antigen (b).

Involvement of the rectum by carcinoma of the prostate is unusual, and it is even more uncommon for prostatic carcinoma to present with signs and symptoms of rectal disease in the absence of, or overshadowing, urinary symptoms. In such cases the rectal disease presents as a stricture, anterior rectal ulcer or anterior submucosal mass [550,551]. Histopathologically, the differential diagnosis of metastatic carcinoma of the prostate from colorectal carcinoma is not often a diagnostic challenge. The distinction from rectal endocrine tumours may not be so easy because both tumours may show a nested or pseudo-glandular pattern and both tumours can express prostatic acid phosphatase. Expression of PSA by carcinoma of the prostate is much more specific and helpful (Figure 38.32). Among other sources of secondary colorectal cancer are the ovary, kidney [552–554], cervix and lung.

In summary, the pathologist must always be alert for the possibility of secondary carcinoma or endometriosis (see Chapter 40), when assessing large bowel biopsies in which the appearances of the tumour are unusual or unlike ordinary colorectal cancer. This is especially true when considering the diagnosis of the rarer carcinomas of the colon or rectum.

Datasets and reporting standards

Throughout this chapter we have emphasised the importance of establishing an evidence base for reporting of pathological parameters. The number of relevant parameters in both macroscopic and microscopic assessment of colorectal cancer specimens has increased remarkably over the last couple of decades. This has been recognised by professional bodies and reporting guidelines are now a well-accepted feature of clinical life [3]. An important suggestion to emerge from this process is the reporting proforma in which the relevant data items are systematically listed and grouped so that the pathologist is reminded to include all in the final report. Introduction of this approach has been shown to improve completeness of reporting [555]. This finding is given additional weight by a Welsh randomised trial comparing data item-style reporting to free text. The systematic approach led to a 28% higher level of completeness of reporting [556]. Dataset-style reports have the added advantage of being easily read and should vary little between one pathologist and another. The evidence favours abandoning the time-honoured style, although many pathologists are reluctant to do so.

Screening for colorectal cancer

Large bowel cancer is now a major target for population screening. A number of approaches have been adopted. Guiac-based faecal occult blood testing followed by colonoscopy for positive tests has been shown to reduce disease-specific mortality in randomised clinical trials [557]. Once-only flexible sigmoidoscopy has also been used and similarly shown to lead to a reduction in mortality [558]. Colonoscopy and CT colonography have been used as screening techniques in different populations [559]. All approaches ultimately use endoscopic examination with biopsy and polypectomy as the end-point in diagnosis. The process therefore generates a significant workload increase for pathology departments. Endoscopy-based primary screening (sigmoidoscopy, colonoscopy) is particularly prone to producing large numbers of pathological specimens. The other particular challenges are in correctly identifying early cancer in adenomatous polyps, identifying adenoma patients at high risk of future malignancy and determining prognostic features in individuals with early stage screen-detected cancer. A number of national and international guidelines have been produced with a view to standardising and improving pathology reporting [506,507].

References

1. Office of National Statistics. *Cancer Incidence and Mortality in the United Kingdom and Constituent Countries 2003–5*. Newport: Office of National Statistics, 2008.
2. Quirke P, Morris E. Reporting colorectal cancer. *Histopathology* 2007;**50**:103.
3. Williams GT, Quirke P, Shepherd NA. *Standards and Datasets for Reporting Cancers – Dataset for Colorectal Cancer*, 2nd edn. London: The Royal College of Pathologists, 2007.
4. DeCosse JJ, Ngoi SS, Jacobson JS, Cennerazzo WJ. Gender and colorectal cancer. *Eur J Cancer Prev* 1993;**2**:105.
5. Benedix F, Kube R, Meyer F, Schmidt U, Gastinger I, Lippert H. Comparison of 17,641 patients with right- and left-sided colon cancer: differences in epidemiology, perioperative course, histology, and survival. *Dis Colon Rectum* ;**53**:57.
6. Rabeneck L, Davila JA, El-Serag HB. Is there a true 'shift' to the right colon in the incidence of colorectal cancer? *Am J Gastroenterol* 2003;**98**:1400.
7. Vogelstein B, Fearon ER, Hamilton SR, et al. Genetic alterations during colorectal-tumor development. *N Engl J Med* 1988;**319**:525.
8. Tomlinson I, Webb E, Carvajal-Carmona L, et al. A genome-wide association scan of tag SNPs identifies a susceptibility variant for colorectal cancer at 8q24.21. *Nat Genet* 2007;**39**:984.
9. Zanke BW, Greenwood CM, Rangrej J, et al. Genome-wide association scan identifies a colorectal cancer susceptibility locus on chromosome 8q24. *Nat Genet* 2007;**39**:989.
10. Haenszel W, Kurihara M. Studies of Japanese migrants. I. Mortality from cancer and other diseases among Japanese in the United States. *J Natl Cancer Inst* 1968;**40**:43.
11. Correa P, Haenszel W. The epidemiology of large-bowel cancer. *Adv Cancer Res* 1978;**26**:1.
12. McMichael AJ, McCall MG, Hartshorne JM, Woodings TL. Patterns of gastro-intestinal cancer in European migrants to Australia: the role of dietary change. *Int J Cancer* 1980;**25**:431.
13. He J, Wilkens LR, Stram DO, et al. Generalizability and epidemiologic characterization of eleven colorectal cancer GWAS hits in multiple populations. *Cancer Epidemiol Biomarkers Prev* 2011;**20**:70.

14. Wynder EL. The epidemiology of large bowel cancer. *Cancer Res* 1975;**35**(11 Part 2):3388.

15. Larsson SC, Wolk A. Meat consumption and risk of colorectal cancer: a meta-analysis of prospective studies. *Int J Cancer* 2006; **119**:2657.

16. McMichael AJ, Potter JD, Hetzel BS. Time trends in colo-rectal cancer mortality in relation to food and alcohol consumption: United States, United Kingdom, Australia and New Zealand. *Int J Epidemiol* 1979;**8**:295.

17. Burkitt DP. Epidemiology of cancer of the colon and rectum. *Cancer* 1971;**28**:3.

18. Graham S, Dayal H, Swanson M, Mittelman A, Wilkinson G. Diet in the epidemiology of cancer of the colon and rectum. *J Natl Cancer Inst* 1978;**61**:709.

19. Ferguson LR, Harris PJ. Studies on the role of specific dietary fibres in protection against colorectal cancer. *Mutat Res* 1996;**350**:173.

20. Nelson RL, Samelson SL. Inability of the mutagen-blocking agent oleic acid to protect against colon carcinogenesis in the rat. *Mutat Res* 1984;**140**:155.

21. Aries V, Crowther JS, Drasar BS, Hill MJ. Degradation of bile salts by human intestinal bacteria. *Gut* 1969;**10**:575.

22. Moorehead RJ, Campbell GR, Donaldson JD, McKelvey ST. Relationship between duodenal bile acids and colorectal neoplasia. *Gut* 1987;**28**:1454.

23. Reddy BS, Narisawa T, Weisburger JH. Effect of a diet with high levels of protein and fat on colon carcinogenesis in F344 rats treated with 1,2-dimethylhydrazine. *J Natl Cancer Inst* 1976; **57**:567.

24. Wilpart M, Mainguet P, Maskens A, Roberfroid M. Mutagenicity of 1,2-dimethylhydrazine towards *Salmonella typhimurium*, co-mutagenic effect of secondary biliary acids. *Carcinogenesis* 1983;**4**:45.

25. Reddy BS. Dietary fat and colon cancer: animal model studies. *Lipids* 1992;**27**:807.

26. Reddy BS, Hanson D, Mangat S, et al. Effect of high-fat, high-beef diet and of mode of cooking of beef in the diet on fecal bacterial enzymes and fecal bile acids and neutral sterols. *J Nutr* 1980;**110**:1880.

27. Gupta I, Suzuki K, Bruce RW, Krepinsky JJ, Yates P. A model study of fecapentaenes: mutagens of bacterial origin with alkylating properties. *Science* 1984;**225**:521.

28. Szekely J, Gates KS. Noncovalent DNA binding and the mechanism of oxidative DNA damage by fecapentaene-12. *Chem Res Toxicol* 2006;**19**:117.

29. Narahara H, Tatsuta M, Iishi H, et al. K-ras point mutation is associated with enhancement by deoxycholic acid of colon carcinogenesis induced by azoxymethane, but not with its attenuation by all-trans-retinoic acid. *Int J Cancer* 2000;**88**:157.

30. Crowley-Weber CL, Dvorakova K, Crowley C, et al. Nicotine increases oxidative stress, activates NF-kappaB and GRP78, induces apoptosis and sensitizes cells to genotoxic/xenobiotic stresses by a multiple stress inducer, deoxycholate: relevance to colon carcinogenesis. *Chem Biol Interact* 2003;**145**:53.

31. Hursting SD, Thornquist M, Henderson MM. Types of dietary fat and the incidence of cancer at five sites. *Prev Med* 1990; **19**:242.

32. Newmark HL, Wargovich MJ, Bruce WR. Colon cancer and dietary fat, phosphate, and calcium: a hypothesis. *J Natl Cancer Inst* 1984;**72**:1323.

33. Armstrong B, Doll R. Environmental factors and cancer incidence and mortality in different countries, with special reference to dietary practices. *Int J Cancer* 1975;**15**:617.

34. Kune S, Kune GA, Watson LF. Case-control study of dietary etiological factors: the Melbourne Colorectal *Cancer* Study. *Nutr Cancer* 1987;**9**:21.

35. Kune GA. The Melbourne Colorectal *Cancer* Study: reflections on a 30-year experience. *Med J Aust* 2010;**193**:648.

36. Gonzalez CA, Riboli E. Diet and cancer prevention: Contributions from the European Prospective Investigation into *Cancer and Nutrition* (EPIC) study. *Eur J Cancer* 2010;**46**:2555.

37. Alexander DD, Cushing CA. Red meat and colorectal cancer: a critical summary of prospective epidemiologic studies. *Obes Rev* 2010;**12**:e472.

38. Hoeft B, Linseisen J, Beckmann L, et al. Polymorphisms in fatty-acid-metabolism-related genes are associated with colorectal cancer risk. *Carcinogenesis* 2010;**31**:466.

39. Obrador A. Fibre and colorectal cancer: a controversial question. *Br J Nutr* 2006;**96**(suppl 1):S46.

40. Cruse JP, Lewin MR, Clark CG. Failure of bran to protect against experimental colon cancer in rats. *Lancet* 1978;**ii**: 1278.

41. Jass JR. Diet, butyric acid and differentiation of gastrointestinal tract tumours. *Med Hypotheses* 1985;**18**:113.

42. Scharlau D, Borowicki A, Habermann N, et al. Mechanisms of primary cancer prevention by butyrate and other products formed during gut flora-mediated fermentation of dietary fibre. *Mutat Res* 2009;**682**:39.

43. Alberts DS, Tinez ME, Roe DJ, et al. Phoenix Colon Cancer Prevention Physicians' Network. Lack of effect of a high-fiber cereal supplement on the recurrence of colorectal adenomas. *N Engl J Med* 2000;**342**:1156.

44. Schatzkin A, Lanza E, Corle D, et al., Polyp Prevention Trial Study Group. Lack of effect of a low-fat, high-fiber diet on the recurrence of colorectal adenomas. *N Engl J Med* 2000; **342**:1149.

45. Lanza E, Yu B, Murphy G, et al. The polyp prevention trial continued follow-up study: no effect of a low-fat, high-fiber, high-fruit, and -vegetable diet on adenoma recurrence eight years after randomization. *Cancer Epidemiol Biomarkers Prev* 2007;**16**:1745.

46. Sansbury LB, Wanke K, Albert PS, Kahle L, Schatzkin A, Lanza E. The effect of strict adherence to a high-fiber, high-fruit and -vegetable, and low-fat eating pattern on adenoma recurrence. *Am J Epidemiol* 2009;**170**:576.

47. Corfe BM, Williams EA, Bury JP, et al. A study protocol to investigate the relationship between dietary fibre intake and fermentation, colon cell turnover, global protein acetylation and early carcinogenesis: the FACT study. *BMC Cancer* 2009; **9**:332.

48. Little J, Logan RF, Hawtin PG, Hardcastle JD, Turner ID. Colorectal adenomas and energy intake, body size and physical activity: a case-control study of subjects participating in the Nottingham faecal occult blood screening programme. *Br J Cancer* 1993;**67**:172.

49. Lechand L, Wilkens LR, Kolonel LN, Hankin JH, Lyu LC. Associations of sedentary lifestyle, obesity, smoking, alcohol use, and diabetes with the risk of colorectal cancer. *Cancer Res* 1997; **57**:4787.

50. Russo A, Franceschi S, La Vecchia C, et al. Body size and colorectal-cancer risk. *Int J Cancer* 1998;**78**:161.

51. Harriss DJ, Atkinson G, Batterham A, et al. Lifestyle factors and colorectal cancer risk: a systematic review and meta-analysis of associations with leisure-time physical activity. *Colorectal Dis* 2009;**11**:689.

52. Larsson SC, Wolk A. Obesity and colon and rectal cancer risk: a meta-analysis of prospective studies. *Am J Clin Nutr* 2007; **86**:556.

53. Bassett JK, Severi G, English DR, et al. Body size, weight change, and risk of colon cancer. *Cancer Epidemiol Biomarkers Prev* 2010;**19**:2978.

54. Pischon T, Lahmann PH, Boeing H, et al. Body size and risk of colon and rectal cancer in the European Prospective Investigation Into Cancer and Nutrition (EPIC). *J Natl Cancer Inst* 2006;**98**:920.

55. Morois S, Mesrine S, Josset M, Clavel-Chapelon F, Boutron-Ruault MC. Anthropometric factors in adulthood and risk of colorectal adenomas: The French E3N-EPIC prospective cohort. *Am J Epidemiol* 2010;**172**:1166.

56. Reeves GK, Pirie K, Beral V, Green J, Spencer E, Bull D. Cancer incidence and mortality in relation to body mass index in the Million Women Study: cohort study. *BMJ* 2007;**335**:1134.

57. Campbell PT, Jacobs ET, Ulrich CM, et al. Case-control study of overweight, obesity, and colorectal cancer risk, overall and by tumor microsatellite instability status. *J Natl Cancer Inst* 2010;**102**:391.

58. Kang HW, Kim D, Kim HJ, et al. Visceral obesity and insulin resistance as risk factors for colorectal adenoma: a cross-sectional, case-control study. *Am J Gastroenterol* 2010;**105**:178.

59. Limburg PJ, Stolzenberg-Solomon RZ, Vierkant RA, et al. Insulin, glucose, insulin resistance, and incident colorectal cancer in male smokers. *Clin Gastroenterol Hepatol* 2006;**4**:1514.

60. Giouleme O, Diamantidis MD, Katsaros MG. Is diabetes a causal agent for colorectal cancer? Pathophysiological and molecular mechanisms. *World J Gastroenterol* 2011;**17**:444.

61. Rinaldi S, Cleveland R, Norat T, et al. Serum levels of IGF-I, IGFBP-3 and colorectal cancer risk: results from the EPIC cohort, plus a meta-analysis of prospective studies. *Int J Cancer* 2010;**126**:1702.

62. Sung MK, Bae YJ. Linking obesity to colorectal cancer: application of nutrigenomics. *Biotechnol J* 2010;**5**:930.

63. Testino G, Borro P. Alcohol and gastrointestinal oncology. *World J Gastrointest Oncol* 2010;**2**:322.

64. Honjo S, Kono S, Shinchi K, et al. The relation of smoking, alcohol use and obesity to risk of sigmoid colon and rectal adenomas. *Jpn J Cancer Res* 1995;**86**:1019.

65. Boutron MC, Faivre J, Dop MC, Quipourt V, Senesse P. Tobacco, alcohol, and colorectal tumors: a multistep process. *Am J Epidemiol* 1995;**141**:1038.

66. Heineman EF, Zahm SH, McLaughlin JK, Vaught JB. Increased risk of colorectal cancer among smokers: results of a 26-year follow-up of US veterans and a review. *Int J Cancer* 1994;**59**:728.

67. Figueiredo JC, Levine AJ, Lee WH, et al. Genes involved with folate uptake and distribution and their association with colorectal cancer risk. *Cancer Causes Control* 2010;**21**:597.

68. Giovannucci E, Rimm EB, Stampfer MJ, et al. A prospective study of cigarette smoking and risk of colorectal adenoma and colorectal cancer in U.S. men. *J Natl Cancer Inst* 1994;**86**:183.

69. Anderson JC, Pleau DC, Rajan TV, et al. Increased frequency of serrated aberrant crypt foci among smokers. *Am J Gastroenterol* 2010;**105**:1648.

70. Tsoi KK, Pau CY, Wu WK, Chan FK, Griffiths S, Sung JJ. Cigarette smoking and the risk of colorectal cancer: a meta-analysis of prospective cohort studies. *Clin Gastroenterol Hepatol* 2009;**7**:682, e1.

71. Poynter JN, Haile RW, Siegmund KD, et al. Associations between smoking, alcohol consumption, and colorectal cancer, overall and by tumor microsatellite instability status. *Cancer Epidemiol Biomarkers Prev* 2009;**18**:2745.

72. Leufkens AM, Van Duijnhoven FJ, Siersema PD, et al. Cigarette smoking and colorectal cancer risk in the European prospective investigation into cancer and nutrition study. *Clin Gastroenterol Hepatol* 2011;**9**:137.

73. Slattery ML, Curtin K, Anderson K, et al. Associations between cigarette smoking, lifestyle factors, and microsatellite instability in colon tumors. *J Natl Cancer Inst* 2000;**92**:1831.

74. Diergaarde B, Vrieling A, van Kraats AA, van Muijen GN, Kok FJ, Kampman E. Cigarette smoking and genetic alterations in sporadic colon carcinomas. *Carcinogenesis* 2003;**24**:565.

75. Chia VM, Newcomb PA, Bigler J, Morimoto LM, Thibodeau SN, Potter JD. Risk of microsatellite-unstable colorectal cancer is associated jointly with smoking and nonsteroidal anti-inflammatory drug use. *Cancer Res* 2006;**66**:6877.

76. Swede H, Bartos JD, Chen N, et al. Genomic profiles of colorectal cancers differ based on patient smoking status. *Cancer Genet Cytogenet* 2006;**168**:98.

77. Curtin K, Samowitz WS, Wolff RK, Herrick J, Caan BJ, Slattery ML. Somatic alterations, metabolizing genes and smoking in rectal cancer. *Int J Cancer* 2009;**125**:158.

78. Limsui D, Vierkant RA, Tillmans LS, et al. Cigarette smoking and colorectal cancer risk by molecularly defined subtypes. *J Natl Cancer Inst* 2010;**102**:1012.

79. Larsson SC, Orsini N, Wolk A. Vitamin B_6 and risk of colorectal cancer: a meta-analysis of prospective studies. *JAMA* 2010; **303**:1077.

80. Lechand L, White KK, Nomura AM, et al. Plasma levels of B vitamins and colorectal cancer risk: the multiethnic cohort study. *Cancer Epidemiol Biomarkers Prev* 2009;**18**:2195.

81. Figueiredo JC, Levine AJ, Grau MV, et al. Vitamins B_2, B_6, and B_{12} and risk of new colorectal adenomas in a randomized trial of aspirin use and folic acid supplementation. *Cancer Epidemiol Biomarkers Prev* 2008;**17**:2136.

82. Gonzalez MJ, Miranda-Massari JR, Duconge J. Vitamin C and cancer: what can we conclude – 1,609 patients and 33 years later: comment on the article by Cabanillas. *P R Health Sci J* 2010;**29**:410; author reply 1.

83. Kune G, Watson L. Colorectal cancer protective effects and the dietary micronutrients folate, methionine, vitamins B_6, B_{12}, C, E, selenium, and lycopene. *Nutr Cancer* 2006;**56**:11.

84. Rheem DS, Baylink DJ, Olafsson S, Jackson CS, Walter MH. Prevention of colorectal cancer with vitamin D. *Scand J Gastroenterol* 2010;**45**:775.

85. Wallace K, Baron JA, Cole BF, et al. Effect of calcium supplementation on the risk of large bowel polyps. *J Natl Cancer Inst* 2004;**96**:921.

86. Hofstad B, Vatn MH, Andersen SN, Owen RW, Larsen S, Osnes M. The relationship between faecal bile acid profile with or without supplementation with calcium and antioxidants on recurrence and growth of colorectal polyps. *Eur J Cancer Prev* 1998;**7**:287.

87. Weisgerber UM, Boeing H, Owen RW, Waldherr R, Raedsch R, Wahrendorf J. Effect of longterm placebo controlled calcium supplementation on sigmoidal cell proliferation in patients with sporadic adenomatous polyps. *Gut* 1996;**38**:396.

88. Thomas MG, Thomson JP, Williamson RC. Oral calcium inhibits rectal epithelial proliferation in familial adenomatous polyposis. *Br J Surg* 1993;**80**:499.

89. Logan RF, Grainge MJ, Shepherd VC, Armitage NC, Muir KR. Aspirin and folic acid for the prevention of recurrent colorectal adenomas. *Gastroenterology* 2008;**134**:29.

90. Paspatis GA, Karamanolis DG. Folate supplementation and adenomatous colonic polyps. *Dis Colon Rectum* 1994;**37**:1340.

91. Jaszewski R, Misra S, Tobi M, et al. Folic acid supplementation inhibits recurrence of colorectal adenomas: a randomized chemoprevention trial. *World J Gastroenterol* 2008;**14**:4492.

92. Cole BF, Baron JA, Sandler RS, et al. Folic acid for the prevention of colorectal adenomas: a randomized clinical trial. *JAMA* 2007;**297**:2351.

93. Van Guelpen B, Hultdin J, Johansson I, et al. Low folate levels may protect against colorectal cancer. *Gut* 2006;**55**:1461.

94. Flood A, Mason JB, Liu Z, et al. Concentration of folate in colorectal tissue biopsies predicts prevalence of adenomatous polyps. *Gut* 2011;**60**:66.

95. Kennedy DA, Stern SJ, Moretti M, et al. Folate intake and the risk of colorectal cancer: A systematic review and meta-analysis. *Cancer Epidemiol* 2011;**35**:2.

96. Shamberger RJ. Relationship of selenium to cancer. I. Inhibitory effect of selenium on carcinogenesis. *J Natl Cancer Inst* 1970;**44**:931.

97. Soullier BK, Wilson PS, Nigro ND. Effect of selenium on azoxymethane-induced intestinal cancer in rats fed high fat diet. *Cancer Lett* 1981;**12**:343.

98. Hu Y, McIntosh GH, Le Leu RK, Woodman R, Young GP. Suppression of colorectal oncogenesis by selenium-enriched milk proteins: apoptosis and K-ras mutations. *Cancer Res* 2008;**68**:4936.

99. Fang W, Goldberg ML, Pohl NM, et al. Functional and physical interaction between the selenium-binding protein 1 (SBP1) and the glutathione peroxidase 1 selenoprotein. *Carcinogenesis* 2010;**31**:1360.

100. Nelson RL. Is the changing pattern of colorectal cancer caused by selenium deficiency? *Dis Colon Rectum* 1984;**27**:459.

101. Virtamo J, Valkeila E, Alfthan G, Punsar S, Huttunen JK, Karvonen MJ. Serum selenium and risk of cancer. A prospective follow-up of nine years. *Cancer* 1987;**60**:145.

102. Williams CD, Satia JA, Adair LS, et al. Antioxidant and DNA methylation-related nutrients and risk of distal colorectal cancer. *Cancer Causes Control* 2010;**21**:1171.

103. Bristol JB, Emmett PM, Heaton KW, Williamson RC. Sugar, fat, and the risk of colorectal cancer. *BMJ (Clin Res Ed)* 1985;**291**:1467.

104. Macquart-Moulin G, Riboli E, Cornee J, Kaaks R, Berthezene P. Colorectal polyps and diet: a case-control study. *Int J Cancer* 1987;**40**:179.

105. Terry PD, Jain M, Miller AB, Howe GR, Rohan TE. Glycemic load, carbohydrate intake, and risk of colorectal cancer in women: a prospective cohort study. *J Natl Cancer Inst* 2003;**95**:914.

106. Wattenberg LW. Studies of polycyclic hydrocarbon hydroxylases of the intestine possibly related to cancer. Effect of diet on benzpyrene hydroxylase activity. *Cancer* 1971;**28**:99.

107. Arikawa AY, Gallaher DD. Cruciferous vegetables reduce morphological markers of colon cancer risk in dimethylhydrazine-treated rats. *J Nutr* 2008;**138**:526.

108. Nakamura Y, Yogosawa S, Izutani Y, Watanabe H, Otsuji E, Sakai T. A combination of indol-3-carbinol and genistein synergistically induces apoptosis in human colon cancer HT-29 cells by inhibiting Akt phosphorylation and progression of autophagy. *Mol Cancer* 2009;**8**:100.

109. Kim MK, Park JH. Conference on 'Multidisciplinary approaches to nutritional problems'. Symposium on 'Nutrition and health'. Cruciferous vegetable intake and the risk of human cancer: epidemiological evidence. *BMJ* 2009;**68**:103.

110. Ritchie KJ, Walsh S, Sansom OJ, Henderson CJ, Wolf CR. Markedly enhanced colon tumorigenesis in Apc(Min) mice lacking glutathione S-transferase Pi. *Proc Natl Acad Sci U S A* 2009;**106**:20859.

111. Thun MJ, Namboodiri MM, Heath CW Jr. Aspirin use and reduced risk of fatal colon cancer. *N Engl J Med* 1991;**325**:1593.

112. Rosenberg L, Palmer JR, Zauber AG, Warshauer ME, Stolley PD, Shapiro S. A hypothesis: nonsteroidal anti-inflammatory drugs reduce the incidence of large-bowel cancer. *J Natl Cancer Inst* 1991;**83**:355.

113. Logan RF, Little J, Hawtin PG, Hardcastle JD. Effect of aspirin and non-steroidal anti-inflammatory drugs on colorectal adenomas: case-control study of subjects participating in the Nottingham faecal occult blood screening programme. *BMJ* 1993;**307**:285.

114. Rothwell PM, Fowkes FG, Belch JF, Ogawa H, Warlow CP, Meade TW. Effect of daily aspirin on long-term risk of death due to cancer: analysis of individual patient data from randomised trials. *Lancet* 2011;**377**:31.

115. Din FV, Theodoratou E, Farrington SM, et al. Effect of aspirin and NSAIDs on risk and survival from colorectal cancer. *Gut* 2010;**59**:1670.

116. Benamouzig R, Uzzan B, Martin A, et al. Cyclooxygenase-2 expression and recurrence of colorectal adenomas: effect of aspirin chemoprevention. *Gut* 2010;**59**:622.

117. Vatn MH, Stalsberg H. The prevalence of polyps of the large intestine in Oslo: an autopsy study. *Cancer* 1982;**49**:819.

118. O'Brien MJ, Winawer SJ, Zauber AG, et al. The National Polyp Study. Patient and polyp characteristics associated with high-grade dysplasia in colorectal adenomas. *Gastroenterology* 1990;**98**:371.

119. Correa P, Strong JP, Reif A, Johnson WD. The epidemiology of colorectal polyps: prevalence in New Orleans and international comparisons. *Cancer* 1977;**39**:2258.

120. Davidson M, Yoshizawa CN, Kolonel LN. Do sex hormones affect colorectal cancer? *BMJ (Clin Res Ed)* 1985;**290**:1868.

121. Agrez MV, Spencer RJ. Estrogen receptor protein in adenomas of the large bowel. *Dis Colon Rectum* 1982;**25**:348.

122. Jass JR, Young PJ, Robinson EM. Predictors of presence, multiplicity, size and dysplasia of colorectal adenomas. A necropsy study in New Zealand. *Gut* 1992;**33**:1508.

123. Tsilidis KK, Allen NE, Key TJ, et al. Oral contraceptives, reproductive history and risk of colorectal cancer in the European Prospective Investigation into Cancer and Nutrition. *Br J Cancer* 2010;**103**:1755.

124. Bosetti C, Bravi F, Negri E, La Vecchia C. Oral contraceptives and colorectal cancer risk: a systematic review and meta-analysis. *Hum Reprod Update* 2009;**15**:489.

125. Kabat GC, Miller AB, Rohan TE. Oral contraceptive use, hormone replacement therapy, reproductive history and risk of colorectal cancer in women. *Int J Cancer* 2008;**122**:643.

126. Long MD, Martin CF, Galanko JA, Sandler RS. Hormone replacement therapy, oral contraceptive use, and distal large bowel cancer: a population-based case-control study. *Am J Gastroenterol* 2010;**105**:1843.

127. Gao RN, Neutel CI, Wai E. Gender differences in colorectal cancer incidence, mortality, hospitalizations and surgical procedures in Canada. *J Public Health (Oxf)* 2008;**30**:194.

128. Klein I, Parveen G, Gavaler JS, Vanthiel DH. Colonic polyps in patients with acromegaly. *Ann Intern Med* 1982;**97**:27.

129. Rokkas T, Pistiolas D, Sechopoulos P, Margantinis G, Koukoulis G. Risk of colorectal neoplasm in patients with acromegaly: a meta-analysis. *World J Gastroenterol* 2008;**14**:3484.

130. Bertrand C, Kowalski-Chauvel A, Do C, et al. A gastrin precursor, gastrin-Gly, upregulates VEGF expression in colonic epithelial cells through an HIF-1-independent mechanism. *Int J Cancer* 2010;**126**:2847.

131. Kovac S, Xiao L, Shulkes A, Patel O, Baldwin GS. Gastrin increases its own synthesis in gastrointestinal cancer cells via the CCK2 receptor. *FEBS Lett* 2010;**584**:4413.

132. Wu P, Mao JD, Yan JY, et al. Correlation between the expressions of gastrin, somatostatin and cyclin and cyclin-depend kinase in colorectal cancer. *World J Gastroenterol* 2005;**11**:7211.

133. D'Onghia V, Leoncini R, Carli R, et al. Circulating gastrin and ghrelin levels in patients with colorectal cancer: correlation with tumour stage, *Helicobacter pylori* infection and BMI. *Biomed Pharmacother* 2007;**61**:137.

134. Robertson DJ, Sandler RS, Ahnen DJ, et al. Gastrin, *Helicobacter pylori*, and colorectal adenomas. *Clin Gastroenterol Hepatol* 2009; **7**:163.

135. Poulsen ML, Bisgaard ML. MUTYH associated polyposis (MAP). *Curr Genom* 2008;**9**:420.

136. Groden J, Thliveris A, Samowitz W, et al. Identification and characterization of the familial adenomatous polyposis coli gene. *Cell* 1991;**66**:589.

137. Leach FS, Nicolaides NC, Papadopoulos N, et al. Mutations of a mutS homolog in hereditary nonpolyposis colorectal cancer. *Cell* 1993;**75**:1215.

138. Merg A, Howe JR. Genetic conditions associated with intestinal juvenile polyps. *Am J Med Genet C Semin Med Genet* 2004; **129C**:44.

139. Hobert JA, Eng C. PTEN hamartoma tumor syndrome: an overview. *Genet Med* 2009;**11**:687.

140. Jeevaratnam P, Cottier DS, Browett PJ, Van De Water NS, Pokos V, Jass JR. Familial giant hyperplastic polyposis predisposing to colorectal cancer: a new hereditary bowel cancer syndrome. *J Pathol* 1996;**179**:20.

141. Sampson JR, Jones N. MUTYH-associated polyposis. *Best Pract Res Clin Gastroenterol* 2009;**23**:209.

142. Vogt S, Jones N, Christian D, et al. Expanded extracolonic tumor spectrum in MUTYH-associated polyposis. *Gastroenterology* 2009;**137**:1976, e1.

143. Hamilton SR, Liu B, Parsons RE, et al. The molecular basis of Turcot's syndrome. *N Engl J Med* 1995;**332**:839.

144. Weitzer M, Pokos V, Jeevaratnam P, Van De Water NS, Browett PJ, Jass JR. Isolated expression of the Muir-Torre phenotype in a member of a family with hereditary non-polyposis colorectal cancer. *Histopathology* 1995;**27**:573.

145. Laken SJ, Petersen GM, Gruber SB, et al. Familial colorectal cancer in Ashkenazim due to a hypermutable tract in APC. *Nat Genet* 1997;**17**:79.

146. Zauber NP, Sabbath-Solitare M, Marotta S, et al. Clinical and genetic findings in an Ashkenazi Jewish population with colorectal neoplasms. *Cancer* 2005;**104**:719.

147. Azzopardi D, Dallosso AR, Eliason K, et al. Multiple rare nonsynonymous variants in the adenomatous polyposis coli gene predispose to colorectal adenomas. *Cancer Res* 2008;**68**:358.

148. Hitchins M, Williams R, Cheong K, et al. MLH1 germline epimutations as a factor in hereditary nonpolyposis colorectal cancer. *Gastroenterology* 2005;**129**:1392.

149. Hitchins MP, Ward RL. Constitutional (germline) MLH1 epimutation as an aetiological mechanism for hereditary nonpolyposis colorectal cancer. *J Med Genet* 2009;**46**:793.

150. Suter CM, Martin DI, Ward RL. Germline epimutation of MLH1 in individuals with multiple cancers. *Nat Genet* 2004; **36**:497.

151. Houlston RS, Murday V, Harocopos C, Williams CB, Slack J. Screening and genetic counselling for relatives of patients with colorectal cancer in a family cancer clinic. *BMJ* 1990; **301**:366.

152. Kerber RA, O'Brien E. A cohort study of cancer risk in relation to family histories of cancer in the Utah population database. *Cancer* 2005;**103**:1906.

153. Cannon-Albright LA, Skolnick MH, Bishop DT, Lee RG, Burt RW. Common inheritance of susceptibility to colonic adenomatous polyps and associated colorectal cancers. *N Engl J Med* 1988;**319**:533.

154. Burt RW, DiSario JA, Cannon-Albright L. Genetics of colon cancer: impact of inheritance on colon cancer risk. *Annu Rev Med* 1995;**46**:371.

155. Boutron MC, Faivre J, Quipourt V, Senesse P, Michiels C. Family history of colorectal tumours and implications for the adenoma-carcinoma sequence: a case control study. *Gut* 1995; **37**:830.

156. Vasen HF, Taal BG, Griffioen G, et al. Clinical heterogeneity of familial colorectal cancer and its influence on screening protocols. *Gut* 1994;**35**:1262.

157. Jass JR, Pokos V, Arnold JL, et al. Colorectal neoplasms detected colonoscopically in at-risk members of colorectal cancer families stratified by the demonstration of DNA microsatellite instability. *J Mol Med* 1996;**74**:547.

158. Fearnhead NS, Wilding JL, Winney B, et al. Multiple rare variants in different genes account for multifactorial inherited susceptibility to colorectal adenomas. *Proc Natl Acad Sci USA* 2004;**101**:15992.

159. Tenesa A, Farrington SM, Prendergast JG, et al. Genome-wide association scan identifies a colorectal cancer susceptibility locus on 11q23 and replicates risk loci at 8q24 and 18q21. *Nature Genet* 2008;**40**:631.

160. Poynter JN, Figueiredo JC, Conti DV, et al. Variants on 9p24 and 8q24 are associated with risk of colorectal cancer: results from the Colon Cancer Family Registry. *Cancer Res* 2007;**67**: 11128.

161. Li L, Plummer SJ, Thompson CL, et al. A common 8q24 variant and the risk of colon cancer: a population-based case-control study. Cancer epidemiology, biomarkers and prevention: a publication of the American Association for Cancer Research, cosponsored by the American Society of Preventive Oncology. *Cancer Epidemiol Biomarkers Prev* 2008;**17**:339.

162. He J, Wilkens LR, Stram DO, et al. Generalizability and epidemiologic characterization of eleven colorectal cancer GWAS hits in multiple populations. *Cancer epidemiology, biomarkers and prevention: a publication of the American Association for Cancer Research, cosponsored by the American Society of Preventive Oncology.* 2011;**20**:70.

163. Cui R, Okada Y, Jang SG, et al. Common variant in 6q26-q27 is associated with distal colon cancer in an Asian population. *Gut* 2011;**60**:799.

164. Kupfer SS, Anderson JR, Hooker S, et al. Genetic heterogeneity in colorectal cancer associations between African and European Americans. *Gastroenterology* 2010;**139**:1677, e1.

165. Lang NP, Chu DZ, Hunter CF, Kendall DC, Flammang TJ, Kadlubar FF. Role of aromatic amine acetyltransferase in human colorectal cancer. *Arch Surg* 1986;**121**:1259.

166. Ilett KF, David BM, Detchon P, Castleden WM, Kwa R. Acetylation phenotype in colorectal carcinoma. *Cancer Res* 1987;**47**: 1466.

167. Shibuta K, Nakashima T, Abe M, et al. Molecular genotyping for N-acetylation polymorphism in Japanese patients with colorectal cancer. *Cancer* 1994;**74**:3108.

168. Little J, Faivre J. Family history, metabolic gene polymorphism, diet and risk of colorectal cancer. *Eur J Cancer Prev* 1999; **8**(suppl 1):S61.

169. Bell DA, Stephens EA, Castranio T, et al. Polyadenylation polymorphism in the acetyltransferase 1 gene (NAT1) increases risk of colorectal cancer. *Cancer Res* 1995;**55**:3537.

170. Nothlings U, Yamamoto JF, Wilkens LR, et al. Meat and heterocyclic amine intake, smoking, NAT1 and NAT2 polymorphisms, and colorectal cancer risk in the multiethnic cohort study. *Cancer Epidemiol Biomarkers Prev* 2009;**18**:2098.

171. Strange RC, Matharoo B, Faulder GC, et al. The human glutathione S-transferases: a case-control study of the incidence of the GST1 0 phenotype in patients with adenocarcinoma. *Carcinogenesis* 1991;**12**:25.

172. Szarka CE, Pfeiffer GR, Hum ST, et al. Glutathione S-transferase activity and glutathione S-transferase mu expression in subjects with risk for colorectal cancer. *Cancer Res* 1995;**55**:2789.

173. Chenevix-Trench G, Young J, Coggan M, Board P. Glutathione S-transferase M1 and T1 polymorphisms: susceptibility to colon cancer and age of onset. *Carcinogenesis* 1995;**16**:1655.

174. Gao Y, Cao Y, Tan A, Liao C, Mo Z, Gao F. Glutathione S-transferase M1 polymorphism and sporadic colorectal cancer risk: An updating meta-analysis and HuGE review of 36 case-control studies. *Ann Epidemiol* 2010;**20**:108.

175. Chen J, Giovannucci E, Kelsey K, et al. A methylenetetrahydrofolate reductase polymorphism and the risk of colorectal cancer. *Cancer Res* 1996;**56**:4862.

176. Ma J, Stampfer MJ, Giovannucci E, et al. Methylenetetrahydrofolate reductase polymorphism, dietary interactions, and risk of colorectal cancer. *Cancer Res* 1997;**57**:1098.

177. Hubner RA, Houlston RS. MTHFR C677T and colorectal cancer risk: A meta-analysis of 25 populations. *Int J Cancer* 2007;**120**:1027.

178. Kervinen K, Sodervik H, Makela J, et al. Is the development of adenoma and carcinoma in proximal colon related to apolipoprotein E phenotype? *Gastroenterology* 1996;**110**:1785.

179. Mrkonjic M, Chappell E, Pethe VV, et al. Association of apolipoprotein E polymorphisms and dietary factors in colorectal cancer. *Br J Cancer* 2009;**100**:1966.

180. Sivaraman L, Leatham MP, Yee J, Wilkens LR, Lau AF, Lechand L. CYP1A1 genetic polymorphisms and in situ colorectal cancer. *Cancer Res* 1994;**54**:3692.

181. Bethke L, Webb E, Sellick G, et al. Polymorphisms in the cytochrome P450 genes *CYP1A2, CYP1B1, CYP3A4, CYP3A5, CYP11A1, CYP17A1, CYP19A1* and colorectal cancer risk. *BMC Cancer* 2007;**7**:123.

182. Habano W, Gamo T, Sugai T, Otsuka K, Wakabayashi G, Ozawa S. *CYP1B1*, but not *CYP1A1*, is downregulated by promoter methylation in colorectal cancers. *Int J Oncol* 2009;**34**:1085.

183. Jass JR. Classification of colorectal cancer based on correlation of clinical, morphological and molecular features. *Histopathology* 2007;**50**:113.

184. Snover DC. Update on the serrated pathway to colorectal carcinoma. *Hum Pathol* 2011;**42**:1.

185. O'Brien M J. The serrated polyp pathway to colorectal carcinoma. *Diagn Histopathol* 2008;**14**:78.

186. Tops CM, Wijnen JT, Hes FJ. Introduction to molecular and clinical genetics of colorectal cancer syndromes. *Best Pract Res Clin Gastroenterol* 2009;**23**:127.

187. Muto T, Bussey HJ, Morson BC. The evolution of cancer of the colon and rectum. *Cancer* 1975;**36**:2251.

188. Kinzler KW, Nilbert MC, Vogelstein B, et al. Identification of a gene located at chromosome 5q21 that is mutated in colorectal cancers. *Science* 1991;**251**:1366.

189. Bodmer WF, Bailey CJ, Bodmer J, et al. Localization of the gene for familial adenomatous polyposis on chromosome 5. *Nature* 1987;**328**:614.

190. Leppert M, Dobbs M, Scambler P, et al. The gene for familial polyposis coli maps to the long arm of chromosome 5. *Science* 1987;**238**:1411.

191. Galiatsatos P, Foulkes WD. Familial adenomatous polyposis. *Am J Gastroenterol* 2006;**101**:385.

192. Beroud C, Soussi T. *APC* gene: database of germline and somatic mutations in human tumors and cell lines. *Nucleic Acids Res* 1996;**24**:121.

193. Gomez-Fernandez N, Castellvi-Bel S, et al. Molecular analysis of the *APC* and *MUTYH* genes in Galician and Catalonian FAP families: a different spectrum of mutations? *BMC Med Genet* 2009;**10**:57.

194. Hes FJ, Nielsen M, Bik EC, et al. Somatic APC mosaicism: an underestimated cause of polyposis coli. *Gut* 2008;**57**:71.

195. Kaufmann A, Vogt S, Uhlhaas S, et al. Analysis of rare APC variants at the mRNA level: six pathogenic mutations and literature review. *J Mol Diagn* 2009;**11**:131.

196. Nieuwenhuis MH, Bulow S, Bjork J, et al. Genotype predicting phenotype in familial adenomatous polyposis: a practical application to the choice of surgery. *Dis Colon Rectum* 2009;**52**:1259.

197. Will OC, Leedham SJ, Elia G, Phillips RK, Clark SK, Tomlinson IP. Location in the large bowel influences the APC mutations observed in FAP adenomas. *Fam Cancer* 2010;**9**:389.

198. Lamlum H, Ilyas M, Rowan A, et al. The type of somatic mutation at APC in familial adenomatous polyposis is determined by the site of the germline mutation: a new facet to Knudson's 'two-hit' hypothesis. *Nat Med* 1999;**5**:1071.

199. Crabtree M, Sieber OM, Lipton L, et al. Refining the relation between 'first hits' and 'second hits' at the APC locus: the 'loose fit' model and evidence for differences in somatic mutation spectra among patients. *Oncogene* 2003;**22**:4257.

200. Albuquerque C, Breukel C, van der Luijt R, et al. The 'just-right' signaling model: APC somatic mutations are selected based on a specific level of activation of the beta-catenin signaling cascade. *Hum Mol Genet* 2002;**11**:1549.

201. Levy DB, Smith KJ, Beazer-Barclay Y, Hamilton SR, Vogelstein B, Kinzler KW. Inactivation of both APC alleles in human and mouse tumors. *Cancer Res* 1994;**54**:5953.

202. Ichii S, Horii A, Nakatsuru S, Furuyama J, Utsunomiya J, Nakamura Y. Inactivation of both APC alleles in an early stage of colon adenomas in a patient with familial adenomatous polyposis (FAP). *Hum Mol Genet* 1992;**1**:387.

203. Moser AR, Mattes EM, Dove WF, Lindstrom MJ, Haag JD, Gould MN. ApcMin, a mutation in the murine Apc gene, predisposes to mammary carcinomas and focal alveolar hyperplasias. *Proc Natl Acad Sci U S A* 1993;**90**:8977.

204. Aoki K, Taketo MM. Adenomatous polyposis coli (APC): a multi-functional tumor suppressor gene. *J Cell Sci* 2007;**120**(Part 19):3327.

205. Barker N. The canonical Wnt/beta-catenin signalling pathway. *Methods Mol Biol* 2008;**468**:5.

206. Bienz M, Clevers H. Linking colorectal cancer to Wnt signaling. *Cell* 2000;**103**:311.

207. Clevers H. Wnt/beta-catenin signaling in development and disease. *Cell* 2006;**127**:469.

208. Morin PJ, Sparks AB, Korinek V, et al. Activation of beta-catenin-Tcf signaling in colon cancer by mutations in beta-catenin or APC. *Science* 1997;**275**:1787.

209. Polakis P. The oncogenic activation of beta-catenin. *Curr Opin Genet Dev* 1999;**9**:15.

210. Polakis P. The many ways of Wnt in cancer. *Curr Opin Genet Dev* 2007;**17**:45.

211. He TC, Sparks AB, Rago C, et al. Identification of c-MYC as a target of the APC pathway. *Science* 1998;**281**:1509.

212. Wilkins JA, Sansom OJ. C-Myc is a critical mediator of the phenotypes of Apc loss in the intestine. *Cancer Res* 2008;**68**:4963.

213. Wielenga VJ, Smits R, Korinek V, et al. Expression of CD44 in Apc and Tcf mutant mice implies regulation by the WNT pathway. *Am J Pathol* 1999;**154**:515.

214. Janssen KP, Alberici P, Fsihi H, et al. *APC* and oncogenic *KRAS* are synergistic in enhancing Wnt signaling in intestinal tumor formation and progression. *Gastroenterology* 2006;**131**:1096.

215. Fearon ER. Molecular genetics of colorectal cancer. *Annu Rev Pathol* 2011;**6**:479.

216. Bienz M, Hamada F. Adenomatous polyposis coli proteins and cell adhesion. *Curr Opin Cell Biol* 2004;**16**:528.

217. Ashton GH, Morton JP, Myant K, et al. Focal adhesion kinase is required for intestinal regeneration and tumorigenesis downstream of Wnt/c-Myc signaling. *Dev Cell* 2010;**19**:259.

218. Carothers AM, Melstrom KA Jr, Mueller JD, Weyant MJ, Bertagnolli MM. Progressive changes in adherens junction structure during intestinal adenoma formation in Apc mutant mice. *J Biol Chem* 2001;**276**:39094.

219. Nathke I. Cytoskeleton out of the cupboard: colon cancer and cytoskeletal changes induced by loss of APC. *Nat Rev Cancer* 2006;**6**:967.

220. Li Z, Kroboth K, Newton IP, Nathke IS, et al. self-association of the APC molecule affects APC clusters and cell migration. *J Cell Sci* 2008;**121**(Part 11):1916.

221. Mili S, Moissoglu K, Macara IG. Genome-wide screen reveals APC-associated RNAs enriched in cell protrusions. *Nature* 2008;**453**:115.

222. Jaiswal AS, Narayan S. A novel function of adenomatous polyposis coli (APC) in regulating DNA repair. *Cancer Lett* 2008;**271**:272.

223. Beamish H, de Boer L, Giles N, Stevens F, Oakes V, Gabrielli B. Cyclin A/cdk2 regulates adenomatous polyposis coli-dependent mitotic spindle anchoring. *J Biol Chem* 2009;**284**:29015.

224. Rusan NM, Peifer M, Original CIN: reviewing roles for APC in chromosome instability. *J Cell Biol* 2008;**181**:719.

225. Draviam VM, Shapiro I, Aldridge B, Sorger PK. Misorientation and reduced stretching of aligned sister kinetochores promote chromosome missegregation in EB1- or APC-depleted cells. *EMBO J* 2006;**25**:2814.

226. Green RA, Kaplan KB. Chromosome instability in colorectal tumor cells is associated with defects in microtubule plus-end attachments caused by a dominant mutation in APC. *J Cell Biol* 2003;**163**:949.

227. Green RA, Wollman R, Kaplan KB. APC and EB1 function together in mitosis to regulate spindle dynamics and chromosome alignment. *Mol Biol Cell* 2005;**16**:4609.

228. Anderson CB, Neufeld KL, White RL. Subcellular distribution of Wnt pathway proteins in normal and neoplastic colon. *Proc Natl Acad Sci U S A* 2002;**99**:8683.

229. Blaker H, Scholten M, Sutter C, Otto HF, Penzel R. Somatic mutations in familial adenomatous polyps. Nuclear translocation of beta-catenin requires more than biallelic APC inactivation. *Am J Clin Pathol* 2003;**120**:418.

230. Inomata M, Ochiai A, Akimoto S, Kitano S, Hirohashi S. Alteration of beta-catenin expression in colonic epithelial cells of familial adenomatous polyposis patients. *Cancer Res* 1996;**56**:2213.

231. Takayama T, Ohi M, Hayashi T, et al. Analysis of K-ras, APC, and beta-catenin in aberrant crypt foci in sporadic adenoma, cancer, and familial adenomatous polyposis. *Gastroenterology* 2001;**121**:599.

232. Phelps RA, Chidester S, Dehghanizadeh S, et al. A two-step model for colon adenoma initiation and progression caused by APC loss. *Cell* 2009;**137**:623.

233. Obrador-Hevia A, Chin SF, Gonzalez S, et al. Oncogenic KRAS is not necessary for Wnt signalling activation in APC-associated FAP adenomas. *J Pathol* 2010;**221**:57.

234. Pollard P, Deheragoda M, Segditsas S, et al. The Apc 1322T mouse develops severe polyposis associated with submaximal nuclear beta-catenin expression. *Gastroenterology* 2009;**136**:2204, e1.

235. Lewis A, Segditsas S, Deheragoda M, et al. Severe polyposis in Apc(1322T) mice is associated with submaximal Wnt signalling and increased expression of the stem cell marker Lgr5. *Gut* 2010;**59**:1680.

236. Lipkin M. Phase 1 and phase 2 proliferative lesions of colonic epithelial cells in diseases leading to colonic cancer. *Cancer* 1974;**34**(suppl):878.

237. Nakamura S, Kino I, Baba S. Nuclear DNA content of isolated crypts of background colonic mucosa from patients with familial adenomatous polyposis and sporadic colorectal cancer. *Gut* 1993;**34**:1240.

238. Potten CS, Kellett M, Rew DA, Roberts SA. Proliferation in human gastrointestinal epithelium using bromodeoxyuridine in vivo: data for different sites, proximity to a tumour, and polyposis coli. *Gut* 1992;**33**:524.

239. Mills SJ, Shepherd NA, Hall PA, Hastings A, Mathers JC, Gunn A. Proliferative compartment deregulation in the non-neoplastic colonic epithelium of familial adenomatous polyposis. *Gut* 1995;**36**:391.

240. Wasan HS, Park HS, Liu KC, et al. APC in the regulation of intestinal crypt fission. *J Pathol* 1998;**185**:246.

241. Campbell F, Geraghty JM, Appleton MA, Williams ED, Williams GT. Increased stem cell somatic mutation in the non-neoplastic colorectal mucosa of patients with familial adenomatous polyposis. *Hum Pathol* 1998;**29**:1531.

242. Keller JJ, Offerhaus GJ, Polak M, et al. Rectal epithelial apoptosis in familial adenomatous polyposis patients treated with sulindac. *Gut* 1999;**45**:822.

243. Yeung AT, Patel BB, Li XM, et al. One-hit effects in cancer: altered proteome of morphologically normal colon crypts in familial adenomatous polyposis. *Cancer Res* 2008;**68**:7579.

244. Khare S, Chaudhary K, Bissonnette M, Carroll R. Aberrant crypt foci in colon cancer epidemiology. *Methods Mol Biol* 2009;**472**:373.

245. Bird RP. Observation and quantification of aberrant crypts in the murine colon treated with a colon carcinogen: preliminary findings. *Cancer Lett* 1987;**37**:147.

246. Pretlow TP, Barrow BJ, Ashton WS, et al. Aberrant crypts: putative preneoplastic foci in human colonic mucosa. *Cancer Res* 1991;**51**:1564.

247. Roncucci L, Stamp D, Medline A, Cullen JB, Bruce WR. Identification and quantification of aberrant crypt foci and microadenomas in the human colon. *Hum Pathol* 1991;**22**:287.

248. Paulsen JE, Namork E, Steffensen IL, Eide TJ, Alexander J. Identification and quantification of aberrant crypt foci in the colon of Min mice – a murine model of familial adenomatous polyposis. *Scand J Gastroenterol* 2000;**35**:534.

249. Kukitsu T, Takayama T, Miyanishi K, et al. Aberrant crypt foci as precursors of the dysplasia-carcinoma sequence in patients with ulcerative colitis. *Clin Cancer Res* 2008;**14**:48.

250. Jen J, Powell SM, Papadopoulos N, et al. Molecular determinants of dysplasia in colorectal lesions. *Cancer Res* 1994;**54**:5523.

251. Nucci MR, Robinson CR, Longo P, Campbell P, Hamilton SR. Phenotypic and genotypic characteristics of aberrant crypt foci in human colorectal mucosa. *Hum Pathol* 1997;**28**:1396.

252. Rosenberg DW, Yang S, Pleau DC, et al. Mutations in BRAF and KRAS differentially distinguish serrated versus non-serrated hyperplastic aberrant crypt foci in humans. *Cancer Res* 2007;**67**:3551.

253. Beach R, Chan AO, Wu TT, et al. BRAF mutations in aberrant crypt foci and hyperplastic polyposis. *Am J Pathol* 2005;**166**:1069.

254. Gupta AK, Pinsky P, Rall C, et al. Reliability and accuracy of the endoscopic appearance in the identification of aberrant crypt foci. *Gastrointest Endosc* 2009;**70**:322.

255. Gupta AK, Schoen RE. Aberrant crypt foci: are they intermediate endpoints of colon carcinogenesis in humans? *Curr Opin Gastroenterol* 2009;**25**:59.

256. Schoen RE, Mutch M, Rall C, et al. The natural history of aberrant crypt foci. *Gastrointest Endosc* 2008;**67**:1097.

257. Boman BM, Fields JZ, Cavanaugh KL, Guetter A, Runquist OA. How dysregulated colonic crypt dynamics cause stem cell overpopulation and initiate colon cancer. *Cancer Res* 2008;**68**:3304.

258. Ricci-Vitiani L, Pagliuca A, Palio E, Zeuner A, Deia R. Colon cancer stem cells. *Gut* 2008;**57**:538.

259. Leedham SJ, Wright NA. Expansion of a mutated clone: from stem cell to tumour. *J Clin Pathol* 2008;**61**:164.

260. Bjerknes M, Cheng H. Clonal analysis of mouse intestinal epithelial progenitors. *Gastroenterology* 1999;**116**:7.

261. Marshman E, Booth C, Potten CS. The intestinal epithelial stem cell. *Bioessays* 2002;**24**:91.

262. Barker N, van Es JH, Kuipers J, et al. Identification of stem cells in small intestine and colon by marker gene Lgr5. *Nature* 2007;**449**:1003.

263. Brabletz S, Schmalhofer O, Brabletz T. Gastrointestinal stem cells in development and cancer. *J Pathol* 2009;**217**:307.

264. Zeki SS, Graham TA, Wright NA. Stem cells and their implications for colorectal cancer. *Nat Rev Gastroenterol Hepatol* 2011;**8**:90.

265. Kim KM, Calabrese P, Tavare S, Shibata D. Enhanced stem cell survival in familial adenomatous polyposis. *Am J Pathol* 2004;**164**:1369.

266. van de Wetering M, Sancho E, Verweij C, et al. The beta-catenin/TCF-4 complex imposes a crypt progenitor phenotype on colorectal cancer cells. *Cell* 2002;**111**:241.

267. Sansom OJ, Reed KR, Hayes AJ, et al. Loss of Apc in vivo immediately perturbs Wnt signaling, differentiation, and migration. *Genes Dev* 2004;**18**:1385.

268. Boman BM, Walters R, Fields JZ, et al. Colonic crypt changes during adenoma development in familial adenomatous polyposis: immunohistochemical evidence for expansion of the crypt base cell population. *Am J Pathol* 2004;**165**:1489.

269. Preston SL, Wong WM, Chan AO, et al. Bottom-up histogenesis of colorectal adenomas: origin in the monocryptal adenoma and initial expansion by crypt fission. *Cancer Res* 2003;**63**:3819.

270. Barker N, Ridgway RA, van Es JH, et al. Crypt stem cells as the cells-of-origin of intestinal cancer. *Nature* 2009;**457**:608.

271. Greaves LC, Preston SL, Tadrous PJ, et al. Mitochondrial DNA mutations are established in human colonic stem cells, and mutated clones expand by crypt fission. *Proc Natl Acad Sci USA* 2006;**103**:714.

272. Kubota O, Kino I. Minute adenomas of the depressed type in familial adenomatous polyposis of the colon. A pathway to ordinary polypoid adenomas. *Cancer* 1993;**72**:1159.

273. Kubota O, Kino I, Nakamura S. A morphometrical analysis of minute depressed adenomas in familial polyposis coli. *Pathol Int* 1994;**44**:200.

274. Novelli MR, Williamson JA, Tomlinson IP, et al. Polyclonal origin of colonic adenomas in an XO/XY patient with FAP. *Science* 1996;**272**:1187.

275. Thirlwell C, Will OC, Domingo E, et al. Clonality assessment and clonal ordering of individual neoplastic crypts shows polyclonality of colorectal adenomas. *Gastroenterology* 2010;**138**:1441, e1.

276. Lengauer C, Kinzler KW, Vogelstein B. Genetic instabilities in human cancers. *Nature* 1998;**396**:643.

277. Walther A, Houlston R, Tomlinson I. Association between chromosomal instability and prognosis in colorectal cancer: a meta-analysis. *Gut* 2008;**57**:941.

278. Cheng YW, Pincas H, Bacolod MD, et al. CpG island methylator phenotype associates with low-degree chromosomal abnormalities in colorectal cancer. *Clin Cancer Res* 2008;**14**:6005.

279. Thompson SL, Bakhoum SF, Compton DA. Mechanisms of chromosomal instability. *Curr Biol* 2010;**20**:R285.

280. Pino MS, Chung DC. The chromosomal instability pathway in colon cancer. *Gastroenterology* 2010;**138**:2059.

281. Rao CV, Yamada HY, Yao Y, Dai W. Enhanced genomic instabilities caused by deregulated microtubule dynamics and chromosome segregation: a perspective from genetic studies in mice. *Carcinogenesis* 2009;**30**:1469.

282. Muleris M, Salmon RJ, Dutrillaux B. Cytogenetics of colorectal adenocarcinomas. *Cancer Genet Cytogenet* 1990;**46**:143.

283. Sieber OM, Heinimann K, Gorman P, et al. Analysis of chromosomal instability in human colorectal adenomas with two mutational hits at APC. *Proc Natl Acad Sci U S A* 2002;**99**:16910.

284. Fishel R, Lescoe MK, Rao MR, et al. The human mutator gene homolog MSH2 and its association with hereditary nonpolyposis colon cancer. *Cell* 1993;**75**:1027.

285. Papadopoulos N, Nicolaides NC, Wei YF, et al. Mutation of a mutL homolog in hereditary colon cancer. *Science* 1994;**263**:1625.

286. Nicolaides NC, Papadopoulos N, Liu B, et al. Mutations of two PMS homologues in hereditary nonpolyposis colon cancer. *Nature* 1994;**371**:75.

287. Bronner CE, Baker SM, Morrison PT, et al. Mutation in the DNA mismatch repair gene homologue hMLH1 is associated with hereditary non-polyposis colon cancer. *Nature* 1994;**368**:258.

288. Akiyama Y, Sato H, Yamada T, et al. Germ-line mutation of the *hMSH6/GTBP* gene in an atypical hereditary nonpolyposis colorectal cancer kindred. *Cancer Res* 1997;**57**:3920.

289. Peltomaki P. Deficient DNA mismatch repair: a common etiologic factor for colon cancer. *Hum Mol Genet* 2001;**10**:735.

290. Parsons R, Li GM, Longley MJ, et al. Hypermutability and mismatch repair deficiency in RER+ tumor cells. *Cell* 1993;**75**:1227.

291. Poulogiannis G, Frayling IM, Arends MJ. DNA mismatch repair deficiency in sporadic colorectal cancer and Lynch syndrome. *Histopathology* 2010;**56**:167.

292. Fukui K. DNA mismatch repair in eukaryotes and bacteria. *J Nucleic Acids* 2010;2010.

293. Polosina YY, Cupples CG. MutL: conducting the cell's response to mismatched and misaligned DNA. *Bioessays* 2010;**32**:51.

294. Hong Z, Jiang J, Hashiguchi K, Hoshi M, Lan L, Yasui A. Recruitment of mismatch repair proteins to the site of DNA damage in human cells. *J Cell Sci* 2008;**121**(Part 19):3146.

295. Guerrette S, Acharya S, Fishel R. The interaction of the human MutL homologues in hereditary nonpolyposis colon cancer. *J Biol Chem* 1999;**274**:6336.

296. Yuan ZQ, Gottlieb B, Beitel LK, et al. Polymorphisms and HNPCC: PMS2-MLH1 protein interactions diminished by single nucleotide polymorphisms. *Hum Mutat* 2002;**19**:108.

297. Bao F, Panarelli NC, Rennert H, Sherr DL, Yantiss RK. Neoadjuvant therapy induces loss of MSH6 expression in colorectal carcinoma. *Am J Surg Pathol* 2010;**34**:1798.

298. Markowitz S, Wang J, Myeroff L, et al. Inactivation of the type II TGF-beta receptor in colon cancer cells with microsatellite instability. *Science* 1995;**268**:1336.

299. Schwartz S Jr, Yamamoto H, Navarro M, Maestro M, Reventos J, Perucho M. Frameshift mutations at mononucleotide repeats in caspase-5 and other target genes in endometrial and gastrointestinal cancer of the microsatellite mutator phenotype. *Cancer Res* 1999;**59**:2995.

300. Yamamoto H, Sawai H, Perucho M. Frameshift somatic mutations in gastrointestinal cancer of the microsatellite mutator phenotype. *Cancer Res* 1997;**57**:4420.

301. Fang DC, Luo YH, Yang SM, Li XA, Ling XL, Fang L. Mutation analysis of APC gene in gastric cancer with microsatellite instability. *World J Gastroenterol* 2002;**8**:787.

302. Kitaeva MN, Grogan L, Williams JP, et al. Mutations in beta-catenin are uncommon in colorectal cancer occurring in occasional replication error-positive tumors. *Cancer Res* 1997;**57**: 4478.

303. Shimizu Y, Ikeda S, Fujimori M, et al. Frequent alterations in the Wnt signaling pathway in colorectal cancer with microsatellite instability. *Genes Chromosomes Cancer* 2002;**33**:73.

304. Souza RF, Appel R, Yin J, et al. Microsatellite instability in the insulin-like growth factor II receptor gene in gastrointestinal tumours. *Nat Genet* 1996;**14**:255.

305. Rampino N, Yamamoto H, Ionov Y, et al. Somatic frameshift mutations in the *BAX* gene in colon cancers of the microsatellite mutator phenotype. *Science* 1997;**275**:967.

306. Boland CR, Thibodeau SN, Hamilton SR, et al. A National Cancer Institute Workshop on Microsatellite Instability for cancer detection and familial predisposition: development of international criteria for the determination of microsatellite instability in colorectal cancer. *Cancer Res* 1998;**58**:5248.

307. Tomlinson I, Halford S, Aaltonen L, Hawkins N, Ward R. Does MSI-low exist? *J Pathol* 2002;**197**:6.

308. Laiho P, Launonen V, Lahermo P, et al. Low-level microsatellite instability in most colorectal carcinomas. *Cancer Res* 2002;**62**: 1166.

309. Yearsley M, Hampel H, Lehman A, Nakagawa H, de la Chapelle A, Frankel WL. Histologic features distinguish microsatellite-high from microsatellite-low and microsatellite-stable colorectal carcinomas, but do not differentiate germline mutations from methylation of the MLH1 promoter. *Hum Pathol* 2006; **37**:831.

310. Iglesias D, Fernandez-Peralta AM, Nejda N, et al. RIS1, a gene with trinucleotide repeats, is a target in the mutator pathway of colorectal carcinogenesis. *Cancer Genet Cytogenet* 2006;**167**:138.

311. Wright CM, Dent OF, Newland RC, et al. Low level microsatellite instability may be associated with reduced cancer specific survival in sporadic stage C colorectal carcinoma. *Gut* 2005; **54**:103.

312. Kohonen-Corish MR, Daniel JJ, Chan C, et al. Low microsatellite instability is associated with poor prognosis in stage C colon cancer. *J Clin Oncol* 2005;**23**:2318.

313. Nagasaka T, Sasamoto H, Notohara K, et al. Colorectal cancer with mutation in BRAF, KRAS, and wild-type with respect to both oncogenes showing different patterns of DNA methylation. *J Clin Oncol* 2004;**22**:4584.

314. Whitehall VL, Walsh MD, Young J, Leggett BA, Jass JR. Methylation of O-6-methylguanine DNA methyltransferase characterizes a subset of colorectal cancer with low-level DNA microsatellite instability. *Cancer Res* 2001;**61**:827.

315. Konishi M, Kikuchi-Yanoshita R, Tanaka K, et al. Molecular nature of colon tumors in hereditary nonpolyposis colon cancer, familial polyposis, and sporadic colon cancer. *Gastroenterology* 1996;**111**:307.

316. Salahshor S, Kressner U, Pahlman L, Glimelius B, Lindmark G, Lindblom A. Colorectal cancer with and without microsatellite instability involves different genes. *Genes Chromosomes Cancer* 1999;**26**:247.

317. Olschwang S, Hamelin R, Laurent-Puig P, et al. Alternative genetic pathways in colorectal carcinogenesis. *Proc Natl Acad Sci U S A* 1997;**94**:12122.

318. Heinen CD, Richardson D, White R, Groden J. Microsatellite instability in colorectal adenocarcinoma cell lines that have full-length adenomatous polyposis coli protein. *Cancer Res* 1995;**55**:4797.

319. Jass JR, Do KA, Simms LA, et al. Morphology of sporadic colorectal cancer with DNA replication errors. *Gut* 1998;**42**:673.

320. Young J, Leggett B, Gustafson C, et al. Genomic instability occurs in colorectal carcinomas but not in adenomas. *Hum Mutat* 1993;**2**:351.

321. Loukola A, Salovaara R, Kristo P, et al. Microsatellite instability in adenomas as a marker for hereditary nonpolyposis colorectal cancer. *Am J Pathol* 1999;**155**:1849.

322. Iino H, Jass JR, Simms LA, et al. DNA microsatellite instability in hyperplastic polyps, serrated adenomas, and mixed polyps: a mild mutator pathway for colorectal cancer? *J Clin Pathol* 1999;**52**:5.

323. Jass JR, Iino H, Ruszkiewicz A, et al. Neoplastic progression occurs through mutator pathways in hyperplastic polyposis of the colorectum. *Gut* 2000;**47**:43.

324. Toyota M, Ahuja N, Ohe-Toyota M, Herman JG, Baylin SB, Issa JP. CpG island methylator phenotype in colorectal cancer. *Proc Natl Acad Sci U S A* 1999;**96**:8681.

325. You JF, Buhard O, Ligtenberg MJ, et al. Tumours with loss of MSH6 expression are MSI-H when screened with a pentaplex of five mononucleotide repeats. *Br J Cancer* 2010;**103**:1840.

326. Greenson JK, Huang SC, Herron C, et al. Pathologic predictors of microsatellite instability in colorectal cancer. *Am J Surg Pathol* 2009;**33**:126.

327. Boland CR, Goel A. Microsatellite instability in colorectal cancer. *Gastroenterology* 2010;**138**:2073, e3.

328. Hewish M, Lord CJ, Martin SA, Cunningham D, Ashworth A. Mismatch repair deficient colorectal cancer in the era of personalized treatment. *Nat Rev Clin Oncol* 2010;**7**:197.

329. Sinicrope FA, Sargent DJ. Clinical implications of microsatellite instability in sporadic colon cancers. *Curr Opin Oncol* 2009; **21**:369.

330. Des Guetz G, Schischmanoff O, Nicolas P, Perret GY, Morere JF, Uzzan B. Does microsatellite instability predict the efficacy of adjuvant chemotherapy in colorectal cancer? A systematic review with meta-analysis. *Eur J Cancer* 2009;**45**:1890.

331. Ahuja N, Li Q, Mohan AL, Baylin SB, Issa JP. Aging and DNA methylation in colorectal mucosa and cancer. *Cancer Res* 1998; **58**:5489.

332. Herman JG, Baylin SB. Gene silencing in cancer in association with promoter hypermethylation. *N Engl J Med* 2003; **349**:2042.

333. Irizarry RA, Ladd-Acosta C, Wen B, et al. The human colon cancer methylome shows similar hypo- and hypermethylation at conserved tissue-specific CpG island shores. *Nat Genet* 2009;**41**:178.

334. Jass JR. Gastrointestinal polyposes: clinical, pathological and molecular features. *Gastroenterol Clin North Am* 2007;**36**:927, viii.

335. Minoo P, Baker K, Goswami R, et al. Extensive DNA methylation in normal colorectal mucosa in hyperplastic polyposis. *Gut* 2006;**55**:1467.

336. Ward RL, Williams R, Law M, Hawkins NJ. The CpG island methylator phenotype is not associated with a personal or family history of cancer. *Cancer Res* 2004;**64**:7618.

337. Samowitz WS, Albertsen H, Sweeney C, et al. Association of smoking, CpG island methylator phenotype, and V600E BRAF mutations in colon cancer. *J Natl Cancer Inst* 2006;**98**:1731.

338. Morimoto LM, Newcomb PA, Ulrich CM, Bostick RM, Lais CJ, Potter JD. Risk factors for hyperplastic and adenomatous polyps: evidence for malignant potential? *Cancer Epidemiol Biomarkers Prev* 2002;**11**(10 Part 1):1012.

339. Worthley DL, Leggett BA. Colorectal cancer: molecular features and clinical opportunities. *Clin Biochem Rev* 2010;**31**:31.

340. Shen L, Toyota M, Kondo Y, et al. Integrated genetic and epigenetic analysis identifies three different subclasses of colon cancer. *Proc Natl Acad Sci U S A* 2007;**104**:18654.

341. Issa JP, Shen L, Toyota M. CIMP, at last. *Gastroenterology* 2005; **129**:1121.

342. Robertson KD, Jones PA. The human ARF cell cycle regulatory gene promoter is a CpG island which can be silenced by DNA methylation and down-regulated by wild-type p53. *Mol Cell Biol* 1998;**18**:6457.

343. Toyota M, Shen L, Ohe-Toyota M, Hamilton SR, Sinicrope FA, Issa JP. Aberrant methylation of the cyclooxygenase 2 CpG island in colorectal tumors. *Cancer Res* 2000;**60**:4044.

344. Issa JP, Ottaviano YL, Celano P, Hamilton SR, Davidson NE, Baylin SB. Methylation of the oestrogen receptor CpG island links ageing and neoplasia in human colon. *Nat Genet* 1994; **7**:536.

345. Esteller M, Toyota M, Sanchez-Cespedes M, et al. Inactivation of the DNA repair gene O6-methylguanine-DNA methyltransferase by promoter hypermethylation is associated with G to A mutations in K-ras in colorectal tumorigenesis. *Cancer Res* 2000;**60**:2368.

346. Esteller M, Sparks A, Toyota M, et al. Analysis of adenomatous polyposis coli promoter hypermethylation in human cancer. *Cancer Res* 2000;**60**:4366.

347. Feinberg AP, Gehrke CW, Kuo KC, Ehrlich M. Reduced genomic 5-methylcytosine content in human colonic neoplasia. *Cancer Res* 1988;**48**:1159.

348. Goelz SE, Vogelstein B, Hamilton SR, Feinberg AP. Hypomethylation of DNA from benign and malignant human colon neoplasms. *Science* 1985;**228**:187.

349. Cui H, Horon IL, Ohlsson R, Hamilton SR, Feinberg AP. Loss of imprinting in normal tissue of colorectal cancer patients with microsatellite instability. *Nat Med* 1998;**4**:1276.

350. Moran A, Ortega P, de Juan C, et al. Differential colorectal carcinogenesis: Molecular basis and clinical relevance. *World J Gastrointest Oncol* 2010;**2**:151.

351. Fearon ER, Vogelstein B. A genetic model for colorectal tumorigenesis. *Cell* 1990;**61**:759.

352. Pawlik TM, Raut CP, Rodriguez-Bigas MA. Colorectal carcinogenesis: MSI-H versus MSI-L. *Diskers* 2004;**20**:199.

353. Powell SM, Zilz N, Beazer-Barclay Y, et al. APC mutations occur early during colorectal tumorigenesis. *Nature* 1992;**359**:235.

354. Okamoto M, Sasaki M, Sugio K, et al. Loss of constitutional heterozygosity in colon carcinoma from patients with familial polyposis coli. *Nature* 1988;**331**:273.

355. Solomon E, Voss R, Hall V, et al. Chromosome 5 allele loss in human colorectal carcinomas. *Nature* 1987;**328**:616.

356. Ashton-Rickardt PG, Dunlop MG, Nakamura Y, et al. High frequency of APC loss in sporadic colorectal carcinoma due to breaks clustered in 5q21–22. *Oncogene* 1989;**4**:1169.

357. Law DJ, Olschwang S, Monpezat JP, et al. Concerted nonsyntenic allelic loss in human colorectal carcinoma. *Science* 1988; **241**:961.

358. Polakis P. Mutations in the APC gene and their implications for protein structure and function. *Curr Opin Genet Dev* 1995;**5**:66.

359. Stryker SJ, Wolff BG, Culp CE, Libbe SD, Ilstrup DM, MacCarty RL. Natural history of untreated colonic polyps. *Gastroenterology* 1987;**93**:1009.

360. Malumbres M, Barbacid M. RAS oncogenes: the first 30 years. *Nat Rev Cancer* 2003;**3**:459.

361. Jass JR, Baker K, Zlobec I, et al. Advanced colorectal polyps with the molecular and morphological features of serrated polyps and adenomas: concept of a 'fusion' pathway to colorectal cancer. *Histopathology* 2006;**49**:121.

362. Ishii T, Notohara K, Umapathy A, et al. Tubular adenomas with minor villous changes show molecular features characteristic of tubulovillous adenomas. *Am J Surg Pathol* 2011;**35**:212.

363. Burmer GC, Loeb LA. Mutations in the *KRAS2* oncogene during progressive stages of human colon carcinoma. *Proc Natl Acad Sci U S A* 1989;**86**:2403.

364. Vakiani E, Solit DB. *KRAS* and *BRAF*: drug targets and predictive biomarkers. *J Pathol* 2011;**223**:219.

365. Haigis KM, Kendall KR, Wang Y, et al. Differential effects of oncogenic K-Ras and N-Ras on proliferation, differentiation and tumor progression in the colon. *Nat Genet* 2008;**40**:600.

366. Smakman N, Borel Rinkes IH, Voest EE, Kranenburg O. Control of colorectal metastasis formation by K-Ras. *Biochim Biophys Acta* 2005;**1756**:103.

367. Losi L, Benhattar J, Costa J. Stability of K-ras mutations throughout the natural history of human colorectal cancer. *Eur J Cancer* 1992;**28A**:1115.

368. Pritchard CC, Grady WM. Colorectal cancer molecular biology moves into clinical practice. *Gut* 2011;**60**:116.

369. Mehlen P, Fearon ER. Role of the dependence receptor DCC in colorectal cancer pathogenesis. *J Clin Oncol* 2004;**22**:3420.

370. Chen YQ, Hsieh JT, Yao F, et al. Induction of apoptosis and G2/M cell cycle arrest by DCC. *Oncogene* 1999;**18**:2747.

371. Shekarabi M, Kennedy TE. The netrin-1 receptor DCC promotes filopodia formation and cell spreading by activating Cdc42 and Rac1. *Mol Cell Neurosci* 2002;**19**:1.

372. Fazeli A, Dickinson SL, Hermiston ML, et al. Phenotype of mice lacking functional Deleted in colorectal cancer (Dcc) gene. *Nature* 1997;**386**:796.

373. Paradisi A, Mehlen P. Netrin-1, a missing link between chronic inflammation and tumor progression. *Cell Cycle* 2010; **9**:1253.

374. Hahn SA, Schutte M, Hoque AT, et al. *DPC4*, a candidate tumor suppressor gene at human chromosome 18q21.1. *Science* 1996; **271**:350.

375. Miyaki M, Iijima T, Konishi M, et al. Higher frequency of *Smad4* gene mutation in human colorectal cancer with distant metastasis. *Oncogene* 1999;**18**:3098.

376. Lips EH, van Eijk R, de Graaf EJ, et al. Progression and tumor heterogeneity analysis in early rectal cancer. *Clin Cancer Res* 2008;**14**:772.

377. Bevan S, Woodford-Richens K, et al. Screening *SMAD1*, *SMAD2*, *SMAD3*, and *SMAD5* for germline mutations in juvenile polyposis syndrome. *Gut* 1999;**45**:406.

378. Goh AM, Coffill CR, Lane DP. The role of mutant *p53* in human cancer. *J Pathol* 2011;**223**:116.

379. Baker SJ, Preisinger AC, Jessup JM, et al. p53 gene mutations occur in combination with 17p allelic deletions as late events in colorectal tumorigenesis. *Cancer Res* 1990;**50**:7717.

380. Tang R, Wang PF, Wang HC, Wang JY, Hsieh LL. Mutations of *p53* gene in human colorectal cancer: distinct frameshifts among populations. *Int J Cancer* 2001;**91**:863.

381. Petitjean A, Mathe E, Kato S, et al. Impact of mutant *p53* functional properties on TP53 mutation patterns and tumor phenotype: lessons from recent developments in the IARC TP53 database. *Hum Mutat* 2007;**28**:622.

382. Milner J, Medcalf EA. Cotranslation of activated mutant *p53* with wild type drives the wild-type p53 protein into the mutant conformation. *Cell* 1991;**65**:765.

383. Srivastava S, Wang S, Tong YA, Hao ZM, Chang EH. Dominant negative effect of a germ-line mutant *p53*: a step fostering tumorigenesis. *Cancer Res* 1993;**53**:4452.

384. Kern SE, Pietenpol JA, Thiagalingam S, Seymour A, Kinzler KW, Vogelstein B. Oncogenic forms of *p53* inhibit *p53*-regulated gene expression. *Science* 1992;**256**:827.

385. Mills AA. p53: link to the past, bridge to the future. *Genes Dev* 2005;**19**:2091.

386. Pietsch EC, Sykes SM, McMahon SB, Murphy ME. The p53 family and programmed cell death. *Oncogene* 2008;**27**:6507.

387. Lane DP. Cancer. p53, guardian of the genome. *Nature* 1992;**358**:15.

388. Vousden KH, Prives C. Blinded by the light: the growing complexity of p53. *Cell* 2009;**137**:413.

389. Green DR, Kroemer G. Cytoplasmic functions of the tumour suppressor p53. *Nature* 2009;**458**:1127.

390. Hollstein M, Hainaut P. Massively regulated genes: the example of TP53. *J Pathol* 2010;**220**:164.

391. Tasdemir E, Maiuri MC, Galluzzi L, et al. Regulation of autophagy by cytoplasmic p53. *Nat Cell Biol* 2008;**10**:676.

392. Morselli E, Tasdemir E, Maiuri MC, et al. Mutant p53 protein localized in the cytoplasm inhibits autophagy. *Cell Cycle* 2008;**7**:3056.

393. Suzuki HI, Yamagata K, Sugimoto K, Iwamoto T, Kato S, Miyazono K. Modulation of microRNA processing by p53. *Nature* 2009;**460**:529.

394. Livingstone LR, White A, Sprouse J, Livanos E, Jacks T, Tlsty TD. Altered cell cycle arrest and gene amplification potential accompany loss of wild-type p53. *Cell* 1992;**70**:923.

395. Farmer G, Bargonetti J, Zhu H, Friedman P, Prywes R, Prives C. Wild-type p53 activates transcription in vitro. *Nature* 1992;**358**:83.

396. Leslie A, Carey FA, Pratt NR, Steele RJ. The colorectal adenoma–carcinoma sequence. *Br J Surg* 2002;**89**:845.

397. Einspahr JG, Martinez ME, Jiang R, et al. Associations of Ki-ras proto-oncogene mutation and p53 gene overexpression in sporadic colorectal adenomas with demographic and clinicopathologic characteristics. *Cancer Epidemiol Biomarkers Prev* 2006;**15**:1443.

398. Wattenberg LW. A histochemical study of five oxidative enzymes in carcinoma of the large intestine in man. *Am J Pathol* 1959;**35**:113.

399. Chadeneau C, Hay K, Hirte HW, Gallinger S, Bacchetti S. Telomerase activity associated with acquisition of malignancy in human colorectal cancer. *Cancer Res* 1995;**55**:2533.

400. Skinner SA, Frydman GM, O'Brien PE. Microvascular structure of benign and malignant tumors of the colon in humans. *Dig Dis Sci* 1995;**40**:373.

401. Bossi P, Viale G, Lee AK, Alfano R, Coggi G, Bosari S. Angiogenesis in colorectal tumors: microvessel quantitation in adenomas and carcinomas with clinicopathological correlations. *Cancer Res* 1995;**55**:5049.

402. Frank RE, Saclarides TJ, Leurgans S, Speziale NJ, Drab EA, Rubin DB. Tumor angiogenesis as a predictor of recurrence and survival in patients with node-negative colon cancer. *Ann Surg* 1995;**222**:695.

403. Mulcahy HE, Patchett SE, Daly L, O'Donoghue DP. Prognosis of elderly patients with large bowel cancer. *Br J Surg* 1994;**81**:736.

404. Hewitt RE, Powe DG, Griffin NR, Turner DR. Relationships between epithelial basement membrane staining patterns in primary colorectal carcinomas and the extent of tumour spread. *Int J Cancer* 1991;**48**:855.

405. Tan K, Powe DG, Gray T, Turner DR, Hewitt RE. Regional variations of urokinase-type plasminogen activator in human colorectal cancer: a quantitative study by image analysis. *Int J Cancer* 1995;**60**:308.

406. Jass JR, Smith M. Sialic acid and epithelial differentiation in colorectal polyps and cancer – a morphological, mucin and lectin histochemical study. *Pathology* 1992;**24**:233.

407. Pignatelli M, Vessey CJ. Adhesion molecules: novel molecular tools in tumor pathology. *Hum Pathol* 1994;**25**:849.

408. Goh HS, Jass JR. DNA content and the adenoma-carcinoma sequence in the colorectum. *J Clin Pathol* 1986;**39**:387.

409. Cui G, Yuan A, Vonen B, Florholmen J. Progressive cellular response in the lamina propria of the colorectal adenoma-carcinoma sequence. *Histopathology* 2009;**54**:550.

410. Williams GT, Arthur JF, Bussey HJ, Morson BC. Metaplastic polyps and polyposis of the colorectum. *Histopathology* 1980;**4**:155.

411. Rasheed S, Yap T, Zia A, McDonald PJ, Glynne-Jones R. Chemoradiotherapy: an alternative to surgery for squamous cell carcinoma of the rectum – report of six patients and literature review. *Colorectal Dis* 2009;**11**:191.

412. Goldstein NS, Bhanot P, Odish E, Hunter S. Hyperplastic-like colon polyps that preceded microsatellite-unstable adenocarcinomas. *Am J Clin Pathol* 2003;**119**:778.

413. Torlakovic E, Skovlund E, Snover DC, Torlakovic G, Nesland JM. Morphologic reappraisal of serrated colorectal polyps. *Am J Surg Pathol* 2003;**27**:65.

414. Makinen MJ. Colorectal serrated adenocarcinoma. *Histopathology* 2007;**50**:131.

415. Harvey NT, Ruszkiewicz A. Serrated neoplasia of the colorectum. *World J Gastroenterol* 2007;**13**:3792.

416. O'Brien MJ, Yang S, Mack C, et al. Comparison of microsatellite instability, CpG island methylation phenotype, BRAF and KRAS status in serrated polyps and traditional adenomas indicates separate pathways to distinct colorectal carcinoma end points. *Am J Surg Pathol* 2006;**30**:1491.

417. Fujita K, Yamamoto H, Matsumoto T, et al. Sessile serrated adenoma with early neoplastic progression: a clinicopathologic and molecular study. *Am J Surg Pathol* 2011;**35**:295.

418. Barradas M, Gonos ES, Zebedee Z, et al. Identification of a candidate tumor-suppressor gene specifically activated during Ras-induced senescence. *Exp Cell Res* 2002;**273**:127.

419. Minoo P, Jass JR. Senescence and serration: a new twist to an old tale. *J Pathol* 2006;**210**:137.

420. Kaye GI, Fenoglio CM, Pascal RR, Lane N. Comparative electron microscopic features of normal, hyperplastic, and adenomatous human colonic epithelium. Variations in cellular structure relative to the process of epithelial differentiation. *Gastroenterology* 1973;**64**:926.

421. Hayashi T, Yatani R, Apostol J, Stemmermann GN. Pathogenesis of hyperplastic polyps of the colon: a hypothesis based on ultrastructure and in vitro cell kinetics. *Gastroenterology* 1974;**66**:347.

422. Tateyama H, Li W, Takahashi E, Miura Y, Sugiura H, Eimoto T. Apoptosis index and apoptosis-related antigen expression in serrated adenoma of the colorectum: the saw-toothed structure may be related to inhibition of apoptosis. *Am J Surg Pathol* 2002;**26**:249.

423. Yang S, Farraye FA, Mack C, Posnik O, O'Brien MJ. BRAF and KRAS mutations in hyperplastic polyps and serrated adenomas of the colorectum: relationship to histology and CpG island methylation status. *Am J Surg Pathol* 2004;**28**:1452.

424. O'Brien MJ, Yang S, Clebanoff JL, et al. Hyperplastic (serrated) polyps of the colorectum: relationship of CpG island methylator phenotype and K-ras mutation to location and histologic subtype. *Am J Surg Pathol* 2004;**28**:423.

425. Dhir M, Yachida S, Van Neste L, et al. Sessile serrated adenomas and classical adenomas: An epigenetic perspective on premalignant neoplastic lesions of the gastrointestinal tract. *Int J Cancer* 2010;**129**:1889.

426. Spring KJ, Zhao ZZ, Karamatic R, et al. High prevalence of sessile serrated adenomas with BRAF mutations: a prospective

study of patients undergoing colonoscopy. *Gastroenterology* 2006;**131**:1400.

427. Snover DC, Jass JR, Fenoglio-Preiser C, Batts KP. Serrated polyps of the large intestine: a morphologic and molecular review of an evolving concept. *Am J Clin Pathol* 2005;**124**:380.

428. Sandmeier D, Benhattar J, Martin P, Bouzourene H. Serrated polyps of the large intestine: a molecular study comparing sessile serrated adenomas and hyperplastic polyps. *Histopathology* 2009;**55**:206.

429. Pai RK, Hart J, Noffsinger AE. Sessile serrated adenomas strongly predispose to synchronous serrated polyps in nonsyndromic patients. *Histopathology* 2010;**56**:581.

430. Lu FI, van Niekerk de W, Owen D, Tha SP, Turbin DA, Webber DL. Longitudinal outcome study of sessile serrated adenomas of the colorectum: an increased risk for subsequent right-sided colorectal carcinoma. *Am J Surg Pathol* 2010;**34**:927.

431. Oh K, Redston M, Odze RD. Support for hMLH1 and MGMT silencing as a mechanism of tumorigenesis in the hyperplastic–adenoma–carcinoma (serrated) carcinogenic pathway in the colon. *Hum Pathol* 2005;**36**:101.

432. Yachida S, Mudali S, Martin SA, Montgomery EA, Iacobuzio-Donahue CA. Beta-catenin nuclear labeling is a common feature of sessile serrated adenomas and correlates with early neoplastic progression after BRAF activation. *Am J Surg Pathol* 2009;**33**:1823.

433. Sheridan TB, Fenton H, Lewin MR, et al. Sessile serrated adenomas with low- and high-grade dysplasia and early carcinomas: an immunohistochemical study of serrated lesions 'caught in the act'. *Am J Clin Pathol* 2006;**126**:564.

434. Goldstein NS. Serrated pathway and APC (conventional)-type colorectal polyps: molecular–morphologic correlations, genetic pathways, and implications for classification. *Am J Clin Pathol* 2006;**125**:146.

435. Longacre TA, Fenoglio-Preiser CM. Mixed hyperplastic adenomatous polyps/serrated adenomas. A distinct form of colorectal neoplasia. *Am J Surg Pathol* 1990;**14**:524.

436. Matsumoto T, Mizuno M, Shimizu M, Manabe T, Iida M, Fujishima M. Serrated adenoma of the colorectum: colonoscopic and histologic features. *Gastrointest Endosc* 1999;**49**:736.

437. Oka S, Tanaka S, Hiyama T, et al. Clinicopathologic and endoscopic features of colorectal serrated adenoma: differences between polypoid and superficial types. *Gastrointest Endosc* 2004;**59**:213.

438. Torlakovic EE, Gomez JD, Driman DK, et al. Sessile serrated adenoma (SSA) vs. traditional serrated adenoma (TSA). *Am J Surg Pathol* 2008;**32**:21.

439. Chan TL, Zhao W, Leung SY, Yuen ST. *BRAF* and *KRAS* mutations in colorectal hyperplastic polyps and serrated adenomas. *Cancer Res* 2003;**63**:4878.

440. Lee EJ, Choi C, Park CK, et al. Tracing origin of serrated adenomas with *BRAF* and KRAS mutations. *Virchows Arch* 2005;**447**:597.

441. Park SJ, Rashid A, Lee JH, Kim SG, Hamilton SR, Wu TT. Frequent CpG island methylation in serrated adenomas of the colorectum. *Am J Pathol* 2003;**162**:815.

442. Kambara T, Simms LA, Whitehall VL, et al. BRAF mutation is associated with DNA methylation in serrated polyps and cancers of the colorectum. *Gut* 2004;**53**:1137.

443. Dong SM, Lee EJ, Jeon ES, Park CK, Kim KM. Progressive methylation during the serrated neoplasia pathway of the colorectum. *Mod Pathol* 2005;**18**:170.

444. Jass JR. Serrated route to colorectal cancer: back street or super highway? *J Pathol* 2001;**193**:283.

445. Goldstein NS. Clinical significance of (sessile) serrated adenomas: Another piece of the puzzle. *Am J Clin Pathol* 2005;**123**:329.

446. Kim KM, Lee EJ, Kim YH, Chang DK, Odze RD. KRAS mutations in traditional serrated adenomas from Korea herald an aggressive phenotype. *Am J Surg Pathol* 2010;**34**:667.

447. Tuppurainen K, Makinen JM, Marttila O, et al. Morphology and microsatellite instability in sporadic serrated and non-serrated colorectal cancer. *J Pathol* 2005;**207**:285.

448. Laiho P, Kokko A, Vanharanta S, et al. Serrated carcinomas form a subclass of colorectal cancer with distinct molecular basis. *Oncogene* 2007;**26**:312.

449. Shirouzu K, Isomoto H, Morodomi T, Ogata Y, Akagi Y, Kakegawa T. Primary linitis plastica carcinoma of the colon and rectum. *Cancer* 1994;**74**:1863.

450. Sasaki O, Atkin WS, Jass JR. Mucinous carcinoma of the rectum. *Histopathology* 1987;**11**:259.

451. Jass JR, Love SB, Northover JM. A new prognostic classification of rectal cancer. *Lancet* 1987;**i**:1303.

452. Pretlow TP, Keith EF, Cryar AK, et al. Eosinophil infiltration of human colonic carcinomas as a prognostic indicator. *Cancer Res* 1983;**43**:2997.

453. Fernandez-Acenero MJ, Galindo-Gallego M, Sanz J, Aljama A. Prognostic influence of tumor-associated eosinophilic infiltrate in colorectal carcinoma. *Cancer* 2000;**88**:1544.

454. Wang LM, Kevans D, Mulcahy H, et al. Tumor budding is a strong and reproducible prognostic marker in T3N0 colorectal cancer. *Am J Surg Pathol* 2009;**33**:134.

455. Garcia-Solano J, Perez-Guillermo M, Conesa-Zamora P, et al. Clinicopathologic study of 85 colorectal serrated adenocarcinomas: further insights into the full recognition of a new subset of colorectal carcinoma. *Hum Pathol* 2010;**41**:1359.

456. Nasir A, Boulware D, Kaiser HE, et al. Flat and polypoid adenocarcinomas of the colorectum: A comparative histomorphologic analysis of 47 cases. *Hum Pathol* 2004;**35**:604.

457. Watanabe T, Muto T. Colorectal carcinogenesis based on molecular biology of early colorectal cancer, with special reference to nonpolypoid (superficial) lesions. *World J Surg* 2000;**24**:1091.

458. Koga Y, Yao T, Hirahashi M, et al. Flat adenoma-carcinoma sequence with high-malignancy potential as demonstrated by CD10 and beta-catenin expression: a different pathway from the polypoid adenoma–carcinoma sequence. *Histopathology* 2008;**52**:569.

459. Chandler I, Houlston RS. Interobserver agreement in grading of colorectal cancers – findings from a nationwide web-based survey of histopathologists. *Histopathology* 2008;**52**:494.

460. Mandard AM, Dalibard F, Mandard JC, et al. Pathologic assessment of tumor regression after preoperative chemoradiotherapy of esophageal carcinoma. Clinicopathologic correlations. *Cancer* 1994;**73**:2680.

461. Dhadda AS, Dickinson P, Zaitoun AM, Gandhi N, Bessell EM. Prognostic importance of Mandard tumour regression grade following pre-operative chemo/radiotherapy for locally advanced rectal cancer. *Eur J Cancer* 2011;**47**:1138.

462. Dworak O, Keilholz L, Hoffmann A. Pathological features of rectal cancer after preoperative radiochemotherapy. *Int J Colorectal Dis* 1997;**12**:19.

463. Takeuchi H, Toda T, Nagasaki S, et al. Synchronous multiple colorectal adenocarcinomas. *J Surg Oncol* 1997;**64**:304.

464. Salk JJ, Salipante SJ, Risques RA, et al. Clonal expansions in ulcerative colitis identify patients with neoplasia. *Proc Natl Acad Sci U S A* 2009;**106**:20871.

465. Nosho K, Kure S, Irahara N, et al. A prospective cohort study shows unique epigenetic, genetic, and prognostic features

of synchronous colorectal cancers. *Gastroenterology* 2009;**137**: 1609, e1.

466. Viennot S, Deleporte A, Moussata D, Nancey S, Flourie B, Reimund JM. Colon cancer in inflammatory bowel disease: recent trends, questions and answers. *Gastroenterol Clin Biol* 2009;**33**(suppl 3):S190.

467. Mitchard JR, Love SB, Baxter KJ, Shepherd NA. How important is peritoneal involvement in rectal cancer? A prospective study of 331 cases. *Histopathology* 2010;**57**:671.

468. Shepherd NA, Baxter KJ, Love SB. The prognostic importance of peritoneal involvement in colonic cancer: a prospective evaluation. *Gastroenterology* 1997;**112**:1096.

469. Puppa G, Shepherd NA, Sheahan K, Stewart CJ. Peritoneal elastic lamina invasion in colorectal cancer: the answer to a controversial area of pathology? *Am J Surg Pathol* 2011;**35**:465.

470. Warth A, Muley T, Herpel E, et al. A histochemical approach to the diagnosis of visceral pleural infiltration by non-small cell lung cancer. *Pathol Oncol Res* **16**:119.

471. Sobin LH, Gospodarowicz MK, Wittekind C, eds. *UICC TNM Classification of Malignant Tumors*, 7th edn. New York: Wiley-Blackwell, 2009.

472. Faerden AE, Sjo OH, Bukholm IR, et al. Lymph node micrometastases and isolated tumor cells influence survival in stage I and II colon cancer. *Dis Colon Rectum* 2011;**54**:200.

473. Koyanagi K, Bilchik AJ, Saha S, et al. Prognostic relevance of occult nodal micrometastases and circulating tumor cells in colorectal cancer in a prospective multicenter trial. *Clin Cancer Res* 2008;**14**:7391.

474. Doekhie FS, Kuppen PJ, Peeters KC, et al. Prognostic relevance of occult tumour cells in lymph nodes in colorectal cancer. *Eur J Surg Oncol* 2006;**32**:253.

475. van der Zaag ES, Kooij N, van de Vijver MJ, Bemelman WA, Peters HM, Buskens CJ. Diagnosing occult tumour cells and their predictive value in sentinel nodes of histologically negative patients with colorectal cancer. *Eur J Surg Oncol* 2011;**36**:350.

476. Petersen VC, Baxter KJ, Love SB, Shepherd NA. Identification of objective pathological prognostic determinants and models of prognosis in Dukes' B colon cancer. *Gut* 2002;**51**:65.

477. Roxburgh CS, McMillan DC, Anderson JH, McKee RF, Horgan PG, Foulis AK. Elastica staining for venous invasion results in superior prediction of cancer-specific survival in colorectal cancer. *Ann Surg* 2010;**252**:989.

478. Ceyhan GO, Liebl F, Maak M, et al. The severity of neural invasion is a crucial prognostic factor in rectal cancer independent of neoadjuvant radiochemotherapy. *Ann Surg* **252**:797.

479. Cawthorn SJ, Parums DV, Gibbs NM, et al. Extent of mesorectal spread and involvement of lateral resection margin as prognostic factors after surgery for rectal cancer. *Lancet* 1990; **335**:1055.

480. Li MK, Folpe AL. CDX-2, a new marker for adenocarcinoma of gastrointestinal origin. *Adv Anat Pathol* 2004;**11**:101.

481. Hinoi T, Tani M, Lucas PC, et al. Loss of CDX2 expression and microsatellite instability are prominent features of large cell minimally differentiated carcinomas of the colon. *Am J Pathol* 2001;**159**:2239.

482. Moll R, Robine S, Dudouet B, Louvard D. Villin: a cytoskeletal protein and a differentiation marker expressed in some human adenocarcinomas. *Virchows Arch B Cell Pathol Mol Pathol* 1987; **54**:155.

483. Duncan TJ, Watson NF, Al-Attar AH, Scholefield JH, Durrant LG. The role of MUC1 and MUC3 in the biology and prognosis of colorectal cancer. *World J Surg Oncol* 2007;**5**:31.

484. Molaei M, Mansoori BK, Mashayekhi R, et al. Mucins in neoplastic spectrum of colorectal polyps: can they provide predictions? *BMC Cancer* 2010;**10**:537.

485. Dukes CE. The classification of cancer of the rectum. *J Pathol Bacteriol* 1932;**35**:323.

486. Astler VB, Coller FA. The prognostic significance of direct extension of carcinoma of the colon and rectum. *Ann Surg* 1954;**139**:846.

487. Sobin LH, Wittekind C, eds. *UICC TNM Classification of Malignant Tumors*, 5th edn. New York: Wiley-Liss, 1997.

488. Quirke P, Cuvelier C, Ensari A, et al. Evidence-based medicine: the time has come to set standards for staging. *J Pathol* 2010; **221**:357.

489. Fenoglio CM, Kaye GI, Lane N. Distribution of human colonic lymphatics in normal, hyperplastic, and adenomatous tissue. Its relationship to metastasis from small carcinomas in pedunculated adenomas, with two case reports. *Gastroenterology* 1973; **64**:51.

490. Zlobec I, Lugli A. Prognostic and predictive factors in colorectal cancer. *J Clin Pathol* 2008;**61**:561.

491. Moug SJ, Saldanha JD, McGregor JR, Balsitis M, Diament RH. Positive lymph node retrieval ratio optimises patient staging in colorectal cancer. *Br J Cancer* 2009;**100**:1530.

492. Blenkinsopp WK, Stewart-Brown S, Blesovsky L, Kearney G, Fielding LP. Histopathology reporting in large bowel cancer. *J Clin Pathol* 1981;**34**:509.

493. Purdie CA, Piris J. Histopathological grade, mucinous differentiation and DNA ploidy in relation to prognosis in colorectal carcinoma. *Histopathology* 2000;**36**:121.

494. Vass DG, Ainsworth R, Anderson JH, Murray D, Foulis AK. The value of an elastic tissue stain in detecting venous invasion in colorectal cancer. *J Clin Pathol* 2004;**57**:769.

495. Munro AJ, Lain S, Lane DP. P53 abnormalities and outcomes in colorectal cancer: a systematic review. *Br J Cancer* 2005;**92**:434.

496. Plesec TP, Hunt JL. KRAS mutation testing in colorectal cancer. *Adv Anat Pathol* 2009;**16**:196.

497. Andreyev HJ, Norman AR, Cunningham D, et al. Kirsten ras mutations in patients with colorectal cancer: the 'RASCAL II' study. *Br J Cancer* 2001;**85**:692.

498. Bokemeyer C, Bondarenko I, Makhson A, et al. Fluorouracil, leucovorin, and oxaliplatin with and without cetuximab in the first-line treatment of metastatic colorectal cancer. *J Clin Oncol* 2009;**27**:663.

499. Carey FA. Measurement of nuclear DNA content in histological and cytological specimens: principles and applications. *J Pathol* 1994;**172**:307.

500. Sinicrope FA, Rego RL, Halling KC, et al. Prognostic impact of microsatellite instability and DNA ploidy in human colon carcinoma patients. *Gastroenterology* 2006;**131**:729.

501. Lanza G, Gafa R, Santini A, et al. Prognostic significance of DNA ploidy in patients with stage II and stage III colon carcinoma: a prospective flow cytometric study. *Cancer* 1998;**82**:49.

502. Conio M, Ponchon T, Blanchi S, Filiberti R. Endoscopic mucosal resection. *Am J Gastroenterol* 2006;**101**:653.

503. Neary P, Makin GB, White TJ, et al. Transanal endoscopic microsurgery: a viable operative alternative in selected patients with rectal lesions. *Ann Surg Oncol* 2003;**10**:1106.

504. Kikuchi R, Takano M, Takagi K, et al. Management of early invasive colorectal cancer. Risk of recurrence and clinical guidelines. *Dis Colon Rectum* 1995;**38**:1286.

505. Ueno H, Mochizuki H, Hashiguchi Y, et al. Risk factors for an adverse outcome in early invasive colorectal carcinoma. *Gastroenterology* 2004;**127**:385.

506. Bowel Cancer Screening Programme Pathology Group. *Reporting Lesions in the NHS Bowel Cancer Screening Programme.* Sheffield: NHS Cancer Screening Programmes, 2007. Available at: www.cancerscreening.nhs.uk/bowel/publications/nhsbcsp01. pdf (accessed 30 April 2012).

507. Quirke P, Risio M, Lambert R, von Karsa L, Vieth M. Quality assurance in pathology in colorectal cancer screening and diagnosis-European recommendations. *Virchows Arch* 2011;**458**:1.

508. Modlin IM, Sandor A. An analysis of 8305 cases of carcinoid tumors. *Cancer* 1997;**79**:813.

509. Ellis L, Shale MJ, Coleman MP. Carcinoid tumors of the gastrointestinal tract: trends in incidence in England since 1971. *Am J Gastroenterol* 2010;**105**:2563.

510. Hiripi E, Bermejo JL, Sundquist J, Hemminki K. Familial gastrointestinal carcinoid tumours and associated cancers. *Ann Oncol* 2009;**20**:950.

511. Greenstein AJ, Balasubramanian S, Harpaz N, Rizwan M, Sachar DB. Carcinoid tumor and inflammatory bowel disease: a study of eleven cases and review of the literature. *Am J Gastroenterol* 1997;**92**:682.

512. Konishi T, Watanabe T, Kishimoto J, Kotake K, Muto T, Nagawa H. Prognosis and risk factors of metastasis in colorectal carcinoids: results of a nationwide registry over 15 years. *Gut* 2007;**56**:863.

513. Rindi G, Kloppel G, Couvelard A, et al. TNM staging of midgut and hindgut (neuro)endocrine tumors: a consensus proposal including a grading system. *Virchows Arch* 2007;**451**:757.

514. Berardi RS. Carcinoid tumors of the colon (exclusive of the rectum): review of the literature. *Dis Colon Rectum* 1972;**15**:383.

515. Federspiel BH, Burke AP, Sobin LH, Shekitka KM. Rectal and colonic carcinoids. A clinicopathologic study of 84 cases. *Cancer* 1990;**65**:135.

516. O'Briain DS, Dayal Y, DeLellis RA, Tischler AS, Bendon R, Wolfe HJ. Rectal carcinoids as tumors of the hindgut endocrine cells: a morphological and immunohistochemical analysis. *Am J Surg Pathol* 1982;**6**:131.

517. Williams GT. Endocrine tumours of the gastrointestinal tract-selected topics. *Histopathology* 2007;**50**:30.

518. Fiocca R, Rindi G, Capella C, et al. Glucagon, glicentin, proglucagon, PYY, PP and proPP-icosapeptide immunoreactivities of rectal carcinoid tumors and related non-tumor cells. *Regul Pept* 1987;**17**:9.

519. Koura AN, Giacco GG, Curley SA, Skibber JM, Feig BW, Ellis LM. Carcinoid tumors of the rectum: effect of size, histopathology, and surgical treatment on metastasis free survival. *Cancer* 1997;**79**:1294.

520. Kobayashi K, Katsumata T, Yoshizawa S, et al. Indications of endoscopic polypectomy for rectal carcinoid tumors and clinical usefulness of endoscopic ultrasonography. *Dis Colon Rectum* 2005;**48**:285.

521. Mashimo Y, Matsuda T, Uraoka T, et al. Endoscopic submucosal resection with a ligation device is an effective and safe treatment for carcinoid tumors in the lower rectum. *J Gastroenterol Hepatol* 2008;**23**:218.

522. Tsai BM, Finne CO, Nordenstam JF, Christoforidis D, Madoff RD, Mellgren A. Transanal endoscopic microsurgery resection of rectal tumors: outcomes and recommendations. *Dis Colon Rectum* 2010;**53**:16.

523. Gui X, Qin L, Gao ZH, Falck V, Harpaz N. Goblet cell carcinoids at extraappendiceal locations of gastrointestinal tract: an underrecognized diagnostic pitfall. *J Surg Oncol* 2011;**103**:790.

524. Gledhill A, Hall PA, Cruse JP, Pollock DJ. Enteroendocrine cell hyperplasia, carcinoid tumours and adenocarcinoma in long-standing ulcerative colitis. *Histopathology* 1986;**10**:501.

525. Miller RR, Sumner HW. Argyrophilic cell hyperplasia and an atypical carcinoid tumor in chronic ulcerative colitis. *Cancer* 1982;**50**:2920.

526. Yaziji H, Broghamer WL Jr. Primary small cell undifferentiated carcinoma of the rectum associated with ulcerative colitis. *South Med J* 1996;**89**:921.

527. Bernick PE, Klimstra DS, Shia J, et al. Neuroendocrine carcinomas of the colon and rectum. *Dis Colon Rectum* 2004;**47**:163.

528. Stelow EB, Moskaluk CA, Mills SE. The mismatch repair protein status of colorectal small cell neuroendocrine carcinomas. *Am J Surg Pathol* 2006;**30**:1401.

529. Li AF, Li AC, Hsu CY, Li WY, Hsu HS, Chen JY. Small cell carcinomas in gastrointestinal tract: immunohistochemical and clinicopathological features. *J Clin Pathol* 2010;**63**:620.

530. Minkowitz S. Primary squamous cell carcinoma of the rectosigmoid portion of the colon. *Arch Pathol* 1967;**84**:77.

531. Gaston EA, Wilde WL. Epidermoid carcinoma arising in a pilonidal sinus. *Dis Colon Rectum* 1965;**8**:343.

532. Dyson T, Draganov PV. Squamous cell cancer of the rectum. *World J Gastroenterol* 2009;**15**:4380.

533. Gelas T, Peyrat P, Francois Y, et al. Primary squamous-cell carcinoma of the rectum: report of six cases and review of the literature. *Dis Colon Rectum* 2002;**45**:1535.

534. Frizelle FA, Hobday KS, Batts KP, Nelson H. Adenosquamous and squamous carcinoma of the colon and upper rectum: a clinical and histopathologic study. *Dis Colon Rectum* 2001;**44**:341.

535. Williams GT, Blackshaw AJ, Morson BC. Squamous carcinoma of the colorectum and its genesis. *J Pathol* 1979;**129**:139.

536. Mir-Madjlessi SH, Farmer RG. Squamous cell carcinoma of the rectal stump in a patient with ulcerative colitis. Report of a case and review of the literature. *Cleve Clin Q* 1985;**52**:257.

537. Cheng H, Sitrin MD, Satchidanand SK, Novak JM. Colonic squamous cell carcinoma in ulcerative colitis: Report of a case and review of the literature. *Can J Gastroenterol* 2007;**21**:47.

538. Nahas CS, Shia J, Joseph R, et al. Squamous-cell carcinoma of the rectum: a rare but curable tumor. *Dis Colon Rectum* 2007;**50**:1393.

539. Audeau A, Han HW, Johnston MJ, Whitehead MW, Frizelle FA. Does human papilloma virus have a role in squamous cell carcinoma of the colon and upper rectum? *Eur J Surg Oncol* 2002;**28**:657.

540. Kong CS, Welton ML, Longacre TA. Role of human papillomavirus in squamous cell metaplasia-dysplasia-carcinoma of the rectum. *Am J Surg Pathol* 2007;**31**:919.

541. Matsuda A, Takahashi K, Yamaguchi T, et al. HPV infection in an HIV-positive patient with primary squamous cell carcinoma of rectum. *Int J Clin Oncol* 2009;**14**:551.

542. Sotlar K, Koveker G, Aepinus C, Selinka HC, Kandolf R, Bultmann B. Human papillomavirus type 16-associated primary squamous cell carcinoma of the rectum. *Gastroenterology* 2001;**120**:988.

543. Tronconi MC, Carnaghi C, Bignardi M, et al. Rectal squamous cell carcinoma treated with chemoradiotherapy: report of six cases. *Int J Colorectal Dis* 2010;**25**:1435.

544. Cerezo L, Alvarez M, Edwards O, Price G. Adenosquamous carcinoma of the colon. *Dis Colon Rectum* 1985;**28**:597.

545. Weidner N, Zekan P. Carcinosarcoma of the colon. Report of a unique case with light and immunohistochemical studies. *Cancer* 1986;**58**:1126.

546. Shim HJ, Hong YK, Kim SJ, Choi YJ, Kang JG. Carcinosarcoma on ascending colon found by bowel perforation: a case report. *J Korean Soc Coloproctol* 2010;**26**:368.

547. Aramendi T, Fernandez-Acenero MJ, Villanueva MC. Carcinosarcoma of the colon: report of a rare tumor. *Pathol Res Pract* 2003;**199**:345.

548. Klein MS, Sherlock P. Gastric and colonic metastases from breast cancer. *Am J Dig Dis* 1972;**17**:881.

549. Rees BI, Okwonga W, Jenkins IL. Intestinal metastases from carcinoma of the breast. *Clin Oncol* 1976;**2**:113.

550. Davis JM. Carcinoma of the prostate presenting as disease of the rectum. *Br J Urol* 1960;**32**:197.

551. Olsen BS, Carlisle RW. Adenocarcinoma of the prostate simulating primary rectal malignancy. *Cancer* 1970;**25**:219.

552. Shoemaker CP Jr, Hoyle CL, Levine SB, Farman J. Late solitary colonic recurrence of renal carcinoma. *Am J Surg* 1970;**120**:99.

553. Fraser AM, Morgan MN. Secondary carcinoma from the cervix involving the large bowel. *Br J Surg* 1969;**56**:317.

554. Christodoulopoulos JB, Papaioannou AN, Drakopoulou EP, Kontos EK, Razis DV. Carcinoma of the cervix presenting with rectal symptomatology: report of three cases. *Dis Colon Rectum* 1972;**15**:373.

555. Cross SS, Feeley KM, Angel CA. The effect of four interventions on the informational content of histopathology reports of resected colorectal carcinomas. *J Clin Pathol* 1998;**51**:481.

556. Branston LK, Greening S, Newcombe RG, et al. The implementation of guidelines and computerised forms improves the completeness of cancer pathology reporting. The CROPS project: a randomised controlled trial in pathology. *Eur J Cancer* 2002;**38**:764.

557. Scholefield JH, Moss S, Sufi F, Mangham CM, Hardcastle JD. Effect of faecal occult blood screening on mortality from colorectal cancer: results from a randomised controlled trial. *Gut* 2002;**50**:840.

558. Atkin WS, Edwards R, Kralj-Hans I, et al. Once-only flexible sigmoidoscopy screening in prevention of colorectal cancer: a multicentre randomised controlled trial. *Lancet* 2010;**375**:1624.

559. Philip AK, Lubner MG, Harms B. Computed tomographic colonography. *Surg Clin North Am* 2011;**91**:127.

CHAPTER 39

Non-epithelial tumours of the large intestine

Jean-François Fléjou

Hôpital Saint-Antoine, AP-HP; Faculté de Médecine Pierre et Marie Curie, Paris, France

Tumours of lymphoid tissue

The large intestine is well endowed with lymphoid tissue and the prevalence and distribution of lymphoid tumours within the colorectum reflect the physiological distribution of this lymphoid tissue [1,2]. Thus the caecum and anorectum are the most common sites for primary lymphomas of the large bowel. The plentiful lymphoid tissue in the lower rectum and anus has resulted in the epithets of rectal and anal tonsil. Hyperplasia of this lymphoid tissue leads to polypoid lesions which are usually solitary. Throughout the colorectum there are numerous lymphoid aggregates, positioned in the lower mucosa and extending across the muscularis mucosae into the upper submucosa [3]. These lymphoglandular complexes (LGCs) may become hyperplastic and polypoid in several situations. In children hyperplasia causes the dramatic colonoscopic appearances of benign lymphoid polyposis. In adults, polypoid lymphoid hyperplasia occurs usually in response to chronic inflammatory conditions, especially ulcerative colitis, which may be accompanied by prominent lymphoid follicular hyperplasia [4], principally in the rectum. Diversion proctocolitis is also characterised by lymphoid follicular hyperplasia, producing highly distinctive mucosal nodularity at endoscopy [5]. Furthermore, lymphocyte homing mechanisms of mantle cells ensure that LGCs are the site of tumorigenesis for mantle cell lymphoma when it involves the gut, causing the characteristic macroscopic pathology of lymphomatous polyposis [6,7].

Benign lymphoid polyps

Isolated benign lymphoid polyps, representing a localised exaggerated lymphoid response to a largely unrecognised antigenic stimulus and are almost entirely confined to the rectum and around the anorectal junction. Such polyps elsewhere in the colon are exceptional [8]. They present as smooth, round tumours in the lower third of the rectum [9]. They are usually sessile but occasionally pedunculated (Figure 39.1). Most are single but occasionally up to five polypoid nodules are seen. Multiplicity of lymphoid polyps, especially if involving more proximal large bowel, should always raise the suspicion of lymphoma, unless the patient is a child, in which case benign lymphoid polyposis is the most likely diagnosis. However it should also be noted that mucosa-associated lymphoid tissue (MALT) lymphoma can be polypoid and mimic benign lymphoid polyps histologically [10].

Benign lymphoid polyps are slightly more common in men in their third and fourth decades. They are usually asymptomatic, being found incidentally during examination for other conditions. They vary in size from a few millimetres to 50 mm in diameter and only rarely ulcerate [8]. Histologically, benign lymphoid polyps show an intact surface mucosa, either rectal or anal canal type, although this may be compressed or attenuated by the submucosal mass. The body of the polyp within the submucosa and/or the lamina propria is composed of hyperplastic lymphoid tissue with multiple enlarged, geographical, lymphoid

Morson and Dawson's Gastrointestinal Pathology, Fifth Edition. Edited by Neil A. Shepherd, Bryan F. Warren, Geraint T. Williams, Joel K. Greenson, Gregory Y. Lauwers and Marco R. Novelli.

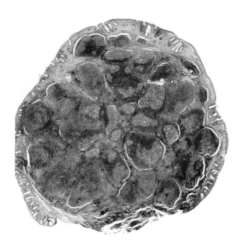

Figure 39.1 Histology of a benign lymphoid polyp of the rectum: the lesion appears pedunculated and is characterised by lymphoid follicular hyperplasia in the submucosa. The overlying mucosa is intact.

centres with prominent germinal centres (Figure 39.1). The appearances are not dissimilar to those of a reactive lymph node apart from the lack of a capsule and sinuses. Sarcoid-like granulomas are sometimes present. Involvement of the muscularis propria is exceptional.

Benign lymphoid polyps show no increased risk of malignant lymphoma. Excision is curative although many regress without resort to excision. On biopsy, differentiation from malignant lymphoma, especially that deriving from MALT, may be difficult [10]. Any diagnostic doubt should encourage excision biopsy to fully refute the diagnosis of lymphoma. Helpful discriminative features of benign lymphoid polyps include their relatively small size, circumscription of the lesion, non-involvement of the muscularis propria, lack of ulceration and an absence of positive features of lymphoma, notably infiltration and destruction of epithelial structures (destructive 'lympho-epithelial lesions') and infiltration of germinal centres by cleaved lymphoid cells. On immunohistochemistry, B cells are largely confined to the follicles, which can be delineated with follicular dentritic cell markers and are *bcl2* negative [9]. On occasion molecular analysis may be required to demonstrate the lack of clonal immunoglobulin gene rearrangement, the characteristic molecular finding in B-cell lymphomas of the gut [10].

Benign lymphoid polyposis

Benign lymphoid polyposis is a loosely defined condition characterised by multiple lymphoid polyps with benign histological features. In adults lymphoid polyposis may be due to hyperplastic LGCs, especially in ulcerative colitis and diversion proctocolitis. However, for the purpose of this discussion, the term is applied only to a rare condition of children in which LGCs show marked hyperplasia and present as a diffuse polyposis of the colorectum. Although the cause is not always known in individual cases, there is evidence that benign lymphoid polyposis is an exaggerated response to viral infection, especially echovirus and adenovirus [11]. A familial trait has been described [12] and the condition may also occur in immunodeficiency syndromes [13]. At colonoscopy, innumerable polyps festoon the intestinal mucosa, appearing as grey nodules measuring 3–6mm in diameter. The polyps show an intact surface mucosa with prominent reactive lymphoid tissue in the underlying submucosa, which often extends into the deep aspect of the overlying mucosa, as do physiological lymphoglandular complexes. These hyperplastic follicles are surrounded by a normal-appearing mantle zone.

In children with colorectal benign lymphoid polyposis, response to steroid therapy is often dramatic, although the condition may regress without specific treatment. There is no propensity for malignant change and therefore major surgical resection is not indicated [14]. Apart from being a possible indicator of immunodeficiency and/or viral infection, the disease's main significance lies in its potential mimicry of other polyposis syndromes, most notably familial adenomatous polyposis (FAP). Cases have been recorded in which colectomy has been carried out for this condition in the erroneous belief that the presence of multiple polyps equated with FAP [15]. The importance of adequate histological sampling of polyposis syndromes cannot be over-emphasised. In adults, a lymphoid polyposis should always raise the suspicion of malignant (multiple) lymphomatous polyposis.

Primary malignant lymphoma

Primary lymphoma of the colon and rectum is defined as extra-nodal lymphoma arising in either the colon or rectum, with the bulk of disease localised to this site [16]. The interested reader is referred to the further discussion concerning primary gastrointestinal lymphoma (see 'Tumours of lymphoid tissue', Chapter 15 and 'Primary malignant lymphoma of the small intestine', Chapter 26) and to specialist texts [16,17]. For the purposes of this discussion, the fourth Word Health Organization (WHO) classification [18] has been used with reorganisation, to reflect the occurrence and prevalence of these diseases in the large bowel. This classification is based on the Revised European–American Classification of Lymphoid Neoplasms (REAL) [19].

Primary lymphoma of the colon and rectum represents only 0.2–0.5% of primary malignant neoplasms at this site but it does represent between 5% and 10% of primary gastrointestinal lymphomas [1,20,21]. As would be expected from the distribution of lymphoid tissue within the large intestine, the most common sites of lymphoma are the caecum and rectum (Figure 39.2) [22–24]. The spectrum of

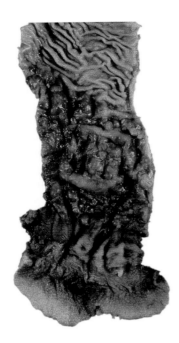

Figure 39.2 A high grade B-cell lymphoma of the rectum: there is characteristic diffuse, long segment involvement of the rectum, lower sigmoid colon and upper anal canal with extensive ulceration. The tumour showed massive involvement of local mesorectal lymph nodes.

disease is somewhat different from primary lymphoma affecting the stomach and small bowel, although the rarity of colorectal disease means that there has been less accurate disease classification compared with its counterparts in the stomach and small intestine. In the colorectum B-cell lymphomas are much more frequent than T-cell lymphomas. Among lymphomas of B-cell phenotype, diffuse large B-cell lymphoma is the most common type, followed by marginal zone B-cell lymphoma of MALT, mantle cell lymphoma, follicular lymphoma and Burkitt's lymphoma [2,24]. Other lymphoma subtypes affecting this part of the alimentary system are distinctly unusual.

Localised primary lymphoma of the large intestine may result as a rare complication of both major types of chronic inflammatory bowel disease (IBD) [25]. Those lymphomas complicating ulcerative colitis are predominantly high grade B-cell lymphomas, although rare cases of marginal zone B-cell lymphomas have been described [26]. As with carcinoma complicating ulcerative colitis, the extent and duration of disease appear to be the major risk factors [25]; however, recent reports suggest that, in ulcerative colitis patients treated with immunotherapy, the mean time to the development of lymphoma has decreased [27]. Colorectal lymphoma may arise in association with Crohn's disease but this is less commonly seen than with ulcerative colitis and Crohn's disease patients are more likely to develop

small intestinal lymphomas. Colorectal lymphomas arising on a background of Crohn's disease are a disparate group of B- and T-cell lymphomas, with a relatively high proportion of Hodgkin's lymphoma [25,28]. Intestinal lymphomas complicating IBD often harbour Epstein–Barr virus (EBV) [29]. Anorectal lymphoma is a common malignancy in HIV-infected patients; however, there has been a decreasing frequency as a result of the use of highly active antiretroviral therapy (HAART) [30]. The gastrointestinal tract is frequently involved in post-transplantation lymphoproliferative disorders (PTLDs) but the small intestine is affected more often than the colon [31]. Radiation and uretero-sigmoidostomy have been complicated by malignant lymphoma of the large bowel [32,33].

Diffuse large B-cell lymphoma

Most patients with diffuse large B-cell lymphoma (DLBCL) are adults, with a slight male predominance. Most cases involve the caecum or ascending colon, followed by the rectum [2,21,23,24,34]. The anorectum is the predominant site of disease in immunodeficient patients infected with HIV. The lesions tend to form large transmural masses with stricture and ulcer formation involving large segments of the colorectum.

DLBCL of the colon is typically composed of centroblastic, large, non-cleaved cells but there may be variation in the cellular morphology (multi-lobulated, monomorphic, polymorphic). A low grade component can be present, suggesting that there has been transformation of a pre-existing low grade lymphoma, which may be either MALT or follicular lymphoma. The immunophenotype is similar to that of gastric DLBCL, with mature B cells expressing CD20 and CD79a. Genetic studies confirm the heterogeneous nature of this disease, in some cases suggesting a follicular origin – t(14;18) translocation – whereas other cases show a t(11;18) translocation consistent with large-cell transformation of marginal-zone lymphoma.

Treatment is often based on a combination of surgery and chemotherapy. The disease is aggressive but potentially curable. As for gastric and small intestinal locations of DLBCL, the prognosis is influenced by the stage of the disease, with a poorer prognosis for patients with large tumours and for lymph-node positive disease [21].

Marginal zone B-cell lymphoma (MALT lymphoma)

In the fourth WHO classification of tumours of lymphoid tissues, MALT lymphoma is defined as a lymphoma composed predominantly of small cells [18]. This implies that the term 'high grade MALT lymphoma' should not be used. Associations between gastric *Helicobacter pylori* infection and lymphoma have been described, with evidence of regression of MALT-type colorectal lymphoma after antibiotic treatment for *H. pylori* [35]. It remains uncertain how strong the relationship is between colorectal lymphoma and gastric *H. pylori*.

MALT lymphoma occurs in adults; both men and women can be affected, it can occur in any part of the large intestine but a high proportion of cases occur in the rectum. Most commonly these lesions present as annular or plaque-like thickenings of the intestinal wall, although many are exophytic and polypoid. Very occasional cases of proven MALT lymphoma present with multi-focal polyposis-like involvement of the colorectum, masquerading as malignant lymphomatous polyposis of mantle cell type [36,37]. Gastrointestinal involvement of more than one anatomical site is frequent.

As with MALT lymphoma elsewhere in the gut, these lymphomas show characteristic microscopic appearances, with large reactive germinal centres, surrounded by the lymphomatous cells [16,18]. Typically, cells show the morphology of marginal zone lymphocytes, with centrocytic features unfortunately similar to those of both mantle cells and follicle centre cells. However, polymorphism, with prominent plasma cell differentiation and an admixture of blast cells, helps to differentiate this tumour from other lymphoma subtypes.

Infiltration and destruction of reactive germinal centres and crypt epithelium of the colorectum are two morphological diagnostic discriminators for MALT lymphoma. The infiltration by and destruction of epithelium produces the characteristic lympho-epithelial lesion (LEL) (Figure 39.3). These are not seen as often in intestinal MALT lymphoma as in their gastric counterpart. Also, lesions mimicking LELs do occur in other intestinal lymphomas, especially mantle-cell lymphoma (see below). The immunopheno-

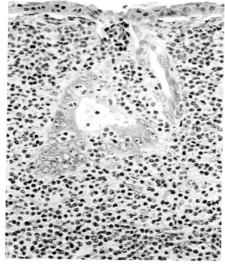

Figure 39.3 Marginal-zone (mucosa-associated lymphoid tissue) lymphoma of the colon: the central crypt is extensively infiltrated by lymphoid cells, producing the distinctive lymphoepithelial lesion.

typic features are similar to those seen in the stomach. Cytokeratin immunohistochemistry may be useful in highlighting the epithelial destruction and LELs. The same genetic alterations can be observed as in gastric MALT lymphoma, with a t(11;18) translocation resulting in the *API2–MALT1* fusion present in some cases and with relatively common trisomy 3 and trisomy 18 [38].

The prognosis of colorectal MALT lymphoma is considered to be less favourable than that of its gastric counterpart; however, it is better than the prognosis of other types of intestinal lymphoma. MALT lymphomas of the colorectum are, in general, amenable to local surgery and this may well be curative, in cases of truly localised disease [23,39].

Mantle-cell lymphoma – malignant lymphomatous polyposis

This distinctive and well-characterised form of lymphoma represents about a quarter of primary lymphomas of the colorectum [2,6,40]. Although it tends to present with large intestinal disease, the lymphoma also extensively involves the small bowel [6,40]. Gastric involvement is less pronounced, presumably because of the lack of lymphoid tissue in the normal stomach. The neoplasm usually presents with the physical effects of multiple polypoid masses in the intestine [40]. Thus mucus diarrhoea, steatorrhoea, protein-losing enteropathy or colopathy, abdominal pain and melaena are all recognised presentations. However, it should be noted that, when random biopsies are taken from the gastrointestinal tract of patients with mantle-cell lymphoma but no intestinal symptoms or endoscopic abnormalities the digestive tract is involved in 80% of the cases [41,42]. This lymphoma is a tumour of mantle cells, B-cell lymphocytes deriving from the mantle region, immediately adjacent to the germinal centre within lymphoid follicles. The tumour was originally termed 'multiple lymphomatous polyposis', a name that is still in regular usage. As polyposis implies the presence of multiple polyps, we believe that this term should be discouraged because of tautology: malignant lymphomatous polyposis (MLP) or simply lymphomatous polyposis would seem, to us, more appropriate to designate the macroscopic appearance in typical cases. MLP was thought to be pathognomonic of mantle-cell lymphoma but other lymphomas can present rarely with the same polyposis pattern on endoscopy, including MALT lymphoma, follicular lymphoma and even T-cell lymphoma [43].

Mantle-cell lymphoma is exclusively a disease of adults, with a median age at presentation of 50 years and a male preponderance. The condition is sporadic and no familial tendency has been recorded. Macroscopically the large intestinal mucosa in mantle-cell lymphoma with MLP shows innumerable, relatively well-circumscribed, polypoid masses (Figure 39.4). These are particularly found in the ileo-caecal region (Figure 39.4) [40]. Indeed the disease

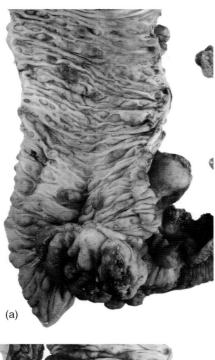

(a)

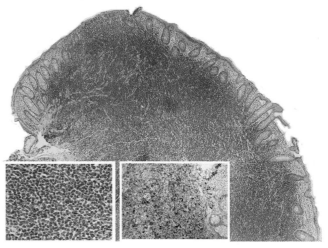

Figure 39.5 Mantle cell lymphoma of the colon: dense and grossly nodular lymphoid infiltrate of lower mucosa and submucosa. On higher power (left inset) monotonous infiltrate of intermediate-sized lymphoid cells that express cyclin-D1 (right inset).

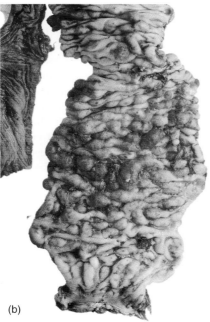

(b)

Figure 39.4 Malignant lymphomatous polyposis of the colon and rectum: (a) the right colon demonstrating a mass lesion in the region of the terminal ileum and caecum with numerous polyps in the proximal colon and local lymph node involvement (at right); (b) the left colon and rectum from the same specimen showing massive polypoid rectal involvement.

may present with an obstructing large mass, centred on the terminal ileum and involvement of the distal colon may be detected only subsequently. The lymphomatous polyps derive from pre-existing lymphoid aggregates and hence Peyer's patches of the small bowel and lymphoglandular complexes of the caecum and rectum are prominent sites of disease. In advanced disease, most of the small and large bowel is involved (Figure 39.4). The polyps appear smooth because of the intact overlying mucosa and usually measure between 5 and 100 mm. The endoscopic appearances are not unlike those of FAP.

Low-power microscopy reveals a characteristic nodular pattern: involvement is primarily in the lower mucosa and upper submucosa (Figure 39.5). In smaller (and hence earlier) lesions, neoplastic mantle cells surround surviving germinal centres [6]. As the lesions become larger, the nodularity may be lost and the infiltrate more diffuse in nature. High-power microscopy shows the relative monotonous infiltrate of small to intermediate-sized lymphoid cells, with cleaved nuclei, inconsequential nucleoli and modest amounts of cytoplasm. Collections of epithelioid histiocytes, sometimes forming well-defined granulomas, are not uncommon. There are morphological variants of mantle-cell lymphoma either blastoid or pleomorphic.

Differentiation of mantle-cell lymphoma from marginal-zone lymphoma (MALT lymphoma) may be difficult, especially on biopsy material. Although the morphological heterogeneity of MALT lymphoma and the presence of LELs may be helpful, these are not specific, e.g. epithelial destruction in mantle-cell lymphoma often produces lesions that cannot be distinguished from classic LELs [6].

The endoscopic appearances are usually the most helpful diagnostic indicator but mantle-cell lymphoma can lack the classic polyposis appearance. Immunohistochemistry and sometimes molecular analysis are required to make a definitive diagnosis. Mantle-cell lymphoma is characterised by CD20+ B lymphocytes that also express CD5 and cyclin-D1. Both these markers are not expressed in MALT lymphoma and hence are useful discriminators of these two diseases. The molecular basis of cyclin-D1 overexpression is a t(11,14) translocation in which the cyclin-D1 (CCND1) gene (on chromosome 11) is translocated to the immunoglobulin IGH gene on chromosome 14 [44]. In rare cases cells may not express CD5 but they remain cyclin-D1 positive.

Mantle-cell lymphoma in general has a poor prognosis and MLP represents a relatively advanced and certainly multifocal stage of the lymphoma [2,40]. Bone marrow involvement is usually present at presentation: systemic disease and leukaemia are characteristic late features of MLP [6,40]. As a result of its multifocal nature, major surgery is usually contraindicated although we have seen a case where the symptoms of colonic involvement (notably excessive mucus loss and electrolyte deficiency) necessitated emergency colectomy. Treatment is primarily by chemotherapy and the prognosis is poor. In one series, despite treatment, most patients were dead in 5 years, with a mean survival of 3 years [45]. Adverse histopathological parameters include blastoid/pleomorphic morphology, a high mitotic rate and a high proportion of Ki67 positive cells [18,21].

Other primary malignant lymphomas of the large intestine

DLBCL, marginal-zone lymphoma and mantle-cell lymphoma make up the vast majority of primary lymphomas in the large bowel. Follicular lymphoma is rare in the colon and rectum; it can be multifocal and in some cases it presents on endoscopy as polyposis [46]. There are isolated reports of plasmacytomas in the large bowel and myelomatous involvement can lead to tumorous masses closely mimicking low and high grade lymphoma [47]. Burkitt's lymphoma can involve the right colon in children but this tumour is primarily of terminal ileal origin and is considered elsewhere (see 'Primary malignant lymphoma of the small intestine', Chapter 26).

Anorectal lymphoma is a recognised complication of HIV infection in heavily immunodeficient patients. Most of these tumours are of high grade type and show the features of DLBCL or Burkitt's disease and Burkitt's disease-like lymphoma [48,49]; a few cases of plasmablastic lymphoma have also been reported, which can be difficult to diagnose because they do not express B-cell markers [50]. There is good evidence that these tumours are driven by EBV infection [49]. Despite the high grade nature of these tumours, they are often confined to the anorectal region at presenta-

tion [49]. Nevertheless, as with extra-nodal lymphoma complicating HIV infection at other sites, the prognosis is extremely poor [51].

T-/natural killer (NK)-cell lymphoma is relatively common in the small intestine but is distinctly unusual in the large bowel, except in Asian countries where it shows a slightly higher incidence [52]. Various types have been reported, including peripheral T-cell lymphoma not otherwise specified, extra-nodal NK/T-cell lymphoma of nasal type, anaplastic large cell lymphoma of both ALK+ and ALK– types and adult T-cell leukaemia/lymphoma. Multifocality is a particular property of T-cell lymphomas in the gut and rarely T-cell lymphoma can present as MLP when involving the colon [43,53]. Reports of primary Hodgkin's disease of the large bowel should be treated with extreme scepticism. Many recorded cases of primary gastrointestinal Hodgkin's disease have been subsequently demonstrated to represent non-Hodgkin's lymphoma, often of T-cell phenotype.

The biopsy diagnosis of lymphoid tumours of the colorectum

The differentiation of benign lymphoid polyp/polyposis from malignant lymphoma is of critical importance. Endoscopic appearances and size are useful discriminators between benign and malignant lesions. However, MALT lymphomas in the rectum can be small and polypoid; they may also mimic benign lymphoid polyps histologically [10]. Ulceration is generally only a feature of lymphomas, which are usually appreciably larger than their benign counterparts. If the lesion is relatively small, then excisional biopsy will provide a fully representative, undistorted and well-oriented specimen. The morphological discriminators of MALT lymphoma and mantle-cell lymphoma have been previously described but it is as well to emphasise their histological mimicry. Both lymphomas are characterised by a predominance of cells with centrocyte-like morphology and both may show lymphomatous destruction of epithelium. Their division, on biopsy material, can be difficult and attention should paid to the clinical and colonoscopic features. Even then occasional cases of MALT lymphoma can manifest as polyposis [36,37]. It is advisable to perform immunohistochemistry on all such cases: CD5 and cyclin-D1 immunostaining providing a definitive diagnosis in nearly all cases. As favourable-stage MALT lymphoma is most appropriately treated by excisional surgery with or without chemotherapy and surgery is generally contraindicated in MLP, the importance of this distinction is indisputable.

Leukaemia in the large intestine

Acute myeloblastic leukaemia may cause tumorous masses in the large bowel simulating carcinoma. On occasion such myeloid (granulocytic) sarcomas may be the presenting feature of the disease, before the leukaemic phase [54]. The tumour cells have relatively plentiful eosinophilic cytoplasm, often with an eccentric nucleus. The cells themselves may mimic plasma cells or other primitive lymphoid cells and may lead to an erroneous diagnosis of malignant lymphoma, plasmacytoma or myelomatous involvement of the gut. Demonstration of myeloperoxidase, lysozyme, CD117 and CD34 on immunohistochemistry serves to confirm the diagnosis. A single case of mast cell sarcoma has been reported in the ascending colon [55].

Connective tissue tumours

Despite the amount of connective tissue in the large bowel, these tumours are relatively unusual compared with their counterparts in other parts of the gut and with epithelial tumours of the colorectum. Lipomas are undoubtedly the most common connective tissue tumours in the large bowel but they are usually discovered incidentally and do not, on the whole, cause symptoms. Most other connective tissue tumours of the colorectum present with the symptoms and signs of a mass effect. Of these, gastrointestinal stromal tumours (GISTs) are the most common but even these are unusual compared with GISTs arising in the stomach and small bowel.

Gastrointestinal stromal tumours

It is now apposite to consider most, if not all, tumours in the gut, with a spindle cell morphology and without identifying features indicating an origin from specific connective cells, as GISTs, arising from interstitial cells of Cajal. This rethink has been prompted by the ready availability of immunohistochemistry for CD34 and then for CD117 (KIT) and by molecular evidence [56–59]. It is not appropriate to recapitulate a comprehensive account of the histogenesis and morphological features of GISTs here because this subject has been dealt with elsewhere (see 'Gastrointestinal stromal tumours', Chapters 14 and 25). Although some have suggested that stromal tumours of the oesophagus and the colorectum, especially the rectum, are more likely to demonstrate specific features of smooth muscle tumours and should be largely considered as such [60], in general we prefer the broader brush approach (for the intestines at least) and to refer to all of these tumours, whatever their site of origin and morphology, as GISTs. In this treatise, therefore, tumours that do not have the morphological features of specific entities such as schwannoma, neurofibroma or granular cell tumour have been regarded as GISTs. We do not deny that, rarely, tumours indistinguishable from leiomyomas elsewhere (e.g. in the uterus) do occur in the large bowel, specifically the rectum but it is abundantly clear that such tumours are very rare

in the colon and most of these tumours are therefore most conveniently regarded as GISTs.

GISTs are rare in the colon, compared with their gastric and small intestinal counterparts [58]. For this reason, there are relatively few data on their histogenetic features, behaviour and prognosis. Of particular importance is the fact that there is a much higher proportion of malignant GISTs, among colorectal tumours, compared with GISTs in the stomach and small intestine.

Colonic GISTs represent about 1% of all GISTs and their most common location is the sigmoid colon, followed the by transverse colon [61]. Although rarely cases consist of small firm whitish nodules involving the serosal aspect of the colonic wall, most tumours are large intramural masses, usually >50 mm in diameter and often in excess of 100 mm. Most cases are composed of spindle cells but some show an epithelioid cell morphology. Skeinoid fibres can be present. Nuclear palisading is a common feature, whereas perinuclear vacuolisation is not prominent. On immunohistochemistry, colorectal GISTs are consistently positive for KIT, DOG1 and CD34 and can express smooth muscle actin. They are negative for S-100 protein [62,63]. The KIT mutation spectrum is similar to small intestinal GISTs with a majority of mutations occurring in exon 11 [61]. Although some of these tumours share the morphological features of the apparently benign tumours, more characteristic of the stomach and small intestine, it is notoriously difficult to predict the probable behaviour in these tumours. Time-honoured macroscopic and morphological features may be helpful. Size, the presence of necrosis, cellularity and tumour necrosis may be of some help. However, as with GISTs elsewhere, the mitotic rate supplies the most useful guide to likely behaviour and in its presence other parameters appear not to provide additional prognostic information. A rate of more than 5 mitoses/5 mm^2 will identify GISTs at high risk of malignancy [61,64]. Although pleomorphism is relatively uncommon among this group of tumours, occasional bizarre cells with grossly enlarged nuclei do occur in otherwise benign tumours and some care is advisable in assessing tumours with such cells, especially if they have low mitotic activity.

Frankly malignant GISTs, often termed 'pleomorphic sarcomas', are particularly aggressive, with high rates of metastatic disease (Figure 39.6) [65,66]. These tumours characteristically cause blood-borne metastases; local lymph node involvement is an unusual feature [67]. One feature of such tumours, which is relatively specific to the colon, is that they may grow as confluent nodules in a longitudinal fashion, with a dominant mass and multinodular thickening of the adjacent colonic wall, a feature that is virtually never seen elsewhere in the gut [68]. This appearance is different from so-called leiomyomatosis of the colon, in which there are well-separated nodules of spindle cell tumour [69], a lesion that is also seen in the

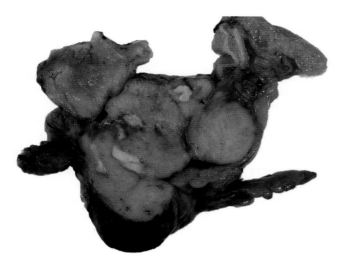

Figure 39.6 Stromal tumour of the rectum: large multinodular mass with areas of necrosis.

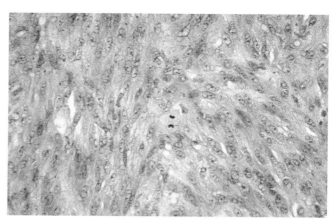

Figure 39.7 A deep stromal tumour of the rectum: the tumour is spindle celled but with marked nuclear anaplasia and a high mitotic activity. The tumour recurred after local excision and ultimately the patient died of metastatic disease.

oesophagus. Whether this extremely rare lesion is truly of smooth muscle derivation remains uncertain.

The most significant features of colonic GISTs are their rarity, high risk of malignancy and poorly defined management strategies. We cannot over-emphasise the lack of predictability of biological behaviour in many of these lesions: cases of small tumours with low mitotic activity have been described that have subsequently metastasised, often many years after the primary tumour has been excised. We would regard any colonic GIST as a potentially malignant lesion and would generally advise relatively radical surgery, if clinically indicated.

Stromal tumours in the rectum

Despite the concept of GISTs and the intentions of many to regard all spindle-cell tumours of the gastrointestinal tract within this broad umbrella term, there is evidence that primary smooth muscle tumours do occur in the large bowel and that these are almost entirely restricted to the rectum and distal sigmoid colon [68]. Most tumours showing such definitive evidence of smooth muscle derivation derive from the muscularis mucosae. Indeed the rectum is the only part of the gut where tumours arise from the muscularis mucosae with any frequency [68]. These leiomyomas present as small intramucosal and submucosal nodules visible to the endoscopist as a small elevation [70]. They are usually incidental findings, only about 5 mm in diameter, although occasionally they may reach a size of 15 mm [70]. Although these occur at any age, they are slightly more common in men, with a male:female ratio of 1.8:1 [70]. Apart from the oesophageal leiomyoma, this rectal lesion is the only tumour of the gut characterised by morphologically typical (albeit apparently hypertrophic) smooth muscle cells with the typical bundling morphology [68]. They are almost universally benign [68,70].

Although the leiomyomatous polyp, arising from the muscularis mucosae, is undoubtedly the most common spindle-cell tumour of the rectum, there is a further spindle-cell tumour of the lower rectum and anus with distinctive features. This tumour, previously known as the deep intramural stromal tumour of the rectum [68,71], is now considered an anorectal GIST [72,73]. Therefore, the rectum is the third most common site for GIST, after stomach and small intestine. Anorectal GISTs comprise 4% of all GISTs and show a marked male predominance. They occur in any segment, arise from the deep tissues of the rectum and anal canal and appear to derive from the muscularis propria (Figure 39.6). Local recurrence is a characteristic feature of this tumour (in about half the cases) and late metastatic disease is also a considerable problem. It is possible that the high rate of metastatic disease, often after a considerable time period since primary surgery, relates to the inadequacy of that surgery, because this tumour is often treated initially by local excision only [57,59,60].

Anorectal GISTs are usually moderately large at presentation, because of their deep position in the anorectal wall and often measure in excess of 50 mm in diameter. Histologically they tend to be composed of relatively regular spindle cells with darkly staining nuclei in a fascicular pattern, which can show palisading (Figure 39.7) [68,72,73]. There are no skeinoid fibres. The immunohistochemical pattern and the *KIT* mutational spectrum is similar to that observed in colonic GISTs. Those tumours that locally recur, or metastasise, are typically more cellular, with very closely packed spindle cells and have the higher mitotic activity, with a cut-off value of 5 mitoses/5 mm^2 as in colonic tumours [72,73]. These tumours should be treated aggressively because of their propensity for local recurrence. However, reports would suggest that, although radicality may prevent local recurrence, it may not materially affect the potential for metastatic disease and overall survival [68,70]. Aside from anorectal GISTs, rare cases of intramural leiomyomas and true leiomyosarcomas, can be observed that are actin positive and KIT negative [73].

Tumours of adipose tissue

Lipoma

Although clinically significant lipomas are uncommon, small submucosal lipomas are not so very unusual as an incidental finding at colonoscopy. The right side of the colon is the most common site (Figure 39.8) [74,75]. Such lesions are seen at colonoscopy or in resection specimens as small (usually <20mm), yellow, circumscribed nodules with an intact overlying mucosa. Only in larger lesions is there surface ulceration: this may be a mechanical effect and does not necessarily imply any likelihood of malignancy (Figure 39.8). Much larger lesions, especially in the right colon, may present because of a mass lesion, or characteristically with intussusception (Figure 39.8). Angiographic mimicry of angiodysplasia (angio-ectasia) of the proximal colon by lipoma has been described because

lipomas have a large feeder vessel and produce a blush of smaller vessels similar to those seen in angiodysplasia [75].

Colorectal lipomas are usually single but are on occasion multiple. The term 'lipomatosis' infers the presence of multiple lipomas. There are occasional case reports of lipomatosis occurring in the colonic submucosa [76], also involving the small bowel [77], the appendices epiploicae [78] and the pelvic connective tissues [79]. Such lipomatosis can result in multiple polyps in the colon and has been referred to as lipomatous polyposis [80]. As with other rare polyposis syndromes, there is potential mimicry of the more common and clinically significant polyposis syndromes. It is probable that multiplicity of these fatty tumours is a hamartomatous phenomenon rather than a neoplastic one: there is no malignant potential of either solitary lipomas or lipomatosis.

Microscopically, the appearances of lipoma are those of simple adipose tissue, with circumscribed masses of adipocytes compressing the adjacent muscularis mucosae (Figure 39.9) and, sometimes, the underlying muscularis propria. Lipomatosis is usually accompanied by an increase in submucosal fat. Necrosis and haemorrhage may occur if there are secondary mechanical effects, such as intussusception. Some lesions in this situation show much granulation tissue formation and this can be disconcerting to the diagnostic pathologist. Atypical features, akin to those seen in lipomas of the subcutis, can be seen; these lesions have been termed 'atypical lipoma' [81]. However frank liposarcoma is an extreme rarity in the colon and should be

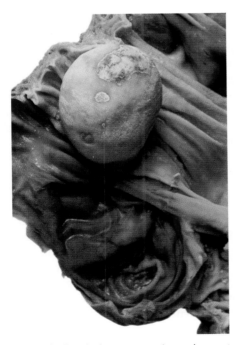

Figure 39.8 A right hemicolectomy specimen demonstrating an intussuscepted lipoma of the proximal colon. The surface ulceration is a mechanical effect and does not indicate malignancy in this case.

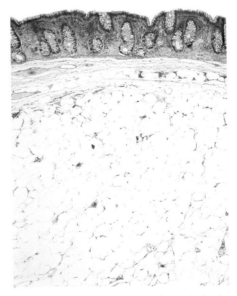

Figure 39.9 A colonic lipoma showing the typical submucosal position with the compressed but otherwise normal overlying mucosa.

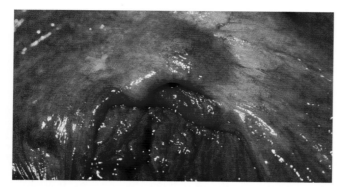

Figure 39.10 Lipohyperplasia of the ileo-caecal valve: the appearance has been likened to a pouting cervix uteri.

diagnosed only when lipoblasts are definitively demonstrated [81,82].

Lipohyperplasia of the ileo-caecal valve

This condition, also known as lipomatosis and lipomatous hypertrophy of the ileo-caecal valve, is characterised by an excess of adipose tissue in the submucosa of the ileo-caecal valve producing thickening and pouting of the valve. which protrudes into the caecum [83]. The thickening of the valve may produce narrowing of the lumen and the appearances of the valve have been likened to those of prolapsed haemorrhoids or a pouting cervix uteri (Figure 39.10). In our experience mild lipohyperplasia of the ileo-caecal valve is extremely common. Less commonly, especially in association with prolapse into the caecal lumen, the neoplasm-like prominence of the valve can masquerade as a malignant tumour on barium enema. Right hemicolectomy has been performed, on occasion, in the mistaken belief that a malignant tumour had been demonstrated radiologically. It may give rise, rarely, to symptoms of subacute obstruction and is but one cause of the ileo-caecal valve syndrome [84].

The condition is, unsurprisingly, closely associated with obesity and histological examination reveals an excess of histologically normal adipose tissue in the submucosa. This accumulation is not encapsulated and gradually diminishes on either side of the valve. Occasionally the adipotic valve becomes congested and eroded with ulceration and bleeding. The lesion, which we believe is best termed 'lipohyperplasia' because it is simply an increase in fatty tissue within the valve, should not be confused with lipoma or true intestinal lipomatosis.

Vascular tumours of the large intestine

Haemangiomas

Most 'haemangiomas' are not true neoplasms at all but are merely malformations or hamartomas. Nevertheless they may present as mass lesions and are appropriately considered here. They usually present with rectal bleeding or mechanical effects such as intussusception. Most haemangiomas of the large bowel are of cavernous type [85], most often in the sigmoid colon and/or rectum. Here they may involve a relatively long segment whereas involvement of the whole colon has been reported [86]. The angiomatous abnormality involves the entire blood supply, including perirectal or pericolic tissues as well as vessels within the bowel wall. We have seen cases where there is also extensive involvement of the ischiorectal fossa and the musculature of the buttock, unilaterally. Such involvement makes surgical treatment very difficult. Angiographic embolisation has been attempted with some success, although there are dangers of causing necrosis of the bowel wall and other important structures.

Macroscopically, the colonic or rectal mucosa has a plum-coloured appearance but is intact and otherwise normal. Huge, tortuous vascular spaces can be seen in the bowel wall and adjacent tissues. These often contain easily recognisable phleboliths that show up radiographically and are a useful diagnostic sign. The microscopic appearance is similar to that of haemangiomas elsewhere, often with intravascular thrombosis as a prominent feature.

Multiplicity of haemangiomas can be seen in several conditions, some well defined and others less so. The blue rubber bleb naevus syndrome [87] is associated with cutaneous vascular naevi and prominent, often life-threatening, gastrointestinal haemorrhage. The lesions are small (<5 mm) and have a blue wrinkled surface. In the colon, the haemangiomas are more likely to be left sided and in the rectum. The Klippel–Trenaunay–Weber syndrome associates soft tissue and bone hypertrophy, varicose veins and port wine haemangiomas with vascular malformations of the gut. An apparent forme fruste of Peutz–Jeghers syndrome, due to incomplete penetrance of the gene, may also result in multiple intestinal haemangiomas [87]. Histological assessment of these lesions, unless at the time of colonic resection, is not usually undertaken due to the considerable risks of inducing severe haemorrhage. Most of these lesions simply show the features of cavernous haemangiomas [88].

Other vascular tumours of the large intestine

Haemagiopericytomas [89] and glomus tumours [68,90] do occur in the colon and rectum but both are distinctly unusual. They show similar macroscopic and microscopic pathology to those seen elsewhere. Angiosarcoma affecting the colon is very uncommon and can be difficult to diagnose, with frequent epithelioid differentiation [91]. A case of post-irradiation angiosarcoma of the rectum has been reported in a patient treated for rectal adenocarcinoma [92].

Much more common, typically in the context of AIDS, is Kaposi's sarcoma of the colon, rectum and anus. In the gut, small intestinal involvement is most common in necropsy practice but gastric and colorectal involvement are more likely to be seen in clinical practice [93]. The disease is often multifocal and affects several parts of the gut. The presence of Kaposi's sarcoma in the intestines reflects advanced immunosuppression. The disease itself does not necessarily imply a poor prognosis but the advanced immunosuppression of which it is a marker may do so [93,94].

It is predominantly a disease of homosexual men with AIDS but cases have been reported in other immunosuppressed patients, including organ transplant recipients and patients with ulcerative colitis under immunosuppressive drugs [95,96]. The very high prevalence initially reported in the AIDS epidemic has been markedly reduced since the introduction of HAART [93,94]. Kaposi's sarcoma presents colonoscopically in diverse forms. It may appear as a macular bluish lesion but polypoid, eruptive and papular variants are also described [93,97]. Kaposi's sarcoma masquerading as ulcerative colitis is also well recognised [98]. The neoplasm, now convincingly linked to human herpesvirus 8 (HHV8) [99,100] is characterised histologically by pleomorphic spindle cells, with adjacent clefts in which red cells are enmeshed. Haemorrhage, both old and recent, is usually demonstrated and hyaline droplets are characteristic features within the cytoplasm of the tumour cells. Immunohistochemical expression of HHV8 is a highly sensitive and specific diagnostic marker of Kaposi's sarcoma.

Lymphangioma

Lymphangiomas of the colon and rectum are very uncommon and usually found coincidentally during investigations for unassociated symptomatology [101]. There is a confusing plethora of terminology, including lymphatic cyst, mesenteric cyst and cystic hygroma, which all probably represent the same spectrum of pathology. Along with haemangioma in the intestines, it is likely that lymphangioma is not a true neoplasm at all but rather a developmental abnormality or acquired as a hamartoma-like lesion. Lymphangiomas are more likely to involve the mesenteric tissues than the bowel wall itself. They may occur as polypoid lesions of the colonic submucosa, on a broad base, although more often they are ill-defined diffuse lesions in the colonic wall [101]. Their cut surfaces show cystic spaces from which lymph may exude. Histologically they are composed of widely dilated lymphatic spaces within which lymphocytes can be identified. These lesions should not be confused with lymphangiectasia, a condition that much more diffusely involves the intestinal mucosa and submucosa. Although lymphangiectasia is usually small intestinal and associated with protein-losing enteropathy, colonic variants have been rarely described [102,103].

Neurogenic tumours

Before initiating discussion on neurogenic tumours of the large intestine, it is appropriate to reaffirm the concept of GISTs. Although rare, it is possible that GISTs in the large bowel, especially the colon, whether benign or malignant, may show some evidence of neural differentiation, particularly by immunohistochemistry. If such lesions conform to the general morphological descriptions of GISTs given elsewhere (see 'Gastrointestinal stromal tumours', Chapters 14 and 25), then such lesions are appropriately considered as GISTs with their attendant (often uncertain) management strategies and prognosis. This section considers those tumours with definitive morphological and immunohistochemical evidence of an origin in neural tissue within the large bowel. This group of tumours of neural origin has been enriched by newly described types of tumours presenting as small mucosal polyps, designated by various names and usually discovered during colonoscopy performed for colorectal screening in asymptomatic patients.

Solitary benign neurofibroma of the rectum or colon is very rare as an isolated lesion. It usually presents incidentally as a small submucosal tumour that may diffusely involve the overlying mucosa. This is not a feature in itself to indicate any aggressive behaviour but is more part of the character of diffuse-type neurofibromas seen elsewhere. The appearance has been likened to that of an early juvenile polyp in the colonic mucosa [68]. Even a solitary neurofibroma in the rectum may yet presage the presence of von Recklinghausen's disease [104] and it is wise always to raise this possibility when reporting such lesions. Gastrointestinal involvement is common in von Recklinghausen's disease [105], although the colon seems to be involved less frequently than the small intestine [106]. To add to the confusion concerning neurogenic differentiation and GISTs, tumours with the morphological features of GISTs are relatively common features of von Recklinghausen's disease [106]. The neurofibromas of von Recklinghausen's disease may present with either obstruction or, more commonly, bleeding [107,108]. Carcinoid tumours and spindle-cell sarcomas are both recognised complications of colorectal neurofibromatosis [106,109].

Schwannomas (neurilemmomas) appear to be excessively rare in the large intestine. They present as intraluminal polypoid masses with mural involvement, often with mucosal ulceration [110,111]. Whether small polypoid neural lesions of the colon, recently described as mucosal benign epithelioid nerve sheath tumor [112] and mucosal Schwann cell hamartoma [113], represent early mucosal schwannomas or separate forms of benign intramucosal Schwann cell proliferation remains to be determined. These two benign lesions predominate in the distal colon and present as isolated small sessile polyps, with no associated inherited syndrome. Histologically, they are composed of a diffuse proliferation of uniform bland spindle cells, strongly expressing S-100 protein, with no other marker expressed. Another type of small polyp of the colorectum composed of bland-looking spindle cells has been described

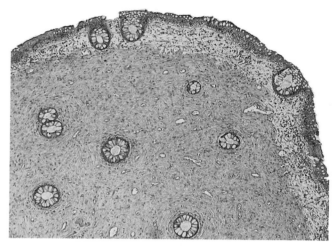

Figure 39.11 A colonic peri-neurioma: diffuse proliferation of uniform bland spindle cells with entrapped crypts.

as intestinal perineuroma, and initially as benign fibroblastic polyp (Figure 39.11) [114–119]; it predominates in women and is often localised in the rectosigmoid. A striking feature is the almost constant presence within the lesion of serrated glands intermixed with the mesenchymal proliferation [116,119]. Contrary to Schwann cells, the spindle cells show positivity for perineural cell markers (epithelial membrane antigen, claudin-1, collagen IV) and do not express S-100 protein.

Granular cell tumours, demonstrated to be tumours of nerve sheath origin, are rare lesions in the large intestine, with a predilection for the ascending colon and rectum [120,121]. They are morphologically identical to their more common counterparts in the skin and at other sites.

Ganglioneuroma and ganglioneuromatosis represent the ends of a spectrum of neurogenic lesions that contain Schwann cell, ganglion cell and neurite derivatives. Solitary ganglioneuroma of the colorectum is very rare and is much more likely to be seen in the retroperitoneum. It has been confusingly described as localised ganglioneuromatosis [122]. Ganglioneuromatosis itself represents a spectrum of disease from diffuse colorectal involvement to disease that is predominantly submucosal and results in polypoid masses in the large bowel. Diffuse intestinal ganglioneuromatosis, medullary carcinoma of the thyroid, phaeochromocytoma and multiple mucosal neuromas together comprise the inherited syndrome now known as multiple endocrine neoplasia (MEN) type 2b [122,123]. Although phaeochromocytoma and von Recklinghausen's disease frequently coexist, the neural tumours in neurofibromatosis and MEN-2b differ in their distribution and histological appearances. Neurofibromas are made up of loose fibrous tissue, with cells having their characteristic wavy appearance interspersed with occasional nerve fibres.

The absence of ganglion cells would be consistent with a defect involving the sympathetic nerve supply to the gut. Diffuse ganglioneuromatosis, on the other hand, involves the nerves and nerve cell bodies (ganglion cells) of nerve plexuses and has no connective tissue component. The defect here may involve the parasympathetic nerve supply or non-adrenergic, non-cholinergic enteric nerves. Polypoid ganglioneuromatosis differs from diffuse intestinal ganglioneuromatosis in that the neural proliferation lies within the lamina propria and gives rise to mucosal polyps. There are recognised associations between polypoid ganglioneuromatosis, on the one hand and juvenile polyposis and Cowden's syndrome, on the other [124–126]. This demonstrates that the genetic defects associated with these polyposis syndromes affect many tissue types other than epithelium.

On occasion traumatic neuroma may be seen after previous surgery in the colon [127]. It is likely that primary neurofibrosarcomas of the large bowel do exist but it is probable that such tumours have been and will be, regarded as malignant GISTs unless evidence of their neural derivation is compelling.

Miscellaneous tumours of the colorectum and retrorectal space

Very rarely other sarcomas have been described in the colon and rectum, including fibrosarcoma and rhabdomyosarcoma but it is likely that many of these represent secondary involvement of the large bowel. Tumours arising in the retrorectal space may manifest as anorectal masses. Benign lesions include retrorectal cystic hamartomas (tailgut cysts – see Chapter 33) and benign cystic teratomas. Chordoma and myxopapillary ependymoma, arising in or close to the sacrum, may secondarily involve the rectum. The 'Ivalon tumour' produces confounding histological appearances to the unwary [128,129]. Rectopexy, performed for rectal prolapse, using Ivalon, a sponge-like material, may result in a mass effect, often several years after the primary surgery. Removal of the mass and submission for histopathology have confused many a pathologist. This is because the Ivalon itself has an appearance not unlike osteoid and the incitement of a histiocytic and giant cell reaction, the latter resembling osteoclasts, further enhances the mimicry of a bone tumour. Viewing the lesion under cross-polarised light identifies the foreign material within the lesion and prevents the dispatching of a potentially embarrassing pathology report.

References

1. Richards MA. Lymphoma of the colon and rectum. *Postgrad Med J* 1986;**62**:615.
2. Shepherd NA, Hall PA, Coates PJ, Levison DA. Primary malignant lymphoma of the colon and rectum. A histopathological

and immunohistochemical analysis of 45 cases with clinico-pathological correlations. *Histopathology* 1988;**12**:235.

3. O'Leary AD, Sweeney EC. Lymphoglandular complexes of the colon: structure and distribution. *Histopathology* 1986;**10**:267.

4. Flejou JF, Potet F, Bogomoletz WV, et al. Lymphoid follicular proctitis. A condition different from ulcerative proctitis? *Dig Dis Sci* 1988;**33**:314.

5. Yeong ML, Bethwaite PB, Prasad J, Isbister WH. Lymphoid follicular hyperplasia – a distinctive feature of diversion colitis. *Histopathology* 1991;**19**:55.

6. Lavergne A, Brouland JP, Launay E, Nemeth J, Ruskone-Fourmestraux A, Galian A. Multiple lymphomatous polyposis of the gastrointestinal tract. An extensive histopathologic and immunohistochemical study of 12 cases. *Cancer* 1994;**74**:3042.

7. Geissmann F, Ruskoné-Fourmestraux A, Hermine O, et al. Homing receptor alpha4beta7 integrin expression predicts digestive tract involvement in mantle cell lymphoma. *Am J Pathol.* 1998;**153**:1701.

8. Cornes JS, Wallace MH, Morson BC. Benign lymphomas of the rectum and anal canal. *J Pathol Bacteriol* 1961;**82**:371.

9. Farris AB, Lauwers GY, Ferry JA, Zukerberg LR. The rectal tonsil: a reactive lymphoid proliferation that may mimic lymphoma. *Am J Surg Pathol* 2008;**32**:1075.

10. Kojima M, Itoh H, Motegi A, Sakata N, Masawa N. Localized lymphoid hyperplasia of the rectum resembling polypoid mucosa-associated lymphoid tissue lymphoma: a report of three cases. *Pathol Res Pract.* 2005;**201**:757.

11. Atwell JD, Burge D, Wright D. Nodular lymphoid hyperplasia of the intestinal tract in infancy and childhood. *J Pediatr Surg* 1985;**20**:25.

12. Louw JH. Polypoid lesions of the large bowel in children with particular reference to benign lymphoid polyposis. *J Pediatr Surg* 1968;**3**:195.

13. Shaw EB, Hennigar GR. Intestinal lymphoid polyposis. *Am J Clin Pathol* 1974;**61**:417.

14. Benchimol D, Frileux P, Herve de Sigalony JP, Parc R. Benign lymphoid polyposis of the colon. Report of a case in an adult. *Int J Colorectal Dis* 1991;**6**:165.

15. Berk T, Cohen Z, McLeod RS, Cullen JB. Surgery based on misdiagnosis of adenomatous polyposis. The Canadian Polyposis Registry experience. *Dis Colon Rectum* 1987;**30**:588.

16. Isaacson PG. Gastrointestinal lymphomas of T- and B-cell type. *Mod Pathol* 1999;**12**:151.

17. Crump M, Gospodarowicz M, Shepherd NA. Lymphoma of the gastrointestinal tract. *Semin Oncol* 1999;**26**:324.

18. Swerdlow SH, Campo E, Harris NL, et al., eds. *WHO Classification of Tumours of Haematopoietic and Lymphoid Tissues.* Lyon: IARC, 2008.

19. Isaacson PG. The revised European-American lymphoma (REAL) classification [editorial]. *Clin Oncol (R Coll Radiol)* 1995; **7**:347.

20. Gurney KA, Cartwright RA, Gilman EA. Descriptive epidemiology of gastrointestinal non-Hodgkin's lymphoma in a population-based registry. *Br J Cancer* 1999;**79**:1929.

21. Müller-Hermelink HK, Delabie J, Ko YH, Jaffe ES, van Krieken JH, Nakamura S. B-cell lymphoma of the colon and rectum. In: Bosman FT, Carneiro F, Hruban RH, Theise ND (eds), *WHO Classification of Tumours of Haematopoietic and Lymphoid Tissues.* Lyon: IARC, 2010: 178.

22. Zighelboim J, Larson MV. Primary colonic lymphoma. Clinical presentation, histopathologic features, and outcome with combination chemotherapy. *J Clin Gastroenterol* 1994;**18**:291.

23. Koch P, del Valle F, Berdel WE, et al. Primary gastrointestinal non-Hodgkin's lymphoma: I. Anatomic and histologic distribution, clinical features, and survival data of 371 patients registered in the German Multicenter Study GIT NHL 01/92. *J Clin Oncol.* 2001;**19**:3861.

24. Kohno S, Ohshima K, Yoneda S, Kodama T, Shirakusa T, Kikuchi M. Clinicopathological analysis of 143 primary malignant lymphomas in the small and large intestines based on the new WHO classification. *Histopathology* 2003;**43**:135.

25. Shepherd NA, Hall PA, Williams GT, et al. Primary malignant lymphoma of the large intestine complicating chronic inflammatory bowel disease. *Histopathology* 1989;**15**:325.

26. Holubar SD, Dozois EJ, Loftus EV Jr, et al. Primary intestinal lymphoma in patients with inflammatory bowel disease: A descriptive series from the prebiologic therapy era. *Inflamm Bowel Dis* 2010;**17**:1557.

27. Farrell R, Ang Y, Kileen P, et al. Increased incidence of non-Hodgkin's lymphoma in inflammatory bowel disease patients on immunosuppressive therapy but overall risk is low. *Gut* 2000;**47**:514.

28. Kumar S, Fend F, Quintanilla-Martinez L, et al. Epstein–Barr virus-positive primary gastrointestinal Hodgkin's disease: association with inflammatory bowel disease and immunosuppression. *Am J Surg Pathol* 2000;**24**:66.

29. Wong NA, Herbst H, Herrmann K, et al. Epstein–Barr virus infection in colorectal neoplasms associated with inflammatory bowel disease: detection of the virus in lymphomas but not in adenocarcinomas. *J Pathol.* 2003;**201**:312.

30. Raphaël M, Said J, Borisch B, Cesarman E, Harris NL. Lymphomas associated with HIV infection. In: Swerdlow SH, Campo E, Harris NL, et al. (eds), *WHO Classification of Tumours of Haematopoietic and Lymphoid Tissues.* IARC: Lyon, 2008: 340.

31. Aigner F, Boeckle E, Albright J. Malignancies of the colorectum and anus in solid organ recipients. *Transpl Int.* 2007;**20**:497.

32. Sibly TF, Keane RM, Lever JV, Southwood WF. Rectal lymphoma in radiation injured bowel. *Br J Surg* 1985;**72**:879.

33. Ghanem AN, Perry KC. Malignant lymphoma as a complication of ureterosigmoidostomy. *Br J Surg* 1985;**72**:559.

34. Wong MTC, Eu KW. Primary colorectal lymphomas. *Colorectal Dis* 2006;**8**:586.

35. Matsumoto T, Iida M, Shimizu M. Regression of mucosa-associated lymphoid-tissue lymphoma of rectum after eradication of *Helicobacter pylori. Lancet* 1997;**350**:115.

36. Yatabe Y, Nakamura S, Nakamura T, et al. Multiple polypoid lesions of primary mucosa-associated lymphoid-tissue lymphoma of colon. *Histopathology* 1998;**32**:116.

37. Breslin NP, Urbanski SJ, Shaffer EA. Mucosa-associated lymphoid tissue (MALT) lymphoma manifesting as multiple lymphomatosis polyposis of the gastrointestinal tract. *Am J Gastroenterol* 1999;**94**:2540.

38. Hosaka S, Akamatsu T, Nakamura S, et al. Mucosa-associated lymphoid tissue (MALT) lymphoma of the rectum with chromosomal translocation of the t(11;**18**)(q21;q21) and an additional aberration of trisomy 3. *Am J Gastroenterol* 1999;**94**:1951.

39. Romaguera J, Hagemeister FB. Lymphoma of the colon. *Curr Opin Gastroenterol.* 2004;**21**:80.

40. Isaacson PG, MacLennan KA, Subbuswamy SG. Multiple lymphomatous polyposis of the gastrointestinal tract. *Histopathology* 1984;**8**:641.

41. Romaguera J, Medeiros LJ, Hagemeister FB, et al. Frequency of gastrointestinal involvement and its clinical significance in mantle cell lymphoma. *Cancer* 2003;**97**:586.

42. Salar A, Juanpere N, Bellosillo B, et al. Gastrointestinal involvement in mantle cell lymphoma: a prospective clinic, endoscopic, and pathologic study. *Am J Surg Pathol* 2006;**30**:1274.

43. Hokama A, Tomoyose T, Yamamoto Y, et al. Adult T-cell leukemia/lymphoma presenting multiple lymphomatous polyposis. *World J Gastroenterol* 2008;**14**:6584.

44. Kumar S, Krenacs L, Otsuki T, et al. bcl-1 rearrangement and cyclin D1 protein expression in multiple lymphomatous polyposis. *Am J Clin Pathol* 1996;**105**:737.

45. Ruskone-Fourmestraux A, Aegerter P, Delmer A, Brousse N, Galian A, Rambaud JC, Groupe d'Etude des Lymphomes Digestifs. Primary digestive tract lymphoma: a prospective multicentric study of 91 patients. *Gastroenterology* 1993;**105**:1662.

46. Shia J, Teruya-Feldstein J, Pan D, et al. Primary follicular lymphoma of the gastrointestinal tract. A clinical and pathologic study of 26 cases. *Am J Surg Pathol* 2002;**26**:216.

47. Griffiths AP, Shepherd NA, Beddall A, Williams JG. Gastrointestinal tumour masses due to multiple myeloma: a pathological mimic of malignant lymphoma. *Histopathology* 1997;**31**:318.

48. Reynolds P, Saunders LD, Layefsky ME, Lemp GF. The spectrum of acquired immunodeficiency syndrome (AIDS)-associated malignancies in San Francisco 1980–1987. *Am J Epidemiol* 1993;**137**:19.

49. Ioachim HL, Antonescu C, Giancotti F, Dorsett B, Weinstein MA. EBV-associated anorectal lymphomas in patients with acquired immune deficiency syndrome. *Am J Surg Pathol* 1997;**21**:997.

50. Chetty R, Hlatswayo N, Muc R, Sabaratnam R, Gatter K. Plasmablastic lymphoma in HIV+ patients: an expanding spectrum. *Histopathology* 2003;**42**:605.

51. Cappell MS, Botros N. Predominantly gastrointestinal symptoms and signs in 11 consecutive AIDS patients with gastrointestinal lymphoma: a multicenter, multiyear study including 763 HIV-seropositive patients. *Am J Gastroenterol* 1994;**89**:545.

52. Kim YH, Lee JH, Yang SK, et al. Primary colon lymphoma in Korea: a KASID (Korean Association for the Study of Intestinal Diseases) study. *Dig Dis Sci* 2005;**50**:2243.

53. Hirakawa K, Fuchigami T, Nakamura S, et al. Primary gastrointestinal T-cell lymphoma resembling multiple lymphomatous polyposis. *Gastroenterology* 1996;**111**:778.

54. Catalano MF, Levin B, Hart RS, Troncoso P, DuBrow RA, Estey EH. Granulocytic sarcoma of the colon. *Gastroenterology* 1991;**100**:555.

55. Kojima M, Nakamura S, Itoh H, et al. Mast cell sarcoma with tissue eosinophilia arising in the ascending colon. *Mod Pathol* 1999;**12**:739.

56. Rubin BP. Gastrointestinal stromal tumours: an update. *Histopathology* 2006;**48**:83.

57. Miettinen M, Lasota J. Gastrointestinal stromal tumors. Review on morphology, molecular pathology, prognosis, and differential diagnosis. *Arch Pathol Lab Med* 2006;**130**:1466.

58. Miettinen M, Lasota J. Gastrointestinal stromal tumors: pathology and prognosis at different sites. *Semin Diagn Pathol* 2006;**23**:70.

59. Lasota J, Miettinen M. Clinical significance of oncogenic KIT and PDGFRA mutations in gastrointestinal stromal tumours. *Histopathology* 2008;**53**:245.

60. Ueyama T, Guo KJ, Hashimoto H, Daimaru Y, Enjoji M. A clinicopathologic and immunohistochemical study of gastrointestinal stromal tumors. *Cancer* 1992;**69**:947.

61. Miettinen M, Sarlomo-Rikala M, Sobin LH, Lasota J. Gastrointestinal stromal tumors and leiomyosarcomas in the colon. A clinicopathologic, immunohistochemical, and molecular genetic study of 44 cases. *Am J Surg Pathol* 2000;**24**:1339.

62. Miettinen M, Sobin LH, Sarlomo-Rikala M. Immunohistochemical spectrum of GISTs at different sites and their differential diagnosis with a reference to CD117 (KIT). *Mod Pathol* 2000;**13**:1134.

63. Miettinen M, Wang ZF, Lasota J. DOG1 antibody in the differential diagnosis of gastrointestinal stromal tumors. A study of 1840 cases. *Am J Surg Pathol* 2009;**33**:1401.

64. Tworek JA, Goldblum JR, Weiss SW, et al. Stromal tumors of the abdominal colon: A clinicopathologic study of 20 cases. *Am J Surg Pathol* 1999;**23**:937.

65. Meijer S, Peretz T, Gaynor JJ, et al. Primary colorectal sarcoma. A retrospective review and prognostic factor study of 50 consecutive patients. *Arch Surg* 1990;**125**:1163.

66. Moyana TN, Friesen R, Tan LK. Colorectal smooth-muscle tumors. A pathobiologic study with immunohistochemistry and histomorphometry. *Arch Pathol Lab Med* 1991;**115**:1016.

67. Akwari OE, Dozois RR, Weiland LH, Beahrs OH. Leiomyosarcoma of the small and large bowel. *Cancer* 1978;**42**:1375.

68. Appelman HD. Mesenchymal tumors of the gastrointestinal tract. In: Ming S, Goldman H (eds), *Pathology of the Gastrointestinal Tract*. Baltimore, MA: Williams & Wilkins, 1998: 361.

69. Freni SC, Keeman JN. Leiomyomatosis of the colon. *Cancer* 1977;**39**:263.

70. Walsh TH, Mann CV. Smooth muscle neoplasms of the rectum and anal canal. *Br J Surg* 1984;**71**:597.

71. Haque S, Dean PJ. Stromal neoplasms of the rectum and anal canal. *Hum Pathol* 1992;**23**:762.

72. Tworek JA, Goldblum JR, Weiss SW, et al. Stromal tumors of the anorectum: A clinicopathologic study of 22 cases. *Am J Surg Pathol* 1999;**23**:946.

73. Miettinen M, Furlong M, Sarlomo-Rikala M, Burke A, Sobin LH, Lasota J. Gastrointestinal stromal tumors, intramural leiomyomas, and leiomyosarcomas in the rectum and anus. A clinicopathologic, immunohistochemical, and molecular genetic study of 144 Cases. *Am J Surg Pathol* 2001;**25**:1121.

74. Michowitz M, Lazebnik N, Noy S, Lazebnik R. Lipoma of the colon. A report of 22 cases. *Am Surg* 1985;**51**:449.

75. Ryan J, Martin JE, Pollock DJ. Fatty tumours of the large intestine: a clinicopathological review of 13 cases. *Br J Surg* 1989;**76**:793.

76. Santos-Briz A, Garcia JP, Gonzales C, Colina F. Lipomatous polyposis of the colon. *Histopathology* 2001;**38**:81.

77. Climie AR, Wylin RF. Small-intestinal lipomatosis. *Arch Pathol Lab Med* 1981;**105**:40.

78. Swain VA, Young WF, Pringle EM. Hypertrophy of the appendices epiploicae and lipomatous polyposis of the colon. *Gut* 1969;**10**:587.

79. Jones DJ, Dharmeratnam R, Langstaff RJ. Large bowel obstruction due to pelvic lipomatosis. *Br J Surg* 1985;**72**:309.

80. Yatto RP. Colonic lipomatosis. *Am J Gastroenterol* 1982;**77**:436.

81. Snover DC. Atypical lipomas of the colon. Report of two cases with pseudomalignant features. *Dis Colon Rectum* 1984;**27**:485.

82. Amato G, Martella A, Ferraraccio F, et al. Well differentiated 'lipoma-like' liposarcoma of the sigmoid mesocolon and multiple lipomatosis of the rectosigmoid colon. Report of a case. *Hepatogastroenterology* 1998;**45**:2151.

83. Boquist L, Bergdahl L, Andersson A. Lipomatosis of the ileocecal valve. *Cancer* 1972;**29**:136.

84. Gazet JC. The ileocaecal valve syndrome. *Br J Surg* 1964;**51**:371.

85. Mills CS, Lloyd TV, Van Aman ME, Lucas J. Diffuse hemangiomatosis of the colon. *J Clin Gastroenterol* 1985;**7**:416.

86. Westerholm P. A case of diffuse haemangiomatosis of the colon and rectum. *Acta Chir Scand* 1966;**109**:173.

87. Camilleri M, Chadwick VS, Hodgson HJ. Vascular anomalies of the gastrointestinal tract. *Hepatogastroenterology* 1984;**31**:149.

88. Boley SJ, Brandt LJ, Mitsudo SM. Vascular lesions of the colon. *Adv Intern Med* 1984;**29**:301.

89. Genter B, Mir R, Strauss R, et al. Hemangiopericytoma of the colon: report of a case and review of literature. *Dis Colon Rectum* 1982;**25**:149.

90. Oliphant R, Gardiner S, Reid R, McPeake J, Porteous C. Glomus tumour of the ascending colon. *J Clin Pathol* 2007;**60**:846.

91. Allison KH, Yoder BJ, Bronner MP, Goldblum JR, Rubin BP. Angiosarcoma involving the gastrointestinal tract: a series of primary and metastatic cases. *Am J Surg Pathol* 2004;**28**:298.

92. Tardío JC, Nájera L, Alemany I, Martín T, Castaño A, Pérez-Regadera JF. Rectal angiosarcoma after adjuvant chemoradiotherapy for adenocarcinoma of the rectum. *J Clin Oncol* 2009; **27**:e116.

93. Parente F, Cernuschi M, Orlando G, Rizzardini G, Lazzarin A, Bianchi PG. Kaposi's sarcoma and AIDS: frequency of gastrointestinal involvement and its effect on survival. A prospective study in a heterogeneous population. *Scand J Gastroenterol* 1991; **26**:1007.

94. Friedman SL. Kaposi's sarcoma and lymphoma of the gut in AIDS. *Baillière's Clin Gastroenterol* 1990;**4**:455.

95. Svrcek M, Tiret E, Bennis M, Guyot P, Fléjou JF. KSHV/HHV8-associated intestinal Kaposi's sarcoma in patient with ulcerative colitis receiving immunosuppressive drugs: report of a case. *Dis Colon Rectum* 2009;**52**:154.

96. Rodríguez-Peláez M, Fernández-García MS, Gutiérrez-Corral N, et al. Kaposi's sarcoma: an opportunistic infection by human herpesvirus-8 in ulcerative colitis. *J Crohn's Colitis.* 2010;**4**:586.

97. Weprin L, Zollinger R, Clausen K, Thomas FB. Kaposi's sarcoma: endoscopic observations of gastric and colon involvement. *J Clin Gastroenterol* 1982;**4**:357.

98. Weber JN, Carmichael DJ, Boylston A, et al. Kaposi's sarcoma of the bowel – presenting as apparent ulcerative colitis. *Gut* 1985;**26**:295.

99. Mesri EA, Cesarman E, Boshoff C. Kaposi's sarcoma and its associated herpesvirus. *Nat Rev Cancer* 2010;**10**:707.

100. Strickler HD, Goedert JJ, Bethke FR, et al. Human herpesvirus 8 cellular immune responses in homosexual men. *J Infect Dis* 1999;**180**:1682.

101. Nakagawara G, Kojima Y, Mai M, Akimoto R, Miwa K. Lymphangioma of the transverse colon treated by transendoscopic polypectomy: report of a case and review of literature. *Dis Colon Rectum* 1981;**24**:291.

102. Schaefer JW, Griffen WO Jr. Colonic lymphangiectasis associated with a potassium depletion syndrome. *Gastroenterology* 1968;**55**:515.

103. Ivey K, DenBesten L, Kent TH, Clifton JA. Lymphangiectasia of the colon with protein loss and malabsorption. *Gastroenterology* 1969;**57**:709.

104. Grodsky L. Neurofibroma of the rectum in a patient with von Recklinghausen's disease. *Am J Surg* 1958;**95**:474.

105. Raszkowski HJ, Hufner RF. Neurofibromatosis of the colon: a unique manifestation of von Recklinghausen's disease. *Cancer* 1971;**27**:134.

106. Fuller CE, Williams GT. Gastrointestinal manifestations of type 1 neurofibromatosis (von Recklinghausen's disease). *Histopathology* 1991;**19**:1.

107. Petersen JM, Ferguson DR. Gastrointestinal neurofibromatosis. *J Clin Gastroenterol* 1984;**6**:529.

108. Waxman BP, Buzzard AJ, Cox J, Stephens MJ. Gastric and intestinal bleeding in multiple neurofibromatosis with cardiomyopathy. *Aust N Z J Surg* 1986;**56**:171.

109. Hough DR, Chan A, Davidson H. Von Recklinghausen's disease associated with gastrointestinal carcinoid tumors. *Cancer* 1983; **51**:2206.

110. Miettinen M, Shekitka KM, Sobin LH. Schwannomas in the colon and rectum: a clinicopathologic and immunohistochemical study of 20 cases. *Am J Surg Pathol* 2001;**25**:846.

111. Hou YY, Tan YS, Xu JF, et al. Schwannoma of the gastrointestinal tract : a clinicopathological, immunohistochemical, and ultrastructural study of 33 cases. *Histopathology* 2006;**48**:536.

112. Lewin MR, Dilworth HP, Abu Alfa AK, et al. Mucosal benign epithelioid nerve sheath tumors. *Am J Surg Pathol* 2005;**29**:1310.

113. Gibson JA, Hornick JL. Mucosal Schwann cell 'hamartoma': clinicopathologic study of 26 neural colorectal polyps distinct from neurofibromas and mucosal neuromas. *Am J Surg Pathol* 2009;**33**:781.

114. Eslami-Varzaneh F, Washington K, Robert ME, et al. Benign fibroblastic polyps of the colon: a histologic, immunohistochemical, and ultrastructural study. *Am J Surg Pathol* 2004; **28**:374.

115. Groisman GM, Polak-Charcon S. Fibroblastic polyp of the colon and colonic perineurioma: 2 names for a single entity? *Am J Surg Pathol* 2008;**32**:1088.

116. Groisman GM, Polak-Charcon S, Appelman HD. Fibroblastic polyp of the colon: clinicopathological analysis of 10 cases with emphasis on its common association with serrated crypts. *Histopathology* 2006;**48**:431.

117. Hornick JL, Fletcher CD. Intestinal perineuriomas: clinicopathologic definition of a new anatomic subset in a series of 10 cases. *Am J Surg Pathol* 2005;**29**:859.

118. Agaimy A, Märkl B, Kitz J, et al. Peripheral nerve sheath tumors of the gastrointestinal tract: a multicenter study of 58 patients including NF1-associated gastric schwannoma and unusual morphologic variants. *Virchows Arch* 2010;**456**:411.

119. Agaimy A, Stoehr R, Vieth M, Hartmann A. Benign serrated colorectal fibroblastic polyps/intramucosal perineuriomas are true mixed epithelial-stromal polyps (hybrid hyperplastic polyp/mucosal perineurioma) with frequent BRAF mutations. *Am J Surg Pathol* 2010;**34**:1663.

120. Johnston J, Helwig EB. Granular cell tumors of the gastrointestinal tract and perianal region: a study of 74 cases. *Dig Dis Sci* 1981;**26**:807.

121. Singhi AD, Montgomery EA. Colorectal granular cell tumor: a clinicopathologic study of 26 cases. *Am J Surg Pathol* 2010;**34**:1186.

122. Shekitka KM, Sobin LH. Ganglioneuromas of the gastrointestinal tract. Relation to von Recklinghausen disease and other multiple tumor syndromes. *Am J Surg Pathol* 1994;**18**:250.

123. Carney JA, Go VL, Sizemore GW, Hayles AB. Alimentary-tract ganglioneuromatosis. A major component of the syndrome of multiple endocrine neoplasia, type 2b. *N Engl J Med* 1976; **295**:1287.

124. Mendelsohn G, Diamond MP. Familial ganglioneuromatous polyposis of the large bowel. Report of a family with associated juvenile polyposis. *Am J Surg Pathol* 1984;**8**:515.

125. Weidner N, Flanders DJ, Mitros FA. Mucosal ganglioneuromatosis associated with multiple colonic polyps. *Am J Surg Pathol* 1984;**8**:779.

126. Lashner BA, Riddell RH, Winans CS. Ganglioneuromatosis of the colon and extensive glycogenic acanthosis in Cowden's disease. *Dig Dis Sci* 1986;**31**:213.

127. Chandrasoma P, Wheeler D, Radin DR. Traumatic neuroma of the intestine. *Gastrointest Radiol* 1985;**10**:161.

128. Jass JR, Shepherd NA, Maybee J. Tumours of the retrorectal space. In: Jass JR, Shepherd NA, Maybee J (eds), *Atlas of Surgical Pathology of the Colon, Rectum and Anus*. Edinburgh: Churchill Livingstone, 1989: 220.

129. Thomas R, Deasy J, Royston D. Retrorectal pseudotumour induced by Ivalon. *Histopathology* 2001;**39**:640.

CHAPTER 40

Miscellaneous disorders of the large intestine

Adrian C. Bateman

Southampton General Hospital, Southampton, UK

Amyloid

Amyloid is an abnormally folded fibrillar protein that on structural examination is represented by the β-pleated sheet, a complex network of fibrils varying in diameter from 7.5 nm to 10 nm that can be identified by electron microscopy. In routine diagnostic biopsies light microscopic examination will show amyloid deposition when stained with haematoxylin and eosin as an eosinophilic thickening either of vessel walls or as an eosinophilic deposit in the extracellular matrix (Figure 40.1a). The special staining characteristics of amyloid, when examined histochemically, are conveyed by the coupling of amyloid to glycoproteins. Congo red stains these amyloid-associated glycoproteins (and other proteins) red (Figure 40.1b), and the specificity for amyloid is given by the added apple green birefringence that is found when the sections are viewed in polarised light. About 20 different unrelated proteins can form amyloid fibrils in vivo. Some of these are natural wild-type proteins that are inherently amyloidogenic and cause amyloidosis in old age or if present for long periods at abnormally high concentration, whereas others are acquired or inherited variants that aggregate into amyloid deposits [1]. In addition to the fibrils, amyloid deposits always contain the non-fibrillar pentraxin plasma protein, serum amyloid P component (SAP), that probably stabilises amyloid fibrils by retarding their clearance. Although Congo red staining remains the most useful and cost-efficient diagnostic technique, histological diagnosis and classification of amyloid are greatly facilitated by the use of immunohistochemistry using antibodies directed at

SAP (as a 'general' marker of amyloid) and the different possible protein components.

Amyloid deposition in the gastrointestinal tract is most commonly found in systemic type AA (reactive) amyloidosis, which complicates a range of chronic inflammatory disorders such as rheumatoid arthritis, chronic infections such as tuberculosis and certain malignant tumours of different lineages [2]. Occasionally the underlying disease itself is centred on the gastrointestinal tract, e.g. Crohn's disease. The most common sites for AA amyloid deposition are the blood vessels, particularly in the submucosa, and lamina propria of the mucosa [3]. Systemic AL amyloid, due to proliferative abnormalities of B cells and plasma cells, is more often found in the muscular layers of the bowel wall, although it is also frequently deposited in vessel walls. Senile amyloidosis, due to fibrillary deposits of transthyretin, is typically found in vessels and in the submucosa [4], whereas dialysis-associated amyloidosis due to β2-microglobulin shows particularly heavy deposition in the submucosa and muscularis propria [5,6]. However, these patterns of amyloid deposition should in no way be considered exclusive for any one form of disease and are no substitute for immunohistochemical characterisation in the classification of the disease. Involvement of the gastrointestinal tract by hereditary systemic amyloidosis is extremely rare but may occur in some non-neuropathic (Ostertag-type) forms [1]. Generally speaking, amyloid deposition in systemic amyloidosis is more prevalent in the stomach and duodenum than the large bowel, and upper gastrointestinal biopsy is likely to be a more sensitive method of diagnosing amyloidosis than rectal biopsy [3]

Morson and Dawson's Gastrointestinal Pathology, Fifth Edition. Edited by Neil A. Shepherd, Bryan F. Warren,
Geraint T. Williams, Joel K. Greenson, Gregory Y. Lauwers and Marco R. Novelli.

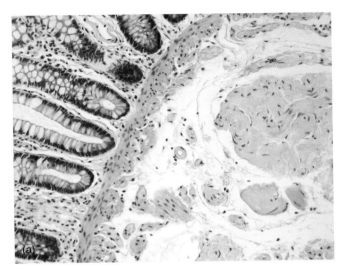

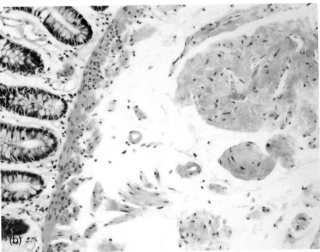

Figure 40.1 Rectal biopsy in amyloidosis showing hyaline eosinophilic material that (a) is particularly evident within the walls of small submucosal blood vessels and (b) is highlighted with Congo red staining.

– although clinicians investigating a patient for possible amyloidosis still commonly request examination of the latter.

Amyloid deposition localised to the gastrointestinal tract is uncommon. It may occasionally be found in elderly people [4] and there are case reports of localised amyloid tumours (amyloidomas) within the gastrointestinal tract [7,8]. In the latter the deposited protein frequently induces a foreign body-type giant cell reaction.

The clinical effects of amyloid deposition depend mainly on where the amyloid is deposited within the bowel. Although most patients with gastrointestinal amyloidosis are asymptomatic, severe haemorrhage may result when fragile, amyloid-infiltrated blood vessels rupture. Discrete ulcers and masses (amyloidoma) are more common in the

stomach and colon than in the small bowel, which may be affected by a protein-losing enteropathy. Focal ulcers, sometimes leading to perforation, may occur in any part of the gastrointestinal tract and often represent multi-focal localised ischaemia due to vascular deposition of amyloid in the submucosa and deeper in the bowel wall. Abnormalities of gut motility may result from amyloid within the muscularis propria and nerves of the myenteric plexus. This may result in pyloric obstruction, small intestinal stasis with bacterial overgrowth and malabsorption, large intestinal pseudo-obstruction or severe constipation.

A number of conditions enter the differential diagnosis of amyloidosis in the large bowel and it is prudent to use the Congo red stain or immunostaining for SAP whenever an eosinophilic vascular or connective tissue deposit is encountered. Subepithelial deposition of amyloid may be confused with a thickened subepithelial collagen plate in collagenous colitis. The latter is 'fenestrated' by lymphocytes and capillaries and often shows a characteristic artefact where the surface epithelium appears to peel off the underlying subepithelial collagen band: features that are not usually seen in association with subepithelial amyloid deposition. A connective tissue stain such as haematoxylin–van Gieson can be very helpful in this situation as a means of confirming that the subepithelial collagen plate is truly thickened. Occasionally eosinophilic arteriosclerotic changes and fibrin may present diagnostic difficulty, especially after radiotherapy, whereas eosinophilic collagen deposition within the muscularis propria in systemic sclerosis or familial visceral myopathies can cause confusion in full-thickness biopsies taken for the evaluation of intestinal pseudo-obstruction.

Endometriosis

Endometriosis of the large bowel is not uncommon. It is one of the most common extra-genitourinary sites of involvement, occurring in 15–20% of all cases [9–11]. Despite this, bowel symptoms are relatively uncommon and most cases are discovered as incidental histological findings in colorectal specimens resected for other reasons. Symptoms of colorectal endometriosis, when present, are a frequent source of confusion with more serious colorectal conditions. They include bleeding, pain and obstruction. Bleeding and pain are classically cyclical, giving a clue to the diagnosis. Endometriotic lesions almost never ulcerate and when ulceration is seen it is usually a consequence of repeated mucosal biopsies. Most endometriotic lesions are on the left side of the colon. Occasional caecal endometriomas have been associated with intussusception [12].

It is often not appreciated clinically that endometriosis may occur in postmenopausal women, especially in those receiving hormone replacement therapy. This may cause clinical and histological confusion. We have seen a number

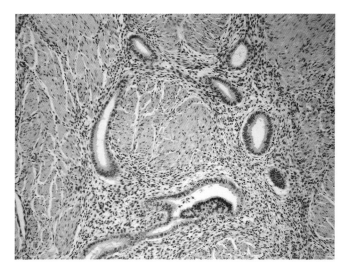

Figure 40.2 Endometriosis evidenced by the presence of endometrial glands and stroma within the muscularis propria of the colon.

of cases of colorectal adenocarcinoma accompanied by endometriosis within the bowel wall and subserosa that had led to radiological and macroscopic over-staging of the carcinoma.

The histological diagnosis of endometriosis depends on the finding of at least two of the following: endometrial glands, endometrial-type stroma and haemosiderin (Figure 40.2). In small colorectal biopsies, differential cytokeratin immunohistochemistry can be useful, in that it highlights cytokeratin 7-positive endometrial glands in contrast to cytokeratin 20-positive colonic crypts. CD10 immunohisto-chemistry may also be valuable as a means of highlighting the presence of endometrial stroma (Figure 40.3). In post-menopausal women, the endometriotic lesions may be characterised by very bland glandular structures and inconspicuous stroma, therefore it is important not to over-look the possibility of this diagnosis when examining spec-imens from women of this age.

Melanosis coli

Melanosis coli describes an accumulation of a brown granu-lar pigment within histiocytes in the lamina propria of the colorectum (Figure 40.4). It is closely related to increased epithelial cell apoptosis, both in laboratory animals and in humans [13,14]. Melanosis coli resembles lipofuscin in its staining characteristics and shows positivity with both peri-odic acid–Schiff (PAS) stain and the Masson–Hamperl reac-tion [15]. Post mortem studies have revealed a prevalence of up to 60%, and anecdotal experience indicates that very mild degrees of melanosis are commonly seen within color-ectal biopsies taken during investigations for possible colitis. However, it is our impression that the condition is decreasing in frequency in the UK. Melanosis coli affects the

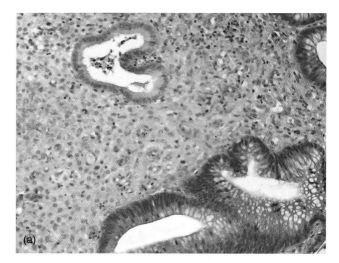

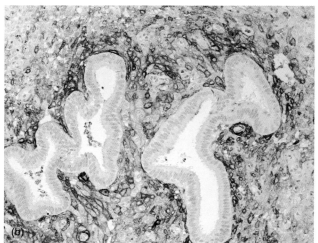

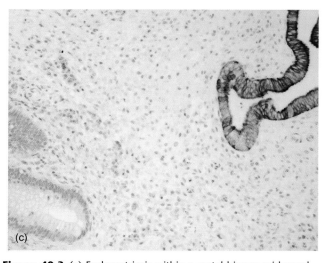

Figure 40.3 (a) Endometriosis within a rectal biopsy evidenced by bland endometrial glands within subtle pseudo-decidualised endometrial stroma. (b) The stroma is highlighted with CD10 immunohistochemistry whereas (c) the endometrial glands are highlighted with cytokeratin 7 immunohistochemistry.

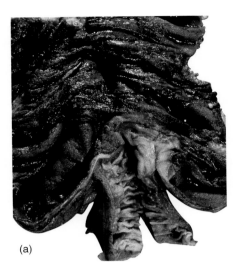

(a)

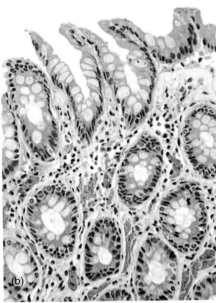

(b)

Figure 40.4 Melanosis coli: (a) diffuse black mucosal pigmentation of the proximal colon contrasts with the unaffected normal mucosa of the terminal ileum. (b) Mucosal biopsy showing pigment-containing histiocytes within the lamina propria.

right side of the colon more than the left, and it is seen in the appendix but not in the terminal ileum [16,17]. The lymphoid follicles in the colonic mucosa are not affected and may stand out as pale spots on endoscopy. Paradoxically, pigment-containing histiocytes may be found in the sinuses of lymph nodes draining an area of melanosis coli [18].

The important histological differential diagnosis is mucosal haemosiderosis, a feature of chronic ischaemic colitis (see Chapter 36), and Perls' stain is often useful in the distinction. Although melanosis coli remains an important marker for anthraquinone laxative abuse, it has to be remembered that it is an end-product of apoptosis and several other drugs cause excess apoptosis and melanosis

coli. The most frequent of these are non-steroidal anti-inflammatory drugs [14,19]. On the other hand, not all conditions characterised by increased apoptosis are associated with melanosis coli – it is not seen in graft-versus-host disease and HIV colitis. This may imply that a longstanding (rather than acute) increase in apoptotic activity is necessary in the aetiology of melanosis coli. Melanosis is also seen in some patients with ulcerative colitis [20]. Some such patients with distal ulcerative colitis present with constipation and the melanosis may represent laxative use. In other patients with ulcerative colitis, active disease is associated with increased epithelial cell and lymphocyte apoptosis [20]. Another possible explanation is the use of sulphasalazine, which induces microscopic colitis (and presumed increased epithelial apoptosis) in a small number of patients.

Muciphages

Muciphages were first described as mucin-containing macrophages in the colorectal lamina propria by Azzopardi and Evans in 1966 [21]. They may occur in normal and abnormal colorectal mucosal biopsies [22] and they not regarded as pathological in themselves: they can be found in up to 50% of rectal biopsies [21]. Muciphages are probably related to previous epithelial damage, usually subtle and clinically insignificant, that releases mucin into the lamina propria. They must not be mistaken for the characteristic macrophages of Whipple's disease [23], metastatic malignant cells [24] or macrophages containing *Mycobacterium avium-intracellulare*. *Mycobacterium avium-intracellulare*-containing PAS-positive macrophages may be distinguished from PAS-positive muciphages by the use of a Ziehl–Neelsen stain. Table 40.1 highlights the histochemical features of a range of conditions that enter the differential diagnosis of colorectal muciphages, which can be supplemented by judicious use of immunohistochemistry for markers of cell lineage.

Pneumatosis coli

This condition in the colon is identical to pneumatosis cystoides intestinalis of the small intestine and the aetiology is discussed in Chapter 27. It is characterised by gas cysts in the submucosal and subserosal layers of the large bowel wall and can affect the entire colon and rectum or just one part [26]. The disease is often symptomless but can present with diarrhoea, rectal bleeding due to mucosal erosion over the cysts or rarely pneumo-peritoneum from rupture of a gas cyst into the peritoneal cavity. It is also possible that pneumatosis coli can lead to intestinal obstruction and clinical simulation of a neoplastic stricture, especially if the mucosa is also involved (i.e. pseudo-lipomatosis – see below).

The macroscopic appearances are characteristic. The mucosal surface has a coarse cobblestone appearance due

Table 40.1 Mucosal accumulations in the colorectum

	Cytoplasmic composition	Diagnostic histochemical features	Clinical significance
Muciphages	Mucin	Tinctorial properties of mucin	None
Melanosis coli	Lipofuscin-like pigment	PAS +ve Melanin −ve	Drug ingestion
Pseudo-lipomatosis	Gas	No histiocytic lining to gas cysts	Effects of endoscopy
Pneumatosis coli[a]	Gas	Histiocytic and giant cell lining to gas cysts	Association with psychiatric and chronic lung diseases [21]
Haemosiderosis	Iron-related compounds	Perls positive	Marker of ischaemia, torsion and trauma
Barium granuloma[a]	Barium sulphate	Refractile crystals	Previous barium studies with mucosal severance
Whipple's disease	*Tropheryma whipplei* bacteria	PAS +ve, bacilli on EM, PCR positive	Multi-system disorder
Signet ring cell carcinoma	Mucin	Tinctorial properties of mucin	Primary or metastatic carcinoma
Atypical mycobacteriosis	*Mycobacterium avium-intracellulare*	PAS +ve but ZN reveals innumerable acid-fast bacilli	Immunosuppression, especially AIDS
Malakoplakia[a]	MG bodies and lysosomes	MG bodies are PAS/Alcian blue and von Kossa +ve	May accompany other conditions, especially colorectal cancer
Langerhans cell histiocytosis[a]	Lysosomes	Normal properties of histiocytes, especially EM	Multi-system disorder
Chronic granulomatous disease	Lipofuscin-like pigment	PAS +ve, lipid +ve	Multi-system disorder in children
Glycolipid storage diseases	Various lipids	Dependent on disorder type	Multi-system disorders

Reproduced from Shepherd NA (2000). What is the significance of muciphages in colorectal biopsies? Histopathology, 36; 559.
[a]These diseases are primarily submucosal accumulations but may be seen within the lamina propria.
EM, electron microscopy; MG, Michaelis–Guttmann; PAS, periodic acid–Schiff; PCR, polymerase chain reaction; ZN, Ziehl–Neelsen.

to large numbers of submucosal cysts, the apices of which may show intramucosal haemorrhage. The gas seems to be under some pressure, because rupture of the cysts during endoscopic biopsy or in fresh surgical specimens may cause a popping sound. The biopsy appearances are distinctive. Cystic spaces in the submucosa are lined by endothelial cells, macrophages and multinucleate macrophage giant cells with eosinophilic cytoplasm (Figure 40.5). The connective tissue between the cysts, which are often multi-locular, shows little inflammation. The covering mucosa is attenuated, sometimes contains small haemorrhages and may show architectural distortion similar to that seen in inflammatory bowel disease (Figure 40.5). The appearances are most likely to be confused with lymphangioma (see Chapter 39), oleogranuloma (see Chapter 44) or possibly a granulomatous process such as infection or Crohn's disease [27].

Pseudo-lipomatosis

This is a mucosal accumulation of microscopic gas bubbles, manifested as multiple spherical empty spaces of variable size in the lamina propria that resemble fat cells in paraffin sections. There is no epithelial or histiocytic lining to the spaces and some are seen within lymphoid aggregates [28]. Large amounts result in a typical appearance endoscopically resembling 'muciphage mucosa' [28]. Pseudo-lipomatosis is effectively part of the spectrum of changes seen in pneumatosis coli [29,30,31]. The gas spaces are thought usually to arise as a consequence of air entering the lamina propria through minute breaches in the surface epithelium during insufflation at endoscopy. Although this may sometimes occur in normal mucosa, it may be that atrophic mucosa such as that found in inactive longstanding inflammatory bowel disease is more susceptible.

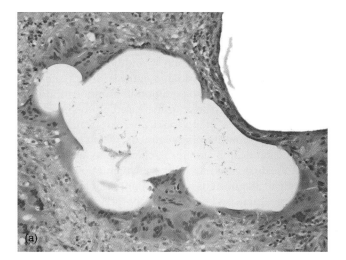

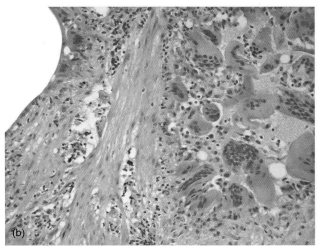

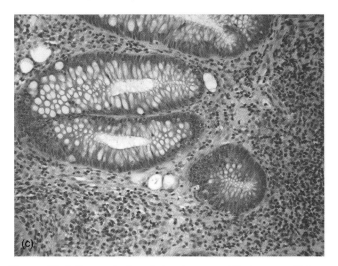

Figure 40.5 Pneumatosis coli showing a gas-filled space within the submucosa of the colon, partly lined by (a) multinucleate giant cells that form (b) sheets in some areas. (c) The overlying mucosa may show architectural distortion reminiscent of that seen in conditions such as inflammatory bowel disease.

Pseudo-lipomatosis has also been described after inadequate washing of endoscopes following hydrogen peroxide endoscope disinfection, when residual peroxide reacts with normal tissues to release oxygen [29,32].

Stercoral ulceration

Stercoral ulcers result from pressure of abnormally hard faecal masses on the mucosa of the large bowel, most commonly at the rectosigmoid junction where there is a narrow lumen whose expansion is restricted by the presence of neighbouring structures. They are usually a consequence of intractable constipation and are an uncommon cause of perforation and faecal peritonitis, which may be initiated with straining at stool. Non-absorbable antacids containing aluminium salts and cation exchange resins, used to treat hyperkalaemia in renal patients, appear to be contributory [33,34]. Stercoral ulcers appear as well demarcated, irregular, longitudinal tears and perforations through which hard stool may be seen to protrude. The adjacent tissues appear necrotic or gangrenous. Histologically the appearances are of ulceration with focal ischaemic features and intense acute and chronic inflammation penetrating the bowel wall [35]. The differential diagnosis may include diverticular disease and the latter should be excluded, primarily by very careful macroscopic examination of the resection specimen.

Graft-versus-host disease

Graft-versus-host disease (GVHD) occurs when donor lymphocytes bearing different HLA types from the host are given to an immunosuppressed individual, usually in the context of bone marrow transplantation. The large bowel (along with the skin, remainder of the gastrointestinal tract and biliary system) is a well recognised site of involvement in affected individuals, usually resulting in watery diarrhoea or rectal bleeding, and rectal biopsy is often used as a convenient method of confirming the clinical diagnosis. General features of the pathology of the condition are described in Chapter 16.

The histological hallmark of GVHD in the colorectum is increased apoptosis of the epithelial cells in the proliferative zone at the base of crypts [36,37]. In early cases this may be the only abnormality and, as it may be patchy, several levels taken through the biopsy may be necessary to identify it with confidence. Typically the apoptotic cells are seen within lacunae along the crypt basement membrane (Figure 40.6). There may also be more overt epithelial cell necrosis in the upper reaches of the crypt and on the luminal surface, which may result in crypts lined by flattened degenerate cells and distended by necrotic cells. This may induce an acute neutrophil infiltrate, and in florid

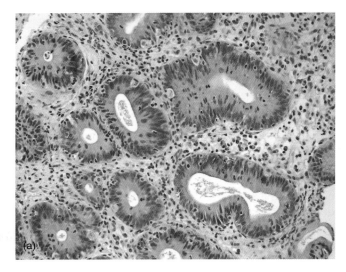

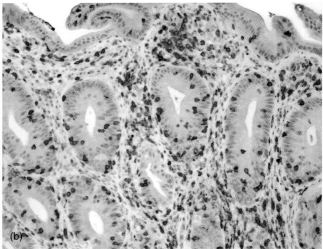

Figure 40.6 (a) Graft-versus-host disease showing prominent intra-epithelial lymphocytes (IELs) and crypt epithelial cell apoptosis. (b) The IELs are highlighted and confirmed as T-cells using CD3 immunohistochemistry.

acute GVHD there may be total mucosal loss and ulceration. Chronic inflammatory cells in the lamina propria may be slightly increased, but this is rarely pronounced.

As the disease progresses towards chronic GVHD the crypts with stem cells damaged by the immunological attack are wiped out, leaving only 'gravestones' composed of isolated clusters of epithelial cells in the lamina propria. These clusters are often composed entirely of endocrine cells, probably reflecting the slower turnover of this cell population compared with colonocytes and goblet cells [38]. Residual crypts undergo regeneration by epithelial proliferation and crypt fission, resulting in a markedly distorted mucosal architecture that may suggest longstanding inactive chronic ulcerative colitis. However, in chronic

GVHD it is often accompanied by fibrosis of the lamina propria, an unusual feature of ulcerative colitis, and this, the increased apoptotic activity and the clinical history all serve to make the distinction. Conditions that are more important in the differential diagnosis are cytomegalovirus colitis, which is also common in immunosuppressed patients and may give rise to increased epithelial apoptosis, and the effects of pre-bone marrow transplantation chemotherapy-conditioning regimens, which may produce virtually identical histological changes to acute GVHD during the first 3 weeks after transplantation. Confident histological diagnosis is virtually impossible during this time frame. Increased epithelial apoptosis is also a feature of HIV colitis (see Chapter 35).

Chronic GVHD may also give rise to submucosal and even transmural fibrosis of the intestinal wall, and can lead to bowel strictures [39].

Cord colitis syndrome

This term has recently been given to a newly recognised condition characterised by culture-negative diarrhoea (usually watery), fever and weight loss that occurs in approximately 10% of recipients of haematopoietic stem cell transplants, specifically with umbilical cord blood [40]. It has not been reported after allogeneic peripheral blood or bone marrow transplantations. The condition typically occurs 3–9 months after cord blood therapy and, despite the failure to identify any obvious infective agent, responds well to antibiotic therapy. Sometimes relapses occur, but these are also antibiotic responsive. The condition appears to be clinically and pathologically distinct from GVHD. Colorectal biopsies typically show a chronic active colitis of variable degree with a mixed inflammatory cell infiltrate in the lamina propria, focal neutrophilic cryptitis and Paneth cell metaplasia, but little crypt distortion. Granulomas, either compact epithelioid forms or looser histiocytic collections related to ruptured crypts, are common. Epithelial apoptosis, the hallmark of GVHD, is inconspicuous. Ileal biopsies from one recorded patient had pseudo-pyloric metaplasia, suggesting that there may also be a chronic ileitis. In view of the dramatic response to antibiotic therapy, the possibility remains that cord colitis is caused by a hitherto unrecognised infective agent.

Effects of bowel preparation

Old-fashioned hyperosmolar bowel preparations for colonoscopy have been recorded to cause considerable oedema and mucin depletion in the absence of inflammation [41]. The newer ones may cause focal acute colitis in the proximal colon, leading to an erroneous diagnosis of Crohn's disease [42–45].

Torsion of appendices epiploicae

Appendices epiploicae come to the notice of histopathologists when they undergo torsion. This results in infarction and haemorrhage, occasionally with resolution. There may be intestinal stenosis, but this is rare. They may also autoamputate and present as peritoneal loose bodies (see Chapter 48). Fat necrosis, hyalinisation and calcification are seen histologically.

Barium granuloma

Barium granulomas result from extravasation of radiological contrast material into the bowel wall via mucosal tears or diverticula. They may present as polypoid or ulcerated lesions that can closely mimic a tumour endoscopically, especially when they are not discovered until some considerable time after the causative barium enema examination. The rectum is most commonly involved and macroscopically the raised lesions may vary from white to grey–pink in colour; they may be ulcerated with yellow plaque-like areas. On rare occasions they may penetrate into the bowel wall, resulting in barium abscesses and barium peritonitis (see Chapter 46). Barium granulomas are made up of macrophages containing light green/grey barium sulphate crystals that may vary in size and shape from small granular crystals to large rhomboidal forms. They are anisotropic in polarised light and may be identified histochemically by the rhodizonate method and characterised further by energy dispersive X-ray analysis [46].

Malakoplakia

Malakoplakia involving the large intestine may be seen in association with ulcerative colitis, in patients with coexisting debilitating illnesses or malignancy, or rarely in isolation. It may present as ulcers with sentinel polyps, as a tumour-like mass or even as diffuse thickening of the bowel wall. Histologically malakoplakia is composed of sheets of large macrophages with eosinophilic granular cytoplasm (Hansemann's cells) containing characteristic PAS-positive iron and copper-containing calculospherules (Michaelis–Gutmann bodies) [47,48].

Squamous metaplasia of the colorectum

Squamous metaplasia occurring within the colon and rectum is rare. Squamous metaplasia has been observed in patients with ulcerative colitis [49,50] and Crohn's disease [51], as well as in Hirschsprung's disease [52] and within the ileo-anal pouch (where progression to squamous cell carcinoma has been described) [53]. Squamous metaplasia has also been described within colonic adenomas, and both adenosquamous and pure invasive squamous cell carcinoma may rarely arise within the large bowel [54]. These tumours, and the possible role of human papillomavirus in their causation, are discussed in Chapter 38.

References

1. Pepys MB. Pathogenesis, diagnosis and treatment of systemic amyloidosis. *Philos Trans R Soc Lond B Biol Sci* 2001;**356**:203.
2. Tan SY, Pepys MB. Amyloidosis. *Histopathology* 1994;**25**:403.
3. Yamada M, Hatakeyama S, Tsukagoshi H. Gastrointestinal amyloid deposition in AL (primary or myeloma-associated) and AA (secondary) amyloidosis. *Hum Pathol* 1985;**16**:1206.
4. Rocken C, Saeger W, Linke RP. Gastrointestinal amyloid deposits in old age. *Pathol Res Pract* 1994;**190**:641.
5. Borczuk A, Mannion C, Dickson D, Alt E. Intestinal pseudoobstruction and ischemia secondary to both β2-microglobulin and serum A amyloid deposition. *Mod Pathol* 1995;**8**:577.
6. Jimenez RE, Price DA, Pinkus GS, et al. Development of gastrointestinal beta2-microglobulin amyloidosis correlates with time on dialysis. *Am J Surg Pathol* 1998;**22**:729.
7. Senapati A, Fletcher C, Bultitude MI, Jackson BT. Amyloid tumour of the rectum. *J R Soc Med* 1995;**88**:48.
8. Deans GT, Hale RJ, McMahon RFT, Brough WA. Amyloid tumour of the colon. *J Clin Pathol* 1995;**48**:592.
9. Tagart REB. Endometriosis of the large intestine. *Br J Surg* 1959;**47**:27.
10. Spjut HJ, Perkins DE. Endometriosis of the sigmoid colon and rectum. *Am J Roentgenol* 1969;**82**:1070.
11. Davis C, Alexander RW, Buenger EG. Surgery of endometrioma of the ileum and colon. *Am J Surg* 1963;**105**:250.
12. Fujimoto A, Osuga Y, Tsutsumi O, Fuji T, Okagaki R, Taketani Y. Successful laparoscopic treatment of ileo-cecal endometriosis producing large bowel obstruction. *J Obstet Gynecol Res* 2001;**27**:221.
13. Walker NI, Smith MM, Smithers BM. Ultrastructure of human melanosis coli with reference to its pathogenesis. *Pathology* 1993;**25**:120.
14. Byers RJ, Marsh p, Parkinson D, Haboubi NY. Melanosis coli is associated with an increase in colonic epithelial apoptosis and not with laxative abuse. *Histopathology* 1997;**30**:160.
15. Walker NI, Bennett RE, Axelsen RA. Melanosis coli. A consequence of anthraquinone-induced apoptosis of colonic epithelial cells. *Am J Pathol* 1988;**131**:465.
16. Ming SC, Goldman H. Disorders common to the gastrointestinal tract. In: *Pathology of the Gastrointestinal Tract*, 2nd edn. Baltimore, MA: Williams & Wilkins, 1998: 410.
17. Rutty GN, Shaw PA. Melanosis of the appendix: prevalence, distribution and review of the pathogenesis of 47 cases. *Histopathology* 1997;**30**:319.
18. Hall M, Eusebi V. Yellow-brown spindle bodies in mesenteric lymph nodes: a possible relationship with melanosis coli. *Histopathology* 1978;**2**:47.
19. Lee FD. The importance of apoptosis in the histopathology of drug related lesions of the large intestine. *J Clin Pathol* 1993;**46**:118.
20. Pardi DS, Tremaine WJ, Rothenberger HJ, Batts KP. *J Clin Gastroenterol* 1998;**26**:167.
21. Azzopardi JG, Evans DJ. Mucoprotein containing histiocytes (muciphages) in the rectum. *J Clin Pathol* 1966;**19**:368.
22. Salto-Tellez M, Price AB. What is the significance of muciphages in colorectal biopsies? *Histopathology* 2000;**36**:556.
23. Caravati CM, Litch M, Weisiger BB, et al. Diagnosis of Whipple's disease by rectal biopsy with report of 3 additional cases. *Ann Intern Med* 1963;**58**:166.

24. Talbot IC, Price AB. Assessment of abnormalities: diagnostic signposts. In: *Biopsy Pathology in Colorectal Disease.* London: Chapman & Hall 1995: 54.

25. Shepherd NA. What is the significance of muciphages in colorectal biopsies? *Histopathology* 2000;**36**:559.

26. Galandiuk S, Fazio VW. Pneumatosis cystoides intestinalis. *Dis Colon Rectum* 1986;**29**:358.

27. Koreishi A, Lauwers GY, Misdraji J. Pneumatosis intestinalis – a challenging biopsy diagnosis. *Am J Surg Pathol* 2007;**31**:1469.

28. Snover DC, Sandstad J, Hutton S. Mucosal pseudolipomatosis of the colon. *Am J Clin Pathol* 1985;**84**:575.

29. Waring JP, Manne RK, Wadas DD, Sanowski RA. Mucosal pseudolipomatosis: an air pressure related colonoscopy complication. *Gastrointest Endosc* 1989;**35**:93.

30. Gagliardi G, Thompson IW, Hershman MJ, Forbes A, Hawley PR, Talbot IC. Pneumatosis coli: a proposed pathogenesis based on study of 25 cases and review of the literature. *Int J Colorectal Dis* 1996;**11**:111.

31. Nakasono M, Hirokawa M, Muguruma N, et al. Colonic pseudolipomatosis, microscopically classified into two groups. *J Gastroenterol Hepatol* 2006;**21**:65.

32. Ryan CK, Potter GD. Disinfectant colitis. Rinse as well as you wash. *J Clin Gastroenterol* 1995;**21**:6.

33. Aquilo JJ, Zinche H, Woods JE, Buckingham JM. Intestinal perforation due to faecal impaction after renal transplantation. *J Urol* 1976;**116**:153.

34. Archibald SD, Jirsch DW, Bear RA. Gastrointestinal complications of renal transplantation: 2 the colon. *Can Med Assoc J* 1978;**119**:1301.

35. Huttunen R, Heikkinen E, Larmi TKI. Stercoraceous and idiopathic perforations of the colon. *Surg Gynecol Obstet* 1975;**140**:756.

36. Bombi JA, Nadal A, Carreras E, et al. Assessment of histopathologic changes in the colonic biopsy in acute graft-versus-host disease. *Am J Clin Pathol* 1995;**103**:690.

37. Snover DC. Graft versus host disease of the gastrointestinal tract. *Am J Surg Pathol* 1991;**14**(suppl 1):101.

38. Lampert IA, Thorpe P, van Noorden S, et al. Selective sparing of enterochromaffin cells in graft versus host disease affecting the colonic mucosa. *Histopathology* 1985;**9**:875.

39. Shulman HM, Sullivan KM, Weiden PL, et al. Chronic graft-versus-host syndrome in man: a long-term clinicopathologic study of 20 Seattle patients. *Am J Med* 1980;**69**:204.

40. Herrera AF, Soriano G, Bellizzi AM, et al. Cord colitis syndrome in cord-blood stem-cell transplantation. *N Engl J Med* 2011;**365**:815.

41. Leriche M, Devroede G, Sanchez G, et al. Changes in the rectal mucosa induced by hypertonic enemas. *Dis Col Rectum* 1978;**21**:227.

42. Saunders DR, Sillery J, Rachmilewitz D, et al. Effect of bisacodyl on the structure and function of rodent and human intestine. *Gastroenterology* 1977;**72**:849.

43. Meisel JL, Bergman D, Graney D, et al. Human rectal mucosa: proctoscopic and morphological changes caused by laxatives. *Gastroenterology* 1977;**72**:1274.

44. Pockros PJ, Foroozan P. Golytely lavage versus a standard colonoscopy preparation: effect on a normal colonic mucosal histology. *Gastroenterology* 1985;**88**:545.

45. Pike BF, Phillipi PJ, Lawson EH. Soap colitis. *N Engl J Med* 1971;**285**:217.

46. Levison DA, Crocker PR, Smith A, Blackshaw AJ, Bartram CI. Varied light and scanning electron microscopic appearances of barium sulphate in smears and histological sections. *J Clin Pathol* 1984;**37**:481.

47. Lewin K, Harell J, Lee A, Crowley L. An electron microscopic study: demonstration of bacilliform organisms in malakoplakic macrophages. *Gastroenterology* 1974;**66**:28.

48. Radin DR, Chandrosoma P, Halls JM. Colonic malakoplakia. *Gastrointest Radiol* 1984;**9**:359.

49. Cheng H, Sitrin MD, Satchidanand SK, Novak JM. Colonic squamous cell carcinoma in ulcerative colitis: report of a case and review of the literature. *Can J Gastroenterol* 2007;**21**:47.

50. Fu K, Tsujinaka Y, Hamahata Y, Matsuo K, Tsutumi O. Squamous metaplasia of the rectum associated with ulcerative colitis diagnosed using narrow-band imaging. *Endoscopy* 2008;**40**(suppl 2):E45.

51. Langner C, Wenzl HH, Bodo K, Petritsch W. Squamous metaplasia of the colon in Crohn's disease. *Histopathology* 2007;**51**:556.

52. Mahesha V, Sehgal K, Saikia UN, Rao KL. Squamous metaplasia of the rectum in a case of Hirschprung's disease: a coincidence or an association. *J Clin Pathol* 2006;**59**:889.

53. Schaffzin DM, Smith LE. Squamous-cell carcinoma developing after an ileoanal pouch procedure: report of a case. *Dis Colon Rectum* 2005;**48**:1086.

54. Williams GT, Blackshaw AJ, Morson BC. Squamous carcinoma of the colorectum and its genesis. *J Pathol* 1979;**129**:139.

PART

6

The Anal Region

Normal anal region: anatomy, histology relevant to pathological practice and specimen handling

Kevin P. West

University Hospitals of Leicester NHS Trust, Leicester Royal Infirmary, Leicester, UK

Normal anal region: anatomy, histology relevant to pathological practice and specimen handling

Anatomy

Although there is general agreement that the anus constitutes the distal 30–40 mm of the gastrointestinal tract, the definition of the anal canal is a subject of some debate. In general terms it is an anteroposterior slit situated between the rectum above and the perianal skin below [1]. Different groups tend to use different anatomical landmarks to define the precise upper and lower limits of the rectum, e.g. pathologists use the upper and lower borders of the internal anal sphincter [2]. Surgeons and physicians, however, usually regard the level of the levator ani muscle as the upper limit and the anal orifice as the lower limit. Anatomists, on the other hand, use the levels of the anal valves and the anal orifice, respectively, to mark the upper and lower borders of the anus [3].

The anal canal is separated from the tip of the coccyx by a mass of fibromuscular tissue known as the anococcygeal ligament. Lying immediately anterior to the anus is the perineal body, beyond which are the membranous part of the urethra and the bulb of the penis in the male or the lower end of the vagina in the female.

The mucosa in the upper half of the anal canal forms 6–12 vertical folds known as the anal columns. The lower ends of these are joined at approximately the mid-point of the internal sphincter by the anal valves, which are small transverse crescents of mucosa marking the position of the pectinate or dentate line. The recesses created by the anal valves are known as anal sinuses. Faecal material may become impacted within them leading to inflammation.

Below the dentate line the anal canal has a smooth lining and this area is referred to as the pecten (Figure 41.1). The submucosal tissue of the pecten is dense and firmly anchors the epithelium to the underlying internal sphincter. This is believed to be important in limiting the spread of cancer. Above the dentate line, however, the submucosal connective tissue is loose, which allows prolapse to occur.

The arterial supply to the anus comes from the superior middle and inferior rectal arteries. There is considerable variation in the anatomical detail [4]. The internal rectal venous plexus lies beneath the mucosa in the upper two-thirds of the anal canal. In the left lateral, right anterior and right posterior zones the plexus is modified into three specialised vascular anal cushions, consisting of submucosal and anastomosing networks of arterioles and venules with arteriovenous communications showing similar features to erectile tissue. When the vessels of the anal cushions become engorged and prolapse downwards they give rise to haemorrhoids [5].

The anus is drained by the superior, middle and inferior rectal veins. It was previously believed that the internal rectal plexus drained into the portal system via the superior rectal vein, whereas the external venous plexus drained into the systemic circulation by the middle and inferior rectal veins. However, more recent studies suggest that there are usually free communications of the superior, middle and inferior rectal veins and that the venous drainage from the anal cushions is primarily to the systemic circulation [6,7].

Morson and Dawson's Gastrointestinal Pathology, Fifth Edition. Edited by Neil A. Shepherd, Bryan F. Warren, Geraint T. Williams, Joel K. Greenson, Gregory Y. Lauwers and Marco R. Novelli.

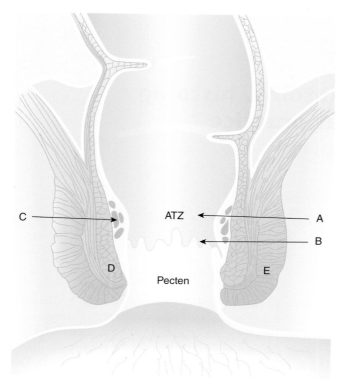

Figure 41.1 Diagram of the normal anatomy of the anorectal region. ATZ, anal transitional zone; A, anal columns; B, dentate line; C, submucosal vascular cushions; D, internal anal sphincter; E, external anal sphincter.

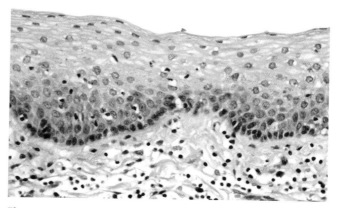

Figure 41.2 Squamous zone of anal canal.

The lymphatic drainage of the anal canal above the dentate line passes to the superior rectal group of lymph nodes. Lymphatic drainage below the dentate line passes to the superficial inguinal lymph nodes.

Embryologically the anus is derived from part of the cloaca and the anal pit. These are separated by the anal membrane in the fetus. The dentate line was thought to represent the site of the anal membrane. However more recent studies suggest that the attempt to separate precisely different parts of the anus on embryological grounds is artificial and it is better regarded as a single, albeit complex, structure [8].

There are differences in innervation of the anus above and below the dentate line. The mucosa below the dentate line has a somatic type of nerve supply in keeping with its ectodermal origin. It is, therefore, extremely sensitive to touch and pain. The anal mucosa above the dentate line is insensitive with an autonomic nerve supply typical of endodermally derived tissues.

The internal anal sphincter is composed of smooth muscle and represents an enlargement of the circular muscle of the rectum, with which it is in continuity. The external anal sphincter is composed of striated muscle and it has been described as having three parts: subcutaneous,

superficial and deep. These are, in fact, barely distinguishable from each other and their existence as distinct entities has been questioned. The internal and external sphincters and the puborectalis muscle are responsible for maintaining continence, providing what has been described as triple security. It is likely that these three structures act in a coordinated manner with each serving slightly different roles [9].

Histology

Three histological zones can be identified in the anus [2,10]. The uppermost of these is the colorectal zone which differs from the normal rectal mucosa by virtue of a predominance of sialo-mucins over sulpho-mucins and the splaying of the fibres of the muscularis mucosae, which extend upwards into the lamina propria between crypts. In the rectum these features are associated with mucosal prolapse but in the colorectal zone of the anus they may be regarded as normal.

The lowermost part of the anal canal is the squamous zone lined by non-keratinising stratified squamous epithelium (Figure 41.2). Sweat glands and pilo-sebaceous units are absent. The squamous zone merges with the perianal skin below.

Between the colorectal and squamous zones is the anal transitional zone. This is covered predominantly by stratified squamous epithelium but columnar cells producing small quantities of mucin are frequent (Figure 41.3). Polygonal cells and flattened cells may also be found, giving the mucosa an appearance reminiscent of transitional epithelium in the urinary tract (Figure 41.4). Occasional melanocytes and endocrine cells may also be found [11].

There is wide variation between the histological zones of the anus and the gross anatomical landmarks. The lower limit of the transitional zone usually coincides with the dentate line. The lower pecten of the anal canal corresponds

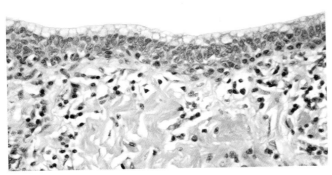

Figure 41.3 Anal transitional zone showing pseudo-stratified columnar epithelium with surface cells containing small amounts of mucin.

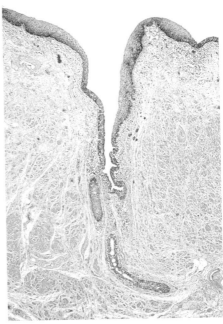

Figure 41.5 Anal crypt lined by transitional epithelium and anal duct lined by columnar epithelium.

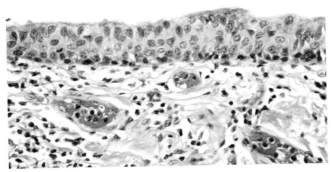

Figure 41.4 Urothelial-like epithelium of the anal transitional zone.

with the histological squamous zone. In about 10% of cases, however, the transitional zone is higher and lies entirely above the dentate line or lower, straddling the dentate line. In a small minority of cases the transitional zone is absent or very limited in extent. The columnar cells of the anal transitional zone and the anal glands produce a mixture of sulpho-mucins and sialo-mucins but unlike those of the large bowel mucosa they are not O-acetylated [12].

Six to ten anal glands arise from the mucosa of the transitional zone. Their orifices open behind the cusps of the anal valves. Branching ducts pass downwards and outwards through the submucosa (Figure 41.5), often extending into or even through the muscle of the internal anal sphincter [12]. They act as a potential channel for infection, allowing it to reach the perianal tissues and ischiorectal fossa. The lining epithelium is identical to the epithelium of the anal transitional zone but tiny intra-epithelial micro-cysts are frequent [2]. Neoplasms have been described reflecting all the various cell types found in the anal canal [13].

Specimen handling

The entire anus is received as part of an abdomino-perineal excision of the rectum for rectal adenocarcinoma. The handling of such specimens is described elsewhere. Chemoradiotherapy is the favoured treatment option for carcinomas of the anus and resection is usually reserved for recurrent disease [13]. The resection may be accompanied by inguinal lymph nodes. T staging incorporates tumour size and depth of invasion [14]. Completeness of excision must also be assessed and may be facilitated by inking the surgical margins.

Sampling of excisional biopsies for suspected invasive or *in situ* neoplasia should also be aimed at determining adequacy of excision. Incisional biopsies should be embedded on edge.

Representative blocks should be taken from samples of fissures, fistulae and abscesses. Adenocarcinomas have been reported in fistula specimens [15]. There is debate about the value of undertaking histological examination of routine haemorrhoidectomy specimens, with some authors suggesting that histology should be reserved for cases where the surgeon regards the clinical appearance as atypical [16].

References

1. Parks AG. Modern concepts of the anatomy of the anal canal. *Postgrad Med J* 1958;**34**:360.

2. Fenger C. The anal transitional zone. *Acta Pathol Microbiol Scand A* 1987;**95**:1.

3. Nivatvongs S, Stern HS, Fryd DS. The length of the anal canal. *Dis Colon Rectum* 1981;**24**:600.

4. Thomson WHF. The nature of haemorrhoids. *Br J Surgery* 1975; **62**:542.

5. Aigner F, Gruber H, Conrad F, et al. Revised morphology and hemodynamics of the anorectal vascular plexus: impact on the course of hemorrhoidal disease. *Int J Colorectal Dis* 2009;**24**:105.

6. Stelzner F. Die Haemorrhoiden und andere Kranheiten des Corpus cavernosum recti und des Analkanals. *Dtsch Med Wochenschr* 1963;**88**:689.

7. Gibbons CP, Trowbridge EA, Bannister JJ, Read NW. Role of anal cushions in maintaining continence. *Lancet* 1986;**i**:886.

8. Fritsch H, Aigner F, Ludwikowski B, et al. Epithelial and muscular regionalization of the human developing anorectum. *Anat Rec* 2007;**11**:1449.

9. Raizada V, Mittal RK. Pelvic floor anatomy and applied physiology. *Gastroenterol Clinics North Am* 2008;**37**:493.

10. Fenger C. Histology of the anal canal. *Am J Surg Pathol* 1988;**12**:41.

11. Fenger C, Lyon H. Endocrine and melanin-containing cells in the anal canal epithelium. *Histochem J* 1982;**14**:631.

12. Fenger C. The anal transitional zone. Location and extent. *Acta Pathol Microbiol Scand A* 1979;**87**:379.

13. Klas JV, Rothenberger DA, Wong MD, Madoff RD. Malignant tumours of the anal canal; the spectrum of disease, treatment and outcomes. *Cancer* 1999;**85**:1686.

14. Sobin LH, Gospodarowicz MK, Wittekind C, eds. *UICC/TNM Classification of Malignant Tumors*, 7th edn. New York: Wiley-Blackwell, 2009.

15. Gaertner WB, Hagerman GF, Finne CO, et al. Fistula-associated anal adenocarcinoma; good results with aggressive therapy. *Dis Colon Rectum* 2008;**7**:1061.

16. Lemarchand N, Tanne F, Aubert M, et al. Is routine pathologic evaluation of haemorrhoidectomy specimens necessary? *Gastroenterol Clin Biol* 2004;**28**:659.

CHAPTER 42

Inflammatory disorders of the anal region

Alison M. Winstanley and Marco R. Novelli
University College Hospital, London, UK

Miscellaneous inflammatory conditions

Anal/Rectal tonsil

Mucosa-associated lymphoid tissue (MALT) is normally present throughout the large intestine but there is marked variation in the density and distribution of such tissue. Lympho-epithelial complexes are more commonly seen in the left than the right colon and are particularly frequent in the anus just above the dentate line. These complexes vary markedly in size but in the anorectum, particularly in young children and adolescents, they may become enlarged and polypoid, forming a discrete mass known as the anal/ rectal tonsil [1]. In most cases the aetiology of this lymphoid hyperplasia is uncertain but there is evidence to suggest that in some cases it arises secondary to an anorectal infection (e.g. chlamydial infection [2]). As well as raising the possibility of an atypical proctitis these lesions may also be mistaken for lymphoproliferative disease.

Anal fissure

Anal fissure can be classified into acute (<6 weeks' duration) and chronic (>6 weeks' duration), primary (iatrogenic) or secondary [3]. Secondary fissures are linked with known disorders such as Crohn's disease, leukaemia, primary syphilis or anal carcinoma. They can also result as sequelae of anal surgery or parturition.

The typical anal fissure is found predominantly in the midline posteriorly and is very infrequent in other quadrants of the anal canal, except in children when anal fissures are often lateral rather than posterior [4].

Anal fissures form an elongated triangular ulcer in the squamous mucosa of the lower anal canal overlying the internal sphincter and the subcutaneous part of the external sphincter. The posterior midline is supplied by end-arterioles that pass through the internal anal sphincter. There is evidence to suggest that the blood supply to the posterior midline of the anus is supplied by end-arterioles [5]. The increased maximum resting anal pressure seen in patients with anal fissures is thought to compress these end-arterioles, reducing blood flow and resulting in the formation of the fissure [5, 6]. An important priority for medical and surgical therapy for acute and chronic anal fissures is aimed at reducing anal pressure in an attempt to improve blood flow [7]. The microscopic appearances of anal fissures are those of non-specific inflammation. The edges of chronic fissures are often thickened and the tissues immediately adjacent are oedematous and heavily infiltrated by lymphocytes and plasma cells. Granulation tissue can be scarce. In a proportion of cases the oedematous skin at the lower end of the fissure may form a polypoid projection known as a 'sentinel tag'.

Anal abscess and anal fistula

An anal abscess usually begins with an infection of the anal glands [8], which lie in the submucosa of the anal canal with branches penetrating through the internal sphincter into the potential space between the internal and

Morson and Dawson's Gastrointestinal Pathology, Fifth Edition. Edited by Neil A. Shepherd, Bryan F. Warren,
Geraint T. Williams, Joel K. Greenson, Gregory Y. Lauwers and Marco R. Novelli.

external sphincter. Their ducts open into the anal crypts at the level of the dentate line. In many cases the glands also penetrate into and through the external sphincter. Infection within these glands can track in several directions depending on the complexity of their branching.

An anorectal fistula arises as the result of an anal abscess developing a communication with the lumen of the anus/rectum and/or with perianal skin. Despite their name, some fistulae *in ano* are really sinuses because they connect to only one epithelial surface. The classification of anal fistula is based on knowledge of the anatomy of the anal glands. The main anatomical varieties of fistula are [9,10]:

• *Inter-sphincteric*: the track runs between the internal and external sphincteric muscle. It is deemed low if it runs distally to the skin and high if it runs proximally to open into the rectum.
• *Trans-sphincteric*: the track runs through the external sphincter and the ischiorectal fossa to the perianal skin.
• *Supra-sphincteric*: the track passes upwards into the inter-sphincteric space, above the external sphincter and back into the ischiorectal fossa to the perianal skin.
• *Extra-sphincteric*: these fistulae are secondary to pelvic sepsis rather than anal gland infection and discharge through the ischiorectal fossa to the skin.

Of 769 anal fistulae reviewed at St Mark's Hospital, the relative frequencies of the various sub-types was: inter-sphincteric 55.9%, trans-sphincteric 21.3%, supra-sphincteric 3.4% and extra-sphincteric 3.0%; 16.4% were classified as superficial in association with chronic anal fissures and sentinel tags [11].

Most anal abscesses and therefore fistulae are thought to be idiopathic or secondary to Crohn's disease. Idiopathic abscesses/fistulae are considered to be the result of cryptoglandular inflammation and probably the most common type [8]. It seems likely that stasis and secondary infection of the gland are generally due to obstruction resulting from inflammation, either of the gland itself, or the rectal tonsil [1,12].

It has been suggested that the chronicity of anal fistulae is due to persistence of anal gland epithelium in the part of the tract adjoining the internal opening, keeping the tract patent and preventing healing [13]. Infection does not of itself explain the persistence of anal fistulae [14].

Most fistulae are treated by fistulotomy [15]. During the exploration and surgical treatment of anal fistulae and abscesses, tissue is usually sent for histological examination to exclude malignancy, a rare but well-recognised complication, particularly on a background of Crohn's disease [16]. Anal fistulae and sinuses can show a variety of histological patterns (Figure 42.1). In the great majority of cases sections will show an ordinary pyogenic type of inflammatory reaction. Careful examination is important to exclude the small risk of a haematological malignancy because, in

one series, 6% of haematological malignancies had anal lesions, a fifth of these cases initially presenting with the anal lesion [17]. Giant cells of the foreign body type are frequently encountered – presumably a reaction to the presence of faecal material within the track (Figure 42.1a) – although an oleogranulomatous reaction can be seen in some cases (Figure 42.1b). It is important that a foreign body reaction should be distinguished from the well-formed non-caseating epithelioid granulomas seen in Crohn's disease (Figure 42.1c), or the confluent caseating epithelioid granulomas of tuberculosis (Figure 42.1d). Miliary tuberculosis can also present as an anal abscess [18]. The spread of infection in and around fistulous tracks can provoke tissue damage such as fat necrosis, secondary vasculitis and degenerative changes in striated muscle, with the formation of giant hyperchromatic nuclei. Occasionally *Trichuris* sp. and *Enterobius vermicularis* may be the cause of an anal canal abscess [19,20] and there is a report describing actinomycosis occurring as a secondary infection [21].

Pilonidal sinus

Pilonidal sinuses consist of single or multiple sinus tracts that typically open on to the skin crease of the natal cleft and extend into subcutaneous abscess tracks. The tracks branch, most often in a cephalad direction and laterally into the buttocks but occasionally towards the anus. Pilonidal sinuses are most common in young men. Hirsutism, chronic irritation and intertrigo are precipitating factors. Pilonidal sinuses are thought to be caused by puncture of the skin of the natal cleft by ingrowing hair shafts [22]. An inflammatory reaction results, leading to the formation of a tract lined by squamous epithelium and granulation tissue into which more hair and skin debris accumulates. Further secondary infection causes the formation of subcutaneous abscess tracks. Microscopic examination of surgically excised pilonidal sinuses shows granulation tissue-lined sinus tracks, which usually, although not invariably, contain numerous hair shafts around which there is a florid foreign body giant cell reaction (Figure 42.2). They may occur at any site of hair growth and have even been described in the anal canal [23,24]. Squamous cell carcinoma complicating pilonidal sinuses has been reported, although it is extremely rare [25,26].

Hidradenitis suppurativa

Hidradenitis suppurativa (Verneuil's disease) is a chronic inflammatory condition that usually affects the skin and subcutaneous tissues of those parts of the body where apocrine sweat glands are found, namely the axilla, areola of the breast, umbilicus, genitalia and perianal area. Perianal hidradenitis is an uncommon condition which is more frequent in females than males (female:male ratio as high as 4:1) [27,28]. The affected area of skin has a red and white

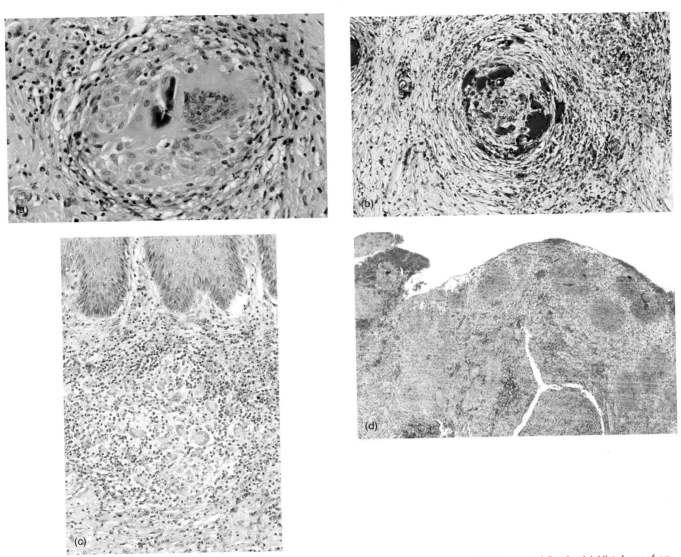

Figure 42.1 (a) Foreign body giant cell reaction in an anal fistula. (b) Oleogranulomatous reaction in an anal fistula. (c) Histology of an anal lesion of Crohn's disease showing a sarcoid-like granuloma beneath the perianal skin. (d) Tuberculous anal fistula showing granulomatous reaction with caseation.

blotchy appearance and is thickened and oedematous with watery pus seen draining from multiple sinus track openings. The persistent chronic nature of this disease leads to ulceration and scarring [29]. Lesions may be localised or involve large areas of perianal skin extending on to the buttocks but differ from anal fistulae in being superficial to the sphincteric muscle and not connected to the intersphincteric plane [29]. Microscopic examination of excised specimens shows a mixed inflammatory exudate with abscess and sinus track formation. Foreign body-type giant cells may be present but well-formed epithelioid granulomas are very seldom seen and, if present, should raise the possibility of perianal Crohn's disease [30].

The distribution of hidradenitis suppurativa suggests that it results from a primary infection of apocrine glands. However, some consider that these glands are infected secondarily to keratin plugging of hair follicles and a pilosebaceous folliculitis and that hidradenitis can affect skin in sites other than apocrine gland-bearing areas [31]. The cause of the disease is not understood but, similar to acne, it seems to have some relationship to hormonal activity [27] and there may be a genetic component. Studies have reported a positive family history (up to 38% in one study) [27,32,33]. Other aetiological factors suggested include excessive local moisture in apposing skin surfaces and the difficulty of maintaining cleanliness in the regions involved.

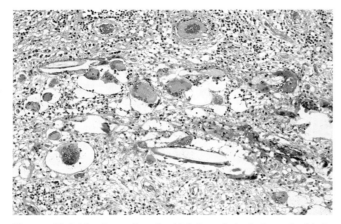

Figure 42.2 Histology of a pilonidal sinus: hair shafts embedded in granulation tissue.

Hidradenitis most commonly involves the axillary area, where it is self-limiting and rarely requires surgery. However, perineal, perianal and gluteal hidradenitis usually require surgical intervention [34,35]. Malignant change, although rare, has been reported [36].

Infectious disease of the anorectum

Anorectal tuberculosis

Tuberculosis (TB) of the anorectal region is rare [37] and may be associated with abdominal TB either by direct extension or secondary spread via lymphatics [38]. Anorectal TB most frequently presents as anal fistulae [39] but may also present with sinuses, ulceration, fissures, strictures and inguinal lymphadenopathy. Typically the predominant histological features are those of caseating granulomatous inflammation but necrotising granulomas are not always present and histological diagnosis may be difficult, especially the distinction from Crohn's disease (see Figure 42.1c,d). A diagnosis of anorectal TB can be confirmed by culture of fresh tissue, the demonstration of acid-fast bacilli in Ziehl–Neelsen-stained tissue sections or using *Mycobacterium tuberculosis*-specific polymerase chain reaction (PCR) [40].

Histoplasmosis, leishmaniasis and schistosomiasis

Anal involvement by histoplasmosis [41,42,43] and leishmaniasis [44] is extremely uncommon and typically occurs on a background of HIV infection, with only a handful of case reports in the literature. In a review of 77 cases of gastrointestinal histoplasmosis, none involved the anus [45]. Schistosomiasis may also rarely involve the anus [46].

Sexually transmitted infections

Since the introduction of highly active anti-retroviral therapies in the late 1990s, there has been an increasing incidence of sexually transmitted infections involving the anal region. This increase has been particularly marked in the male homosexual community [47] but occasional cases are also seen in female patients. Syphilis, gonorrhoea, chancroid, herpes simplex, lymphogranuloma venereum and granuloma inguinale may all involve the anorectum and present with non-specific anal ulceration [48,49].

Syphilis

Both primary and secondary stages of syphilis can affect the anus. Primary anorectal syphilis presents with an anal chancre, a small indurated papule that eventually ulcerates and heals without treatment in 2–4 weeks [50]. The primary chancre is painful and associated with painless inguinal lymphadenopathy. Chancres may be single or multiple and situated on the perianal skin or within the anal canal. The clinical appearance of primary anal syphilis typically resembles and may be mistaken for, other inflammatory conditions of the anus, particularly fissure *in ano* [51,52]. Secondary syphilis results from the haematogenous dissemination of untreated syphilis and is associated with condyloma latum – spirochaete-filled, moist, reddened, hypertrophic papular lesions which appear adjacent to the primary chancre. The histological appearances of anorectal syphilis are non-specific, with mucosal ulceration, prominent vascular proliferation and a mixed inflammatory cell infiltrate rich in plasma cells. Loose epithelioid granulomas may be present and there may also be a non-specific active chronic proctitis. The combination of these histological appearances may potentially lead to a misdiagnosis of Crohn's disease. In histological material the diagnosis of syphilis may be confirmed by directly visualising the spirochaetes using either histochemical (Warthin–Starry) or immunohistochemical stains, or indirectly by PCR analysis.

Gonorrhoea

Anorectal gonorrhoea is usually acquired by anoreceptive intercourse although direct spread from gonococcal cervicitis can occur in women [53]. External examination of the anus is often unremarkable; however, anal erythema and ulceration may be evident and thick purulent discharge can usually be expressed from the anal crypts on external pressure [48]. A clinical diagnosis is typically confirmed by anal swabbing with direct visualisation of the organism using a Gram stain, culture or PCR analysis.

Granuloma inguinale

Granuloma inguinale (donovanosis) is generally regarded as a sexually transmitted infection [54]. It is widespread in the tropics [55]. The causative organism, *Calymmatobacterium granulomatis*, has recently been cultured and phylogenetic analysis showed similarities more closely related to the genus *Klebsiella* than *Calymmatobacterium* [56]. Classically there are four types of lesion: (1) ulcerogranulomatous – beefy red, non-tender ulcers that bleed easily; (2) hypertrophic or verrucous ulcer; (3) necrotic with a foul-smelling deep ulcer; and (4) dry, sclerotic or cicatricial lesion. Histologically the lesions show pseudo-epitheliomatous hyperplasia of the squamous epithelium, with a prominent inflammatory cell infiltrate composed of plasma cells, neutrophils and some lymphocytes. Diagnostic Donovan bodies can be demonstrated by Leishman, Giemsa or Warthin–Starry stains. Carcinoma is a rare complication.

Lymphogranuloma venereum

Lymphogranuloma venereum (LGV) is caused by *Chlamydia trachomatis*. Anorectal LGV is usually acquired through receptive anal intercourse. Symptomatic proctitis and anorectal disease are typically associated with LGV serovars L1–3 [57]. Patients may present with a proctocolitis with clinical and endoscopic features that closely mimic inflammatory bowel disease (IBD). The anal manifestations include confluent nodules with fissuring, multiple anal fistulae, stricturing and perianal elephantiasis. Local lymphadenopathy is characteristic with masses of matted nodes occurring in the iliac, perirectal, inguinal or femoral regions. The histological features of anorectal LGV are also very similar to those of IBD, with non-specific ulceration, cryptitis, crypt abscess formation and granuloma formation. Crypt architectural distortion also occurs but is said to be less marked than that seen in IBD [57] (Figure 42.3). As the histological features are non-specific, diagnosis depends on a high clinical index of suspicion supported by chlamydia serology and confirmed by PCR analysis of rectal swabs.

Chancroid

This condition, which is rare in developed countries, is caused by *Haemophilus ducreyii* and can produce multiple painful perianal ulcers. Painful unilateral inguinal lymphadenopathy is often present due to abscesses forming in the draining lymph nodes. The histological appearances are those of non-specific ulceration. A clinical diagnosis was traditionally made from identification of organisms in an ulcer swab and subsequent culture but these methods have now largely been superseded by PCR-based methodologies.

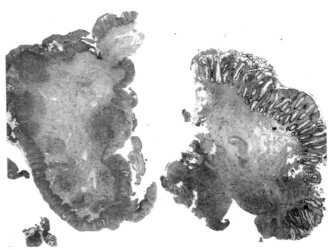

Figure 42.3 Anorectal lymphogranuloma venereum infection. Anorectal mucosa showing non-specific inflammatory type changes including mild crypt architectural distortion with crypt hypertrophy, patchy non-specific active chronic inflammation and an area of ulceration. Close examination of the squamous mucosa on the left of the picture shows concomitant AIN3, the presence of which should increase the index of suspicion for an atypical infective proctocolitis.

Virally related causes of anal ulceration

Herpes simplex is the one of the most common sexually transmitted infections worldwide [58]. Anal herpes simplex infection is most commonly acquired by anoreceptive intercourse or ano-oral sex but can also result from contiguous spread from a pre-existing genital lesion. Historically anogenital herpes has been associated with herpes simplex virus type 2 infection but an increasing proportion of cases are now caused by HSV type 1 [59]. The histological appearances of anal herpes simplex infection are those of non-specific ulceration but in most cases typical herpetic inclusions can be seen in keratinocytes at the edges of ulcers. Immunohistochemistry can be used to confirm the presence of HSV-1/-2.

Cytomegalovirus (CMV) may also cause anal ulceration in immunocompromised patients although this is rare [60].

Inflammatory bowel disease involving the anorectum

Crohn's disease

The anus is an important site of disease activity in Crohn's disease (see also 'The differential diagnosis of Crohn's disease and ulcerative colitis', Chapter 35) [61]. The frequency of anal lesions in Crohn's disease varies from 25% to 80% [62, 63]. This range partly reflects the site of primary involvement, anal lesions being more common with more distal Crohn's disease but there is also a lack of consensus on what constitutes a perianal complication of Crohn's disease, with perianal skin irritation being considered a complication by some but dismissed by others. Up to 5% of patients with Crohn's disease present with anal disease [64] and intestinal involvement may not manifest for up to 10 years. The spectrum of Crohn's disease-related anal lesions includes fissures, skin tags, cavitating ulcers, fistulae, strictures and abscesses. In approximately 5% of cases these pathologies are sufficiently debilitating to warrant rectal excision [65].

A clinical diagnosis of anorectal Crohn's disease may be confirmed in targeted biopsy material from patients suspected of having Crohn's disease but may also be made by chance in unsuspected cases during routine histopathological evaluation of surgically resected anal lesions (e.g. fibroepithelial polyps and fistulae). The classic histological features of perianal Crohn's disease include oedema with dilated lymphatics, patchy active chronic inflammation with lymphoid aggregates and well-formed epithelioid granulomas, the granulomas often seen in close apposition to, or lying within, lymphatic channels or at the dermo-epidermal junction. However, the histological features of anorectal Crohn's disease are not always specific, with classic sarcoid-like granulomas being present in only around 60% of cases. There are also a number of other conditions, in particular atypical infections, that may mimic anorectal Crohn's disease both clinically and histologically, many of which may also show granulomatous inflammation. As the clinical features of Crohn's disease are not always distinctive and granulomatous histology is absent in some 40% of cases, in many cases anal Crohn's disease continues to remain unrecognised until abdominal disease becomes apparent.

There is a well-documented association between perianal Crohn's disease and carcinomas in the anal region. Adenocarcinomas may arise in the glandular epithelium of the anorectal junction or in association with fistulae [66]. Squamous cell carcinomas of the anal canal have also been described [66,67].

Ulcerative colitis

Ulcerative colitis typically involves the colorectal zone of the anus because it involves the rectum. In patients who have undergone restorative proctocolectomy, with either ileo-rectal anastomosis or ileo-anal pouch formation, there is often a short segment of persistent colorectal zone mucosa the 'anal cuff'. This area of residual colonic type mucosa may continue to be involved by ulcerative colitis,

which has been termed 'cuffitis' [68]. In patients with ileo-anal pouches such inflammation may cause clinical symptoms that mimic pouchitis, in particular causing frequency of defecation. There is also a small long-term risk of dysplasia and malignancy developing in the anal cuff [69].

Although lesions of the lower anal canal do occur in patients with ulcerative colitis, they are less frequent than and have a different character from, the anal lesions seen in Crohn's disease. Ordinary anal and rectovaginal fistulae are seen but the inflammatory changes in the anal canal and anal margin are usually more superficial, presenting as an acute anal fissure or excoriation of the skin around the anus. Whereas chronic anal lesions are characteristic of Crohn's disease, acute perianal or ischiorectal abscesses are more frequent in ulcerative colitis. The histology of these shows no specific features that help in the diagnosis of ulcerative colitis.

References

1. Farris AB, Lauwers GY, Ferry JA, Zukerberg LR. The rectal tonsil: a reactive lymphoid proliferation that may mimic lymphoma. *Am J Surg Pathol* 2008;**32**:1075.
2. Cramer SF, Romansky S, Hulbert B, Rauh S, Papp JR, Casiano-Colon AE. The rectal tonsil: a reaction to chlamydial infection? *Am J Surg Pathol* 2009;**33**:483.
3. Crapp AR, Alexander-Williams J. Fissure-in-ano and anal stenosis. *Clin Gastroenterol* 1975;**43**:619.
4. Kleinhaus S. Miscellaneous anal disorders. In: Ravitch MM (ed.), *Paediatric Surgery*, 3rd edn. Chicago: Year Book Medical Publishers, 1979.
5. Klosterhalfen B, Vogel P, Rixen H, Mittermayer C. Topography of the inferior rectal artery: A possible cause of chronic, primary anal fissure. *Dis Colon Rectum* 1969;**32**:43.
6. Schouten WR, Breil JW, Auwerda JJ. Relationship between anal pressure and anodermal blood flow. The vascular pathogenesis of anal fissures. *Dis Colon Rectum* 1994;**37**:664.
7. McCallion K, Gardiner KR. Progress in the understanding and treatment of chronic anal fissure. *Postgrad Med J* 2001;**77**:753.
8. Parks AG. Pathogenesis and treatment of fistula-in-ano. *BMJ* 1961;**i**:463.
9. Parks AG, Gordon PH, Hardcastle JD. A classification of fistula-in-ano. *Br J Surg* 1976;**63**:1.
10. Fazio VW. Complex anal fistulae. *Gastroenterol Clinics North Am* 1987;**16**:93.
11. Marks CG, Ritchie JK. Anal fistulae at St Marks Hospital. *Br J Surg* 1977;**64**:84.
12. Parks AG, Morson BC. Fistula-in-ano. *Proc R Soc Med* 1962;**55**:751.
13. Hawley PR. Anorectal fistula. *Clin Gastroenterol* 1975;**4**:635.
14. Lunniss PJ, Faris B, Rees HC, Heard S, Phillips RKS. Histological and microbiological assessment of the role of microorganisms in chronic anal fistula. *Br J Surg* 1993;**80**:1072.
15. Davies M, Harris D, Lohana P, et al. The surgical management of fistula-in-ano in a specialist colorectal unit. *Int J Colorectal Dis* 2008;**23**:833.
16. Thomas M, Bienkowski R, Vandermeer TJ, Trostle D, Cagir B. Malignant transformation in perianal fistulas of Crohn's disease: a systematic review of literature. *J Gastrointest Surg* 2010;**14**:66.
17. Vanheuverzwyn R, Delannoy A, Michaux JL, Dive C. Anal lesions in haematologic disease. *Dis Colon Rectum* 1980;**23**:310.

18. O'Donohue MK, Waldron RP, O'Malley E. Miliary tuberculosis presenting as an acute perianal abscess. *Dis Colon Rectum* 1987; **30**:697.

19. Mortensen NJ, Thompson JP. Perianal abscess due to *Enterobius vermicularis*. *Dis Colon Rectum* 1984;**27**:677.

20. Feigen GM. Suppurative anal cryptitis associated with *Trichuris trichiura*. *Dis Colon Rectum* 1987;**30**:620.

21. Alvarado-Cerna R, Bracho-Riquelme R. Perianal actinomycosis – A complication of a fistula-in-ano. Report of a case. *Dis Colon Rectum* 1994;**37**:378.

22. Weale FE. A comparison of Barber's and post-anal pilonidal sinuses. *Br J Surg* 1964;**51**:513.

23. Ortiz H, Marti J, DeMiguel M, Carmona A, Cabanas IP. Hair-containing lesions within the anal canal. *Int J Colorectal Dis* 1987; **2**:153.

24. Taylor BA, Hughes LE. Circumferential perianal pilonidal sinuses. *Dis Colon Rectum* 1984;**27**:120.

25. Gaston EA, Wilde WL. Epidermoid carcinoma arising in a pilonidal sinus. *Dis Colon Rectum* 1965;**8**:343.

26. Lineaweaver WC, Brumsom MB, Smith JF, Franzini DA, Rumley TO. Squamous carcinoma arising in a pilonidal sinus. *J Surg Oncol* 1984;**27**:239.

27. Shah N. Hidradenitis suppurativa: a treatment challenge. *Am Fam Physn* 2005;**72**:1547.

28. Kagan RJ, Yakuboff KP, Arner P, Warden GD. Surgical treatment of hidradenitis suppurativa: a 10-year experience. *Surgery* 2005; **138**:734.

29. Culp CE. Chronic hidradenitis suppurativa of the anal canal. *Dis Colon Rectum* 1983;**26**:669.

30. Attanoos RL, Appleton MAC, Hughes LE, et al. Granulomatous hidradenitis suppurativa and cutaneous Crohn's disease. *Histopathology* 1993;**23**:111.

31. Anderson MJ, Dockerty MB. Perianal hidradenitis suppurativa. *Dis Colon Rectum* 1958;**1**:23.

32. Von der Werth JM, Williams HC. The natural history of hidradenitis suppurativa. *J Eur Acad Dermatol Venerol* 2000;**14**:389.

33. Von der Werth JM, Williams HC, Raeburn JA. The clinical genetics of hidradenitis suppurativa revisited. *Br J Dermatol* 2000; **142**:947.

34. Balik E, Eren T, Bulut T, Büyükuncu Y, Bugra D, Yamaner S. Surgical approach to hidradenitis suppurativa in the perineal/perianal and gluteal regions. *World J Surg* 2009;**33**:481.

35. Bocchini SF, Habr-Gama A, Kiss DR, Imperiale AR, Araujo SE. Gluteal and perianal hidradenitis suppurativa: surgical treatment by wide excision. *Dis Colon Rectum* 2003;**46**:944.

36. Humphrey LJ, Playforth H, Leavell VW. Squamous cell carcinoma arising in hidradenitis suppurativum. *Arch Dermatol* 1969; **100**:59.

37. Maartens G, Wilkinson RJ. Tuberculosis. *Lancet* 2007;**370**:2030.

38. Barnes PF, Barrows SA. Tuberculosis in the 1990's. *Ann Intern Med* 1993;**119**:400.

39. Gupta PJ. Ano-perianal tuberculosis – solving a clinical dilemma. *Afr Health Sci* 2005;**5**:345.

40. Nopvichai C, Sanpavat A, Sawatdee R, et al. PCR detection of *Mycobacterium tuberculosis* in necrotising non-granulomatous lymphadenitis using formalin-fixed paraffin-embedded tissue: a study in Thai patients. *J Clin Pathol* 2009;**62**:812.

41. Recondo G, Sella A, Ro JY, Dexeus FH, Amato R, Kilbourn R. Perianal ulcer in disseminated histoplasmosis. *South Med J* 1991; **84**:931.

42. Winburn GB, Yeh KA. Severe anal ulceration secondary to *Histoplasma capsulatum* in a patient with HIV disease. *Am Surg* 1999;**65**:321.

43. Earle JHO, Highman JH, Lockey E. A case of disseminated histoplasmosis. *BMJ* 1960;**i**:607.

44. Pérez-Molina JA, Fortún J, López-Vélez R. Anal ulcer and chronic diarrhoea as manifestations of visceral leishmaniasis in a patient infected with human immunodeficiency virus. *Trans R Soc Trop Med Hyg* 1997;**91**:436.

45. Cappell MS, Mandell W, Grimes MM, Neu HC. Gastrointestinal histoplasmosis. *Dig Dis Sci* 1988;**33**:353.

46. Gholam P, Autschbach F, Hartschuh W. Schistosomiasis in an HIV-positive patient presenting as an anal fissure and giant anal polyp. *Arch Dermatol* 2008;**144**:950.

47. Truong HM, Kellogg T, Klausener JD, et al. Increases in sexually transmitted infections and sexual risk behaviour without a concurrent increase in HIV incidence among men who have sex with men in San Francisco: a suggestion of HIV serosorting? *Sex Transm Infect* 2006;**82**:461.

48. Whitlow CB. Bacterial sexually transmitted diseases. *Clin Colon Rectal Surg* 2004;**17**:209.

49. McMillan A, Smith IW. Painful anal ulceration in homosexual men. *Br J Surg* 1984;**71**:215.

50. Goligher JC. Sexually transmitted diseases. In: Goligher JC (ed.), *Diseases of the Anus, Rectum and Colon*, 5th edn. London: Baillière Tindall, 1985: 1033.

51. Samenius B. Primary syphilis of the anorectal region. *Dis Colon Rectum* 1968;**11**:462.

52. Quinn TC, Lukehart SA, Goodell S, et al. Rectal mass caused by *Treponema pallidum*: Confirmation by immunofluorescent staining. *Gastroenterology* 1982;**82**:135.

53. Hook EW III, Hansfield HH. Gonococcal infection in the adult. In: Holmes KK, Sparling PR, Mardh PA (eds), *Sexually Transmitted Diseases*. New York: McGraw-Hill, 1999: 451.

54. Goldberg J. Studies on Granuloma inguinale V, Isolation of a bacterium resembling donovania granulomatis from the faeces of a patient with granuloma inguinale. *Br J Vener Dis* 1962;**38**:99.

55. Greenblatt RB, Dienst RB, Baldwin KR. Lymphogranuloma venereum and granuloma inguinale. *Med Clinics North Am* 1959;**43**:1493.

56. Carter JS, Bowden FJ, Bastian I, Myers GM, Sriprakash KS, Kemp DJ. Phylogenetic evidence for reclassification of *Calymmatobacterium granulomatis* as *Klebsiella granulomatis* comb. nov. *Int J Syst Bacteriol* 1999;**49**:1695.

57. Soni S, Srirajaskanthan R, Lucas SB, Alexander S, Wong T, White JA. Lymphogranuloma venereum proctitis masquerading as inflammatory bowel disease in 12 homosexual men. *Aliment Pharmacol Ther* 2010;**32**:59.

58. Corey L, Wald A. Genital herpes. In: Holmes KK, Sparling PF, Mardh PA, et al. (eds), *Sexually Transmitted Diseases*. New York: McGraw-Hill, 1999: 285.

59. Ryder N, Jin F, McNulty AM, Grulich AE, Donovan B. Increasing role of herpes simplex virus type 1 in first-episode anogenital herpes in heterosexual women and younger men who have sex with men, 1992–2006. *Sex Transm Infect* 2009;**85**:416.

60. Cohen SM, Schmitt SL, Lucas FV, Wexner SD. The diagnosis of anal ulcers in AIDS patients. *Int J Colorect Dis* 1994;**9**:169.

61. Cohen Z, McLeod RS. Perianal Crohn's disease. *Gastroenterol Clinics North Am* 1987;**16**:175.

62. Fielding JF. Perianal lesions in Crohn's disease. *J R Coll Surg* 1972;**17**:32.

63. Lockhart-Mummery HE, Morson BC. Crohn's disease of the large intestine. *Gut* 1964;**5**:493.

64. Lockhart-Mummery HE. Crohn's disease: anal lesions. *Dis Colon Rectum* 1975;**18**:200.

65. Buchmann P, Keighley MRB, Allan RN, Thompson H, Alexander-Williams J. Natural history of perianal Crohn's disease. *Am J Surg* 1980;**140**:642.

66. Connell WR, Sheffield JP, Kamm MA, et al. Lower gastrointestinal malignancy in Crohn's disease. *Gut* 1994;**35**:347.

67. Lumley JW, Stitz RW. Crohn's disease and anal carcinoma: an association? A case report and review of the literature. *Aust N Z J Surg* 1991;**61**:76.

68. Thompson-Fawcett MW, Mortensen NJ, Warren BF. 'Cuffitis' and inflammatory changes in the columnar cuff, anal transi-tional zone, and ileal reservoir after stapled pouch-anal anasto-mosis. *Dis Colon Rectum* 1999;**42**:348.

69. Chambers WM, McC Mortensen NJ. Should ileal pouch-anal anastomosis include mucosectomy? *Colorectal Dis* 2007;**9**:384.

CHAPTER 43

Tumours and tumour-like conditions of the anorectal region

Thomas Guenther

St Mark's Hospital, North West London Hospitals NHS Trust, London, UK; Otto-von-Guericke University, Magdeburg, Germany

Epithelial tumours of the anal canal are all uncommon and comprise a diverse collection of histological types. This reflects the many different varieties of epithelium seen in this area. A detailed knowledge of the histology of the epithelial lining of the anorectal region is an essential prerequisite to the classification of anorectal tumours.

A distinction should be made between malignant tumours of the anal canal and those of the anal margin. The former are mostly non-keratinising variants of squamous cell carcinoma arising from the mucous membrane. The latter are keratinising squamous cell carcinomas of the perianal skin with a generally better prognosis and requiring less aggressive treatment. Apart from the exceptional occurrence of lymphomas and connective tissue tumours in the anorectal region, consideration must also be given to tumours of the ischiorectal fossae and presacral tumours.

Benign epithelial tumours and pre-cancerous lesions of the anorectal region

This section encompasses a heterogeneous group of lesions, some arising in the anal canal, some in the perianal skin and some within both sites. Squamous cell papillomas arising from the epithelium of the anal canal, both below and above the dentate line, are encountered only rarely. They may be related to viral warts even when human papillomavirus immunohistochemistry is negative.

Fibro-epithelial polyps

Also known as skin tags, these common lesions have been viewed as burnt-out, thrombosed haemorrhoids but may represent a primary hyperplasia of the subepithelial connective tissue of the anal mucosa [1]. The polyps consist of a myxoid or collagenous stroma covered by squamous epithelium (Figure 43.1). The stromal fibroblasts or myofibroblasts may be multi-nucleated and occasionally show atypical nuclear features [1]. The same cells may be found in normal subepithelial connective tissue of the anal canal mucosa. Mast cells are also present and may be implicated in the pathogenesis of these lesions through the production of fibrogenic factors [1]. Vacuolation of the superficial keratinocytes is another feature of these lesions [2]. Inflammation of the stroma, usually inconspicuous, is mainly caused by trauma but can also be related to a nearby fissure or fistula opening. If there is granulomatous inflammation the possibility of Crohn's disease or anorectal tuberculosis has to be excluded. A dense lymphoplasmocytic cellular infiltrate may indicate secondary syphilis (condylomata lata).

Although CD34-positive stromal cells can occur in the anal submucosal tissue and haemorrhoids, there seems to be an increase in fibro-epithelial polyps related to their size. This finding suggests that CD34-positive stromal cells have the capability for tissue repair and overgrowth [3]. Fibro-epithelial polyps vary in size but are usually small, causing no significant clinical problems. So-called giant fibro-epithelial polyps are rare and an anecdotal case of a fibro-epithelial polyp complicated by obstructive ileus has been reported [4].

Inflammatory cloacogenic polyp

The inflammatory cloacogenic polyp (proctitis cystica profunda) is the polypoid variant of mucosal prolapse (see

Morson and Dawson's Gastrointestinal Pathology, Fifth Edition. Edited by Neil A. Shepherd, Bryan F. Warren, Geraint T. Williams, Joel K. Greenson, Gregory Y. Lauwers and Marco R. Novelli.

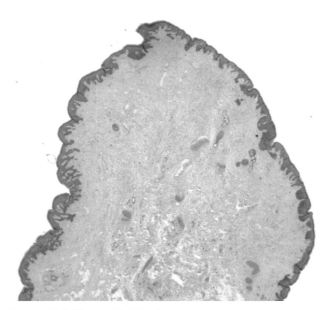

Figure 43.1 Fibro-epithelial polyp.

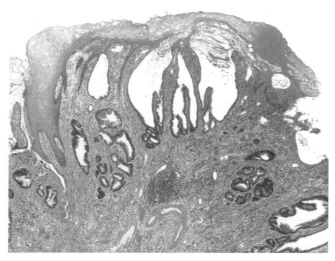

Figure 43.2 Inflammatory cloacogenic polyp.

'Mucosal prolapse and the solitary ulcer syndrome', Chapter 34) and shares the histological features seen in the solitary rectal ulcer of the anterior rectal wall, the inflammatory myoglandular polyp of the colon and prolapsing mucosal folds in diverticular colitis (crescentic fold disease) [5,6]. The polyps are covered by a combination of rectal, transitional and anal squamous mucosa [7,8]. There is often erosion with underlying fibrosis of the lamina propria, and reactive and regenerative changes of the epithelium lining with hyperplastic, elongated and distorted crypts. As in all forms of colorectal prolapse, there is a characteristic arborising extension of smooth muscle fibres from the muscularis mucosae into the lamina propria (Figure 43.2). Prolapsing

haemorrhoids may show similar epithelial changes [9]. Inflammatory cloacogenic polyps have been described in children [10].

Clinically the polyp can be mistaken for a neoplastic lesion because of its macroscopic appearance. Even the histology of biopsies from an inflammatory cloacogenic polyp may be misinterpreted because the reactive epithelium can mimic dysplasia and the surrounding dense fibrotic stroma may resemble desmoplastic stroma. Crypts completely surrounded by vertically oriented smooth muscle fibres and misplaced glandular structures in the submucosa may also look like stromal invasion.

Squamous hyperplasia (leukoplakia)

A variety of pathological lesions may present clinically as a white plaque. A common cause is squamous metaplasia and hyperkeratosis of the transitional mucosa, at the lower pole of prolapsing internal haemorrhoids, or upgrowth of thickened squamous mucosa from the anal canal over ulcerating haemorrhoids. There is no evidence that such white plaques are pre-cancerous. However, pre-cancerous epithelial dysplasia may present as a white plaque in the anal canal. Specific dermatological conditions, such as lichen planus and lichen sclerosus (et atrophicus), may affect lower anal canal mucosa and perianal skin, and present clinically as a white plaque. Any prolonged irritation in the perianal region may lead to a chronic, non-specific dermatitis characterised histologically by hyperkeratosis and chronic inflammatory cell infiltration of the dermis.

When the above causes of white plaque have been excluded, there remains a specific condition occurring in the lower anal canal and perianal skin. Leukoplakia is a clinical term and no longer acceptable as a histopathological diagnosis and the following lesion, analogous to terminology applied to the vulva, is described as anal hyperplasia (generally without dysplasia). Clinical inspection shows a white thickened and sometimes circumferential anal lesion (Figure 43.3). Microscopically, there is hyperkeratosis, focal parakeratosis and acanthosis. Wispy spikes of epithelium project into the underlying connective tissue in which there is a dense lymphocytic and plasma cell infiltrate. The infiltrate often follows the saw-tooth contour of the dermoepidermal junction in a band-like manner, and invades the lower epidermis (Figure 43.4). The appearances thereby closely mimic lichen planus, except for the greater degree of acanthosis and the presence of parakeratosis. Epithelial dysplasia is seen in a minority of cases only. At St Mark's Hospital, patients have been treated by local excision, which in some instances has required skin grafting [11]. The lesion has been observed to recur and progression to malignancy has been recorded, the cancers generally being well differentiated squamous cell carcinomas. In other patients squamous hyperplasia and carcinoma have been

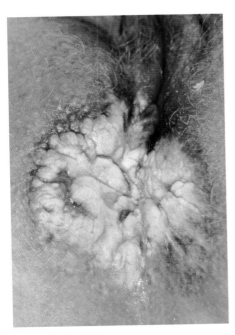

Figure 43.3 Anal leukoplakia.

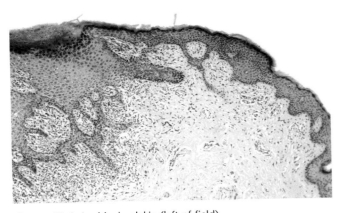

Figure 43.4 Anal leukoplakia (left of field).

synchronous presentations. One patient was treated by excision of the rectum and developed recurrent disease around the colostomy. The lesion is therefore a distinct clinico-pathological entity with a definite risk of cancer but the aetiology remains obscure.

Anal intra-epithelial neoplasia

Anal intra-epithelial neoplasia (AIN) of the anal canal is found in the transitional epithelium above the dentate line more frequently than in the squamous mucous membrane of the lower anal canal [12–14]. This observation corresponds with the relative incidence of invasive carcinoma

above and below the dentate line (see 'Malignant epithelial tumours of the anal canal' below). Although the incidence of AIN remains unknown, it can be assumed that the incidence is increasing, especially in high-risk individuals (predominantly male homosexuals) [15]. In a meticulous examination of a consecutive series of minor surgical specimens, dysplasia was an incidental finding in 2.3% but was severe in only 1 of 306 cases [16]. Patients with dysplasia were younger than a corresponding series of patients with established anal canal carcinoma. In a systematic examination of the anal region in 139 surgical specimens for anal cancer, rectal cancer or inflammatory bowel disease, 16 squamous cell carcinomas of the anal canal were discovered. Severe dysplasia was present in 13 of these but in none of the other specimens. Dysplasia occurred patchily and away from the cancers as well as in the immediately adjacent epithelium [17]. Such observations give strong support to the concept that anal cancer frequently develops on a background of epithelial dysplasia and that the risk of cancer is greatest for high grade dysplasia.

The natural history of low grade AIN is uncertain but progression of AIN III to carcinoma has been reported by Scholefield et al. [18]. Subsequently it has been shown by the same group that three of their six immunosuppressed patients with AIN III developed invasive anal squamous cell carcinoma. However, no malignant transformation was seen in immunocompetent AIN III patients [19]. Now it seems clear that patients at high risk for malignant transformation of AIN are those who are either immunocompromised or have genital intra-epithelial field change [20].

Histological examination reveals a thickened epithelium in which undifferentiated cells with a high nucleocytoplasmic ratio extend from their usual basal position towards the mucosal surface (Figure 43.5). Maturation abnormalities with varying degrees of nuclear pleomorphism and increased mitotic activity are the most characteristic features of AIN. Similar to the grading system of cervical and vulval intraepithelial neoplasia (CIN and VIN), the AIN grading is based on the degree of dysmaturation, which in AIN I involves only the lower third of the epithelium, in AIN II the lower two-thirds and in AIN III more than two-thirds of the epithelium. The AIN III category also includes full-thickness intra-epithelial neoplastic transformation and has made the old term 'carcinoma *in situ*' obsolete.

As a result of the morphological similarities of the AIN, CIN and VIN changes (usually the non-keratinising small cell or basaloid type), it had been assumed that the same group of sexually transmitted agents was implicated in these disorders. This is supported by observations of concomitant genital and anal neoplasia [21], similar epidemiology of anal and genital neoplasia [22,23] and the association between anal cancer and homosexual activity, in particular receptive anal intercourse [24,25]. The principal contender for a role in such transmission is the group of small DNA

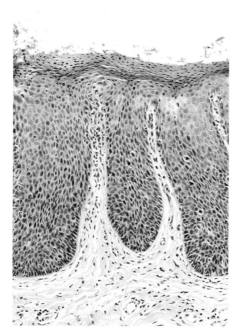

Figure 43.5 Severe dysplasia or grade III intra-epithelial neoplasia of the anal canal.

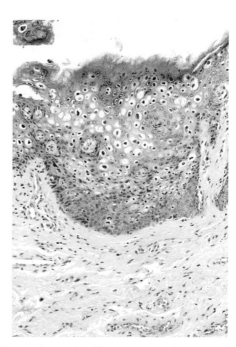

Figure 43.6 Koilocytosis within grade I anal intra-epithelial neoplasia.

viruses known collectively as human papillomavirus (HPV). Indeed, AIN may show squamous maturation, individual cell dyskeratosis and koilocytosis, histopathological features that are indicative of HPV infection (Figure 43.6). There is often concomitant hyperkeratosis and the lesion then presents as a white plaque (Figure 43.7). Infection with the high-risk HPV types 16 and 18 is strongly associated with AIN III and anal squamous cell carcinoma [26–28]. The grading of AIN is subject to considerable inter-observer variation especially when based on conventional haematoxylin and eosin (H&E) histology alone. Therefore it has been suggested that only two grades (low and high) should be used [29–31]. In the two-tiered system, AIN I and AIN II are subsumed to low grade AIN and AIN III is termed 'high grade AIN' [32]. The interobserver agreement can be further improved by using immunohistochemistry to detect the gene product of the cyclin-dependent kinase inhibitor p16 [33] and the assessment of the proliferative activity with the Ki-67 marker [34,35]. As p16 expression correlates with the HPV integration into the genome of the affected cells, the combination of p16 immunohistochemistry and HPV subtyping by *in situ* hybridisation seems to provide a useful tool to distinguish intra-epithelial neoplastic transformation from benign transitional-zone epithelium that can mimic neoplastic transformation [36].

Given the risk of high grade AIN transforming into invasive neoplasia, high-risk patients should be screened and anal cytology has been introduced as a screening method [37–39].

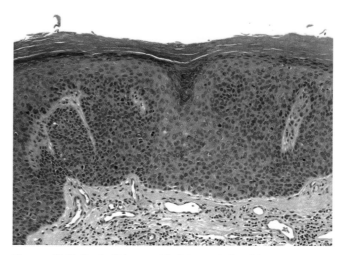

Figure 43.7 Grade III intra-epithelial neoplasia with hyperkeratosis.

In addition to known genetic alterations of tumour-suppressor genes and oncogenes in anal intra-epithelial and invasive neoplasias, epigenetic events have been observed in AIN and anal squamous cell carcinomas. Methylation of *IGSF4* and *DAPK1* has been described as specific for high grade intra-epithelial anal lesions as well as in anal squamous cell carcinomas. DNA methylation was less common in low grade AIN and normal mucosa [40].

Viral warts (condylomata acuminata)

These papilliferous, warty growths are found in the peri-anal region as well as other parts of the perineum, vulva and penis. They are often multiple, covering a wide area of perianal skin and may extend into the anal canal but do not involve rectal mucosa. They are caused by members of the HPV family, of which over 50 types have now been identified [41]. Types 6 and 11 have been implicated in the aetiology of anogenital warts, whereas types 16 and 18 (sometimes in association with 6 and 11) are associated with anogenital squamous carcinoma [42]. Genital warts are being seen with increasing frequency and anal warts are especially common in male homosexuals and females who practice anal intercourse. Anal dysplasia and carcinoma are also being described in male homosexuals, both with and without the acquired immune deficiency syndrome (AIDS) [31,43,44]. Such observations, as well as reports of malignant transformation within viral warts [45,46], strongly support the concept of an oncogenic role for particular HPV types.

Low power microscopy reveals the characteristic acuminate or saw-tooth outline that is due to marked papillomatosis involving a thickened or acanthotic epithelium (Figure 43.8). Other features include hyperplasia of the prickle cells, parakeratosis, hyperkeratosis and an underlying chronic inflammatory cell infiltrate. The most notable feature is vacuolation or koilocytosis of cells in the upper layers of the epidermis (Figure 43.9). The nuclei of these cells give a positive immunohistochemical reaction with HPV antibodies (Figure 43.10). An occasional dyskeratotic cell is seen, especially if the wart has been treated with podophyllin. This should not be equated with dysplasia.

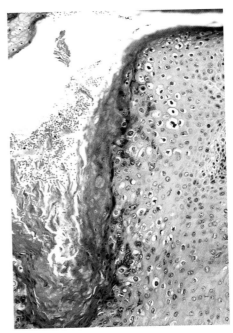

Figure 43.9 Koilocytosis in condyloma acuminatum.

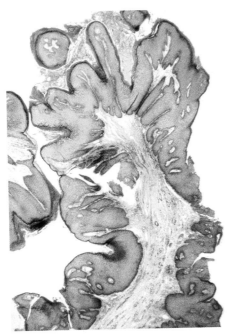

Figure 43.8 Condyloma acuminatum or viral wart.

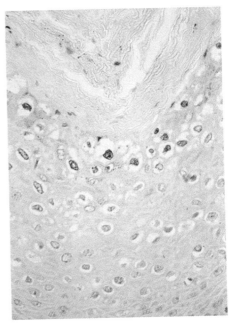

Figure 43.10 Wart virus coat antigen within nuclei of vacuolated cells (immunoperoxidase).

Verrucous carcinoma (giant condyloma of Buschke and Löwenstein)

It is now generally accepted that verrucous carcinoma and giant condyloma of Buschke and Löwenstein are identical lesions and the terms are used synonymously [47].

In the past, the term 'verrucous carcinoma' has been used in two ways: one to describe the lesion under discussion and the other to describe the well differentiated end of the spectrum of squamous cell carcinoma. The latter use has been a source of confusion and should not be continued.

Giant condyloma of Buschke and Löwenstein is a rare penile or vulval lesion that presents as a large, warty, cauliflower-like growth (Figure 43.11) and characteristically penetrates and burrows into the deeper tissues. Similar lesions occur even more rarely in the perianal and anorectal region [46,48–52]. Cases have been described showing extensive erosion of the soft tissues around the anus with invasion of the ischiorectal fossae, perirectal tissues and even the pelvic cavity [53]. These tumours may not only become ulcerated but may be complicated by the formation of fistulous tracks and sinuses. The lesion is resistant to treatment with podophyllin. In spite of its locally aggressive behaviour, verrucous carcinoma shows limited metastatic potential. Lymph node metastases have been described after transformation to a conventional squamous cell carcinoma [54]. Total excision is therefore usually curative but in advanced cases this may only be achieved by abdomino-perineal excision (and sometimes more radical surgery) [53,55].

Lesions are generally insensitive to radiotherapy but useful tumour shrinkage may be produced by means of preoperative chemoradiotherapy [56]. There is no evidence that radiotherapy can transform giant condyloma/ verrucous carcinoma into a more aggressive tumour. The microscopic features are similar to those of the typical anal wart, including the presence of vacuolated cells [46]. The major difference is the presence of endophytic or downward growth but the advancing tongues of epithelium are bulbous and pushing, with an intact basement membrane (Figure 43.12). HPV-6 and -11 are found in giant condyloma/ verrucous carcinoma, as in simple viral warts. Subtypes of HPV-6 with variations in non-coding (regulatory) DNA may account for the differing behaviour of giant condyloma [57,58]. The progression to dysplasia and squamous cell carcinoma has been documented [46]. In a review of 33 cases, 14 (42%) were considered to show malignant transformation [55]. The molecular basis for this transformation is unknown. Additional infection with HPV-16/-18 could be one mechanism.

Rapid progression of a Buschke–Löwenstein tumour into a metastasising squamous cell carcinoma has been described in a HIV-infected patient [59]. Case reports have described Buschke–Löwenstein tumours in children [60,61].

Kerato-acanthoma

This is not a premalignant lesion but is mentioned at this juncture because an incision biopsy can easily be misdiag-

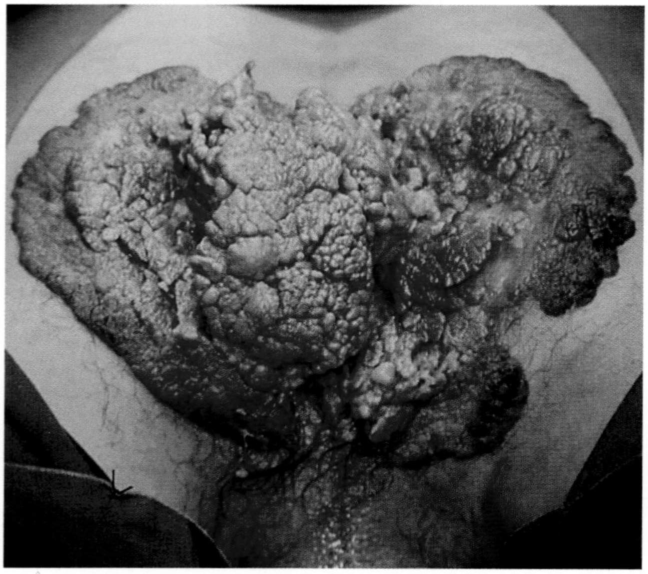

Figure 43.11 Giant condyloma of Buschke–Löwenstein. (Courtesy of Professor John MA Northover, St Mark's Hospital London.)

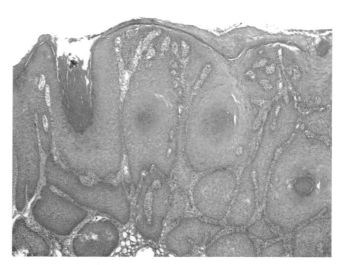

Figure 43.12 Giant condyloma of Buschke–Löwenstein: endophytic component composed of well differentiated squamous epithelium. (Courtesy of Dr Eduardo Calonje, St John's Institute of Dermatology, St Thomas's Hospital, London.)

nosed as a well differentiated squamous cell carcinoma. Its rare occurrence in the perianal region should therefore be appreciated [62,63] The pilar tumour, more usually associated with the scalp, can be mistaken for both kerato-acanthoma and squamous cell carcinoma but is an extremely rare occurrence in the perianal skin.

Bowen's disease

This is essentially a form of carcinoma *in situ* that typically affects the skin of the head and neck and the upper and lower limbs but is very rarely found in the perianal skin [64–66]. When occurring in the anogenital region, Bowen's disease is sometimes termed 'erythroplasia'. It presents as a red, encrusted plaque with irregular edges. The lesion can be multi-focal. The presence of ulceration usually indicates that invasive carcinoma has developed. Microscopically the changes are no different from those found in the common sites of Bowen's disease. Dyskeratotic and mitotically active cells with large, atypical nuclei are seen within an acanthotic epithelium, sometimes showing hyperkeratosis and parakeratosis.

For non-invasive anal neoplastic transformation the AIN categories are widely accepted and AIN III covers high grade intra-epithelial neoplasia including carcinoma *in situ*. This makes the use of the term 'Bowen's disease' obsolete. Unlike Bowen's disease of the skin, which is usually actinic or rarely arsenic induced, anal and perianal intra-epithelial neoplasia share the high-risk type of HPV-related pathogenesis [67,68]. Therefore it has been suggested that the term 'Bowen's disease' should be avoided even for perianal high grade intraepithelial neoplasia [19,69]. The recommendation follows the classification for VIN which has also abandoned all older terms for full-thickness dysplasia such as Bowen's disease and erythroplasia of Queyrat [70]. Clearly Bowen's disease is not a single clinical entity [71,72].

Bowenoid papulosis

This presents as a papular eruption in the anogenital region, usually in young to middle-aged adults. Cases of perianal bowenoid papulosis have also been described in children, suggesting that there is potential for development of the disease in young patients, particularly those with HIV infection [73,74]. The histology somewhat resembles Bowen's disease but the scattered dyskeratotic cells are set against a background of near normal epithelial maturation. A 'salt-and-pepper' effect is imparted by a random scattering of dyskeratotic and mitotically active cells (Figure 43.13). Unlike Bowen's disease, bowenoid papulosis apparently shows little propensity for malignant invasion and no association with internal malignancy [75] and it is therefore controlled by conservative means and might even regress

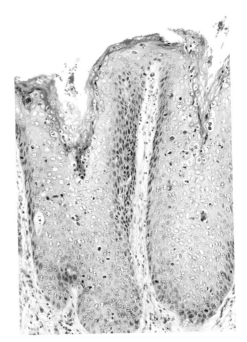

Figure 43.13 Bowenoid papulosis.

spontaneously. However, it has been shown that there is a potential risk for HIV patients to develop invasive squamous neoplasia in bowenoid papulosis [76].

Multiple HPV types have been implicated in the aetiology of this disease: 16, 18, 31, 32, 34, 35, 39, 42, 48 and 51–54 [77,78]. Recurrence has been described [79].

As with Bowen's disease it has been suggested that bowenoid papulosis might represent a subtype of AIN and the term should also be avoided [69]. However, there are clear clinical differences between these conditions suggesting that bowenoid papulosis is a distinct entity.

Sweat gland tumours

Sweat gland tumours of the anus are rare, the most common type being the hidradenoma papilliferum, a tumour derived from apocrine sweat glands [80]. This benign lesion usually occurs in middle-aged women and presents as a circumscribed, firm nodule rarely >10mm in diameter. On sectioning it is often cystic. Microscopically the tumour shows a papillary pattern in which two cell types can be discerned. A columnar cell layer with apical blebs rests upon a layer of cuboidal cells with eosinophilic cytoplasm (Figure 43.14). The latter contain periodic acid–Schiff (PAS)-positive, diastase-resistant material. Tumours arising from anogenital mammary-like glands can show mixed histological features, in which apocrine and exocrine differentiation can occur next to structures resembling mammary intracanalicular fibroadenomas (Figure 43.15) [81,82].

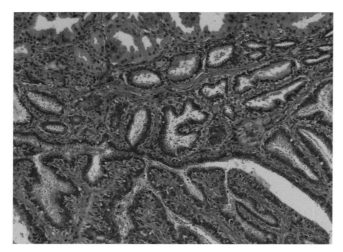

Figure 43.14 Hidradenoma papilliferum with apocrine metaplasia (top of field).

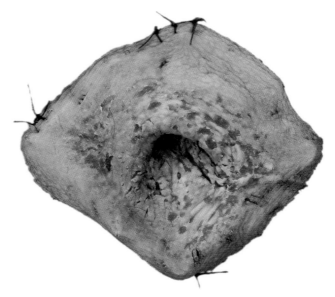

Figure 43.16 Paget's disease of perianal skin.

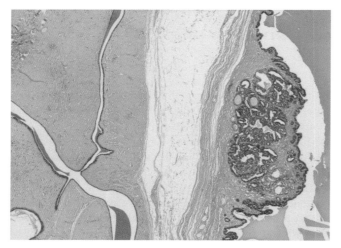

Figure 43.15 Anogenital mammary-like gland tumour with mixed histological features (apocrine and exocrine differentiation – right of field and fibroadenoma-like appearance – left of field)

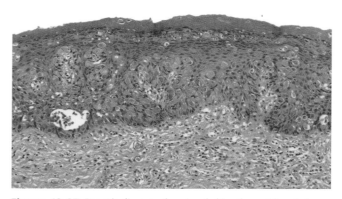

Figure 43.17 Paget's disease of perianal skin: the epidermis is infiltrated by clear Paget's cells.

Extra-mammary Paget's disease

Paget's disease of the perianal skin is a rare neoplastic condition that presents clinically as a slightly raised, red, scaly and moist area [83–86] (Figure 43.16). The condition primarily affects elderly men and women and is indistinguishable histologically from Paget's disease of the breast [87]. The diagnosis is established by biopsy, which reveals the characteristic Paget's cells in an epidermis that may show pseudo-epitheliomatous hyperplasia. The cells occur singly or in small groups and are concentrated mainly within the basal region of the epidermis. They may invade the ducts of sweat glands or the epithelium lining hair follicles. The typical Paget's cell is large with foamy, vacu-

olated cytoplasm and a vesicular nucleus that is sometimes displaced towards the periphery of the cell (Figure 43.17). The cells secrete mucus that is PAS, diastase and Alcian blue positive.

The histogenesis of perianal Paget's disease is not fully understood but ultrastructural and immunohistochemical studies have helped to clarify the debate [88,89]. As well as secreting mucus, Paget's cells express other glandular phenotypes including epithelial membrane antigen (EMA) [89], carcinoembryonic antigen [88–90] and low-molecular-weight cytokeratins [88–91]. These findings highlight the differences between Paget's cells and squamous epithelium and are consistent with the concept that Paget's cells originate within glandular skin appendages. An alternative hypothesis implicating pluripotential intraepidermal cells cannot be excluded [92] but firm evidence for such a histogenesis is lacking. Immunohistochemical studies have indicated similar antigenic profiles between perianal and mammary Paget's disease, notably the expression of human milk fat globule glycoprotein antigens [89], casein [92] and gross cystic disease fluid protein (GCDFP) [88,89, 93]. However, higher expression of c-erbB-2 and nm23 oncoproteins is seen in mammary Paget's disease [93].

In a more recent study a dual cell population has been identified in extra-mammary Paget's disease: large polygonal Paget's cells uniformly expressing CK19- and associated CK15-positive small keratinocytes. This cytokeratin immunoprofile typical for follicular differentiation suggests a proliferation of adnexal stem cells from the infundibulo-sebaceous unit of hair follicles [94].

Perianal Paget's disease (unlike mammary but similar to other forms of extra-mammary Paget's disease occurring in the vulva, axilla, eyelid, external ear and oesophagus) is not usually associated with an underlying malignancy.

It has been suggested that extra-mammary Paget's cells arise from the ducts of apocrine glands and show selective diffuse infiltration of the adjoining squamous epithelium by virtue of their extraordinary epidermotropism.

The widespread or multifocal nature of the disease means that local excision is often followed by recurrence [95]. Conceivably this might be prevented by wide local excision with frozen section control [96,97].

Some cases of perianal Paget's disease are associated with an underlying malignancy [83,98] but the latter is usually a mucin-secreting adenocarcinoma rather than a typical apocrine malignancy [99]. In this context it is important to distinguish between genuine Paget's disease and downward pagetoid spread by signet-ring cells from a primary anorectal adenocarcinoma [100]. Signet-ring cells usually secrete more mucus than Paget's cells and invade the epidermis singly and diffusely with no predilection for the basal zone. Unfortunately, many of the markers expressed by Paget's cells of putative apocrine origin are also expressed by signet-ring cell carcinomas of the large bowel [100]. A useful exception is the specific apocrine marker GCDFP, which is positive in classic Paget's disease. The expression of CK20 favours an underlying colorectal primary [100–103]. CK7 is a sensitive but non-specific antibody in Paget's cells [102]. These markers will, however, ably distinguish epithelial Paget's cells from pagetoid melanotic malignant melanoma and Bowen's disease of the perianal skin, both of which may mimic Paget's disease histologically.

Occasionally Paget's cells express prostate-specific antigen (PSA) suggesting a pagetoid tumour infiltration of a prostatic primary. However, it has been shown that PSA positivity can be seen in Paget's disease in up to 50% of cases without underlying prostate adenocarcinoma [104,105].

Malignant epithelial tumours of the anal canal

Squamous cell carcinoma of the anal canal

Anal cancer is currently a rare neoplasia but its incidence is increasing. In the USA the incidence of anal cancer in men increased from 1.06 per 100 000 in 1973–79 to 2.04 per 100 000 in the period 1994–2000. In women it has also increased from 1.39 per 100 000 to 2.06 per 100 000 over the same period. The overall increase is attributed to the increase in the incidence of squamous cell carcinoma. With an incidence of 2.71 per 100 000, black men had the highest rate [106]. In England and Wales anal cancer remains uncommon, probably being responsible for no more than 100 deaths per annum. It is impossible to be precise because cancer of the anal margin may be classified as a malignant neoplasm of the skin and many deaths from anal carcinoma are probably registered under rectal cancer. A better picture of the incidence is obtained from the study of surgical patients in whom anal cancer as a whole accounts for only 3% of all anorectal cancers [107].

A major risk factor for developing anal cancer is a compromised immune system. In a cohort study from Denmark it has been shown that HIV infection, solid organ transplantation, haematological malignancies and specific autoimmune disease are associated with an increased risk of anal cancer [108].

Further risk factors are smoking, receptive anal intercourse and the number of lifetime sexual partners [109,110].

Anal cancer is being seen with increasing frequency among male homosexuals, both with and without HIV infection [25,43,44]. Sexually transmitted HPV has been implicated in the aetiology of anal neoplasia in male homosexuals [111]. HPV-16 and -18 have been identified within squamous cell carcinoma of the anus [28,42,112–114]. These HPV types are associated with E6 and E7 proteins, which have a high binding affinity for tumour-suppressor gene products (retinoblastoma and p53) [115–117].

Immunosuppression associated with the AIDS epidemic is likely to be an important co-factor, accounting for the increasing incidence [44,118]. Large cohort studies have shown that anal squamous cell carcinomas are among the most frequent neoplasias associated with HIV infection [119,120]. In one study an incidence rate of 111.2 per 100 000 person-years in HIV-positive patients was observed, compared with an incidence rate of 7.4 per 100 000 person-years in HIV-negative individuals [121].

Unlike in other HIV-associated tumours, highly active anti-retroviral therapy (HAART) seems to have no protective effect on the development of anal cancer [122]. In fact the incidence of anal neoplasias has increased since the therapy has been introduced [123,124], probably attributed to the overall increased patient survival associated with HAART [125].

Anal cancers in immunosuppressed individuals are more likely to be multi-focal, persistent, recurrent and aggressive [126,127]. Interestingly, AIDS and anal warts appear to be independent risk factors in relation to risk of AIN [118]. Screening for precursor lesions has been advocated in HIV-infected male homosexuals in view of their considerably increased risk [23,128,129]. The possible role of chronic inflammation associated with Crohn's disease [130] and such sexually transmitted infections as syphilis and lymphogranuloma venereum should also not be forgotten. Minor inflammatory lesions probably play little part in the causation of anal cancer [131].

Squamous cell carcinoma of the anal margin is relatively common in parts of South America and the Indian subcontinent where conditions of extreme poverty are found. Under these circumstances carcinoma of the penis, vulva and cervix, as well as of anus, are more prevalent.

The importance of distinguishing between squamous carcinoma of the anal canal and that of the anal margin was emphasised many years ago [132]. These two types of cancer differ in their epidemiology, pathology and behaviour. Anal canal carcinoma is almost three times more common than cancer of the anal margin in the population of England and Wales. The age incidence is the same (average 57 years) but anal canal cancer is more common in women than men (3:2), whereas anal margin carcinoma is more frequent in men (4:1) [133].

Site

Most squamous carcinomas of the anal canal arise above, or mainly above, the dentate line and within the region of the transitional zone [133,134]. Probably only about a quarter arise from the squamous mucous membrane of the lower anal canal (Figure 43.18). Moreover, direct spread in continuity is preferentially upwards in the submucosal plane, because downward spread is limited by the way in which the dentate line is tethered to the underlying internal sphincter, thus obliterating the submucosal layer. This also explains why most anal canal cancers present clinically as tumours of the lower rectum.

Histology

Squamous carcinomas of the anal canal show a diversity of histological appearances that reflects the variability and instability of the epithelium in this area. They have been divided into two principal types, which occur with roughly equal frequency. The first has been given a variety of names: 'basaloid', 'cloacogenic', 'transitional' or the more descriptive term 'non-keratinising, small cell squamous carcinoma' [12,135–137]. This tumour is found in the upper anal canal and arises from the epithelium of the junctional or cloacogenic zone. The second is the ordinary or large cell

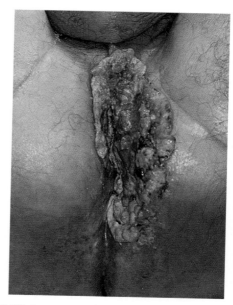

Figure 43.18 Recurrent anal squamous cell carcinoma. (Courtesy of Professor John MA Northover, St Mark's Hospital, London.)

squamous cell carcinoma. This may show some keratinisation but extensively keratinising squamous cell carcinomas are more common in the perianal skin. Muco-epidermoid carcinoma of the upper anal canal has been described but is rare [138,139]. Careful histological examination will show that most, if not all, can be distinguished from salivary gland muco-epidermoid carcinoma and would be better designated as squamous carcinoma with mucinous microcysts [140]. This pattern has also been described as ductal differentiation [133].

The distinction between basaloid and squamous cell carcinoma is subjective [133]. Mixed types commonly occur and the clinical outcome for the two types is the same [141–144]. Pure basaloid carcinomas appear to be uncommon [133]. Some find the presence of HPV not to be correlated with this histological type [112] but others associate prominent basaloid features with high-risk HPV subtypes [145]. Keratin expression matches the morphological heterogeneity, with both simple and keratinocyte keratins occurring in the same lesion [133]. In view of the preceding points, it is recommended that basaloid and squamous cell carcinoma should not be regarded as distinct entities. The generic term 'squamous cell carcinoma' should be employed and qualified by a description of the histopathological features [146]. However, it is important to appreciate the range of histological types of squamous cell carcinoma that may be encountered in the anal canal so that they can be distinguished from other malignancies arising in the anorectal region. The most important differential diagnoses are small and large cell undifferentiated carcinoma of rectal origin, malignant melanoma, basal cell carcinoma of the anal

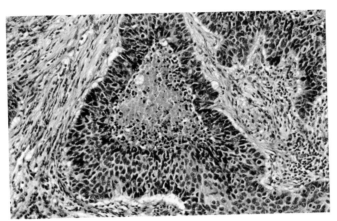

Figure 43.19 Basaloid or small cell, non-keratinising squamous cell carcinoma of the anal canal. Peripheral nuclear palisading and a central necrotic zone are typical findings.

margin, endocrine tumours and direct spread from a primary tumour of the female genital tract.

Squamous cell carcinomas showing basaloid features may resemble basal cell carcinoma of hair-bearing skin. Features common to both include the formation of islands of small cells with basophilic cytoplasm and a distinctive pattern of nuclear palisading at the periphery of the clumps of tumour cells (Figure 43.19). There may be some differentiation towards squamous cells in small concentric whorls and sharply defined plugs of keratin may be scattered throughout the tumour. One feature, unlike basal cell carcinoma, is the presence of masses of eosinophilic necrosis surrounded by a relatively narrow rim of tumour cells, giving a 'Swiss cheese' appearance under the low power of the microscope. Immunohistochemistry can be helpful to distinguish the two lesions. In the skin basal cell carcinomas strongly express Ber-EP4 whereas most squamous cell carcinomas show a positive reaction with anti-EMA [147]. Ber-EP4 is, however, not a completely reliable marker because areas with squamoid features in basal cell carcinomas fail to express this antigen [148]. The usually strong BCL-2 expression in basal cell carcinomas is again not an entirely consistent marker for the differential diagnosis because a positive reaction can occasionally also be seen in squamous cell carcinomas [149]. In occasional cases there can be a striking likeness to transitional cell carcinoma of the bladder.

As anal cancer is rare, most series have been retrospective and relatively small. Most reports have stated that poor differentiation influences prognosis adversely [12,150,151] but this effect is insignificant in the presence of variables relating to tumour stage [150,152]. However, radiotherapy and chemoradiotherapy are the preferred primary forms of treatment [66,153–155]; detailed pathological staging then, of course, becomes impossible. Under these circumstances the main role of the pathologist is to

establish the correct diagnosis and comment on the type and grade of the tumour as obtained by an incisional biopsy. This information may not only be useful for stratifying patients in therapeutic trials but also have a direct bearing on management, e.g. sphincter-saving local excision is the treatment of choice for tumours <20 mm in diameter but is inappropriate if the carcinoma is poorly differentiated [150]. A particular type of poorly differentiated squamous cell carcinoma is characterised by small cells, nuclear moulding, a high mitotic rate and diffuse infiltration [152]. Squamous cell carcinoma with mucinous microcysts is also associated with a poor prognosis [152]. Nevertheless, a superficial biopsy may not always be representative of the tumour as a whole. DNA aneuploidy as demonstrated by flow cytometry has been shown to be an independent prognostic factor [152]. Aneuploidy and proliferation are both correlated with the presence of HPV [41]. The small cell undifferentiated ('oat cell') carcinoma is rare but it is important that this entity is recognised when it occurs. Radical surgery invariably fails because, similar to the pulmonary counterpart, the disease is generalised at the time of diagnosis [150].

In biopsies it can be extremely difficult to distinguish poorly differentiated squamous cell carcinomas from a poorly differentiated adenocarcinoma with a solid growth pattern or an endocrine carcinoma. However, in view of the different clinical management a correct classification is crucial. The immunohistochemical detection of the p63 protein in squamous cell carcinomas has been shown to be a highly specific and useful tool to establish a confident diagnosis [156].

Cytogenetics and molecular pathology

Deletion of chromosomes 11q and 3p are described in anal canal squamous cell carcinoma [157]. Immunohistochemical evidence of p53 overexpression has been demonstrated in AIN as well as invasive cancer and did not correlate with HPV type [158]. Mutant p53 is more common in actinic-related squamous cell carcinoma [159] and rare in anal squamous cell carcinoma [160]. MDM2 accumulation has also been found in anal squamous cell carcinomas positively associated with phosphorylated AKT expression [160]. K-ras mutations are uncommon in anal cancer and limited to those that are non-HPV-associated [161]. The role of E6 and E7 HPV proteins is noted above.

Spread and prognosis

Squamous cell carcinoma of the anal canal shows preferential direct spread upwards into the lower third of the rectum, which explains why many squamous carcinomas (and giant condylomas) of the anal canal present clinically as tumours of the lower rectum. This is probably because the line of least resistance is upwards in the submucous layer. Anal canal carcinoma also spreads to the superior haemorrhoidal lymph nodes and to nodes on the lateral wall of the pelvis, as well as to the inguinal glands. Haemorrhoidal lymph node involvement has been found in about 43% of major operation specimens of anal cancer seen at St Mark's Hospital. Clinical and pathological evidence of inguinal gland metastases is recorded in about 36% of cases. There is clinical evidence that, in anal canal carcinoma, the inguinal nodes are involved at a later stage than the haemorrhoidal glands, the malignant cells possibly spreading backwards from within the pelvis [134,151, 162]. The presence of lymph node metastases has an important adverse effect on prognosis, as does the size of the tumour and the depth of invasion [142]. Measurements of depth of invasion should be made using the easily identified outer border of the internal anal sphincter as a point of reference.

Most surgical series report corrected 5-year survival rates of between 50 and 65% [151] and the results of radiotherapy appear to be equally good [143]. In a large National Cancer Database analysis 19 199 patients with anal squamous cell carcinoma were identified with an overall 5-year survival rate of 58%, ranging from 69.5% in stage I lesions to 18.7% in stage IV tumours. Patients had a higher risk of death if they were male, ≥65 years old, black, living in lower median income areas and had more advanced TNM stage [163]. In another recently published study the ultimately free of disease (UNED) rate was strongly associated with the T and N stage and also with the tumour mobility on palpation. Patients with a mobile tumour had a 5-year UNED rate of 89.2% ± 4.6% compared with 59.3% ± 6.1% for those with fixed tumours [164].

Treatment

For a long time abdomino-perineal resection has been the therapy of choice in anal cancer, accepting a high morbidity and a permanent colostomy with significant loss of quality of life. Despite radical surgery the high local recurrence rate and relatively poor 5-year survival rates were frustrating [165]. A new era of managing anal cancer started when a conservative approach was introduced in the mid-1970s [166]. Based on various randomised trials, the gold standard of therapy now is sphincter-saving combined modality therapy, leaving surgery only for patients with persistent disease or local recurrence [167]. The current standard non-surgical management is based on radiotherapy in combination with 5-fluorouracil and mitomycin chemotherapy. Other chemotherapy protocols combined with radiation treatment are part of various trials [168–171]. In the high-risk group of HIV-infected patients, standard chemoradiation is poorly tolerated and a higher rate of treatment failure has been documented [172,173]. HIV-positive patients might benefit from a less toxic chemotherapy regimen and relatively recently implemented intensity-modulated radiotherapy [174,175].

The fact that anal squamous cell carcinomas universally express the epidermal growth factor receptor implies the possibility of targeted treatment options [176,177]. As *K-ras* does not seem to play a major role in anal squamous cell carcinomas [161,178], anti-epidermal growth factor receptor monoclonal (EGFR), antibody-based treatments (e.g. cetuximab) could be a valuable treatment option. The first promising results came from a study in which patients with metastatic anal squamous cell carcinoma had been treated with cetuximab [179].

Although local excision might be a therapeutic option for tumours <20 mm in diameter [153], it has been suggested that small cancers could be treated by adjuvant moderate-dose radiotherapy [180]. Detailed pathological staging will obviously be impossible for patients treated by modalities other than radical surgery and there is a need for an internationally agreed system of clinico-pathological staging so that the results of therapeutic trials performed in different centres can be compared.

Malignant melanoma

Malignant melanoma of the anal canal is uncommon, 1 case presenting for every 8 squamous cell carcinomas of this region and 1 for every 250 rectal adenocarcinomas [181]. Only 1.5% of malignant melanomas develop at this site, a proportion that is likely to decrease as the number of solar-associated cutaneous melanomas goes on increasing. Of all mucosal malignant melanomas, anal tumours account for about 22% [182]. The age incidence is about the same as for cancer of the rectum and the sexes are affected equally in most studies [183–187]. Epidemiological data from the USA, however, showed a male:female ratio of 1 : 1.72, with a lower mean age of male patients and an increasing incidence in males aged <45 years. There was some evidence that HIV infection might be a risk factor [188].

Patients present with bleeding or an altered bowel habit and a protuberant or polypoid mass is seen in the lower rectum, anal canal and sometimes projecting downwards beyond the anal verge. The lesion can resemble thrombosed piles, especially if pigment is present (Figure 43.20). However, pigment is not always obvious on macroscopic observation. An association with neurofibromatosis type 1 has been reported [189].

Malignant melanoma invariably arises from the transitional zone above the dentate line. Melanocytes are normally found in this location and the tumour is therefore classified among the melanomas of mucous membranes. The diagnosis is made by biopsy but the distinction from lymphoma, undifferentiated carcinoma of the rectum and poorly differentiated squamous carcinoma of the anal canal can be difficult unless obvious pigmentation is present (Figure 43.21). The microscopic appearances are variable [190]. The conventional histomorphology of anal malig-

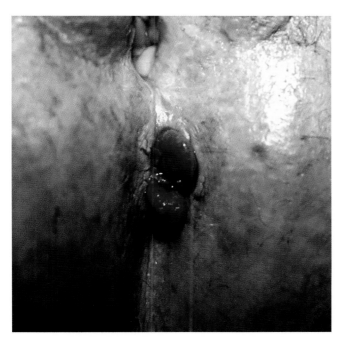

Figure 43.20 Polypoid malignant melanoma of the anal canal. (Courtesy of Professor John MA Northover, St Mark's Hospital, London.)

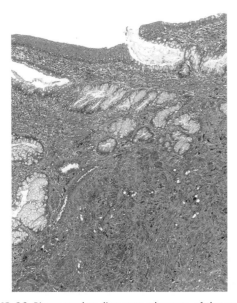

Figure 43.21 Pigmented malignant melanoma of the anal canal undermining the anorectal junction.

nant melanomas is similar to cutaneous melanomas and other mucosal melanomas and no difference has been seen in the expression of the classic melanoma markers S-100 protein, HMB45 and Melan A [191].

The tumours are often very invasive, with a marked degree of pleomorphism that usually comes with large numbers of mitotic figures. One of the most common appearances is that of polygonal cells with eosinophilic cytoplasm, each with a large slightly eccentric nucleus and prominent single nucleolus. The cells are arranged in packets or more diffuse sheets. Spindle-cell forms also occur, requiring careful distinction from spindle-cell squamous carcinoma (pseudo-sarcoma) of the anal canal [192]. Sometimes the appearance may closely mimic carcinoid tumours. Tumour giant cells, when present, are a helpful indication towards the correct diagnosis and the presence of junctional change, which may present at the lower pole of the growth, will facilitate the diagnosis of a primary anal malignant melanoma. However, areas of junctional change are often destroyed by ulceration. Pigmentation can be found in about half of all cases if searched for carefully. Silver staining methods and the identification of melanosomes at the ultrastructural level were useful special techniques but have now mostly been replaced by a variety of immunohistochemical antibodies as diagnostic tools.

Malignant melanoma of the anal canal spreads rapidly in the anorectal tissues and may even ulcerate on to the perianal skin through the ischiorectal fossae. The superior haemorrhoidal group of lymph nodes is involved early in the course of the disease with later spread to the glands on the lateral wall of the pelvis, the para-aortic nodes and the inguinal glands. Death occurs from widespread blood-borne metastases, mostly to the liver and lungs. Anal malignant melanoma has an extremely poor prognosis and the survival rate after surgical excision is measured in months rather than years. Long-term survival is very rare [193]. In a series of nine amelanotic anorectal melanomas a tumour thickness of <4 mm correlated with long-term disease-free survival [194]. Patients with anal malignant melanomas showing a lower proliferative activity (*Ki-67* <40%, *PCNA* <80%) had a survival advantage over those with tumours showing higher proliferation [195].

Although the H&E histomorphology and the immunohistochemical expression are similar in anal and cutaneous malignant melanomas, they show a different pattern of molecular alterations, which seems to define these two lesions as different entities. In cutaneous malignant melanomas and naevi, activating *BRAF* mutations targeting exon 15 are a common event [196,197]. The typical *V599E* mutation of cutaneous melanomas has, however, not been detected in anal malignant melanomas [198]. It has also been shown that anal malignant melanomas express the protein deleted in malignant brain tumours 1 (DMBT1) frequently, whereas in cutaneous malignant melanomas DMBT1 expression is rare. Given the rather distinct molecular changes it seems likely that the two lesions follow different pathways [191].

Adenocarcinoma

Columnar epithelium lines the transitional zone of the anal canal and must obviously be prone to neoplastic change.

However, as all malignancies in this site invade upwards and present as rectal tumours, there is no way of distinguishing adenocarcinoma of the anal canal from adenocarcinoma of the lower rectum. For this reason all typical adenocarcinomas of the anorectal region are grouped as cancers of the lower third of the rectum at St Mark's Hospital. However, two special forms of adenocarcinoma peculiar to this region deserve special mention: adenocarcinoma of the anal ducts or glands and mucinous adenocarcinoma associated with anorectal fistulae [199].

Adenocarcinoma of anal ducts and glands

Acceptable examples of adenocarcinoma of the anal ducts or glands are extremely rare [200,201]. These tumours are flat, mainly submucosal growths, which tend to spread widely within the tissues of the anal canal producing stenosis. Microscopically they are adenocarcinomas in which the neoplastic glandular epithelium bears a close resemblance to normal anal ducts with well differentiated small glands and scant mucin production. There are, however, also reports on mucinous adenocarcinomas arising from anal ducts or glands [202,203] (Figure 43.22). There may be associated pagetoid spread [202]. For the diagnosis to be established for certain, it is necessary to demonstrate a transition from anal canal duct epithelium to carcinoma through an *in situ* stage. Otherwise the distinction from adenocarcinoma of the rectum, squamous cell carcinoma of the anal canal with mucinous microcysts (glandular differentiation) and apocrine carcinoma of the perianal skin can be difficult if not impossible. Anal duct carcinomas should be separated from mucinous carcinomas arising in anorectal fistulae (see below). There is evidence that mucin histochemistry may be useful in distinguishing between anal duct or gland carcinoma and other adenocarcinomas of the anorectal region. Goblet cells of the rectum and anal canal transitional zone secrete *O*-acetyl-sialomucin and this type of mucus is at least partially retained in adenocarcinomas of the lower rectum. On the other hand, sialomucin in anal gland adenocarcinomas lacks *O*-acetyl groups. *O*-Acetyl groups can be demonstrated indirectly through the acquisition of PAS reactivity which accompanies their removal after saponification with potassium hydroxide. Such a test is positive for rectal and negative for anal gland adenocarcinoma [204].

Unlike rectal adenocarcinomas the immunohistochemistry of anal gland adenocarcinomas reveals a cytokeratin (CK) expression profile positive for CK7 but negative for CK20 [205].

Mucinous adenocarcinoma in anorectal fistulae

In this condition patients present with anorectal fistulae or recurrent abscesses around the anus. Mucus can sometimes be clearly seen within abscesses or fistulous tracks but there is no visible mucosal lesion within the rectum (Figure 43.23). Microscopic examination of biopsies obtained during surgical treatment shows fragments of mucinous carcinoma, which may be so well differentiated that the diagnosis of adenocarcinoma is not even considered (Figure 43.24). Awareness of the condition is important because the diagnosis may otherwise be unsuspected by both clinician and pathologist.

It has been suggested that these unusual tumours arise in duplications of the lower end of the hindgut [206]. Support for this view is provided by the fact that some of the fistulous tracks are lined by entirely normal rectal mucosa, including muscularis mucosae [206]. Furthermore, it may be possible to demonstrate that rectal mucosa lines the upper part of the track, giving way to squamous epi-

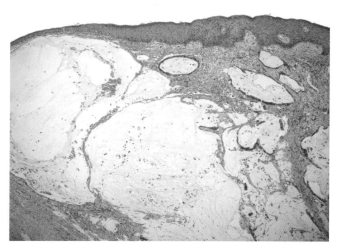

Figure 43.22 Adenocarcinoma of the anal ducts and glands with mucinous pools.

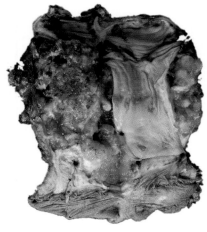

Figure 43.23 Mucinous adenocarcinoma in anorectal fistula.

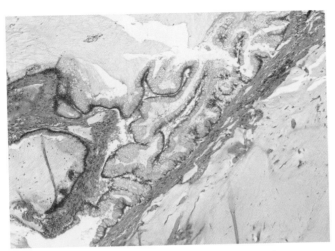

Figure 43.24 Well differentiated mucinous adenocarcinoma within anorectal fistula.

thelium at the appropriate line of the anal valves. Others suggest that these tumours arise in pre-existing anal sinuses or fistulae [207]. Examples of this condition have been observed in association with Crohn's disease [130, 208].

The tumours are well differentiated and characterised by the presence of pools of mucin which dissect and infiltrate the stromal tissues of the perianal and perirectal regions. There are two important differential diagnoses. Anal fistulae can sometimes be lined by essentially normal rectal mucosa. Innocent misplacement of this epithelium may occur, closely mimicking a well differentiated mucinous carcinoma. Misplacement of epithelium may also complicate solitary ulcer syndrome ('colitis cystica profunda'). The clinical setting should help in the differentiation of these conditions.

Recently another group of extra-luminal adenocarcinomas of the anal region has been described in patients who had a pull-through procedure for imperforate anus. Similar to adenocarcinomas arising from anorectal fistulae, the tumours of the two cases were of mucinous type. The histogenesis of these tumours remains unclear but, given the immunoprofile, which is identical to that of colorectal adenocarcinomas, it is believed that these tumours arise in a remnant of rectal mucosa [209].

Malignant epithelial tumours of the anal margin

Squamous cell carcinoma of the anal margin

Squamous cell carcinomas of the anal margin mostly arise at the junction of the squamous mucous membrane of the lower end of the anal canal with the hair-bearing perianal skin [210]. This junctional origin, the appearance of the

tumours, their histology and behaviour suggest a comparison with squamous carcinoma of the lip. At both sites one usually encounters a slowly growing, keratinising squamous cell carcinoma, which metastasises to regional lymph nodes at a late stage in its natural history.

Squamous cell carcinoma of the anal margin is about a third as frequent as anal canal carcinoma [134,211]. It is more common in men than in women (4:1) but there is no significant difference in age incidence compared with adenocarcinoma of the rectum or squamous cell carcinoma of the anal canal. There are case reports of squamous cell carcinoma arising in the anal skin tags of a patient with Crohn's disease [212] and in association with perianal hidradenitis suppurativa [213]. Verrucous carcinoma arising in a pilonidal sinus has also been described [214]. Macroscopically, the lesion presents as either an ulcer or a cauliflower-like growth. Microscopically it is usually a well differentiated, keratinising squamous cell carcinoma [162]. Poorly differentiated tumours are very rare.

Inguinal lymph node metastases are found in about 20% of cases [153]. Well-to-moderately differentiated T1 carcinomas often undergo local excision only, whereas more advanced lesions are treated with radiotherapy. Adjuvant chemotherapy is indicated for T3/4 tumours and/or cases with involved lymph nodes [215–217]. In advanced cases that have been treated by radical removal of the rectum, involvement of the haemorrhoidal group of lymph nodes is exceptional.

The 5-year survival figures for anal margin cancer show the prognosis to be more favourable than for disease of the anal canal [151]. Size, extensive local invasion (T3 or T4) and inguinal lymph node involvement are adverse prognostic features [153].

Basal cell carcinoma

Basal cell carcinoma of the perianal skin is rare and accounts for only 0.2% of tumours in the anorectal region [218]. In a series of 34 patients the median age was 68 (range 43–86) and the sexes were affected equally [218]. The macroscopic and microscopic features are no different from those seen in rodent ulcers occurring elsewhere. It is important to distinguish basal cell carcinoma from basaloid squamous cell carcinoma of the anal canal. Histological features that would support a diagnosis of basal cell carcinoma include prominent nuclear palisading, formation of a characteristic stroma, clefting between the epithelial islands and surrounding stroma, low invasiveness and little nuclear pleomorphism. The macroscopic appearances, including the difference in location, will also be important guides to the correct diagnosis. In the series referred to above, the death rate was not higher than the normal population of the same age and sex and in fact no death was due to basal cell carcinoma [218].

Miscellaneous tumours

We have seen a few examples of adenocarcinoma of the perianal apocrine glands without any evidence of extramammary Paget's disease. They were ulcerating growths and microscopic examination showed glands lined by columnar epithelium containing PAS-positive apical secretions.

Smooth muscle tumours arising from the internal sphincter are very rare. Perianal rhabdomyosarcoma has been reported [219–221] and a rhabdomyoma has been described in a neonate [222]. Benign lymphoid polyps are not infrequently found in the upper anal canal just above the dentate line, although they are more common in rectal mucosa. Malignant lymphoma of the anal canal is rare [223,224] but it is not uncommon for perianal abscess to be a presenting sign of leukaemia [225]. There has been a recent increase in anorectal B-cell lymphoma in individuals with AIDS, particularly male homosexuals [226,227]. There is a report of a cutaneous T-cell lymphoma presenting initially as a perianal lesion [228]. Langerhans' cell histiocytosis has been reported in children [229,230] and an adult [231]. Perianal Kaposi's sarcoma has been described in HIV-infected individuals [232]. In a series of 74 cases of benign granular cell 'myoblastoma' of the gastrointestinal tract, 16 were reported to occur in the perianal region [233]. Lipoma, liposarcoma, fibrosarcoma and aggressive angiomyxoma [234] are seen in the ischiorectal fossa. Secondary carcinoma can occasionally present in the anal canal as a manifestation of spread by implantation from an adenocarcinoma of the colon or rectum. The internal haemorrhoidal plexus is a rare site of metastatic spread from a primary neoplasm of the lung [235].

Presacral tumours

A wide variety of conditions can present as a presacral tumour. Most of them fall into one of four categories: congenital abnormalities, bone tumours, neurogenic tumours and a miscellaneous group of lesions including secondary carcinoma and connective tissue tumours. Among the congenital anomalies dermoid cysts, teratomas, meningocele and pelvic kidney can be included. Among bone and connective tissue tumours found at this site are chordoma, osteochondroma, giant cell tumour, Ewing's sarcoma and myeloma. Neurofibroma, schwannoma, ependymoma and primitive neuro-ectodermal tumours are also seen [236,237].

Rectrorectal cyst hamartoma

This rare condition may be discovered incidentally or present in a variety of ways, including large bowel obstruction, abscesses and recurrent fistulae due to complicating

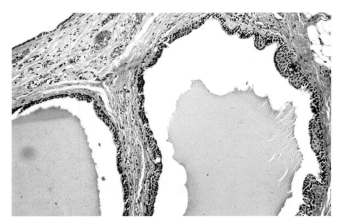

Figure 43.25 Retrorectal cyst hamartoma.

infection, or with complaints such as pain and tenesmus [238,239]. In a larger series only about 50% of the patients were symptomatic, some due to a mass effect and others with pain in the lower back, rectal region and/or during defecation [240]. It is unclear whether the condition is acquired as a result of cystic change and misplacement of anal gland epithelium after an episode of inflammation, or represents a congenital anomaly. It is possible that small examples discovered incidentally are acquired, whereas the larger presacral masses are congenital defects arising from remnants of the embryonic postanal segment or tailgut [238]. The latter hypothesis receives support from the fact that the lesion arises in the posterior midline of the anococcygeal and rectrorectal areas, which are defined by the peritoneal reflection superiorly and the levators ani and coccygeus muscles inferiorly. At the lateral aspect the area is defined by the ureters and iliac vessels. Specimens comprise multi-locular cysts lined by squamous, transitional, columnar and ciliated columnar epithelium (Figure 43.25). The cysts are filled with fluid, varying from clear thin fluid to a brown pasty substance and the variation of the epithelial lining occurs not only among the multiple cystic spaces but also within individual cysts [240]. Bundles of smooth muscle occupy the surrounding connective tissue but unlike in a duplication cyst, a double layer of muscle or neural plexus are not present [240].

Occasionally glomus bodies are found in the wall of the lesion. Immature structures and neural elements are never seen in retrorectal cystic hamartomas. The differential diagnosis includes simple anal gland cysts, teratoma, dermoid cyst, duplication cysts of the rectum and well differentiated adenocarcinoma of the anal glands. There are reports of adenocarcinoma developing in rectrorectal cyst hamartoma [241,242], emphasising the need to achieve complete surgical removal.

References

1. Groisman GM, Polak-Charcon S. Fibroepithelial polyps of the anus. A histologic, immunohistochemical, and ultrastructural study, including comparison with the normal anal subepithelial layer. *Am J Surg Pathol* 1998;**22**:70.

2. Beer TW, Carr NJ. Fibroepithelial polyps of the anus with epithelial vacuolation. *Am J Surg Pathol* 1999;**23**:488.

3. Sakai Y, Matsukuma S. CD34+ stromal cells and hyalinized vascular changes in the anal fibroepithelial polyps. *Histopathology* 2002;**41**:230.

4. Galanis I, Dragoumis D, Tsolakis M, Zarampoukas K, Zarampoukas T, Atmatzidis K. Obstructive ileus due to a giant fibroepithelial polyp of the anus. *World J Gastroenterol* 2009;**15**:3687.

5. Nakamura S, Kino I, Akagi T. Inflammatory myoglandular polyps of the colon and rectum. A clinicopathological study of 32 pedunculated polyps, distinct from other types of polyps. *Am J Surg Pathol* 1992;**16**:772.

6. Gore S, Shepherd NA, Wilkinson SP. Endoscopic crescentic fold disease of the sigmoid colon: the clinical and histopathological spectrum of a distinctive endoscopic appearance. *Int J Colorectal Dis* 1992;**7**:76.

7. Lobert PF, Appelman HD. Inflammatory cloacogenic polyp. A unique inflammatory lesion of the anal transitional zone. *Am J Surg Pathol* 1981;**5**:761.

8. Chetty R, Bhathal PS, Slavin JL. Prolapse-induced inflammatory polyps of the colorectum and anal transitional zone. *Histopathology* 1993;**23**:63.

9. Kaftan SM, Haboubi NY. Histopathological changes in haemorrhoid associated mucosa and submucosa. *Int J Colorect Dis* 1995;**10**:15.

10. Bass J, Soucy P, Walton M, Nizalik E. Inflammatory cloacogenic polyps in children. *J Pediatr Surg* 1995;**30**:585.

11. Donaldson DR, Jass JR, Mann CV. Anal leukoplakia. *Gut* 1987;**28**:A1368.

12. Klotz RG, Pamukcoglu T, Souillard H. Transitional cloacogenic carcinoma of the anal canal. *Cancer* 1967;**20**:1727.

13. Grodsky L. Current concepts on cloacogenic transitional cell anorectal cancer. *JAMA* 1969;**207**:2057.

14. Foust RL, Dean PJ, Stoler MH, Moinuddin SM. Intraepithelial neoplasia of the anal canal in hemorrhoidal tissue: a study of 19 cases. *Hum Pathol* 1991;**22**:528.

15. Palefsky JM, Holly EA, Hogeboom CJ, et al. Virologic, immunologic, and clinical parameters in the incidence and progression of anal squamous intraepithelial lesions in HIV-positive and HIV-negative homosexual men. *J Acquir Immune Defic Syndr Hum Retrovirol* 1998;**17**:314.

16. Fenger C, Nielsen VT. Dysplastic changes in the anal canal epithelium in minor surgical specimens. *Acta Pathol Microbiol Immunol Scand A* 1981;**89**:463.

17. Fenger C, Nielsen VT. Precancerous changes in the anal canal epithelium in resection specimens. *Acta Pathol Microbiol Immunol Scand A* 1986;**94**:63.

18. Scholefield JH, Ogunbiyi OA, Smith JHF, Rogers K, Sharp F. Treatment of anal intraepithelial neoplasia. *Br J Surg* 1994;**81**:1238.

19. Scholefield JH, Castle MT, Watson NF. Malignant transformation of high-grade anal intraepithelial neoplasia. *Br J Surg* 2005;**92**:1133.

20. Watson AJ, Smith BB, Whitehead MR, Sykes PH, Frizelle FA. Malignant progression of anal intra-epithelial neoplasia. *Austr NZ J Surg* 2006;**76**:715.

21. Schlaerth JB, Morrow CP, Nalick RH, Gaddis O. Anal involvement by carcinoma *in situ* of the perineum in women. *Obstet Gynecol* 1984;**64**:406.

22. Zbar AP, Fenger C, Efron J, Beer-Gabel M, Wexner SD. The pathology and molecular biology of anal intraepithelial neoplasia: comparisons with cervical and vulvar intraepithelial carcinoma. *Int J Colorectal Dis* 2002;**17**:203.

23. Melbye M, Rabkin C, Frisch M, Biggar RJ. Changing patterns of anal cancer incidence in the United States, 1940–1989. *Am J Epidemiol* 1994;**139**:772.

24. Peters RK, Mack TM, Bernstein L. Parallels in the epidemiology of selected anogenital carcinomas. *J Natl Cancer Inst* 1984;**72**:609.

25. Daling JR, Weiss NS, Klopfenstein LL, et al. Correlates of homosexual behaviour and the incidence of anal cancer. *JAMA* 1982;**247**:1988.

26. Palmer JG, Shepherd NA, Jass JR, Crawford LV, Northover JM. Human papillomavirus type 16 DNA in anal squamous cell carcinoma. *Lancet* 1987;**ii**:42.

27. Youk EG, Ku JL, Park JG. Detection and typing of human papillomavirus in anal epidermoid carcinomas: sequence variation in the E7 gene of human papillomavirus Type 16. *Dis Colon Rectum* 2001;**44**:236.

28. Hoots BE, Palefsky JM, Pimenta JM, Smith JS. Human papillomavirus type distribution in anal cancer and anal intraepithelial lesions. *Int J Cancer* 2009;**124**:2375.

29. Colquhoun P, Nogueras JJ, Dipasquale B, Petras R, Wexner SD, Woodhouse S. Interobserver and intraobserver bias exists in the interpretation of anal dysplasia. *Dis Colon Rectum* 2003;**46**:1332.

30. Lytwyn A, Salit IE, Raboud J, et al. Interobserver agreement in the interpretation of anal intraepithelial neoplasia. *Cancer* 2005;**103**:1447.

31. Carter PS, Sheffield JP, Shepherd N, et al. Interobserver variation in the reporting of the histopathological grading of anal intraepithelial neoplasia. *J Clin Pathol* 1994;**47**:1032.

32. Scholefield JH. Anal intraepithelial neoplasia. *Br J Surg* 1999;**86**:1363.

33. Bean SM, Meara RS, Vollmer RT, et al. p16 improves interobserver agreement in diagnosis of anal intraepithelial neoplasia. *J Low Genit Tract Dis* 2009;**13**:145.

34. Bean SM, Eltoum I, Horton DK, Whitlow L, Chhieng DC. Immunohistochemical expression of p16 and Ki-67 correlates with degree of anal intraepithelial neoplasia. *Am J Surg Pathol* 2007;**31**:555.

35. Walts AE, Lechago J, Bose S. P16 and Ki67 immunostaining is a useful adjunct in the assessment of biopsies for HPV-associated anal intraepithelial neoplasia. *Am J Surg Pathol* 2006;**30**:795.

36. Bernard JE, Butler MO, Sandweiss L, Weidner N. Anal intraepithelial neoplasia: correlation of grade with p16INK4a immunohistochemistry and HPV in situ hybridization. *Appl Immunohistochem Mol Morphol* 2008;**16**:215.

37. Palefsky JM, Holly EA, Hogeboom CJ, Berry JM, Jay N, Darragh TM. Anal cytology as a screening tool for anal squamous intraepithelial lesions. *J Acquir Immune Defic Syndr Hum Retrovirol* 1997;**14**:415.

38. Friedlander MA, Stier E, Lin O. Anorectal cytology as a screening tool for anal squamous lesions: cytologic, anoscopic, and histologic correlation. *Cancer* 2004;**102**:19.

39. Mathews WC, Sitapati A, Caperna JC, Barber RE, Tugend A, Go U. Measurement characteristics of anal cytology, histopathology, and high-resolution anoscopic visual impression in an anal dysplasia screening program. *J Acquir Immune Defic Syndr* 2004;**37**:1610.

40. Zhang J, Martins CR, Fansler ZB, Ret al. DNA methylation in anal intraepithelial lesions and anal squamous cell carcinoma. *Clin Cancer Res* 2005 **15**;11:6544.
41. Noffsinger AE, Hui YZ, Suzuk L, et al. The relationship of human papillomavirus to proliferation and ploidy in carcinoma of the anus. *Cancer* 1995;**75**:958.
42. Palmer JG, Scholefield JH, Coates PJ, et al. Anal cancer and human papillomaviruses. *Dis Colon Rectum* 1989;**32**:1016.
43. Croxson T, Chabon B, Rorat E, Barash M. Intraepithelial carcinoma of the anus in homosexual men. *Dis Colon Rectum* 1984; **27**:325.
44. Breese PL, Judson FN, Penley KA, Douglas JM. Anal human papillomavirus infection among homosexual and bisexual men: Prevalence of type-specific infection and association with human immunodeficiency virus. *Sex Transm Dis* 1995;**22**:7.
45. Lee SH, McGregor DH, Kuziez MN. Malignant transformation of perianal condyloma acuminatum: a case report with review of the literature. *Dis Colon Rectum* 1981;**24**:462.
46. Bogomoletz WV, Potet F, Molas G. Condylomata acuminata, giant condyloma acuminatum (Buschke–Lowenstein tumour) and verrucous squamous cell carcinoma of the perianal and anorectal region: a continuous precancerous spectrum? *Histopathology* 1985;**9**:1155.
47. Fenger C, Frisch M, Marti MC, Parc R. Tumours of the anal canal. In: Hamilton SR, Aaltonen LA (eds), *World Health Organization Classification of Tumours. Pathology and genetics of the digestive system.* Lyons: IARC Press, 2000: 147.
48. Knoblich R, Failing JF. Condyloma acuminatum (Buschke–Lowenstein tumour) of the rectum. *Am J Clin Pathol* 1967;**48**:389.
49. Judge JR. Giant condyloma acuminatum involving vulva and rectum. *Arch Pathol* 1969;**88**:46.
50. Gingrass PJ, Bubrick MP, Hitchcock CR, Strom RL. Anorectal verrucose squamous cell carcinoma; report of two cases. *Dis Colon Rectum* 1978;**21**:210.
51. Elliot MS, Werner ID, Immelman EJ, Harrison AC. Giant condyloma acuminatum (Buschke–Lowenstein tumour) of the anorectum. *Dis Colon Rectum* 1979;**22**:497.
52. Drut R, Ontiveros S, Cabral DH. Perianal verrucose carcinoma spreading to the rectum. *Dis Colon Rectum* 1975;**18**:516.
53. Grassegger A, Hopfl R, Hussl H, Wicke K, Fritsch P. Buschke–Loewenstein tumour infiltrating pelvic organs. *Br J Dermatol* 1994;**130**:221.
54. Marsh RW, Agaliotis D, Killeen RJ. Treatment of invasive squamous cell carcinoma complicating anal Buschke–Lowenstein tumor: a case history. *Cutis* 1995;**55**:358.
55. Bertram P, Treutner KH, Rubben A, Hauptmann S, Schumpelick V. Invasive squamous-cell carcinoma in giant anorectal condyloma (Buschke–Lowenstein tumor). *Langenbecks Arch Chir* 1995; **380**:115.
56. Hyacinthe M, Karl R, Coppola D, et al. Squamous-cell carcinoma of the pelvis in a giant condyloma acuminatum: Use of neoadjuvant chemoradiation and surgical resection. *Dis Colon Rectum* 1998;**41**:1450.
57. Boshart M, zur Hausen H. Human papillomaviruses in Buschke–Lowenstein tumors: physical state of the DNA and identification of a tandem duplication in the noncoding region of a human papillomavirus 6 subtype. *J Virol* 1986;**58**:963.
58. Rando RF, Sedlacek T, Hunt J, et al. Verrucous carcinoma of the vulva associated with an unusual type 6 human papillomavirus. *Obstet Gynecol* 1986;**67**:708.
59. Handisurya A, Rieger A, Bago-Horvath Z, et al. Rapid progression of an anal Buschke–Lowenstein tumour into a metastasising squamous cell carcinoma in an HIV-infected patient. *Sex Transm Infect* 2009;**85**:261.
60. Ambriz-González G, Escobedo-Zavala LC, Carrillo de la Mora F, et al. Buschke–Löwenstein tumor in childhood: a case report. *J Pediatr Surg* 2005;**40**:e25.
61. Schneider A, Lacreuse I, Moog R, Kauffmann I, Becmeur F. Buschke–Löwenstein anal tumour in children: two case reports. *Eur J Pediatr Surg* 2009;**19**:330.
62. Elliot GB, Fisher BK. Perianal keratoacanthoma. *Arch Dermatol* 1967;**95**:81.
63. Maruani A, Michenet P, Lagasse JP, et al. Keratoacanthoma of the anal margin. *Gastroenterol Clin Biol* 2004;**28**(10 Part 1):906.
64. Grodsky L. Bowen's disease of the anal region (squamous cell carcinoma-*in-situ*): report of three cases. *Am J Surg* 1954;**88**:710.
65. Scoma JA, Levy EI. Bowen's disease of the anus. *Dis Colon Rectum* 1975;**18**:137.
66. Beck DE, Karulf RE. Combination therapy for epidermoid carcinoma of the anal canal. *Dis Colon Rectum* 1994;**37**:1118.
67. Bensaude A, Parturier-Albot M. Anal localization of Bowen's disease. *Proc R Soc Med* 1971;**64**:3.
68. Ikenberg H, Gissmann L, Gross G, et al. Human papillomavirus type 16-related DNA in genital Bowen's disease and in bowenoid papulosis. *Int J Cancer* 1983;**32**:563.
69. Shepherd NA. Anal intraepithelial neoplasia and other neoplastic precursor lesions of the anal canal and perianal region. *Gastroenterol Clinics North Am* 2007;**36**:969.
70. Hart WR. Vulvar intraepithelial neoplasia: historical aspects and current status. *Int J Gynecol Pathol* 2001;**20**:16.
71. Marchesa P, Fazio VW, Oliart S, Goldblum JR, Lavery C. Perianal Bowen's disease: a clinicopathologic study of **47** patients. *Dis Colon Rectum* 1997;**40**:1286.
72. Sarmiento JM, Wolff BG, Burgart LJ, Frizelle FA, Illstrup DM. Perianal Bowen's disease: associated tumors, human papillomavirus, surgery, and other controversies. *Dis Colon Rectum* 1997;**40**:912.
73. Halacz C, Silvers D, Crum CP. Bowenoid papulosis in three-year-old girl. *J Am Acad Dermatol* 1986 **14**(2 Part 2): 326.
74. Godfrey JC, Vaughan MC, Williams JV. Successful treatment of bowenoid papulosis in a 9-year-old girl with vertically acquired human immunodeficiency virus. *Pediatrics* 2003;**112** (1 Part 1):e73.
75. Patterson JW, Kao GF, Graham JH, Helwig EB. Bowenoid papulosis. A clinicopathologic study with ultrastructural observations. *Cancer* 1986;**57**:823.
76. Rüdlinger R, Buchmann P. HPV 16-positive bowenoid papulosis and squamous-cell carcinoma of the anus in an HIV-positive man. *Dis Colon Rectum* 1989;**32**:1042.
77. Cobb MW. Human papillomavirus infection. *J Am Acad Dermatol* 1990;**22**:547.
78. Rudlinger R, Grob R, Yu YX, et al. Human papillomavirus-35-positive bowenoid papulosis of the anogenital area and concurrent human papillomavirus-35-positive verruca with bowenoid dysplasia of the periungual area. *Arch Dermatol* 1989; **125**:655.
79. Grussendorf CE. Anogenital premalignant and malignant tumors (including Buschke–Lowenstein tumors). *Clin Dermatol* 1997;**15**:377.
80. Meeker JH, Neubecker RD, Helwig EB. Hidradenoma papilliferum. *Am J Clin Pathol* 1962;**37**:182.
81. Assor D, Davis JB. Multiple apocrine fibroadenomas of the anal skin. *Am J Clin Pathol* 1977;**68**:397.
82. Kazakov DV, Spagnolo DV, Stewart CJ, et al. Fibroadenoma and phyllodes tumors of anogenital mammary-like glands: a series of 13 neoplasms in 12 cases, including mammary-type juvenile fibroadenoma, fibroadenoma with lactation changes, and neurofibromatosis-associated pseudoangiomatous stromal

hyperplasia with multinucleated giant cells. *Am J Surg Pathol* 2010;**34**:95.

83. Helwig EB, Graham JH. Anogenital (extramammary) Paget's disease. *Cancer* 1963;**16**:387.

84. Grodsky L. Extramammary Paget's disease of the perianal region. *Dis Colon Rectum* 1960;**3**:502.

85. Linder JM, Myers RT. Perianal Paget's disease. *Am Surg* 1970; **36**:342.

86. Goldman S, Ihre T, Lagerstedt U, Svensson C. Perianal Paget's disease: report of five cases. *Int J Colorect Dis* 1992;**7**:167.

87. Potter B. Extramammary Paget's disease. *Acta Dermatol Venereol* 1967;**47**:259.

88. Mazoujian G, Pinkus GS, Haagensen DE. Extramammary Paget's disease – evidence for an apocrine origin. An immunoperoxidase study of gross cystic disease fluid protein-15, carcinoembryonic antigen and keratin proteins. *Am J Surg Pathol* 1984;**8**:43.

89. Ordonez NG, Awalt H, Mackay B. Mammary and extramammary Paget's disease. An immunocytochemical and ultrastructural study. *Cancer* 1987;**59**:1173.

90. Kariniemi A-L, Forsman L, Wahlstrom T, Vesterinen E, Andersson L. Expression of differentiation antigens in mammary and extramammary Paget's disease. *Br J Dermatol* 1984;**110**:203.

91. Nagle RB, Lucas DO, McDaniel KM, Clark VA, Schmalzel GM. Paget's cells. New evidence linking mammary and extramammary Paget cells to a common cell phenotype. *Am J Clin Pathol* 1985;**83**:431.

92. Bussolati G, Pich A. Mammary and extramammary Paget's disease. An immunocytochemical study. *Am J Pathol* 1975;**80**:117.

93. Nakamura G, Shikata N, Shoji T, et al. Immunohistochemical study of mammary and extramammary Paget's disease. *Anticancer Res* 1995;**15**:467.

94. Regauer S. Extramammary Paget's disease – a proliferation of adnexal origin? *Histopathology* 2006;**48**:723.

95. Marchesa P, Fazio VW, Oliart S, et al. Long-term outcome of patients with perianal Paget's disease. *Ann Surg Oncol* 1997;**4**:475.

96. Stacy D, Burrell MO, Franklin EW. Extramammary Paget's disease of the vulva and anus: use of intraoperative frozen-section margins. *Am J Obstet Gynecol* 1986;**155**:519.

97. McCarter MD, Quan SHQ, Busam K, Paty PP, Wong D, Guillem JG. Long-term outcome of perianal Paget's disease. *Dis Colon Rectum* 2003;**46**:612.

98. Minicozzi A, Borzellino G, Momo R, Steccanella F, Pitoni F, de Manzoni G. Perianal Paget's disease: presentation of six cases and literature review. *Int J Colorectal Dis* 2010;**25**:1.

99. Sasaki M, Terada T, Nakanuma Y, et al. Anorectal mucinous adenocarcinoma associated with latent perianal Paget's disease. *Am J Gastroenterol* 1990;**85**:199.

100. Armitage NR, Jass JR, Richman PI, Thomson JPS, Phillips RKS. Paget's disease of the anus: a clinicopathological study. *Br J Surg* 1989;**76**:60.

101. Battles OE, Page DL, Johnson JE. Cytokeratins, CEA, and mucin histochemistry in the diagnosis and characterization of extramammary Paget's disease. *Am J Clin Pathol* 1997;**108**:6.

102. Goldblum JR, Hart WR. Perianal Paget's disease: a histologic and immunohistochemical study of 11 cases with and without associated rectal adenocarcinoma. *Am J Surg Pathol* 1998;**22**:170.

103. Nowak MA, Guerriere KP, Pathan A, Campbell TE, Deppisch LM. Perianal Paget's disease: distinguishing primary and secondary lesions using immunohistochemical studies including gross cystic disease fluid protein-15 and cytokeratin 20 expression. *Arch Pathol Lab Med* 1998;**122**:1077.

104. Inoguchi N, Matsumura Y, Kanazawa N, et al. Expression of prostate-specific antigen and androgen receptor in extramammary Paget's disease and carcinoma. *Clin Exp Dermatol* 2007; **32**:91.

105. Hammer A, Hager H, Steiniche T. Prostate-specific antigen-positive extramammary Paget's disease – association with prostate cancer. *APMIS* 2008;**116**:81.

106. Johnson LG, Madeleine MM, Newcomer LM, Schwartz SM, Daling JR. Anal cancer incidence and survival: The Surveillance, Epidemiology, and End Results experience, 1973–2000. *Cancer* 2004;**101**:281.

107. Morson BC. The polyp-cancer sequence in the large bowel. *Proc R Soc Med* 1974;**67**:451.

108. Sunesen K, Nørgaard M, Thorlacius-Ussing O, Laurberg S. Immunosuppressive disorders and risk of anal squamous cell carcinoma: A nationwide cohort study in Denmark, 1978–2005. *Int J Cancer* 2009;**127**:675.

109. Daling JR, Madeleine MM, Johnson LG, et al. Human papillomavirus, smoking, and anal sexual practices in the etiology of anal cancer. *Cancer* **101**:270.

110. Daling JR, Weiss NS, Hislop TG, et al. Sexual practices, sexually transmitted diseases, and the incidence of anal cancer. *N Engl J Med* 1987;**317**:973.

111. Frazer IH, Medley G, Crapper RM, Brown TC, Mackay IR. Association between anorectal dysplasia, human papillomavirus, and human immunodeficiency virus infection in homosexual men. *Lancet* 1986;**ii**:657.

112. Shroyer KR, Brookes CG, Markham NE, Shroyer AL. Detection of human papillomavirus in anorectal squamous cell carcinoma. Correlation with basaloid pattern of differentiation. *Am J Clin Pathol* 1995;**104**:299.

113. Noffsinger A, Witte D, Fenoglio-Preiser CM. The relationship of human papillomaviruses to anorectal neoplasia. *Cancer* 1992; **70**:1276.

114. Zaki SR, Judd R, Coffield LM, et al. Human papillomavirus infection and anal carcinoma. Retrospective analysis by in situ hybridization and the polymerase chain reaction. *Am J Pathol* 1992;**140**:1345.

115. Dyson H, Howley PM, Munger K, Harlow E. The human papillomavirus-16 E7 oncoprotein is able to bind to the retinoblastoma gene product. *Science* 1989;**243**:934.

116. Munger K, Werness BA, Dyson N, et al. Complex formation of human papillomavirus E7 proteins with the retinoblastoma tumor suppressor gene product. *EMBO J* 1989;**8**:4099.

117. Werness BA, Levine AJ, Howley PM. Association of human papillomaviorus type 16 and 18 E6 proteins with p53. *Science* 1990;**248**:76.

118. Carter PS, de Ruiter A, Whatrup C, et al. Human immunodeficiency virus infection and genital warts as risk factors for anal intraepithelial neoplasia in homosexual men. *Br J Surg* 1995;**82**:474.

119. Hessol NA, Pipkin S, Schwarcz S, Cress RD, Bacchetti P, Scheer S. The impact of highly active antiretroviral therapy on non-AIDS-defining cancers among adults with AIDS. *Am J Epidemiol* 2007;**165**:1143.

120. Patel P, Hanson DL, Sullivan PS, et al., Adult and Adolescent Spectrum of Disease Project and HIV Outpatient Study Investigators. Incidence of types of cancer among HIV-infected persons compared with the general population in the United States, 1992–2003. *Ann Intern Med* 2008;**148**:728.

121. Bedimo RJ, McGinnis KA, Dunlap M, Rodriguez-Barradas MC, Justice AC. Incidence of non-AIDS-defining malignancies in HIV-infected versus noninfected patients in the HAART era: impact of immunosuppression. *J Acquir Immune Defic Syndr* 2009;**52**:203.

122. Abramowitz L, Benabderrahmane D, Ravaud P, et al. Anal squamous intraepithelial lesions and condyloma in HIV-infected

heterosexual men, homosexual men and women: prevalence and associated factors. *AIDS* 2007;**21**:1457.

123. Fox P, Stebbing J, Portsmouth S, et al. Lack of response of anal intra-epithelial neoplasia to highly active antiretroviral therapy. *AIDS* 2003;**17**:279.

124. Diamond C, Taylor TH, Aboumrad T, Bringman D, Anton-Culver H. Increased incidence of squamous cell anal cancer among men with AIDS in the era of highly active antiretroviral therapy. *Sex Transm Dis* 2005;**32**:314.

125. Fagan SP, Bellows CF 3rd, Albo D, et al. Length of human immunodeficiency virus disease and not immune status is a risk factor for development of anal carcinoma. *Am J Surg* 2005; **190**:732.

126. McMillan A, Bishop PE. Clinical course of anogenital warts in men infected with human immunodeficiency virus. *Genitourin Med* 1989;**65**:225.

127. Sillman FH, Sedlis A. A anogenital papillomavirus infection and neoplasia in immunodeficient women: an update. *Dermatol Clinics* 1991;**9**:353.

128. Goldie SJ, Kuntz KM, Weinstein MC, et al. The clinical effectiveness and cost-effectiveness of screening for anal squamous intraepithelial lesions in homosexual and bisexual HIV-positive men. *JAMA* 1999;**281**:1822.

129. Palefsky JM, Holly EA, Ralston ML, et al. High incidence of anal high-grade squamous intra-epithelial lesions among HIV-positive and HIV-negative homosexual and bisexual men. *AIDS* 1998;**12**:495.

130. Connell WR, Sheffield JP, Kamm MA, et al. Lower gastrointestinal malignancy in Crohn's disease. *Gut* 1994;**35**:347.

131. Frisch M, Olsen JH, Bautz A, Melbye M. Benign anal lesions and the risk of anal cancer. *N Engl J Med* 1994;**331**:300.

132. Gabriel WB. Squamous cell carcinoma of the anus and anal canal. An analysis of 55 cases. *Proc R Soc Med* 1941;**34**:139.

133. Williams GR, Talbot IC. Anal carcinoma – a histological review. *Histopathology* 1994;**25**:507.

134. Morson BC. The pathology and results of treatment of squamous cell carcinoma of the anal canal and anal margin. *Proc R Soc Med* 1960;**53**:416.

135. Lone F, Berg JW, Stearns MW. Basaloid tumours of the anus. *Cancer* 1960;**13**:907.

136. Pang LSC, Morson BC. Basaloid carcinoma of the anal canal. *J Clin Pathol* 1967;**20**:28.

137. Jass JR, Sobin LH. Histological typing of intestinal tumours. In: *WHO International Classification of Tumours*. Berlin: Springer-Verlag, 1989.

138. Berg JW, Lone F, Stearns MW. Mucoepidermoid anal cancer. *Cancer* 1960;**13**:914.

139. Morson BC, Volkstadt H. Mucoepidermoid tumours of the anal canal. *J Clin Pathol* 1963;**16**:200.

140. Dougherty BG, Evans HL. Carcinoma of the anal canal: a study of 69 cases with special attention to histologic grading. *Am J Clin Pathol* 1984;**81**:696.

141. Clark J, Petrelli N, Herrera L, Mittelman A. Epidermoid carcinoma of the anal canal. *Cancer* 1986;**57**:400.

142. Frost DB, Richards PC, Montague ED, Giacco GG, Martin RG. Epidermoid cancer of the anorectum. *Cancer* 1984;**53**:1285.

143. Salmon RJ, Zafrani B, Labib A, Asselain B, Girodet J. Prognosis of cloacogenic and squamous cancers of the anal canal. *Dis Colon Rectum* 1986;**29**:336.

144. Greenall MJ, Quan SHQ, De Cosse JJ. Epidermoid cancer of the anus. *Br J Surg* 1985;**72**:97.

145. Frisch M, Fenger C, van-den-Brule AJ, et al. Variants of squamous cell carcinoma of the anal canal and perianal skin and their relation to human papillomaviruses. *Cancer Res* 1999;**59**:753.

146. Fenger C, Frisch M, Jass JR, Williams GT, Hilden J. Anal cancer subtype reproducibility study. *Virchows Arch* 2000;**436**:229.

147. Beer TW, Shepherd P, Theaker JM. Ber EP4 and epithelial membrane antigen aid distinction of basal cell, squamous cell and basosquamous carcinomas of the skin. *Histopathology* 2000; **37**:218.

148. Yu L, Galan A, McNiff JM. Caveats in BerEP4 staining to differentiate basal and squamous cell carcinoma. *J Cutan Pathol* 2009;**36**:1074.

149. Swanson PE, Fitzpatrick MM, Ritter JH, Glusac EJ, Wick MR. Immunohistologic differential diagnosis of basal cell carcinoma, squamous cell carcinoma, and trichoepithelioma in small cutaneous biopsy specimens. *J Cutan Pathol* 1998;**25**:153.

150. Boman BM, Moertel CG, O'Connell, et al. Carcinoma of the anal canal. A clinical and pathologic study of 188 cases. *Cancer* 1984;**54**:114.

151. Hardcastle JD, Bussey HJR. Results of surgical treatment of squamous cell carcinoma of the anal canal and anal margin seen at St. Mark's Hospital 1928. *Proc R Soc Med* 1968;**61**:27.

152. Shepherd NA, Scholefield JH, Love SB, England J, Northover JMA. Prognostic factors in anal squamous carcinoma: a multivariate analysis of clinical, pathological and flow cytometric parameters in 235 cases. *Histopathology* 1990;**16**:545.

153. Deans GT, McAleer JJA, Spence RAJ. Malignant anal tumours. *Br J Surg* 1994;**81**:500.

154. Touboul E, Schlienger M, Buffat L, et al. Epidermoid carcinoma of the anal margin: 17 cases treated with curative-intent radiation therapy. *Radiother Oncol* 1995;**34**:195.

155. Schlag PM, Hunerbein M. Anal cancer: multimodal therapy. *World J Surg* 1995;**19**:282.

156. Owens SR, Greenson JK. Immunohistochemical staining for p63 is useful in the diagnosis of anal squamous cell carcinomas. *Am J Surg Pathol* 2007;**31**:285.

157. Muleris M, Salmon R-J, Girodet J, Zafrani B, Dutrillaux B. Recurrent deletions of chromosomes 11q and 3p in anal canal carcinoma. *Int J Cancer* 1987;**39**:595.

158. Walts AE, Koeffler HP, Said JW. Localization of p53 protein and human papillomavirus in anogenital squamous lesions: Immunohistochemical and in situ hybridization studies in benign, dysplastic, and malignant epithelia. *Hum Pathol* 1993;**24**:1238.

159. Coulter LK, Wolber R, Tron VA. Site-specific comparison of p53 immunostaining in squamous cell carcinomas. *Hum Pathol* 1995;**26**:531.

160. Patel H, Polanco-Echeverry G, Segditsas S, et al. Activation of AKT and nuclear accumulation of wild type TP53 and MDM2 in anal squamous cell carcinoma. *Int J Cancer* 2007 **15**;121:2668.

161. Hiorns LR, Scholefield JH, Palmer JG, Shepherd NA, Kerr IB. Ki-ras oncogene mutations in non-HPV-associated anal carcinoma. *J Pathol* 1990;**161**:99.

162. Morson BC, Pang LSC. Pathology of anal cancer. *Proc R Soc Med* 1968;**61**:623.

163. Bilimoria KY, Bentrem DJ, Rock CE, Stewart AK, Ko CY, Halverson A. Outcomes and prognostic factors for squamous-cell carcinoma of the anal canal: analysis of patients from the National Cancer Data Base. *Dis Colon Rectum* 2009;**52**:624.

164. Myerson RJ, Outlaw ED, Chang A, et al. Radiotherapy for epidermoid carcinoma of the anus: thirty years' experience. *Int J Radiat Oncol Biol Phys* 2009;**75**:428.

165. Boman BM, Moertel CG, O'Connell MJ, et al. Carcinoma of the anal canal. A clinical and pathologic study of 188 cases. *Cancer* 1984;**54**:114.

166. Nigro ND, Vaitkevicius VK, Considine B Jr. Combined therapy for cancer of the anal canal: a preliminary report. *Dis Colon Rectum* 1974;**17**:354.

167. Akbari RP, Paty PB, Guillem JG, et al. Oncologic outcomes of salvage surgery for epidermoid carcinoma of the anus initially managed with combined modality therapy. *Dis Colon Rectum* 2004;**47**:1136.

168. UKCCCR Anal Cancer Trial Working Party. Epidermoid anal cancer: results from the UKCCCR randomised trial of radiotherapy alone versus radiotherapy, 5-fluorouracil, and mitomycin. *Lancet* 1996;**348**:1049.

169. Czito BG, Willett CG. Current management of anal canal cancer. *Curr Oncol Rep* 2009;**11**:186.

170. Chan E, Kachnic LA, Thomas CR Jr. Anal cancer: progress on combined-modality and organ preservation. *Curr Probl Cancer* 2009;**33**:302.

171. Ajani JA, Winter KA, Gunderson LL, et al. Fluorouracil, mitomycin, and radiotherapy vs fluorouracil, cisplatin, and radiotherapy for carcinoma of the anal canal: a randomized controlled trial. *JAMA* 2008;**299**:1914.

172. Kim JH, Sarani B, Orkin BA, et al. HIV-positive patients with anal carcinoma have poorer treatment tolerance and outcome than HIV-negative patients. *Dis Colon Rectum* 2001;**44**:1496.

173. Holland JM, Swift PS. Tolerance of patients with human immunodeficiency virus and anal carcinoma to treatment with combined chemotherapy and radiation therapy. *Radiology* 1994;**193**:251.

174. Wexler A, Berson AM, Goldstone SE, et al. Invasive anal squamous-cell carcinoma in the HIV-positive patient: outcome in the era of highly active antiretroviral therapy. *Dis Colon Rectum* 2008;**51**:73.

175. Salama JK, Mell LK, Schomas DA, et al. Concurrent chemotherapy and intensity-modulated radiation therapy for anal canal cancer patients: a multicenter experience. *J Clin Oncol* 2007;**25**:4581.

176. Lê LH, Chetty R, Moore MJ. Epidermal growth factor receptor expression in anal canal carcinoma. *Am J Clin Pathol* 2005;**124**:20.

177. Walker F, Abramowitz L, Benabderrahmane D, et al. Growth factor receptor expression in anal squamous lesions: modifications associated with oncogenic human papillomavirus and human immunodeficiency virus. *Hum Pathol* 2009;**40**:1517.

178. Zampino MG, Magni E, Sonzogni A, Renne G. K-ras status in squamous cell anal carcinoma (SCC): it's time for target-oriented treatment? *Cancer Chemother Pharmacol* 2009;**65**:197.

179. Lukan N, Ströbel P, Willer A, et al. Cetuximab-based treatment of metastatic anal cancer: correlation of response with KRAS mutational status. *Oncology* 2009;**77**:293.

180. Ortholan C, Ramaioli A, Peiffert D, et al. Anal canal carcinoma: early-stage tumors ≤10 mm (T1 or Tis): therapeutic options and original pattern of local failure after radiotherapy. *Int J Radiat Oncol Biol Phys* 2005 1;**62**:479.

181. Morson BC, Volkstadt H. Malignant melanoma of the anal canal. *J Clin Pathol* 1963;**16**:126.

182. Sutherland CM, Chmiel JS, Henson DE, Winchester DP. Patient characteristics, methods of diagnosis, and treatment of mucous membrane melanoma in the United States of America. *J Am Coll Surg* 1994;**179**:561.

183. Bolivar JC, Harris JW, Branch W, Sherman RT. Melanoma of the anorectal region. *Surg Gynecol Obstet* 1982;**154**:337.

184. Quan SHQ, White JE, Deddish MR. Malignant melanoma of the anorectum. *Dis Colon Rectum* 1959;**2**:275.

185. Brady MS, Kavolius JP, Quan SH. Anorectal melanoma. A 64-year experience at Memorial Sloan-Ketteirng Cancer Center. *Dis Colon Rectum* 1995;**38**:146.

186. Konstadoulakis MM, Ricaniadis N, Walsh D, Karakousis CP. Malignant melanoma of the anorectal region. *J Surg Oncol* 1995;**58**:118.

187. Goldman S, Glimelius B, Pahlman L. Anorectal malignant melanoma in Sweden. Report of 49 patients. *Dis Colon Rectum* 1990;**33**:874.

188. Cagir B, Whiteford MH, Topham A, Rakinic J, Fry RD. Changing epidemiology of anorectal melanoma. *Dis Colon Rectum* 1999;**42**:1203.

189. Ben-Izhak O, Groisman GM. Anal malignant melanoma and soft-tissue malignant fibrous histiocytoma in neurofibromatosis type 1. *Arch Pathol Lab Med* 1995;**119**:285.

190. Mason JK, Helwig EB. Anorectal melanoma. *Cancer* 1966;**19**:39.

191. Helmke BM, Renner M, Poustka A, Schirmacher P, Mollenhauer J, Kern MA. DMBT1 expression distinguishes anorectal from cutaneous melanoma. *Histopathology* 2009;**54**:233.

192. Kalogeropoulous NK, Antonakopoulos GN, Agapitos MB, Papacharalampous NX. Spindle cell carcinoma (pseudosarcoma) of the anus: a light electron microscopic and immunocytochemical study of a case. *Histopathology* 1985;**9**:987.

193. Berkley JL. Melanoma of the anal canal: report of a case of five-year survival after abdominoperineal resection. *Dis Colon Rectum* 1960;**3**:159.

194. Hillenbrand A, Barth TF, Henne-Bruns D, Formentini A. Anorectal amelanotic melanoma. *Colorectal Dis* 2008;**10**:612.

195. Ben-Izhak O, Bar-Chana M, Sussman L, et al. Ki67 antigen and PCNA proliferation markers predict survival in anorectal malignant melanoma. *Histopathology* 2002;**41**:519.

196. Davies H, Bignell GR, Cox C, et al. Mutations of the *BRAF* gene in human cancer. *Nature* 2002;**417**:949.

197. Gorden A, Osman I, Gai W, et al. Analysis of *BRAF* and *N-RAS* mutations in metastatic melanoma tissues. *Cancer Res* 2003;**63**:3955.

198. Helmke BM, Mollenhauer J, Herold-Mende C, et al. *BRAF* mutations distinguish anorectal from cutaneous melanoma at the molecular level. *Gastroenterology* 2004;**127**:1815.

199. Tarazi R, Nelson RL. Anal adenocarcinoma: a comprehensive review. *Semin Surg Oncol* 1994;**10**:235.

200. Basik M, Rodriguez-Bigas MA, Penetrante R, Petrelli NJ. Prognosis and recurrence patterns of anal adenocarcinoma. *Am J Surg* 1995;**169**:233.

201. Wellman KF. Adenocarcinoma of anal duct origin. *Can J Surg* 1962;**5**:311.

202. Wong AY, Rahilly MA, Adams W, Lee CS. Mucinous anal gland carcinoma with perianal Pagetoid spread. *Pathology* 1998;**30**:1.

203. Fenoglio-Preiser CM, Noffsinger AE, Stemmermann GN, Lantz PE, Isaacson PG. Neoplastic lesions of the anus. In: *Gastrointestinal Pathology: An atlas and text*, 3rd edn. Philadelphia, PA: Wolters Kluwer Lippincott Williams & Wilkins, 2008: 1079.

204. Fenger C, Filipe MI. Mucin histochemistry of the anal canal epithelium. Studies of normal and mucosa and mucosa adjacent to carcinoma. *Histochem J* 1981;**13**:921.

205. Hobbs CM, Lowry MA, Owen D, Sobin LH. Anal gland carcinoma. *Cancer* 2001;**92**:2045.

206. Jones EA, Morson BC. Mucinous adenocarcinoma in anorectal fistulae. *Histopathology* 1984;**8**:279.

207. Anthony T, Simmang C, Lee EL, Turnage RH. Perianal mucinous adenocarcinoma. *J Surg Oncol* 1997;**64**:218.

208. Ky A, Sohn N, Weinstein MA, Korelitz BI. Carcinoma arising in anorectal fistulas of Crohn's disease. *Dis Colon Rectum* 1998;**41**:992.

209. Symons NR, Guenther T, Gupta A, Northover JM. Paraneorectal mucinous adenocarcinoma following childhood pull-through procedure for imperforate anus. *Colorectal Dis* 2010;**12**:262.

210. Greenall MJ, Quan SHQ, Stearns MW, Urmacher C, DeCosse JJ. Epidermoid cancer of the anal margin. Pathologic features, treatment and clinical results. *Am J Surg* 1985;**149**:95.

211. Kuehn PG, Beckett R, Eisenberg H, Reed JF. Epidermoid carcinoma of the perianal skin and anal canal. A review of 157 cases. *N Engl J Med* 1964;**270**:614.

212. Somerville KW, Langman MJS, Da Cruz DJ, Balfour TW, Sully L. Malignant transformation of anal skin tags in Crohn's disease. *Gut* 1984;**25**:1124.

213. Shukla VK, Hughes LE. A case of squamous cell carcinoma complicating hidradenitis suppurativa. *Eur J Surg Oncol* 1995;**21**:106.

214. Anscombe AM, Isaacson P. An unusual variant of squamous cell carcinoma (inverted verrucous carcinoma) arising in a pilonidal sinus. *Histopathology* 1983;**7**:123.

215. Newlin HE, Zlotecki RA, Morris CG, Hochwald SN, Riggs CE, Mendenhall WM. Squamous cell carcinoma of the anal margin. *J Surg Oncol* 2004;**86**:55.

216. Sahai A, Kodner IJ. Premalignant neoplasms and squamous cell carcinoma of the anal margin. *Clin Colon Rectal Surg* 2006;**19**:88.

217. Chapet O, Gerard JP, Mornex F, et al. Prognostic factors of squamous cell carcinoma of the anal margin treated by radiotherapy: the Lyon experience. *Int J Colorectal Dis* 2007;**22**:191.

218. Nielsen OV, Jensen SL. Basal cell carcinoma of the anus – a clinical study of 34 cases. *Br J Surg* 1981;**68**:856.

219. Fagundes LA. Embryonal rhabdomysarcoma (sarcoma botryoides) of the anus. *Gastroenterology* 1963;**44**:351.

220. Raney Jr RB, Crist W, Hays D, et al. Soft tissue sarcoma of the perineal region in childhood. A report from the Intergroup Rhabdomyosarcoma Studies I and II, 1972 through 1984. *Cancer* 1990;**65**:2787.

221. Kessler KJ, Kerlakian GM, Welling RE. Perineal and perirectal sarcomas: report of two cases. *Dis Colon Rectum* 1996;**39**:468.

222. Lapner PC, Chou S, Jimenez C. Perianal fetal rhabdomyoma: case report. *Pediatr Surg Int* 1997;**12**:544.

223. Steele RJC, Eremin O, Krajewski AS, Ritchie GL. Primary lymphoma of the anal canal presenting as perianal suppuration. *BMJ* 1985;**291**:311.

224. Porter AJ, Meagher AP, Sweeney JL. Anal lymphoma presenting as a perianal abscess. *Austr NZ J Surg* 1994;**64**:279.

225. Kott I, Urca I. Perianal abscess as a presenting sign of leukaemia. *Dis Colon Rectum* 1969;**11**:213.

226. Heise W, Arasteh K, Mostertz P, et al. Malignant gastrointestinal lymphomas in patients with AIDS. *Digestion* 1997;**58**:218.

227. Ioachim HL, Antonescu C, Giancott F, Dorsett B, Weinstein MA. EBV-associated anorectal lymphomas in patients with acquired immune deficiency syndrome. *Am J Surg Pathol* 1997;**21**:997.

228. Hill VA, Hall-Smith P, Smith NP. Cutaneous T-cell lymphoma presenting with atypical perianal lesions. *Dermatology* 1995;**190**:313.

229. Grapin C, Audry G, Josset P, et al. Histiocytosis X revealed by complex anal fistula. *Eur J Pediatr Surg* 1994;**4**:184.

230. Kader HA, Ruchelli E, Maller ES. Langerhans' cell histiocytosis with stool retention caused by a perianal mass. *J Pediatr Gastroenterol Nutr* 1998;**26**:226.

231. Conias S, Strutton G, Stephenson G. Adult cutaneous Langerhans cell histiocytosis. *Australas J Dermatol* 1998;**39**:106.

232. Barrett WL, Callahan TD, Orkin BA. Perianal manifestations of human immunodeficiency virus infection: experience with 260 patients. *Dis Colon Rectum* 1998;**41**:606.

233. Johnston J, Helwig EB. Granular cell tumors of the gastrointestinal tract and perianal region. *Dig Dis Sci* 1981;**26**:807.

234. Fetsch JF, Laskin WB, Lefkowitz M, Kindblom LG, Meis KJ. Aggressive angiomyxoma: a clinicopathologic study of 29 female patients. *Cancer* 1996;**78**:79.

235. Ger R, Reuben J. Squamous cell carcinoma of the anal canal: a metastatic lesion. *Dis Colon Rectum* 1968;**11**:213.

236. Genna M, Leopardi F, Fambri P, Postorino A. Neurogenic tumors of the ano-rectal region. *Ann Ital Chir* 1997;**68**:351.

237. Webber EM, Fraser RB, Resch L, Giacomantonio M. Perianal ependymoma presenting in the neonatal period. *Pediatr Pathol Lab Med* 1997;**17**:283.

238. Edwards M. Multilocular retrorectal cystic disease – cyst–hamartoma. *Dis Colon Rectum* 1961;**4**:103.

239. Mills SE, Walker AN, Stallings RG, Allen S. Retrorectal cyst hamartoma. *Arch Pathol Lab Med* 1984;**108**:737.

240. Hjermstad BM, Helwig EB. Tailgut cysts. Report of 53 cases. *Am J Clin Pathol* 1988;**89**:139.

241. Marco V, Autonell J, Farre J, Fernandez-Layos M, Doncel F. Retrorectal cyst hamartomas. Report of two cases with adenocarcinoma developing in one. *Am J Surg Pathol* 1982;**6**:707.

242. Hjermstad BM, Tailgut cyst and carcinoma. *Military Med* 1985;**150**:218.

Miscellaneous conditions of the anal region

Manuel Salto-Tellez

Centre for Cancer Research and Cell Biology, Queen's University Belfast, Belfast, UK

Haemorrhoids

The term 'haemorrhoids' derives from the Greek *haima* (blood) and *rhois* (flowing). Humans have suffered with haemorrhoids since at least Ancient Greek times, with Hippocrates making reference to 'veins in the rectum' in 400 BC. They are now one of the most common anal pathologies, with approximately one million new cases presenting each year in the USA alone. In some histopathology practices they represent one of the most common routine surgical specimens. Opinion remains divided concerning the utility of their routine histological examination but there may be a number of pathologies arising either within or associated with them [1,2].

Haemorrhoids are caused by the prolapse of the vascular anal submucosal cushions at the anorectal junction. These cushions are normal erectile tissue structures composed of arterioles, venules and arteriovenous communications, which are predominantly situated in the left lateral, right anterior and right posterior parts of the anal canal and exercise a primary protective function. Providing a link between the portal and systemic venous structures, haemorrhoid-related veins are devoid of valves.

Although these protective cushions are present from birth, their pathological engorgement usually occurs during adult life, most commonly in the third decade. The factors leading to prolapse of the anal cushions and the development of haemorrhoids are not well understood. Two 'mechanical' causes have been suggested: loosening of the mucosal attachment to the outer bowel wall resulting in prolapse and tightening of the anal canal, leading to

compression of the anal cushion with subsequent vascular engorgement [3]. A key structure in the pathophysiology of haemorrhoids is the perianal connective tissue, which is linked to the internal sphincter and associated longitudinal muscles [4]. This tissue becomes fibrotic with age [5], resulting in a tight anus and subsequent prolapse [6,7]. There may also be associated changes in the anal canal and related anatomical structures, including a change of the muscle fibre subtype in the internal sphincter and neuronal hyperplasia [8,9]. The notion that haemorrhoids are always varicosities of the inferior rectal veins due to venous hypertension is not entirely accurate because there is no evidence that they occur more frequently in patients with portal hypertension [10,11].

A history of straining at defecation due to constipation is common, which may by itself directly move the cushions out of the anal canal, or cause venous engorgement of the cushions and thus indirectly make their displacement during defecation more likely [12]. The association of haemorrhoids with a low dietary fibre intake [13] may be related to the straining required to expel hard faeces. It has been hypothesised that chronic straining might disrupt connective tissues surrounding the anal canal but, although the association of straining and haemorrhoids [14] is intuitively appealing, epidemiological studies have failed to show that one leads to the other [15,16]. Pregnancy has also been associated with haemorrhoids, with the suggestion that they occur on a background of raised intra-abdominal pressure and pelvic venous engorgement; but despite this haemorrhoids remain more common in men that in women [17]). Spasm of the anal sphincters [18] and hereditary predisposition have also been suggested as potential aetiological factors.

Complications of haemorrhoids include thrombosis, bleeding, infection and strangulation. Bleeding from haemorrhoids is usually of arteriolar origin and, although the blood loss is rarely of significance, it may give rise to chronic anaemia. Conditions associated with portal hypertension also tend to be associated with a coagulopathy, which may explain the excessive haemorrhoidal bleeding in some of these patients [19]. In a similar fashion anticoagulant therapy can lead to profuse haemorrhoidal bleeding [20].

Microscopically, haemorrhoids are composed of a collection of dilated vascular spaces (Figure 44.1), generally with more smooth muscle in their walls than that found in ordinary veins. Varying degrees of haemorrhage and thrombosis are usually noted. Recanalisation of thrombus is common and occasionally causes prominent endothelial hyperplasia – an appearance that can closely resemble a cavernous haemangioma – and has rarely been confused with angiosarcoma. Immunohistochemistry and molecular pathology studies show evidence of neovascularisation, suggesting that haemorrhoids may represent a biologically more complex process than mere venous engorgement [21]. As in any prolapsing and/or protruding structure in the gastrointestinal tract, mucosal prolapsed-type changes in over-lying colonic type mucosa are not infrequent. These changes include mucosal thickening, crypt elongation and tortuosity, fibromuscularisation of the lamina propria and surface erosion, which, on occasions, can lead to an inflam-

matory cap polyp-type appearance. Entrapment of glands in a hypertrophied muscularis mucosae may also be seen, a feature that could potentially be misinterpreted as invasive adenocarcinoma. These changes are associated with a variable degree of inflammation, which is usually related to ulceration rather than thrombosis. Squamous metaplasia of the overlying transitional zone may also occur, a feature of no clinical significance [22]. There may also be widespread fibrosis involving the submucosa and muscularis propria, which is also one of the main histological features seen in association with anal incontinence (see below). In general, the stromal changes appear rather bland but rarely fibroblastic cells may become enlarged and somewhat atypical; however, they are usually evenly distributed throughout the lesion and are considered reactive in nature [23]. Mast cells may be very prominent around haemorrhoidal vessels [24].

As already noted the utility of the routine histological examination of haemorrhoids has been disputed, with some studies suggesting that it is unnecessary [1,2] but others supporting such routine examination [25,26]. However, it should be noted that haemorrhoids may be associated with a number of pathologies and that suboptimal or lack of histological examination may result in delayed diagnosis or misdiagnosis, with clear prognostic and therapeutic implications [27,28]. These associations include, among others, rectal cancer [29] (sometimes haemorrhoids may be the first manifestation), condylomata and human papillomavirus (HPV)-related anal intra-epithelial neoplasia [30], cytomegalovirus infection [31], anal duct carcinomas, carcinoid

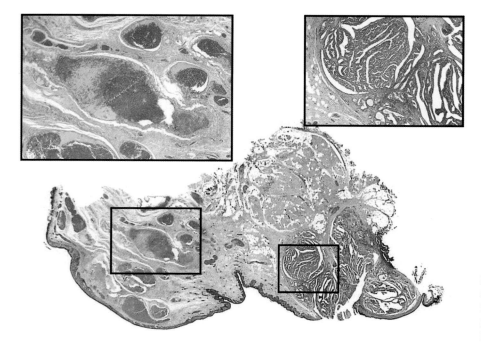

Figure 44.1 Low power appearance of a resection specimen showing a haemorrhoid (left) and a hidradenoma papilliferum (right). Insets show the two lesions at higher power.

tumors, lymphomas, melanomas [32], gastrointestinal stromal tumors [33], Kaposi's sarcoma [34], tuberculosis, anal adenofibroma [35], renal cell carcinoma [36] and hidradenoma papilliferum (see Figure 44.1). Reported associations of haemorrhoids with trauma or leaking aortic aneurysm may be coincidental [37]. On the other hand, skin tags and/or fibrous polyps in the anal region may be the end-result of thrombosis and organisation of an internal haemorrhoid [38]. The differential diagnosis with other vascular lesions is also of importance [39].

Macroscopically similar to haemorrhoids, perianal hematomas can present as a tender lump beneath the skin of the anal verge, which can lead to rupture, bleeding and thrombosis. However, these conditions are aetiologically unrelated.

Oleogranuloma

Oleogranulomas and other related lesions such as oleomas or paraffinomas, are pseudo-tumors most frequently associated with sclerosing substances used to obliterate haemorrhoids. Oleogranuloma represents a foreign body reaction to non-absorbable oily agents in the tissues. These lesions are always benign but may grossly simulate an anorectal neoplasm.

Such lesions are typically iatrogenic in nature and include a foreign body reaction to the oil used as a vehicle in the injection treatment of haemorrhoids [40,41], paraffin-containing ointments applied topically [42] and oil dressings applied after surgery [40]. Interestingly, occasionally oleogranulomas appear for no obvious reason [43].

Oleogranulomas usually present as a circumscribed, submucosal mass in the lower rectum or in the anal canal above the dentate line. On occasions, their clinical presentation can be rather atypical, including the extension of the reaction into deeper layers of the anal canal (Figure 44.2), or the clinical appearance as an annular and ulcerating lesion [44,45], which may evoke an important differential diagnosis including malignancy. Indeed, in such cases, awareness of this condition and a diagnostic biopsy may prevent unnecessary radical surgery [46].

The histological degree of the tissue reaction may depend on the type of oil used. Vegetable oils produce the least severe reaction, followed by animal fats, with mineral oils causing the most extensive changes. The early stages of oleogranuloma formation show an acute inflammatory response. As the lesion evolves, a variable degree of inflammation and fibrosis develop, at which point, the most characteristic appearance of this condition can be identified: circular, well-demarcated spaces lined by large mononuclear cells and multinucleated histiocytes (Figure 44.2). The spaces are filled with the oily agents described before, which usually do not survive conventional pathological tissue processing.

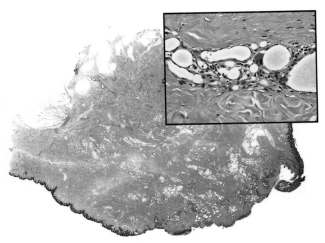

Figure 44.2 Low power appearance showing a deeply extending oleogranuloma. Inset shows the characteristic multinucleated appearance around the oil-related spaces.

Although histological diagnosis is usually straightforward in some cases, particularly those with a paucity of multinucleated giant cells, there is a differential diagnosis including lymphangioma [47], cystic pneumatosis and sclerosing liposarcoma [48].

Ectopic tissue

Ectopic tissue occurs at many anatomical sites and may lead to diagnostic confusion. The anus is no exception, with both ectopic prostatic tissue [49] and endometriosis [50] being described at this site.

Anal incontinence

Anal continence is maintained by the internal and external anal sphincters and the musculature of the pelvic floor [51]. Puborectalis forms a muscular sling around the rectum, creating a functional valve which on muscular relaxation opens, allowing defecation [52]. Although considered functionally important, the role of the external anal sphincter is less well defined [53,54]. In addition, other factors such as rectal and anal sensation [55], the consistency of the stool and the overall capacity of the rectum [56] are of importance.

In a small proportion of cases anal incontinence may be secondary to a pathology of the distal colon or rectum; examples include anorectal neoplasia, inflammatory bowel disease, faecal impaction (primarily in elderly people), pelvic trauma (including surgical [57] and obstetric trauma) and neurological lesions [58]. However, in most cases faecal incontinence is idiopathic. Many of the patients in this idiopathic group have coexisting rectal prolapse or 'perineal descent', whereas others are probably due to damage of the peripheral nerve supply [59,60].

Histological examination of the muscles included in the resection specimen of patients with anal incontinence exhibit atrophy with fatty or fibrous replacement in differing degrees. The remaining, intact muscle fibres show fibre type grouping, indicative of denervation, as well as other muscle changes secondary to denervation. Endoneurial fibrosis of the intermuscular nerves [59,60] is frequently seen, suggesting that pelvic floor nerve damage may be a leading cause of incontinence. Most of these changes related to primary incontinence are difficult to see in a biopsy specimen and only become evident to the pathologist in retrospect, in resection specimens or in postmortem material.

References

1. Lemarchand N, Tanne F, Aubert M, et al. Is routine pathologic evaluation of haemorrhoidectomy specimens necessary? *Gastroenterol Clin Biol* 2004;**28**:659.
2. Cataldo PA, MacKeigan JM. The necessity of routine pathologic evaluation of hemorrhoidectomy specimens. *Surg Gynaecol Obstet* 1992;**174**:302.
3. Alexander-Williams J. The nature of piles. *BMJ* 1982;**285**:1064.
4. Haas PA, Fox TA, Haas GP. The pathogenesis of haemorrhoids. *Dis Colon Rectum* **1984 27**:442.
5. Haqqani MT, Hancock BD. Internal sphincter and haemorrhoids: a pathological study. *J Clin Pathol* 1978;**31**:268.
6. Gass OC, Adams J. Haemorrhoids: aetiology and pathology. *Am J Surg* 1950;**79**:40.
7. Hass PA. Fox TA. Age-related changes and scar formation of perianal connective tissue. *Dis Colon Rectum* 1980;**23**:160.
8. Teramoto T, Parks AG, Swash M. Hypertrophy of the external and sphincter in haemorrhoids: a histometric study. *Gut* 1981;**22**:45.
9. Fenger C, Schrøder HD. Neuronal hyperplasia in the anal canal. *Histopathology* 1990;**16**:481.
10. Bernstein WC. What are haemorrhoids and what is their relationship to the portal venous system? *Dis Colon Rectum* 1983;**26**:829.
11. Weinshel E, Chen W, Falkenstein DB, Kessler R, Raicht RF. Hemorrhoids or rectal varices: defining the cause of massive rectal hemorrhage in patients with portal hypertension. *Gastroenterology* 1986;**90**:744.
12. Thomson WHF. The nature of haemorrhoids. *Br J Surg* 1975;**62**:542.
13. Burkitt DP. Varicose veins, DVT and haemorrhoids: epidemiology and suggested aetiology. *BMJ* 1972;**ii**:556.
14. Dehn TC, Kettlewell MG. Haemorrhoids and defaecatory habits. *Lancet* 1989;**i**:54.
15. Gibbons CP, Bannister JJ, Read NW. Role of constipation and anal hypertonia in the pathogenesis of haemorrhoids. *Br J Surg* 1988;**75**:656.
16. Johanson JF, Sonnenberg A. The prevalence of hemorrhoids and chronic constipation. An epidemiologic study. *Gastroenterology* 1990;**98**:380.
17. Thomson H. Haemorrhoids and all that. *Practitioner* 1982;**226**:619.
18. Hancock BD. The internal sphincter and anal fissure. *Br J Surg* 1977;**64**:92.
19. Bernstein WC. What are haemorrhoids and what is their relationship to the portal venous system? *Dis Colon Rectum* 1983;**26**:829.
20. Ozdil B, Akkiz H, Sandikci M, Kece C, Cosar A. Massive lower gastrointestinal hemorrhage secondary to rectal hemorrhoids in elderly patients receiving anticoagulant therapy: case series. *Dig Dis Sci* 2010;**55**:2693.
21. Chung YC, Hou YC, Pan AC. Endoglin (CD105) expression in the development of haemorrhoids. *Eur J Clin Invest* 2004;**34**:107.
22. Adair C. Pathology of the anus. In: Iacobuzio-Donahue CA, Montgomery E, Goldblum JR (eds), *Gastrointestinal and Liver Pathology*. New York: Churchill Livingstone, 2005: 395.
23. Shanmugam V, Watson AJ, Chapman AD, Binnie NR, Loudon MA. Pathological audit of stapled haemorrhoidopexy. *Colorectal Dis* 2005;**7**:172.
24. Taweevisit M, Wisadeopas N, Phumsuk U, Thorner PS. Increased mast cell density in haemorrhoid venous blood vessels suggests a role in pathogenesis. *Singapore Med J* 2008;**49**:977.
25. Lohsiriwat V, Vongjirad A, Lohsiriwat D. Value of routine histopathologic examination 25 of three common surgical specimens: appendix, gallbladder, and hemorrhoid. *World J Surg* 2009;**33**:2189.
26. Matthyssens LE, Ziol M, Barrat C, Champault GG. Routine surgical pathology in general surgery. *Br J Surg* 2006;**93**:362.
27. Lemarchand N, Tanne F, Aubert M, et al. Is routine pathologic evaluation of hemorrhoidectomy specimens necessary? *Gastroenterol Clin Biol* 2004;**28**:659.
28. Winburn GB. Anal carcinoma or 'just hemorrhoids'? *Am Surg* 2001;**67**:1048.
29. Cataldo PA, MacKeigan JM. The necessity of routine pathologic evaluation of hemorrhoidectomy specimens. *Surg Gynecol Obstet* 1992;**174**:302.
30. Foust RL, Dean PJ, Stoler MH, Moinuddin SM. Intraepithelial neoplasia of the anal canal in hemorrhoidal tissue: a study of 19 cases. *Hum Pathol* 1991;**22**:528.
31. Khosravi M, Nobakht A, Nikokar AR Cytomegalovirus disease with atypical presentation in a renal transplant patient: case report. *Exp Clin Transplant* 2006;**4**:458.
32. Zhang S, Gao F, Wan D. Effect of misdiagnosis on the prognosis of anorectal malignant melanoma. *J Cancer Res Clin Oncol* 2010;**136**:1401.
33. Firoozmand E, Binder S, Thompson A, Hoffman GH. A gastrointestinal stromal tumor discovered in a resected hemorrhoidal donut after stapled hemorrhoidopexy: report of a case. *Am Surg* 2005;**71**:155.
34. Khan AA, Ravalli S, Vincent RA, Chabon AB. Primary Kaposi's sarcoma simulating hemorrhoids in a patient with acquired immune deficiency syndrome. *Am J Gastroenterol* 1989;**84**:1592.
35. Choi WW, Tadros TS, Majmudar B. Anal fibroadenoma: report of a common tumor type in an unusual location. *South Med J* 2007;**100**:914.
36. Sawh RN, Borkowski J, Broaddus R. Metastatic renal cell carcinoma presenting as a hemorrhoid. *Arch Pathol Lab Med* **2002 1**;26:856.
37. Antrum RM. Perianal haematoma: an unusual feature of a leaking aortic aneurysm. *Br J Surg* 1984;**71**:649.
38. Gao XH, Fu CG, Nabieu PF. Residual skin tags following procedure for prolapse and hemorrhoids: differentiation from recurrence. *World J Surg* 2010;**34**:344.
39. Sylla P, Deutsch G, Luo J, et al. Cavernous, arteriovenous, and mixed hemangioma-lymphangioma of the rectosigmoid: rare causes of rectal bleeding – case series and review of the literature. *Int J Colorectal Dis* 2008;**23**:653.

40. Susnow DA. Oleogranuloma of the rectum. *Am J Surg* 1952;**83**:496.
41. Graham-Stewart CW. Injection treatment of haemorrhoids. *BMJ* 1962;**i**:213.
42. Greaney MG, Jackson PR. Oleogranuloma of the rectum produced by Lasonil ointment. *BMJ* 1977;**ii**:997.
43. Bennett DHJ. Rectal paraffinoma. *Proc R Soc Med* 1969;**62**:818.
44. Webb AJ. Oleocysts presenting as rectal tumours. *Br J Surg* 1966; **53**:410.
45. Hernandez V, Hernandez IA, Berthrong M. Oleo-granuloma simulating carcinoma of the rectum. *Dis Colon Rectum* 1967;**10**:205.
46. Symmers WSC. Simulation of cancer by oil granulomas of therapeutic origin. *BMJ* 1955;**ii**:1536.
47. Dalton ML, Gronvall JA. Lymphangioma of the rectum. *Dis Colon Rectum* 1963;**6**:385.
48. Whitehead R. The anal canal. In: *Gastrointestinal and Oesophageal Pathology*, 2nd edn. Edinburgh: Churchill Livingstone, 1995: 713.
49. Morgan MB. Ectopic prostatic tissue of the anal canal. *J Urol* 1992;**147**:165.
50. Sayfan J, Benosh L, Segal M, Orda R. Endometriosis in episiotomy scar with anal sphincter involvement. Report of a case. *Dis Colon Rectum* 1991;**34**:713.
51. Duthie HL. Progress report: anal continence. *Gut* 1971;**12**:844.
52. Parks AG. Anorectal incontinence. *Proc R Soc Med* 1975;**68**:681.
53. Henry MM. Current concepts in anorectal physiology. *Br J Hosp Med* 1986;**35**:238.
54. Bartolo DCC, Read NW, Jarratt JA, et al. Differences in anal sphincter function and clinical presentation in patients with pelvic floor descent. *Gastroenterology* 1983;**85**:68.
55. Bajwa A, Emmanuel A. The physiology of continence and evacuation. *Best Pract Res Clin Gastroenterol* 2009;**23**:477.
56. Bharucha AE, Fletcher JG, Harper CM, et al. Relationship between symptoms and disordered continence mechanisms in women with idiopathic faecal incontinence. *Gut* 2005;**54**:546.
57. Yamada K, Ogata S, Saiki Y, Fukunaga M, Tsuji Y, Takano M. Long-term results of intersphincteric resection for low rectal cancer. *Dis Colon Rectum* 2009;**52**:1065.
58. Butler ECB. Complete rectal prolapse following removal of tumours of the cauda equina. *Proc R Soc Med* 1954;**47**:521.
59. Parks AG, Swash M, Urich H. Sphincter denervation in anorectal incontinence and rectal prolapse. *Gut* 1977;**18**:656.
60. Swash M. Idiopathic faecal incontinence: histopathological evidence on pathogenesis. *Clin Gastroenterol* 1980;**1**:71.

PART 7

Peritoneum

CHAPTER 45

The normal peritoneum

Geraint T. Williams
Cardiff University, Cardiff, UK

Anatomy

The peritoneum is a smooth, elastic membrane that lines the whole of the abdominal cavity, with the exception of the ostia of the fallopian tubes in the female. It is divided into the *visceral peritoneum*, covering the abdominal viscera and the surface of their supporting mesenteries, and the *parietal peritoneum*, which lines the abdominal wall, the pelvis, the inferior surface of the diaphragm and the anterior surface of the retroperitoneum [1]. Embryologically of mesodermal origin, the peritoneal cavity arises from the intra-embryonic coelom by a complex mechanism of coalescence and re-partitioning of primitive coelomic spaces, which also gives rise to the pericardial and pleural cavities and, in the male, to the tunica vaginalis of the testis [2]. Failure of this process leads to abnormal communications between the various cavities, usually termed 'congenital hernias'. By far the most common of these is the congenital inguinal hernia, where failure to obliterate the processus vaginalis after testicular descent into the scrotum leads to a persistent communication between the peritoneal cavity and the tunica vaginalis [3]. Congenital diaphragmatic hernia, due to incomplete partitioning of the peritoneal and pleural cavities by maldevelopment of the diaphragm, is another example (see Chapter 2) [4].

The peritoneal cavity, although a single continuous space, can usefully be divided into four anatomical zones or compartments by the mesenteries of the small and large intestines, which form incomplete barriers. As these mesenteries arise as serosal folds from the posterior wall of the peritoneum, the four zones are best delineated posteri-

orly. The *supracolic space*, which is the uppermost zone, is situated between the inferior surface of the diaphragm above and the transverse colon and its mesocolon below. It is sometimes further subdivided into right and left subphrenic spaces, the sub-hepatic space and the so-called lesser sac of the peritoneum (the omental bursa) [1]. The *pelvic cavity*, as the name suggests, is the lowermost part of the peritoneal cavity and comprises that part contained within the anatomical pelvis. The *left* and *right infracolic spaces* occupy the intervening zone, between the transverse colon and mesocolon above and the pelvic brim below. They are separated from each other by the small bowel mesentery that passes downwards, obliquely and to the right, from a position underneath the transverse mesocolon, just left of the midline, to the right iliac fossa. The right infracolic space is therefore widest above and tapers down to the right lower quadrant, whereas the left infracolic space is narrowest above and broadens out below, where it is continuous with the pelvic cavity. Other anatomical barriers, such as the greater omentum and the intra-abdominal viscera themselves, further compartmentalise the normal peritoneal cavity and when post-inflammatory peritoneal adhesions occur the abdominal cavity may become subdivided even more. The importance of these various barriers, even though they are usually incomplete, is that they greatly influence the direction of movement of fluids from one part of the abdominal cavity to another, and therefore govern the spread of infection and neoplasia within the peritoneum, e.g. gravitational pooling of infected fluids in the sub-phrenic or sub-hepatic spaces or in the pelvic cavity, especially in supine patients, is responsible

Morson and Dawson's Gastrointestinal Pathology, Fifth Edition. Edited by Neil A. Shepherd, Bryan F. Warren,
Geraint T. Williams, Joel K. Greenson, Gregory Y. Lauwers and Marco R. Novelli.
© 2013 Blackwell Publishing Ltd. Published 2013 by Blackwell Publishing Ltd.

for the frequent occurrence of localised intra-abdominal abscesses in these zones.

The arterial blood supply, and venous and lymphatic drainage of the peritoneum differ between the parietal and visceral layers. The parietal peritoneal vasculature is of systemic 'somatic' type, in common with that of the overlying abdominal wall, whereas the visceral peritoneum has a splanchnic circulation, receiving its blood supply from the mesenteric arteries and draining into the portal venous system. At the junctions of the parietal and visceral peritoneum, therefore, there are potential anastomoses between the systemic and portal venous circulations and, when there is portal hypertension, venous varices may occur at these sites, especially around the diaphragm. The peritoneal lymphatics follow the corresponding blood vessels and drain to the coeliac lymph nodes. Frequent anastomoses between the lymphatics of the parietal peritoneum and with those of the parietal pleura, on either side of the diaphragm, may be responsible for the spread of infection and malignant disease between the two cavities. Particulate matter in the peritoneal cavity may find its way by this route to the intrathoracic lymph nodes [5]. The nervous innervation of the parietal and visceral peritoneum mirrors the vascular supply. In common with the overlying abdominal wall, the parietal peritoneum has a somatic innervation that mediates, among other sensations, pain. The visceral peritoneum, on the other hand, receives a splanchnic autonomic nerve supply and although insensitive to pain it is exquisitely responsive to stretching.

Microscopic appearances

The peritoneum consists of a sheet of flat mesothelial cells overlying a zone of dense connective tissue in which elastic fibres are prominent. The thickness of this zone varies considerably between visceral and parietal peritoneum (typically being 5–10 μm in visceral and 25–75 μm in parietal peritoneum), and between different parts of the abdomen and pelvis. It contains abundant glycosaminoglycans that are rich in hyaluronic acid, along with scattered spindle-shaped sub-mesothelial cells. Underneath this there is looser connective tissue containing a sprinkling of mononuclear inflammatory cells, variable quantities of fat, usually reflecting the overall degree of obesity of the individual, a plexus of small blood vessels, lymphatics and nerves. The elastic fibres are oriented parallel to the mesothelial surface, often forming a discrete 'elastic lamina'. Invasion of this lamina has recently been shown to be an independent prognostic factor in stage II colorectal cancer [6].

The intestinal mesenteries and omenta are essentially folds of visceral peritoneum with no special histological features. However, in addition to the connective tissue components described above, the mesenteries contain large blood vessels and nerves that supply the intestines, lymph

nodes and smaller lymphoid and histiocytic aggregates surrounding dilated vascular sinusoids; these can sometimes be recognised macroscopically as so-called 'milk spots' [7]. These are sites of transit of leukocytes between the blood and the peritoneal cavity. They contain B cells, T cells and dendritic cells [8], are most commonly found in young children and are usually distributed around the portal vascular tree. It has been suggested that they play an important role in the development of gastrointestinal immunity in infancy and they may re-appear when there is peritoneal inflammation.

At light microscopy resting mesothelial cells appear as elongated, regular cells with an attenuated cytoplasm that is more abundant around the nucleus [9]. This may stain with Alcian blue but not with periodic acid–Schiff (PAS). On electron microscopy the cytoplasm contains ribosomes, rough endoplasmic reticulum, micro-pinocytotic vesicles and some mitochondria but the most striking feature is the presence of long surface microvilli that protrude from the serosal surface of the cell into the peritoneal cavity (Figure 45.1). The microvilli appear to be especially well developed on mesothelial cells covering serosal surfaces that move actively, causing speculation that they may trap macromolecules of mucopolysaccharide on the cell surface, thus making the peritoneal surfaces more slippery and reducing friction [10]. Mesothelial cells also secrete a number of factors that are important in host defence against infection and in the regulation of peritoneal permeability to a wide range of molecules. They lie on a basal lamina, but do not themselves form a complete sheet over the peritoneal surface; although there is widespread contact between adjacent cells with the formation of specialised junctional complexes, intercellular gaps (stomata) exist through which

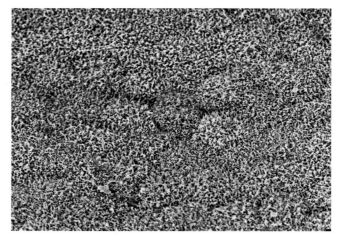

Figure 45.1 Scanning electron micrograph of the surface of normal human parietal peritoneum showing abundant microvilli.

molecules diffuse [11] and inflammatory cells, notably bone marrow-derived macrophages [12], may migrate. This may explain the avidity with which substances injected intraperitoneally enter the systemic circulation, and hence the clinical usefulness of peritoneal dialysis for the treatment of renal failure.

In normal peritoneum the spindle-shaped submesothelial cells have the ultrastructural characteristics of fibroblasts, but there is growing evidence to suggest that they are specialised multipotent cells that have the potential to proliferate and differentiate after injury to contribute to the mesothelial lining cells [13,14]. Indeed, there is some evidence that transdifferentiation in the opposite direction, from epithelioid mesothelial cells to spindle-shaped submesothelial cells, is also possible [15]. On immunocytochemistry, normal mesothelial lining cells express both high-and low-molecular-weight cytokeratins whereas the sub-mesothelial cells express only vimentin. However, when there is reactive mesothelial hyperplasia, proliferating subserosal cells also express cytokeratins, supporting the view that they have a lineage in common with mesothelial cells [14]. Other immunohistochemical markers of mesothelial differentiation include calretinin, cytokeratin 5/6, thrombomodulin, Wilms' tumour gene 1 (*WT1*) protein, mesothelin and D2-40. The degree of immunoreactivity varies with cell maturity, and in 'reactive' conditions there may also be expression of desmin and muscle-specific actin. For this reason a panel of antibody markers is strongly recommended for the investigation of cell lineage in tumours and other proliferative lesions involving the peritoneum (see Chapter 47).

The peritoneal cavity normally contains some 100 ml of clear, straw-coloured fluid containing a little protein and acid mucopolysaccharides, which lubricates the peritoneal surfaces as they glide over each other. The peritoneal fluid is largely a transudate of plasma and there is considerable exchange of water, electrolytes and other molecules of up to 5000 Da in size across the peritoneal membrane. Nevertheless, active transport also occurs, and there is active secretion of the acid mucopolysaccharides by mesothelial cells. Dispersed within the fluid are a number of cell types, which can be recognised when normal peritoneal fluid is examined cytologically. Apart from red cells, which are presumed to represent accidental contamination, the pre-

dominant cells are macrophages, exfoliated mesothelial cells and forms that appear morphologically intermediate between macrophages and mesothelial cells. Lymphocytes are also present in smaller numbers, and sometimes a few granulocytes (usually eosinophils).

References

1. Standring S, ed. Peritoneum and peritoneal cavity. In: *Gray's Anatomy*, 40th edn. Edinburgh, Churchill Livingstone-Elsevier, 2008: 1099.
2. Carlson BM. *Human Embryology and Developmental Biology*, 3rd edn. Philadelphia, PA: Mosby, 2004: 353.
3. Clatworthy HW Jr, Gilbert M, Clement A. The inguinal hernia, hydrocoele and undescended testicle problem in infants and children. *Postgrad Med J* 1957;**22**:122.
4. Snyder WH Jr, Greaney EM Jr. Congenital diaphragmatic hernia: 77 consecutive cases. *Surgery*, 1965;**57**:576.
5. Yoffey JM, Courtice FC. *Lymphatics, Lymph and the Lymphomyeloid Complex*. London: Academic Press, 1970: 295.
6. Kojima M, Nakajima K, Ishii G, Saito N, Ochiai A. Peritoneal elastic laminal invasion of colorectal cancer: the diagnostic utility and clinicopathologic relationship. *Am J Surg Pathol* 2010; **34**:1351.
7. Shimotsuma M, Takahashi T, Kawata M, Dux K. Cellular subsets of the milky spots in the human greater omentum. *Cell Tissue Res* 1991;**264**:599.
8. Carlow DA, Gold MR, Ziltener HJ. Lymphocytes in the peritoneum home to the omentum and are activated by resident dendritic cells. *J Immunol* 2009;**183**:1155.
9. Michailova KN, Usunoff KG. Serosal membranes (pleura, pericardium, peritoneum): normal structure, development and experimental pathology, *Adv Anat Embryol Cell Biol* 2006;**183**:1.
10. Andrews PM, Porter KR. The ultrastructural morphology and possible functional significance of mesothelial microvilli. *Anat Rec* 1973;**177**:409.
11. Cotran RS, Karnovsky MJ. Ultrastructural studies on the permeability of the mesothelium to horseradish peroxidase. *J Cell Biol* 1968;**37**:123.
12. Murch AR, Grounds MD, Papadimitriou JM. Improved chimaeric mouse model confirms that resident peritoneal macrophages are derived solely from bone marrow precursors. *J Pathol* 1984; **144**:81.
13. Raftery AT. Regeneration of parietal and visceral peritoneum: an electron microscopical study. *J Anat* 1973;**115**:375.
14. Bolen JW, Hammar SP, McNutt MA. Reactive and neoplastic serosal tissue. A light-microscopic, ultrastructural, and immunocytochemical study. *Am J Surg Pathol* 1986;**10**:34.
15. Yanez-Mo M, Lara-Pezzi E, Selgas R et al. Peritoneal dialysis and epithelial-to-mesenchymal transition of mesothelial cells. *N Engl J Med* 2003;**348**:403.

CHAPTER 46

Inflammatory disorders of the peritoneum

Maurice B. Loughrey

Royal Victoria Hospital, Queen's University Belfast, Belfast, UK

Despite the widespread availability of antibacterial agents in recent decades, acute peritonitis continues to be a common condition causing much morbidity and mortality worldwide. In the vast majority of cases inflammation of the peritoneum is a consequence of some other intra-abdominal disease, so-called primary peritonitis being extremely uncommon. Spread of infective organisms from the alimentary tract, usually as a result of primary gastrointestinal disease, is by far the most common cause, although secondary pelvic peritonitis from gynaecological infections has increased in frequency: this may occur by direct spread into the peritoneal cavity via the ostia of the fallopian tubes (through which the peritoneal cavity is in direct continuity with the lumina of the uterus and vagina), or by spread of infective agents through the wall of the uterus or uterine tubes. Infection of the peritoneum may also arise from the external surface of the body as a result of paracentesis, laparotomy or penetrating trauma. Blood-borne infection is rare.

Acute diffuse peritonitis

In western countries, the three major causes of acute diffuse peritonitis are appendicitis, perforated peptic ulcer and colonic diverticulitis. In appendicitis and diverticulitis, severe generalised peritoneal inflammation usually results from perforation of the inflamed viscus, when the peritoneal cavity is suddenly flooded with faecal organisms, tissue debris and foreign matter, resulting in abdominal pain and shock. A mixture of the organisms that form the normal flora of the alimentary tract, with anaerobic bacte-

ria and coliforms predominating, is therefore found on microbiological examination of the peritoneal contents [1]. Perforation of the bowel wall is not essential to produce peritonitis – virulent bacteria may pass through the diseased wall of the bowel to the serosa when there are lesser degrees of intestinal inflammation.

The initial peritoneal inflammation after perforation of a peptic ulcer, on the other hand, is the result of the irritant 'chemical' effects of the gastric or duodenal contents, including gastric juice, bile, pancreatic juice and partly digested food, although this is commonly followed later by bacterial infection. Other well recognised causes of peritonitis include perforation of gastrointestinal neoplasms, inflammatory bowel disease, intestinal infections, ischaemia or obstruction, perforation of the gallbladder in acute cholecystitis and pancreatitis. The alimentary viscera are usually the source of peritonitis in childhood also, although in newborn infants direct spread of umbilical infection is well recognised. Gynaecological causes of acute diffuse peritonitis include rupture of a pyosalpinx or a tubo-ovarian abscess, septic abortion, puerperal sepsis and endometritis associated with the presence of an intra-uterine contraceptive device. A variety of organisms may be responsible, aerobic and anaerobic, including gonococci, *Chlamydia* spp., *Actinomyces* spp. and fungi [1]. Less commonly, peritonitis may result from disorders of the urinary tract, such as intra-abdominal rupture of the bladder, perforation of a renal abscess or, in the male, prostatitis.

The organisms causing peritonitis of extraneous origin after perforating abdominal trauma are also varied. As might be expected, staphylococci are frequently incrimi-

Morson and Dawson's Gastrointestinal Pathology, Fifth Edition. Edited by Neil A. Shepherd, Bryan F. Warren, Geraint T. Williams, Joel K. Greenson, Gregory Y. Lauwers and Marco R. Novelli.
© 2013 Blackwell Publishing Ltd. Published 2013 by Blackwell Publishing Ltd.

nated but, as abdominal trauma frequently involves damage to the gastrointestinal viscera, infection by enteric organisms often dominates the microbiological picture.

Abdominal surgery and peritoneal dialysis are important iatrogenic causes of infective peritonitis. Although the introduction of preoperative sterilisation of the intestinal contents with antibiotics has greatly reduced the frequency of acute diffuse peritonitis after gastrointestinal surgery, faecal soiling of the abdominal cavity remains a serious complication of emergency procedures and of elective surgery complicated by breakdown of an intestinal anastomosis, due to either infection or ischaemia. Peritonitis resulting from acute peritoneal dialysis may result from damage to intra-abdominal viscera during cannulation, when it is caused by the release of enteric bacteria, or when there is failure to adhere to the most meticulous aseptic technique, as a result of which infection by hospital-acquired, antibiotic-resistant organisms can ensue. In recent decades there has been increasing use of chronic ambulatory peritoneal dialysis for the long-term management of renal failure, when intra-abdominal cannulae are kept in place for many weeks or months. The risk of infection, especially from skin-derived Gram-positive cocci, is particularly high in these patients [2].

Haemorrhage into the peritoneal cavity (haemoperitoneum) may also result in an acute diffuse peritonitis. The clinical features of peritonitis are seldom dramatic in such cases, and the inflammatory reaction is not pronounced unless there is an additional infective element. On the other hand, the spillage of bile [3] or pancreatic juice, the latter especially in acute pancreatitis, produces a severe acute chemical peritonitis with fat necrosis, which frequently results in shock.

The development of acute diffuse peritonitis without obvious cause, so-called 'primary peritonitis' or 'spontaneous bacterial peritonitis', occurs much more commonly than previously considered [4,5]. Usually encountered in adults in the setting of advanced cirrhosis with high volume ascites, spontaneous bacterial peritonitis, when under-diagnosed and under-treated, is associated with a high mortality. Now it is considered a treatable complication of cirrhosis, albeit with a high risk of recurrence [6]. Pathogenesis relates to the increased permeability of the gut in patients with advanced cirrhosis, allowing translocation of enteric bacteria to mesenteric lymph nodes, lymph and eventually ascitic fluid [7]. The inability of macrophages and neutrophils in ascitic fluid to kill the virulent bacteria results in uncontrolled bacterial growth [8]. Unlike secondary peritonitis from overt gastrointestinal disease, when culture of the peritoneal fluid reveals a mixed flora of enteric-type bacteria, the infection in primary peritonitis is caused by a single type of bacterium, usually *Escherichia coli* or *Klebsiella* spp. Appropriate antibiotic therapy is typically curative but, given the high rate of recurrence of up

to 70% at 1 year [9], prophylactic antibiotic therapy is recommended in selected patients [10].

Macroscopic and microscopic appearances

The earliest macroscopic manifestations of acute diffuse peritonitis are engorgement of the subserosal capillary blood vessels and dulling of the normally glistening peritoneal surface. These are soon followed by the exudation into the peritoneal cavity of a protein-rich fluid containing fibrinogen, which is rapidly converted into a thin film of fibrin covering the serosal surfaces. Fibrin has a stringy, sticky consistency that causes adjacent loops of bowel to adhere to each other and the parietal peritoneum. In severe cases the exudate may be haemorrhagic or even frankly purulent. Histological examination in the early stages of the inflammatory reaction shows first swelling and then desquamation of the mesothelial cells, so that the serosal surface becomes covered by a layer of fibrin enclosing many neutrophils and cellular debris, leading to the formation of granulation tissue. In the less inflamed areas mesothelial cells undergo marked regenerative hyperplasia (Figure 46.1a). Pleomorphism and mitotic activity in mesothelial cells, and in subserosal mononuclear cells, may be sufficiently marked to suggest a malignant infiltrate (Figure 46.1b).

Cytological examination of peritoneal fluid obtained directly by aspiration [11,12], or after lavage [13], is a useful rapid method for confirming the diagnosis of peritonitis in an emergency. The fluid contains large numbers of neutrophil polymorphs, many of which are degenerate, and variable numbers of bacteria and red blood cells. It is important to scan smears of these purulent deposits, because the presence of squamous cells is clear evidence of a leak or rupture in the gastrointestinal tract, permitting swallowed saliva to reach the peritoneal cavity.

Complications of acute peritonitis

Acute diffuse peritonitis is frequently complicated by the development of clinical shock, the severity of which is related to the virulence of the causative agent. A number of factors may be responsible for circulatory collapse, including severe pain, systemic bacteraemia (or toxaemia), respiratory embarrassment due to diaphragmatic malfunction and excess catecholamine release, but the most important factor is an acute reduction in the circulating blood volume. This occurs for two reasons: an exudation of fluid from the vascular compartment into the inflamed abdominal cavity, as is found in any acute inflammatory reaction, and a loss of fluid into the lumen of the intestine as a result of paralytic ileus (adynamic ileus), resulting from a failure of peristaltic motility of the intestine.

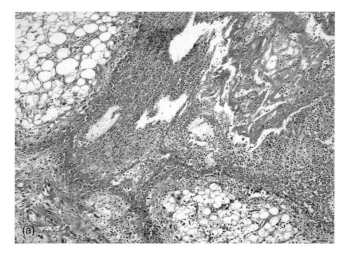

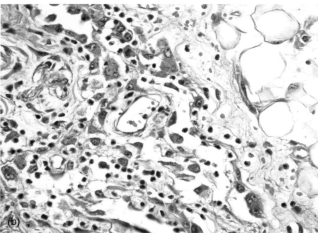

Figure 46.1 (a) Acute peritonitis in a patient with perforated sigmoid diverticulitis, showing mesothelial hyperplasia and a serosal coating of fibrin and neutrophilic inflammatory debris. (b) High power showing marked reactive atypia of mesothelial cells, including multinucleate forms.

The development of ileus within hours or days of the onset of acute peritonitis is common but poorly understood [14]. It may affect much of the small intestine, although commonly it is confined to a short length of ileum or colon that has lain in a pool of purulent exudate in the pelvis. Damage to Auerbach's plexus by toxins absorbed through the inflamed serosa of the intestine may be one cause of the muscular paralysis; other possibilities include impaired contractility of enteric smooth muscle resulting from disturbances in electrolyte balance, sympathetic stimulation and partial anoxia related to blood stasis, which is frequently present. Whatever its cause, the ileus results in a functional complete intestinal obstruction, producing distension of both the affected segment and the proximal bowel loops by gas and intestinal secretions, and resulting

in a series of physiological disturbances, the effects of which are most profound on the circulatory system. Gaseous distension of the intestine increases the intramural tension and leads to impairment of its blood supply. This in turn causes increased absorption of toxic materials from the gut lumen, themselves causing further circulatory embarrassment, so that a vicious circle of intestinal damage and cardiovascular impairment ensues. Furthermore, in the adynamic segment, there is both failure of intestinal fluid absorption (despite continued secretion of digestive juices) and active exudation into the gut lumen, resulting in a significant loss of fluid, sometimes litres in volume, from the effective extracellular fluid compartment and contributing greatly to the circulatory collapse. Urgent correction of this, by intravenous rehydration, is a very important component of the emergency treatment of peritonitis.

Once acute peritonitis has been established, its spread throughout the abdominal cavity is promoted by the free movement of infected fluids over the surface of the peritoneum under the influence of gravity, posture, respiratory and bowel movements, and by dissemination in the subserosal lymphatics. Portal pyaemia may occur in severe cases, leading to the spread of infection to the liver and beyond and to septic thrombosis of mesenteric veins. If the patient recovers from the acute stage of peritonitis, two serious complications may result: the formation of localised abscesses and the creation of peritoneal adhesions.

Intra-abdominal abscess

Intra-abdominal abscesses after acute diffuse peritonitis arise from the pooling of purulent exudate in the dependent parts of the peritoneal cavity, notably the rectovesical pouch, paracolic gutters and sub-phrenic region. Sometimes they are multiple. Their location is generally related to the site of the primary disease, e.g. after perforation of a peptic ulcer, pus tends to accumulate in the sub-phrenic spaces or in the lesser sac of the peritoneum, whereas after appendicitis and colonic diverticulitis a pelvic or paracolic collection of pus is more usual [15]. However, not all intra-abdominal abscesses follow acute diffuse peritonitis: some develop as a result of localised spread of infection around a diseased intra-abdominal organ, such as peri-appendiceal abscess complicating appendicitis.

Subphrenic abscess was traditionally said to be more common on the right side than on the left, although earlier surgery for appendicitis has reduced the incidence of right sub-phrenic abscess from this cause in recent decades [16]. Nevertheless, in children appendicitis is still the most common cause [17]. In adults, sub-phrenic abscesses are seen most often as a complication of upper abdominal surgery, especially that of the biliary tree or the stomach [18], although a significant proportion follow perforated peptic ulcer, cholecystitis, diverticulitis, pancreatitis or appendicitis. The condition develops insidiously, pus collecting in one of the anatomical compartments bounded by the diaphragm, liver and falciform ligament, and becoming sealed off from the abdominal cavity by adhesions. The abscess may occasionally resolve spontaneously, although surgical drainage is usually necessary to prevent complications such as rupture into the peritoneal or pleural cavities or extension into adjacent structures. Pelvic abscesses are most commonly of large intestinal or gynaecological origin. Pus accumulates in the recto-vesical or recto-uterine pouches, where it becomes walled off by adhesions. Small collections may resolve spontaneously but the majority, if untreated, rupture into the rectum, bladder or vagina.

Microbiological culture of pus from intra-abdominal abscesses usually reveals a mixture of bacteria, with anaerobic Gram-negative bacilli predominating. The pathogens found reflect the origin of the infection, enteric organisms being by far the most common.

Peritoneal adhesions

In most cases of acute diffuse peritonitis, resolution of the fibrinous or purulent inflammatory exudate results in reconstitution of a smooth serosal surface by a process that appears to differ in important respects from the healing of epithelial surfaces such as the skin [19]. The inflamed surface, denuded of mesothelium and covered by fibrin and pus cells, becomes infiltrated by macrophages, which phagocytose the cell debris and, in concert with plasminogen activators released from mesothelial cells, initiate fibrinolysis [20]. A layer of newly formed mesothelium, most probably derived from subserosal mesenchymal cells, soon covers the defect, and fibroblasts in the underlying zone complete the healing process by the synthesis of new collagen.

The removal of fibrin from the damaged serosa is crucial to the complete resolution of peritonitis [21,22]. When this is impaired the fibrinous exudate becomes converted into granulation tissue in which progressive fibroblastic proliferation and collagen synthesis eventually lead to dense fibrosis. As the initial fibrinous material frequently causes adjacent peritoneal surfaces to adhere to each other, it is not surprising that fibrous organisation of this fibrin results in the formation of dense fibrous adhesions, especially between adjacent loops of bowel or between the intestine and the parietal peritoneum [23]. Experimental studies have shown that after severe and widespread mesothelial damage there is commonly complete healing without the formation of fibrous adhesions, provided that there is no ischaemia of the serosa. It is only when areas of the peritoneal surface are devascularised that adhesions are consistently produced. How ischaemia has this profound effect on peritoneal healing is uncertain but there is evidence that it is often accompanied by a depression of fibrinolytic activity lasting for several days [21]. It is possible that, during this time, when there is inadequate clearing of the fibrinous exudate on the serosal surface, adhesion formation may be initiated, perhaps irreversibly. The use of surgical sutures in the peritoneum can produce localised areas of serosal ischaemia and this may explain the fact that adhesions occur much more commonly after abdominal surgery, even for minor procedures, than after a severe diffuse peritonitis when presumably there is widespread serosal denudation but little ischaemia.

Peritoneal adhesions may be localised or generalised. Although most are dense, fibrous and irreversible, some may be temporary and gradually disappear. Intestinal obstruction, by constricting or strangling a segment of bowel, is their important complication. In the developed world, they are the most common cause of acute intestinal obstruction [24].

Localised peritonitis

In most cases of acute peritonitis the unlimited spread of inflammation within the abdominal cavity results in diffuse involvement of the peritoneal serosa. Nevertheless, peritonitis may occasionally remain localised to the vicinity of the lesion that has given rise to it, especially if there are adhesions or other anatomical barriers to limit the normal movements of intra-abdominal fluids. Peritonitis resulting from perforation of a peptic ulcer, for example, may be localised to the epigastric region by the presence of adhesions (pre-existing or newly formed) and by the enveloping action of the greater omentum, a structure that probably plays a particularly important role in limiting the spread of intra-abdominal infection. Two features of the greater omentum facilitate this: its large size and its frequent changes in position relative to other viscera, resulting from intestinal movements and alterations in posture, which allow it to come into contact with many sites of inflammation and to be anchored there by the fibrinous exudate that forms on its serosal surface. Thus the greater omentum is frequently found adherent to an acutely inflamed appendix, the colon in complicated diverticulitis, the ileum in Crohn's disease or portions of infarcted bowel. It is also occasionally found extending into inguinal hernial sacs, where it becomes attached to any inflamed bowel that is present.

Special forms of peritonitis

Tuberculous peritonitis

Tuberculous peritonitis, a frequently fatal complication of intestinal or pulmonary tuberculosis (TB) before the era of anti-tuberculous chemotherapy, remains common in developing countries but is now rare in the western world, outwith the setting of urban immigrant populations and patients with HIV infection [25,26]. Patients undergoing peritoneal dialysis are at increased risk of acquiring myco-bacterial infection [27], as are those receiving anti-tumour necrosis factor (TNF) therapy [28]. Tuberculous peritonitis may be primary or arise by spread from a primary focus elsewhere in the body [29]. Pulmonary TB, usually due to *Mycobacterium tuberculosis*, is the most common source but other primary sites include the intestine, mesenteric lymph nodes and female genital tract, when other mycobacteria may be involved.

Peritoneal TB is characterised by the studding of the serosal membrane with glistening tubercles, initially of pin-head size but later enlarging and coalescing to form plaques or even caseous masses (Figure 46.2a). The greater omentum is often extensively affected and may appear post mortem as an elongated, retracted, fibrocaseous mass lying trans-versely across the abdomen. The nature of the accompany-ing inflammatory reaction varies considerably between

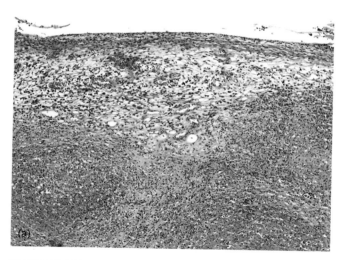

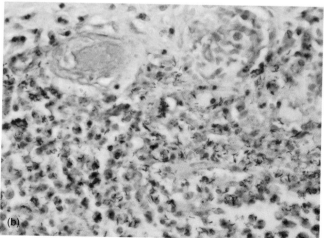

Figure 46.2 (a) Tuberculous peritonitis: confluent subserosal granulomas with caseous necrosis. (b) High power showing numerous mycobacteria with Ziehl–Neelsen staining.

cases. Sometimes, in the so-called 'dry' form of the disease, there is a dense fibrinous exudate that mats together the intestinal loops and abdominal viscera into a firm, doughy mass. More commonly, there is exudation of large quanti-ties of protein-rich, sometimes blood-stained, ascites – the 'wet' or ascitic form of tuberculous peritonitis. Either form can mimic disseminated malignancy, in particular advanced ovarian cancer [30]. Persistent fibrous adhesions are a fre-quent complication, leading to recurrent attacks of acute and subacute intestinal obstruction.

The diagnosis of tuberculous peritonitis is best made by peritoneal biopsy, in which typical caseating granuloma-tous inflammation is seen, in which mycobacteria may be recognisable on Ziehl–Neelsen staining [31] (Figure 46.2b). The specimen may be taken at laparoscopy or laparotomy or by blind peritoneal biopsy. Culture of the biopsy tissue should always be undertaken in order to confirm the diag-nosis and establish the antibiotic sensitivity of the organ-isms. Cytological examination alone of ascitic fluid in the wet form of the disease does not allow a confident diagno-sis of TB to be made, although culture of the fluid fre-quently gives a positive result. The fluid contains a mixed inflammatory cell population including many lymphocytes, although these do not necessarily dominate the picture as they do in tuberculous pleurisy. Macrophages, neutrophils, lympho-plasmacytoid cells and small numbers of mesothe-lial cells may also be found but epithelioid cells and Lang-hans' giant cells are unusual in tuberculous effusions.

Actinomycotic peritonitis

Actinomycotic peritonitis occurs secondary to infection of the gastrointestinal tract, notably the appendix, or after infection of the female genital tract, when the condition is usually associated with the presence of an intra-uterine contraceptive device [32]. Almost always the infection remains localised within the affected region of the perito-neal cavity, usually the pelvis, by the formation of dense fibrotic adhesions, resulting in an extensive inflammatory mass involving the appendix or a tubo-ovarian abscess [33]. Fistulae with adjacent viscera or the abdominal wall may form, to discharge the characteristic actinomycotic pus containing so-called sulphur granules. In recent years there have been reports of peritonitis secondary to the closely related filamentous bacterium, *Nocardia* spp., usually in the setting of chronic peritoneal dialysis [34].

Fungal peritonitis

Peritonitis due to fungal organisms is uncommon and is typically associated with immunosuppression or patients on long-term peritoneal dialysis [35]. *Candida albicans* is the most common causative agent [36]. *C. albicans* peritonitis has been described after intestinal perforation [37]. Cryptococcal peritonitis has been associated with chronic liver disease [38] whereas coccidioidomycotic, blastomycotic and histoplasmic infections are rare causes of peritonitis in endemic areas [39,40].

Metazoal peritonitis

Metazoal peritonitis is uncommon and may present clinically with a variety of symptoms and signs. The most innocuous form, which is virtually always asymptomatic and found either incidentally during laparotomy for some unrelated condition or post mortem, is a chronic pelvic peritonitis in women caused by the pinworm (threadworm) *Enterobius vermicularis* [41]. The macroscopic appearances do not immediately suggest peritonitis in that there are numerous nodules scattered over the peritoneal surface that measure <10 mm in diameter, are white or yellow in colour and consist of a firm, fibrous capsule surrounding a necrotic core. The serosa covering the pelvic viscera is affected predominantly but very rarely there is a more generalised involvement of the peritoneal cavity. The lesions are often mistaken for tumour deposits, tuberculosis or foci of endometriosis [41]. Microscopic examination of the nodules shows a brisk, often granulomatous, inflammatory reaction, rich in neutrophil and eosinophil leukocytes, surrounding either an adult female worm or its ova (Figure 46.3) and enveloped by a dense collagenous capsule.

Ascaris lumbricoides is another rare metazoal cause of chronic serositis that develops covertly without producing the typical clinical features of peritonitis. It is the ascaris ova, rather than the adult worms, that are mainly responsible for the inflammatory reaction, which is more fibrotic than that found in pinworm peritonitis and consequently

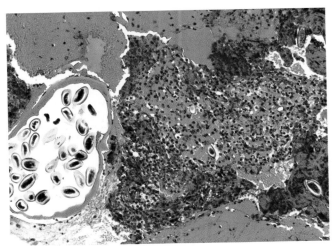

Figure 46.3 Metazoal peritonitis caused by the pinworm *Enterobius vermicularis*. Peritoneal biopsy revealed a gravid worm (left) and numerous eggs lying within a fibrino-purulent exudate.

associated with the frequent formation of adhesions. Although some cases are diagnosed incidentally at laparotomy for unrelated conditions, a significant number present with intestinal obstruction. Macroscopically the picture may resemble the dry form of tuberculous peritonitis, in that there are pale nodules or 'tubercles' scattered over the serosal surfaces and adhesions. Histological examination of the nodules gives the diagnosis and reveals a granulomatous reaction within which the characteristic ascarid ova, with their coarsely mamillate outer shell, can be recognised [42].

Other metazoal causes of chronic peritonitis that may lead to the formation of adhesions or an omental inflammatory mass include the larvae of *Strongyloides stercoralis* or the herring-worm *Anisakis* spp. [43] and schistosomiasis [44], which may involve the peritoneal cavity by secondary spread from the gastrointestinal or urinary tracts. In each of these conditions there is an eosinophil-rich granulomatous peritonitis, within which the causative organisms may be detected. Hydatid cysts, with their characteristic histological appearances, are occasionally found in the omentum or mesenteries, or scattered throughout the peritoneal cavity, the latter situation usually resulting from intra-abdominal rupture of a hepatic cyst [45].

Traumatic peritonitis

Trauma to the peritoneal membrane, classically during abdominal surgery, usually results in local mesothelial damage with an acute inflammatory reaction. In uncomplicated circumstances this is followed by healing, by the process described above, when the serosal lining returns to normal. Quite frequently, however, there is undue proliferation of fibrous tissue leading to the formation of intra-abdominal adhesions. Experimental studies have identified a number of factors predisposing to the formation of adhesions following trauma, including the persistence of blood in the peritoneal cavity, the prolonged drying of the mesothelium during laparotomy [21,46], local ischaemia of the peritoneum (discussed above) and the persistence of any non-degradable irritant, especially of exogenous origin such as suture material or talc (see below) [19,47]. It is a remarkable paradox, therefore, that large defects in the peritoneal membrane after surgery regularly heal to their original pristine state whereas defects that are meticulously closed by sutures often heal with the formation of adhesions, the result of chronic irritation by foreign materials and focal ischaemia of the mesothelium caused by stretching or suturing [19].

Peritonitis caused by foreign bodies

Foreign bodies enter the peritoneal cavity as a consequence of visceral rupture, surgical laparotomy or laparoscopy, or trauma. The nature of the ensuing inflammatory reaction depends on the physico-chemical properties of the foreign body, and in particular its irritant effect. Some foreign materials, such as silicone rubber dialysis catheters, cause very little peritoneal reaction whereas foreign bodies that are infected, as is almost invariable after trauma and is frequently the case with retained surgical swabs, produce an acute diffuse peritonitis. Less irritant agents result in a more localised foreign-body granulomatous reaction of the serosa that, although often clinically silent in its early course, may come to light later when post-inflammatory peritoneal adhesions cause intestinal obstruction. Most foreign bodies that cause a granulomatous peritonitis are of microscopic dimensions and can be identified only by light microscopy of biopsy material, supplemented if necessary by polarisation or electron microscopy [48]. Nevertheless, in a few instances, e.g. after uterine perforation by an intra-uterine contraceptive device or when a sterile gauze swab has been left inadvertently in the abdominal cavity, the nature of the foreign material is obvious on gross examination at laparotomy.

When granulomatous peritonitis follows visceral perforation, the most common source of the foreign material is the alimentary tract. Perforations of the uterus or bladder are infrequent events and when they occur they are often the result of surgical instrumentation. A remarkable number and variety of foreign bodies may escape into the peritoneal cavity after gastrointestinal perforation, and granulomatous reactions after such events may contain a variety of materials of vegetable or meat origin or of an amorphous or crystalline nature. Sometimes these granulomas contain central necrosis surrounded by epithelioid cells and Langhans-type giant cells that can mimic tuberculosis (Figure 46.4a). Food-starch particles are usually birefringent and a proportion may show a characteristic 'Maltese-cross' pattern of polarisation (Figure 46.4b), although this can be lost after tissue degradation. They are periodic acid–Schiff (PAS) positive, often variable in shape and size and usually extremely resistant to salivary diastase digestion [49,50], features that may allow food-derived starch in granulomas to be distinguished from the round diastase-digestible starch particles found in iatrogenic starch granulomatosis that may follow abdominal surgery (see below). Barium sulphate is another foreign material that may escape into the abdominal cavity to produce a granulomatous reaction, typically as a complication of lower or, less commonly, upper gastrointestinal contrast investigation [51]. In such cases there is almost always an initial bacterial peritonitis due to the release of faecal organisms that necessitates laparotomy to repair the perforation and to wash out the contaminating material from the abdominal cavity. Any residual barium sulphate is ingested by macrophages to produce a foreign body granulomatous reaction within which barium sulphate particles may be recognised

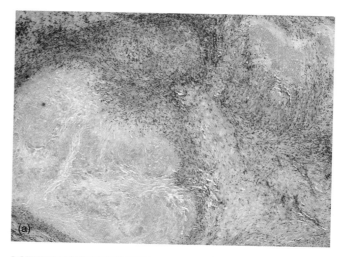

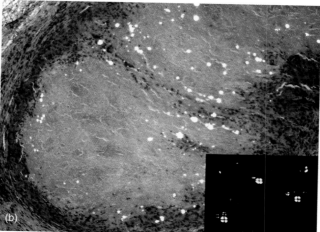

Figure 46.4 (a) Starch granulomatosis of the peritoneum after previous surgery. The necrotising granulomatous reaction mimics tuberculosis. (b) Examination under polarised light reveals abundant starch granules within the necrotic material with the characteristic Maltese-cross appearance evident under high power (inset).

[52]. They have a variety of appearances when examined by polarised light, depending on the particulate constitution of the radiological contrast medium used [53]. Barium granulomas are rarely complicated by significant fibrosis, and consequently barium sulphate peritonitis is virtually never complicated by adhesions with their serious clinical consequences.

In previous decades, among the best recognised chronic inflammatory reactions after surgical laparotomy caused by peritoneal foreign bodies was that due to talcum powder, which was used formerly as a lubricant on surgeons' gloves. It produced a chronic peritoneal reaction that in some patients, led to the development of extensive peritoneal adhesions and intestinal obstruction. Talc is a mixture

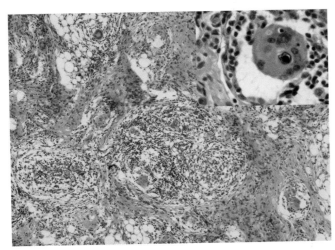

Figure 46.5 Talc peritonitis: florid foreign-body-type granulomatous reaction with talc particles seen on high power within giant cells (inset).

of magnesium silicate and calcium and magnesium carbonates with crystals that are readily demonstrated by polarisation microscopy in the multi-nucleated foreign-body-type giant cells conspicuous in talc granulomas (Figure 46.5) [54]. Epichlorhydrin-treated Indian corn or rice starch was used to lubricate surgeons' gloves more recently. It was originally introduced because studies in experimental animals had suggested that absorption of the starch from the peritoneal cavity would abolish glove powder peritonitis. Unfortunately this did not occur in the humans and starch became known as a rare but important cause of postoperative peritonitis that led to the formation of a granulomatous inflammatory reaction and dense adhesions in a minority of individuals [55]. Histologically, the granulomas consisted of macrophages and multinucleate giant cells, often in a palisade arrangement, enclosing foci of necrosis that on casual inspection could mimic tuberculosis. Polarisation microscopy demonstrated the starch granules by their 'Maltese-cross' pattern of birefringence (see Figure 46.4b) [56]. The hazards of glove powder have resulted in a move towards powder-free surgical gloves in recent decades [57].

Other foreign materials that may be introduced into the peritoneal cavity at laparotomy and that may lead to a granulomatous peritonitis with adhesion formation include insoluble antibiotic preparations, various oily substances such as liquid paraffin and cellulose fibres from disposable surgical gowns and drapes [58]. Other described causes of foreign-body granulomatous peritonitis include intra-peritoneal leakage of Ivalon, used to plug the site of percutaneous liver biopsy in patients with impaired coagulation [59], and spillage of gallstones into the peritoneal cavity at laparoscopic cholecystectomy [60].

Meconium peritonitis

Spillage of meconium into the peritoneal cavity in the fetus or newborn infant as a result of intra-uterine or neonatal intestinal perforation results in a distinctive clinico-pathological syndrome known as meconium peritonitis [61,62]. Most patients present within 48 hours of birth with non-specific features of peritonitis but occasionally the condition is clinically silent for months or years, when the ensuing chronic inflammatory reaction with fibrosis leads to the formation of a palpable abdominal mass or to intestinal obstruction from adhesions. Intestinal perforation in fetal and early neonatal life may be due to obstruction from congenital atresias and stenoses, intussusception, volvulus, duplication, hernia or the abnormally viscid meconium of cystic fibrosis, or ischaemia of the fetal or neonatal intestine [63]. Such intra-uterine perforations frequently seal spontaneously, however, so that in some cases of meconium peritonitis it is impossible to establish the precise site of meconium leakage.

Normal meconium consists of swallowed amniotic fluid (with its contained hair and desquamated squames), mucus, biliary, pancreatic and intestinal secretions, and it is the last that are particularly irritant to the peritoneum, causing an intense peritonitis with fat necrosis. If the infant survives this early stage, a florid granulomatous peritonitis develops, often progressing to the formation of extensive adhesions. The whole of the peritoneal cavity is involved diffusely in most cases, although sometimes the inflammatory reaction is localised by intestinal loops to form a thick-walled inflammatory cyst. Calcification within fat necrosis and within the mucinous component of the meconium occurs frequently and may be sufficiently marked to allow the diagnosis to be made on a plain abdominal radiograph. Histological examination in the early stages of meconium peritonitis shows a florid inflammatory reaction with fat necrosis and foreign-body giant cells. Biopsies taken later show loose fibrous tissue surrounding mucinous material, derived from meconium containing amorphous or granular calcification, haemosiderin deposition, histiocytes and foreign-body giant cells (Figure 46.6). Occasionally fetal hairs, derived from amniotic fluid, may be observed. Further fibrosis eventually results in the formation of a fibrous, calcified nodule.

Meconium peritonitis may extend from the peritoneal cavity into the tunica vaginalis in boys (so-called meconium vaginalitis or meconium periorchitis) [64,65]. Indeed in rare instances it appears to be confined to the tunica vaginalis, clinically occult until the late stage, when it presents as a scrotal nodule that can mimic a tumour, especially if a history of an acute episode of peritonitis in the neonatal period is not obtained [65]. Many such infants have a congenital hydrocele, presumably representing the early manifestations of meconium irritation, and this is an important

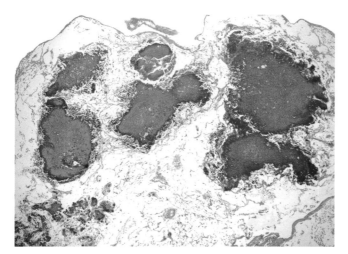

Figure 46.6 Meconium peritonitis: heavily calcified amorphous masses with a surrounding foreign-body-type giant cell inflammatory reaction.

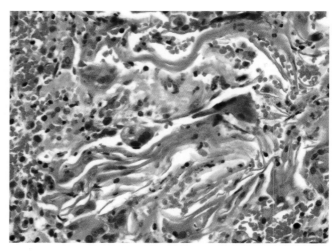

Figure 46.7 Peritoneal keratin granuloma in a patient with a ruptured benign cystic teratoma of the ovary (dermoid cyst).

clue to the correct diagnosis in young males presenting with a scrotal mass. Even rarer is extension of meconium from the abdomen into the thoracic cavity through a congenital diaphragmatic defect, a complication recognised by abnormal calcification on chest radiology [66].

Vernix caseosa peritonitis and keratin granulomatous peritonitis in women

Very rarely, a granulomatous peritonitis similar to meconium peritonitis has been described in women due to spillage of amniotic fluid into the maternal peritoneal cavity during a caesarean section, a condition referred to as maternal vernix caseosa peritonitis [67,68]. The organising inflammatory exudate may contain visible masses of cheesy yellow–white vernix caseosa on gross inspection and on histological examination the diagnosis is confirmed by the recognition of effete squamous cells and/or lanugo hairs within the granulomatous reaction. Several cases of antenatal leakage of amniotic fluid have been reported, causing maternal peritonitis characterised by an acute inflammatory response [69]. Why the condition is so uncommon, despite the frequent contamination of the maternal peritoneal cavity with amniotic fluid at caesarean section, is not clear.

Granulomatous peritonitis due to intra-abdominal keratin debris has been described after rupture of a dermoid ovarian cyst (benign cystic teratoma) (Figure 46.7) [70] and in women undergoing surgery for endometrial or ovarian adenocarcinomas with squamous differentiation [71,72]. In the latter it is important to sample the lesions thoroughly to look for neoplastic cells, because if they are absent the lesions do not appear to be associated with a poor prognosis.

Necrotic granulomatous peritoneal nodules in endometriosis

Peritoneal endometriosis can usually be recognised easily by the presence of endometrial glands and stroma, often with attendant haemosiderin-laden macrophages due to haemorrhage (see Chapter 47). However on rare occasions degeneration in endometriotic foci may give rise to small peritoneal nodules composed of a central necrotic focus surrounded by macrophages with eosinophilic or foamy cytoplasm, ceroid or haemosiderin pigment and hyaline fibrosis [73,74]. Such necrotic pseudo-xanthomatous nodules tend to be found in older women and can cause confusion with other granulomatous peritoneal lesions, especially when the underlying endometriosis is inconspicuous or absent from the lesion under study. In most cases, however, the recognition of more typical endometriosis elsewhere within the pelvis clarifies the diagnosis.

Peritonitis in the systemic connective tissue diseases

Peritonitis may occur in patients with collagen diseases, especially polyarteritis nodosa, rheumatoid arthritis and systemic lupus erythematosus (SLE), in three situations. By far the most common is secondary peritonitis after gastrointestinal ulceration or infarction, due either to vasculitis or therapy with steroids or to non-steroidal anti-inflammatory drugs. However, immunosuppressed patients with SLE may develop a primary Gram-negative bacterial peritonitis [75], and a primary low grade non-infective serositis may occur in others. This, by giving rise to painless ascites, may be the first manifestation of SLE [76,77].

Familial Mediterranean fever

Familial Mediterranean fever (recurrent hereditary polyserositis, periodic disease) is an autosomal recessive disorder occurring predominantly in Turks, Armenians, Arabs and Sephardic Jews but with occasional sporadic cases in other ethnic groups [78,79]. The disease usually presents during the first two decades of life with recurrent episodes of abdominal pain and fever, clinically indistinguishable from acute diffuse peritonitis and lasting for 24–48 hours. There may also be pleuritis, an asymmetrical arthritis of large joints, skin lesions, myalgia and, less frequently, features of pericarditis or myocarditis, hepatosplenomegaly or lymphadenopathy [80]. The most important complication of the disease is amyloidosis, causing renal failure. Although the precise pathogenesis remains unknown, the causative gene was isolated in 1997 and encodes a protein, named pyrin, that resembles cytokines, agents that can down-regulate inflammation [81]. Pyrin is expressed mainly in leukocytes and it has been postulated that inactivating mutations inhibit the anti-inflammatory activity of the protein. However, there is only limited phenotype–genotype correlation and it appears that other genetic and environmental modifiers influence the expression of the disease [78]. The drug colchicine has been shown to be very useful in the prevention of the acute inflammatory attacks in most patients and appears to prevent the development of amyloidosis [82]. Clinical manifestations of peritonitis frequently result in laparotomy being undertaken, revealing a diffuse fibrinous serositis. There are no specific histopathological features although rarely amyloid deposition may be recognised in mesenteric blood vessels, leading to the correct diagnosis.

Sclerosing peritonitis

Sclerosing peritonitis, or encapsulating peritoneal sclerosis, was originally used to describe a dense, progressive fibrosis of the peritoneal cavity in a minority of patients taking the β-adrenergic-blocking agent practolol in the 1970s [83,84]. This affected the peritoneum of the small bowel predominantly, enclosing the ileum in a shiny fibrotic 'cocoon' and leading to intestinal obstruction. Histologically the picture was one of featureless laminated fibrous tissue deposited immediately deep to the mesothelium, with mild underlying mononuclear inflammatory cell infiltrates (Figure 46.8). Despite subsequent single case reports attributing the condition to other β blockers, the evidence for this class association is unconvincing [85].

An identical clinical picture was then reported as a rare but serious complication in patients on chronic peritoneal dialysis [86] and this is now the most common clinical setting, having an approximate overall prevalence of 2.5% among peritoneal dialysis patients [87]. Prevalence increases

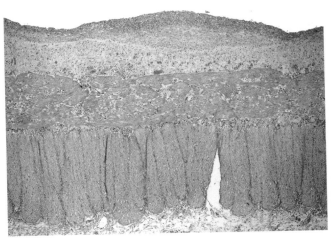

Figure 46.8 Sclerosing peritonitis affecting the colon of a patient on chronic peritoneal dialysis, showing featureless sub-mesothelial laminated fibrous tissue with mild associated chronic inflammation in the upper third of the image. The colonic muscularis propria (below) is unremarkable.

with number of years on peritoneal dialysis therapy and many cases develop after cessation of therapy. The initial stimulus for sclerosing peritonitis is most probably injury to, or irritation of, the peritoneal lining in susceptible individuals. Continual exposure to non-physiological dialysis fluid and intermittent episodes of acute bacterial peritonitis [88] are likely to be important factors. Mesothelial cells produce cytokines and growth factors in response to irritants in dialysis fluid, and this may promote angiogenesis, fibroblastic proliferation and collagen deposition [89,90]. Moreover, chronic exposure to the hypertonic, glucose-rich nature of the dialysis fluid appears to initiate a hyalinising obliterative venulopathy within the superficial vessels of the peritoneal membrane (Figure 46.9) that may aggravate the tissue damage and fibrosis [91].

Although sclerosing peritonitis typically has a chronic evolution, it may arise rapidly after treatment of acute bacterial peritonitis [92]. Reduction in acute peritonitis with improvement in aseptic techniques has not reduced the incidence of sclerosing peritonitis [93] and >80% of patients on peritoneal dialysis for >15 years do not develop sclerosing peritonitis [87]. It is therefore likely that there are other risk factors involved and multiple genetic and environmental 'hits' are required to develop the condition.

Sclerosing peritonitis has also been described in association with luteinised thecomas of the ovaries [94,95], in patients with liver cirrhosis, with and without associated peritoneal–venous shunting [96,97], rarely in patients with SLE [98] and in two children as a complication of long-standing ventriculoperitoneal shunt placement to treat hydrocephalus [99].

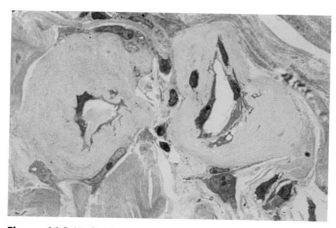

Figure 46.9 Hyalinising obliterative venulopathy within blood vessels in the superficial peritoneal membrane, in a patient on chronic peritoneal dialysis (toluidine blue).

Polyserositis

Polyserositis (Concato's disease) is a condition affecting the peritoneal, pericardial and pleural surfaces, characterised by pearly white subserosal thickening and the formation of effusions with the biochemical features of a transudate. In the peritoneum this thickening may produce either discrete plaques or an almost continuous sheet over the serosal surface of the liver, spleen and the underpart of the diaphragm, accompanied by an ascitic transudate. The aetiology and pathogenesis of polyserositis are obscure. It has been regarded by some as a complication of tuberculosis but there is no good evidence to support this view. Similar lesions are occasionally found accompanying asbestosis.

Eosinophilic peritonitis

Examples of peritonitis in which the predominant inflammatory cell type is the eosinophil leukocyte are uncommon. Some are associated with metazoal infection [100] (see above), malignant disease or eosinophilic gastroenteritis [101], but the most common setting now is in patients undergoing chronic peritoneal dialysis [102,103]. Its pathogenesis is unknown but a hypersensitivity reaction to plasticisers or other constituents of dialysis bags, lines or catheters may be responsible.

Peritoneal malakoplakia

Malakoplakia of the pelvic peritoneum has been described at caesarean section in a woman who had had a coliform urinary tract infection earlier in the pregnancy [104]. Macroscopically the pelvic organs were covered in a brown film containing brown tomato seed-like nodules and histology showed the characteristic granular histiocytes containing Michaelis–Gutmann bodies.

Sclerosing mesenteritis

Sclerosing mesenteritis is used to describe a variety of previously reported entities with similar or overlapping clinical and pathological features, including retractile mesenteritis, mesenteric panniculitis, mesenteric lipodystrophy [105], liposclerotic mesenteritis, xantho-granulomatous mesenteritis and mesenteric lipogranuloma. It represents a rare fibrosing tumefactive process primarily involving the small bowel mesentery, with variable degrees of associated inflammation and fat necrosis, reflecting the spectrum of descriptive terms applied. The aetiology is unknown. The condition is more common in males and a wide age range is affected, with the median in the seventh decade [105,106]. The clinical presentation is variable. Non-specific symptoms of abdominal pain, vomiting, pyrexia or weight loss are prominent in some whereas in others the inflammatory process is clinically silent, the condition being recognised only during routine clinical abdominal examination or at laparotomy for some unrelated reason. A minority of cases present at a late stage, when florid post-inflammatory mesenteric fibrosis produces intestinal obstruction or mesenteric venous thrombosis. Progression from the inflammatory to the sclerotic form is not inevitable, however, and some cases show apparent complete spontaneous resolution.

The macroscopic appearances in the inflammatory phase of sclerosing mesenteritis are of ill-circumscribed oedematous or rubbery thickening of the mesentery or omentum, most notably at the root of the small intestinal mesentery. The extent of involvement varies. In some cases the condition affects a segment of the mesentery diffusely whereas in others one or more discrete inflammatory mesenteric masses are found. Cystic spaces containing liquefied fat or chyle may be seen, the latter resulting from lymphatic obstruction. Later, in the fibrotic phase, there is sclerotic thickening of the mesentery with retraction and distortion of the bowel and formation of adhesions. The histological appearances in the early stages of the disease are those of mesenteric fat necrosis with neutrophil polymorphs, clusters of lipophages, foreign body-type giant cells and cholesterol clefts. There is an overlying serositis with reactive mesothelial hyperplasia. The more commonly encountered later stage demonstrates pauci-cellular dense mesenteric fibrosis and variable degrees of non-specific chronic inflammation, fat necrosis and calcification (Figure 46.10a). Lymphocytic venulitis, often associated with complete luminal occlusion (obliterative phlebitis), is identifiable in many cases (Figure 46.10b). Secondary ischaemic change may be evident in adjacent bowel. The differential diagnoses to consider on morphology include mesenteric fibromatosis,

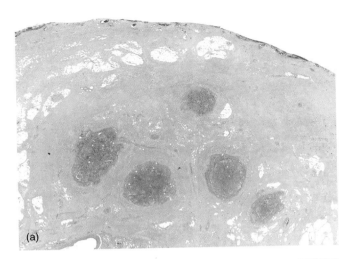

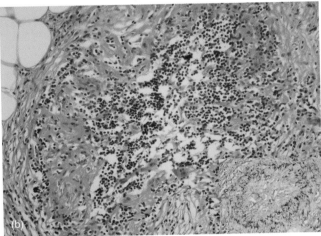

Figure 46.10 (a) Sclerosing mesenteritis: low power view showing lymph nodes entrapped within dense mesenteric fibrosis. (b) A focus of obliterative phlebitis with complete luminal occlusion, demonstrated by orcein stain for elastin (inset).

gastrointestinal stromal tumour and inflammatory myofibroblastic tumour (see Chapter 47).

Neoplastic infiltration of the mesentery may lead to mesenteric fibrosis resembling sclerosing mesenteritis. Any form of malignancy can produce the effect but the mimicry is greatest in cases of well differentiated endocrine carcinomas of the midgut (so-called carcinoid tumours), which may elicit a particularly dense fibrotic reaction when they invade the mesentery, leading to retraction and kinking [107]. This mesenteric fibrosis, along with a distinctive elastic vascular sclerosis of the mesenteric blood vessels induced by such endocrine tumours, may result in intestinal ischaemia or even frank infarction [108,109]. When involving the pancreatic region, sclerosing mesenteritis can closely mimic pancreatic cancer [110]. Given the often marked desmoplastic stromal reaction and low cellularity

of typical pancreatic ductal carcinoma, endoscopically derived biopsy material may not allow confident distinction and a high index of suspicion must be maintained before issuing a diagnosis of malignancy. A lymphoma, of Hodgkin's or non-Hodgkin's type, can also be difficult to confidently distinguish from sclerosing mesenteritis, especially on a biopsy specimen, and requires the judicious use of ancillary immunohistochemical and/or molecular assays if any suspicious lymphoid population is identified. There have been several individual reports of lymphomas and sclerosing mesenteritis arising separately in the same patient, associated with a poor prognosis [111,112].

Occasional examples of sclerosing mesenteritis are associated with a more widespread panniculitis such as the Pfeifer–Weber–Christian syndrome (relapsing non-suppurative nodular panniculitis) [113], whereas in other cases the condition extends into the retro-peritoneum to overlap with idiopathic retro-peritoneal fibrosis [114,115]. The relationship between sclerosing mesenteritis and the family of IgG4-related sclerosing disorders, including idiopathic retro-peritoneal fibrosis, has been investigated [106,111,116]. Lymphocytic venulitis is a morphological feature shared with this group of conditions [111]. Although based on small numbers of cases examined, it would appear that a minority of cases of sclerosing mesenteritis shows significant infiltration by IgG4-positive plasma cells, or increased IgG4:total IgG immunostaining ratio, raising the possibility that a subset is IgG4 mediated [106,111].

In the absence of secondary intestinal complications and with the confident exclusion of any underlying malignancy, sclerosing mesenteritis usually follows a benign course [105,106,117]. Aggressive surgery is therefore not indicated in the treatment of this condition, with medical therapy in the form of oral steroids and tamoxifen more appropriate, and surgical intervention reserved for complications [106,117].

Fat necrosis after pancreatitis

Intra-abdominal leakage of pancreatic enzymes in pancreatitis may lead to fat necrosis, not only of the peri-pancreatic tissues but also of the omentum, mesenteries or retroperitoneum. Although this is easily recognised both macroscopically and microscopically in the acute phase, it may be more difficult later, when the original pancreatitis has settled, but the areas of fat necrosis remain to become organised into markedly fibrotic tumour-like masses. Often there is calcification but this is not specific for fat necrosis resulting from pancreatitis. One feature that may point to a diagnosis of pancreatic fat necrosis is the presence of strongly birefringent crystalloids of saponified free fatty acids within the ghost adipocytes, often accompanied by basophilic debris [118]. Such crystalloids are not found in traumatic fat necrosis.

References

1. Levison ME, Pontzer RE. *Peritonitis and other intra-abdominal infections.* In: Mandell GL, Douglas RG Jr, Bennett JE (eds), *Principles and Practice of Infectious Diseases*, 2nd edn. New York: Wiley, 1985: 476.
2. Working Party of the British Society for Antimicrobial Chemotherapy. Diagnosis and management of peritonitis in continuous ambulatory peritoneal dialysis. *Lancet* 1987;**i**:845.
3. Ellis H, Adair HM. Bile peritonitis – a report of fifteen patients. *Postgrad Med J* 1974;**50**:713.
4. Garcia-Tsao G. Spontaneous bacterial peritonitis: a historical perspective. *J Hepatol* 2004;**41**:522.
5. Conn HO. Spontaneous peritonitis and bacteremia in Laennec's cirrhosis caused by enteric organisms. A relatively common but rarely recognized syndrome. *Ann Intern Med* 1964;**60**:568.
6. Sheer TA, Runyon BA. Spontaneous bacterial peritonitis. *Dig Dis* 2005;**23**:39.
7. Runyon BA, Squier S, Borzio M. Translocation of gut bacteria in rats with cirrhosis to mesenteric lymph nodes partially explains the pathogenesis of spontaneous bacterial peritonitis. *J Hepatol* 1994;**21**:792.
8. Runyon BA. Patients with deficient ascitic fluid opsonic activity are predisposed to spontaneous bacterial peritonitis. *Hepatology* 1988;**8**:632.
9. Rimola A, Garcia-Tsao G, Navasa M, et al., International Ascites Club. Diagnosis, treatment and prophylaxis of spontaneous bacterial peritonitis: a consensus document. *J Hepatol* 2000;**32**:142.
10. Ghassemi S, Garcia-Tsao G. Prevention and treatment of infections in patients with cirrhosis. *Best Pract Res Clin Gastroenterol* 2007;**21**:77.
11. Baker WN, Mackie DB, Newcombe JF. Diagnostic paracentesis in the acute abdomen. *BMJ* 1967;**iii**:146.
12. Stewart RJ, Gupta RK, Purdie GL, Isbister WH. Fine-catheter aspiration cytology of peritoneal cavity improves decision-making about difficult cases of acute abdominal pain. *Lancet* 1986;**ii**:1414.
13. Evans C, Rashid A, Rosenberg IL, Pollock AV. An appraisal of peritoneal lavage in the diagnosis of the acute abdomen. *Brit J Surg* 1975;**62**:119.
14. Ellis H. *Intestinal Obstruction.* New York: Appleton-Century-Crofts, 1982.
15. Altemeier WA, Culbertson WR, Fullen WD, Shook CD. Intra-abdominal abscesses. *Am J Surg* 1973;**125**:70.
16. Sanders RC. The changing epidemiology of subphrenic abscess and its clinical and radiological consequences. *Br J Surg* 1970;**57**:449.
17. Mackenzie M, Fordyce J, Young DG. Subphrenic abscess in children. *Br J Surg* 1975;**62**:305.
18. Wang SM, Wilson SE. Subphrenic abscess. The new epidemiology. *Arch Surg* 1977;**112**:934.
19. Ellis H. Wound repair. Reaction of the peritoneum to injury. *Ann R Coll Surg Engl* 1978;**60**:219.
20. Whitaker D, Papadimitriou JM, Walters M. The mesothelium: its fibrinolytic properties. *J Pathol* 1982;**136**:291.
21. Ryan GB, Grobety J, Majno G. Mesothelial injury and recovery. *Am J Pathol* 1973;**71**:93.
22. Buckman RF, Woods M, Sargent L, Gervin AS. A unifying pathogenetic mechanism in the etiology of intraperitoneal adhesions. *J Surg Res* 1976;**20**:1.
23. Ellis H. The cause and prevention of postoperative intraperitoneal adhesions. *Surg Gynecol Obstet* 1971;**133**:497.
24. Menzies D, Ellis H. Intestinal obstruction from adhesions – how big is the problem? *Ann R Coll Surg Engl* 1990;**72**:60.
25. Kapoor VK, Sharma LK. Abdominal tuberculosis. *Br J Surg* 1988;**75**:2.
26. Palmer KR, Patil DH, Basran GS, Riordan JF, Silk DB. Abdominal tuberculosis in urban Britain – a common disease. *Gut* 1985;**26**:1296.
27. Akpolat T. Tuberculous peritonitis. *Perit Dial Int* 2009;**29**(suppl 2):S166.
28. Verhave JC, van Altena R, Wijnands MJ, Roerdink HT. Tuberculous peritonitis during infliximab therapy. *Neth J Med* 2008;**66**:77.
29. Manohar A, Simjee AE, Haffejee AA, Pettengell KE. Symptoms and investigative findings in 145 patients with tuberculous peritonitis diagnosed by peritoneoscopy and biopsy over a five year period. *Gut* 1990;**31**:1130.
30. Elmore RG, Li AJ. Peritoneal tuberculosis mimicking advanced-stage epithelial ovarian cancer. *Obstet Gynecol* 2007;**110**:1417.
31. Schofield PF. Abdominal tuberculosis. *Gut* 1985;**26**:1275.
32. Dawson JM, O'Riordan B, Chopra S. Ovarian actinomycosis presenting as acute peritonitis. *Aust N Z J Surg* 1992;**62**:161.
33. Berardi RS. Abdominal actinomycosis. *Surg Gynecol Obstet* 1979;**149**:257.
34. Li SY, Yu KW, Yang WC, Chen TW, Lin CC. Nocardia peritonitis – a case report and literature review. *Perit Dial Int* 2008;**28**:544.
35. Matuszkiewicz-Rowinska J. Update on fungal peritonitis and its treatment. *Perit Dial Int* 2009;**29**(suppl 2):S161.
36. Bayer AS, Blumenkrantz MJ, Montgomerie JZ, Galpin JE, Coburn JW, Guze LB. Candida peritonitis. Report of 22 cases and review of the English literature. *Am J Med* 1976;**61**:832.
37. Solomkin JS, Flohr AB, Quie PG, Simmons RL. The role of *Candida* in intraperitoneal infections. *Surgery* 1980;**88**:524.
38. Albert-Braun S, Venema F, Bausch J, Hunfeld KP, Schafer V. *Cryptococcus neoformans* peritonitis in a patient with alcoholic cirrhosis: case report and review of the literature. *Infection* 2005;**33**:282.
39. Phillips P, Ford B. Peritoneal coccidioidomycosis: case report and review. *Clin Infect Dis* 2000;**30**:971.
40. Perez-Lasala G, Nolan RL, Chapman SW, Achord JL. Peritoneal blastomycosis. *Am J Gastroenterol* 1991;**86**:357.
41. Pearson RD, Irons RP, Sr., Irons RP, Jr. Chronic pelvic peritonitis due to the pinworm *Enterobius vermicularis*. *JAMA* 1981;**245**:1340.
42. Cooray GH, Panabokke RG. Granulomatous peritonitis caused by ascaris ova. *Trans R Soc Trop Med Hyg* 1960;**54**:358.
43. Rushovich AM, Randall EL, Caprini JA, Westenfelder GO. Omental anisakiasis: a rare mimic of acute appendicitis. *Am J Clin Pathol* 1983;**80**:517.
44. Konstantinidou E, Alexiou C, Demonakou M, Sakellaridis T, Fotopoulos A, Antsaklis G. Schistosomal peritonitis: a rare cause of acute abdomen. *Trans R Soc Trop Med Hyg* 2009;**103**:1068.
45. Beyrouti MI, Beyrouti R, Abbes I, et al. [Acute rupture of hydatid cysts in the peritoneum: 17 cases.] *Presse Med* 2004;**33**:378.
46. Ryan GB, Grobety J, Majno G. Postoperative peritoneal adhesions. A study of the mechanisms. *Am J Pathol* 1971;**65**:117.
47. Duron JJ, Olivier L. Foreign bodies and intraperitoneal postoperative adhesions. *J Long Term Eff Med Implants* 1997;**7**:235.
48. Crocker PR, Doyle DV, Levison DA. A practical method for the identification of particulate and crystalline material in paraffin – embedded tissue specimens. *J Pathol* 1980;**131**:165.
49. Davies JD, Ansell ID. Food-starch granulomatous peritonitis. *J Clin Pathol* 1983;**36**:435.

50. Veress B, Alafuzoff I, Juliusson G. Granulomatous peritonitis and appendicitis of food starch origin. *Gut* 1991;**32**:718.

51. Karanikas ID, Kakoulidis DD, Gouvas ZT, Hartley JE, Koundourakis SS. Barium peritonitis: a rare complication of upper gastrointestinal contrast investigation. *Postgrad Med J* 1997;**73**:297.

52. Kay S. Tissue reaction to barium sulfate contrast medium; histopathologic study. *AMA Arch Pathol* 1954;**57**:279.

53. Levison DA, Crocker PR, Smith A, Blackshaw AJ, Bartram CI. Varied light and scanning electron microscopic appearances of barium sulphate in smears and histological sections. *J Clin Pathol* 1984;**37**:481.

54. Postlethwait RW, Howard HL, Schanher PW. Comparison of tissue reaction to talc and modified starch glove powder. *Surgery* 1949;**25**:22.

55. Neely J, Davies JD. Starch granulomatosis of the peritoneum. *BMJ* 1971;**iii**:625.

56. Davies JD, Neely J. The histopathology of peritoneal starch granulomas. *J Pathol* 1972;**107**:265.

57. Edlich RF, Long WB 3rd, Gubler DK, et al. Dangers of cornstarch powder on medical gloves: seeking a solution. *Ann Plast Surg* 2009;**63**:111.

58. Tinker MA, Burdman D, Deysine M, Teicher I, Platt N, Aufses AH Jr. Granulomatous peritonitis due to cellulose fibers from disposable surgical fabrics: laboratory investigation and clinical implications. *Ann Surg* 1974;**180**:831.

59. Thompson NP, Scheuer PJ, Dick R, Hamilton G, Burroughs AK. Intraperitoneal ivalon mimicking peritoneal malignancy after plugged percutaneous liver biopsy. *Gut* 1993;**34**:1635.

60. Warren CW, Wyatt JI. Gallstones split at laparoscopic cholecystectomy: a new cause of intraperitoneal granulomas. *J Clin Pathol* 1996;**49**:84.

61. Forouhar F. Meconium peritonitis. Pathology, evolution, and diagnosis. *Am J Clin Pathol* 1982;**78**:208.

62. Tibboel D, Molenaar JC. Meconium peritonitis – a retrospective, prognostic analysis of 69 patients. *Z Kinderchir* 1984;**39**:25.

63. Tibboel D, Gaillard JL, Molenaar JC. The importance of mesenteric vascular insufficiency in meconium peritonitis. *Hum Pathol* 1986;**17**:411.

64. Dehner LP, Scott D, Stocker JT. Meconium periorchitis: a clinicopathologic study of four cases with a review of the literature. *Hum Pathol* 1986;**17**:807.

65. Regev RH, Markovich O, Arnon S, Bauer S, Dolfin T, Litmanovitz I. Meconium periorchitis: intrauterine diagnosis and neonatal outcome: case reports and review of the literature. *J Perinatol* 2009;**29**:585.

66. Patole S, Whitehall J, Almonte R, Stalewski H, Lee-Tannock A, Murphy A. Meconium thorax: a case report and review of literature. *Am J Perinatol* 1998;**15**:53.

67. Selo-Ojeme D. Vernix caseosa peritonitis. *J Obstet Gynaecol* 2007;**27**:660.

68. George E, Leyser S, Zimmer HL, Simonowitz DA, Agress RL, Nordin DD. Vernix caseosa peritonitis. An infrequent complication of cesarean section with distinctive histopathologic features. *Am J Clin Pathol* 1995;**103**:681.

69. Davis JR, Miller HS, Feng JD. Vernix caseosa peritonitis: report of two cases with antenatal onset. *Am J Clin Pathol* 1998;**109**:320.

70. Waxman M, Boyce JG. Intraperitoneal rupture of benign cystic ovarian teratoma. *Obstet Gynecol* 1976;**48**(1 suppl):9S.

71. Kim KR, Scully RE. Peritoneal keratin granulomas with carcinomas of endometrium and ovary and atypical polypoid adenomyoma of endometrium. A clinicopathological analysis of 22 cases. *Am J Surg Pathol* 1990;**14**:925.

72. van der Horst C, Evans AJ. Peritoneal keratin granulomas complicating endometrial carcinoma: a report of two cases and review of the literature. *Int J Gynecol Cancer* 2008;**18**:549.

73. Carey M, Kirk ME. Necrotic pseudoxanthomatous nodules of the omentum and peritoneum: a peculiar reaction to endometriotic cyst contents. *Obstet Gynecol* 1993;**82**(4 Part 2 suppl):650.

74. Clement PB, Young RH, Scully RE. Necrotic pseudoxanthomatous nodules of ovary and peritoneum in endometriosis. *Am J Surg Pathol* 1988;**12**:390.

75. Lipsky PE, Hardin JA, Schour L, Plotz PH. Spontaneous peritonitis and systemic lupus erythematosus. Importance of accurate diagnosis of gram-positive bacterial infections. *JAMA* 1975;**232**:929.

76. Jones PE, Rawcliffe P, White N, Segal AW. Painless ascites in systemic lupus erythematosus. *BMJ* 1977;**i**:1513.

77. Weinstein PJ, Noyer CM. Rapid onset of massive ascites as the initial presentation of systemic lupus erythematosus. *Am J Gastroenterol* 2000;**95**:302.

78. Orbach H, Ben-Chetrit E. Familial mediterranean fever – a review and update. *Minerva Med* 2001;**92**:421.

79. Cook GC. Periodic disease, recurrent polyserositis, familial Mediterranean fever, or simply 'FMF'. *Q J Med* 1986;**60**:819.

80. Sohar E, Gafni J, Pras M, Heller H. Familial Mediterranean fever. A survey of 470 cases and review of the literature. *Am J Med* 1967;**43**:227.

81. The International FMF Consortium. Ancient missense mutations in a new member of the *RoRet* gene family are likely to cause familial Mediterranean fever. *Cell* 1997;**90**:797.

82. Zemer D, Pras M, Sohar E, Modan M, Cabili S, Gafni J. Colchicine in the prevention and treatment of the amyloidosis of familial Mediterranean fever. *N Engl J Med* 1986;**314**:1001.

83. Brown P, Baddeley H, Read AE, Davies JD, McGarry J. Sclerosing peritonitis, an unusual reaction to a beta-adrenergic-blocking drug (practolol). *Lancet* 1974;**ii**:1477.

84. Marshall AJ, Baddeley H, Barritt DW, et al. Practolol peritonitis. A study of 16 cases and a survey of small bowel function in patients taking beta adrenergic blockers. *Q J Med* 1977;**46**:135.

85. Marigold JH, Pounder RE, Pemberton J, Thompson RP. Propranolol, oxprenolol, and sclerosing peritonitis. *BMJ (Clin Res Ed)* 1982;**284**:870.

86. Bradley JA, McWhinnie DL, Hamilton DN, et al. Sclerosing obstructive peritonitis after continuous ambulatory peritoneal dialysis. *Lancet* 1983;**ii**:113.

87. Kawanishi H, Kawaguchi Y, Fukui H, et al. Encapsulating peritoneal sclerosis in Japan: a prospective, controlled, multicenter study. *Am J Kidney Dis* 2004;**44**:729.

88. Nakamoto H, Kawaguchi Y, Suzuki H. Encapsulating peritoneal sclerosis in patients undergoing continuous ambulatory peritoneal dialysis in Japan. *Adv Perit Dial* 2002;**18**:119.

89. Topley N, Williams JD. Effect of peritoneal dialysis on cytokine production by peritoneal cells. *Blood Purif* 1996;**14**:188.

90. Ha H, Cha MK, Choi HN, Lee HB. Effects of peritoneal dialysis solutions on the secretion of growth factors and extracellular matrix proteins by human peritoneal mesothelial cells. *Perit Dial Int* 2002;**22**:171.

91. Williams JD, Craig KJ, Topley N, et al. Morphologic changes in the peritoneal membrane of patients with renal disease. *J Am Soc Nephrol* 2002;**13**:470.

92. Courtney AE, Doherty CC. Fulminant sclerosing peritonitis immediately following acute bacterial peritonitis. *Nephrol Dial Transplant* 2006;**21**:532.

93. Rigby RJ, Hawley CM. Sclerosing peritonitis: the experience in Australia. *Nephrol Dial Transplant* 1998;**13**:154.

94. Clement PB, Young RH, Hanna W, Scully RE. Sclerosing peritonitis associated with luteinized thecomas of the ovary. A clinicopathological analysis of six cases. *Am J Surg Pathol* 1994;**18**:1.

95. Staats PN, McCluggage WG, Clement PB, Young RH. Luteinized thecomas (thecomatosis) of the type typically associated with sclerosing peritonitis: a clinical, histopathologic, and immunohistochemical analysis of 27 cases. *Am J Surg Pathol* 2008;**32**:1273.

96. Cudazzo E, Lucchini A, Puviani PP, et al. [Sclerosing peritonitis. A complication of LeVeen peritoneovenous shunt.] *Minerva Chir* 1999;**54**:809.

97. Yamamoto S, Sato Y, Takeishi T, Kobayashi T, Hatakeyama K. Sclerosing encapsulating peritonitis in two patients with liver cirrhosis. *J Gastroenterol* 2004;**39**:172.

98. Odama UO, Shih DJ, Korbet SM. Sclerosing peritonitis and systemic lupus erythematosus: a report of two cases. *Perit Dial Int* 1999;**19**:160.

99. Sigaroudinia MO, Baillie C, Ahmed S, Mallucci C. Sclerosing encapsulating peritonitis – a rare complication of ventriculoperitoneal shunts. *J Pediatr Surg* 2008;**43**:E31.

100. Lambroza A, Dannenberg AJ. Eosinophilic ascites due to hyperinfection with *Strongyloides stercoralis*. *Am J Gastroenterol* 1991;**86**:89.

101. Yun MY, Cho YU, Park IS, et al. Eosinophilic gastroenteritis presenting as small bowel obstruction: a case report and review of the literature. *World J Gastroenterol* 2007;**13**:1758.

102. Gokal R, Ramos JM, Ward MK, Kerr DN. 'Eosinophilic' peritonitis in continuous ambulatory peritoneal dialysis (CAPD). *Clin Nephrol* 1981;**15**:328.

103. Quinlan C, Cantwell M, Rees L. Eosinophilic peritonitis in children on chronic peritoneal dialysis. *Pediatr Nephrol* 2010;**25**:517.

104. Rose G, Morrison EA, Kirkham N, Machling R. Malakoplakia of the pelvic peritoneum in pregnancy. Case report. *Br J Obstet Gynaecol* 1985;**92**:170.

105. Emory TS, Monihan JM, Carr NJ, Sobin LH. Sclerosing mesenteritis, mesenteric panniculitis and mesenteric lipodystrophy: a single entity? *Am J Surg Pathol* 1997;**21**:392.

106. Akram S, Pardi DS, Schaffner JA, Smyrk TC. Sclerosing mesenteritis: clinical features, treatment, and outcome in ninety-two patients. *Clin Gastroenterol Hepatol* 2007;**5**:589; quiz 523.

107. O'Rourke MG, Lancashire RP, Vattoune JR. Carcinoid of the small intestine. *Aust N Z J Surg* 1986;**56**:405.

108. Anthony PP, Drury RA. Elastic vascular sclerosis of mesenteric blood vessels in argentaffin carcinoma. *J Clin Pathol* 1970;**23**:110.

109. Strobbe L, D'Hondt E, Ramboer C, Ceuppens H, Hinnekens P, Verhamme M. Ileal carcinoid tumors and intestinal ischemia. *Hepatogastroenterology* 1994;**41**:499.

110. Scudiere JR, Shi C, Hruban RH, et al. Sclerosing mesenteritis involving the pancreas: a mimicker of pancreatic cancer. *Am J Surg Pathol* 2010;**34**:447.

111. Chen TS, Montgomery EA. Are tumefactive lesions classified as sclerosing mesenteritis a subset of IgG4-related sclerosing disorders? *J Clin Pathol* 2008;**61**:1093.

112. Hiridis S, Hadgigeorgiou R, Karakitsos D, Karabinis A. Sclerosing mesenteritis affecting the small and the large intestine in a male patient with non-Hodgkin lymphoma: a case presentation and review of the literature. *J Med Case Reports* 2008;**2**:388.

113. Milner RD, Mitchinson MJ. Systemic Weber–Christian disease. *J Clin Pathol* 1965;**18**:150.

114. Binder SC, Deterling RA Jr, Mahoney SA, Patterson JF, Wolfe HJ. Systemic idiopathic fibrosis. Report of a case of the concomitant occurrence of retractile mesenteritis and retroperitoneal fibrosis. *Am J Surg* 1972;**124**:422.

115. Lim CS, Singh Ranger G, Tibrewal S, Jani B, Jeddy TA, Lafferty K. Sclerosing mesenteritis presenting with small bowel obstruction and subsequent retroperitoneal fibrosis. *Eur J Gastroenterol Hepatol* 2006;**18**:1285.

116. Belghiti H, Cazals-Hatem D, Couvelard A, Guedj N, Bedossa P. [Sclerosing mesenteritis: can it be a IgG4 dysimmune disease?] *Ann Pathol* 2009;**29**:468.

117. Durst AL, Freund H, Rosenmann E, Birnbaum D. Mesenteric panniculitis: review of the literature and presentation of cases. *Surgery* 1977;**81**:203.

118. Keen CE, Buk SJ, Brady K, Levison DA. Fat necrosis presenting as obscure abdominal mass: birefringent saponified fatty acid crystalloids as a clue to diagnosis. *J Clin Pathol* 1994;**47**:1028.

CHAPTER 47

Tumours and tumour-like lesions of the peritoneum

Richard L. Attanoos
University Hospital Llandough, Penarth, UK

Introduction

The peritoneum is site to a wide spectrum of tumours and tumour-like conditions. The nomenclature of many of these conditions has evolved over recent years but there persist many morphological and immunophenotypic similarities between the tumours and non-neoplastic lesions.

Primary tumours of the peritoneum are regarded as those with primary peritoneal manifestation in the absence of a visceral origin. They may be classified according to their likely histogenetic cell of origin: mesothelial, subserosal mesenchymal and uncertain (from putative uncommitted pluripotent stem cells). In each compartment there are reported tumours with biological behaviour ranging from benign to malignant. The World Health Organization (WHO) formulated a classification of tumours of the peritoneum in 2003 [1]. Since that time more conditions have emerged and, although there is no perfect classification scheme for tumours of the peritoneum, Table 47.1 summarises a pragmatic approach.

Tumour-like lesions arising in the peritoneum encompass a variety of cysts of the omentum and mesentery, pseudo-tumours, as well as diverse metaplastic conditions. Some are developmental, others post-inflammatory in nature, but for some the precise nature of the lesion is not known. These tumour-like conditions may mimic both primary and secondary peritoneal neoplasms and therefore accurate diagnosis is important. This chapter presents a review of the various conditions with particular emphasis on the diagnostic features and the role of ancillary investigations that may be of value in discriminating between them.

Mesothelial hyperplasia and mesothelial tumours

Mesothelial hyperplasia

The normal peritoneum is lined by flat, bland and monotonous mesothelial cells with underlying fibrovascular connective tissue devoid of inflammation. Any inflammatory process or serosal injury may induce mesothelial proliferations that range from mild cuboidal cell change to florid multi-layering with cytonuclear atypia and mitoses [2,3]. The presence of reactive mesothelial hyperplasia is common in association with pelvic inflammatory disease, endometriosis [4], hernial sacs or ascites, or in people with abdominal neoplasia [5]. Reactive mesothelial hyperplasia must be distinguished from müllerian endosalpingiosis or endometriosis, and this is usually straightforward on morphological grounds alone. Reactive papillary mesothelial hyperplasia (Figure 47.1) requires distinction from well differentiated papillary mesothelioma, malignant mesothelioma and serous papillary müllerian neoplasms. Consideration of the clinical factors is essential. Cytological features such as multi-nucleation, pleomorphism and mitoses, and the presence or absence of inflammation, have been found to be insufficient for the confident separation of reactive and malignant mesothelial proliferations [6]. The most reliable criterion of mesothelial malignancy is the presence of frank stromal invasion into subserosal mesenchymal tissue and fat. This morphological feature is accentuated by immunohistochemical labelling with broad-spectrum cytokeratin. Morphologically, additional features

Morson and Dawson's Gastrointestinal Pathology, Fifth Edition. Edited by Neil A. Shepherd, Bryan F. Warren,
Geraint T. Williams, Joel K. Greenson, Gregory Y. Lauwers and Marco R. Novelli.
© 2013 Blackwell Publishing Ltd. Published 2013 by Blackwell Publishing Ltd.

Table 47.1 Classification of primary peritoneal tumours

Mesothelial tumours
Adenomatoid tumour
Well differentiated papillary mesothelioma
Multicystic mesothelioma
Diffuse malignant mesothelioma

Epithelial tumours
Primary peritoneal müllerian borderline tumour (specify type)
Primary peritoneal müllerian adenocarcinoma (specify type)

Subserosal mesenchymal tumours
Solitary fibrous tumour
Desmoid tumour
Inflammatory myofibroblastic tumour/omental mesenteric myxoid 'hamartoma'
Vascular neoplasms
Epithelioid haemangio-endothelioma
Angiosarcoma
Synovial sarcoma

Other tumours
Gastrointestinal stromal tumour
Desmoplastic small round cell tumour
Lymphoma

Primary effusion lymphoma

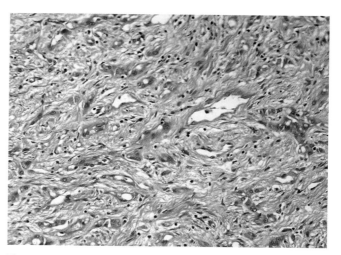

Figure 47.2 Adenomatoid tumour comprising vacuolated epithelioid mesothelial cells forming tubular structures in a loose matrix.

pressed in neoplastic mesothelium, whereas desmin is preferentially expressed in reactive mesothelium [7]. Equivocal cases should be termed 'atypical mesothelial proliferation' and further biopsies sought to determine the underlying disease process.

Nodular histiocytic mesothelial hyperplasia

Nodular histiocytic/mesothelial hyperplasia (NHMH) is a rare tumour-like condition seen in the peritoneum and in hernial sacs [8]. It is composed of a mixture of histiocytes, reactive mesothelial cells, lymphocytes and fibrin. The lesions are considered to be related to local irritation and inflammation. Macroscopically, these lesions may mimic malignancy. Pathologically, NHMH may also mimic metastatic carcinoma, haematological malignancy and Langerhans cell histiocytosis. Immunohistochemistry confirms the histiocytic (CD68+) and mesothelial (AE1/3+, calretinin+) cell components. Epithelial markers such carcinoembryonic antigen (CEA) and Ber-EP4 should be negative.

Adenomatoid tumour

Adenomatoid tumour, formerly termed 'benign mesothelioma', is a localised benign mesothelial proliferation primarily arising from the male or female genital tract [9]. Occasional cases have been reported in the omentum and mesentery, and rarely in extra-abdominal sites. There is no association with asbestos exposure. Adenomatoid tumours are nearly always incidental findings, occurring as small (<10 mm), grey–white or tan-coloured nodules. Microscopically, they are composed of a proliferation of epithelioid mesothelial cells arranged in solid cellular sheets, gland-like structures, trabeculae or microcysts (Figure 47.2). The

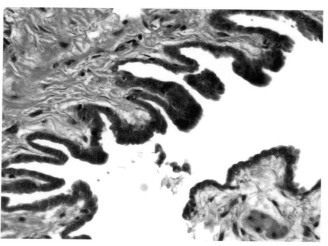

Figure 47.1 Reactive papillary mesothelial hyperplasia: the mesothelial unilayer comprises cuboidal cells with small nucleoli.

favouring malignancy are delicate papillary mesothelial proliferations and necrosis, when devoid of inflammation and outwith the setting of tuberculosis or connective tissue disease.

Immunohistochemistry has an important role in distinguishing reactive and neoplastic mesothelial proliferations in serous cytology and histological samples. Epithelial membrane antigen and nuclear p53 are preferentially ex-

intervening stroma may be fibrotic or contain smooth muscle. The mesothelial cells may exhibit cytoplasmic vacuolation and a signet ring-like appearance, whereas in more cystic lesions they may be flattened and mimic a vasoformative neoplasm. Some adenomatoid tumours have elements akin to well differentiated papillary mesothelioma [10], others may be reminiscent of multicystic mesothelioma, outlining their common histogenesis [11], but cytonuclear atypia is not seen. The mesothelial nature of the lesional cells may be confirmed by immunohistochemistry (calretinin, cytokeratin 5/6) and, if necessary, by electron microscopy (long slender microvilli, numerous tight junctions).

Adenomatoid tumours are always benign. However, they may have ill-defined margins and appear infiltrative in nature. The differential diagnosis includes metastatic adenocarcinoma, vascular tumours (particularly epithelioid haemangioendothelioma) and localised malignant mesothelioma. An immunohistochemical panel including the above-stated mesothelial markers together with epithelial/carcinoma markers (CEA, Ber-EP4) and vascular markers (CD31, CD34) greatly facilitates the differential diagnosis. Although microcystic or adenomatoid areas may be seen in malignant mesothelioma, this is almost always a diffuse serosal neoplasm. Moreover, marked cytonuclear atypia, mitoses and necrosis are not features of benign adenomatoid tumour.

Well differentiated papillary mesothelioma

This is an uncommon tumour arising predominantly in the female peritoneum or less frequently in the tunica vaginalis testis in men [12]. More recently similar tumours have been reported in the pericardium and pleura [13]. There is no epidemiological evidence linking well differentiated papillary mesothelioma with asbestos, although a history of asbestos exposure has been reported in anecdotal cases [13,14]. Clinically most cases are asymptomatic and incidental findings, although occasionally torsion of pedunculated tumours may cause abdominal pain. In general, well differentiated papillary mesotheliomas follow either a benign indolent or low grade malignant course with progressive disease extending over a 5- to 10-year period [15]. Individuals with localised tumours at presentation have a more favourable prognosis than those with multifocal or multi-cavitary disease. Macroscopically, the tumours often appear as multiple, firm, pale nodules <10mm over the pelvic peritoneum or omentum. Microscopically, they have a distinctive papillary architecture and a superficial growth pattern (Figure 47.3). The single-layered epithelioid mesothelial cells often contain large subnuclear vacuoles, show mild atypia and have inconspicuous mitotic activity. The papillary cores are mostly fibrovascular or hyaline; some are inflammatory with foam cells, others myxoid in nature

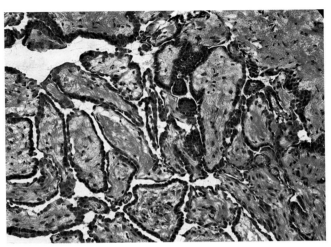

Figure 47.3 Well differentiated papillary mesothelioma: delicate mesothelial cell proliferation with distinct fibrous stroma.

[16]. Psammoma bodies may be seen. Occasional cases may show superficial peritoneal fat invasion, although this must not be a prominent feature and is probably a poor prognostic sign heralding a progressive course. In such cases there is dispute about whether well differentiated papillary mesothelioma undergoes malignant transformation anew or whether the underlying disease represents genuine diffuse malignant mesothelioma.

The differential diagnosis includes reactive papillary mesothelial hyperplasia, diffuse malignant mesothelioma and a spectrum of serous müllerian neoplasms, as well as metastatic peritoneal carcinomatosis from a variety of primary papillary adenocarcinomas. Immunohistochemistry is of use in confirming the mesothelial nature of the lesion (with expression of broad-spectrum cytokeratins and the mesothelial markers calretinin and cytokeratin 5/6), but is of limited value in resolving the differential diagnosis further. One exception is that epithelial membrane antigen (EMA) is positive (with membranous expression) in well differentiated papillary mesothelioma and malignant mesothelioma and often negative in wholly reactive mesothelial proliferations. The clinical and macroscopic features are important. Rapidly progressive disease points to an underlying malignant neoplasm. Diffuse peritoneal disease is frequently seen in disseminated metastatic carcinoma, serous peritoneal carcinoma and malignant mesothelioma, but it is uncommon for well differentiated papillary mesothelioma to exhibit such a diffuse appearance. Morphologically, it is recognised that genuine malignant mesotheliomas may exhibit areas that are essentially indistinguishable from typical well differentiated papillary mesotheliomas. Although the presence of solid elements, malignant mesenchymal components or florid frank invasion of viscera points to the diagnosis of malignant mesothelioma, such features are often not obvious. For this reason caution should be exercised in making a confident diagnosis of either condition on small biopsies and diagnosis based on cytology alone should be avoided. The epithelial cells of serous peritoneal and ovarian papillary carcinomas display more overtly malignant features than well differentiated papillary mesothelioma and marked cytonuclear atypia, mitotic activity and adjacent tissue invasion are common. In complex cases of papillary peritoneal tumours, the most reliable discriminating factor in separating well differentiated papillary mesothelioma from the other malignant neoplasms is the clinical course.

Multicystic mesothelioma and mesothelial cysts

Cysts of mesothelial origin have been termed 'peritoneal inclusion cysts' and 'benign multicystic mesothelioma'. The terminological confusion underpins the uncertainty about the nature of these lesions. Some cases are reported to be associated with prior pelvic surgery, endometriosis or pelvic inflammatory disease and to have an indolent behaviour. These may be reactive mesothelial hyperplastic proliferations and best called either benign mesothelial or peritoneal inclusion cysts [17]. Other morphologically similar lesions may be associated with local recurrences or a progressive course and have been regarded as low grade or borderline malignant neoplasms of the peritoneal serosa. These are best termed 'multicystic' or 'cystic' mesotheliomas [18]. A genetic or familial link has been suggested in those cases arising in people with familial Mediterranean fever [19]. They are all uncommon and typically arise in the pelvic peritoneum of young and middle-aged women, although cases have been reported over all ages, in men and arising in the pleura. In contrast to diffuse malignant mesothelioma, multicystic mesothelioma is not associated with asbestos exposure.

Macroscopically, mesothelial cysts/multicystic mesotheliomas may show considerable variation in size. Asymptomatic cases may appear as small single or multiple thin-walled cysts with a translucent appearance, often forming grape-like clusters. Larger lesions may exceed 200 mm in diameter and cause pelvic or abdominal pain, urinary disturbances or constipation. The cyst contents are mostly serous or occasionally mucinous in nature. Microscopically, the cysts are lined by attenuated flat or cuboidal epithelioid mesothelial cells (Figure 47.4). There is no significant atypia, although occasional mitoses may be present and in some cases the mesothelial lining may show proliferative changes with papillary and microcystic (adenomatoid) features [20]. Squamous metaplasia is seen in up to a third of cases. The cyst wall is composed of fibrovascular stroma devoid of smooth muscle (this contrasts with cystic lymphangioma) and may show haemorrhagic,

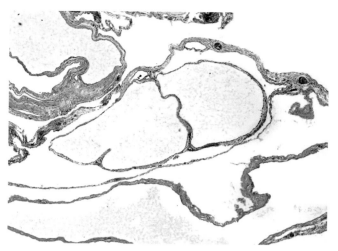

Figure 47.4 Multicystic mesothelioma–peritoneal inclusion cyst: multiloculated cyst lined by attenuated cuboidal mesothelial cells.

inflammatory or reparative granulation tissue change. Less frequently foreign body type granulomas, sparse foam cells or florid xantho-granulomatous mural nodules are observed [21].

The mesothelial nature of the cyst lining cells may be confirmed by immunohistochemistry with expression of broad-spectrum cytokeratins and mesothelial markers (cytokeratin 5/6, calretinin). EMA, p53 and desmin show variable expression and are diagnostically unhelpful. The differential diagnosis in multicystic mesothelioma is with cystic lymphangioma, cystic endosalpingiosis and other müllerian cystic lesions including neoplasms and (diffuse) malignant peritoneal mesothelioma. Diffuse malignant mesothelioma may occasionally display cystic areas but can easily be distinguished from multicystic mesothelioma on account of the gross appearance, cytonuclear atypia and cellularity. Cystic lymphangiomas express vascular markers (CD31, CD34 and von Willebrand factor), which are negative in multicystic mesothelioma. It is important to be mindful that the markers D2-40, thrombomodulin and WT-1 may be expressed on both vascular and mesothelial cells and have no utility in separating the two conditions. Cystic endosalpingiosis differs from multicystic mesothelioma on morphological grounds with the presence of tubal type epithelium with peg cells, ciliated and secretory cell types.

Malignant mesothelioma

Malignant mesothelioma is the most common primary malignant neoplasm arising from the serosa. Peritoneal mesothelioma comprises some 10–20% all malignant mesotheliomas [22]. Currently, the annual incidence of malignant mesothelioma in the UK is an estimated 2000 cases, approximating to 400 primary peritoneal mesotheliomas per year.

The single most important aetiological factor for the development of malignant mesothelioma is asbestos. Diffuse malignant peritoneal mesotheliomas are associated with prior asbestos exposure in approximately 60% cases [23] (compared with 90% in the pleural counterpart) and are typically associated with high cumulative asbestos exposures and exposures to commercial amphiboles (blue crocidolite and brown amosite asbestos forms). There is no epidemiological link between malignant peritoneal mesothelioma and chrysotile exposure. Asbestos-related malignant mesotheliomas characteristically develop after a long latent period (the time from first asbestos exposure to appearance of disease), >15 years in almost all cases with no upper limit [24].

Peritoneal mesotheliomas have also been related to chronic peritonitis, some with familial Mediterranean fever [25], radiation treatment [26], cholangiography with Thorotrast [27] and exposure to the fibrous zeolite mineral erionite [28]. A significant number arising in females are probably spontaneous or sporadic in nature [29]. Genetic predisposition exists, with some familial cases recorded.

Malignant peritoneal mesothelioma usually presents in individuals aged >50 years although childhood cases have been reported [30]. The mortality ratio for malignant peritoneal mesothelioma shows an approximate 2:1 male:female preponderance. This is considerably less than the 10:1 male:female ratio observed in pleural mesothelioma. The clinical symptoms are usually non-specific and insidious, consisting of abdominal pain and distension with weight loss or gain and intractable constipation. In advanced cases an abdominal mass may be palpable and ascites may be present [31]. Some presentations are atypical with localised disease [32], nodal metastasis [33], multiple intestinal polyps [34] and a so-called Sister Mary Joseph's umbilical nodule [35]. The prognosis of malignant peritoneal mesothelioma is poor and most individuals die within 1 year of presentation (44% 1-year survival rate) [36]. Anecdotal case reports detail long-term survival in exceptional cases [37,38]; most of these are probably examples of well differentiated papillary mesothelioma. Indeed, caution must be exercised in accepting a diagnosis of diffuse malignant peritoneal mesothelioma in people who survive >5 years. The North American SEER (Surveillance, Epidemiology and End Results) database, collated over 27 years, reports an age-adjusted relative survival rate of 16% (10% in males, 22% in females) [36]. However, in recent years multi-modality regimens (involving cytoreductive surgery, external beam radiation and hyperthermic intraperitoneal chemotherapy) have enhanced survival in selected patients with good performance status, favourable histology type and resectable disease [39,40].

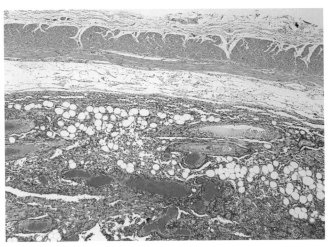

Figure 47.5 Malignant peritoneal mesothelioma: diffuse serosal growth along the mesocolon with minimal visceral invasion.

The typical macroscopic features of malignant mesothelioma show involvement of the entire parietal and visceral peritoneal surfaces. Usually, the peritoneum and omentum appear grossly thickened with myriads of varying sized grey–white tumour nodules, ranging from several millimetres up to large coalescent masses. At post mortem the tumour is usually seen to encase the abdominal viscera but with limited infiltration of the bowel wall, liver, spleen and pancreas (Figure 47.5). Less commonly, malignant peritoneal mesothelioma metastasises to regional lymph nodes and the lung. The macroscopic appearance of malignant peritoneal mesothelioma may be identical to peritoneal carcinomatosis, a condition that is far more common.

Microscopically, malignant peritoneal mesothelioma displays a varied histological appearance. The 2004 WHO classification recognises three major histological subtypes: epithelioid, biphasic and sarcomatoid (including the desmoplastic form). In the peritoneum, approximately 75% of cases are epithelioid in type, approximately 20% are biphasic and <5% are of pure sarcomatoid subtype [41,42]. Primary peritoneal mesothelioma of pure desmoplastic subtype is exceptional. Nevertheless, the WHO classification represents a gross oversimplification of the variety of morphological variants reported in the literature [43–45] (Table 47.2).

Epithelioid and sarcomatoid subtypes may occur in pure forms or in any variety of morphological combination in biphasic or mixed subtype tumours. Cytonuclear atypia and mitotic activity varies from mild to marked in different variant forms. The most common morphological pattern in malignant peritoneal mesothelioma is the pure epithelioid subtype with tubulo-papillary elements (Figure 47.6) and there is morphological resemblance to various müllerian-type tumours (either primary peritoneal or ovarian) and metastatic gastrointestinal tract carcinomas. Other common

Table 47.2 Morphological variants of malignant mesothelioma

Epithelioid	Sarcomatoid
Tubulopapillary	Malignant fibrous histiocytoma like
Microcystic	Desmoplastic
Solid	Leiomyoid
Small cell	Heterologous
Pleomorphic	
Lymphohistiocytoid	
Deciduoid	
Clear cell	
Transitional	

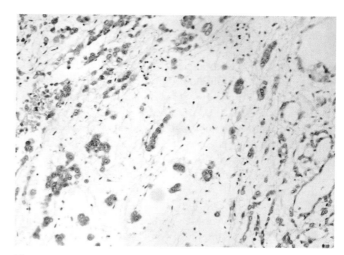

Figure 47.7 Malignant peritoneal mesothelioma, epithelioid subtype: microcystic–adenomatoid subtype.

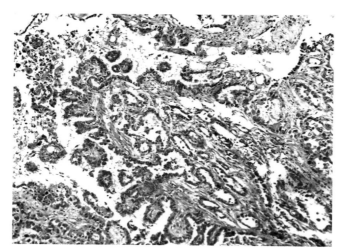

Figure 47.6 Malignant peritoneal mesothelioma, epithelioid subtype with tubulopapillary elements.

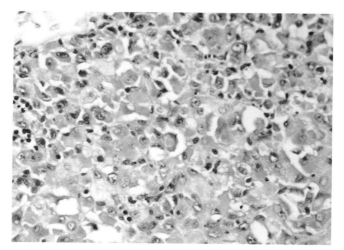

Figure 47.8 Malignant peritoneal mesothelioma, epithelioid subtype: the tumour cells have a solid epithelioid–deciduoid pattern.

cyto-architectural varieties include microcystic (or adenomatoid) tumours with vacuolated (sometimes signet-ring) cells (Figure 47.7) and solid epithelioid sheets of polygonal tumour cells that may have a deciduoid appearance (Figure 47.8). In contrast to early reports, this is not now considered to be a clinically significant feature [46,47]. Some epithelioid mesotheliomas are composed of sheets of small hyperchromatic tumour cells akin to small cell carcinoma (but without nuclear fragility or 'smudging' and karyorrhexis), and here there may be morphological similarity with desmoplastic small round cell tumour (see below). The clear cell variant of epithelioid mesothelioma may mimic metastatic renal cell carcinoma, although the cytoplasmic membranes and vascularity are less distinct in malignant mesothelioma. The poorly differentiated or ple-

omorphic variant of epithelioid mesothelioma may mimic any anaplastic tumour with markedly pleomorphic tumour cells and atypical mitoses.

In some cases the distinction between epithelioid and sarcomatoid cell forms is unclear, warranting the term transitional mesothelioma (Figure 47.9). Pure sarcomatoid mesotheliomas of the peritoneum (Figure 47.10) are very rare – only 2% of 326 sarcomatoid mesotheliomas in one series were peritoneal [48]. They are composed of hypercellular pleomorphic spindle cells with elongated nuclei and mitoses, with an indistinct fascicular arrangement or storiform pattern. The hypocellular, hyalinised, desmoplastic variant (Figure 47.11) is exceptional in the peritoneum, as is the heterologous variant that shows malignant osteo-cartilaginous elements. Lympho-histiocytoid mestheli-

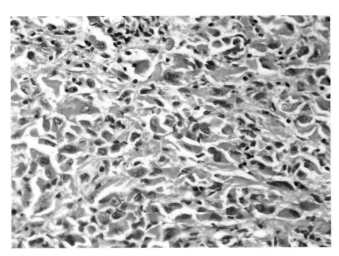

Figure 47.9 Malignant peritoneal mesothelioma: this form, termed a 'transitional variant', contains malignant epithelioid and sarcomatoid elements with transitional cell forms.

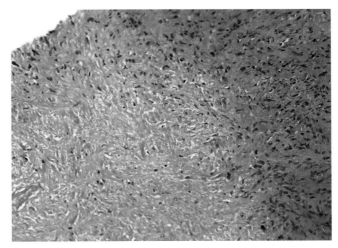

Figure 47.11 Malignant mesothelioma, sarcomatoid subtype: this desmoplastic variant comprises mostly hypocellular tumour with areas of infarctive necrosis.

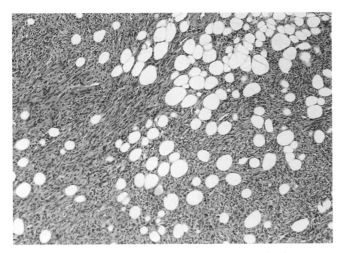

Figure 47.10 Malignant mesothelioma, sarcomatoid subtype: the malignant spindle cells are haphazardly arranged and infiltrate serosal fat.

oma, in which the tumour cells are obscured by a dense infiltrate of lymphocytes, plasma cells and histiocytes, is a pattern seen in <0.5% all mesotheliomas. It may mimic either an inflammatory process or lymphoma.

The differential diagnosis in malignant mesothelioma is, to a large extent, dictated by the gender of the patient and the site and morphology of the tumour. In the peritoneum, malignant epithelioid mesothelioma requires differentiation from reactive conditions such as florid mesothelial hyperplasia, benign (adenomatoid tumour), low grade malignant (well differentiated papillary mesothelioma) and secondary tumours. Distinction of most of these entities from malignant mesothelioma has already been described above. The most common primary tumours

causing carcinomatosis peritonei are lower gastrointestinal tract and ovarian adenocarcinomas. An accurate diagnosis is facilitated by a multi-modal approach incorporating all the available clinical, imaging and pathological information. The pathology involves consideration of tumour morphology, mucin histochemistry and immunohistochemistry. A history of asbestos exposure is not a diagnostic criterion for mesothelioma and should be discounted.

The role of mucin histochemistry has diminished over recent years with the recognition of its limitations and the expansion of immunohistochemistry. The combined acid and neutral mucin stain still remains as a simple and invaluable technique as a first-line investigation. Malignant mesotheliomas typically produce acid mucopolysaccharides detectable by Alcian blue staining at pH 2.5. However, acid mucus glycoproteins are soluble in aqueous fixatives and may not be detectable in routinely fixed tissue. Similar glycoproteins are occasionally found in other non-mesothelial tumours so the reaction has limited specificity. Neutral periodic acid–Schiff (PAS)-positive, diastase-resistant mucins are detectable in most adenocarcinomas and not seen in most epithelioid mesotheliomas. However, the presence of crystalline hyaluronate in 5% of epithelioid mesotheliomas may produce granular intracellular deposits of PAS-positive, diastase-resistant material (Figure 47.12). This reaction may be abolished by hyaluronidase pre-treatment. Such so-called 'mucin-positive' epithelioid mesotheliomas may prove challenging for the unwary pathologist because cases have also been observed to express polyclonal CEA, an epithelial marker. An awareness of this facilitates the accurate diagnosis [49,50]. In most cases a broad immunohistochemical panel is required.

Immunohistochemistry has an important role in the diagnosis of malignant mesothelioma in three areas:

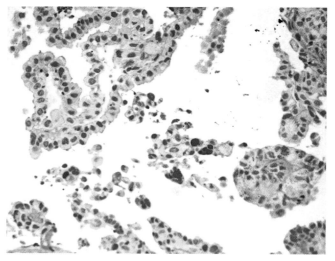

Figure 47.12 Malignant peritoneal mesothelioma, epithelioid subtype: this so-called 'mucin-positive' epithelioid mesothelioma has tumour cells containing diastase-resistant periodic acid–Schiff (PAS) material, a potential diagnostic pitfall (PAS with diastase pre-treatment).

Table 47.3 Useful mesothelial/epithelial immunohistochemical markers

Mesothelial	Epithelial
Calretinin	Carcinoembryonic antigen (CEA)
Cytokeratin 5/6	CD15
WT-1	TAG-72
D2-40	Ber-EP4
Thrombomodulin	MOC-31
Mesothelin	TTF-1 (lung and thyroid)

1. Distinguishing malignant epithelioid mesothelioma from metastatic epithelioid neoplasia
2. Distinguishing malignant sarcomatoid mesothelioma from other spindle-cell tumours
3. Distinguishing neoplastic from reactive mesothelial proliferations.

Many studies have investigated the value of immunohistochemistry in distinguishing malignant epithelioid mesothelioma from adenocarcinoma. Pan-cytokeratin markers are useful, despite being non-discriminatory, because an absence of cytokeratin points to other tumours such as anaplastic lymphoma, amelanotic melanoma or an epithelioid variant sarcoma. The common tissue-specific markers used are listed in Table 47.3.

To distinguish metastatic colorectal adenocarcinoma from malignant peritoneal mesothelioma, monoclonal CEA and CDX-2, a marker of intestinal differentiation, may be used together with the epithelial markers listed and the

first-line mesothelial markers calretinin, cytokeratin 5/6 and WT-1. In the female peritoneum, distinguishing malignant epithelioid mesothelioma from serous papillary carcinoma may be particularly problematic. The combination of calretinin with Ber-EP4 and TAG-72 is the favoured panel [51–53].

The role of immunohistochemistry in distinguishing malignant sarcomatoid mesothelioma from other primary or metastatic spindle-cell tumours is more limited. The demonstration of pan-cytokeratin in a diffuse peritoneal spindle-cell tumour favours malignant mesothelioma, but this may be seen in metastatic sarcomatoid lung or renal carcinoma, synovial sarcoma, leiomyosarcoma and epithelioid variant sarcomas. Consideration of the macroscopic tumour distribution is important. Specific mesothelial markers are unreliable in malignant sarcomatoid mesothelioma because they are usually negative.

Immunohistochemistry has an important role in distinguishing reactive from neoplastic mesothelial proliferations, as described above.

Epithelial tumours and metaplastic tumour-like lesions of the peritoneum

The peritoneal mesothelium and subserosal connective tissue exhibit a diverse plasticity to undergo florid reactive metaplastic and neoplastic transformation with epithelial and mesenchymal spindle-cell differentiation. Embryologically, the peritoneal mesothelium and the müllerian duct derivatives share a common coelomic ancestry [54,55], and the serosal tissues that line the female peritoneal cavity are continuous with the surface covering of the ovary.

Primary peritoneal tumours of müllerian type are those that histologically resemble primary epithelial–stromal tumours of ovarian origin. The most common are serous adenocarcinomas but all müllerian (mucinous, endometrioid clear cell, transitional) and mixed müllerian tumour types (benign, borderline and malignant) have been reported as primary peritoneal tumours. Such neoplastic peritoneal lesions are histologically indistinguishable from their primary ovarian counterparts [1,56–71]. The Gynaecological Oncology Group criteria for primary peritoneal müllerian tumours require that (1) both ovaries are normal in size or enlarged by a benign process, (2) the extra-ovarian involvement must be greater than the ovarian surface involvement and (3) any ovarian component must be confined to the ovarian surface without stromal invasion *or* involve the cortical stroma with tumour measuring no more than $5 \times 5\,mm$ [1].

Primary peritoneal serous carcinoma

Primary peritoneal serous carcinomas are estimated to account for 15% of all pelvic serous adenocarcinomas

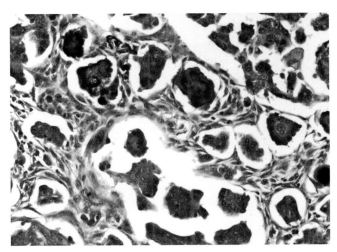

Figure 47.13 Serous adenocarcinoma, high nuclear grade: the tumour infiltrates peritoneal fat.

(Figure 47.13) [1]. They arise anew almost exclusively from the pelvic peritoneum of women as single or multiple tumours and are identical to their ovarian counterparts. There are a few case reports of similar tumours arising in men. Presentation is most common in the fifth decade of life with abdominal pain and distension, or gastrointestinal or genitourinary symptoms. Ascites is common. Patients harbouring germline mutations of the breast cancer gene *BRCA-1* are prone to develop multifocal tumours with a distinct molecular signature [70,71].

Macroscopically, primary peritoneal serous carcinoma usually forms multiple peritoneal tumour nodules, sometimes with extensive omental 'caking'. Most tumours are histologically complex with a variable papillary, glandular and solid architecture, high nuclear grade features and prominent mitotic activity. Psammoma bodies are frequently present. The clinical behaviour is dependent on stage and similar to primary ovarian serous carcinoma. Cytoreductive surgery is advocated with or without platinum-based chemotherapy, dependent on tumour stage. Rarer examples have low grade nuclear features and resemble serous borderline tumours, except for the presence of stromal invasion. Peritoneal psammocarcinoma represents a subset of low grade serous carcinoma in which there are abundant psammoma bodies (involving at least 75% of the papillae or nests); such low grade tumours are generally associated with a relatively favourable prognosis [65,66,68].

Primary peritoneal borderline tumours and peritoneal implants

These peritoneal tumours are identical to borderline ovarian tumours [69]. Most are serous type neoplasms and by definition show no invasion of omental fat or subserosal mesenchyme. Primary peritoneal serous borderline tumours typically occur in young women who often present with abdominal pain or infertility, although the peritoneal lesions may be found incidentally at laparotomy. The typical surgical findings are adhesions or granularity of the peritoneal surfaces, with masses only rarely encountered. Histologically, primary peritoneal serous borderline tumours show epithelial cellular stratification and tufting, detachment of cell groups, mild-to-moderate cytological atypia and mitotic activity, but there is no stromal invasion. The features are similar to non-invasive peritoneal implants of epithelial or desmoplastic type. Primary peritoneal borderline tumours are usually treated by surgery and have a good prognosis.

Around two-thirds of primary ovarian serous borderline tumours are associated with peritoneal implants and the nature of these implants is of prognostic significance: non-invasive implants have no adverse affect on prognosis, in contrast to invasive implants. Non-invasive peritoneal implants are usually located on the surface of the omentum and are further divided on histological grounds into epithelial and desmoplastic types. By definition, they show no stromal invasion but may extend along the surfaces of omental fissures and septa – care must be taken to distinguish this phenomenon from direct invasion of omental adipose tissue. Epithelial implants consist mainly of epithelial cells and typically have a complex, branching, papillary architecture, similar to that seen in the primary ovarian tumour. Psammoma bodies may be present. They do not induce any stromal reaction. Desmoplastic implants, on the other hand, comprise epithelial nests, glands or papillae in a granulation tissue-like or fibrous stroma. Although the presence of such epithelial structures within a cellular stroma may give an initial impression of invasive tumour, these implants have a circumscribed contour, show no true infiltration of the underlying or surrounding tissue and frequently appear to be 'stuck on' to the peritoneal surface.

Invasive peritoneal implants show overt infiltration of the sub-mesothelial connective tissue or omentum and usually resemble low grade serous adenocarcinoma. Assessment of invasion requires examination of the sub-mesothelial tissue. If this is not present in a superficial biopsy specimen, it may be reasonable to classify a peritoneal implant as non-invasive on the assumption that it has been easily stripped from the underlying tissue (Figure 47.14).

Endometriosis

Endometriosis is a common condition that may affect any part of the visceral and parietal peritoneum in women. It is defined as the presence of functional extra-uterine endometrial stroma, with or without glands [72]. The

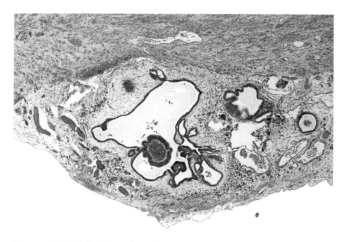

Figure 47.14 Peritoneal implant, non-invasive type: the serous epithelium shows papillary architecture and the lesion has a 'stuck-on' appearance in the peritoneum.

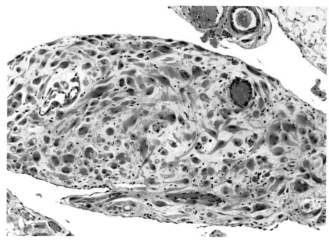

Figure 47.15 Deciduosis in the meso-appendix: a degree of nuclear atypia is possible although mitoses should not be seen.

histogenesis of endometriosis is controversial. Three theories have been proposed to explain its origin: retrograde menstruation and implantation of endometrium in the peritoneal cavity; metaplastic differentiation of the serosal surfaces; and induction of undifferentiated pluripotent mesenchymal cells. It is estimated to occur in approximately 10% of women of childbearing age. Many affected women are asymptomatic, although pelvic pain, dysmenorrhoea, dysfunctional uterine bleeding and infertility are not uncommon. Pelvic adhesions and implants on the peritoneal surfaces of the bowel and bladder may cause various gastrointestinal problems (see Chapters 31 and 40) and intermittent haematuria. Macroscopically, endometriosis appears as red–brown nodules, cysts or haemorrhage on the peritoneal surfaces. Long-standing lesions typically induce peritoneal fibrous adhesions and some may induce intestinal obstruction. Microscopy confirms the presence of endometrial-type glands and stroma, as well as haemosiderin-laden macrophages. Endometriosis can undergo metaplastic, hyperplastic and neoplastic change. Prominent smooth muscle hyperplasia may be present (endomyometriosis). Rarely, malignant transformation may arise in endometriotic foci; most cases have reported endometrioid–clear cell adenocarcinomas [73].

Endosalpingiosis

Endosalpingiosis is a common and usually incidental microscopic finding that occurs almost exclusively in women of reproductive age. It is a metaplastic process usually involving the pelvic peritoneal surfaces and ovaries, although the process may also involve lymph nodes. Endosalpingiosis describes the presence of glands lined by a single layer of ciliated columnar epithelial cells, or a mixture of ciliated cells, secretory cells and peg cells, as seen in the normal fallopian tube. Occasional papillae and psammoma bodies are seen. No stromal desmoplastic reaction is present. Florid endosalpingiosis may mimic neoplasia [74].

Deciduosis

Deciduosis is the presence of typical decidualised cells in the subserosal tissues, most commonly in the pelvic peritoneum during pregnancy. The process is mostly asymptomatic and macroscopically inconspicuous, being seen incidentally on histological examination of tubal pregnancies or in appendectomy specimens from pregnant women [75]. Deciduosis may appear as multiple small, grey, peritoneal nodules or, in florid cases, may suggest a malignant process. Microscopically, the groups of decidual cells have abundant pale, eosinophilic, granular cytoplasm and may show nuclear atypia (Figure 47.15). There may be mimicry of metastatic squamous cell carcinoma or malignant deciduoid mesothelioma [46,47]. Unlike decidua, both of these malignant tumours will be cytokeratin positive. Deciduosis may be seen alongside endometriosis and leiomyomatosis peritonealis disseminata.

Leiomyomatosis peritonealis disseminata

Leiomyomatosis peritonealis disseminata is characterised by the presence of multiple nodules of proliferating smooth muscle over the peritoneal surface (Figure 47.16) [76]. The macroscopic features mimic disseminated malignancy. This condition occurs mostly in women of reproductive age and has been associated with oral contraceptive use and pregnancy. In some patients there are uterine leiomyomas

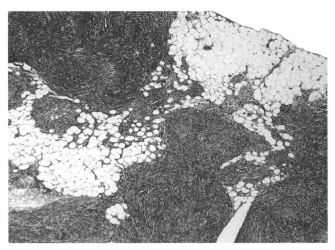

Figure 47.16 Leiomyomatosis peritonealis disseminata – multiple nodules of proliferating smooth muscle are seen within the omental fat. This may be a mimic of disseminated malignancy.

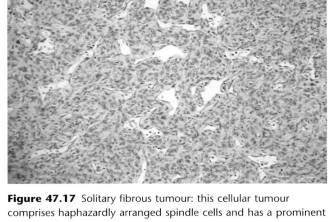

Figure 47.17 Solitary fibrous tumour: this cellular tumour comprises haphazardly arranged spindle cells and has a prominent vascular pattern.

and in others oestrogen-secreting ovarian tumours. Histologically the peritoneal nodules develop in the immediate submesothelial region as well defined whorls of mature smooth muscle cells. There is no mitotic activity and minimal atypia. The precise nature of the condition is subject to debate. It likely represents metaplastic change in subserosal mesenchymal cells, and to support this it has been reported alongside other metaplastic processes such as ectopic decidua [75], endometriosis, endometriosis and peritoneal inclusion cysts/multicystic mesothelioma [77]. However, analysis of methylation status using the human androgen receptor gene reported multicentric clonal proliferations [78]. Malignant transformation has been reported [79]. However, in most cases, spontaneous regression has been reported after the cause of the oestrogenic stimulation has been removed. Cases have also been successfully treated by gonadotrophin-releasing hormone agonists [80].

Gliomatosis peritonei

Gliomatosis peritonei describes the presence of numerous peritoneal (omental–mesenteric) implants of glial tissue [81,82]. The pathogenesis of the condition is postulated to relate to either trans-coelomic spread from a primary germ-cell tumour [83] or glial metaplasia from pluripotent müllerian stem cells in the peritoneum. Cases have been reported in association with ventriculo-peritoneal shunts placed early in infancy, where it is postulated that neural growth factors normally present in cerebrospinal fluid induce glial differentiation within the peritoneum [84]. Macroscopically, gliomatosis peritonei may mimic disseminated carcinoma but microscopy shows multiple nests of mature glial

tissue throughout the peritoneum. Gliomatosis peritonei is a benign condition with an excellent prognosis.

Primary tumours arising from the subserosal mesenchyme

Solitary fibrous tumour

Solitary fibrous tumours of the peritoneum are rare compared with their pleural counterparts [85,86]. They are considered to arise from fibroblasts of the sub-mesothelial connective tissue. Some are associated with symptomatic hypoglycaemia (Doege–Potter syndrome) due to production of an insulin-like growth factor. Macroscopically, solitary fibrous tumours are usually well defined solid mass lesions. Histologically, they are spindle-celled lesions that vary in cellularity: some are composed of haphazardly arranged spindle cells with a so-called 'patternless pattern', some have a distinctive haemangio pericytic pattern (Figure 47.17), some are sclerotic and others are myxoid in nature. Most behave benignly, although malignant forms are well recognised and associated with large tumour size (>100 mm), increased mitotic frequency (>4 mitoses/10 high power fields [hpf]), abnormal mitoses, marked cytonuclear pleomorphism and macronucleoli, necrosis and the lack of a tumour pedicle. The differential diagnosis includes localised sarcomatoid mesothelioma, gastrointestinal stromal tumour (GIST), inflammatory myofibroblastic tumour, desmoid tumour (fibromatosis) and various sarcomas. Solitary fibrous tumours typically express CD34, bcl-2 and CD99, although this is not specific. They are not cytokeratin or mesothelial marker positive, lack CD117 and *ALK*-1 translocations, which helps in their distinction from mesothelioma, GIST and inflammatory myofibroblastic tumour, respectively. Desmoid tumours and sarcomas are more widely infiltrative than solitary fibrous tumours.

Desmoid tumour (omental–mesenteric fibromatosis)

Desmoid tumours most often develop in the mesentery of the small intestine, although the mesocolon, omentum and retro-peritoneum are reported sites. There is a slight male preponderance and peak onset is in the third to fourth decades. A common presentation is with abdominal pain or a mass, depending on the anatomical site. Macroscopically, lesions appear well circumscribed but microscopically have infiltrative margins. Histologically, mesenteric fibromatosis is indistinguishable from fibromatosis arising elsewhere in the body [87]. The lesions may be variably cellular, composed of cytologically bland spindle cells within a dense fibrous stroma. Keloid-like collagenous areas may be seen. There is little mitotic activity or atypia. Mesenteric fibromatosis is typically locally aggressive and recurrent and wide local excision is the treatment of choice. The development of mesenteric fibromatosis (desmoid tumour) may be sporadic, related to trauma or hyper-oestrogenic states, or may arise in patients with familial adenomatous polyposis (FAP), especially those with germline mutations in the 3'-region of the *APC* gene (see Chapter 37). Desmoid tumours in patients with FAP typically develop 1–2 years after intestinal surgery and are more prone to recurrence [88]. The main differential diagnosis is with extra-gastrointestinal stromal tumours (eGIST), where caution is necessary because some desmoid tumours express CD34 and CD117 (but not DOG-1). Nuclear expression of β-catenin in fibromatosis is diagnostically useful and not found in eGIST [89].

Soft tissue tumours and sarcomas

Rare reports of primary soft tissue tumours of the peritoneum, including cases termed 'smooth muscle tumours', 'nerve sheath tumours' and 'omental liposarcomas', may represent forms of what is now regarded as eGIST [90,91]. Nevertheless, genuine cases do occur, albeit rarely. Vascular sarcomas, both epithelioid haemangioendotheliomas and angiosarcomas, have been reported in the peritoneum [92,93]. Their appearances resemble those tumours arising in counterpart soft tissues and can be distinguished from malignant peritoneal mesothelioma by their expression of CD31, CD34 and/or von Willebrand factor. Synovial sarcoma has also been reported within the peritoneal cavity, and on account of its monophasic and biphasic features needs to be distinguished from malignant peritoneal mesothelioma. It is usually a localised tumour, as opposed to the diffuse nature of malignant mesothelioma. Cytoge-netic analysis to detect the t(X;18) present in >90% synovial sarcomas may be required, because there are no reliable immunohistochemical markers that can distinguish the tumour from mesothelioma [94].

Inflammatory myofibroblastic tumour

Inflammatory myofibroblastic tumours have been reported in various anatomical sites and termed 'plasma cell granuloma', 'inflammatory pseudo-tumour', 'hyalinising granuloma' and 'fibrous histiocytoma' [95–97]. In the peritoneum they have been reported in young adults as mesenteric–omental mass lesions associated with various constitutional symptoms such as pyrexia, weight loss, hypochromic/microcytic anaemia, thrombocytosis and polyclonal hyper-gammaglobulinaemia. They are neoplasms that are either benign or have intermediate malignant potential. Most are effectively treated by surgical excision with spontaneous resolution of constitutional symptoms after excision. Macroscopically, they are solitary, well circumscribed, grey–white or tan coloured. Microscopically, they are composed of a mixture of spindled mesenchymal cells, vascularised fibrous tissue and inflammation. The varying proportions of each component have probably prompted the different terms for the same lesion. Immunohistochemical and ultrastructural studies have confirmed the myofibroblastic nature of the constituent spindled mesenchymal cells, being positive for vimentin, smooth muscle and muscle-specific actins. The spindle cells are negative for cytokeratins and S-100.

The aetiology of inflammatory myofibroblastic tumours is unknown. Some appear to follow abdominal injury or surgery. Others have been suggested to represent so-called IgG4 disease [98]. Some have distinct *ALK* gene translocations [99] and abnormalities of *ALK*, *p80* and chromosomal rearrangements of 2p23 occur in >50% of abdominal cases, particularly those arising in infancy and childhood, and are associated with more recurrent disease [100]. Most cases over-express ALK protein on immunostaining with diffuse cytoplasmic elaboration and this appears to be a favourable prognostic factor. ALK-negative inflammatory myofibroblastic tumours appear to occur in an older age group, exhibit subtle morphological changes of hypercellularity, cytonuclear atypia and mitotic activity, and are associated with a more aggressive behaviour with higher risk of metastatic disease.

A distinct form of intra-abdominal inflammatory myofibroblastic tumour has been reported with male predilection. This so-called epithelioid inflammatory myofibroblastic sarcoma has epithelioid or prominent round-cell elements. Necrosis may be seen and a higher mitotic count (>4/10 hpf) observed. The inflammatory elements of neutrophils and plasma cells are often absent. Most cases show nuclear membranous or perinuclear ALK expression and are reported to have a more aggressive course [101].

The differential diagnosis is dependent on the morphology. Those lesions with inflammatory-rich elements resemble reactive inflammatory conditions, those more cellular spindle lesions resemble fibrosarcoma and fibromatosis, whereas those with vascular-rich elements resemble vasoformative tumours. The presence of necrosis and mitoses is very unusual in inflammatory myofibroblastic tumour and argues against the diagnosis.

Omental–mesenteric myxoid hamartoma

This is a rare benign infantile condition characterised by the development of multiple peritoneal (omental and mesenteric) nodules with distinct morphology and mimicry of a variety of benign and malignant tumours [102–105]. Macroscopically, the lesions are pink to grey–white in colour and range from 10 mm to 100 mm in size. Microscopically, there are plump myofibroblastic spindle cells, abundant loose, myxoid stroma, numerous capillaries and an inflammatory cell infiltrate in varying proportions. Mitoses are inconspicuous. The myxoid stroma is strongly positive for acid mucopolysaccharides and Alcian blue at pH 2.5. Although originally considered to be hamartomatous lesions, it is likely that omental–mesenteric myxoid lesions more accurately fall within the spectrum of inflammatory myofibroblastic tumours described in the preceding paragraph [102]. Surgical excision is the mainstay of treatment.

Extra-gastrointestinal stromal tumours (eGISTs)

Extra-gastrointestinal stromal tumours of the omental–mesenteric tissues are uncommon, representing <3% of all GISTs [106]. They usually present during adult life with a median age of 50–60 years and are rare in childhood. eGISTs are usually large (>100 mm) at presentation, probably as a result of a prolonged clinically asymptomatic growth phase. Most are solid, grey–tan in colour with variable areas of haemorrhage and cyst formation. Microscopically, 70% are of spindle-cell morphology, 20% epithelioid and 10% mixed phenotype. Spindle-cell tumours may have fusiform cells arranged in short fascicles interspersed in a fine fibrillary collagenous matrix. Some have distinct nuclear palisading (mimicking neural tumours) and others show prominent perivascular hyalinisation. Skeinoid fibres may be seen. Epithelioid tumours may show prominent (but artefactual) cell vacuolation that may mimic signet-ring cell adenocarcinoma or liposarcoma but typically lack intracellular mucin and lipid. eGISTs are immunophenotypically similar to GISTs, usually expressing CD117 (*KIT*), DOG-1, often expressing CD34, and with variable expression of smooth muscle actin and S-100.

Cytokeratin and desmin are nearly always negative and they do not express oestrogen receptor, a feature that can be helpful in the distinction from stromal tumours of gynaecological origin. Similar to their conventional GIST counterparts (see Chapters 14 and 25) they are histogenetically related to the interstitial cells of Cajal [107], have a prognosis that is related to tumour size and mitotic index [108], and frequently have *KIT* or *PDGFRA* gene mutations that may determine their response to treatment with tyrosine kinase inhibitors such as imatinib. One analysis of 95 omental eGISTs suggested two distinct clinico-pathological and prognostic groups [106]. Solitary omental forms resembled gastric GISTs, had a more favourable prognosis (median survival 129 months) and were usually amenable to resection. On the other hand, multiple omental eGISTs more often resembled small intestinal GISTs and had a worse prognosis (median survival 8 months). Indeed it has been postulated that these may represent multiple metastatic omental tumour deposits or parasitised tumours from inconspicuous intestinal tumours.

Tumours of uncommitted stem cells or uncertain histogenesis

Desmoplastic small round cell tumour

Desmoplastic small round cell tumour is a rare, clinically aggressive malignancy with approximately 85% affecting adolescent and young adult males [1,109]. The tumour presents as a single mass or multiple nodules in the abdominal cavity, pelvic peritoneum or para-testicular tissue, and ascites is common. Microscopy shows nests of small ovoid tumour cells set in a cellular desmoplastic stroma. Mitoses are conspicuous. The immunohistochemical phenotype shows divergent differentiation, with expression of epithelial and various mesenchymal markers (Figure 47.18) [110,111]: cytokeratin, EMA, polyclonal CEA and CD15, vimentin and desmin. Neuron-specific enolase is positive

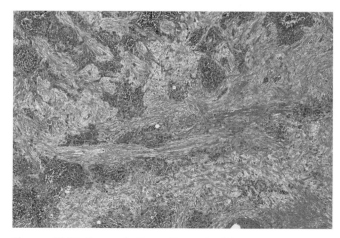

Figure 47.18 Desmoplastic small round-cell tumour.

but not specific. Chromogranin A is occasionally positive whereas mesothelial markers are generally negative. WT-1 immuno-expression is also present, due to the chimaeric protein product of the characteristic translocation of t(11;22) (p13;q12) that results in the fusion of Ewing's tumour gene (*EWS*) and Wilms' tumour gene (*WT-1*) [112,113]. Accordingly, cytogenetic analysis is useful in the diagnosis of this tumour and its distinction from other small round cell tumours. Despite multi-modality therapy with surgical debulking, external beam radiation and chemotherapy, the prognosis is poor.

Primary effusion lymphoma

This is a distinct subtype of clinically aggressive non-Hodgkin's lymphoma that presents as a serous effusion with involvement of one or multiple body cavities (pleural, pericardial and peritoneal), usually without discernible tumour masses [114–116]. Most reported cases have occurred in the context of HIV infection. The lymphoma cells have large immunoblastic or plasmablastic features with prominent nucleoli and basophilic cytoplasm. Primary effusion lymphoma cells usually express leukocyte common antigen (CD45), plasma cell-related markers (CD138, VS38c) (Figure 47.19) and activation-associated markers including CD30, CD38 and EMA. Despite their postulated origin from post-germinal centre B cells, primary effusion lymphoma cells are negative for B-cell markers such as CD19, CD20 and CD79a: the tumour cells are of either null phenotype or aberrantly express the pan-T-cell marker CD3. An awareness of this should prevent misdiagnosis of peripheral T-cell lymphoma. Surface immunoglobulin is undetectable but cytoplasmic immunoglobulins are demonstrable in about 20% of cases. The tumour cells typically contain human herpes virus 8 (HHV-8)/Kaposi's sarcoma herpes virus (KSHV) DNA and most cases are co-infected with Epstein–Barr virus. Molecular genetic studies show clonal rearrangements of immunoglobulin genes, confirming that these primary effusion lymphomas are monoclonal B-cell neoplasms. The disease course is extremely aggressive, irrespective of treatment, with a median survival at <6 months.

Tumour-like conditions of the peritoneum

Omental and mesenteric cysts

Most cysts arising within the omentum and mesentery may be classified according to their aetiology or their pathological appearances. The aetiological approach divides mesenteric cysts into four groups: embryonic and developmental; acquired and traumatic; infective/post-inflammatory; and neoplastic. The pathological approach is to classify cysts by

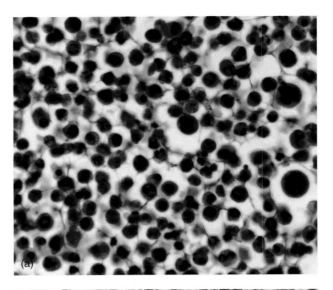

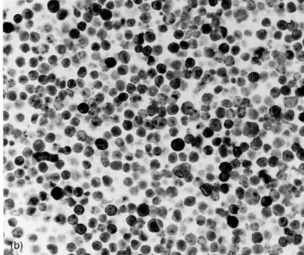

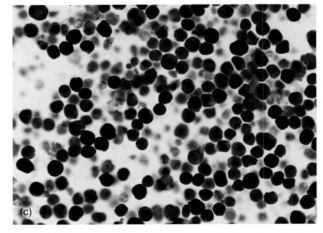

Figure 47.19 Primary effusion lymphoma: (a) the dissociated cells have an immunoblastic/plasmablastic appearance; (b) CD138-positive cells; (c) Kaposi's sarcoma virus-positive tumour cells (100 ×).

histogenetic type: lymphatic, mesothelial, enteric (enterogenous), urogenital, metaplastic or infective/post-inflammatory 'pseudo-cysts'. In all cases it is important to separate the purely benign conditions from the variety of primary cystic neoplasms that arise in the peritoneum (see above) [117].

Cystic lymphangioma

Synonymous with chylous cyst and cystic hygroma, cystic lymphangioma represents the most common 'tumour' arising in the omentum and mesentery of children [118]. Most arise in either the mesentery of the terminal ileum or the jejunum, or less frequently in the omentum or the mesocolon. In children most become symptomatic within the first 2 years of life and may be associated with abdominal pain, distension or even acute abdomen due to obstruction, torsion, haemorrhage or infection. Lesions in adults are usually asymptomatic and found incidentally at abdominal surgery. The treatment is surgical excision. Grossly, they vary greatly in size and the cysts may be uni-locular or multilocular with a smooth and thin-walled lining filled by milky chylous fluid. By light microscopy, the cyst wall is composed of smooth muscle and fibrovascular tissue with a chronic inflammatory cell infiltrate, often with well-formed lymphoid follicles and active germinal centres, and is lined by flattened endothelial cells [119], the lymphatic vascular nature of which may be confirmed by CD31, CD34 and D2-40 (podoplanin) immunoreactivity. Fluid cytology of cyst contents reveals abundant foamy macrophages.

Most cystic lymphangiomas are regarded as developmental anomalies of the lymphatic system arising secondary to agenesis and obstruction. Unlike their counterparts in the neck, there is no recognised association of intra-abdominal lesions with Turner's syndrome or any other genetic disorder. Indeed, some mesenteric lymphangiomas have been considered to be acquired lesions secondary to chronic intermittent volvulus, especially when located near the duodeno-jejunal junction [120].

In a minority of patients with coeliac disease, particularly those with refractory sprue, severe ulcerating mucosal disease and splenic atrophy and enteropathy-associated T-cell lymphoma, mesenteric lymph nodes may undergo cystic cavitation and fibrosis with distension by milky fluid (see Chapter 21). Distinct from cystic lymphangioma, the cystic spaces do not have an endothelial lining. The pathogenesis of this change is unknown but it is associated with poor prognosis [121].

Peritoneal melanosis

This is a rare condition characterised by focal or diffuse brown peritoneal pigmentation that may form tumour-like nodules in the omentum or pelvis [122]. Cases have been associated with ovarian cystic teratomas, ovarian serous tumours and enteric duplication cysts. The serosal surfaces show brown–black discoloration. Histologically, there are pigment-laden macrophages. The pigment is sometimes true melanin, sometimes a product of underlying peritoneal haemorrhage with abundant iron and lipid contents. Macroscopically, metastatic malignant melanoma may have a similar appearance, although it tends to form larger masses, and histologically contains the characteristic tumour cells.

Calcifying fibrous tumour

Calcifying fibrous tumour is rare in the peritoneum, mostly presenting as a solitary mass in children or young adults [123]. Familial multifocal cases have been reported [124]. Pathologically, much of the lesion is composed of pauci-cellular hyalinised collagen with numerous dispersed psammoma bodies. Chronic lymphoplasmacytic inflammatory cell infiltrates aggregate around the periphery (Figure 47.20). The pathogenesis of the lesion is unclear but some authors postulate a link with inflammatory myofibroblastic tumour [125]. Surgical excision is usually curative although recurrences may occur. The differential diagnosis includes fibrous plaques of the peritoneum, solitary fibrous tumour and, when multifocal, malignant desmoplastic mesothelioma. The constituent spindle cells in calcifying fibrous tumour are vimentin positive but cytokeratin and CD34 negative, contrasting with mesothelioma and solitary fibrous tumour, respectively. There is no association between calcifying fibrous tumour and asbestos. The entity reactive nodular fibrous pseudo-tumour of the mesentery has emerged in the literature and may represent a non-calcifying variant of this condition [126].

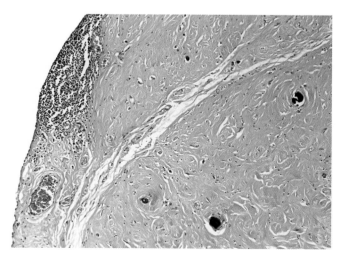

Figure 47.20 Calcifying fibrous tumour: the lesion is mostly composed of bland pauci-cellular collagen with dystrophic calcification and small lymphocytic aggregates.

Secondary tumours

Peritoneal involvement by secondary tumours is common and may arise by direct extension, lymphovascular permeation or trans-coelomic dissemination (Figure 47.21). Metastatic carcinoma from primary ovarian, gastrointestinal tract, pancreas, lung and breast tumours are most common although serosal involvement from disseminated lymphomas, sarcomas and germ-cell tumours may also occur [127]. The macroscopic appearances of these tumours vary considerably. Secondary tumours arising from direct extension tend to form localised masses. Those arising from lymphovascular permeation may appear as a network of fine white lines beneath the serosal surface secondary to lymphatic obstruction and later form chylous ascites. Trans-coelomic spread may appear as miliary serosal implants. Secondary seedlings of the peritoneum may occur during surgery or biopsy when there is tumour spillage into the peritoneal cavity. Tumour cells tend to coalesce in gravity-dependent pelvic recesses as well in the subdiaphragmatic spaces. Ultimately, the visceral and parietal tumour nodules coalesce and the omental fat is replaced by tumour and fibrosis with encasement of the abdominal viscera. This appearance may macroscopically mimic malignant peritoneal mesothelioma, miliary tuberculosis and the rare condition leiomyomatosis peritonealis disseminata, and is resolved only by histology.

Pseudomyxoma peritonei

Pseudomyxoma peritonei (PP) is a condition in which there is abundant accumulation of mucinous material secondary to peritoneal spread of a mucinous neoplasm. In the vast majority of cases, the primary tumour is a mucinous appendiceal neoplasm (Figure 47.22) [128–130] and this is discussed fully in Chapter 30. Cases of PP not associated with an appendiceal neoplasm have been reported, with mucinous tumours arising elsewhere in the gastrointestinal tract, pancreas, biliary tract or ovary. The natural history of PP is governed by the underlying disease process, cases resulting from low grade mucinous lesions (sometimes called disseminated peritoneal adenomucinosis) being less aggressive than peritoneal mucinous carcinomatosis from higher grade mucinous (colloid) adenocarcinomas (Figure 47.23). Traditionally, treatment has essentially been palliative and conservative. However, more recently radical

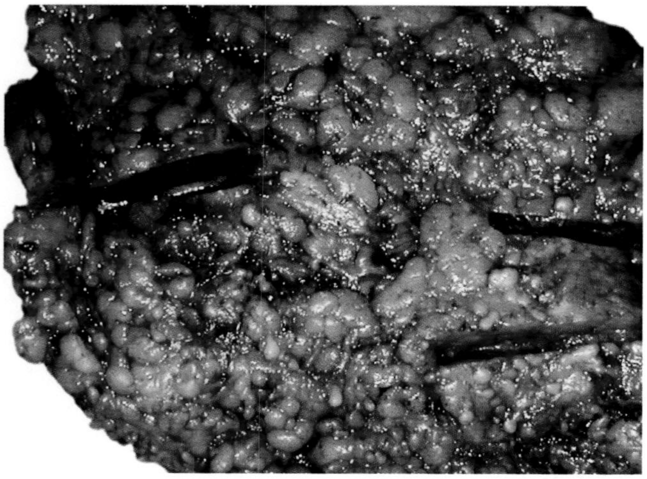

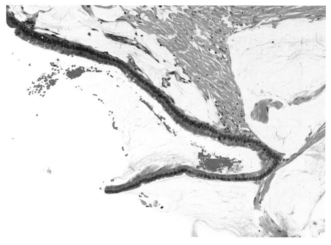

Figure 47.22 Appendiceal mucinous neoplasm, low grade with occasional strips of neoplastic glandular epithelium admixed with abundant mucin. The patient had pseudomyxoma peritonei.

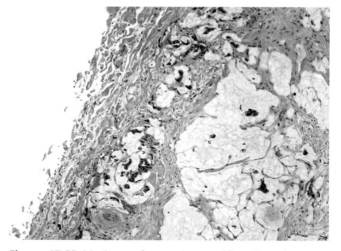

Figure 47.23 Mucinous adenocarcinoma with peritoneal involvement: small groups of hyperchromatic neoplastic cells within colloid stroma. There was an underlying primary colonic adenocarcinoma in this individual.

![Figure 47.21]

Figure 47.21 Carcinomatosis peritonei from a primary ovarian malignancy.

cytoreductive surgery with or without perioperative hyperthermic intraperitoneal chemotherapy has yielded encouraging results in selected patients with low grade tumours [131,132].

References

1. Mok SC, Schorge JO, Welch WR, et al. Peritoneal tumours. In: Tavasolli FA, Devilee P (eds), *World Health Organization Classification of Tumours. Pathology and genetics. Tumours of the breast and female genital organs.* Lyon: IARC Press, 2003: 197.

2. McCaughey WTE, Al-Jabi M. Differentiation of serosal hyperplasia and neoplasia in biopsies. *Pathol Annu* 1986;**21**:271.

3. Bolen JW, Hammar SP, McNutt MA. Reactive and neoplastic serosal tissue a light-microscopic, ultrastructural, and immunocytochemical study. *Am J Surg Pathol* 1986;**10**:34.

4. Oparka R, McCluggage WG, Herrington CS. Peritoneal mesothelial hyperplasia associated with gynaecological disease: a potential diagnostic pitfall that is commonly associated with endometriosis. *J Clin Pathol* 2011;**64**:313.

5. Clement PB, Young RH. Florid mesothelial hyperplasia associated with ovarian tumors: a potential source of error in tumor diagnosis and staging. *Int J Gynecol Pathol* 1993;**12**:51.

6. Churg A, Colby TV, Cagle P, et al. The separation of benign and malignant mesothelial proliferations. *Am J Surg Pathol* 2000;**24**:1183.

7. Attanoos RL, Griffin A, Gibbs AR. The use of immunohistochemistry in distinguishing reactive from neoplastic mesothelium: the novel use for desmin and comparative evaluation with epithelial membrane antigen, p53, platelet derived growth factor receptor, p-glycoprotein and Bcl-2. *Histopathology* 2003;**43**:231.

8. Rosai J, Dehner LP. Nodular mesothelial hyperplasia in hernia sacs. A benign reactive condition stimulating a neoplastic process. *Cancer* 1975;**35**:165.

9. Craig JR, Hart WR. Extragenital adenomatoid tumour. Evidence for the mesothelial theory of origin. *Cancer* 1979;**43**:1678.

10. Hanrahan JB. A combined papillary mesothelioma and adenomatoid tumour of the omentum. *Cancer* 1963;**16**:1497.

11. Zamecnik M, Gomolcak P. Composite multicystic mesothelioma and adenomatoid tumour of the ovary: additional observations suggesting common histogenesis of both lesions. *Cesk Patol* 2000;**36**:160.

12. Daya D, McCaughey WTE. Well differentiated papillary mesothelioma of the peritoneum. A clinicopathologic study of 22 cases. *Cancer* 1990;**65**:292.

13. Butnor KJ, Sporn TA, Hammar SP, Roggli VL. Well differentiated papillary mesothelioma. *Am J Surg Pathol* 2001;**10**:1304.

14. Galateau-Salle F, Vignaud JM, Burke L, et al. Well differentiated papillary mesothelioma of the pleura: a series of 24 cases. *Am J Surg Pathol* 2004;**28**:534.

15. Churg A, Roggli VL, Galateau-Salle F, et al. Tumours of the pleura. In: Travis WD, Brambilla E (eds), *World Health Organization. Pathology and genetics of tumours of the lung, pleura, thymus, and heart.* Lyon: IARC Press, 2004: 125.

16. Diaz LK, Okonkwo A, Solans EP, et al. Extensive myxoid change in well differentiated papillary mesothelioma of the pelvic peritoneum. *Ann Diagn Pathol* 2002;**6**:164.

17. Ross MJ, Welch WR, Scully RE. Multilocular peritoneal inclusion cysts (so-called cystic mesotheliomas). *Cancer* 1989;**64**:1336.

18. Weiss SW, Tavassoli FA. Multicystic mesothelioma: an analysis of pathological findings and biological behavior in 37 cases. *Am J Surg Pathol* 1988;**50**:1615.

19. Gentiloni N, Febbaro S, Barone C. Peritoneal mesothelioma in recurrent familial peritonitis. *J Clin Gastroenterol* 1997;**24**:276.

20. McFadden DE, Clement PB. Peritoneal inclusion cysts with mural mesothelial proliferation. A Clinicopathological analysis of six cases. *Am J Surg Pathol* 1986;**10**:844.

21. Brustmann H. Multilocular peritoneal inclusion cyst with extensive xanthogranulomatous stromal changes: a differential diagnosis of cystic pelvic tumours in women. *Ann Diagn Pathol* 2000;**4**:308.

22. Peto J, Hodgson JT, Matthews FE, Jones JR. Continuing increase in mesothelioma mortality in Britain. *Lancet* 1995;**345**:535.

23. Roggli VL, Sharma A, Butnor KJ, et al. Malignant mesothelioma and occupational exposure to asbestos: a clinicopathological correlation of 1445 cases. *Ultrastruct Pathol* 2002;**26**:55.

24. Britton M. The epidemiology of mesothelioma. *Semin Oncol* 2002;**29**:18.

25. Riddell RH, Goodman MJ, Moossa AR. Peritoneal malignant mesothelioma in a patient with recurrent peritonitis. *Cancer* 1981;**48**:134.

26. Gilks B, Hegedus C, Freeman H, et al. Malignant peritoneal mesothelioma after remote abdominal radiation. *Cancer* 1988;**61**:2019.

27. Maurer R, Egloff B. Malignant peritoneal mesothelioma after cholangiography with Thorotrast. *Cancer* 1975;**36**:1381.

28. Suzuki Y, Kohyama N. Malignant mesothelioma induced by asbestos and zeolite in the mouse peritoneal cavity. *Environ Res* 1984;**35**:277.

29. Peterson JT Jr, Greenberg SD, Bufflier PA. Non-asbestos related malignant mesothelioma. A review. *Cancer* 1984;**54**:951.

30. Berry PJ, Favara BE, Odom LF. Malignant peritoneal mesothelioma in a child. *Pediatr Pathol* 1986;**5**:397.

31. Verschraegen CF, Key CR, Hassan R. Clinical presentation and natural history of mesothelioma: Abdominal. In: Pass HI, Vogelzang NJ, Carbone M (eds), *Malignant Mesothelioma.* New York: Springer, 2005: 391.

32. Fukayama M, Takizawa T, Koike M, et al. Malignant peritoneal mesothelioma as a pelvic mass. *Acta Pathol Jpn* 1987;**37**:1149.

33. Sussman J, Rosai J. Lymph node metastasis as the initial manifestation of malignant mesothelioma. Report of six cases. *Am J Surg Pathol* 1990;**14**:818.

34. Mayall FG, Gibbs AR. Malignant peritoneal mesothelioma giving rise to multiple intestinal polyps. *Histopathology* 1991;**18**:480.

35. Boyde AM, Attanoos RL. Sister Mary Joseph's nodule in malignant peritoneal mesothelioma. *Histopathology* 2003;**43**:303.

36. Connelly RR, Spirtas R, Myers MH, et al. Demographic patterns for mesothelioma in the United States. *J Natl Cancer Inst* 1987;**78**:1053.

37. Brenner J, Sordillo PP, Magill GB. Seventeen year survival in a patient with malignant peritoneal mesothelioma. *Clin Oncol* 1981;**7**:249.

38. Norman PE, Whitaker D. Nine year survival in a case of untreated peritoneal mesothelioma. *Med J Aust* 1989;**150**:43.

39. Feldman AL, Libutt SK, Pingpark JF, et al. Analysis of factors associated with outcome in patients with malignant peritoneal mesothelioma undergoing surgical debulking and intraperitoneal chemotherapy. *J Clin Oncol* 2003;**21**:4560.

40. Wagmiller JA, Keohan M-L, Chabot JA, et al. Peritoneal mesothelioma: The Columbia experience. In: Pass HI, Vogelzang NJ, Carbone M (eds), *Malignant Mesothelioma.* New York: Springer, 2005: 723.

41. Churg A, Roggli VL, Galateau-Salle F, et al. Tumours of the pleura. In: Travis WD, Brambilla E (eds), World Health Organization. Pathology and genetics of tumours of the lung, pleura, thymus, and heart. Lyon: IARC Press, 2004.

42. Kannerstein, M, Churg J. Peritoneal mesothelioma. *Hum Pathol* 1977;**8**:83.

43. Attanoos, RL, Gibbs, AR. Pathology of malignant mesothelioma. *Histopathology* 1997;**30**:403.

44. Roggli VL, Kolbeck, J, Sanfilippo F. Pathology of human mesothelioma. Aetiology and diagnostic considerations. *Pathol Annu* 1987;**22**:91.

45. International Mesothelioma Panel. Classification and histological features of mesothelioma. In: Galateau-Salle F (ed.), *Pathology of Malignant Mesothelioma*. New York: Springer, 2006: 68.

46. Nascimento AG, Keeney GL, Fletcher CDM. Deciduoid peritoneal mesothelioma. An unusual phenotype affecting young females. *Am J Surg Pathol* 1994;**18**:439.

47. Shanks JH, Harris M, Banerjee SS. Mesotheliomas with deciduoid morphology: A morphological spectrum and a variant not confined to young females. *Am J Surg Pathol* 2000;**24**:285.

48. Klebe S, Brownlee N, Mahar A, et al. Sarcomatoid mesothelioma: a clinical–pathologic correlation of 326 cases. *Mod Pathol* 2010;**23**:470.

49. Hammar SP, Bockus DE, Remington FL. Mucin positive epithelial mesotheliomas: a histochemical, immunohistochemical and ultra-structural comparison with mucin producing pulmonary adenocarcinoma. *Ultrastruct Pathol* 1996;**20**:293.

50. Cook DS, Attanoos RL, Jalloh SS. 'Mucin positive' epithelial mesothelioma of the peritoneum: an unusual diagnostic pitfall. *Histopathology* 2000;**17**:33.

51. Bollinger DJ, Wick MR, Dehner LP, Mills SE, Swanson PE, Clarck RE. Peritoneal malignant mesothelioma versus serous papillary adenocarcinoma. A histochemical and immunohistochemical comparison. *Am J Surg Pathol* 1989;**13**:659.

52. Ordonez N G. The diagnostic utility of immunohistochemistry and electron microscopy in distinguishing between peritoneal mesotheliomas and serous carcinomas: a comparative study. *Mod Pathol* 2006;**19**:34.

53. Attanoos RL, Webb R, Dojcinov SD, et al. Value of mesothelial and epithelial antibodies in distinguishing diffuse peritoneal mesothelioma in females from serous papillary carcinoma of the ovary and peritoneum. *Histopathology* 2002;**40**:237.

54. Lauchlan SC. Review: The secondary mullerian system. *Obstet Gynecol Surv* 1972;**27**:133.

55. Blaustein A, Lee H. Surface cells of the ovary and pelvic peritoneum. A histochemical and ultrastructural comparison. *Gynecol Oncol* 1979;**8**:34.

56. Raju, U, Fine, G, Greenawald KA, Ohorodnik JM. Primary Papillary serous neoplasia of the peritoneum: a clinicopathologic and ultrastructural study of eight cases. *Hum Pathol* 1989;**20**:426.

57. Wick MR, Mills SE, Dehner LP, Bollinger DJ, Fechner RE. Serous papillary carcinomas arising from the peritoneum and ovaries. *Int J Gynecol Pathol* 1989;**8**:179.

58. Dalrymple J C, Bannatyne P, Russell P, et al. Extraovarian peritoneal serous papillary carcinomas. A clinicopathologic study of 31 cases. *Cancer* 1989;**64**:110.

59. Truong LD, Maccato ML, Awalt H, et al. Serous surface carcinoma of the peritoneum: a clinicopathologic study of 22 cases. *Hum Pathol* 1990;**21**:99.

60. Shen D, Khoo U, Xue W, et al. Primary peritoneal malignant mixed Mullerian tumours. A clinicopathologic, immunohistochemical and genetic study. *Cancer* 2001;**91**:1052.

61. Sumathi VP, Murnaghan M, Dobbs SP, et al. Extragenital Mullerian carcinosarcoma arising from the peritoneum: a report of two cases. *Int J Gynecol Cancer* 2002;**12**:764.

62. Evans H, Yates WA, Palmer WE, et al. Clear cell carcinoma of the sigmoid mesocolon: a tumour of the secondary Mullerian system. *Am J Obstet Gynecol* 1990;**162**:161.

63. Lee KR, Verma U, Belinson J. Primary clear cell carcinoma of the peritoneum. *Gynecol Oncol* 1991;**41**:259.

64. Clark JE, Wood H, Jaffurs WJ. Endometrioid type cystadenocarcinoma arising in the myosalpinx. *Obstet Gynecol* 1979;**54**:656.

65. Gilks CB, Bell DA, Scully RE. Serous psammocarcinoma of the ovary and peritoneum. *Int J Gynecol Pathol* 1990;**9**:110.

66. McCaughey WTE, Schryer MJP, Lin X, et al. Extraovarian pelvic serous tumour with marked calcification. *Arch Pathol Lab Med* 1986;**110**:78.

67. August CZ, Murad TM, Newton M. Multiple focal extraovarian serous carcinoma. *Int J Gynecol Pathol* 1985;**4**:11.

68. Chen KTK, Flam MS. Peritoneal papillary serous carcinoma with long term survival. *Cancer* 1986;**58**:1371.

69. Bell DA, Scully RE. Benign and borderline serous lesions of the peritoneum in women. *Am J Surg Pathol* 1990;**14**:230.

70. Bandera CA, Muto MG, Schorge JO, et al. *BRCAI* gene mutations in women with papillary serous carcinoma of the peritoneum. *Obstet Gynecol* 1998;**92**:596.

71. Schorge JO, Muto MG, Lee SJ, et al. *BRCAI*-related papillary serous carcinoma of the peritoneum has a unique molecular pathogenesis. *Cancer Res* 2000;**60**:1361.

72. Clement PB. Endometriosis, lesions of the secondary Mullerian system and pelvic mesothelial proliferations. In: Kurman RJ (ed.), *Blaustein's Pathology of the Female Genital Tract*, 5th edn. New York: Springer Verlag, 2002: 729.

73. Heaps JM, Nieberg RK, Berek JS. Malignant neoplasms arising in endometriosis. *Obstet Gynecol* 1990;**75**:1023.

74. Clement PB, Young RH. Florid cystic endosalpingiosis with tumor-like manifestations: a report of four cases including the first case of transmural endosalpingiosis of the uterus. *Am J Surg Pathol* 1999;**23**:166.

75. Buttner A, Bassler R, Theele CH. Pregnancy associated ectopic decidua (deciduosis) of the greater omentum. An analysis of 60 biopsies with cases of fibrosing deciduosis and leiomyomatosis peritonealis disseminate. *Pathol Res Pract* 1993;**189**:352.

76. Tavassoli FA, Norris H J. Peritoneal leiomyomatosis (leiomyomatosis peritonealis disseminata): a clinicopathologic study of 20 cases with ultrastructural observations. *Int J Gynecol Pathol* 1982;**1**:59.

77. Vilos GA, Volisan Haebe JJ. Leiomyomatosis peritonealis disseminated endometriosis and multicystic mesothelioma: an unusual association. *Int J Gynecol Pathol* 1998;**17**:178.

78. Quade BJ, McLachlin CM, Soto-Wright V, et al. Disseminated peritoneal leiomyomatosis. Clonality analysis by X chromosome inactivation and cytogenetics of a clinically benign smooth muscle proliferation. *Am J Pathol* 1997;**150**:2153.

79. Raspagliesi F, Quattrone P, Grosso G, et al. Malignant degeneration in leiomyomatosis peritonealis disseminata. *Gynecol Oncol* 1996;**61**:272.

80. Hales HA, Peterson CM, Jones KP, et al. Leiomyomatosis peritonealis disseminata treated with a gonadotropin-releasing hormone agonist. *Am J Obstet Gynecol* 1992;**167**:512.

81. Truong LD, Jurco S, McGavran MH. Gliomatosis peritonei. Report of two cases and reviews of the literature. *Am J Surg Pathol* 1982;**6**:443.

82. Nielsen SMJ, Scheithauer BW, Gaffey TA. Gliomatosis peritonei. *Cancer* 1985;**56**:2499.

83. Ordonez NG, Manning JT, Ayala AG. Teratoma of the omentum. *Cancer* 1983;**51**:955.

84. Hill DA, Dehner LP, White FV, Langer JC. Gliomatosis peritonei as a complication of a ventriculoperitoneal shunt: case report and review of the literature. *J Pediatr Surg* 2000;**35**:497.

85. Young RH, Clement PB, McCaughey WTE. Solitary fibrous tumors ('fibrous mesotheliomas') of the peritoneum: a report of three cases. *Arch Pathol Lab Med* 1990;**114**:493.

86. Fukunaga M, Naganuma H, Ushigome S, et al. Malignant solitary fibrous tumour of the peritoneum. *Histopathology* 1996;**28**:463.

87. Burke AP, Sobin LH, Shekitka KM. Mesenteric fibromatosis. A follow up study. *Arch Pathol Lab Med* 1990;**114**:832.

88. Gurbuz AK, Giardiello FM, Peterson GM, et al. Desmoid tumours in familial adenomatous polyposis. *Gut* 1994;**35**:377.

89. Li C, Bapat B, Alman BA. Adenomatous polyposis coli gene mutation alters proliferation through its β catenin-regulatory function in aggressive fibromatosis (desmoid tumour). *Am J Pathol* 1998;**153**:709.

90. Mack T M. Sarcomas and other malignancies of soft tissue, retroperitoneum, peritoneum, pleura, heart, mediastinum and spleen. *Cancer* 1995;**75**(suppl 51):211.

91. Stout AP, Hendry J, Purdie FJ. Primary solid tumours of the great omentum. *Cancer* 1963;**16**:231.

92. Lin BT, Colby T, Gown AM, et al. Malignant vascular tumors of the serous membranes mimicking mesothelioma. A report of 14 cases. *Am J Surg Pathol* 2002;**20**:1431.

93. Attanoos RL, Dallimore NS, Gibbs AR. Primary epithelioid haemangioendothelioma of the peritoneum: an unusual mimic of diffuse malignant mesothelioma. *Histopathology* 1997;**30**:375.

94. Helliwell TR, King AP, Raraty M, et al. Biphasic synovial sarcoma in the small intestinal mesentery. *Cancer* 1995;**75**:2862.

95. Coffin CM, Watterson J, Priest JR, Dehner LP. Extrapulmonary inflammatory myofibroblastic tumor (inflammatory pseudotumor). A Clinicopathological and immunohistochemical study of 84 cases. *Am J Surg Pathol* 1995;**19**:859.

96. Meis JM, Enzinger FM. Inflammatory fibrosarcoma of the mesentery and retroperitoneum. *Am J Surg Pathol* 1991;**15**:1146.

97. Day DL, Sane S, Dehner LP. Inflammatory pseudotumour of the mesentery and small intestine. *Pediatr Radiol* 1986;**16**:210.

98. Zen Y, Fujii T, Sato Y, et al. Pathological classification of hepatic inflammatory pseudotumor with respect to IgG4-related disease. *Mod Pathol* 2007;**20**:884.

99. Coffin CM, Patel A, Perkins S, Elenitoba-Johnson KS, Perlman E, Griffin CA. ALK1 and p80 expression and chromosomal rearrangements involving 2p23 in inflammatory myofibroblastic tumor. *Mod Pathol* 2001;**14**:569.

100. Coffin CM, Hornick JL, Fletcher CD. Inflammatory myofibroblastic tumor: comparison of clinicopathologic, histologic, and immunohistochemical features including ALK expression in atypical and aggressive cases. *Am J Surg Pathol* 2007;**37**:509.

101. Mariño-Enríquez A, Wang WL, Roy A, et al. Epithelioid inflammatory myofibroblastic sarcoma: An aggressive intra-abdominal variant of inflammatory myofibroblastic tumor with nuclear membrane or perinuclear ALK. *Am J Surg Pathol* 2011;**35**:135.

102. Coffin CM, Fletcher JA. Inflammatory myofibroblastic tumour. In: Fletcher CDM, Unni KK, Mertens (eds), *Pathology and Genetics of Tumours of Soft Tissue and Bone.* Lyon: IARC Press, 2002:91.

103. Gonzalez-Crussi F, De Mello DE, Sotelo-Avila C. Omental–mesenteric myxoid hamartomas. Infantile lesions simulating malignant tumors. *Am J Surg Pathol* 1983;**7**:567.

104. Gonzalez-Crussi F, Sotelo-Avila C, De Mello DE. Primary peritoneal, omental and mesenteric tumors in childhood. *Semin Diagn Pathol* 1986;**3**:122.

105. Shukla S. Omental myxoid hamartomas – a case report and review of the literature. *Trop Gastroenterol* 2009;**30**:49.

106. Miettinen M, Sobin LH, Lasota J. Gastrointestinal stromal tumours presenting as omental masses – a clinicopathologic analysis of 95 cases. *Am J Surg Pathol* 2009;**33**:1267.

107. Kindblom LG, Remotti HE, Aldenborg F, et al. Gastrointestinal pacemaker cell tumor (GIPACT): Gastrointestinal stromal tumors show phenotypic characteristics of the interstitial cells of Cajal. *Am J Pathol* 1998;**158**:1259.

108. Miettinen M, Lasota J. Gastrointestinal stromal tumors: pathology and prognosis at different sites. *Semin Diagn Pathol* 2006;**23**:70.

109. Gerald WL, Miller HK, Battifora H, et al. Intra-abdominal desmoplastic small round cell tumor. *Am J Surg Pathol* 1991;**15**:499.

110. Schroder S, Padberg B. Desmoplastic small cell tumor of the peritoneum with divergent differentiation: immunocytochemical and biochemical findings. *Am J Clin Pathol* 1993;**99**:353.

111. Dorsey BV, Benjamin LE, Rauscher F III, et al. Intra-abdominal desmoplastic small cell tumor: expansion of the pathological profile. *Mod Pathol* 1996;**9**:703.

112. Brodie SG, Stocker SJ, Wardlaw TC, et al. EWS and WT-1 gene fusion in desmoplastic small round cell tumor of the abdomen. *Hum Pathol* 1995;**26**:1370.

113. Antonescu CR, Gerald WL, Magid MS, et al. Molecular variants of the *EWS–WT1* gene fusion in desmoplastic small round cell tumor. *Diagn Mol Pathol* 1998;**7**:24.

114. Cesarman E, Chang Y, Moore PS, et al. Kaposi's sarcoma-associated herpesvirus-like DNA sequences in AIDS-related body-cavity based lymphomas. *N Engl J Med* 1995;**332**:1186.

115. RG Nador, E Cesarman, A Chadburn, et al. Primary effusion lymphoma: a distinct clinicopathologic entity associated with the Kaposi's sarcoma-associated herpes virus. *Blood* 1996;**88**:645.

116. Boulanger E, Hermine O, Fermand JP, et al. Human herpesvirus-8 (HHV8)-associated peritoneal primary effusion lymphoma (PEL) in two HIV negative elderly patients. *Am J Haematol* 2004;**76**:88.

117. Walker AR, Putnam TL. Omental, mesenteric and retroperitoneal cysts. *Ann Surg* 1973;**178**:13.

118. Takiff H, Calabria R, Yin L, Stabile BE. Mesenteric cysts and intra-abdominal cystic lymphangiomas. *Arch Surg* 1986;**120**:1266.

119. Losanoff JE, Richman BW, El-Sherif A, Rider KD, Jones JW. Mesenteric cystic lymphangioma *J Am Coll Surg* 2002;**196**:598.

120. Weeda VB, Booij KAC, Aronson DC. Mesenteric cystic lymphangioma: a congenital and an acquired anomaly? Two cases and a review of the literature. *J Pediatr Surg* 2008;**43**:1206.

121. Matuchansky C, Colin R, Hemet J, et al. Cavitation of mesenteric lymph nodes, splenic atrophy, and a flat small intestinal mucosa. *Gastroenterology* 1984;**87**:606.

122. Fukushima M, Sharpe L, Okagaki T. Peritoneal melanosis secondary to benign dermoid cyst of the ovary: a case report with ultrastructural study. *Int J Gynecol Pathol* 1984;**2**:403.

123. Kocova L, Michal M, Sulk CM. Calcifying fibrous pseudotumour of visceral peritoneum. *Histopathology* 1997;**31**:182.

124. Chen K T K. Familial peritoneal multifocal calcifying fibrous tumor. *Am J Clin Pathol* 2003;**119**:811.

125. Sigel JE, Smith TA, Reith JD, et al. Immunohistochemical analysis of anaplastic lymphoma kinase expression in deep soft tissue calcifying fibrous pseudotumour:evidence of a late sclerosing stage of inflammatory myofibroblastic tumour? *Ann Diagn Pathol* 2001;**5**:10.

126. Yantiss RK, Nielsen GP, Lauwers GY, et al. Reactive nodular fibrous pseudotumor of the gastrointestinal tract and mesentery *Am J Surg Pathol* 2003;**27**:532.

127. Abu-Rustum NR, Aghajanian CA, Venkatraman ES, et al. Metastatic breast carcinoma to the abdomen and pelvis. *Gynecol Oncol* 1997;**66**:41.

128. Young RH, Gilks CB, Scully RE. Mucinous tumors of the appendix associated with mucinous tumors of the ovary and pseudomyxoma peritonei. A clinicopathological analysis of 22 cases supporting an origin in the appendix. *Am J Surg Pathol* 1991;**15**:415.

129. Ronnett BM, Zahn CM, Kurman RJ, et al. Disseminated peritoneal adenomucinous and peritoneal mucinous carcinomatosis. A clinicopathological analysis of 109 cases with emphasis on distinguishing pathologic features, site of origin, prognosis and relationship to 'pseudomyxoma peritonei'. *Am J Surg Pathol* 1995;**19**:1930.

130. Bradley RF, Stewart JH 4th, Russell GB, et al. Pseudomyxoma peritonei of appendiceal origin: a clinicopathologic analysis of 101 patients uniformly treated as a single institution, with literature review. *Am J Surg Pathol* 2006;**30**:551.

131. Miner TJ, Shia J, Jaques DP, et al. Long term survival following treatment of pseudomyxoma peritonei: an analysis of surgical therapy. *Ann Surg* 2005;**241**:300.

132. Sugarbaker PH, Chang D. Results of treatment of 385 patients with peritoneal surface spread of appendiceal malignancy. *Ann Surg Oncol* 1999;**6**:727.

CHAPTER 48

Miscellaneous conditions of the peritoneum

Geraint T. Williams
Cardiff University, Cardiff, UK

Ascites

Ascites is the accumulation of fluid within the peritoneal cavity. Broadly speaking it may occur by one of two processes, transudation and exudation, although sometimes there are additional factors such as peritoneal extravasation of lymph. The underlying mechanisms govern the biochemical characteristics of the fluid, so that a transudate has a protein content of up to $25\,g/l$ and a specific gravity of up to 1.016, whereas an exudate has a protein content of $>25\,g/l$ and its specific gravity is >1.016. Transudates are usually formed as a result of reduced plasma colloid osmotic pressure or portal hypertension, or a combination of both. Exudative ascites is usually the result of peritoneal inflammation or infiltration. In all cases of ascites there is a continuous dynamic exchange of fluid between the peritoneal cavity and the capillary bed: it has been estimated that about half of the volume of ascitic fluid in cirrhosis enters and leaves the peritoneal cavity every hour [1].

The major conditions associated with ascitic transudates are liver disease (especially cirrhosis), malnutrition, renal disease and cardiac failure (especially due to constrictive pericarditis). In the first three of these a reduced plasma osmotic pressure due to hypo-albuminaemia is thought to play a crucial role in the formation of the transudate, whereas in cardiac failure a raised capillary pressure is probably causative. Ascites due to cirrhosis results from a combination of hypoproteinaemia, portal venous hypertension and renal sodium (and water) retention consequent on a reduced effective circulating blood volume [1,2] that

arises from pooling of fluid in a vasodilated splanchnic circulation. It has been suggested that obstruction to the hepatic venous outflow by regenerative hepatic nodules also contributes by causing an increased production of hepatic lymph that is extravasated into the peritoneal cavity. Such lymph extravasation appears to be particularly important in the ascites occurring in the Budd–Chiari syndrome (hepatic veno-occlusive disease); it may be responsible for the high ascitic fluid protein content that is characteristic of a condition that would otherwise be expected to produce a transudative type of ascites [1].

Peritoneal transudates are usually clear, straw coloured, light green or bile stained. Cytological examination reveals a low cell count, typically consisting mainly of macrophages and degenerating mesothelial cells. These cells may swell up and produce large foamy or signet-ring forms – knowledge of the latter phenomenon is important in avoiding the misdiagnosis of signet-ring carcinoma in the cytopathological evaluation of serous effusions; the lack of intracytoplasmic mucin in mesothelial cells can be useful in distinguishing the two. In liver failure the cytological picture tends to be less typical of a pure transudate, with more numerous lymphocytes and lymphoplasmacytoid cells, possibly reflecting an autoimmune response. In patients with jaundice the macrophages may contain bile pigment, usually amorphous and most easily seen in unstained preparations. Some authors emphasise that in liver failure the mesothelial cells can be especially pleomorphic and liable to be mistaken for neoplastic cells [3]. Immunocytochemical staining can be very useful in such cases (see Chapter 47).

Morson and Dawson's Gastrointestinal Pathology, Fifth Edition. Edited by Neil A. Shepherd, Bryan F. Warren, Geraint T. Williams, Joel K. Greenson, Gregory Y. Lauwers and Marco R. Novelli.

An exudative type of ascites occurs in malignant infiltration of the peritoneum, both with primary mesothelioma and in metastatic carcinomatosis, and when there is a relatively low grade chronic peritonitis, e.g. in tuberculous peritonitis and the collagen diseases, or with peritonitis due to particulate non-infectious materials such as talc (see Chapter 46). In acute suppurative peritonitis the exudate, being more florid, is more fibrino-purulent than fluid, although a marked exudative ascites rich in amylase sometimes occurs in acute pancreatitis. It has been suggested that the fluid exudation that accompanies peritoneal carcinomatosis is caused not by the neoplastic cells themselves but by local alterations in vascular permeability consequent on tumour infiltration, and by the inflammatory reaction induced by the malignant infiltrate.

Peritoneal fluid from exudative ascites is cloudy, turbid and often blood stained. Cytological examination reveals a high cell count, usually with conspicuous reactive mesothelial cells and inflammatory cells of different types, in addition to more specific cell types such as epithelioid cells and giant cells in granulomatous peritonitis, and neoplastic cells when there is malignant infiltration of the peritoneum. Microbiological investigation, including Gram and Ziehl–Neelsen staining and culture of the ascitic fluid, gives invaluable information.

A third variety of ascites, chylous ascites, occurs when there is intra-peritoneal rupture of lymphatics, usually distended lacteals, with leakage of turbid, milky chyle into the abdominal cavity. Obstruction of the cisterna chyli or the main lymphatic ducts, either by tumours or from post-inflammatory scarring due to tuberculosis, filariasis or previous radiotherapy, is the most common cause but traumatic damage to the main lymphatics may rarely be responsible. Recurrent chylous ascites, with chylous pleural effusions, may be found in young women with lymphangioleiomyomatosis, when proliferation of smooth muscle in the walls of lymphatics causes obstruction and eventually leakage of chyle [4]. The condition, which often affects the lungs more than the abdominal cavity, is related to tuberous sclerosis.

Pneumo-peritoneum

By far the commonest causes of free gas within the peritoneal cavity are surgical laparotomy and gastrointestinal perforation. However pneumo-peritoneum has also been described in association a number of other conditions [5], including air insufflation of the female genital tract, rupture of gas cysts in pneumatosis of the colon (see chapter 40), during mechanical respiratory ventilation, when air is believed to leak into the peritoneal cavity from ruptured alveoli [6], and in status epilepticus when pneumo-peritoneum may occur as a result of oesophageal tearing [7].

Intra-peritoneal loose bodies

Loose bodies within the peritoneal cavity, sometimes called peritoneal mice, are uncommon and asymptomatic. They usually consist of small, often spherical firm white bodies covered by a glistening serosa, although rarely they may reach egg-sized proportions [8]. Occasionally they may calcify. Most are formed by torsion or infarction and detachment of appendices epiploicae [8,9] although some originate from small, pedunculated subserosal uterine fibroids. Microscopically they consist of a thick capsule of hyalinised fibrous tissue, with a central core that may show a ghost-like architecture of infarcted adipose or myomatous tissue, sometimes with foci of foamy or haemosiderin-containing macrophages indicative of previous haemorrhage with fat necrosis. Loose cysts measuring up to 60 mm in diameter have also been described in the peritoneal cavity of women [10]. Their origin is uncertain.

Torsion and segmental infarction of the greater omentum

Torsion of the greater omentum is an uncommon condition that usually presents clinically with right-sided abdominal pain mimicking acute appendicitis or cholecystitis [11]. In most cases it is a complication of intra-peritoneal adhesions but examples of so-called primary omental torsion are reported, often in obese patients with an unusually redundant, mobile segment of omentum on the right side. It is this segment that usually undergoes torsion; twisting of the entire greater omentum, although recorded, is exceptionally rare. Although the cause of primary omental torsion is often unclear, it is sometimes precipitated by trauma or hyper-peristalsis after a large meal [11]. Segmental resection of the affected omentum is curative.

A related condition has been called spontaneous segmental infarction of the greater omentum [12]. Clinically identical to omental torsion, laparotomy in this condition reveals an infarcted segment of the greater omentum, almost always wedge shaped and involving its inferior border on the right side, with no obvious cause. Local peritonitis causes adherence of the infarcted tissue to the caecum, ascending colon and anterior parietal peritoneum with a sero-sanguineous exudate. Histological examination of the affected tissue confirms infarction with haemorrhage, fat necrosis and venous thrombosis. The aetiology of segmental infarction of the omentum is unclear. Patients of all ages may be affected, including children [13]. Sometimes a history of recent trauma is obtained and in a few cases a hernial sac, within which torsion or strangulation of the omentum could occur, has been found. Similar to omental torsion, segmental omental infarction is associated with obesity and frequently affects the right side of the omentum, which is larger and more mobile than the left. It

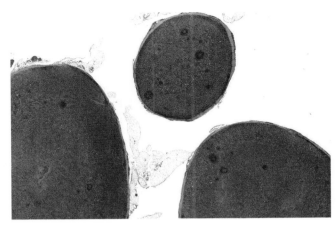

Figure 48.1 Peritoneal splenosis – multiple nodules of normal-appearing splenic tissue are present within the peritoneal tissue. The patient had undergone removal of the spleen 20 years earlier because of rupture in a road traffic accident.

is possible, therefore, that some cases result from partial or reversible torsion of a segment of omentum. However, a satisfactory explanation is not forthcoming in most.

Peritoneal pigmentation

Peritoneal lipofuscinosis, in which sheets of lipofuscin-containing macrophages are found beneath the mesothelium, has been described in association with peritoneal deciduosis [14]. Peritoneal melanosis is discussed in Chapter 47.

Splenosis

Multiple dark-red deposits of histologically normal-appearing splenic tissue, sometimes measuring a few centimetres in diameter (Figure 48.1), may be found scattered throughout the abdominal peritoneal tissue some months or years after traumatic rupture of the spleen [15]. Not surprisingly, they can mimic multiple tumour deposits on radiology or at surgery. They are asymptomatic and incidental findings.

Trophoblastic implants

Peritoneal implants of trophoblastic tissue may occur on the omentum or in the pelvis after surgery for ectopic tubal pregnancy. They may cause abdominal pain or haemorrhage, and may give rise to raised serum human chorionic gonadotrophin levels. Histologically they may appear as intermediate trophoblast or contain overt chorionic villi [16].

Cartilaginous metaplasia

This very rare appearance of nodules of mature cartilage within the peritoneum has been recorded in women who had undergone previous abdominal surgery [17].

References

1. Sherlock S, Dooley J. *Diseases of the Liver and Biliary System*, 12th edn. Oxford: Wiley-Blackwell, 2011.
2. Epstein M. The sodium retention of cirrhosis: a reappraisal. *Hepatology* 1986;**6**:312.
3. Butler EB, Stanbridge CM. *Cytology of Body Cavity Fluids*. London: Chapman & Hall, 1986.
4. Carrington CB, Cugell DW, Gaensler EA, et al. Lymphangioleiomyomatosis: physiologic–pathologic–radiologic correlations. *Am Rev Respir Dis* 1977;**116**:977.
5. Mularski RA, Sippel JM, Osborne ML. Pneumoperitoneum: a review of nonsurgical causes. *Crit Care Med* 2000;**28**:2638.
6. Turner W, Fry WJ. Pneumoperitoneum complicating mechanical ventilation therapy. *Arch Surg* 1977;**112**:723.
7. Richard C, Guiochon A, Rimailho A, Ricome JL, Auzepy P. Pneumo-peritoneum complicating status epilepticus. *N Engl J Med* 1981;**305**:1651.
8. Vuong PN, Guyot H, Moulin G, et al. Pseudotumoral organization of a twisted epiploic fringe or 'hard-boiled egg' in the peritoneal cavity. *Arch Pathol Lab Med* 1990;**114**:531.
9. Elliott GB, Freigang B. Aseptic necrosis, calcification and separation of appendices epiploicae. *Ann Surg* 1962;**155**:501.
10. Lascano EF, Villamayor RD, Llauro JL. Loose cysts of the peritoneal cavity. *Ann Surg* 1960;**152**:836.
11. Adams JT. Primary torsion of the omentum. *Am J Surg* 1973;**126**:102.
12. Schnur PL, McIlrath DC, Carney JA, Whittaker LD. Segmental infarction of the greater omentum. *Mayo Clin Proc* 1972;**47**: 751.
13. Crofoot DD. Spontaneous segmental infarction of the greater omentum. *Am J Surg* 1980;**139**:262.
14. White J, Chan Y-F. Lipofuscinosis peritonei associated with pregnancy-related ectopic decidua. *Histopathology* 1994;**25**: 83.
15. Carr NJ, Turk EP. The histological features of splenosis. *Histopathology* 1992;**21**:549.
16. Doss BJ, Jacques SM, Qureshi F, et al. Extratubal secondary trophoblastic implants: clinico-pathologic correlation and review of the literature. *Hum Pathol* 1998;**29**:184.
17. Fadare O, Bifulco C, Carter D, et al. Cartilaginous differentiation in peritoneal tissues – a report of two cases and a review of the literature. *Mod Pathol* 2002;**15**:777.

Index

Note: Page numbers in *italics* refer to figures. Page numbers in **bold** refer to tables. Sorting is in word-by-word order, ignoring hyphens. Thus, for example, "T cells" comes before "taeniae coli" while "T-cell lymphoma" comes after "taxanes".

Morson and Dawson's Gastrointestinal Pathology, Fifth Edition. Edited by Neil A. Shepherd, Bryan F. Warren, Geraint T. Williams, Joel K. Greenson, Gregory Y. Lauwers and Marco R. Novelli.
© 2013 Blackwell Publishing Ltd. Published 2013 by Blackwell Publishing Ltd.